MILADY®
STANDARD

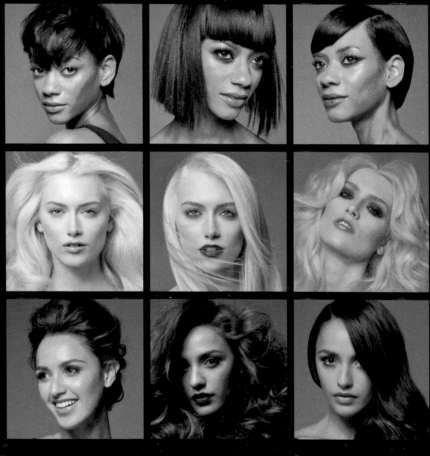

COSMETOLOGY

CONTRIBUTORS FOR 13th EDITION

Jason Backe   Carlos Cintron   C. Jeanine Fulton   Diane DaCosta   Dr. Roychen Joseph   Mary Ann Kilgore
Dr. Mark Lees   Veronique Morrison   Aliesh Pierce   Alisha Rimando Botero   Leslie Roste   Ronald Williams

CREATIVE DIRECTOR FOR 2016 EDITION

Ted Gibson

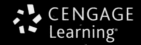

CENGAGE
Learning®

Australia • Brazil • Mexico • Singapore • United Kingdom • United States

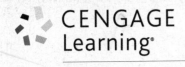

Milady Standard Cosmetology
Milady

Executive Director, Milady: Sandra Bruce

Product Director: Corina Santoro

Product Manager: Philip I. Mandl

Senior Content Developer: Jessica Mahoney

Content Developer: Maria Lynch

Product Assistants: Sarah Prediletto
   and Michelle Whitehead

Director, Marketing & Training:
   Gerard McAvey

Senior Production Director: Wendy Troeger

Production Director: Patty Stephan

Senior Content Project Managers:
   Stacey Lamodi and Nina Tucciarelli

Senior Art Director: Benj Gleeksman

Cover images:

   Hair by Ted Gibson

   Photography by Yuki and Joseph Paradiso

   Makeup Artist: Valenté Frazier

For product information and technology assistance, contact us at
Cengage Learning Customer & Sales Support, 1-800-354-9706
For permission to use material from this text or product,
submit all requests online at **www.cengage.com/permissions.**
Further permissions questions can be e-mailed to
permissionrequest@cengage.com

Library of Congress Control Number: 2014950279

ISBN: 978-1-2857-6941-7 (hard cover)
ISBN: 978-1-2857-6943-1 (soft cover)

Milady
20 Channel Center Street
Boston, MA 02210
USA

Cengage Learning is a leading provider of customized learning solutions with office locations around the globe, including Singapore, the United Kingdom, Australia, Mexico, Brazil, and Japan. Locate your local office at: **international.cengage.com/region**

Cengage Learning products are represented in Canada by Nelson Education, Ltd.

For your lifelong learning solutions, visit **milady.cengage.com**

Purchase any of our products at your local college store or at our preferred online store **www.cengagebrain.com**

Visit our corporate website at cengage.com.

Notice to the Reader

Printed in the United States of America
Print Number: 02   Print Year: 2015

PART 6

BUSINESS SKILLS | 1022

Preface

Milady Standard Cosmetology

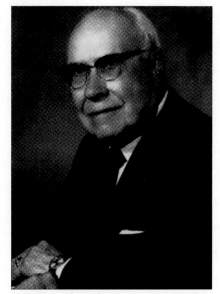

Mr. Nicholas F. Cimaglia, Founder of Milady Publishing Company

Congratulations! You are about to begin a journey that can take you in many directions and that holds the potential to make you a confident, successful professional in cosmetology. As a cosmetologist, you will become a trusted professional—the person your clients rely on to provide ongoing services that enable them to look and feel their best. You will become as personally involved in your clients' lives as their physicians or dentists, and with study and practice, you will have the opportunity to showcase your artistic and creative talents for the entire world to see!

You and your school have chosen the perfect course of study to accomplish all of this and more. *Milady Standard Cosmetology* was the creation of Nicholas F. Cimaglia, founder of Milady Publishing Company, in 1927. The very first edition of *Milady Standard Cosmetology* was published in 1938, and since that time, many of the world's most famous, sought-after, successful, and artistic professional cosmetologists have studied this very book!

Milady employs experts from all aspects of the beauty profession—hair care, skin care, nail care, massage, makeup, infection control, and business development—to write for and consult on every textbook published. Since the field of cosmetology is always changing, progressing, and discovering new technologies, services, and styles, Milady keeps a close eye on its content and is committed to investing the time, energy, resources, and efforts to revising its educational offerings to provide the beauty industry with the most up-to-date and all-encompassing tools available.

So you see, by studying the *Milady Standard Cosmetology*, you have not simply opened the cover of a textbook, you've been adopted by a family of the most well-known and highly respected professional cosmetology educators in the world!

The Industry Standard

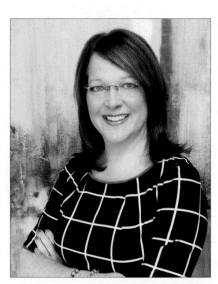

Sandra Bruce, Executive Director for Milady

Since 1927, Milady has been committed to quality education for beauty professionals. Tens of millions of licensed cosmetologists began their career studying from the industry leading *Milady Standard Cosmetology*.

We at Milady are dedicated to providing the most comprehensive learning solutions in the widest possible formats to serve YOU, today's student. The newest edition of *Milady Standard Cosmetology* is available to you in a variety of formats such as the traditional print version, an eBook version, as well as included within an online course that also provides hours of video. Since we know today's student is always "on the go," we also have an app that helps you prepare for the state board exam.

Milady would like to thank the hundreds of educators and professionals who participated in surveys and reviews to identify what needed to be changed, added, or deleted from the previous edition. We are honored to bring you current information from industry icons like Ted Gibson, Jason Backe, and Carlos Cintron.

Thank you for trusting Milady to give you invaluable information that will help build the foundation of your career. Our content combined with your passion, creativity, dedication to hard work, and commitment to customer service will set you on a path to a lifetime of success in the beauty industry. Congratulations for taking the first step toward having a beautiful career!

Sandra Bruce
Executive Director, Milady

New to this Edition

In response to the suggestions of the cosmetology educators and professionals who reviewed the *Milady Standard Cosmetology* and to those submitted by students who use this text, this edition includes many new features and learning tools.

Design

Milady and Ted Gibson joined forces to dramatically transform the cover and interior design of the textbook—it now has a classic, inspirational, sophisticated feel—to reflect the timeless, innovative, and fun hair styles, cuts, and makeup found in the beauty business. Using feedback by students, the designers used fewer background colors to provide more white space for you to take notes on the pages themselves.

Photography and Art

Milady conducted a photo shoot in New York City with a wide network of hairstylists and models, to capture more than 700 new, four-color photographs to appear throughout the book, in both chapter content and step-by-step procedures. In addition, all of the new procedure photographs were taken using live models, instead of mannequins. The part opener image in Part 3 and many of the chapter openers features one of the stunning photos taken at the photo shoot. Ted Gibson and his assistants perfected the hair on each model, while EMMY award-winning makeup artist, Valenté Frazier finessed the makeup.

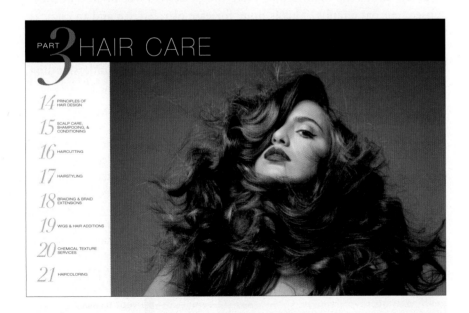

Pre- and Post-Service Procedures

To drive home the point that pre-service cleaning, disinfecting, and preparing for the client are important, you will find that a unique Pre-Service Procedure has been created to specifically address the individual

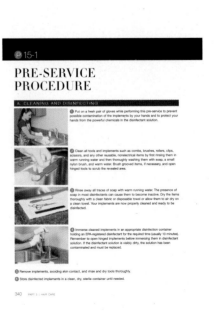

needs of each part—hair care, skin care, and nail care. Additionally, a Post-Service Procedure has been created to address cleaning, disinfecting, and organizing after servicing a client. Both the Pre-Service and Post-Service Procedures appear in every part of the text for you to quickly and easily refer to and follow.

Left-Handed Instruction

Based on feedback from previous editions, Milady continues to include left-handed procedures in the haircutting and hairstyling chapters with full color photography. A great feature for left-handed students, as they will see professionals using their left hand to hold and manipulate the hair and tools.

Study Tools

In order to test your knowledge, you will find a section at the end of every chapter dedicated to Study Tools. This is a reminder that you have resources in addition to your printed textbook to evaluate and practice your own skills. The online course for cosmetology includes an interactive eBook, online quizzes, exercises, PowerPoint® slides, discussion questions, video, and study notes to bring concepts you are learning in the classroom to life.

Learning Objectives

At the beginning of each chapter is a list of learning objectives that tell you what important information you will be expected to know after studying the chapter. Throughout the chapter, learning objectives also originate above the main topic where the objectives will be met in the subsequent paragraphs. This is done for ease of reference and to reinforce the main competencies that are critical to learn in each chapter to prepare for licensure. This duplication is an indication to the reader that the objective can be accurately measured by reading, understanding, and practicing to achieve all of the outcomes for the lesson.

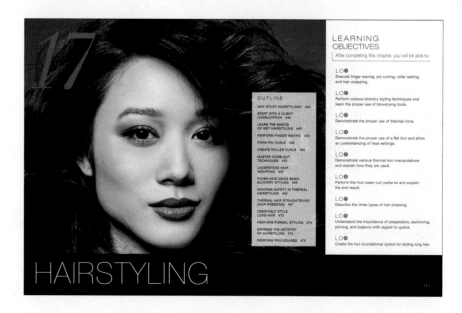

Combination of Key Terms and Glossary List

A complete list of key terms now appears as part of the glossary located at the end of each chapter. In addition to the key terms, you will find the *page reference* for where the key terms are defined and discussed in the chapter material. *Phonetic spellings* for difficult terms are included along with the glossary definition. The combined key term and chapter glossary is a way to learn important terms that are used in the beauty industry and in preparation for licensure. This list is a one–stop resource to create flash cards or study for quizzes on a particular chapter.

All key terms are included in the ***Chapter Glossary***, as well as in the ***Glossary/Index*** at the end of the text.

New Organization of Chapters

The information in this text, along with your teachers' instruction, will enable you to develop the abilities you need to build a loyal and satisfied clientele. To help you locate information more easily, the chapters are grouped into six main parts.

PART *1* ORIENTATION

Orientation consists of four chapters that cover the field of cosmetology and the personal skills you will need to become successful. Chapter 1, History and Career Opportunities, outlines how the profession of cosmetology came into being and where it can take you. In Chapter 2, Life Skills, the ability to set goals and maintain a good attitude is emphasized, along with the psychology of success. Chapter 3, Your Professional Image, stresses the importance of inward beauty and health as well as outward appearance, and Chapter 4, Communicating for Success, describes the important process of building client relationships based on trust and effective communication.

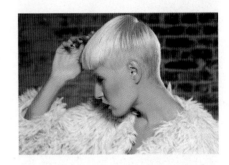

PART *2* GENERAL SCIENCES

General Sciences includes important information you need to know in order to keep yourself and your clients safe and healthy. Chapter 5, Infection Control: Principles and Practices, offers the most current, vital facts about hepatitis, HIV, and other infectious viruses and bacteria and explains how to prevent their spread in the salon. Additional content discuss the types of foot spas and best practices for cleaning and disinfecting the various pedicure units. The remaining chapters in Part 2—General Anatomy and Physiology; Skin Structure, Growth, and Nutrition; Skin Disorders and Diseases; Nail Structure and Growth; Nail Disorders and Diseases; Properties of the Hair and Scalp; Basics of Chemistry; and Basics of Electricity—provide essential information that will affect how you interact with clients and how you use service products and tools.

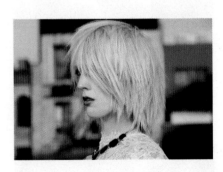

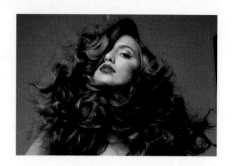

PART 3 HAIR CARE

Hair Care offers information on every aspect of hair. Chapter 14, Principles of Hair Design, explores the ways hair can be sculpted to enhance a client's facial shape. The foundation of every hair service is covered in Scalp Care, Shampooing, and Conditioning, followed by an updated Haircutting chapter, complete with step-by-step procedures for core cuts with fantastic new glamour shots to show the finished look. Step-by-step procedures are also found in Hairstyling, which includes information on new tools and techniques. Another revised chapter, Braiding and Braid Extensions, is followed by Wigs and Hair Additions, and both Chemical Texture Services and Haircoloring reflect the most recent advances in these areas.

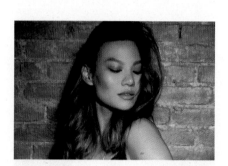

PART 4 SKIN CARE

Skin Care focuses on another area in which new advances have altered the way students must be trained. This part begins with a chapter on Hair Removal, which covers waxing, tweezing, and other popular methods of removing unwanted hair from the face and body. Lip waxing is now covered as a full step-by-step procedure. Next, the basics of skin care is covered in Facials and makeup application in Facial Makeup. These two chapters offer the critical information you'll need for these increasingly requested services in the expanding field of esthetics. Procedures are included for many of the services offered in salons and day spas.

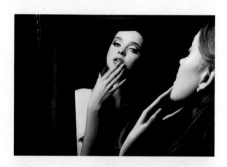

PART 5 NAIL CARE

Nail Care contains completely revised chapters including Manicuring, Pedicuring, Nail Tips and Wraps, Monomer Liquid and Polymer Powder Nail Enhancements, and the Light Cured Gels chapter, with expanded information on nail art. The UV Gels chapter was renamed for this edition as Light Cured Gels to include both UV and LED gels.

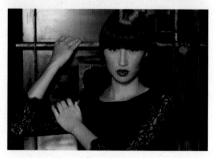

PART 6 BUSINESS SKILLS

Business Skills opens with the updated chapter title, Preparing for Licensure and Employment. This chapter prepares students for licensure exams and job interviews, and it explains how to create a resume and a portfolio. What you will be expected to know and do as a newly licensed cosmetologist is described in On the Job. This chapter offers tips on how to make the most of your first job—including the importance of learning all you can. The final chapter, The Salon Business, exposes students to the numerous types of salons and salon ownerships available to them.

Additional Features of this Edition

As part of this edition, many features are available to help you master key concepts and techniques.

FOCUS ON

Throughout the text, short paragraphs in the outer column draw attention to various skills and concepts that will help you reach your goal. The **Focus On** pieces target sharpening technical and personal skills, ticket upgrading, client consultation, and building your client base. These topics are key to your success as a student and as a professional.

DID YOU KNOW?

This feature provides interesting information that will enhance your understanding of the material in the text and call attention to a special point.

ACTIVITY

The **Activity** boxes describe hands-on classroom exercises that will help you understand the concepts explained in the text.

HERE'S A TIP

These helpful tips draw attention to situations that might arise and provide quick ways of doing things. Look for these tips throughout the text.

CAUTION

Some information is so critical for your safety and the safety of your clients that it deserves special attention. Be sure to direct your attention to the information in the **Caution** boxes.

STATE REGULATORY ALERT!

This feature alerts you to check the laws in your region for procedures and practices that are regulated differently from state to state. It is important, while you are studying, to contact state boards and provincial regulatory agencies to learn what is allowed and not allowed. Your instructor will provide you with contact information.

WEB RESOURCES

The **Web Resources** provide you with Web addresses where you can find more information on a topic and references to additional sites for more information.

FOCUS ON
Being a Good Teammate

While each individual may be concerned with getting ahead and being successful, a good teammate knows that no one can be successful alone. You will be truly successful if your entire salon is successful!

DID YOU KNOW?
Autoclaves penetrate contaminated instruments better than liquid disinfectants and offer complete destruction of all bacterial, viral, and fungal contamination.

ACTIVITY
Research the Web for local and state procedures for licensing electrical, light, and laser therapy devices. Also look at the labels, precautions, and warning labels on various styling tools in your class and home. Discuss your observations in class.

HERE'S A TIP
Remember: Salon professionals are not allowed to treat or recommend treatments for infections, diseases, or abnormal conditions. Clients with such problems should be referred to their physicians.

CAUTION
Do not use negative galvanic current on skin with broken capillaries or pustular acne conditions or on clients with high blood pressure or metal implants.

STATE REGULATORY ALERT!
Always be certain that you are in compliance with your state's regulations for licensing and use of electric current devices.

WEB RESOURCES
For more information on electricity and energy, visit the U.S. Energy Information Administration's website at eia.doe.gov or the Library of Congress' website at loc.gov and enter the search words *electricity* or *energy*.

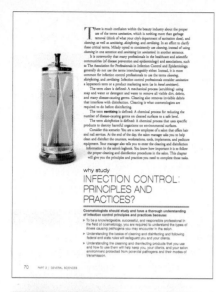

why study
INFECTION CONTROL:
PRINCIPLES AND
PRACTICES?

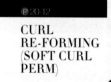

CURL
RE-FORMING
(SOFT CURL
PERM)

Why Study This?

Milady knows, understands, and appreciates how excited students are to delve into the newest and most exciting haircutting, styling, and coloring trends, and we recognize that students can sometimes feel restless spending time learning the basics of the profession. To help you understand why you are learning each chapter's material, and to help you see the role it will play in your future career as a cosmetologist, Milady added this section to each chapter. The section includes bullet points that tell you why the material is important and how you will use the material in your professional career.

Procedures

All step-by-step procedures offer clear, easy-to-understand directions and multiple photographs for learning the techniques. At the beginning of each procedure, you will find a list of the needed implements and materials, along with any preparation that must be completed before the procedure begins. At the introduction of several procedures, you will find photographs showing the finished result.

In previous editions, the procedures interrupted the flow of the main content, often making it necessary for readers to flip through many pages before continuing their study. In order to avoid this interruption, all of the procedures have been moved to a special **Procedures** section at the end of each chapter.

For those students who may wish to review a procedure at the time it is mentioned in the main content, Milady added Procedural Icons. These icons appear where each procedure is mentioned within the main content of the chapter, and they direct you to the page number where the entire procedure appears.

Review Questions

Each chapter ends with questions designed to test your understanding of the chapter's information. Your instructor may ask you to write the answers to these questions as an assignment or to answer them orally in class. If you have trouble answering a chapter review question, go back to the chapter to review the material and then try again. The answers to the **Review Questions** are in your instructor's *Course Management Guide.*

Meet the Team

Creative Director

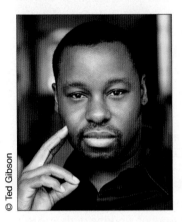

© Ted Gibson

Ted Gibson

"Beauty is individual"

Ted Gibson is one of the most sought-after editorial, runway, and celebrity hair stylists in the business. His work has appeared in publications such as *Vogue, Harper's Bazaar, Elle, Marie Claire, Vanity Fair, People StyleWatch, W,* and *Allure* and at runway shows such as Chanel, Prada, and Dolce & Gabbana. He is also a huge influence and presence at both fall and spring New York Fashion Week styling some of the top American fashion designer labels including Rachel Roy, Carmen Marc Valvo, and Lela Rose. Ted is perhaps most known for toiling over the tresses of top celebrities including Lupita Nyong'o, Anne Hathaway, Debra Messing, Angelina Jolie, Ashley Greene, Joy Bryant, Zoe Saldana, Emma Watson, Gabrielle Union, and many more.

Considering his background, it's not surprising that Ted's incredibly successful Flatiron salon in New York City is frequented by models, actresses, fashion and beauty insiders, and influential women who love its modern vibe and its discreet, down-to-earth flavor of chic. The Fort Lauderdale, Florida is the newest ted gibson salon located in the W Hotel and opened November 2011. Ted was also the resident hair guru on TLC's *What Not To Wear* until

2013, and responsible for the participants life-changing makeovers.

On top of all this, his luxurious product line offers unique, innovative products that have developed a loyal following, as well as being honored with industry accolades and awards. His products, including shampoos, conditioners, and styling products were an immediate success and sold out within hours on QVC. The Ted Gibson hair sheets have become a cult product and beauty closet staple amongst celebrities, editors, and salon clients all over the world.

Born in Texas and raised in a military family, Ted moved from one exotic location to another, living in Germany, Hawaii, and Japan. This experience opened up a whole new world for Ted, as he learned at an early age to appreciate the beauty of different cultures. Upon returning to the Lone Star State, Ted followed his passion and pursued his dream career.

An influential style maker, Ted is a regular contributor on *The Today Show* and has also appeared on *Oprah, The Insider, Good Morning America, Inside Edition, Entertainment Tonight, The Early Show,* FOX News, CNN American Morning, and ABC News.

Today, Ted divides his time between working with clients, managing the ted gibson salons, and creating new products. His career as a fashion, runway, editorial, and celebrity stylist continues to thrive taking him around the world, where the beauty of different cultures inspires him, and where exciting new projects continue to challenge and fulfill him.

Contributors

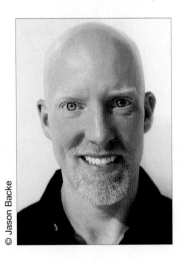

© Jason Backe

Jason Backe

Chapter 21 Haircoloring
Chapter 32 The Salon Business

Over the span of his career, Jason Backe has established himself as a highly accomplished color artist. He is one of the most sought after hair colorists in New York and Florida, and his appointment book at ted gibson salons, which he

co-owns with partner Ted Gibson, is always full. Jason considers hair color an artistic expression of personal beauty and takes great pride in his attention to detail and commitment to impeccable customer care. Jason has worked with celebrities such as Renée Zellweger, Anne Hathaway, Ashley Greene, Christina Ricci, Elettra Wiedemann Rosselini, and Lake Bell.

Jason began his career studying and working at the Aveda Institute Minneapolis where he traveled the world educating stylists, salon owners, and managers in both hair cutting and coloring techniques and business building. He was recently named Celebrity Colorist for L'Oreal Professionnel and was one of the first colorists to adopt their revolutionary ammonia-free INOA hair color. He is on the Color Advisory Board for The Colorist and is a part of Intercoiffure America/Canada Color Council. Today, he also guides and motivates his own staff at ted gibson salon. As CEO of tedgibsonbeauty, Jason is intimately involved with the creation of new ted gibson products, which are fast gathering a devoted following. Known for uniqueness and innovation, the line has been honored with several industry accolades and awards from esteemed publications such as *Women's Wear Daily* and *Redbook*.

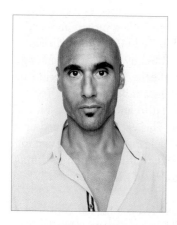

Carlos Cintron

Chapter 1 History & Career Opportunities
Chapter 16 Haircutting
Chapter 17 Hairstyling

Recognized for his exceptional hairdressing and presentation skills, Carlos Cintron is among the world's foremost hair stylist. He rose to prominence at the beginning of the millennium by becoming the 2002–2003 Hairdresser of the Year at the world renowned Toni&Guy™.

Carlos's career in hair was formed at Toni&Guy™, where he began as an assistant to the late Guy Mascolo. He swiftly progressed through the company's legendary training schemes to become part of the International Creative Team, where he brought his expertise and creative ideas to hairdressers across the world.

Carlos was later asked to join the TIGI Session Team where Guy's younger brother mentored him, three-time winner of British Hairdresser of the Year, Anthony Mascolo. He worked Fashion Week for some of the world's top fashion designers and traveled the globe sharing the latest collections and trends inspired by fashion. Additionally, Carlos has worked at some of the top runway shows as both stylist and consultant, including Badgley Mischka, Narciso Rodriguez, Custo Barcelona, Christopher Kane, Millie, Richard Chai, Lacoste, Catherine Malandrino, Nicole Miller, Pringles, Halston, among others. His clients have included celebrities and some of the fashion industry's top models.

In 2011, Carlos won the Texture category at the North America Hairstyling Awards and was a finalist for Hairstylist of the Year. He has appeared on national television creating makeovers, and his work has been published in high fashion and editorial magazines such as *Numero, Nylon, Marie Claire,* and *Vogue España* (Spanish), among others.

Diane DaCosta

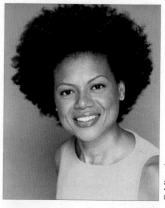

© Mizani

Chapter 18 Braiding & Braid Extensions
Chapter 19 Wigs & Hair Additions

Diane DaCosta is a curly textured expert and author of *Textured Tresses, The Ultimate Guide to Maintaining and Styling Natural Hair* (Simon & Schuster, June 2004) and contributor to *Milady Standard Natural Hair Care and Braiding* (Milady, a part of Cengage Learning®, 2014).

With over 25 years in the beauty business, Diane has brought innovative curly styles to the forefront of today's multi-textured hair movement. A celebrity hair designer to the stars, she has had the pleasure of working with artists and celebrities, including seven-time Grammy winner Lauryn Hill, the Fugees, critically acclaimed actor Blair Underwood, rock star Lenny Kravitz, and many more.

Diane's cutting-edge styles have graced the pages of *The New York Times, EBONY, ESSENCE, British Elle, French Vogue, Heart & Soul, JUICY, The Source, InStyle, Latin Girl, Latina.com, O Magazine, Rolling Stone, Sophisticates Black Hair, Vibe,* and *UPTOWN* magazines. She was also the first hair editor of *Honey* magazine. Diane is currently the owner and creative director of Simplee BEAUTIFUL, a luxury beauty hairstyling and accessory boutique in Westchester, New York.

Diane is also the founder and principal executive of Beautiful Fund, LLC. Beautiful Fund, LLC, is a creative consulting and marketing firm that provides expert beauty and conceptual development, publicity and promotional branding, guest appearances, inspirational speaking, and educational development. Most recently, Diane was named brand stylist for Carol's Daughter and was part of the expert panel behind the Carol's Daughter Transition Me Beautiful Contest. In this new role, Diane develops content for the Carol's Daughter Transitioning Movement website, devoted to supporting the transitioning lifestyle.

C. Jeanine Fulton

Chapter 2 Life Skills
Chapter 3 Your Professional Image
Chapter 4 Communicating For Success

C. Jeanine Fulton impacts thousands of professionals each year through her passion for writing and speaking. She possesses a unique ability to relate to audiences of all ages. Working by the motto, "Fun Education is the Best Motivation!" Jeanine teaches and creates professional performance and motivational programs for schools,

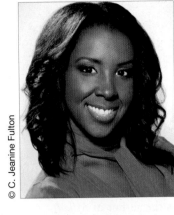

universities, corporations, and non-profit organizations.

After completing her Bachelor of Science degree in Marketing in 1994, Jeanine pursued a career in the field of cosmetology. She also received a Master of Business Administration degree from Nova Southeastern University in 1999. Jeanine combined her marketing and cosmetic flair, and became a consultant for one the world's leading salon services companies.

In 2004, Jeanine started Persona Market Enterprises, a company that focuses on improving brands through education and training. Jeanine is also the author of *Industry In:Site, 101 Top Beauty Careers*, a one-of-a-kind career guide.

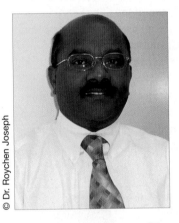

Dr. Roychen Joseph

Chapter 11 Properties of the Hair & Scalp
Chapter 12 Basics of Chemistry
Chapter 13 Basics of Electricity

Dr. Roychen Joseph is the vice president of research and development at Farouk Systems, Inc., in Houston, TX. He has more than 17 years of experience in the personal care industry in formulation and manufacturing. During his career, he has introduced hundreds of innovative products into the U.S. and international personal care market.

Dr. Joseph obtained a Bachelor of Science degree in Chemistry, Master of Science in Organic Chemistry, Master of Science in Industrial Polymers, and a PhD in Chemistry from reputed universities in India and Oklahoma State University. He has several research publications in peer journals. He is an active member of American Chemical Society (ACS) and Society of Cosmetic Chemists (SCC).

Mary Ann Kilgore

Chapter 30 Preparing for Licensure and Employment
Chapter 31 On the Job

Mary Ann Kilgore is a licensed and experienced cosmetologist and holds a Master's Degree in Industrial/

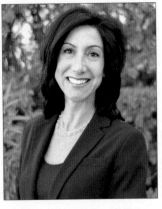

Organizational Psychology. She opened a full-service salon five years after graduating. With salon ownership experience and over a dozen years of dedication as a hair designer, she can clearly relate to the role of being a manager in a creative industry.

In 1999, Mary Ann transitioned her career into the corporate arena and still maintained a small hair clientele. With over 12 years of corporate training experience, Mary Ann has designed and delivered a wide range of learning solutions for teams in Fortune 500 companies in areas such as finance, human resources, customer service, operations, and manufacturing.

In 2010, Mary Ann returned to the beauty industry in the role of International Training Manager for Minx Nails, Inc. She now works as a nail technologist in her studio in Laguna Beach, California and is a contract educator for Minx Nails.

Mary Ann has been involved with Milady since 2010, contributing to training design for the online platform. As a writer of manuscripts for subjects pertaining to beauty sales and leadership, she has also acted as a contributor for two core textbooks, *Milady Standard Cosmetology* (Milady, a part of Cengage Learning®, 2012) and *Milady Standard Nail Technology* (Milady, a part of Cengage Learning®, 2015). In 2012, she completed a revision of the professional product, *Retail Management for Salons and Spas* (Milady, a part of Cengage Learning®, 2012).

Dr. Mark Lees

Chapter 7 Skin Structure, Growth, and Nutrition
Chapter 22 Hair Removal
Chapter 23 Facials

Dr. Mark Lees is one of the country's most noted skin care specialists and an award-winning speaker and product developer. He has been actively practicing clinical skin care for over 20 years at his multi-award-winning, CIDESCO-accredited Florida salon, which has been awarded many honors by the readers of the *Pensacola News-Journal*, including *Best Facial*, *BestMassage*, and *Best Pampering Place*.

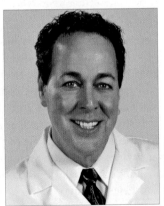

His professional awards are numerous and include Esthetician of the Year from *American Salon Magazine*, the Les Nouvelles Esthétiques Crystal Award, the Dermascope Legends Award, the Rocco Bellino Award for Outstanding Education from the Chicago Cosmetology Association, Best Educational Skin Care Classroom from the Long Beach International Beauty Expo, and, recently, the 2012 Esthetics International Humanitarian Award from The Southern Spa and Salon Conference. Dr. Lees has also been inducted into the National Cosmetology Association's Hall of Renown.

Dr. Lees is a member of the Society of Cosmetic Chemists, and is author of the popular book *Skin Care: Beyond the Basics*, now in its fourth edition; *The Skin Care Answer Book;* and the recently released *Clearing Concepts: A Guide to Acne Treatment.*

Dr. Lees holds a PhD in Health Sciences, a Master of Science in Health, and a CIDESCO International Diploma. He is licensed to practice in both Florida and Washington State. His line of products for problem, sensitive, and sun-damaged skin is available at finer salons and clinics throughout the United States.

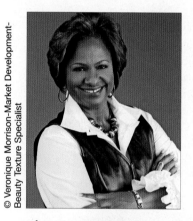

Veronique Morrison

Chapter 14 Principles of Hair Design
Chapter 15 Scalp Care, Shampooing, & Conditioning

Veronique Morrison is a 20-plus year industry professional with successes driven by advanced education, opportunity, creative and technical skills, and her passion for the beauty business.

Veronique's technical and creative skill sets combine advanced knowledge and talent in natural hair chemistry, curl reformation, cutting, and styling. Her commentaries can be found on the editorial and tutorial pages of industry publications such as *Modern Salon*, Behind the Chair.com's *On Paper*, *Sophisticates Black Hair*, and *Essence* magazines, along with various online media sources including Naturally Curly.com, Behind the Chair.com, and Essence.com.

Coupled with ensuring advanced technical expertise, she works to enhance the creative presentation of the professional stylist. Her fervor is training and building skills and consumer awareness in the textured hair market. "I want most to be part of the success story of building more progressive hair stylists, more informed consumers, and more sustainable salon businesses," says Veronique.

Aliesh Pierce

Chapter 24 Facial Makeup

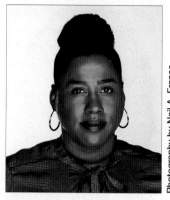

Aliesh Pierce has a diverse educational background, including having studied business management at Fisk University, Art History at the University of Houston, and Italian Language at The School for International Studies. She is the author of *Milady's Aesthetician Series: Treating Diverse Pigmentation* (Milady, a part of Cengage Learning®, 2013). With over 25 years of experience in the beauty industry, Aliesh is a makeup artist, esthetician, and consultant for cosmetic manufacturers. Her work has appeared in a variety of magazines, such as *Italian Elle*, *Vogue*, *Essence*, and *Les Nouvelles Esthetique*. Aliesh regularly shares her expertise with estheticians at various conventions like the International Congress of Esthetics and Spa, The Spa and Resort Expo, as well as the Cosmetology Educators Alliance. As a consultant, she helped Jafra Cosmetics International expand their color range by creating a product line for the African American market, launching the new products in the United States and Europe. Aliesh continues to work as a freelance consultant, lending her expertise to established and emerging brands.

Alisha Rimando Botero

Chapter 9 Nail Structure & Growth
Chapter 10 Nail Disorders & Diseases
Chapter 25 Manicuring
Chapter 26 Pedicuring
Chapter 27 Nail Tips & Wraps
Chapter 28 Monomer Liquid & Polymer Powder Nail Enhancements
Chapter 29 Light Cured Gels

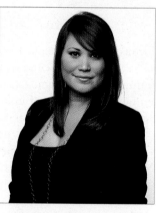

Alisha Rimando Botero is recognized as one of the nail industry's leading experts in training and education. In her first two years as an educator, Alisha taught classes in over 100 beauty schools and vo-techs across the United States. As she expanded internationally, her focus turned to Asia, where she dedicated eight years to implementing artistic training programs and marketing strategies that resulted in the opening of over 100 nail salons and seven schools in Japan, growing that market to become the industry leader in nail art techniques.

Over her 19 years of experience, she has been a platform artist and motivational speaker for thousands of promotional and educational events and has competed in over 100 nail competitions around the globe, winning a World Championship in 2005. She has been featured in multiple training videos and in more than 150 beauty and trade publications and blog spots worldwide.

Through the years, Alisha has garnered the attention of large industry manufacturers, small business entrepreneurs, salon franchises, and nail and beauty associations. She has worked with Research and Development chemists to develop artificial nail enhancement products, nanotechnology skin care and cuticle treatments, polish collections, and natural nail treatments. One of her innovative product lines was awarded an industry ABBIE for best packaging, and several others have been recognized with readers' choice awards for best new products.

Alisha's current position as Executive Vice President for Artistic Nail Design allows her to continue her passion for product development as well as develop a world-renowned education team and training programs for nail artists across the globe.

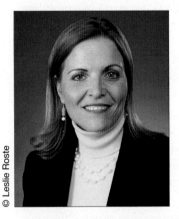

Leslie Roste

Chapter 5 Infection Control: Principles and Practices
Chapter 6 Anatomy & Physiology
Chapter 8 Skin Disorders & Diseases

Leslie Roste, RN, BSN, graduated from the University of Kansas, where she studied Nursing and Microbiology. She worked in various nursing positions including Obstetrical Nursing and Infection Control in the Kansas City area prior to beginning work in the cosmetology industry. Her main focus in the industry has been on health and safety in the professional beauty environment and general education about the sciences involved. She has written many articles for publication such as *Modern Salon* and *NAILS Magazine* and has spoken to audiences large and small on infection control in the work environment, minimum health and safety standards, and safety-based licensure. She is very involved with the industry at all levels, from students to legislators, in making sure that professional beauty industry services are performed safely.

Leslie currently serves on the NACCAS National Career Programs Standardization Committee, The Professional Beauty Coalition for Legislative Education & Reform, and the NIC Education Committee. She also spends a large portion of her time working with individual states on updating and revising rules and/or legislation surrounding Infection Control in the Professional Beauty Industry. She recently wrote and launched a free web-based Infection Control certification that has already certified over 9,000 professionals and students and is being widely used in the schools.

Ronald Williams

Chapter 20 Chemical Texture Services

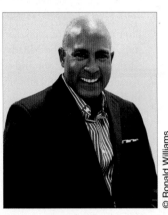

Ronald Williams (also known as Dr. Ron) is sought after by celebrities, socialites, and prestige hair care companies for his experience and knowledge regarding hair relaxing and aftercare. He is the beauty editors' and bloggers go-to guy for hair care advice. Dr. Ron travels throughout the United States and Latin America teaching from a science perspective with technical hair design principles. His motto for hair care is simple: "Well cared for hair is the standard for which good hair design and style becomes a reality for all women." He authored technical journals and researched projects about textured and relaxed hair throughout his 30-year career.

Dr. Ron's print media includes, but is not limited to, *Essence, Ladies Home Journal, People Style Watch, Modern Salon, People, Juicy,* and *Elle.* His online presence is endless and impressive, including his training videos at brand name cosmetics companies.

Dr. Ron holds a doctorate in education, a master's in science, and a bachelor of arts' degree in communication. He is licensed to practice cosmetology in the state of New York.

Contributors for Previous Edition of Milady Standard Cosmetology

Catherine M. Frangie	Frank Shipman
Colleen Hennessy	Bonnie Sanford
Dr. Mark Lees	Victoria Wurdinger
Alisha Rimando Botero	

Acknowledgments

Milady recognizes, with gratitude and respect, the many professionals who have offered their time to contribute to this edition of *Milady Standard Cosmetology* and wishes to extend enormous thanks to the following people who have played an invaluable role in the creation of this edition:

- *Milady would like to offer our special thanks to Ted Gibson and the staff at ted gibson salon for their incredible support and beautiful styling and coloring on the cover models. The end result of the cover and the chapter openers is proof of the advanced and versatile skills the team truly has. Thank you to Natalie Di Benedetto, Courtney Nischan, and many more for a successful photo shoot.*

- Phyto Universe of New York, NY, who, along with their staff, welcomed the Milady team in order to conduct this edition's photo shoot and who were whole-heartedly accommodating and hospitable to all of our crew, models, and stylists!

- The dynamic duo, Yuki and Joseph Paradiso, for their brilliant photography and artistic vision that captured the essence of every model and hair style. Thank you for your dedication to the project by attending casting calls and studio walk-throughs in preparation for an amazing shoot. Your guidance, professionalism, and creativity resonate in every image.

- Tom Carson, professional photographer, for his wonderful finished haircut and styling photos, which truly enhance these pages and are sure to inspire readers.

- The previous edition's professional photographer, Yanik Chauvin, whose photographic expertise helped bring many of these pages to life.

- Dino Petrocelli, Joseph Schuyler, and Paul Castle, professional photographers, for their photographic expertise for many of the photos in the nail technology and communication chapters.

- Margina Dennis, professional makeup artist, for her artfully inspired makeup applications in the interior and procedural photos to enhance the finished hair styles.

- Valenté Frazier, EMMY award-winning and celebrity makeup artist, for an amazing collaboration of creative energies with Milady and ted gibson beauty to transform models into a wide variety of looks for the chapter openers and cover photos.

- Ianthe Foushee, James Le Bosquet, Ron Williams, and Angela Carroll for their on- and off-camera haircutting and styling work, innovative approach, and love for the beauty industry.

- Jason Backe and Jennifer McDougall for their enthusiasm for their work and innovative approach to haircoloring.

- Carlos Cintron for his on-camera haircutting and styling work, authoring abilities, and his passion for cosmetology education.

- Diane DaCosta and Courtney Harris, professional stylists, for their creative braiding styles that are featured in this edition.

- Aliesh Pierce and Neil France for their collaboration on shooting the makeup application photos that are brand new to this edition.

- Alyssa Hardy, fashion stylist at the photo shoot, for spending a great deal of time selecting and prepping outfits and jewelry accessories to create the overall presentation for the finished model looks.

- Carmen Marc Valvo, top fashion designer, for graciously allowing us use of gorgeous outfits and accessories showcased as part of the cover and chapter opener photos.

- A big thank you to the numerous models that graciously allowed us to cut, style, and transform them into their finished looks to help educate future beauty professionals. We are grateful to you for your assistance in making this happen!

Product Suppliers

- **CosmoProf Beauty Supply** for many of the tools, implements, and supplies used and pictured throughout this edition.

- **WELLA SCHOOL PROGRAMS, The Salon Professional Division of P&G**, for generously providing styling aids and backbar product used during the 2016 edition photo shoot.

- **L'Oréal Professionnel USA** for generously providing haircolor, backbar, and on-camera talent for the 2016 edition photo shoot.

- **ted gibson beauty** for providing backbar and talented technicians at the 2016 edition shoot.

- **4420 Hand Crafted Precision Shears**® and Micheal Mailman for generously providing the shears and cutting implements used and pictured at the 2016 edition photo shoot.

- **Sally Beauty Company**® for providing many of the tools, implements, and supplies used and pictured throughout this edition.

- **KERATAGE**® and Carlos Cintron for providing backbar and styling aids during this edition's photo shoot.

- **Jane Carter Solution** for providing the natural hair products, such as nourishing shampoos, conditioners, serums, curl defining sprays, and more.

- **Ebony Styles Beauty Salon**, Manhattan, NY, for quick delivery chemical texture service products at a moment's notice.

- **The Burmax Company** for providing mannequins, many of the tools, implements, and supplies used and pictured throughout this edition.

- **The Shark Fin Shear Company** and *Randy Ferman* for generously providing some of the shears and cutting implements used and pictured throughout this edition.
- **CARMEN MARC VALVO** for graciously allowing us use of timeless fashion and accessories showcased as part of the cover and chapter opener photos.
- **Cinderella Hair Extensions** for providing a variety of hair extensions that are featured in Chapter 18, Braiding and Braid Extensions.

Reviewers of Milady Standard Cosmetology 13th Edition

Arrojo Team, Arrojo Education, New York, NY

Barbara Acello, Innovations in Health Care, Denton, TX

Frances Archer, The South Carolina Association of Cosmetic Arts, Columbia, SC

Cynthia L. Brink, Halo Salon, Costa Mesa, CA

Jenny Bubloni, Lake County High Schools Technology Campus, Round Lake Beach, IL

Krystal A. Buscko, Cosmetology Careers Unlimited College of Hair Skin and Nails, Cloquet, MN

Peggy Braswell, Southeastern Technical College, Swainsboro, GA

Robin Roberts Cochran, Gadsden State Community College-Ayers Campus, Anniston, AL

Lisa W. Crawford, Bellefonte Academy of Beauty, Maysville, KY

Chandra Crosby, Evergreen Beauty College, Lynnwood, WA

Kimberly Cutter, Savannah Technical College, Savannah, GA

Lara Dellomodarme, Tricoci University of Beauty Culture, Vernon Hills, IL

Corrine Denise Edwards, Couture Hair Design & Training, LLC, Temple Hills, MD

Janice Fenner, Central Carolina Community College, Raleigh, NC

Eric Fisher, Eric Fisher Academy and Eric Fisher Salons, Wichita, KS

Lauren Geller, Evergreen Beauty College, Everett, WA

Regina Gilliland, Salon Institute of Northeast Alabama Community College, Cleveland, AL

Laureen Gillis, Kent Career College, Grand Rapids, MI

Jennifer Hain, Columbia Montour AVTS, Middleburg, PA

Linda B. Hairr, Southeastern Technical College, Swainsboro, GA

Donna Haynes, Houston Training Schools, Missouri City, TX

Cindy Heidemann, ABC School of Cosmetology, Esthetics & Nail Technology Inc., Lake in the Hills, IL

Jean Hoffer, Capital Region Career and Technical School, Saratoga Springs, NY

Donna Joy, Ocean County Vocational School, Dundee, NY

Mike Kennamer, Kennamer Media Group, Inc., Henager, AL

Shimika Kennison, Entourage Institute of Beauty, Leaawood, KS

Becky Kunc, College of Hair Design, Lincoln, NE

Danielle Lawson, Innovations Styling Group, Columbia, SC

Patricia Lemke, Mid-State Technical College, Stevens Point, WI

Kelly M. Lisa, Cutting Edge Academy, Vernon, NJ

Patricia Marlene, Eric Fisher Academy and Eric Fisher Salons, Wichita, KS

Yolanda R. Matthews, Eye's of Distinction Beauty & Spa Therapy Institute, Houston, TX

Janet McCormick, Medinail Learning Center, Frostproof, FL

Julie Mead, EQ School of Hair Design, Omaha, NE

Sandra Alexcae Moren, Chiron Marketing Inc. Alberta, Calgary, Canada

Linda Mottishaw, The School of Hairstyling (Pocatello Beauty Academy, Inc.), Chubbuck, ID

Ernestine J. Peete, Tennessee Technology Center at Memphis, Memphis, TN

Sandra Peoples, Pickens Technical College, Aurora, CO

Leslie Roste, King Research, Prairie Village, KS

Wendy Schalk-Cooke, Arts & Technology Centre, Selkirk, Manitoba, Canada

Nancy Schmidt, Capital Region Career and Technical School Schoharie Campus, Pattersonville, NY

Linda Schoenberg, Regency Beauty Institute, St Cloud, MN

Yvette Seils, Continental School of Beauty, Henrietta, NY

Donna Simmons, Tulsa Tech, Collinsville, OK

Madeline Udod, Retired Eastern Suffolk BOCES, Farmingville, NY

Tamara Yusupoff, Bellus Academy, San Diego, CA

Milady's Infection Control Advisory Panel

Special thanks to the following panel members for reviewing and contributing to Chapter 5, Infection Control: Principles and Practices:

- Barbara Acello, M.S., R.N., Denton, TX
- Mike Kennamer, Ed.D., Director of Workforce Development & Skills Training, Northeast Alabama Community College, AL
- Janet McCormick, M.S., Cidesco, FL
- Leslie Roste, R.N., National Director of Education & Market Development, King Research/Barbicide, WI
- Robert T. Spalding, Jr., DPM, TN
- David Vidra, CLPN, WCC, MA, President Health Educators, Inc., OH

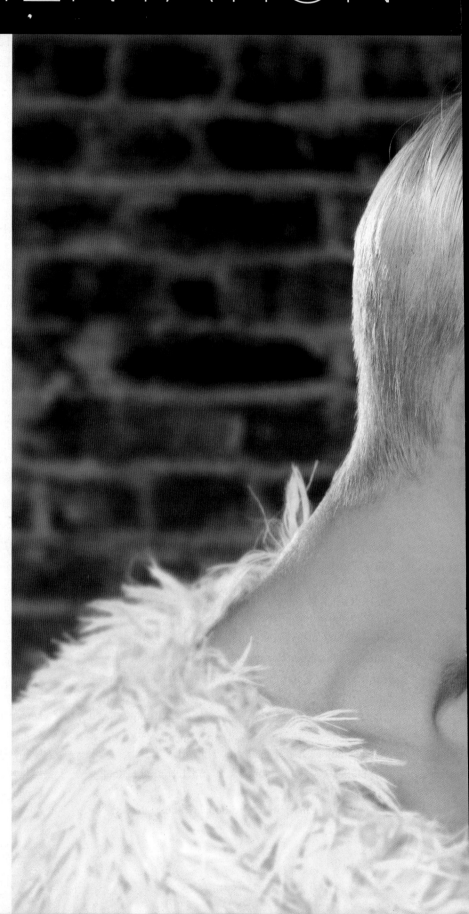

PART *1* ORIENTATION

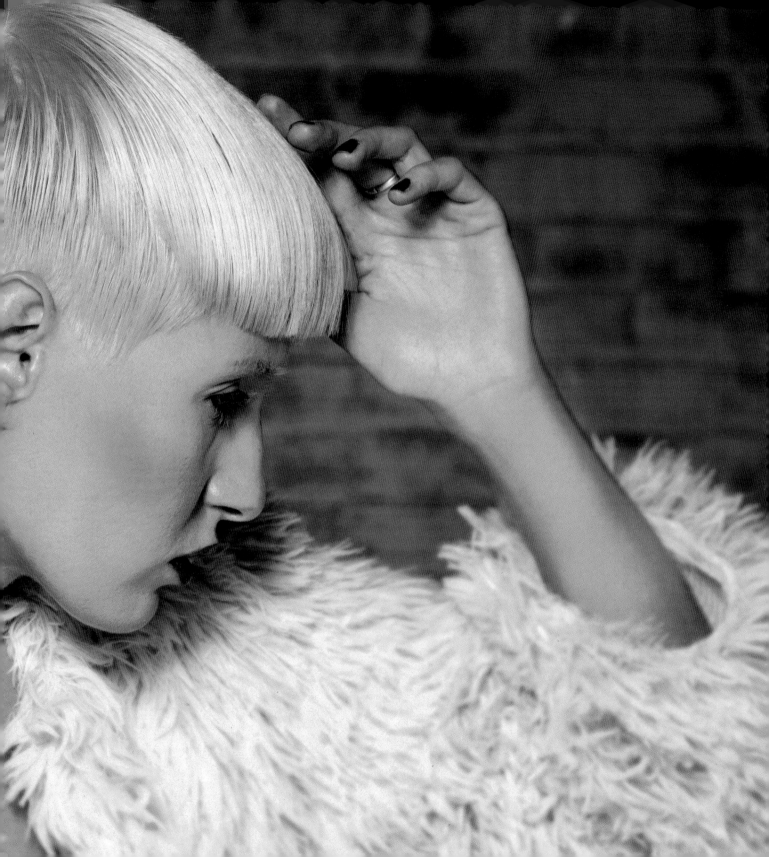

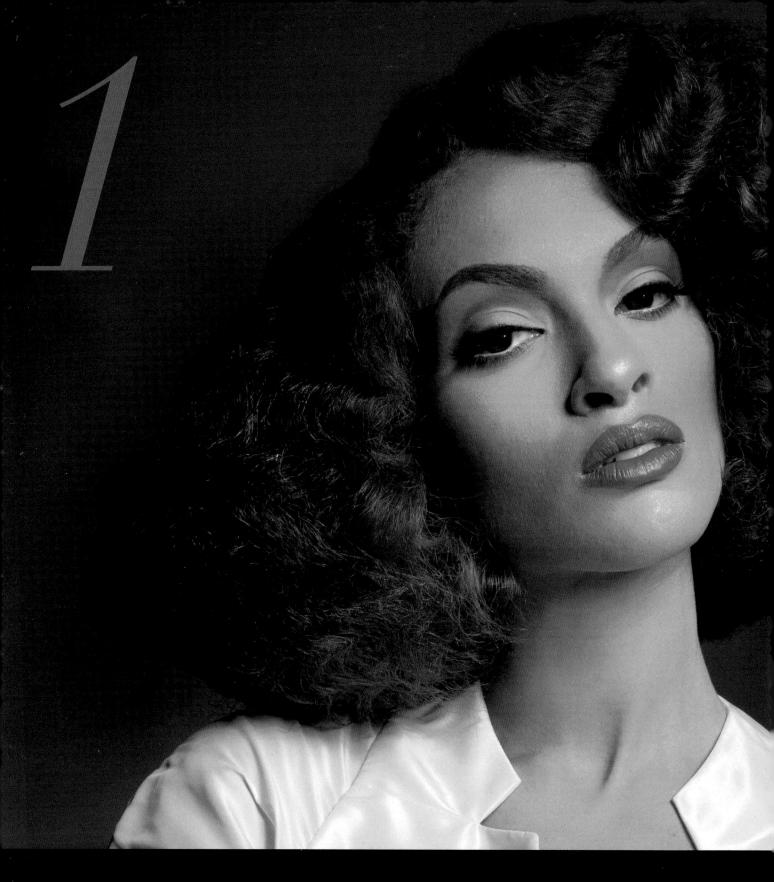

1

HISTORY & CAREER
OPPORTUNITIES

LEARNING OBJECTIVES

After completing this chapter, you will be able to:

LO❶
Describe appearance enhancement and how it relates to cosmetology.

LO❷
Recognize how trends are influenced by the history of cosmetology.

LO❸
List several career opportunities available to a licensed beauty practitioner.

LO **1**   Describe appearance enhancement and how it relates to cosmetology.

A term used to encompass a broad range of specialty areas, including hairstyling, nail technology, and esthetics is **cosmetology** (kahz-muh-TAHL-uh-jee), also described as **appearance enhancement**. Cosmetology is defined as the art and science of beautifying and improving the skin, nails, and hair and includes the study of cosmetics and their application. The term comes from the Greek word *kosmetikos*, meaning skilled in the use of cosmetics. Archaeological studies reveal that haircutting and hairstyling were practiced in some form as early as the Ice Age.

The simple but effective cosmetic implements used at the dawn of history were shaped from sharpened flints, oyster shells, or bone. Animal sinew or strips of hide were used to tie the hair back or as adornment. Ancient people around the world used coloring matter on their hair, skin, and nails, and they practiced tattooing. Pigments were made from berries, tree bark, minerals, insects, nuts, herbs, leaves, and other materials. Many of these colorants are still used today.

why study
COSMETOLOGY HISTORY AND CAREER OPPORTUNITIES?

Cosmetologists should study and have a thorough understanding of the history of cosmetology and the career opportunities available because:

> Many very old methods have evolved into techniques still used today. Studying the origin of these techniques can be useful in fully understanding how to use them.

> Knowing the history of your profession can help you predict and understand upcoming trends.

> Understanding the importance of education will give you clear direction to a successful career.

> By learning about many possible career paths, you'll see the wide range of opportunities open to cosmetologists.

ACTIVITY

Research how *cosmetology* is defined in your state. For instance, the definition of *cosmetology* as described by the NYS Department of State Division of Licensing Services is as follows:

The practice of "Cosmetology" means providing the services to the hair, head, face, neck, or scalp of a human being, including but not limited to shaving, trimming, and cutting the hair or beard either by hand or mechanical appliances and

the application of antiseptics, powders, oils, clays, lotions or applying tonics to the hair, head, or scalp, and in addition includes providing, for a fee or any consideration or exchange, whether direct or indirect, services for the application of dyes, reactive chemicals, or other preparations to alter the color or to straighten, curl, or alter the structure of the hair of a human being[1].

After reading the next few sections, you will be able to:

LO ❷ Recognize how trends are influenced by the history of cosmetology.

Understand the History of Cosmetology

The Africans

African civilization had a variety of hairstyles and they were used as a symbol of tribal traditions and conveyed a message of age, marital status, power, and rank. Many tribes colored the hair with red earth, and wore elaborate hairstyles and head dressing as a symbol of stature (figure 1-1).

In Central and West Africa hairstyles told the story of their status in their respective communities from Kuba of the Democratic Republic of the Congo, the Chokwe of Angola and Zambia, and the Bangwa and Kom chiefdoms of the Cameroon grassfields.

In Southwest African societies, teenage girls and boys underwent initiation rites as part of the journey to adulthood. The young Mbalantu women of Namibia have some of the most intricate hair designs that identified their pre- and post-induction status to the rest of the community. It has been clear from the earliest images of African people that their hair was a preeminent reflection of the state of their well-being and existence in the world. Adorning the head with elaborate hairstyles was and still is considered a sacred place in the African aesthetic.[ii]

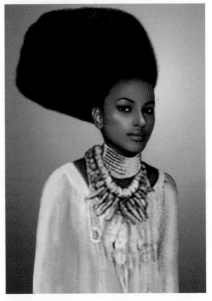

figure 1-1
Africans created grooming aids from materials found in their natural environment.

The Egyptians

Concurrently, in North Africa the Egyptians were the first to cultivate beauty in an extravagant fashion. They used cosmetics as part of their personal beautification habits, religious ceremonies, and preparation of the deceased for burial.

As early as 2630 BC, Egyptians used minerals, insects, and berries to create makeup for their eyes, lips, and skin. Henna was used to stain their hair and nails a rich, warm red. They were also the first civilization to infuse essential oils from the leaves, bark, and blossoms of plants for use as perfumes and for purification purposes. Queen Nefertiti (circa 1400 BC) stained her nails red by dipping her fingertips in henna, wore lavish makeup designs, and used custom-blended essential oils as signature scents. Queen Cleopatra (circa 50 BC) took this dedication to beauty to an entirely new level by erecting a personal cosmetics factory next to the Dead Sea (figure 1-2).

Ancient Egyptians are also credited with creating kohl makeup—originally made from a mixture of ground galena (a black mineral), sulfur, and animal fat—to heavily line the eyes, alleviate eye inflammation, and protect the eyes from the glare of the sun.

In both ancient Egypt and Rome, military commanders stained their nails and lips in matching colors before important battles.

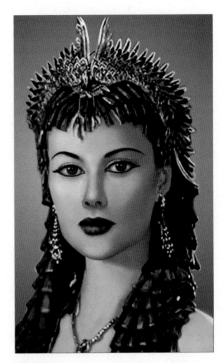

figure 1-2
The Egyptians wore elaborate hairstyles and cosmetics.

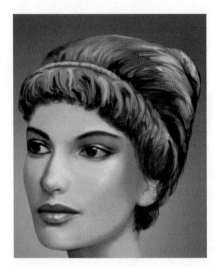

figure 1-3
The Greeks advanced grooming and skin care.

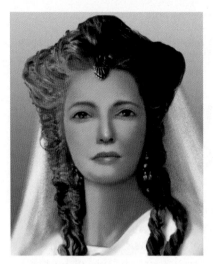

figure 1-4
The Romans applied various preparations to the skin.

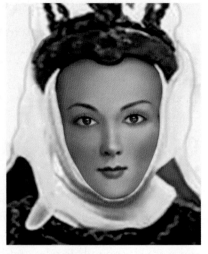

figure 1-5
The Middle Ages show towering headdresses, intricate hairstyles, and the use of cosmetics on skin and hair.

The Chinese

History also shows that during the Shang Dynasty (circa 1600 BC), Chinese aristocrats rubbed a tinted mixture of gum arabic, gelatin, beeswax, and egg whites onto their nails to color them crimson or ebony. Throughout the Zhou Dynasty, also known as Chou Dynasty (circa 1100 BC), gold and silver were the royal colors. During this early period in Chinese history, nail tinting was so closely tied to social status that commoners caught wearing a royal nail color faced a punishment of death.

The Greeks

During the Golden Age of Greece (circa 500 BC), hairstyling became a highly developed art. The ancient Greeks made lavish use of perfumes and cosmetics in their religious rites, in grooming, and for medicinal purposes. They built elaborate baths and developed excellent methods of dressing the hair and caring for the skin and nails. Greek women applied preparations of white lead onto their faces, kohl around their eyes, and vermillion upon their cheeks and lips. Vermillion is a brilliant red pigment, made by grinding cinnabar (a mineral that is the chief source of mercury) to a fine powder. It was mixed with ointment or dusted on the skin in the same way cosmetics are applied today (figure 1-3).

The Romans

Roman women lavishly used fragrances and cosmetics. Facials made of milk and bread or fine wine were popular. Other facials were made of corn with flour and milk, or from flour and fresh butter. A mixture of chalk and white lead was used as a facial cosmetic. Women used hair color to indicate their class in society. Noblewomen tinted their hair red, middle-class women colored their hair blond, and poor women dyed their hair black (figure 1-4).

The Middle Ages

The Middle Ages is the period of European history between classical antiquity and the Renaissance, beginning with the downfall of Rome, circa AD 476, and lasting until about 1450. Beauty culture is evidenced by tapestries, sculptures, and other artifacts from this period. All of these show towering headdresses, intricate hairstyles, and the use of cosmetics on skin and hair (figure 1-5). Women wore colored makeup on their cheeks and lips, but not on their eyes. Around AD 1000, a Persian physician and alchemist named Avicenna refined the process of steam distillation. This ushered in the modern era of steam-distilled essential oils that we use today.

The Renaissance

This is the period in history during which Western civilization made the transition from medieval to modern history. Paintings and written records tell us a great deal about the grooming practices of the time. One of the most unusual practices was the shaving of the eyebrows and the hairline to show a greater expanse of forehead. A brow-less forehead was thought to give women a look of greater intelligence. During this period, both men and women took great pride in their physical appearance and wore elaborate, elegant clothing. Fragrances and cosmetics were used, although highly colored preparations of the lips, cheeks, and eyes were discouraged (figure 1-6).

The Victorian Age

The reign of Queen Victoria of England, between 1837 and 1901, was known as the Victorian age. Fashions in dress and personal grooming were drastically influenced by the social mores of this austere and restrictive period in history. To preserve the health and beauty of the skin, women used beauty masks and packs made from honey, eggs, milk, oatmeal, fruits, vegetables, and other natural ingredients. Victorian women are said to have pinched their cheeks and bitten their lips to induce natural color rather than use cosmetics, such as rouge or lip color (figure 1-7).

The Twentieth Century

In the early twentieth century, the invention of motion pictures coincided with an abrupt shift in American attitudes. As viewers saw pictures of celebrities with flawless complexions, beautiful hairstyles, and manicured nails, standards of feminine beauty began to change. This era also signaled the spread of industrialization, which brought a new prosperity to the United States. Beauty applications began to follow the trends set by celebrities and society figures (figure 1-8).

1901–1910

In 1904, Max Faktor emigrated from Lodz, Poland, to the United States. By 1908, he had Americanized his name to Max Factor and moved to Los Angeles, where he began making and selling makeup. His makeup was popular with movie stars because it wouldn't cake or crack, even under hot studio lights.

On October 8, 1906, Charles Nessler invented a heavily wired machine that supplied electrical current to metal rods around which hair strands were wrapped. These heavy units were heated during the waving process. They were kept away from the scalp by a complex system of counterbalancing weights that were suspended from an overhead chandelier mounted on a

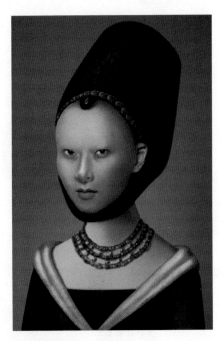
figure 1-6
During the Renaissance, shaving or tweezing of the eyebrows and hairline to show a greater expanse of the forehead was thought to make women appear more intelligent.

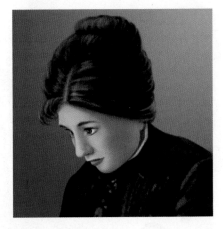
figure 1-7
During the Victorian age, makeup and showy clothing were discouraged except in the theater.

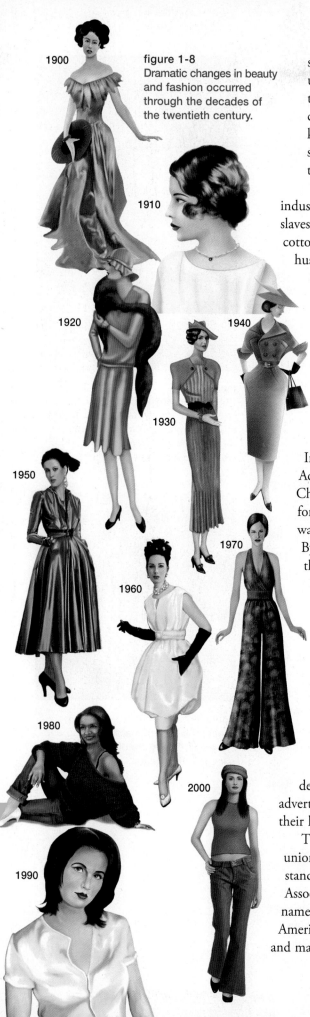

figure 1-8
Dramatic changes in beauty
and fashion occurred
through the decades of
the twentieth century.

1900

1910

1920

1930

1940

1950

1960

1970

1980

1990

2000

stand. Two methods were used to wind hair strands around the metal units. Long hair was wound from the scalp to the ends in a technique called spiral wrapping. After World War I, when women cut their hair into the short bobbed style, the croquignole (KROH-ken-yohl) wrapping technique was introduced. In this method, shorter hair was wound from the ends toward the scalp. The hair was then styled into deep waves with loose end-curls.

One of the most notable success stories of the cosmetology industry is that of Sarah Breedlove. She was the daughter of former slaves and was orphaned at age seven when she went to work in the cotton fields of the Mississippi delta. In 1906, Sarah married her third husband, C. J. Walker, and became known as Madame C. J. Walker. Sarah suffered from a scalp condition and began to lose her hair, which caused her to experiment with store-bought products and homemade remedies. She began to sell her scalp conditioning and healing treatment called "Madam Walker's Wonderful Hair Grower." She devised sophisticated sales and marketing strategies and traveled extensively to give product demonstrations. In 1910, she moved her company to Indianapolis where she built a factory, hair salon, and training school. As she developed new products, her empire grew. She devoted much time and money to a variety of causes in Indianapolis, including the National Association for the Advancement of Colored People (NAACP) and the Young Men's Christian Association (YMCA). In 1917, she organized a convention for her Madam C. J. Walker Hair Culturists Union of America. This was one of the first national meetings for businesswomen ever held. By the time of her death, she had established herself as a pioneer in the modern African American hair care and cosmetics industry.

In 1872, Marcel Grateau (AKA François Marcel) invented the first curling iron—tongs heated by a gas burner. Later, around 1923, he created an electric version. Because he introduced several electric versions, the actual date of the invention remains in dispute. Grateau went on to develop a permanent wave machine, barbers clippers, a safety razor, and other devices.

1920s

The cosmetics industry grew rapidly during the 1920s. Advertising expenditures in radio alone went from $390,000 in 1927 to $3.2 million in 1930. At first, many women's magazines deemed cosmetics improper and refused to print cosmetic advertisements, but by the end of the 1920s, cosmetics provided one of their largest sources of advertising revenue.

The 1920s were also an era of change for cosmetology; the unionizing and practice of barbering ushered in a whole new set of standards that upgraded the practice of cosmetology. In 1924, the Associated Master Barbers of America was organized in Chicago. The name was later changed to Associated Master Barbers and Beauticians of America (AMBBA) and represented barbershop and beauty salon owners and managers. By 1925, the AMBBA established the National Education

Council with the goal of standardizing requirements for barber schools and barber instructor training, establishing a curriculum, and set forth the state licensing laws. By 1929, AMBBA adopted a Barber Code of Ethics to promote professional responsibility in the trade.

1930s

In 1931, the preheat-perm method was introduced. First, hair was wrapped using the croquignole method. Then, clamps that had been preheated by a separate electrical unit were placed over the wound curls (**figure 1-9**). An alternative to the machine perm was introduced in 1932 when chemists Ralph L. Evans and Everett G. McDonough pioneered a method that used heat generated by chemical reaction: Small flexible pads containing a chemical mixture were wound around hair strands. When the pads were moistened with water, a chemical heat was released that created long-lasting curls. Thus the first machineless permanent wave was born. Salon clients were no longer subjected to the dangers and discomforts of the Nessler machine.

In 1932, nearly 4,000 years after the first recorded nail-color craze, Charles Revson of Revlon fame marketed the first nail polish—as opposed to a nail stain—using formulas that were borrowed from the automobile paint industry. This milestone marked a dramatic shift in nail cosmetics as women finally had an array of nail lacquers available to them. The early screen sirens Jean Harlow and Gloria Swanson glamorized this hip new nail fashion in silent pictures and early talkies by appearing in films wearing matching polish on their fingers and toes.

Also in 1932, Lawrence Gelb, a New York chemist, introduced the first permanent haircolor product and founded a company called Clairol. In 1935, Max Factor created pancake makeup to make actors' skin look natural on color film. In 1938, Arnold F. Willatt invented the cold wave that used no machines or heat. The cold wave is considered to be the precursor to the modern perm.

1940s

In 1941, scientists developed another method of permanent waving that used waving lotion. Because this perm did not use heat, it was also called a cold wave. Cold waves replaced virtually all predecessors and competitors. In fact, the terms *cold waving* and *permanent waving* became practically synonymous. Modern versions of cold waves, usually referred to as alkaline perms, are very popular today. The term texture services is used today to refer to the variety of permanent waving and straightening services available for various hair types and conditions.

1951–2000

The second half of the twentieth century saw the introduction of tube mascara, improved hair care and nail products, and the boom and then death of the weekly salon appointment. In the late 1960s, Vidal Sassoon turned the hairstyling world on its ear with his revolutionary geometric cuts.

The 1970s saw a new era in highlighting when French hairdressers introduced the art of hair weaving using aluminum foil. Iconic hairdresser Trevor Sorbie opened his first salon in Covent Garden, England in 1979.

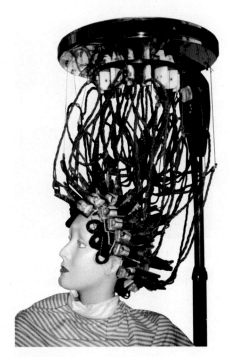

figure 1-9
Antique perm machine

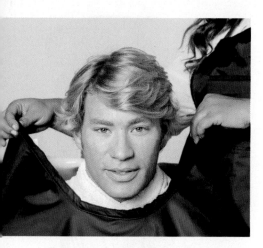

figure 1-10
Men-only specialty spas and barber spas have also grown in popularity.

His creativity and forward thinking have made him one of the most influential hairdressers of all time.[iii] In the 1980s, makeup went full circle, from barely there to heavily made-up "cat-eyes" and the heavy use of eye shadows and blush. In 1985 hairdresser Farouk Shami, led by his passion for his craft and the environment revolutionized the beauty industry by inventing the world's first ammonia-free haircolor.[iv] The first year the North American Hairstyling Awards (NAHA) were held was 1989 and there were only five categories. This event gave hairdressers an opportunity to compete and showcase their talents amongst the best in the industry. Today it is still the most coveted hairstyling award in North America, now with 14 categories to compete in. In the 1990s, haircolor became gentler, allowing all ethnicities to enjoy being blonds, brunettes, or redheads. In 1998, Creative Nail Design introduced the first spa pedicure system to the professional beauty industry.

The Twenty-First Century

Today, hairstylists have far gentler, no-fade haircolor. Estheticians can noticeably rejuvenate the skin, as well as keep disorders such as sunspots and mild acne at bay. The beauty industry has also entered the age of specialization. Now cosmetologists frequently specialize either in haircolor, texture, or in haircutting; estheticians specialize in esthetic or medical-aesthetic services; and nail technicians either offer a full array of services or specialize in artificial nail enhancements, natural nail care, or even pedicures.

Since the late 1980s, the salon industry has evolved to include day spas, a name that was first coined by beauty legend Noel DeCaprio. Day spas now represent an excellent employment opportunity for beauty practitioners.

Men-only specialty spas and barber spas have also grown in popularity. These spas provide exciting new opportunities for men's hair, nail, and skin-care specialists (**figure 1-10**). **Table 1-1** on page 14 is a timeline of significant events in the cosmetology industry.

After reading the next few sections, you will be able to:

LO③ **List several career opportunities available to a licensed beauty practitioner.**

Learn the Importance of Continuing Education

Continuing education is important to your career's future and it holds the key to individual development and personal motivation, gives you knowledge and confidence, and also provides you the best opportunity to advance your career and achieve real success. Hairdressing is an ever-changing profession and education will keep you current with trends, the latest innovations, and newest techniques. Your clients come to you expecting and deserving a knowledgeable professional, and if you are not able to fulfill their needs, chances are, they will not return.

Continuing education gives you the opportunity to observe, practice, and execute the techniques and trends necessary to add value to your skillset. There are many educational resources available to you. Take advantage of the vast range of hands-on classes offered by advanced academies or mentor programs. The educators are typically highly trained experienced professionals willing to help you develop your craft and reach your full potential. Most advanced academies have websites where you can learn about their methods of teaching, courses offered, the educators, and tuition costs. In addition, "look and learn" by getting inspiration from attending trade shows, looking through industry magazines, reading articles, watching instructional videos, viewing websites, and more to show you what's new, including upcoming events to attend. Commitment to perfecting your skills not only advances your technical abilities, but it enhances your professional reputation, increases your earning potential through add-on services, keeps you on the cutting edge of the industry, and allows for networking opportunities with potential employers.

Discover the Career Paths for Cosmetologists

Once you have completed your schooling and are licensed, you will be amazed at how many career opportunities will open up to you. The possibilities can be endless for a hard-working professional cosmetologist who continues their education and approaches her or his career with a strong sense of personal integrity. Within the industry there are numerous opportunities, such as the following:

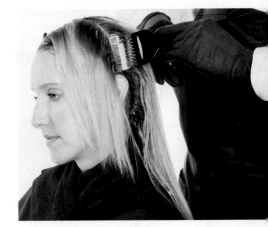

figure 1-11
Haircolor specialists are in great demand.

- **Haircolor specialist.** Once you have received additional training and experience in haircolor, you may be responsible for training others in your salon to perform color services or work for a product manufacturer, where you will be expected to train other professionals how best to perform color services according to the company's guidelines and product instructions (**figure 1-11**).

- **Texture specialist.** Once you have received additional training and experience in texture services, you may be responsible for training others to perform texture services in the salon or work for a manufacturer where you will be expected to train others on how best to perform texture services according to your company's guidelines and product instructions. A subspecialty, curly hair specialist, focuses on maintaining natural curl (**figure 1-12**).

- **Haircutting specialist.** This position requires a dedicated interest in learning various cutting styles and techniques. After perfecting your own skills and developing your own method of cutting (everyone develops his or her own cutting technique), you may want to study with other reputable haircutters to learn and adopt their systems and techniques. This training will allow you to perform top-quality haircutting in your own salon, as well as to coach those around you, helping them to hone their skills.

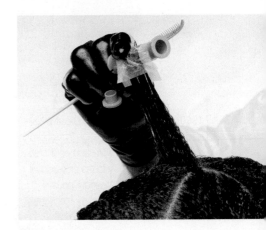

figure 1-12
A texture specialist trains others on how best to perform texture services.

table 1-1

A TIMELINE OF MILESTONES IN THE PROFESSIONAL BEAUTY INDUSTRY.

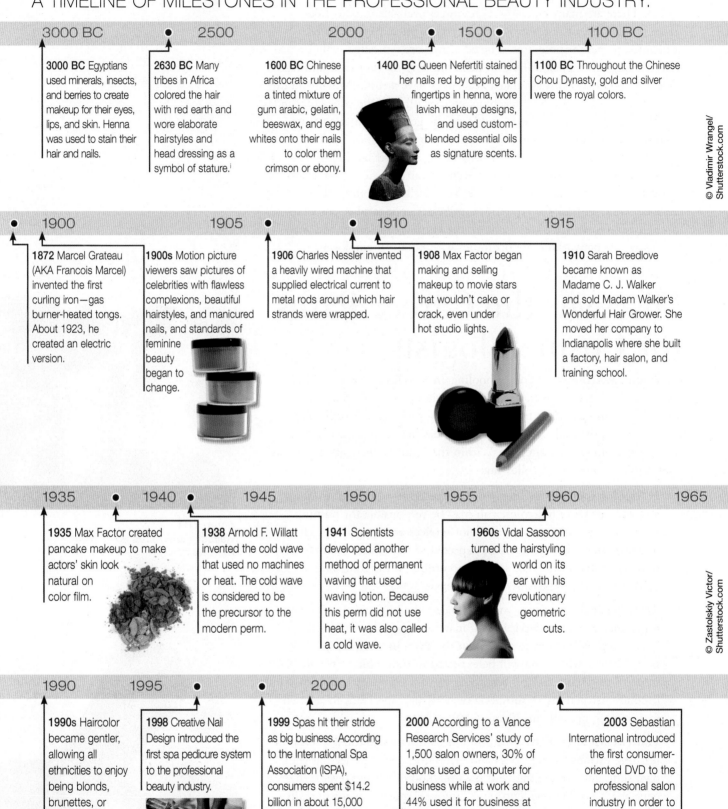

3000 BC   **2500**   **2000**   **1500**   **1100 BC**

3000 BC Egyptians used minerals, insects, and berries to create makeup for their eyes, lips, and skin. Henna was used to stain their hair and nails.

2630 BC Many tribes in Africa colored the hair with red earth and wore elaborate hairstyles and head dressing as a symbol of stature.[i]

1600 BC Chinese aristocrats rubbed a tinted mixture of gum arabic, gelatin, beeswax, and egg whites onto their nails to color them crimson or ebony.

1400 BC Queen Nefertiti stained her nails red by dipping her fingertips in henna, wore lavish makeup designs, and used custom-blended essential oils as signature scents.

1100 BC Throughout the Chinese Chou Dynasty, gold and silver were the royal colors.

© Vladimir Wrangel/ Shutterstock.com

1900   **1905**   **1910**   **1915**

1872 Marcel Grateau (AKA Francois Marcel) invented the first curling iron—gas burner-heated tongs. About 1923, he created an electric version.

1900s Motion picture viewers saw pictures of celebrities with flawless complexions, beautiful hairstyles, and manicured nails, and standards of feminine beauty began to change.

1906 Charles Nessler invented a heavily wired machine that supplied electrical current to metal rods around which hair strands were wrapped.

1908 Max Factor began making and selling makeup to movie stars that wouldn't cake or crack, even under hot studio lights.

1910 Sarah Breedlove became known as Madame C. J. Walker and sold Madam Walker's Wonderful Hair Grower. She moved her company to Indianapolis where she built a factory, hair salon, and training school.

1935   **1940**   **1945**   **1950**   **1955**   **1960**   **1965**

1935 Max Factor created pancake makeup to make actors' skin look natural on color film.

1938 Arnold F. Willatt invented the cold wave that used no machines or heat. The cold wave is considered to be the precursor to the modern perm.

1941 Scientists developed another method of permanent waving that used waving lotion. Because this perm did not use heat, it was also called a cold wave.

1960s Vidal Sassoon turned the hairstyling world on its ear with his revolutionary geometric cuts.

© Zastolskiy Victor/ Shutterstock.com

1990   **1995**   **2000**

1990s Haircolor became gentler, allowing all ethnicities to enjoy being blonds, brunettes, or redheads.

1998 Creative Nail Design introduced the first spa pedicure system to the professional beauty industry.

1999 Spas hit their stride as big business. According to the International Spa Association (ISPA), consumers spent $14.2 billion in about 15,000 destination and day spas.

2000 According to a Vance Research Services' study of 1,500 salon owners, 30% of salons used a computer for business while at work and 44% used it for business at home. 65% of respondents had home Internet access, while just 17% had it in their salons.

2003 Sebastian International introduced the first consumer-oriented DVD to the professional salon industry in order to speak directly to the consumer.

500 BC	50	AD 1000	1500	1850

500 BC During the Golden Age of Greece, hairstyling became a highly developed art. Greek women applied preparations of white lead onto their faces, kohl around their eyes, and vermillion upon their cheeks and lips.

50 BC Queen Cleopatra took dedication to beauty to an entirely new level by erecting a personal cosmetics factory next to the Dead Sea.

AD 1000 Persian physician and alchemist, Avicenna, refined the process of steam distillation. This ushered in the modern era of steam-distilled essential oils that we use today.

1837–1901 To preserve the health and beauty of the skin, women used beauty masks and packs made from honey, eggs, milk, oatmeal, fruits, vegetables, and other natural ingredients.

© iStockphoto/lucato

1920	1925	1930	

1917 Madame Walker organized a convention for her Madam C. J. Walker Hair Culturists Union of America. This was one of the first national meetings for businesswomen ever held.

1920s The cosmetics industry grew rapidly. Advertising expenditures in radio alone went from $390,000 in 1927 to $3.2 million in 1930.

1931 The preheat perm method was introduced. Hair was wrapped using the croquignole method. Clamps, preheated by a separate electrical unit, were then placed over the wound curls.

1932 Chemists Ralph L. Evans and Everett G. McDonough pioneered the first machineless permanent wave.

Also that year, Charles Revson of Revlon fame marketed the first nail polish.

Lawrence Gelb, a New York Chemist, introduced the first permanent haircolor product and founded a company called Clairol.

1970	1975	1980	1985	

1970s French hairdressers introduced the art of hair weaving using aluminum foil.

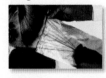

1979 was the year iconic hairdresser Trevor Sorbie opened his first salon in Covent Garden, England.

1980s Makeup went full circle, from barely there to heavily made-up "cat-eyes" and the heavy use of eye shadows and blush. Also, the salon industry evolved to include day spas, a name that was first coined by beauty legend Noel DeCaprio.

1985 Farouk Sami invented the world's first ammonia free haircolor.

1989 The first year the North American Hairstyling Awards was held.[ii]

2005				2013

2005 Most salons had their own websites and used e-mail to communicate. Point-of-sale software and computerized appointment scheduling were in widespread use.

2007 Haircolor became the largest hair care category in terms of in-salon, back bar, and take-home color refresher product sales. The green movement takes off in salons, with many positioning themselves as eco salons and spas striving for sustainability. In April, the first American television reality-competition show for salons, *Shear Genius*, debuted.

2008 There was an explosion in salons using social networking sites to do business. Twitter, which was introduced in March 2006, became the next big thing in social networking with clients.

2009 Many beauty manufacturers had mobile versions of their websites. Access to instant online technical education and color formulas became common.

2013 A Questex/ American Salon Better Business Network Survey found that 72.7% of salons in the U.S. offer complementary Wi-Fi to clients.

- **Salon trainer.** Many companies, such as manufacturers and salon chains, hire experienced salon professionals and train them to educate others. This kind of training can take many forms, from technical training to management and interpersonal relationship training. A salon educator usually reports to the art director or technical director, who oversees the quality of education being implemented in the salon. A salon educator can work with small salons, as well as large organizations and trade associations, to help develop the beauty industry's most valuable resource—salon staff and personnel.

- **Distributor sales consultant.** The salon industry depends heavily on its relationships with product distributors in order to stay abreast of what is occurring in the marketplace. Distributor sales consultants (DSCs) provide information about new products, new trends, and new techniques. This specialty provides an excellent opportunity for highly skilled and trained cosmetology professionals. The DSC is the salon and its staff's link with the rest of the industry, and this relationship represents the most efficient method that outside companies use to reach the salon stylist.

- **Manufacturer educator.** Most manufacturers hire their own educators to train stylists and salon staff to understand and use the company's hair care, haircolor, and chemical-service products. Mastery of the company's product lines is a must for manufacturer educators. An accomplished educator who is a good public speaker can advance to field educator, regional educator, or even platform educator, appearing on stage at shows in the U.S. and around the world.

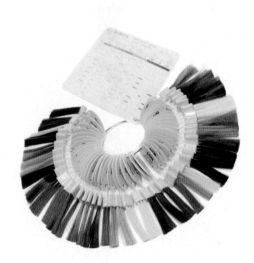

- **Artistic director.** This position establishes the standard for a salon or manufacturer's image. The artistic director's responsibility is to inspire hairdressers and create trends. Being qualified to do this this takes experience and confidence. Investing in continuing education and mastering classic and advanced cutting techniques will establish a great foundation to start. Although there are other skills that are equally as important such as communication, presentation, and leadership. There are many successful artistic directors in the industry and they can be seen performing platform artistry at trade shows representing salons or manufacturers. An important part of this career path is to start early, find a mentor, and ask for tips. Once you've learned all the necessary tools, the following are some of the opportunities available for you on both a salon and manufacturer level: platform artist, manufacturer spokesperson, freelance artist, and salon or manufacturer artistic director.

- **Education director.** Most manufacturers consider this role an integral part of their business. An education director is the liaison between brand and hairdresser, setting the company's standards by creating education that drives sales. This position is only available to cosmetologist with five or more years of experience, and a wealth of continuing education in their resumé is a must. Some of the requirements to qualify for this role are: excellent hairdressing skills, leadership in your prior career role, effective communication and presentation skills, the ability to create budgets and work with spreadsheets, and product knowledge of the company's brand and competitors. The opportunity to contribute to the success of a company can be rewarding in many ways.

- **Cosmetology instructor.** Have you ever wondered how your instructor decided to start teaching? Many instructors had fantastic careers in salons before dedicating themselves to teaching new professionals the tricks of the trade. If this career path interests you, spend some time with your school's instructors and ask them why they went into education. Educating new cosmetologists can be very trying, but it can also be very rewarding.

- **Film, theatrical, or editorial stylist.** Working behind the scenes at magazine and Internet photo shoots or backstage on movie and TV sets all starts with volunteering to assist. Even someone right out of school can volunteer by calling agencies, networking with photographers, and asking other hairdressers who work behind the scenes for advice. The days are long—up to 18 hours on soap opera sets—but once you clock the specific number of hours required by your state of residence, you can join the local union, which opens many doors. All you need are persistence, networking skills, reliability, team spirit, and attention to detail (figure 1-13). This field requires constant continuing education, particularly in working with wigs, hairpieces, and makeup.

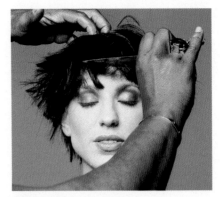

figure 1-13
Film, theatrical or editorial stylist is fast-paced and sometimes has long days.

- **Creative director.** This is one of the most respected and rewarding positions in the industry. Once you have established yourself as a successful hairdresser, with 10 or more years of experience in all facets of hairdressing, this position can be obtainable. Most manufacturers consider this an executive level position and the driving force behind brand success. There can be different position tiers, and some companies have both an international and a global creative director. The responsibilities are to oversee, coach, mentor, and lead all of the company's educators to ensure the highest standards of professionalism. The hairdressers that have made their mark in the industry, through achievements and hard work, hold most of these positions. The privilege of being called *Creative Director* means that you have committed yourself to elevating the standard of education and professionalism of all hairdressers.

Salon Management

After many years of working in the business several hairdressers will take on the responsibility of salon manager. You will find that management opportunities in the salon and spa industry are quite diverse. In addition to your duties as a professional hairstylist, you will assume the duties of: inventory manager, department head, educator, special events manager (promotions), assistant manager, and general manager. With experience, you can also add salon owner to this list of career possibilities. To ensure your success, it is wise to enroll in business classes to learn more about managing products, departments, and—above all—people.

Salon manager is a potential career path for a cosmetologist, but it requires a very different skill set. As a result, some managers of large operations are not cosmetologists. Salon managers must have an aptitude for math and accounting and be able to read documents such as profit and loss statements. They should understand marketing, including the roles of advertising, public relations and promotions, and what makes these programs successful. Much of management involves the business side of the

? DID YOU KNOW?
Although cosmetologists who work in salons and spas do not have to join a union to be considered for work or to be entitled to certain benefits of employment, to work on films, television shows, and theater you may need to join a union. The unions have different names. One of the largest is the Makeup Artists and Hair Stylists Union, also known as the International Alliance of Theatrical Stage Employees, Moving Picture Technicians, Artist and Allied Crafts of the United States and Canada, AFL-CIO, CLC (IA). You may also need to join the Makeup Artists and Hair Stylists Guild, or the Actors' Union.

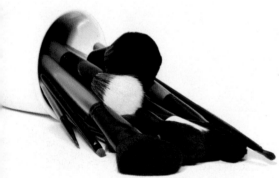

salon—making it profitable—while keeping clients and employees happy. Titles and the accompanying responsibilities vary widely from salon to salon, and it is always possible to learn on the job. However, supplementing your experience with formal business education is also an effective path to success.

Every licensed cosmetologist has the opportunity to expand his or her career. As students you must never forget that no matter what path you choose you control your own destiny. Keep developing your skills in the specialties that interest you, and you'll soon be building and enjoying an extremely creative and rewarding career.

Beyond choosing a specialty, you must decide on the type of facility where you will work. Many options are available:

- Specialty salons
- Full-service salons (offering hair, skin, and nail services)
- Photo, video, or film sets (preparing models and actors for camera appearances)
- Day spas (offering services that emphasize both beauty and wellness)

To learn more about the various types of salon business models, see Chapter 32, The Salon Business. There you will find a wealth of choices, including national and regional chains and low- and high-end salon opportunities.

REVIEW QUESTIONS

1. What are the origins of appearance enhancement?

2. What were some of the male hairstyles during ancient times?

3. What are some of the advancements made in cosmetology during the nineteenth, twentieth, and early twenty-first centuries?

4. What are the benefits of continuing education?

5. What are some of the career opportunities available to licensed beauty practitioners?

STUDY TOOLS

- **Reinforce what you just learned:** Complete the activities and exercises in your Theory or Practical Workbook, or your Study Guide.

- **Expand your knowledge:** Search for websites about the topics in this chapter and make a list of additional resources.

- **Study and prepare for your quiz:** Take the chapter test in your Exam Review or your Milady U: Online Licensing Prep.

- **Re-Test your knowledge:** Take the Chapter 1 *Quizzes*!

- **Learn even more:** Look up in a dictionary or search the internet for the definitions of any additional terms you want to learn about.

CHAPTER GLOSSARY

appearance enhancement	p. 6	A term used to encompass a broad range of specialty areas, including hairstyling, nail technology, and esthetics.
continuing education	p. 12	Education that is employment or license related; used to motivate, enrich, update skill sets, satisfy licensing requirements, or further your career.
cosmetology kahz-muh-TAHL-uh-jee	p. 6	The art and science of beautifying and improving the skin, nails, hair and includes the study of cosmetics and their application.

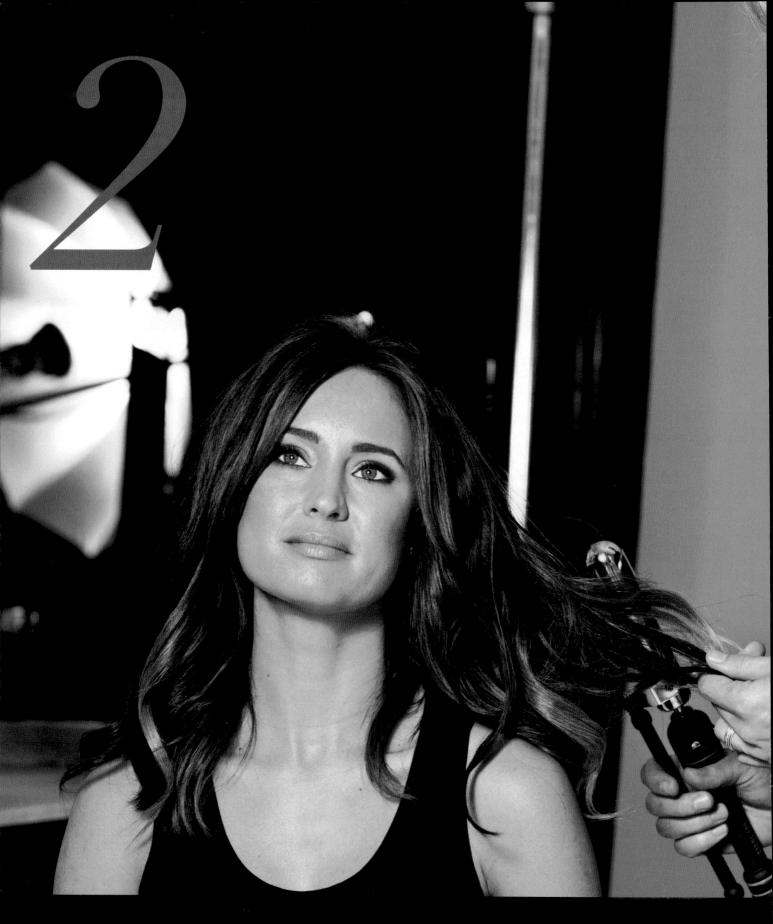

2

LIFE SKILLS

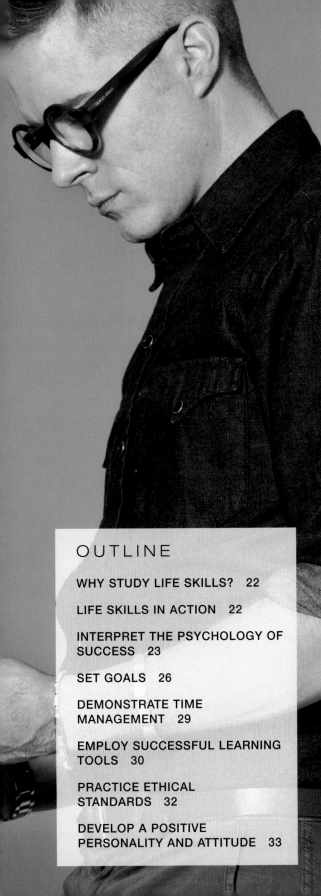

LEARNING OBJECTIVES

After completing this chapter, you will be able to:

LO❶
List the principles that contribute to personal and professional success.

LO❷
Create a mission statement.

LO❸
Explain long-term and short-term goals.

LO❹
Discuss the most effective ways to manage time.

LO❺
Demonstrate good study habits.

LO❻
Define ethics.

LO❼
List the characteristics of a healthy, positive attitude.

While good technical skills are extremely important to master, learning and applying sound life skills are just as important. The salon is a creative workplace where individuals are expected to exercise artistic talent. In addition, a successful salon or spa atmosphere is a highly social environment which influences workers to develop exceptional communication, decision-making, image-building, customer service, self actualization, goal-setting, and time management skills. These life skills are the foundation of success for students and professionals.

why study
LIFE SKILLS?

Cosmetologists should study and have a thorough understanding of life skills because:

> Practicing good life skills will lead to a more satisfying and productive beauty career. Beauty professionals work with many different types of clients, and having good life skills can help keep those interactions positive in any situation.

> The ability to deal with difficult circumstances comes from having well developed life skills.

> Having good life skills builds self-esteem, which helps individuals achieve goals.

Life Skills in Action

Some of the most important life skills for you to remember and practice include:

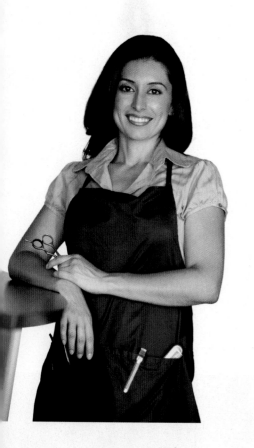

- Being helpful and caring to others.
- Making good friends.
- Feeling good about oneself.
- Having a sense of humor.
- Maintaining a cooperative attitude.
- Approaching work with a strong sense of responsibility.
- Being consistent in your work.
- Adapting successfully to different situations.
- Sticking to a goal and seeing a job through to completion.
- Mastering techniques to become more organized.
- Developing sound decision-making skills.

After reading the next few sections, you will be able to:

LO ❶ List the principles that contribute to personal and professional success.

Interpret the Psychology of Success

Success has been defined in many ways over the years. What is your definition of success? Take a few minutes to think about your answer and write it down. The process of **self actualization**, fulfilling one's full potential, requires lifelong commitment. Stay the course and fuel your passion by following proven success building steps (figure 2-1).

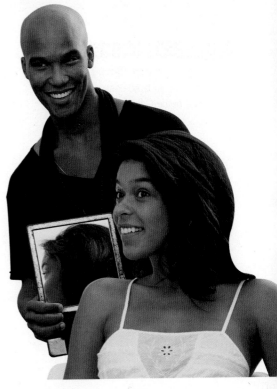

figure 2-1
Loving your work is critical to your success.

Action Steps for Success

Being successful requires hard work and effort. Continually focusing on the following action steps will create a solid foundation for achieving your goals.

- **Build self-esteem.** Self-esteem is based on inner strength and begins with trusting your ability to achieve set goals. It is essential to begin developing high self-esteem while in school. Reading positive affirmations is a great way to start building self-esteem.

- **Visualize success.** Imagine yourself working in your dream salon. You are competently handling clients, loving the job and the environment of the salon. The more you practice visualization, the more easily you will turn your vision into reality.

- **Build on your strengths.** Practice doing whatever helps you maintain a positive self-image. If you are good at doing something (e.g., playing the guitar, running, cooking, gardening, or singing), the time you invest in this activity will allow you to feel good about yourself (figure 2-2). Remember that there may be things you are good at that you may not realize. You may be a good listener, for instance, or a caring and considerate friend.

- **Be kind to yourself.** Eliminate self-critical or negative thoughts that are counterproductive. If you make a mistake, view it as a learning opportunity to improve and get it right.

- **Stay true to yourself.** Be yourself and be professional! Being unique is a valuable asset of beauty professionals. It takes too much time and effort to be someone that you're not.

- **Practice new behaviors.** Because creating success is a skill, you can develop it by practicing positive new behaviors such as speaking with confidence, standing tall, and using proper grammar.

- **Keep your personal life separate from your work.** Talking about your personal life at work is counterproductive and can cause the whole salon to suffer.

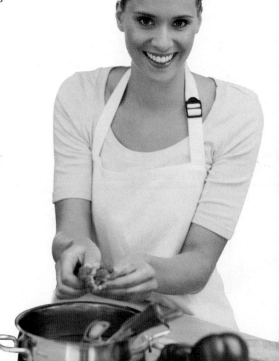

figure 2-2
Spend time on things you do well.

milady pro **LEARN MORE!**

Optional info on **Goal Setting** can
be found at miladypro.com
Keyword: *FutureCosPro*

- **Keep your energy up.** Successful cosmetologists take care of themselves. Get the proper amount of sleep, eat healthy foods, and manage your time wisely. Also, create balance by spending time with family and friends, having hobbies, and enjoying recreational activities.

- **Respect others.** Make a conscious effort to respect everyone. Exercise good manners with others by using words like *please, thank you,* and *excuse me.* Practice being a good listener and remember not to interrupt others when they are speaking.

- **Stay productive.** There are three bad habits that can keep you from maintaining peak performance: (1) procrastination, (2) perfectionism, and (3) lack of a game plan. You will see an almost instant improvement in your productivity when you eliminate these troublesome tendencies.

  1. **Procrastination** (PRO-crass-tin-aye-shun) is putting off until tomorrow what you can do today. (For example, I'll study tomorrow instead of today.) This thought process may be attributed to scheduling too many tasks at one time, which is a symptom of faulty organization.

  2. **Perfectionism** (PUR-fek-shun-izm) is an unhealthy compulsion to do things perfectly. Success is not defined as doing everything perfectly. In fact, someone who never makes a mistake may not be taking the necessary risks for growth and improvement.

  3. **Lacking a game plan.** Having a **game plan** is the conscious act of planning your life, instead of just letting things happen. While an overall game plan is usually organized into large blocks of time (five or ten years), it is just as important to set daily, monthly, and yearly goals. Where do you want to be in your career five years from now? What do you have to do this week, this month, and this year to move closer to that goal?

Motivation and Self-Management

Starting something new can be both exciting and intimidating. For example, many students feel nervous about starting cosmetology school. Despite what emotions a person feels, motivation and self-management skills will help people move to the next level in their career. To achieve success, you need more than an external push; you must feel a sense of personal excitement and a good reason for staying the course. You are the one in charge of managing your own life and learning. To do this successfully, use creativity.

Your Creative Capability

Creativity means having a talent such as painting, acting, cutting hair, applying makeup, or doing artificial nails. Creativity is also an unlimited inner resource of ideas and solutions. To enhance your creativity, keep these guidelines in mind:

- **Be positive.** Criticism blocks the creative mind from exploring ideas and discovering solutions to challenges.

- **Look around for creative inspiration.** Tap into the creative energy of art museums, music, fashion shows, and magazines.

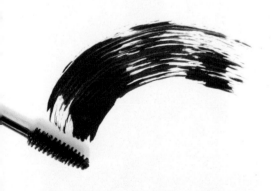

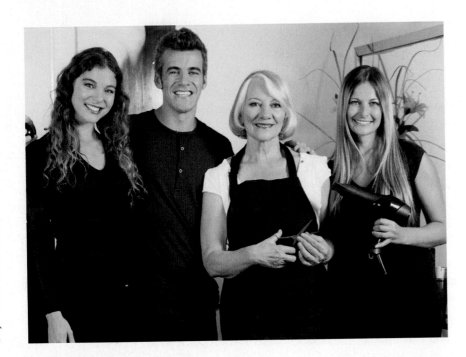

figure 2-3
Build strong relationships for support.

- **Improve your vocabulary.** Build a positive vocabulary by using active problem-solving words like *explore, analyze, determine*.

- **Surround yourself with others who share your passion.** In today's hectic and pressured world, many talented people find that they are more creative in an environment where people work together and share ideas. This is where the value of a strong salon team comes into play (figure 2-3).

After reading the next few sections, you will be able to:

LO❷ **Create a mission statement.**

Design a Mission Statement

An essential part of business is the **mission statement** (MISH-uhn STATE-ment), which establishes the purpose and values for which an individual or institution lives and works by. It provides a sense of direction by defining guiding principles and clarifying goals, as well as how an organization operates. Often you will find the mission statement of a company posted for customers to read. Look for a mission statement next time you're in a hotel, fast food restaurant, or other service-related business. The mission often becomes more than just a statement. It becomes the cultural pulse for organizations. A well thought-out sense of purpose in the form of a mission statement will also help individuals on their journey to success.

Create a mission statement by beginning with your interests. We have created a tool, the Interests Self-Test, to help you get started (figure 2-4).

Next, try to prepare a mission statement in one or two sentences that communicates who you are and what you want for your life. One example of a simple, yet thoughtful, mission statement is: "I am dedicated to pursuing a successful career with dignity, honesty, and integrity." Your mission statement will point you in the right direction and help you feel secure when things temporarily go off course. For reinforcement, keep a copy of your mission statement where you can see it, and read it frequently.

The Interests Self-Test

Your personality is tied to your interests. You've already learned about cosmetology specialties. Why not start thinking about which specialty interests you the most? This quick quiz gives you an idea of where your future might lie, based on your personal preferences.

1. Which subject interests you most?
   A. Chemistry   **B.** Geometry   **C.** Accounting

2. Which of the following would you rather do?
   A. Analyze a problem   **B.** Solve a problem   **C.** Read about a problem

3. When you look at a painting, what do you notice first?
   A. Color   **B.** Shape   **C.** Details

4. When it comes to coworkers, would you prefer to:
   A. Work with one other person on a specific problem   **C.** Work alone or tell teammates
   B. Work with a team to get lots of ideas   what to do

5. When it comes to salon clients, do you think they:
   A. Know exactly what they want, and that's good   **C.** Probably want a good value
   B. Are open to new ideas and suggestions, which is fun

Instructions: Add up the number of As, Bs, and Cs. Then check below to see what might be of most interest to you.

Mostly As. Hair color, which involves chemistry, detail work, and solving specific problems, might be a good choice for you. Of course, color can be creative, too, but you need strong fundamentals and a mind for detail to reach the top. Additionally, clients frequently bring in a photo of a specific hair color, and you must know how to get from point A (their natural color) to point B (their desired color).

Mostly Bs. Hair cutting involves an understanding of geometry, lines, and shapes. Clients may want a certain look but they can't always have it if their hair type doesn't allow it. That's why the ability to gather ideas and make suggestions is important. At the advanced level, there are several different cutting methods to try out.

Mostly Cs. Business demands an attention to details, the ability to crunch numbers, and an understanding of client's desires and consumer trends. While you sometimes work alone, you also have to be able to manage other people, which is an additional consideration. If you like taking responsibility for yourself and others, you might consider focusing on the business of salons.

figure 2-4
The Interests Self-Test

After reading the next few sections, you will be able to:

LO❸ Explain long-term and short-term goals.

Set Goals

Do you have direction, drive, desire, and a dream? If so, do you have a reasonable idea of how to go about meeting your goal(s)?

    Goal setting is the identification of long-term and short-term goals. When you know what you want, you can draw a circle around your destination and chart the best course to get there. By mapping out your goals, you will see where to focus your attention in order to fulfill your dreams.

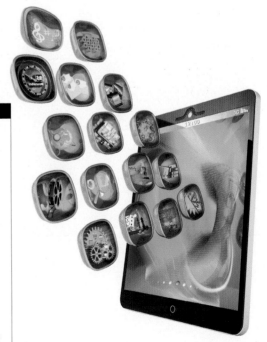

Real-Life Goal Setting:

Goals that salons set are often associated directly with a person's productivity. However, goals that stylists set for themselves are often based on how much money they want to earn. Salon managers will help individuals break down large financial goals into attainable, daily goals. For example, if you want to gross $10,000 more a year, you need to earn an additional $27.39 per day. Of course, you don't work seven days a week. A more realistic number is based on working five days a week, 52 weeks out of the year. You need to gross $38.46 more per day, and fortunately there are many different ways to do it in the salon business. You can sell retail to half your clients; you can up-sell color services and back-bar treatments; or you can get more clients.

How Goal Setting Works

When setting goals, categorize them based on the amount of time it takes to accomplish the goals. An example of a short-term goal is to get through an exam successfully. Another short-term goal is to graduate from cosmetology school. Short-term goals are usually those to be accomplished in a year or less.

Long-term goals are measured in larger increments of time such as two years, five years, ten years, or even longer. An example of a long-term goal is becoming a salon owner in five years.

Once you have organized your thoughts, write them down in short-term and long-term columns and divide each set of goals into workable segments. Now the goals will not seem out of sight or overwhelming. For example, if you are a part-time cosmetology student, one of your long-term goals should be to become a licensed cosmetologist. At first, getting this license might seem to require an overwhelming amount of time and effort. However, when larger aspirations are divided into short-term goals (such as going to class on time, completing homework assignments, and mastering techniques), each step leads to the accomplishment of the larger goal.

Remember to set feasible goals, to create a plan of action, and to revisit the plan often. While adjusting goals and action plans may be necessary from time to time, successful people know that focusing on their goals will move them toward additional successes (figure 2-5 and figure 2-6).

ACTIVITY

It is estimated in the average person's day, four hours are spent checking e-mail, looking at websites, and watching videos. The average teenager sends nearly 80 text messages a day! To find out if you are managing your time well, try this exercise:

• Write down the time in the morning when you first go online, check e-mail, or send a text message.
• Do what you normally do online, then note the time you finish these activities.
• Throughout the day, try to estimate (and add to your list) how much additional time you spend on these activities.
• Add up the total time at the end of your day.

Are you surprised? Time-management experts recommend that people work for the first 45 minutes or hour of the day, avoiding e-mailing, Web browsing, and texting. Instead, use this time to plan the day, review reading materials for school, or do other work. The first hour of the day is often the best time to accomplish something concrete because it is quiet and often interruption-free. Starting the day by being productive helps develop good life-long time-management skills.

figure 2-5
A sample of how to set and track short-term goals

HOW TO SET AND TRACK SHORT-TERM GOALS

Number	Goal Setting Checklist	Completion Date	Done
1.	Read Chapter 2. Action Steps: Read first part at lunch; finish it after dinner.	6/09/2016	✓
2.	Practice speaking to clients in a pleasing voice. Action Steps: Do with family tonight.	6/10/2016	✓
3.	Create my own mission statement. Action Steps: Review sample in Chapter 2; write my own.	6/15/2016	✓
4.	Start learning trends. Action Steps: Search online, read trade and beauty magazines. Make a five-word "trend list."	6/20/2016	✓
5.	Prepare to pass the Chapter 2 exam. Action Steps: Review what I read, ask instructor any questions, have study session with two friends.	7/10/2016	✓
6.	Practice being on time! Action Steps: Set alarm for 15 minutes earlier. Give self $1 every time I get to class 10 minutes early.	Start 6/20 5 days in a row by 7/20	
7.	Build my vocabulary. Action Steps: Buy book or find website. Learn one new word a day.	Daily	

figure 2-6
Photocopy this template and fill in your own goals!

MY GOALS

Number	Goal Setting Checklist	Completion Date	Done
1.			
2.			
3.			
4.			
5.			
6.			
7.			

After reading the next few sections, you will be able to:

LO ④ Discuss the most effective ways to manage time.

Demonstrate Time Management

Each of us has an *inner organizer*. When we pay attention to our inner organizer, we can learn how to manage our time efficiently. This will allow us to reach our goals faster. Here are some of the most effective ways to manage time:

- Learn to **prioritize** (PRIH-or-uh-tize) by ordering tasks on your to-do list from most important to least important.

- When designing your time management system, make sure it will work for you. For example, if you are a person who needs a fair amount of flexibility, schedule some blocks of unstructured time.

- Never take on more than you can handle. Learn to say "no" firmly but kindly, and mean it. It will be easier to complete tasks if activities are limited.

- Learn problem-solving techniques that will save you time and needless frustration.

- Give yourself some downtime whenever you are frustrated, overwhelmed, worried, or feeling guilty. You lose valuable time and energy when you are in a negative state of mind. Unfortunately, there may be situations where you cannot get up and walk away. To handle these difficult times, try practicing the technique of deep breathing. Just fill your lungs as much as you can and exhale slowly. After about five to ten breaths, you will usually find that you have calmed down and your inner balance has been restored.

- Have a notepad, organizer, tablet, or other digital application accessible at all times.

- Make daily, weekly, and monthly schedules that show exam times, study sessions, and any other regular commitments. Plan leisure time around these commitments rather than the other way around (figure 2-7).

> **? DID YOU KNOW?**
> **Real-Life Time Management:**
>
> In a salon environment it takes a team effort to efficiently manage time. Salons book appointments based on the types of services being provided, the clientele, and the salon type. Some salons operate without setting appointments, and instead work on a walk-in or first-come first-serve basis. Both methods require stylists to practice efffective communication with fellow stylists and peers.
>
> Making sure that you arrive on time, start your first client as soon as he or she arrives, and staying on schedule will take you a long way toward success as a stylist. The front desk and salon manager can be a tremendous help if you find yourself falling behind or if you have the opportunity to add-on a color service and need help fitting it into your day. With experience, you'll learn to accommodate late clients and add-on services like a pro.

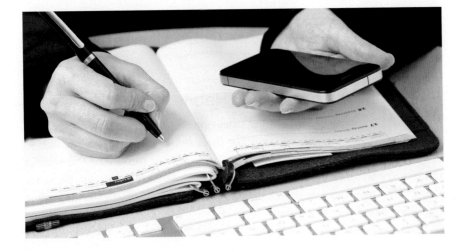

figure 2-7
Keep a schedule for yourself and refer to it frequently.

© Caroline Eibl/Shutterstock.com

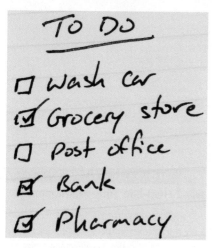

figure 2-8
Use a to-do list to prioritize tasks.

- Identify times during the day when you are energetic and times when you want or need to relax. Plan your schedule accordingly.

- Reward yourself with a special treat or activity for work well done and efficient time management.

- Do not neglect physical activity. Remember that exercise and recreation stimulate clear thinking.

- Schedule at least one block of free time each day. This will be your hedge against events that happen unexpectedly, such as car trouble, baby-sitting problems, helping a friend in need, or other unforeseen circumstances.

- Understand the value of to-do lists for the day and the week. These lists help prioritize tasks and activities, a key element to organizing time efficiently (**figure 2-8**).

- Make effective time management a habit.

After reading the next few sections, you will be able to:

LO⑤ **Demonstrate good study habits.**

Employ Successful Learning Tools

Having a successful career as a beauty professional begins by employing key learning tools while in school. To realize the greatest benefits education can provide, commit yourself to do the following:

- Attend all classes.

- Arrive for class early.

- Have all necessary materials ready.

- Listen attentively to your instructor.

- Take notes.

- Highlight important points.

- Pay close attention during summary and review sessions.

- When something is not clear, ask for clarification. If you are still unsure, ask again for assistance.

Establishing Good Study Habits

If you find studying overwhelming, focus on small tasks one at a time. For example, instead of trying to study for three hours at a time, set the bar lower by studying in smaller chunks of time. If your mind tends to wander in class, try writing down key words or phrases as your instructor discusses them. Any time you lose focus, do not hesitate to stay after class and ask questions based on your notes.

✔ **HERE'S A TIP**

After becoming a licensed professional, seek continuing education opportunities. Never stop learning! The cosmetology industry is constantly changing; there are always new trends, techniques, products, and information. Reading magazines, joining beauty industry associations, attending trade shows, and enrolling in advanced educational classes are all ways to continue learning.

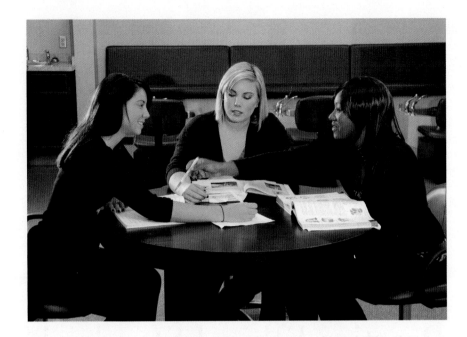

figure 2-9
Studying with a friend can be effective
and fun.

Another study tip is to find other students who are helpful and supportive. Studying in groups can bring positive results for everyone including improved study skills and a better understanding of the material (figure 2-9).

Part of developing good study habits is knowing where, when, and how to study.

Where

- Establish a comfortable, quiet place to study without interruptions.

- Have everything you need—books, pens, paper, proper lighting—prior to studying.

- Remain as alert as possible by sitting upright. Reclining will make you sleepy!

When

- Start out by estimating how much study time you need.

- Study when you feel most energetic and motivated.

- Practice effective time management by studying during blocks of time that would otherwise be wasted—such as while you are waiting in the doctor's office or taking a bus across town.

How

- Study just one section of a chapter at a time and review key points. This method is more effective than reading the entire chapter at once.

- Highlight key words and phrases as you go along.

- Test yourself on each section to ensure that you understand the information.

Remember that every effort you make to follow through on your education is an investment in your future. The progress you make with your learning will increase your confidence. In fact, when you have mastered a range of information and techniques, your self-esteem will soar right along with your grades.

FOCUS ON

The Goal

Determine whether your goal-setting plan is effective by asking yourself these key questions:

- Are there specific skills I will need to learn in order to meet my goals?

- Is the information I need to reach my goals readily available?

- Am I willing to seek out a mentor or a coach to enhance my learning?

- What is the best method or approach that will allow me to accomplish my goals?

- Am I open to finding better ways of putting my plan into practice?

Professional Ethics

Ethical people often embody the following qualities:

- **Self-care.** To be helpful to others, it is essential to take care of yourself. Try The Self-Care Test to assess how you are doing (**figure 2-10**).
- **Integrity.** Maintain your integrity by aligning your behavior and actions to your values. For example, if you believe it is unethical to increase your sales by recommending products that clients don't really need, then do not engage in that behavior. On the other hand, if you feel that a client would benefit from certain products and additional services, it would be unethical not to give the client that information.

- **Discretion.** Do not share your personal issues with clients. Likewise, never breach confidentiality by repeating personal information that clients have shared with you.
- **Communication.** Your responsibility to behave ethically extends to your communications with customers and coworkers. Be aware of what you say and how you say it. Also, be conscious of your nonverbal communication, which is just as important as verbal communication.

After reading the next few sections, you will be able to:

LO ⑥ Define ethics.

Practice Ethical Standards

Ethics (ETH-iks) are the moral principles by which we live and work. In a salon setting, ethical standards should guide your conduct with clients and fellow employees. When your actions are respectful, courteous, and helpful, you are behaving in an ethical manner.

figure 2-10
The Self-Care Test

The Self-Care Test

Some people know intuitively when they need to stop, take a break, or even take a day off. Other people forget when to eat. You can judge how well you take care of yourself by noting how you feel physically, emotionally, and mentally. Here are some questions to ask yourself to see how you rate on the self-care scale.

1. Do you wait until you are exhausted before you stop working?
2. Do you forget to eat nutritious food and substitute junk food on the fly?
3. Do you say you will exercise and then put off starting a program?
4. Do you have poor sleep habits?
5. Are you constantly nagging yourself about not being good enough?
6. Are your relationships with people filled with conflict?
7. When you think about the future are you unclear about the direction you will take?
8. Do you spend most of your spare time watching TV?
9. Have you been told you are too stressed and yet you ignore these concerns?
10. Do you waste time and then get angry with yourself?

Score 5 points for each yes. A score of 0-15 says that you take pretty good care of yourself, but you would be wise to examine those questions you answered yes to. A score of 15-30 indicates that you need to rethink your priorities. A score of 30-50 is a strong statement that you are neglecting yourself and may be headed for high stress and burnout. Reviewing the suggestions in Chapter 2 will help you get back on track.

Practice ethical behavior in the salon by employing these five professional actions:

1. Providing skilled and competent services.

2. Being honest, courteous, and sincere.

3. Avoiding sharing clients' private matters with others—even your closest friends.

4. Participating in continuing education and staying on track with new information, techniques, and skills.

5. Giving clients accurate information about treatments and products.

After reading the next few sections, you will be able to:

LO**7** **List the characteristics of a healthy, positive attitude.**

Develop a Positive Personality and Attitude

Cosmetologists interact with people from all walks of life—every day, all day. It is useful, therefore, to have a sense of how different personality traits work together. Refer regularly to the following characteristics of a healthy, positive attitude:

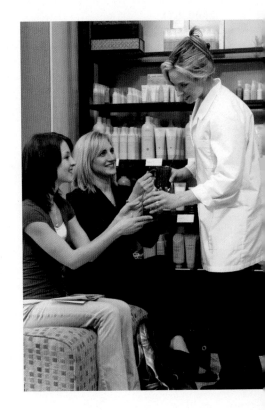

- **Diplomacy.** Being assertive is good because it helps people understand your position. However, it is a short step from assertive to aggressive or even bullying. Take your attitude temperature to see how well you practice the art of diplomacy. Diplomacy—also known as tact—is the ability to deliver truthful, even sometimes critical or difficult, messages in a kind way.

- **Pleasing tone of voice.** The tone of your voice is a personality trait, but if your natural voice is harsh or if you tend to mumble, you can consciously improve by speaking more softly or more clearly. Another technique is to smile when speaking if it is appropriate. This will help the tone of your voice. Practice smiling in person and when talking on the phone.

 FOCUS ON

The Whole Person

An individual's personality is the sum of her or his characteristics, attitudes, and behavioral traits. Attitude improvement is a process that continues throughout life. In both your business and personal life, a pleasing attitude gains more associates, clients, and friends. You will know you have a pleasing attitude when you are able to see the good in difficult situations. People enjoy the company of individuals who can put a positive "spin" on things.

- **Emotional stability.** Learning how to handle a confrontation and how to share your feelings in a professional manner are important indicators of emotional stability.

- **Sensitivity.** Being sensitive means being compassionate and responsive to other people.

- **Values and goals.** Values and goals guide our behavior and give us direction.

- **Receptivity.** Be interested in other people, and responsive to their opinions, feelings, and ideas. Receptivity involves taking the time to really listen to others. Also, be open-minded and willing to work with all personality types. (**figure 2-11**).

- **Effective communication skills.** Commit to practicing effective communication through active listening, non-verbal, and verbal skills. For additional information refer to Chapter 4, Communicating for Success.

figure 2-11
Exercise good listening skills when discussing client requests.

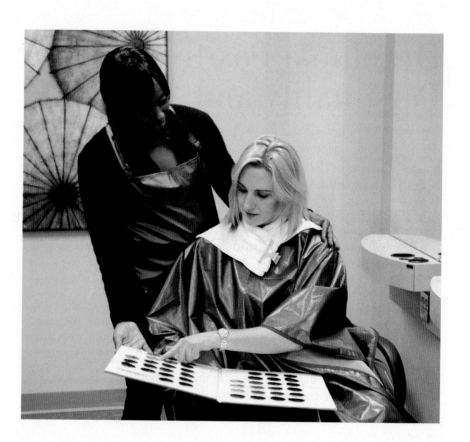

REVIEW QUESTIONS

1. What principles contribute to personal and professional success?

2. How do you create a mission statement? (Give an example.)

3. How do you go about setting long- and short-term goals?

4. What are some of the most effective ways to manage time?

5. How do you describe good study habits?

6. What is the definition of ethics?

7. What are the characteristics of a healthy, positive attitude?

STUDY TOOLS

- **Reinforce what you just learned:** Complete the activities and exercises in your Theory or Practical Workbook, or your Study Guide.

- **Expand your knowledge:** Search for websites about the topics in this chapter and make a list of additional resources.

- **Study and prepare for your quiz:** Take the chapter test in your Exam Review or your Milady U: Online Licensing Prep.

- **Re-Test your knowledge:** Take the Chapter 2 *Quizzes*!

- **Learn even more:** Look up in a dictionary or search the internet for the definitions of any additional terms you want to learn about.

CHAPTER GLOSSARY

ethics ETH-iks	p. 32	The moral principles by which we live and work.
game plan	p. 24	The conscious act of planning your life, instead of just letting things happen.
goal setting	p. 26	The identification of long-term and short-term goals that helps you decide what you want out of life.
mission statement MISH-uhn STATE-ment	p. 25	A statement that establishes the purpose and values for which an individual or institution lives and works by. It provides a sense of direction by defining guiding principles and clarifying goals, as well as how an organization operates.
perfectionism PUR-fek-shun-izm	p. 24	An unhealthy compulsion to do things perfectly.
prioritize PRIH-or-uh-tize	p. 29	To make a list of tasks that need to be done in the order of most-to-least important.
procrastination PRO-crass-tin-aye-shun	p. 24	Putting off until tomorrow what you can do today.
self actualization	p. 23	Fulfilling one's full potential.

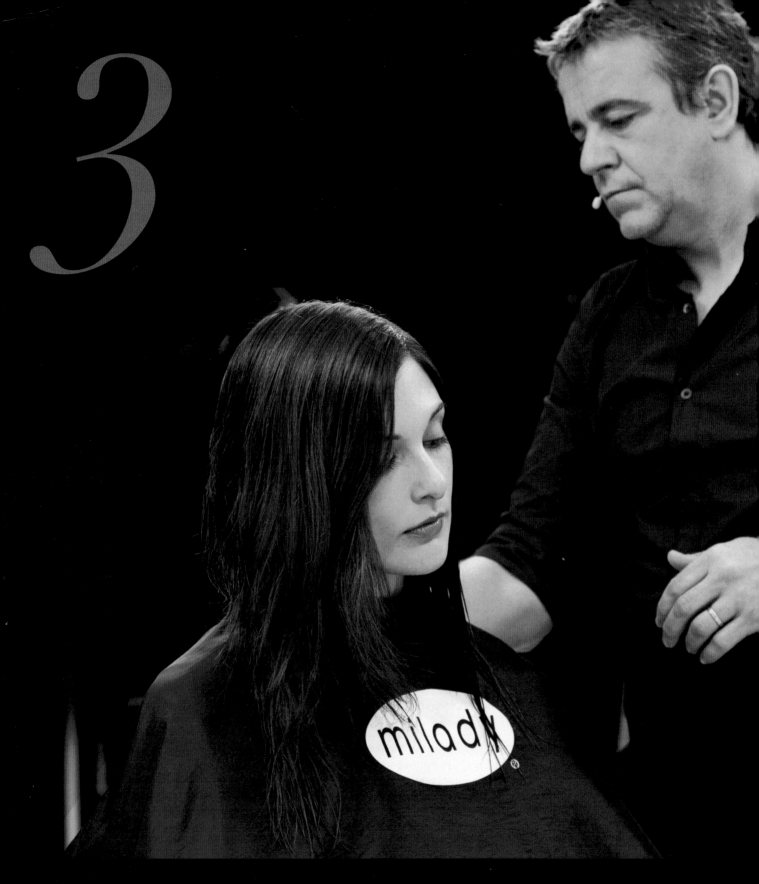

3

YOUR PROFESSIONAL
IMAGE

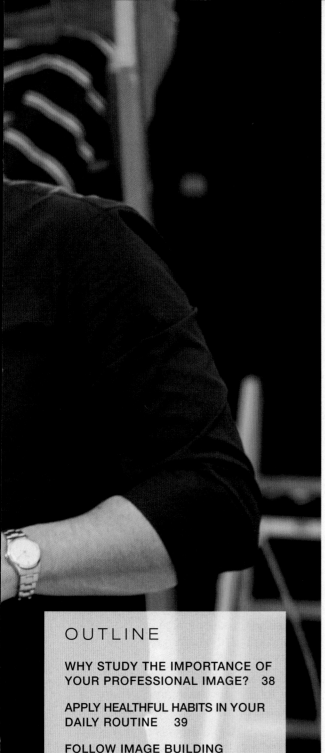

LEARNING OBJECTIVES

After completing this chapter, you will be able to:

LO❶
Name four good personal hygiene habits.

LO❷
Explain the concept of dressing for success.

LO❸
Practice ergonomically correct movement, postures, and principles.

Do you believe that first impressions are important? First impressions are often the gateway to obtaining a job interview, new customers, and to building a professional image. Making a positive impact is essential when working in the business of image building. Beauty professionals are often held to higher image standards by clients because they view beauty professionals as image experts. For this reason alone, it is vital to look and act your absolute best when in public. Letting your image be the standard for clients and peers is a great recipe for success (figure 3-1).

There are many factors that help create a professional image. However, how a person looks is often the first clue to determining if he or she has what it takes to do the job. Professional behavior, a positive attitude, team camaraderie, good communication skills, and proper ergonomics make the recipe for success more flavorful! Ideally, everyone should present a great total package.

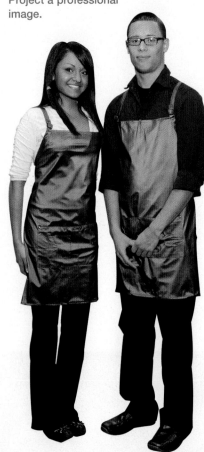

figure 3-1
Project a professional image.

why study
THE IMPORTANCE OF YOUR PROFESSIONAL IMAGE?

Cosmetologists should have a thorough understanding of the importance of their professional image because:

> Clients rely on beauty professionals to look good and be well groomed. Having a professional beauty image helps to build trust with clients and leads to repeat business.

> Finding a salon whose culture complements your image standards and goals is important for career growth and achievements.

> There are consequences to not maintaining a professional image, including loss of clients, a poor reputation, and loss of income.

> Understanding ergonomics can help prevent health issues associated with poor working habits and help professionals stay gainfully employed.

Apply Healthful Habits in Your Daily Routine

Being well groomed begins with looking and smelling fresh. These hygienic characteristics are especially important in the beauty business where practitioners are frequently only inches away from their clients during services.

Personal Hygiene

Basic hygienic practices such as showering or bathing should never be omitted from daily personal care practices. **Personal hygiene** is the daily maintenance of cleanliness by practicing good healthful habits (figure 3-2). When working as a stylist, makeup artist, nail technician, or esthetician, you will be in close proximity to clients. One weak moment of drinking coffee right before performing a service, or wearing something that needs laundering because you did not plan ahead, could be disastrous. Rather than telling you that you smell offensive, most clients will simply not return and may tell others about their bad experience.

As a beauty professional it is imperative to always be clean, neat, and have a pleasant scent.

One of the best ways to ensure that you always smell fresh and clean is to create a hygiene pack to use at work. This pack should include the following items:

- Toothbrush and toothpaste

- Mouthwash

- Sanitizing hand wipes or liquid to clean your hands between clients (when soap and water are not available)

- Dental floss

- Deodorant or antiperspirant and body wipes

Your hygiene pack will be useful in maintaining the following good personal hygiene habits:

- Wash your hands throughout the day as required, including at the beginning of each service.

- Perform self checks, and wash or freshen under the arms as needed.

- Brush and floss your teeth, and use mouthwash or breath mints throughout the day.

- If you smoke cigarettes, *do not* smoke during work hours. Many clients find the lingering smell of smoke offensive. If you smoke during your lunch break, brush your teeth, use mouthwash, and wash your hands afterward!

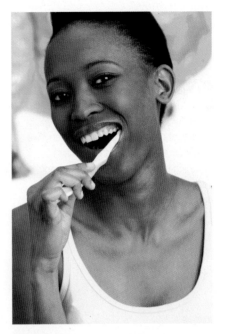

figure 3-2
Practice meticulous personal hygiene every day.

milady pro **LEARN MORE!**

Optional info on **Professionalism** can be found at miladypro.com
Keyword: *FutureCosPro*

Follow Image Building Basics

Being well groomed advertises a beauty professional's commitment to the beauty industry. Consider yourself a walking billboard, and make sure to follow personal grooming habits and to practice professional behavior.

Personal Grooming

Many salon owners and managers view appearance and personality as being just as important as technical knowledge and skills. **Personal grooming** is the process of caring for parts of the body and maintaining an overall polished look. How a person dresses and takes care of his or her hair, skin, and nails reflects one's personal grooming habits.

Dress for Success

While working, your wardrobe selection should express a professional image that is consistent with the image of the salon (figure 3-3). Your **professional image** is the impression you project through both your outward appearance and your conduct in the workplace. Your clothes must be clean—not simply free of the dirt that you can see, but stain free, a feat that is sometimes difficult to achieve in a salon environment. Because you are constantly coming into contact with products and chemicals that can stain fabric, investing in an apron or smock is advised. Be mindful about spills and drips when using chemicals, and avoid leaning on counters in the work area—particularly in the dispensary. Some salons require employees to wear aprons at all times, while others have dress-code rules, such as black and white attire. These requirements are examples of a salon's culture and how stylists can dress for success.

When shopping for work clothes, visualize how you would look in them while performing services. Is the image you will present one that is acceptable to your clients? It is important to consider body type and shape when choosing what to wear to work. Select clothing that looks flattering and be sure to look in the mirror from various angles before leaving for work. Have you ever tried on an item of clothing and wondered if it is too short, too tight, too low cut, or too ugly? Just about everyone has. In these instances, play it safe and choose something more suitable to wear!

Dressing for success does not mean that you have to be someone that you are not. Everyone has a unique personality and it is okay to let your personality speak through clothing, shoes, and accessories. Just remember to tune in to the salon's culture.

While it is important to always follow the employer's dress code, here are some universal wardrobe guidelines:

- Wear clothing that is clean, fresh, and current with fashion.

- Choose clothing that is functional, comfortable, and stylish.

- Invest in supportive and properly fitting undergarments.

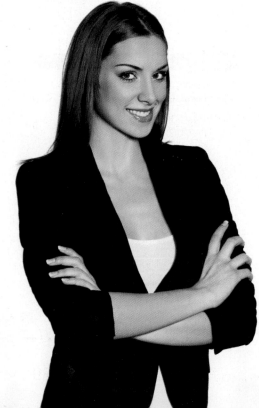

figure 3-3
Be guided by your salon's dress code.

© thuatha/Shutterstock.com

- Accessorize your outfits, but make sure that your jewelry does not jingle while you work because this can irritate fellow professionals and clients.

- Wear shoes that are comfortable, have a low heel, and good arch support. Ill-fitting shoes or high heels are not the best choices to wear when a lot of standing is required (figure 3-4).

Hair Maintenance

Complement your professional wardrobe with an up-to-date hairstyle. It is important to keep your haircut and color fresh. To accomplish this, schedule time for a hair appointment, and possibly barter with other beauty industry professionals for hair care services. Even the pros deserve to be pampered. Remember, you are a walking billboard!

Skin Care and Makeup

Skin care and makeup are exciting for beauty professionals. Just like a smile, proper skin care and makeup application can help promote a professional image. Having and maintaining healthy skin is an ongoing process. Develop a skin care regimen that works best with your skin type. Use protective products on your skin such as sunscreens, and if skin problems occur seek professional advice. Makeup should be used to enhance facial features, so take your time and apply makeup prior to arriving to work or school (figure 3-5). Applying makeup at your station is unprofessional and advertises that you have poor time management skills.

Nail Care

Beauty industry professionals have the privilege of using their hands to make a living, but often neglect their own care. Manicures are a great way to relax hands and thoroughly clean nails. Determine a nail length that suits your personal style and maintain their appearance. Chipped nail polish or broken nails may happen occasionally but should not be a regular occurrence.

Professional Behavior

A positive attitude is one of the foundational principles in developing a professional image. Negative gossip and impolite demeanors can bring an ideal atmosphere to a halt. Always be considerate and treat everyone respectfully. Politeness is the hallmark of professionalism, even under pressure. Cooperating with colleagues is a great way to learn.

Another principle for developing a professional image is communication. A frequent form of communication that can easily be misunderstood is online communication. Establishing a professional online image is an essential image-building attribute. Social media websites, including photo-sharing sites, can quickly diminish a person's reputation if media etiquette is neglected.

DO

- Manage your personal pages/walls.

- Use social media to communicate with peers and clients.

- Post helpful content.

DON'T

- Use profane language.

- Participate in or entertain arguments online.

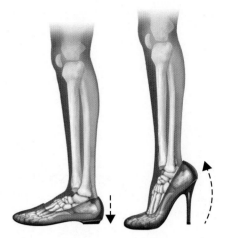

figure 3-4
Working in high heels can throw off the body's balance.

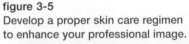

figure 3-5
Develop a proper skin care regimen to enhance your professional image.

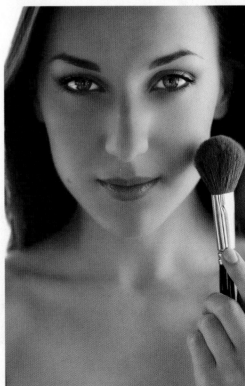

- Post nude or embarrassing photographs.
- Forward spam.

Additional specific communication skills will be discussed in Chapter 4, Communicating for Success.

After reading the next few sections, you will be able to:

LO ③ Practice ergonomically correct movement, postures, and principles.

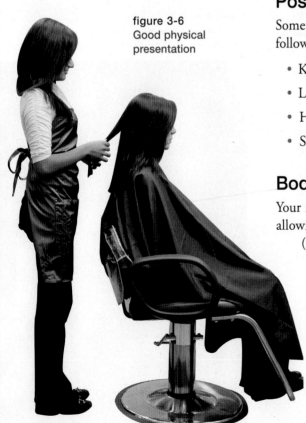

⚠️ **CAUTION**
Not only can wearing inappropriate shoes at work be uncomfortable, it could be dangerous. Flip-flops and open-toed shoes are not safe to wear around electrical tools and sharp implements.

figure 3-6
Good physical presentation

Employ Proper Ergonomics to Protect Your Body

Your **physical presentation** involves your posture and the way you walk and move. Good posture conveys an image of confidence, and can prevent fatigue and many other physical problems. Sitting or standing improperly can put a great deal of stress on your neck, shoulders, back, and legs. Having good posture allows you to get through your day feeling good and doing your best work.

Posture

Some guidelines for achieving and maintaining good posture include the following:

- Keep your neck elongated and balanced directly above the shoulders.
- Lift your upper body so that your chest is out and up (do not slouch).
- Hold your shoulders level and relaxed, not scrunched.
- Sit with your back straight (**figure 3-6**).

Body Movement

Your muscles and bones work together as a musculoskeletal system, allowing you to walk, raise your arms, and use your fingers. **Ergonomics** (UR-go-nom-icks) is the science of designing the workplace as well as its equipment and tools to make specific body movements more comfortable, efficient, and safe.

For example, a hydraulic chair can be raised or lowered to accommodate stylists of different heights, allowing each stylist to service clients without bending over too far. Certain shears are designed to eliminate hand fatigue when cutting hair because repetitive movements are of particular concern.

Each year, hundreds of cosmetology professionals report musculoskeletal disorders, including carpal tunnel syndrome (a wrist injury) and back injuries. Beauty professionals may have to stand or sit all day and perform repetitive movements. This makes them susceptible to problems of the hands, wrists, shoulders, neck, back, feet, and legs.

Prevention is the key to avoiding problems. An awareness of your posture and movements, coupled with good work habits, proper tools, and equipment, will enhance your health and comfort (figure 3-7).

Ergonomics is important to your ability to work and your body's wellness. Repetitive motions have a cumulative effect on the muscles and joints. To avoid problems, monitor yourself as you work to see if you are falling into these bad habits:

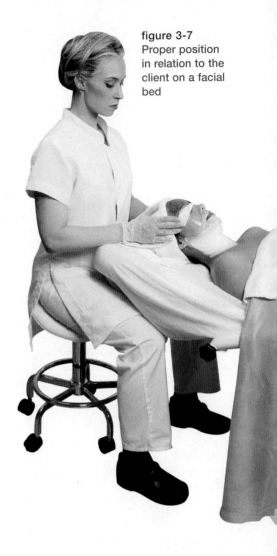

figure 3-7
Proper position in relation to the client on a facial bed

- Gripping or squeezing implements too tightly

- Bending your wrist up or down repeatedly, or contorting your wrist when using the tools of your profession (figure 3-8)

- Holding your arms too far away from your body as you work

- Holding your elbows at more than a 60-degree angle away from your body for extended periods of time. Elbows should be close to the body when cutting.

- Bending forward and/or twisting your body to get closer to your client

To avoid ergonomic-related injuries, follow these guidelines:

- Keep your wrists in a straight or neutral position as much as possible. (figure 3-9).

- When giving a manicure, do not reach across the table; have the client extend his or her hand across the table to you. (figure 3-10).

- Use ergonomically designed implements.

figure 3-8
Improper haircutting position

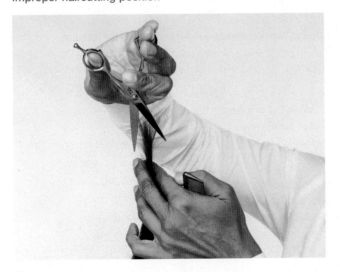

figure 3-9
Correct wrist and hand position for haircutting

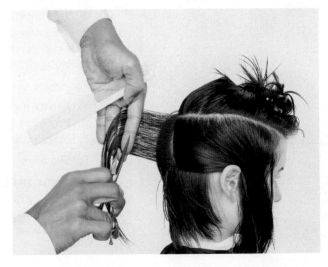

figure 3-10
Follow proper ergonomic techniques
when performing nail services.

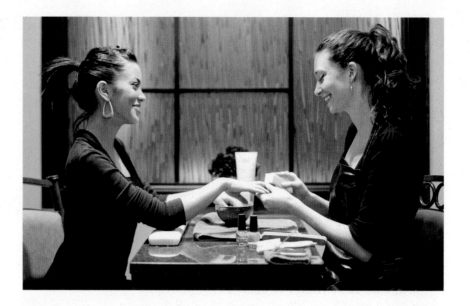

- Keep your back and neck straight.

- Stand on an anti-fatigue mat.

- When standing to cut hair, position your legs hip-width apart, bend your knees slightly, and align your pelvic area with your abdomen.

Counter the negative impact of repetitive motions or long periods spent in one position by stretching and walking around at intervals. Always put your well-being first.

ACTIVITY

Practice these quick exercises, to help you relieve stress from repetitive movements or from standing or sitting in one position for too long:

For Wrists

1. Stand up straight.
2. Raise both of your arms straight out.
3. Bend your wrists so your fingers point upward and hold for five seconds.
4. Hold your wrists steady and turn your hands, so your fingers face the floor and hold for five seconds.
5. Repeat the cycle five times.

For Fingers

1. Get a ball the size of a tennis ball or a tension ball.
2. Grip it tightly for a count of five. Release.
3. Repeat five times.

For Shoulders

1. Stand up straight and shrug your shoulders upward.
2. Roll your shoulders back and hold for a count of five.
3. Reverse direction and roll your shoulders forward for a count of five.
4. Repeat five times.

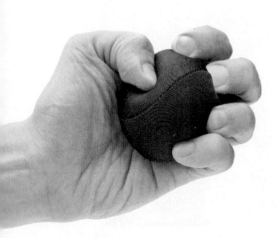

REVIEW QUESTIONS

1. What are four good personal hygiene habits?

2. What is the best way to ensure you are dressed for success?

3. What are four ways you can avoid ergonomic-related injuries?

STUDY TOOLS

- **Reinforce what you just learned:** Complete the activities and exercises in your Theory or Practical Workbook, or your Study Guide.

- **Expand your knowledge:** Search for websites about the topics in this chapter and make a list of additional resources.

- **Study and prepare for your quiz:** Take the chapter test in your Exam Review or your Milady U: Online Licensing Prep.

- **Re-Test your knowledge:** Take the Chapter 3 *Quizzes!*

- **Learn even more:** Look up in a dictionary or search the internet for the definitions of any additional terms you want to learn about.

CHAPTER GLOSSARY

ergonomics UR-go-nom-icks	p. 42	The science of designing the workplace as well as its equipment and tools to make specific body movements more comfortable, efficient, and safe.
personal grooming	p. 40	The process of caring for parts of the body and maintaining an overall polished look.
personal hygiene	p. 39	Daily maintenance and cleanliness by practicing good healthful habits.
physical presentation	p. 42	Your posture, as well as the way you walk and move.
professional image	p. 40	The impression you project through both your outward appearance and your conduct in the workplace.

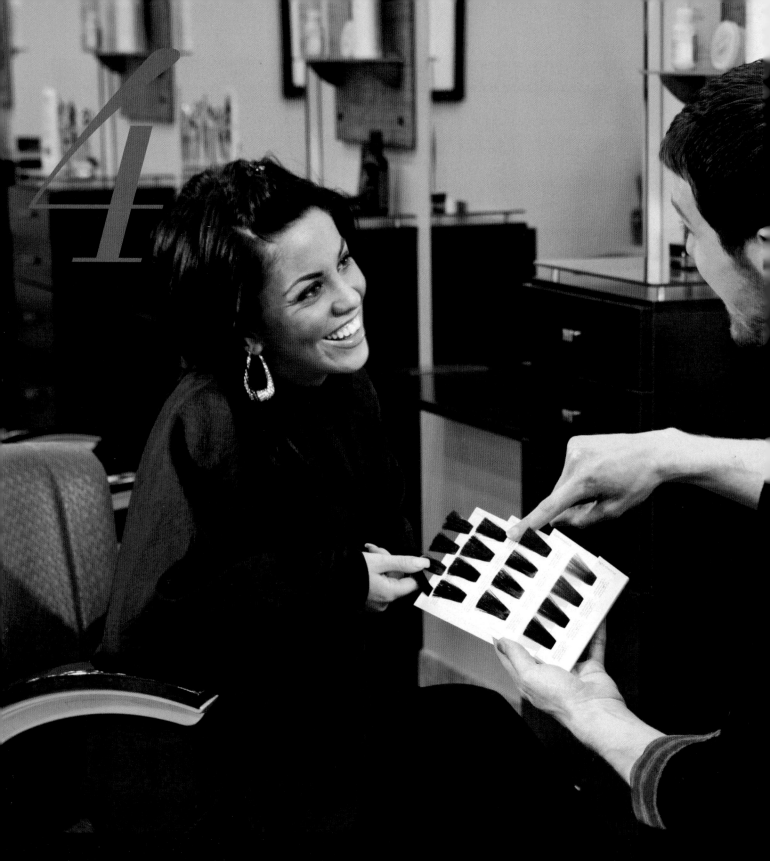

4

COMMUNICATING FOR SUCCESS

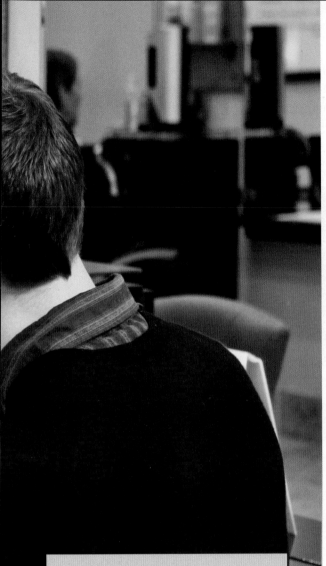

LEARNING OBJECTIVES

After completing this chapter, you will be able to:

LO❶
Take practical steps for effectively communicating in the workplace.

LO❷
Conduct a successful client consultation.

LO❸
Adequately manage tardy clients, schedule mix-ups, and unhappy clients.

LO❹
Build open lines of communication with coworkers.

In order to have a thriving clientele, commit to mastering the art of communication (**figure 4-1**). Effective human relations and communication skills build lasting client relationships, accelerate professional growth, and promote a positive work environment.

figure 4-1
Communication is key in building lasting cosmetologist–client relationships.

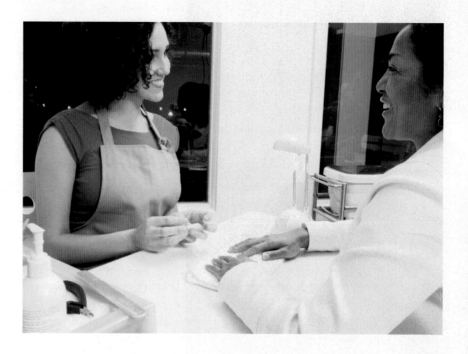

© Blend Images/Shutterstock.com

why study
COMMUNICATING FOR SUCCESS?

Cosmetologists should study and have a thorough understanding of communicating for success because:

> Communicating effectively is the basis of all long-lasting relationships with clients and coworkers.

> The communication process will help stylists perfect the consultation process with clients.

> Effective communication fosters a positive team environment.

> Good communication skills reduce potential workplace conflict.

> Learning how to communicate effectively can help stylists improve retail and service sales.

> Practicing professional communication ensures that clients will enjoy their experience, and encourages their continued patronage.

> Effectively expressing ideas is a necessary skill for career advancement.

LO ❶ Take practical steps for effectively communicating in the workplace.

Practice Communication Skills

The ability to understand people is the key to operating effectively in many industries. It is especially important in cosmetology, where customer service is the cornerstone of success. Most of a stylist's achievements will depend on his or her ability to communicate successfully with a wide range of people: supervisors, coworkers, clients, and various vendors who come into the salon.

Here are practical steps for effectively communicating in the workplace:

- **Respond instead of reacting.** A man was asked why he did not get angry when a driver cut him off. "Why should I let someone else dictate my emotions?" he replied. A wise fellow, don't you think? He may have even saved his own life by not reacting with "an eye for an eye" mentality.

- **Believe in yourself.** When you do, you trust your judgment, uphold your values, and stick to what you believe is right. It is easy to believe in yourself when you have a strong sense of self-worth. Believing in yourself makes you feel strong enough to handle almost any situation in a calm, helpful manner.

- **Talk less, listen more.** There is an old saying that we were given two ears and one mouth for a reason. Listen more than you talk. When you are a good listener, you are fully attentive to what other people are saying.

- **Be attentive.** Each client is different. Some clients are clear about what they want, some are demanding, and still others may be hesitant. If you have an aggressive client, ask your manager for advice. You will likely be advised that what usually calms difficult clients down is agreeing with them. Follow up by asking what you can do to make the service more satisfactory (**figure 4-2**).

milady pro LEARN MORE!

Optional info on **Communication Skills** can be found at miladypro.com
Keyword: *FutureCosPro*

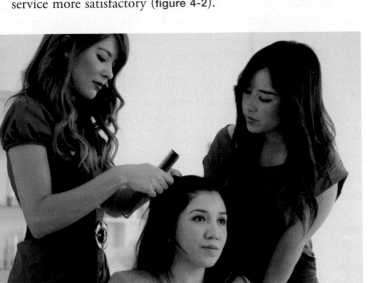

© AntonioDiaz/Shutterstock.com

figure 4-2
Be attentive to your client's needs.

- **Take your temperature.** If you are tired or upset, your interactions with clients may be affected. An important part of succeeding in a service profession is taking care of your personal conflicts first so that you can take the best possible care of your clients.

The Golden Rules of Communication

Keep the following golden rules of communication to build a successful beauty industry career:

- Project a professional demeanor at all times.
- A smile can be your best asset. Wear one every day.
- Be aware of your body language. For example, when listening to clients or team members, don't cross your arms. Instead, nod your head to acknowledge and/or accept their points of view.
- Always remember that listening is the best relationship builder.
- Speak clearly and loudly enough for people to hear. Don't mumble.
- Use correct English.

The Importance of Effective Communication

Effective communication is the act of successfully sharing information between two people (or groups of people) so that the information is understood. You can communicate through words, voice inflections, facial expressions, body language, or visual tools (e.g., a portfolio of your work). When you and your client are both communicating clearly about an upcoming service, your chances of pleasing that client soar.

Meeting and Greeting New Clients

One of the most important encounters you will have is the first time you meet a client. Be polite, genuinely friendly, and inviting. Remember that your clients are coming to you for services and paying for your expertise (figure 4-3). Communicate professionally by using the proper terminology and thoroughly explaining the features and benefits of the products and services.

To earn a client's trust and loyalty, you should:

- Be consistent by always having a positive attitude. Always introduce yourself and use the client's name throughout the service. Set aside a few minutes to take new clients on a quick tour of the salon.
- Introduce clients to people they may have interactions with while in the salon, including potential providers for other services, such as skin care or nail services.

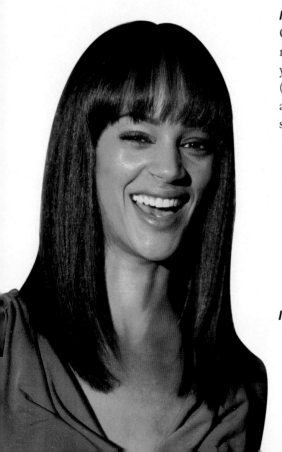

Intake Form   Every new client should fill out a **client intake form**—also called a client questionnaire, consultation card, or health history form. This form can prove to be an extremely useful communication

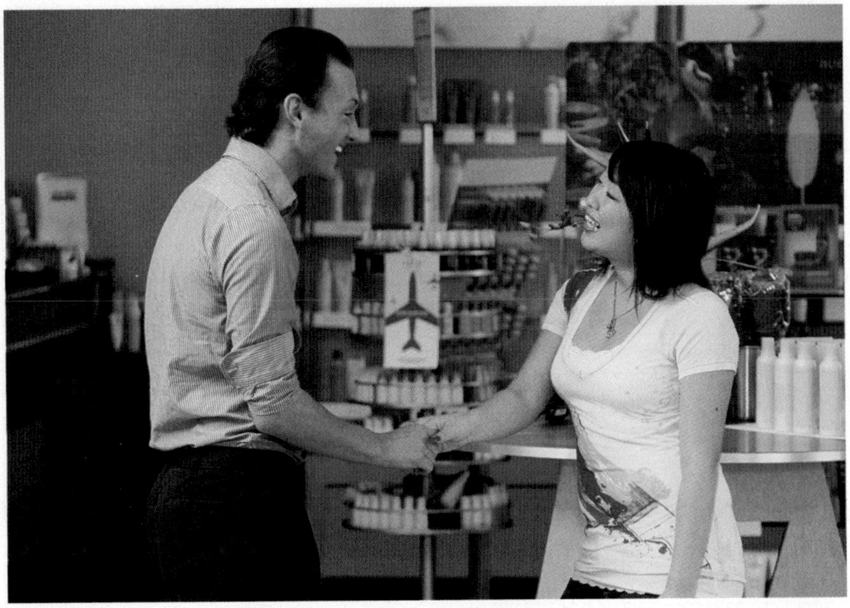

figure 4-3
Welcome your client to the salon.

and business tool (**figure 4-4**). The client intake form is used in beauty and wellness services as a questionnaire that discloses the client's contact information, products they use, hair/nail/skin care needs, preferences, and lifestyle. The form also includes all medications, both topical (applied to the skin) and oral (taken by mouth), along with any known medical issues, skin or scalp disorders, or allergies that might affect services.

Allergies or sensitivities must also be noted, highlighted, and documented on the **service record card**—the client's permanent progress record of services received, results, formulations, and products used during the service or purchased. The service record card is not intended for the client's use, and is completed by the technician or stylist performing the service. It is the technicians' responsibility to update or note changes on this document with each client visit. Some salons use a customer database to record this pertinent information. Examples of a service record card appear in Chapters 21 and 22 related to haircoloring and skin care services.

The amount of information requested on the intake form or questionnaire varies from salon to salon. In cosmetology school, the intake form may be accompanied by a release statement and service notes in which the client acknowledges that the service is being provided by a student who is under instruction. This helps protect the school and the student from legal action.

How to Use the Client Intake Form   The client intake form can be used from the moment a new client calls the salon to make an appointment. When scheduling the appointment, let the client know that you and the salon will require some information before you can begin the service, and that it is important to arrive 15 minutes ahead of the appointment time. Also, allow time in your schedule to do a 5 to 15 minute client consultation.

Client Intake Form

Dear Client,

Our sincerest hope is to provide you with the best hair care services you've ever received! We not only want you to be happy with today's visit, we also want to build a long-lasting relationship with you. In order for us to do so, we would like to learn more about you, your hair care needs, and your preferences. Please take a moment now to answer the questions below as completely and as accurately as possible.

Thank you, and we look forward to building a relationship!

Name: _____

Address: _____

Phone Number: (day) _____ (evening) _____ (cell) _____

E-mail address: _____

Sex: _____ Male _____ Female   Age: _____

How did you hear about our salon? _____

If you were referred, who referred you? _____

Please answer the following questions in the space provided. Thanks!

1.   Approximately when was your last salon visit? _____

2.   In the past year have you had any of the following services either in or out of a salon?

     _____ Haircut   _____ Manicure

     _____ Haircolor   _____ Artificial Nail Services (please describe)

     _____ Permanent Wave or Texturizing Treatment   _____ Pedicure

     _____ Chemical Relaxing or Straightening Treatment   _____ Facial/Skin Treatment

     _____ Highlighting or Lowlighting   _____ Other (please list any other services you've

     _____ Full Head Lightening   enjoyed at a salon that may not be listed here).

3.   What are your expectations for your hair service(s) today?

4.   Are you now, or have you ever been, allergic to any of the products, treatments, or chemicals you've received during any salon service—hair, nails, or skin? (please explain)

     _____

5.   Are you currently taking any medications? (please list)

     _____

6.   Please list all of the products that you use on your hair on a regular basis.

     _____

     _____

7.   What tools do you use at home to style your hair? _____

8.   What is the one thing that you want your stylist to know about you/your hair? _____

9.   Are you interested in receiving a skin care, nail care or makeup consultation? _____

10. Would you like to be contacted via e-mail about upcoming promotions and special events?

     Yes _____ No _____

figure 4-4
The Client Intake Form gives you an opportunity to build an excellent relationship with your clients.

NOTE: If this card were used in a cosmetology school setting, it would include a release form at the bottom such as the one below.

Statement of Release: I hereby understand that supervised cosmetology students render these services for the sole purpose of practice and learning, and that by signing this form, I recognize and agree not to hold the school, its employees, or the student liable for my satisfaction or the service outcome.

Client Signature _____ Date _____

Service Notes

Today's Date:

Today's Services:

Notes:

Today's Date:

Today's Services:

Notes:

Today's Date:

Today's Services:

Notes:

Today's Date:

Today's Services:

Notes:

Today's Date:

Today's Services:

Notes:

---

figure 4-4
(Continued)

⊕ FOCUS ON

Understanding The Total Look Concept

While the enhancement of your client's image should always be your primary concern, it is important to remember that nails, skin, and hair are reflective of an entire lifestyle. How can you help a client make choices that reflect a personal sense of style? Start by doing a little research. Look for books or articles that describe different fashion styles and become familiar with them. This exercise is useful for developing a profile of the broad fashion categories that you can refer to when consulting with clients.

For example, a person may be categorized as having a classic style if simple and sophisticated clothing, monochromatic color, and no bright patterns are preferred. A person who prefers classic styling in her clothing would likely want a simple, elegant, and sophisticated look with respect to her nails, makeup, and hair (**figure 4-5a**).

Someone who prefers a more dramatic look may choose nail designs, hairstyles, clothing, and accessories that require greater attention. These clients are likely to be more willing to try a variety of new products and spend more time having additional services (**figure 4-5b**).

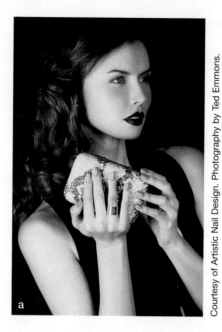

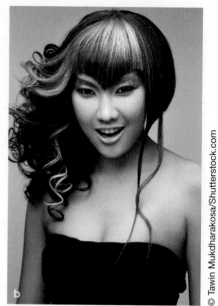

Changes can occur between visits, so remember to have your returning clients refer to their notes on the intake form recorded at their last visit. Any significant changes should be recorded on the service record card as well.

After reading the next few sections, you will be able to:

LO❷ **Conduct a successful client consultation.**

Conducting the Client Consultation

The **client consultation** is the communication with a client that determines the client's needs and how to achieve the desired results. The consultation is one of the most important parts of any service and should always be done before starting the actual service. A consultation should be performed as part of every single service and salon visit. Effective client consultations keep your clientele looking current and stylish, and it will keep them satisfied with your services. A happy client means repeat business for both the salon and you.

Preparing for the Client Consultation

Be well prepared to make the most of this dialogue and have certain important items on hand:

* Have a variety of styling books and/or digital images that your clients can look through.

* Show a variety of style options including various lengths, haircuts, and haircolor.

- Have a portfolio of your work on hand (**figure 4-6**).

- A swatch book or swatch ring is a great tool for discussing haircolor options. These are provided by the companies that manufacture haircolor. They are usually packaged in a book, in a ring, or laid out on a paper chart. Swatches are bundles of hair, dyed to match a particular haircolor shade offered by the manufacturer. Usually made from a synthetic material, swatches are very durable and easy to use in consultations. If the swatch is long enough, it can be held up to the client's face or integrated into his or her own hair to see how it looks.

The Consultation Area

It is the stylist's responsibility to find out the client's needs and to make recommendations accordingly. To do so effectively, you will need a freshly cleaned and uncluttered workspace. Make sure that the product bottles, cans, and jars are also clean. Clients should be able to look at themselves in the mirror without having to compete with sticky product bottles, implements, and tools on the station. While it may take time and effort to make your station esthetically pleasing, the payoff of an effective consultation is worthwhile.

10-Step Consultation Method

Every consultation should be structured so that you cover all the key points that lead to a successful conclusion. While this may seem like a lot of information to memorize, it will become second nature as you become more experienced. To ensure that you cover all the bases, keep a list of the following 10 key points at your station. Modify the list as needed for each actual service:

1. **Review the intake form.** Feel free to make comments that break the ice and initiate conversation with the client. Read the intake

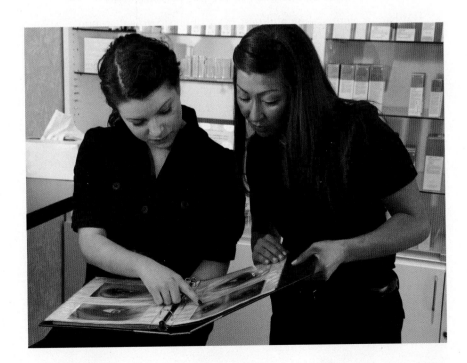

figure 4-6
Use a photo collection to help confirm your client's choice.

form carefully, referring to it often during the consultation process. Also make notes on the service record card (some salons will have a joint intake form and service record card). After the service, record any formulations or products that were used, and include any specific techniques or goals. This information will be needed for future visits.

2. **Perform a needs assessment.** Discover what the client wants and what they need. Start off by assessing the client's current style. Is it soft and unstructured? carefully styled? classic? avant-garde? Is it in sync with her style of clothing and personal image?

3. **Determine and rate the client's preferences.** Using this method will be helpful in determining what services will best help the client. Here is a sample question: How would you rate the manageability of your hair on a scale of 1 to 10, where 1 is poor and 10 is excellent? These numerical values will also serve as a measuring tool for total customer satisfaction. Probing questions like the following will help stylists determine the client's preferences. When was the last time you loved your hair (skin, nails)? What challenges are you having with your hair?

4. **Analyze the client's hair.** Assess your client's hair, including its thickness, texture, manageability, and condition. Is the hair particularly thin on top or at the temples? Check for strong hair growth patterns, including unruly cowlicks. Ask your client what at-home products he or she is using and if the products are effective.

5. **Review the client's lifestyle.** Ask the following questions about career and lifestyle:

   • Do you spend a great deal of time outdoors? Do you swim frequently?

   • What is your occupation? Describe your personal style?

   • What are your styling abilities? How often do you shampoo your hair?

   • How much time do you want to spend styling your hair each day?

6. **Show and tell.** Encourage your client to flip through style books and select styles that he or she likes. Monitor the choices to ensure the styles are feasible for the client's hair type and personal style. Many times, clients desire a specific cut or color that he or she may have seen on a friend or celebrity. If the desired look cannot be achieved, create a plan, offer alternative looks, and set future styling goals.

   In addition, listen to how he or she describes hair length. If the client says they want their hair short, for instance, does that mean shoulder length? above the ears? one-inch long all over the head? When the client's bangs are dry, does he or she want them to still touch their eyebrows? In order to make sure you understand what they are saying, repeat what the client tells you, using specific terms like *chin-length* or *resting on the shoulders*—as opposed to vague terms like *short* or *long*—and reinforce your words both with pictures and by pointing to where the hair would fall. Listening to the client and then repeating, in your own words, what you think the client is telling you is known as **reflective listening**. It is important to focus on the client and not interrupt while he or she is speaking. After the client is finished, restate and confirm what was said. Following this, ask for confirmation to make certain you understand what the client wants or needs.

7. **Make recommendations as part of the needs assessment.** Once you have enough information, ask the client if you may make some recommendations. Before giving any suggestions, wait for him or her to give you permission to do so. Once they have, base your recommendations on the client's needs and desires. Narrow your selections based on the following criteria:

- **Lifestyle.** The styles you choose must fit the client's styling parameters (time and ability), meet your client's needs for business and casual looks, and provide options within those looks.

- **Hair type.** Base your recommendations on whether your client has thick, medium, or thin hair density; fine, medium, or coarse hair texture; straight, wavy, curly, or extremely curly wave patterns.

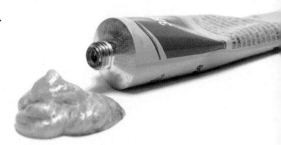

- **Face shape.** Point out hairstyles that would look good with his or her face shape. Is the face narrow across the temple area? If so, you should suggest styles that add a little fullness in this area.

When you make suggestions, qualify them by referencing the above parameters. For example: "I think this hairstyle would work well with the texture of your hair." Tactfully discuss any unreasonable expectations (based on the client's hair and personal needs) that the client expresses. If his or her hair is damaged, address intensive hair treatments, better home-care products, lifestyle changes, and the need to trim damaged ends.

Never hesitate to suggest additional services (be sure to offer two or more services) that will complete the look or improve it in some way. In addition to color, this could be a texture service for added movement or body, a straightening service to tame his or her curls, a makeup lesson to complement your client's new style, and so on.

8. **Make color recommendations.** Unless a client absolutely does not want to talk about color, these recommendations should be part of every consultation service. Almost everyone can use a glossing treatment, have their haircolor enriched, or add some highlights or low lights to make his or her hair (and your work) even more attractive.

Ask if he or she has colored her hair in the past. If the client already has haircolor, find out how long it has been since it was last applied. Have they had color challenges in the past? Does the client color his or her hair at home? Would they like to make a subtle or dramatic hair color change?

When talking about color, be very careful to make sure you and the client are speaking the same language. Hairstylists are accustomed to the technical side of color and tend to use terms like *multidimensional highlighting*, or *no-ammonia, semi permanent tint*. This can be very confusing and misleading to clients. Use pictures as much as possible. The term *blond* to a stylist might be platinum blond, while *blond* to a client may mean a few fine streaks of medium-blond around the hair line. Let photos be your guide.

9. **Discuss upkeep and maintenance.** Counsel every client on the salon maintenance, lifestyle limitations (blond hair and chlorine, for instance, are not a good match), and at-home maintenance that he or she will need to commit to in order to look their best. Let the client know that throughout the service you will be educating them on various products that you would recommend for home use and that at the end of the service they will have an opportunity to choose those home care products that they need.

10. **Review the consultation.** Reiterate everything that you have agreed upon by using a phrase like, "What I heard you say is ..." Make sure to speak in measured, precise terms. Also use visual tools to demonstrate the intended end result. This is the most critical step of the consultation process because it determines the ultimate service(s). Always take your time and be thorough. Pause for your client's confirmation and ask the client for feedback on the consultation process. After a successful consultation it is time to conduct the service.

Concluding the Service

Once the service is finished and the client is satisfied, take a few minutes to record the results on a service record card. Note anything you did that you want to do again, and things you would do differently next time. Also, make note of the final results and any retail products that the client purchased. Be sure to date your notes and file them in the proper place. Depending on your place of work, in some salons the information on each client is entered into a client record database.

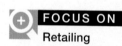

FOCUS ON

Retailing

The best way to make retailing recommendations is to use this three-step plan to discuss the *What, Why,* and *How* of the recommendation:

1. Once you have chosen a product for the client, explain "This is WHAT I recommend...."
2. Next, explain WHY you recommend the product. This is the perfect time to refer back to the concerns the client expressed during the consultation.
3. Finally, describe HOW the client should use the product at home.

Educating clients using these three steps helps them to better understand your recommendations and makes selling the home care products much easier.

LO ❸   Adequately manage tardy clients, schedule mix-ups, and unhappy clients.

Handling Communication Barriers

Although you may do everything in your power to communicate effectively, you will sometimes encounter situations that are beyond your control. Your reactions to situations and your ability to communicate effectively in the face of challenges are critical to being successful in a people profession.

Managing Tardiness

Tardy clients can greatly affect the salon flow. Because beauty professionals depend on appointments and scheduling to maximize working hours, a client who is overly late for an appointment, or one who is habitually late, causes problems. One tardy client can set back an appointment calendar and make stylists late for other services. The pressure involved in making up for lost time can be stressful. Beyond being rushed and feeling harried, you risk inconveniencing the rest of your clients who are prompt for their appointments. Here are a few guidelines on managing late appointments:

- Know and abide by the salon's appointment policy. Many salons set a limit on the amount of time they allow a client to be late before requiring them to reschedule. Generally, if clients are more than 15 minutes late, they should be asked to reschedule. Most clients will accept responsibility and be understanding about the rule, but you may come across a few clients who insist on being serviced immediately. Explain to them that you have other appointments and are responsible to those clients as well. Also explain that rushing through the service would be unacceptable to both of you.

- If a client arrives late and you have the time to take the appointment without jeopardizing other appointments, politely advise the client of the late policy. You can deliver this information diplomatically and still remain pleasant and upbeat.

- As you get to know your clients, you will learn who is habitually late. You may want to schedule such clients for the last appointment of the day or ask them to arrive earlier than their actual appointment time.

- If you are running very late, have the receptionist call your clients and let the client know. The receptionist can give them the opportunity to reschedule or to come a little later than their scheduled time.

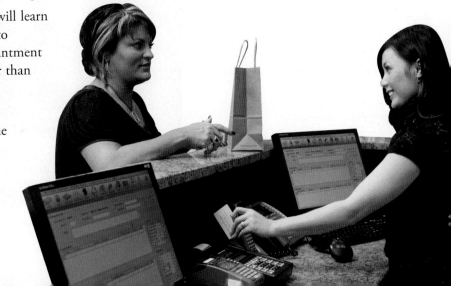

Managing Scheduling Mix-Ups

We are all human, and we all make mistakes. Chances are you have gone to an appointment only to discover that you are in the wrong place at the wrong time. The way you are treated at that moment determines whether you patronize that business again. When you, as a professional, are involved with a scheduling mix-up, always remember to be polite. Never argue about who is correct.

Once you have the chance to consult your appointment book, you can say, "Oh, Mrs. Montez, I have you in my appointment book for 10 o'clock, and unfortunately I already have clients scheduled for 11 and 12 o'clock. I'm so sorry about the mix-up. Can I reschedule you for tomorrow at 10 o'clock?" Even though the client may be fuming, you need to stay detached. Move the conversation away from who is at fault, and squarely into resolving the confusion. Make another appointment for the client and be sure the salon has her telephone number so that the appointment can be confirmed (figure 4-7).

Resolving Unhappy Client Problems

Once in a while you will encounter a client who is dissatisfied. Remember the ultimate goal: Make the client happy. Happy clients build trust with the stylists and will return for future services.

Here are some guidelines:

- Try to find out why the client is unhappy. Ask for specifics.

- If it is possible to change what the client dislikes, do so immediately. If that is not possible, look at your schedule book to see how soon you can fit them in to make the adjustment. You may need to enlist the help of the receptionist if you have to reschedule other appointments.

- If the problem cannot be fixed; honestly and tactfully explain why. The client may not be happy but will usually appreciate your honesty. Sometimes you can offer other options that minimize the client's disappointment.

- Never argue with the client or try to force your opinion.

figure 4-7
Accommodate an unhappy client promptly and calmly.

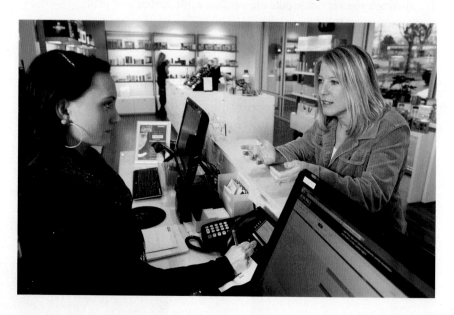

ACTIVITY

At some point in your career you will have a client who is unhappy about something, either related to service or scheduling. The best way to prepare for this scenario is to practice. Role-play with a classmate, taking turns being the client and the stylist.

As you play the role of client:

- Act out different personalities: first shy, then aggressive.
- Act out a problem that was your (the client's) fault. Then evaluate your classmate's (the stylist's) reaction.
- Continue the conversation until you are satisfied.

As you play the role of stylist:

- Pay attention to the tone and level of your voice.
- Make certain you understand the problem.
- Avoid being defensive.
- Offer more than one solution.
- Determine when you should involve a manager.
- Do not hesitate to ask for help from a more experienced stylist or your salon manager. If, after you have tried everything, you are unable to satisfy the client, defer to your manager's advice on how to proceed.
- Confer with your salon manager after the experience. A good manager will not hold the event against you, but will view it instead as an inevitable fact of life from which you can learn. Follow your manager's advice and move on to your next client.

Managing Differences

As a stylist, you'll find the clients you are most likely to attract are similar to yourself in age, style, and taste. On the other hand, you will also service clients who are very different from you; this is a positive element in your career as a stylist. Without both older and younger clients, and ones from different social groups, you won't be able to build a solid client base for future business.

When working with clients who come from a different generation, the basic rules of professionalism should guide you. Older clients, in particular, do not like gum chewing, slang, or the use of *yeah* instead of *yes*. They like to hear *please* and *thank you*. They prefer to keep the topics of conversation professional. Some like to be addressed by the honorific, such as "Mrs. Smith," rather than by their first names. When you meet an older client for the first time, ask how he or she would like to be addressed. Some clients are sensitive to verbiage about aging. When delivering skin care services, do not refer to aging skin; instead, talk about dryness and solutions to remedy the condition.

If these clients are your peers, relate to their image needs but don't act too much like a peer; it is always better to maintain a professional demeanor. When it comes to slang, the same word can have a different meaning across cultures, which is why it is always best to avoid using slang terms. If the word is fashion-related and your client uses it, you can too, indicating that you understand and are aware of current trends. Never use cultural slang words or regionalisms you do not fully understand. When in doubt say, "I have never heard that expression before. What, exactly, do you mean?"

FOCUS ON

Talking Points

Let's imagine a long-time client reveals to you that she and her husband are going through a messy divorce. You care for her and want to be understanding as she reveals increasingly personal details. Other practitioners and their clients are soon listening to every word of this conversation. You want to be helpful and supportive, but this is not the right time or place. What can you do? Decide which of these solutions you might use:

- Tell her you understand that the situation is very difficult, but that while she is in the salon, you want to do everything in your power to give her a break from it. Let her know gently that while she is in your care, you should both concentrate on her enjoyment of the services and not on the things that are stressing her.
- Change the subject. What topic could you shift to that seems the most natural?
- Find a reason to excuse yourself. When you return, change the subject.
- Acknowledge her by saying, "I'm sorry to hear that." Suggest a mini relaxation service the salon is promoting.

Getting Too Personal

Sometimes when a client forms a bond of trust with a stylist, the client can have a hard time differentiating between a professional relationship and a personal one. Manage client relationships tactfully and sensitively, with professionalism and respect. Do not engage in an attempt to fulfill the role of counselor, career guide, parental sounding board, or motivational coach for any of your clients.

If your client gets too far off topic, use neutral subjects to bring the conversation back to beauty needs. If the client tells you about a personal problem, simply listen and tell the client you are sorry. Then ask, "What can we do to make your visit better today?"

If your client is gossiping, change the subject as soon as you can. Try something like, "I just noticed your ends are drier than I thought. We'll do a deep-conditioning treatment after your color." Then describe the treatment and home care.

Books, movies, and celebrities can all be used to move into conversations about a particular look or style. As a rule, avoid discussing religion and politics. When you cannot find a way to move the conversation back to something beauty-related, simply listen; then change the subject.

After reading the next few sections, you will be able to:

LO❹ Build open lines of communication with coworkers.

Guidelines for In-Salon Communication

Behaving in a professional manner is the first step in making meaningful in-salon communication a reality. The salon is a close-knit community in which people spend long hours working side by side. For this reason, it is important to maintain boundaries. Remember, the salon is your place of business and, as such, must be treated respectfully and carefully.

Communicating with Coworkers

In a work environment, you will not have the opportunity to handpick your colleagues. There will always be people you like or relate to better than others. Keep these points in mind as you interact and communicate with coworkers:

- **Treat everyone with respect.** Regardless of whether you like someone, your colleagues are professionals who deserve respect.

- **Remain objective.** Different types of personalities working together over long and intense hours can breed some degree of dissension and disagreement. Make every effort to remain objective. Resist being pulled into spats and cliques.

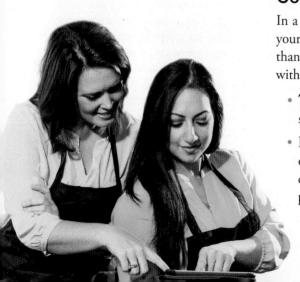

- **Be honest and sensitive.** Many people use the excuse of being honest as a license to say anything to anyone. While honesty is always the best policy, using unkind words or actions at work is never a good idea. Be sensitive, and think before you speak.

- **Remain neutral.** There may be times where you are persuaded to choose sides. Avoid taking sides in a dispute.

- **Avoid gossip.** Gossiping never resolves a problem; it only makes it worse. Participating in gossip can be just as damaging to you as it is to the object of the gossip.

- **Seek help from someone you respect.** If you find yourself at odds with a coworker, seek out someone who is not involved and can be objective, such as the manager. Ask for advice about how to proceed, and then really listen.

- **Do not take things personally.** How many times have you had a bad day, or been thinking about something totally unrelated to work, when a colleague asks you what is wrong, or if you are mad at her? Just because someone is behaving in a certain manner, and you happen to be there, does not mean their behavior involves you. If you are confused or concerned by someone's actions, find a private place and an appropriate time to get clarification.

- **Keep your private life private.** The work environment is never the place to discuss your personal life and relationships.

Communicating During an Employee Evaluation

Salons that are well run make it a priority to conduct frequent and thorough employee evaluations. Sometime during the course of your first few days of work, your salon manager will tell you when to expect your first employee evaluation. If the manager does not mention it, you might

 FOCUS ON

Communicating with Managers

Another important relationship is the one a person will build with their manager. The salon manager is usually the person with the most responsibility regarding the salon's overall operation. The manager's job is a demanding one. Often, in addition to running a hectic salon, he or she also has a personal clientele.

The manager is the person who hires staff and is responsible for training. Managers have a vested interest in the success of staff members. Salon employees might perceive the managers as powerful figures of authority, but it is important to remember that managers are human beings. Staff members should support management and the salon by following the rules and guidelines that are set.

Here are some guidelines for interacting and communicating with your salon manager:

- **Be a problem solver.** When seeking advice about an issue or problem, think of possible solutions beforehand. This will indicate that you are working in the salon's best interest.

- **Get your facts straight.** Make sure that information is accurate before you speak to salon management. This proactive approach to problem solving will save time.

- **Be open and honest.** Advise the salon manager immediately when uncertainty compromises your decision-making skills.

- **Do not gossip or complain about colleagues.** If you are having a legitimate problem with someone, and have tried everything you can to handle the problem with your own resources, only then is it appropriate to go to your manager.

- **Be open to constructive criticism.** It is never easy to hear that you need improvement in any area, but keep in mind that part of your manager's job is to help you achieve professional goals and ensure the salon's success. It is the manager's job to evaluate your skills and offer suggestions on how to improve and expand those skills. Keep an open mind and do not take the criticism personally.

request a copy of the form or list of the criteria on which you will be evaluated. The following are some points to keep in mind as you begin your tenure in the salon:

- Take some time to look over the employee evaluation document. Be mindful that the behaviors and activities most important to the salon are likely to be the ones on which you will be evaluated. You can begin to review and rate yourself in the weeks and months ahead, so you can assess your progress and performance.

- Remember, the criteria are created for the purpose of helping you become a better stylist and to ensure the salon's success. Make the decision to approach the evaluation positively.

- As the time for the evaluation draws near, try filling out the form yourself. In other words, perform a self-evaluation, even if the salon has not asked you to do so. Be objective, and carefully think out your comments.

- Before your evaluation meeting, write down any thoughts or questions so you can share them with your manager. Do not be shy. If you want to know when you can take on more services, when your pay scale might be increased, or when you might be considered for promotion, this meeting is the appropriate time and place to ask. Many beauty professionals never take advantage of this crucial communication opportunity to discuss their future advancement because they are too nervous, intimidated, or unprepared to discuss these issues. Participate proactively in your career and in your success by communicating your desires and interests.

- When you meet with your manager, show him or her your self-evaluation and express that you are serious about your improvement and growth. Your manager will appreciate your input and your initiative. If you are being honest with yourself, there should be no surprises.

- At the end of the meeting, thank your manager for taking the time to do the evaluation and for the feedback and guidance they gave you (figure 4-8).

figure 4-8
Your employee evaluation is a good time to discuss your progress with your manager.

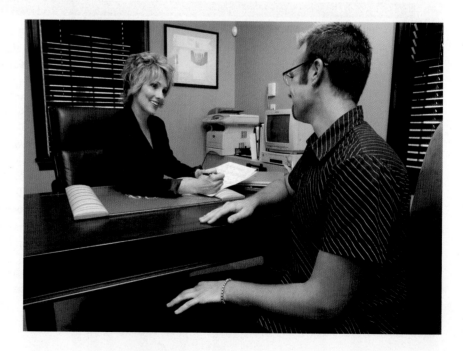

REVIEW QUESTIONS

1. What are the golden rules of communication?

2. What is the definition of effective communication?

3. What are the elements of the 10-Step Consultation Method?

4. How should you handle an unhappy client? (List at least four points to keep in mind.)

5. List at least five things to remember when communicating with your coworkers.

STUDY TOOLS

- **Reinforce what you just learned:** Complete the activities and exercises in your Theory or Practical Workbook, or your Study Guide.

- **Expand your knowledge:** Search for websites about the topics in this chapter and make a list of additional resources.

- **Study and prepare for your quiz:** Take the chapter test in your Exam Review or your Milady U: Online Licensing Prep.

- **Re-Test your knowledge:** Take the Chapter 4 *Quizzes*!

- **Learn even more:** Look up in a dictionary or search the internet for the definitions of any additional terms you want to learn about.

CHAPTER GLOSSARY

client consultation	p. 54	Communication with a client that determines what the client's needs are and how to achieve the desired results.
client intake form	p. 50	Also known as a *client questionnaire*, *consultation card*, or *health history form*; used in beauty and wellness services as a questionnaire that discloses the client's contact information, products they use, hair/nail/skin care needs, preferences and lifestyle. The form also includes all medications, both topical (applied to the skin) and oral (taken by mouth), along with any known medical issues, skin or scalp disorders or allergies that might affect services.
effective communication	p. 50	The act of sharing information between two people (or groups of people) so that the information is successfully understood.
reflective listening	p. 57	Listening to the client and then repeating, in your own words, what you think the client is telling you.
service record card	p. 51	The client's permanent progress record of services received, results, formulations, and products purchased or used.

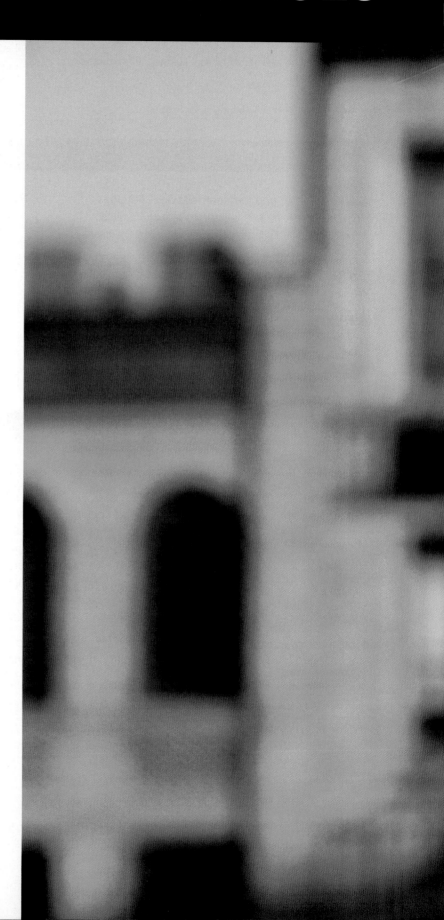

PART 2 GENERAL SCIENCES

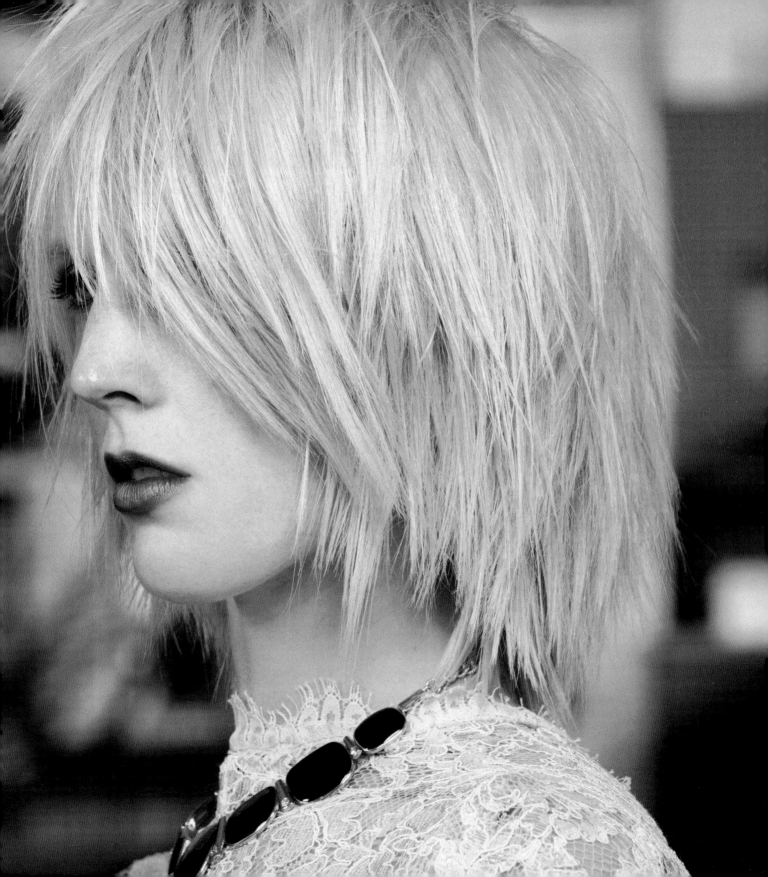

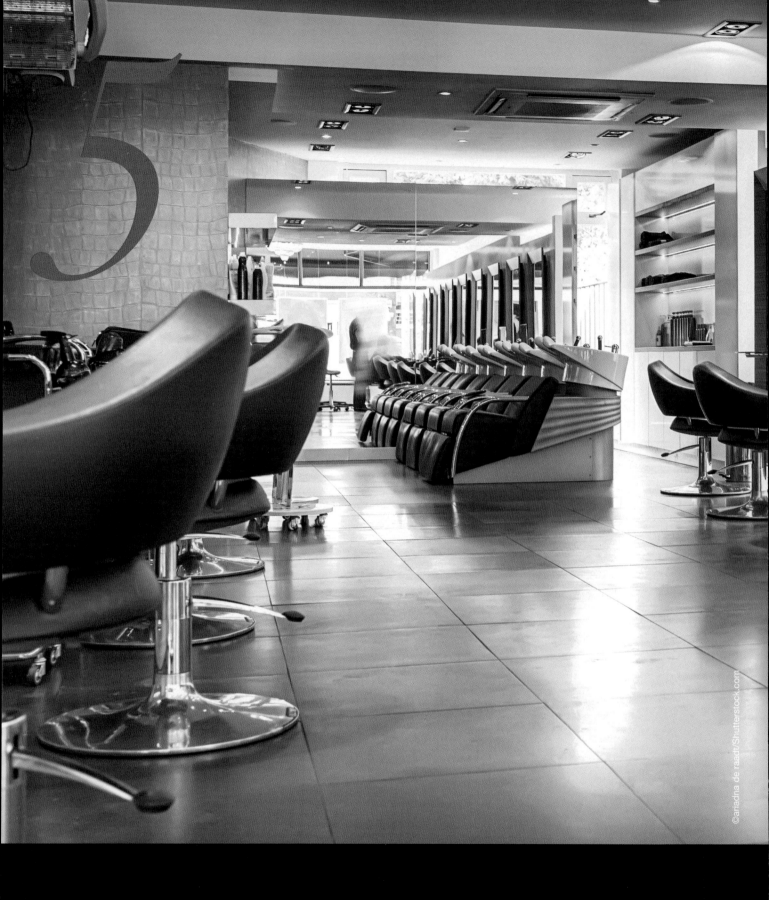

5

INFECTION CONTROL:
PRINCIPLES & PRACTICES

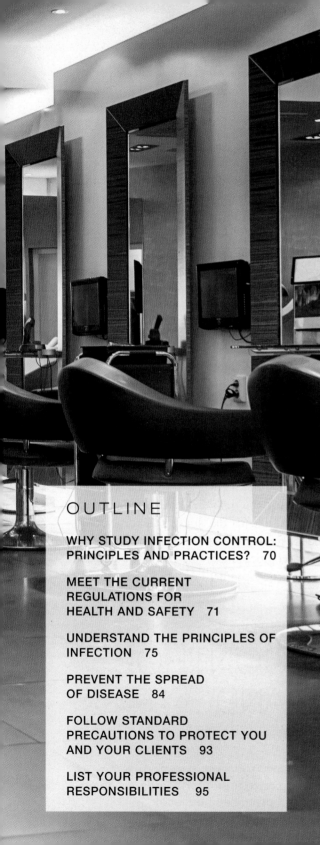

LEARNING OBJECTIVES

After completing this chapter, you will be able to:

LO ❶

List the 16 categories of information required on Safety Data Sheets.

LO ❷

Understand laws and rules and the differences between them.

LO ❸

List the types and classifications of bacteria.

LO ❹

Define bloodborne pathogens and explain how they are transmitted.

LO ❺

Explain the differences between cleaning, disinfecting, and sterilizing.

LO ❻

List the types of disinfectants and the steps to using them properly.

LO ❼

Define Standard Precautions.

LO ❽

List your responsibilities as a salon professional.

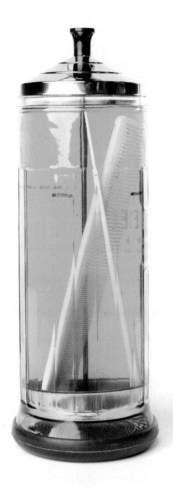

There is much confusion within the beauty industry about the proper use of the terms *sanitation*, which is nothing more than garbage removal (think of what your city's department of sanitation does), and *cleaning*, as well as *sanitizing*, *disinfecting*, and *sterilizing*. In an effort to clarify these critical terms, Milady opted to consistently use *cleaning*, instead of using *cleaning* in one sentence and *sanitizing* (or *sanitation*) in another sentence.

It is noteworthy that many professionals in the healthcare and scientific communities (of disease prevention and epidemiology) and associations, such as The Association for Professionals in Infection Control and Epidemiology, generally do not use the terms interchangeably either. Instead, it is more common for infection control professionals to use the terms *cleaning*, *disinfecting*, and *sterilizing*. Infection control professionals consider *sanitation* a layperson's term or a product marketing term (as in *hand sanitizers*).

The term *clean* is defined: A mechanical process (scrubbing) using soap and water or detergent and water to remove all visible dirt, debris, and many disease-causing germs. Cleaning also removes invisible debris that interferes with disinfection. Cleaning is what cosmetologists are required to do before disinfecting.

The term **sanitizing** is defined: A chemical process for reducing the number of disease-causing germs on cleaned surfaces to a safe level.

The term *disinfection* is defined: A chemical process that uses specific products to destroy harmful organisms on environmental surfaces.

Consider this scenario: You are a new employee of a salon that offers hair and nail services. At the end of the day, the salon manager asks you to help clean and disinfect the counters, workstations, tools, implements, and pedicure equipment. Your manager also tells you to enter the cleaning and disinfection information in the salon's logbook. You know how important it is to follow the proper cleaning and disinfection procedures in the salon. This chapter will give you the principles and practices you need to complete those tasks.

why study
INFECTION CONTROL: PRINCIPLES AND PRACTICES?

Cosmetologists should study and have a thorough understanding of infection control principles and practices because:

> To be a knowledgeable, successful, and responsible professional in the field of cosmetology, you are required to understand the types of illness causing pathogens you may encounter in the salon.

> Understanding the basics of cleaning and disinfecting and following federal and state rules will safeguard you and your clients.

> Understanding the cleaning and disinfecting products that you use and how to use them will help keep you, your clients, and your salon environment protected from potential pathogens and their modes of transmission.

> Understanding and practicing proper infection control within federal, state and local laws/rules will safeguard your business from costly citations for safety violations.

> Respecting the chemicals used in cleaning and disinfecting by reading labels and following manufacturer's instructions is necessary to reduce the risks involved with using any chemical.

Meet the Current Regulations for Health and Safety

Many different federal and state agencies regulate the practice of cosmetology. Federal agencies set guidelines for the manufacturing, sale, and use of equipment and chemical ingredients. These guidelines also provide for monitoring of safety in the workplace and place limits on the types of services you can perform in the salon. State agencies regulate licensing, enforcement, and your conduct when you are working in the salon.

Federal Agencies

Occupational Safety and Health Administration (OSHA)

The Occupational Safety and Health Administration (OSHA) was created as part of the U.S. Department of Labor (DOL) to regulate and enforce safety and health standards to protect employees in the workplace. Regulating employee exposure to potentially toxic substances and informing employees about the possible hazards of materials used in the workplace are key points of the Occupational Safety and Health Act of 1970. This regulation created the Hazard Communication Standard (HCS), which requires that chemical manufacturers and importers assess and communicate the potential hazards associated with their products. The Material Safety Data Sheet (MSDS) was a result of the HCS. In 2012, along with representatives from most nations who participate in the United Nations, OSHA agreed to comply with the Globally Harmonized System of Classification and Labeling of Chemicals System (GHS). This initiative was designed to create label standards to be used around the globe and includes the use of specific pictograms to indicate possible safety concerns, as well as adoption of a 16 category, standard format SDS (Safety Data Sheet) to replace the MSDS. The HCS in 1983 gave workers the "right to know," but the new GHS gives workers the "right to understand."

The standards set by OSHA are important to the cosmetology industry because of the products used in salons. OSHA standards address issues relating to the handling, mixing, storing, and disposing of products; general safety in the workplace; and your right to know about any potentially hazardous ingredients contained in the products you use and how to avoid these hazards. Employees should view OSHA as an agency designed to ensure a safe workplace for all U.S. workers.

WEB RESOURCES

You can find an EPA-approved list of disinfectants by going to the EPA's website at epa.gov and entering a search on the homepage for EPA-registered disinfectants. Disinfectants are not listed as "hospital grade," but instead are listed based on the pathogens they are effective against. Products on list D meet the criteria of most states for "hospital grade" and products on list E meet the criteria for tuberculocidal in those states where that is required.

DID YOU KNOW?

The term *hospital grade* is not a term used by the EPA. The EPA does not grade disinfectants; a product is either approved by the EPA for use as a hospital disinfectant or it is not.

After reading the next few sections, you will be able to:

LO List the 16 categories of information required on Safety Data Sheets.

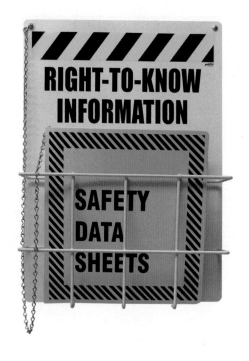

Safety Data Sheet (SDS) Replaces Material Safety Data Sheet (MSDS)

As of June 2015, both federal and state laws require that manufacturers supply a **Safety Data Sheet (SDS)** (previously known as **Material Safety Data Sheet**) for all chemical products manufactured and sold. The SDS contains 16 categories of information and all SDS sheets will be organized identically. The categories are:

1. **Identification:** product identifier; manufacturer or distributor with contact information (including emergency phone number); recommended use of product and restrictions on use

2. **Hazard identification:** all hazards of using the chemical

3. **Composition/Information on ingredients:** includes information on chemical ingredients

4. **First-aid measures:** includes important symptoms/effects—acute and delayed; required treatment

5. **Fire-fighting measures:** lists suitable extinguishing techniques, equipment; chemical hazards from fire

6. **Accidental release measures:** lists emergency procedures, protective equipment; proper methods of containment and clean-up

7. **Handling and storage:** lists precautions for safe handling and storage, including incompatibilities

8. **Exposure controls/personal protection:** lists OSHA's Permissible Exposure Limits (PEL); Personal Protective Equipment (PPE)

9. **Physical and chemical properties:** lists the chemical's characteristics

10. **Stability and reactivity:** lists chemical stability and possibility of hazardous reactions

11. **Toxicology information:** includes routes of exposure, related symptoms, acute and chronic effects

12. **Ecological information:** includes effects on wastewater and environment

13. **Disposal consideration:** includes proper disposal and disposal restrictions

14. **Transport information:** includes restrictions on transportation

15. **Regulatory information:** lists agencies responsible for regulation of product

16. **Revision date:** lists original date of document and any revision

Source: Adapted from United States Department of Labor. (n.d.) *OSHA QuickCard – Hazard Communication Safety Data Sheets.* Retrieved from www.OSHA.gov.

© Travis Klein/Shutterstock.com

In addition, pictograms that are internationally recognized will be used to ensure that information is being communicated in easily recognizable formats (figure 5-1). When necessary, the SDS can be sent to a medical facility so that a doctor can better assess and treat the patient. OSHA and state regulatory agencies require that SDSs be kept available in the salon for all products. Both OSHA and state board inspectors can issue fines to salons for not having SDSs available.

Federal and state laws require salons to obtain SDSs from the chemical product manufacturers and/or distributors for each professional product that is used. SDSs often can be downloaded from the product manufacturer's or the distributor's website. Not having SDSs available poses a health risk to anyone exposed to hazardous materials and violates federal and state regulations. All employees must read the information included on each SDS and verify that they have read it by adding their signatures to a sign-off sheet for the product. These sign-off sheets must be available to state and federal inspectors upon request.

Environmental Protection Agency (EPA)

The Environmental Protection Agency (EPA) registers all types of disinfectants sold and used in the United States. **Disinfectants** (dis-in-FEK-tents) are chemical products that destroy most bacteria (excluding spores), fungi, and viruses on surfaces.

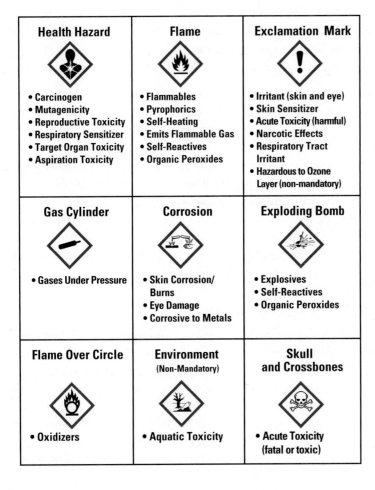

figure 5-1
Pictograms used on SDSs

CAUTION

Disinfectants must be registered with the EPA. Look for an EPA registration number on the label.

- **Hospital disinfectants** (HOS-pih-tal dis-in-FEK-tents) are designated by the EPA as being effective enough to be used in a hospital setting. They can be used on any nonporous surface in the salon. **Nonporous** (nahn-POHW-rus) means that an item is made or constructed of a material that has no pores or openings and cannot absorb liquids. Hospital disinfectants control the spread of **disease** (dih-ZEEZ), an abnormal condition of all or part of the body, or its systems or organs, which makes the body incapable of carrying on normal function. The most commonly used products in this group are quaternary ammonium compounds, commonly known as "quats." They are products made of quaternary ammonium cations and are designed for disinfection on non porous surfaces. They are appropriate for use in non-critical (non-invasive) environments, and are effective against most pathogens of concern in the salon environment.

- **Tuberculocidal disinfectants** (tuh-bur-kyoo-LOH-sy-dahl dis-in-FEK-tents) are proven to kill the bacteria that cause **tuberculosis** (tuh-bur-kyoo-LOH-sus) in addition to the pathogens destroyed through use of hospital disinfectants. Tuberculosis is a disease caused by bacteria that are transmitted through coughing or sneezing, and is not transmitted on surfaces. Tuberculocidal disinfectants are one kind of hospital disinfectants. The fact that tuberculocidal disinfectants are effective against this additional pathogen does not mean that you should automatically reach for them. Some of these products can be harmful to salon tools and equipment, and they may require special methods of disposal. Check the rules of your state to be sure that the product you choose complies with state requirements. Most pathogens of concern in the salon are adequately destroyed by standard EPA registered disinfectants and do not require tuberculocidal disinfectants.

It is against federal law to use any disinfecting product contrary to its labeling. Before a manufacturer can sell a product for disinfecting surfaces, tools, implements, or equipment, they must obtain an EPA registration number that certifies that the disinfectant, when used correctly, will be effective against the pathogens listed on the label. For example, pedicure tub disinfectants must be approved for that specific use or the manufacturer will be breaking federal law by marketing them for disinfecting pedicure tubs. This also means that if you do not follow the label instructions for mixing, contact time, and the type of surface the disinfecting product can be used on, you are not complying with federal law. If there were an injury-related lawsuit, you could be held responsible.

State Regulatory Agencies

State regulatory agencies exist to protect salon professionals and their clients' health and safety while they receive salon services. State regulatory agencies include licensing agencies, state boards of cosmetology, commissions, and health departments. Regulatory agencies require that everyone working in a salon or spa follow specific procedures. Enforcement of the rules through inspections and investigations of consumer complaints is also part of an agency's responsibility. An agency can issue penalties against both the salon owner and the cosmetologist. Penalties vary

HERE'S A TIP

Remember: Salon professionals are not allowed to treat or recommend treatments for infections, diseases, or abnormal conditions. Clients with such problems should be referred to their physicians.

and include warnings, fines, probation, and suspension or revocation of licenses. It is vital that you understand and follow the laws and rules of your state at all times. Your salon's reputation, your license, and everyone's safety depend on it.

After reading the next section, you will be able to:

LO❷ Understand laws and rules and the differences between them.

Laws and Rules—What Is the Difference?

Laws are written by both federal and state legislatures that determine the scope of practice (what each license allows the holder to do) and that establish guidelines for regulatory agencies to make rules. Laws are also called statutes.

Rules and regulations are more specific than laws. Rules are written by the regulatory agency or the state board, and they determine how the law must be applied. Rules establish specific standards of conduct and can be changed or updated frequently. Cosmetologists must be aware of any changes or updates to the rules and regulations, and they must comply with them.

Understand the Principles of Infection

Being a salon professional is fun and rewarding, but it is also a great responsibility. One careless action could cause injury or **infection** (in-FEK-shun), the invasion of body tissues by disease-causing pathogens. If your actions result in an injury or infection, you could lose your license or ruin the salon's reputation. Fortunately, preventing the spread of infection is easy when you know proper procedures and follow them at all times. Prevention begins and ends with *you*.

Infection Control

Infection control refers to the methods used to eliminate or reduce the transmission of infectious organisms. Cosmetologists must understand and remember the following four types of microorganisms:

- Bacteria
- Viruses
- Fungi
- Parasites

Under certain conditions, many of these organisms can cause infectious disease. An **infectious disease** (in-FEK-shus dih-ZEEZ) is caused by pathogenic (harmful) organisms that enter the body. An infectious disease may be spread from one person to another person.

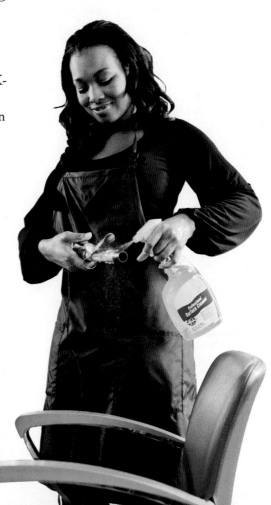

In this chapter, you will learn how to properly clean and disinfect the tools and equipment you use in the salon so they are safe for you and your clients. To **clean** (cleaning) is a mechanical process (scrubbing) using soap and water or detergent and water to remove all visible dirt, debris, and many disease-causing germs from tools, implements, and equipment. The process of **disinfection** (dis-in-FEK-shun) is a chemical process that destroys most, but not necessarily all, harmful organisms on environmental surfaces. The pathogens of concern in the cosmetology industry are effectively destroyed by the disinfection process, which is required in all states.

Cleaning and disinfecting procedures are designed to prevent the spread of infection and disease. Disinfectants used in salons must be **bactericidal** (back-teer-uh-SYD-ul), capable of destroying bacteria; **virucidal** (vy-ru-SYD-ul), capable of destroying viruses; and **fungicidal** (fun-jih-SYD-ul), capable of destroying fungi. Be sure to mix and use these disinfectants according to the instructions on the labels so they are safe and effective.

Infection can be transmitted through contaminated salon tools and equipment if the proper disinfection steps are not taken after every service. You have a professional and legal obligation to protect clients from harm by using proper infection control procedures. If clients are infected or harmed because you perform infection control procedures incorrectly, you may be found legally responsible for their injuries or infections.

After reading the next few sections, you will be able to:

 LO❸ **List the types and classifications of bacteria.**

Bacteria

Bacteria (bak-TEER-ee-ah) (singular: bacterium [back-TEER-ee-um]), are one-celled microorganisms that have both plant and animal characteristics. A **microorganism** (my-kroh-OR-gah-niz-um) is any organism of microscopic or submicroscopic size. Some bacteria are harmful and some are harmless. Bacteria can exist almost anywhere: on skin, in water, in the air, in decayed matter, on environmental surfaces, in body secretions, on clothing, or under the free edge of nails. Bacteria are so small they can only be seen with a microscope.

Types of Bacteria

There are thousands of different kinds of bacteria that fall into two primary types: pathogenic and nonpathogenic.

Most bacteria are **nonpathogenic** (non-path-uh-JEN-ik); in other words, they are harmless organisms that may perform useful functions. They are safe to come in contact with since they do not cause disease or harm. For example, nonpathogenic bacteria are used to make yogurt, cheese, and some medicines. In the human body, nonpathogenic bacteria help the body break down food and protect against infection and stimulate the immune system.

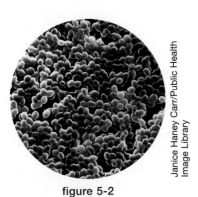

figure 5-2
Cocci

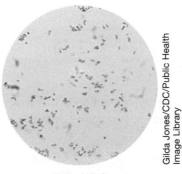

figure 5-3
Staphylococci

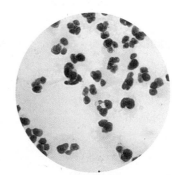

figure 5-4
Streptococci

Pathogenic (path-uh-JEN-ik) bacteria are harmful microorganisms that can cause disease or infection in humans when they invade the body. Salons and schools must maintain strict standards for cleaning and disinfecting at all times to prevent the spread of pathogenic microorganisms. It is crucial that cosmetologists learn proper infection control practices while in school to ensure that you understand the importance of following them throughout your career. **Table 5-1**, Causes of Disease, presents terms and definitions related to pathogens.

Classifications of Pathogenic Bacteria

Bacteria have distinct shapes that help to identify them. Pathogenic bacteria are classified as described below:

- **Cocci** (KOK-sy) are round-shaped bacteria that appear singly (alone) or in groups (**figure 5-2**).

- **Staphylococci** (staf-uh-loh-KOK-sy) are pus-forming bacteria that grow in clusters like bunches of grapes. They cause abscesses, pustules, and boils (**figure 5-3**). Some types of staphylococci (or staph, as many call it) may not cause infections in healthy humans, and others may be deadly.

- **Streptococci** (strep-toh-KOK-sy) are pus-forming bacteria arranged in curved lines resembling a string of beads. They cause infections such as strep throat and blood poisoning (**figure 5-4**).

- **Diplococci** (dip-lo-KOK-sy) are spherical bacteria that grow in pairs and cause diseases such as pneumonia (**figure 5-5**).

- **Bacilli** (bah-SIL-ee) (singular: bacillus) are short, rod-shaped bacteria. They are the most common bacteria and produce diseases such as tetanus (lockjaw), typhoid fever, tuberculosis, and diphtheria (**figure 5-6**).

- **Spirilla** (spy-RIL-ah) are spiral or corkscrew-shaped bacteria. They are subdivided into subgroups, such as syphilis, a sexually transmitted disease (STD), and Lyme disease (**figure 5-7**).

Movement of Bacteria

Different bacteria move in different ways; **motility** (MOH-til-eh-tee) is the term used to describe self-movement. Cocci rarely demonstrate motility and are generally transmitted in the air, in dust, or within the substance in which they settle. Bacilli and spirilla are both capable of movement and use

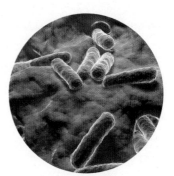

figure 5-5
Diplococci

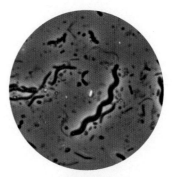

figure 5-6
Bacilli

figure 5-7
Spirilla

table 5-1
CAUSES OF DISEASE

Term	Definition
Bacteria	One-celled microorganisms having both plant and animal characteristics. Some are harmful and some are harmless.
Direct Transmission	Transmission of blood or body fluids through touching (including shaking hands), kissing, coughing, sneezing, and talking.
Fungi	Singular: fungus; single-cell organisms that grow in irregular masses that include molds, mildews, and yeasts.
Indirect Transmission	Transmission of blood or body fluids through contact with an intermediate contaminated object, such as a razor, extractor, nipper, or an environmental surface.
Infection	Invasion of body tissues by disease-causing pathogens.
Germs	Nonscientific synonym for disease-producing organisms.
Microorganism	Any organism of microscopic to submicroscopic size.
Pathogens	Harmful microorganisms that enter the body and can cause disease.
Parasites	Organisms that grow, feed, and shelter on or in another organism (referred to as the host) while contributing nothing to the survival of that organism. Parasites must have a host to survive.
Toxins	Various poisonous substances produced by some microorganisms (bacteria and viruses).
Virus	A submicroscopic particle that infects and resides in cells of biological organisms.

slender, hair-like extensions called **flagella** (fluh-JEL-uh) for locomotion (moving about). You may also hear people refer to **cilia** (SIL-ee-uh) in reference to cell movement, but they are much shorter than flagella and require many more to create movement. Both flagella and cilia move cells, but they have a different motion. Flagella move in a snake-like motion while cilia move in a rowing-like motion.

Bacterial Growth and Reproduction

When seen under a microscope, bacteria look like tiny bags. They generally consist of an outer cell wall that contains liquid called protoplasm. Bacterial cells grow and reproduce. The life cycle of bacteria consists of two distinct phases: the active stage and the inactive or spore-forming stage.

Active stage. During the active stage, bacteria grow and reproduce. Bacteria multiply best in warm, dark, damp, or dirty places. When conditions are favorable, bacteria grow and reproduce. When they reach their largest size, they divide into two new cells. This division is called **binary fission** (BY-nayr-ee FISH-un). The cells that are formed are called daughter cells and are produced every 20 to 60 minutes, depending on the bacteria. The infectious pathogen staphylococcus aureus undergoes cell division every 27 to 30 minutes. When conditions become unfavorable and difficult for them to thrive, bacteria either die or become inactive.

Inactive or spore-forming stage. The stage where a bacteria that is capable of forming a spore to protect itself does so to withstand an environment incompatible with its existence. **Bacterial spore** is the ability of certain types of bacteria to form a hard keratin coating that will protect it until the environment is more favorable.

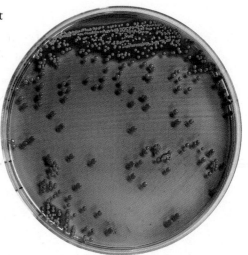

Certain bacteria, such as the bacteria that cause tetanus and botulism, among others, can coat themselves with wax-like outer shells during unfavorable conditions. This makes them able to withstand long periods of famine, dryness, and unsuitable temperatures. In this stage, spores can be blown about and are not harmed by conditions such as extreme heat or cold. Bacterial spores can only be destroyed through sterilization or bleach disinfecting wipes designated as sporacidal. However, none of these spore-forming bacteria are known to present an infectious risk in the salon environment.

When favorable conditions are restored, the spores change into the active form and begin to grow and reproduce.

Bacterial Infections

There can be no bacterial infection without the presence of pathogenic bacteria. Therefore, if pathogenic bacteria are eliminated, clients cannot become infected. You may have a client who has **inflammation** (in-fluh-MAY-shun), a condition in which the body reacts to injury, irritation, or infection. An inflammation may be characterized by redness, heat, pain, and swelling. **Pus** is a fluid containing white blood cells, bacteria, and dead cells, and is the byproduct of the infectious process. The presence of pus can be a sign of a bacterial infection. A **local infection**, such as a pimple or abscess, is confined to a particular part of the body and appears as a lesion containing pus. A **systemic infection** is an infection where the pathogen has distributed throughout the body or a system of the body rather than staying in one body area or organ. Staphylococci are among the most common bacteria that affect humans and are commonly found in our environment, including on our bodies, although most strains do not make us ill. Staph bacteria can be picked up on doorknobs, countertops, and other surfaces, but in the salon they are more frequently spread through skin-to-skin contact (such as shaking hands) or through the use of unclean tools or implements. Although lawsuits are rare considering the number of services performed in a salon, every year many salons are sued for allegedly causing staph infections.

Some types of infectious staph bacteria are highly resistant to conventional treatments due to incorrect doses or choice of antibiotic. An example is the staph infection called **methicillin-resistant Staphylococcus aureus (MRSA)** (mETH-eh-sill-en-ree-ZIST-ent Staf-uh-loh-KOK-us oR-ee-us). Historically, MRSA occurred most frequently among persons with weakened immune systems or among people who had undergone medical procedures. Today, it has become more common in otherwise healthy people. Clients may bring this organism into the salon where it can infect others. Some people carry the bacteria and are not even aware they are harboring a dangerous pathogen. MRSA initially appears as a skin infection, presenting as a pimple, rash, or boil (or cluster of boils) that can be difficult to cure. Without proper treatment, the infection becomes systemic and can have devastating consequences that can result in death. Because of these highly resistant bacterial strains, it is important to clean and disinfect all tools and implements used in the salon. You owe it to yourself and your clients! Also, do not perform services if the client's skin, scalp, neck, hands, or feet show visible signs of abrasion or infection. Cosmetologists are only allowed to work on healthy hair, skin, and nails.

When a disease spreads from one person to another person, it is said to be a **contagious disease** (kon-TAY-jus dih-ZEEZ), also known as *communicable disease* (kuh-MYOO-nih-kuh-bul dih-ZEEZ). Some of the more common contagious diseases that prevent a salon professional from servicing a client are the common cold, ringworm, conjunctivitis (pinkeye), viral infections, and natural nail, toe, or foot infections. The most common way these infections spread is through dirty hands, especially under the fingernails and in the webs between the fingers. Be sure to always wash your hands after using the restroom and before eating. Contagious diseases can also be spread by contaminated implements, cuts, infected nails, open sores, pus, mouth and nasal discharge, shared drinking cups, telephone receivers, and towels. Uncovered coughing or sneezing and spitting in public also spread germs. **Table 5-2**, Terms Related to Disease, lists terms and definitions that are important for a general understanding of disease.

Viruses

A **virus** (VY-rus) (plural: viruses) is a submicroscopic particle that infects and resides in the cells of a biological organism. Viruses are so small that they can only be seen under the most sophisticated and powerful microscopes. They cause common colds and other respiratory and gastrointestinal (digestive tract) infections. Some of the viruses that plague humans are measles, mumps, chicken pox, smallpox, rabies, yellow fever, hepatitis, polio, influenza, and HIV (which causes AIDS).

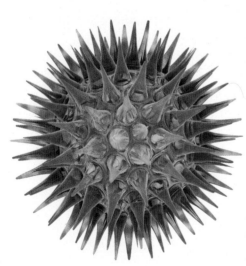

One difference between viruses and bacteria is that a virus can live and reproduce only by taking over other cells and becoming part of them, while bacteria can live and reproduce on their own. Also, bacterial infections can usually be treated with specific antibiotics, but viruses are not affected by antibiotics. In fact, viruses are hard to kill without harming the body's own cells in the process. When available, vaccinations prevent viruses from growing in the body. There are many vaccines available for viruses, but not all viruses have vaccines. There are vaccines available for hepatitis B and varicella (the virus that causes shingles), and you should strongly consider receiving these vaccines, as well as those for the seasonal flu and pneumonia. Discuss with your healthcare provider all of the immunizations to consider.

Biofilm

Researchers are learning that biofilms play a large role in disease and infection. **Biofilms** are colonies of microorganisms that adhere to environmental surfaces, as well as the human body. They secrete a sticky,

table 5-2
TERMS RELATED TO DISEASE

Term	Definition
Allergy	Reaction due to extreme sensitivity to certain foods, chemicals, or other normally harmless substances.
Contagious Disease	Also known as *communicable disease*; a disease that is spread from one person to another person. Some of the more contagious diseases are the common cold, ringworm, conjunctivitis (pinkeye), viral infections, and natural nail or toe and foot infections.
Contamination	The presence, or the reasonably anticipated presence, of blood or other potentially infectious materials on an item's surface or visible debris or residues such as dust, hair, and skin.
Decontamination	The removal of blood or other potentially infectious materials on an item's surface and the removal of visible debris or residue such as dust, hair, and skin.
Diagnosis (dy-ag-NOH-sis)	Determination of the nature of a disease from its symptoms and/or diagnostic tests. Federal regulations prohibit salon professionals from performing a diagnosis.
Disease	An abnormal condition of all or part of the body or its systems or organs that makes the body incapable of carrying on normal function.
Exposure Incident	Contact with non-intact (broken) skin, blood, body fluid, or other potentially infectious materials that are the result of the performance of an employee's duties.
Infectious Disease	Disease caused by pathogenic (harmful) microorganisms that enter the body. An infectious disease may be spread from one person to another person.
Inflammation	Condition in which the body reacts to injury, irritation, or infection. An inflammation is characterized by redness, heat, pain, and swelling.
Occupational Disease	Illnesses resulting from conditions associated with employment, such as prolonged and repeated overexposure to certain products or ingredients.
Parasitic Disease	Disease caused by parasites, such as lice and mites.
Pathogenic Disease	Disease produced by organisms, including bacteria, viruses, fungi, and parasites.
Systemic Disease	Disease that affects the body as a whole, often due to under-functioning or over-functioning internal glands or organs. This disease is carried through the blood stream or the lymphatic system.

protective coating that cements them together and is hard to penetrate. It grows into a complex structure, with many different kinds of microbes. The sticky matrix substance holds communities together, making them very hard to pierce with antisepsis, antimicrobials, and disinfection. It keeps the body in a chronic inflammatory state that is painful and inhibits healing.

Biofilms are usually not visible and must grow very large to be seen with the eyes. Dental plaque is an example of a visible human biofilm. Because biofilms are hard to detect, their presence and effects seem to be underestimated. Biofilm colonies are one of the most significant scientific discoveries of the past few decades. We have much more to learn. Conscientiously using infection control precautions, including standard precautions, cleaning, disinfection, and sterilization, are the best methods of prevention at the present time.

After reading the next few sections, you will be able to:

LO④ Define bloodborne pathogens and explain how they are transmitted.

Bloodborne Pathogens

Disease-causing microorganisms that are carried in the body by blood or body fluids, such as hepatitis and HIV, are called **bloodborne pathogens**. In the salon, the spread of bloodborne pathogens is possible through haircutting, chemical burns, shaving, nipping, clipping, facial treatments, waxing, tweezing, or whenever the skin is broken. Use great care to avoid cutting or damaging clients' skin during any type of service.

Cutting living skin is considered outside the scope of the cosmetologist's licensed and approved practices. Federal law allows only qualified medical professionals to cut living skin, since this is considered a medical procedure. This means that cosmetologists are not allowed to trim or cut the skin around the nail plate. Cutting hardened tissue and removing a callus are both considered medical procedures. Even if the client insists, cosmetologists may not intentionally cut any living skin for any reason.

Hepatitis

Hepatitis (hep-uh-TY-tus) is a bloodborne virus that causes disease and can damage the liver. In general, it is difficult to contract hepatitis. Unlike HIV, hepatitis can live on a surface outside the body for long periods of time. For this reason, it is vital that all surfaces that contact a client are thoroughly cleaned and disinfected.

There are three types of hepatitis that are of concern in the salon: hepatitis A, hepatitis B, and hepatitis C. Hepatitis B is the most difficult to kill on a surface, so check the label of the disinfectant you use to be sure that the product is effective against hepatitis B. Hepatitis B and C are spread from person to person through blood and, less often, through other body fluids, such as semen and vaginal secretions.

HIV/AIDS

Human immunodeficiency virus (HIV) (HYOO-mun ih-MYOO-noh-di-FISH-en-see VY-rus) is the virus that causes **acquired immune deficiency syndrome (AIDS)** (uh-KWY-erd ih-MYOON di-FISH-en-see sin-drohm). AIDS is a disease that breaks down the body's immune system. HIV is spread from person to person through blood and, less often, through other body fluids, such as semen and vaginal secretions. A person can be infected with HIV for many years without having symptoms, but testing can determine whether a person is infected within six months after exposure to the virus. Sometimes people who are HIV-positive have never been tested and do not know they have the potential to infect other people.

The HIV virus is spread mainly through the sharing of needles by intravenous (IV) drug users and by unprotected sexual contact. Less commonly, HIV is spread through accidents with needles in healthcare settings. It is not spread by holding hands, hugging, kissing, sharing food,

---

❓ DID YOU KNOW?

An example of a common viral infection often seen in salons is the **human papilloma virus** (HYOO-mun pap-uh-LOW-ma VY-rus) (abbreviated HPV), a virus that causes warts in humans, but is also the cause of cervical cancer in women. When the virus infects the bottom of the foot and resembles small black dots, usually in clustered groups, it is called plantar warts. However, when it is present in the "bikini" region, it can have no symptoms or can present as genital warts. HPV is highly contagious, difficult to kill, and can be passed in pedicure bowls, wax pots, and from dirty implements. If the client shows signs of HPV infection, do not perform a pedicure service; however, many people have no visible symptoms making infection control for EVERY client even more important!

or using household items such as a telephone or toilet seats. There are no documented cases that indicate the virus can be spread by food handlers, insects, or casual contact during hair, skin, nail, and pedicure salon services.

If you accidentally cut a client, the tool will be contaminated with whatever might be in the client's blood, including HIV. You cannot continue to use the implement without cleaning and disinfecting it. Continuing to use a contaminated implement without cleaning and disinfecting it puts you and others in the salon at risk of infection.

Fungi

Fungi (FUN-jI) (singular: fungus [FUN-gus]) are single-cell organisms that grow in irregular masses that include molds, mildews, and yeasts. They can cause contagious diseases such as ringworm. **Mildew** (MIL-doo), another fungus, affects plants or grows on inanimate objects but does not cause human infections in the salon.

There are several frequently encountered fungal infections resulting from hair services that look similar and are often confused for each other. **Folliculitis barbae** (fah-lik-yuh-LY-tis BAR-bee), also known as *pseudofolliculitis barbae* is an inflammation of hair follicles caused by a bacterial infection often caused by Staphylococcus aureus. Outside of healthcare, this is often referred to as *barbers itch* or *hot tub folliculitis*.

Tinea barbae (TIN-ee-uh BAR-bee) is a superficial fungal infection caused by a variety of dermatophytes that commonly affects the skin. It is primarily limited to the bearded areas of the face and neck or around the scalp. This infection occurs almost exclusively in older adolescent and adult males. A person with tinea barbae may have deep, inflamed or non-inflamed patches of skin on the face or the nape of the neck.

Tinea barbae is similar to **tinea capitis** (TIN-ee-uh KAP-ih-tis), a fungal infection of the scalp characterized by red papules, or spots, at the opening of hair follicles. For more information on tinea capitis, see Chapter 11, Properties of the Hair and Scalp.

Hair stylists must clean and disinfect clipper blades to avoid spreading scalp and skin infections. The risk of spreading skin and scalp infections can be reduced by first removing all visible hair and debris from clippers. This can be done effectively and quickly by using compressed air; then the nonelectrical parts can be cleaned and disinfected properly. Always refer to the manufacturer's directions for proper cleaning and disinfecting methods and recommendations.

Nail infections can be spread by using dirty implements or by not properly preparing the surface of the natural nail before enhancement products are applied. Nail infections can occur on both hands and feet. Fungal infections are much more common on the feet than on the hands, but bacterial infections commonly occur on both hands and feet. The most frequently encountered infection on the foot resulting from nail services is **tinea pedis** (TIN-ee-uh PED-us), a ringworm fungus of the foot. Both bacterial and fungal infections can be spread to an infected client's other nails or to other salon clients unless everything that touches clients is either properly cleaned and disinfected before reuse or is thrown away after use (**figure 5-8**).

? DID YOU KNOW?

Pathogenic bacteria, viruses, or fungi can enter the body through:

- skin: broken or inflamed skin, such as a cut or a scratch. They also can enter through a bruise (weakened tissue) or a rash. Intact skin is an effective barrier to infection.
- mouth: contaminated water, food, fingers, or objects.
- nose: inhaling infectious dust or droplets from a cough or sneeze.
- eye or ears: organisms that reside in water are commonly transmitted this way when swimming.
- genitals: unprotected sex.

The body prevents and controls infections with:

- healthy, uncompromised skin—the body's first line of defense.
- body secretions such as perspiration and digestive juices.
- white blood cells that destroy bacteria.
- antitoxins that counteract the **toxins**, various poisonous substances produced by some microorganisms (bacteria and viruses).

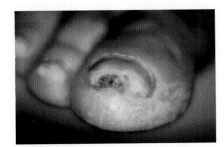

figure 5-8
Nail Fungus

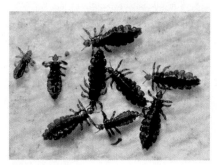

figure 5-9
Head Lice

Courtesy of The National Pediculosis Association® Inc.

Parasites

Parasites are organisms that grow, feed, and shelter on or in another organism (referred to as a host), while contributing nothing to the survival of that organism. They must have a host to survive. Parasites can live on or inside of humans and animals. They also can be found in food, on plants and trees, and in water. Humans can acquire internal parasites by eating fish or meat that has not been properly cooked. External parasites that affect humans on or in the skin include ticks, fleas, and mites.

Head lice are a type of parasite responsible for contagious diseases and conditions (figure 5-9). One condition caused by an infestation of head lice is called pediculosis capitis (puh-dik-yuh-LOH-sis KAP-ih-tus). **Scabies** (SKAY-beez) is also a contagious skin disease and is caused by the itch mite, which burrows under the skin. Contagious diseases and conditions caused by parasites should only be treated by a doctor. Contaminated countertops, tools, and equipment should be thoroughly cleaned and then disinfected with an EPA-registered disinfectant for the time recommended by the manufacturer or with a bleach solution for 10 minutes.

Immunity

Immunity is the ability of the body to destroy, resist, and recognize infection. Immunity against disease can be either natural or acquired and is a sign of good health. **Natural immunity** is partly inherited and partly developed through healthy living. **Acquired immunity** is immunity that the body develops after overcoming a disease, through inoculation (such as flu vaccinations), or through exposure to natural allergens such as pollen, cat dander, and ragweed.

After reading the next few sections, you will be able to:

LO❺ Explain the differences between cleaning, disinfecting, and sterilizing.

Prevent the Spread of Disease

Proper infection control can prevent the spread of disease caused by exposure to potentially infectious materials on an item's surface. Infection control also will prevent exposure to blood and visible debris or residue such as dust, hair, and skin.

Proper infection control requires two steps: cleaning and then disinfecting with an appropriate EPA-registered disinfectant. When these two steps are followed correctly, virtually all pathogens of concern in the salon can be effectively eliminated.

Sterilization (stayr-ih-luh-ZAY-shun), which is the process that destroys all microbial life, can be incorporated but it very rarely mandated.

Effective sterilization typically requires the use of an autoclave to complete—this piece of equipment incorporates heat and pressure. For sterilization to be effective, items must be cleaned prior and the autoclave must be tested and maintained per the manufacturer's specifications. The Centers for Disease Control and Prevention (CDC) requires that autoclaves be tested weekly to ensure they are properly sterilizing implements. The accepted method is called a spore test. Commercial sealed packages containing test organisms are subjected to a typical sterilization cycle and then sent to a contract laboratory that specializes in autoclave performance testing. **Decontamination** (dee-kuhn-tam-ih-NAY-shun) is the removal of blood and all other potentially infectious materials on an item's surface, and the removal of visible debris or residue such as dust, hair, and skin.

? DID YOU KNOW?
Autoclaves penetrate contaminated instruments better than liquid disinfectants and offer complete destruction of all bacterial, viral, and fungal contamination.

Cleaning

As stated, infection control has two steps: cleaning and then disinfecting.

Remember that when you clean, you must remove all visible dirt and debris from tools, implements, and equipment by washing with liquid soap and warm water, and by using a clean and disinfected nail brush to scrub any grooved or hinged portions of the item.

A surface is properly cleaned when the number of contaminants on the surface is greatly reduced. In turn, this reduces the risk of infection. The vast majority of contaminants and pathogens can be removed from the surfaces of tools and implements through proper cleaning. This is why cleaning is an important part of disinfecting tools and equipment. A surface must be properly cleaned before it can be properly disinfected. Using a disinfectant without cleaning first is like using mouthwash without brushing your teeth—it just does not work properly!

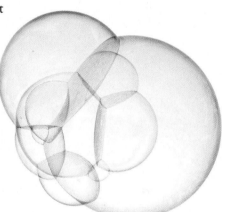

Cleaned surfaces can still harbor small amounts of pathogens, but the presence of fewer pathogens means infections are less likely to be spread. Putting antiseptics on your skin or washing your hands with soap and water will drastically lower the number of pathogens on your hands. However, it does not clean them properly. The proper cleaning of the hands requires rubbing hands together and using liquid soap, warm running water, a nail brush, and a clean towel. (See Procedure 5-4, Proper Hand Washing.) Do not underestimate the importance of proper cleaning and hand washing. They are the most powerful and important ways to prevent the spread of infection.

There are three ways to clean your tools or implements:

1. Washing with soap and warm water, and then scrubbing them with a clean and properly disinfected nail brush.

2. Using an ultrasonic unit.

3. Using a cleaning solvent (e.g., on metal bits for electric files).

Disinfection

The second step of infection control is disinfection. Remember that disinfection is the process that eliminates most, but not necessarily all, microorganisms on nonporous surfaces. This process is not effective against bacterial spores. In the salon setting, disinfection is extremely effective in

While some clients who have impaired immune systems will share that information with you, many will not—either because they do not know it is important, or they do not know that they have a compromised immune system. These people are at very high risk of infection if they come into contact with pathogens in the salon. Keeping in mind that you won't always know who these people are, it is important to practice proper infection control practices before servicing every client! One example is a diabetic whose immune system does not work effectively and also has impaired healing. Most Type 2 diabetics are diabetic for 7 years prior to being diagnosed, which means that even if you ask, they will say "no" because they have not yet been diagnosed! Another example is clients on medication for things like asthma, rheumatoid arthritis, and fibromyalgia—these medications are designed to dull the immune system such that it makes these clients particularly susceptible to infection. Remember, you don't know everyone who sits in your chair, so treat everyone as though they deserve the best in disinfection!

⚠ CAUTION

Read labels carefully! Manufacturers take great care to develop safe and highly effective products. However, when used improperly, many otherwise safe products can be dangerous. If you do not follow proper guidelines and instructions, any professional salon product can be dangerous. As with all products, disinfectants must be used exactly as the label instructs.

⚠ CAUTION

Improper mixing of disinfectants—to be weaker or more concentrated than the manufacturer's instructions—can dramatically reduce their effectiveness. Always add the disinfectant concentrate to the water when mixing and always follow the manufacturer's instructions for proper dilution.

Safety glasses and gloves should be worn to avoid accidental contact with eyes and skin.

controlling microorganisms on surfaces such as shears, nippers, and other multiuse tools and equipment (multiuse and single-use tools are discussed later in this chapter). Any disinfectant used in the salon should carry an EPA-registration number and the label should clearly state the specific organisms the solution is effective in killing when used according to the label instructions.

Remember that disinfectants are products that destroy most bacteria, fungi, and viruses (but not spores) on surfaces. Disinfectants are not for use on human skin, hair, or nails. Never use disinfectants as hand cleaners since this can cause skin irritation and **allergy** (AL-ur-jee), a reaction due to sensitivity to certain foods, chemicals, or other normally harmless substances. All disinfectants clearly state on the label that you should avoid skin contact. Do not put your fingers directly into any disinfecting solution. Disinfectants can be harmful if absorbed through the skin. If you mix a disinfectant in a container that is not labeled by the manufacturer, the container must be properly labeled with the contents and the date it was mixed. All concentrated disinfectants must be diluted exactly as instructed by the manufacturer on the container's label.

Choosing a Disinfectant

You must read and follow the manufacturer's instructions whenever you are using a disinfectant. Mixing ratios (dilution) and **contact time** (the amount of visibly moist time required to be effective against pathogens listed on product label) are very important and can vary widely based on the manufacturer and delivery method. For example, most concentrates have a 10 minute contact time, whereas some wipes have a 2 minute contact time. Not all disinfectants have the same concentration, so be sure to mix the correct proportions according to the instructions on the label. If the label does not have the word concentrate on it, the product is already mixed and must be used directly from the container and must not be diluted. All EPA-registered disinfectants will specify a contact time in their directions for use. Disinfectants must have **efficacy** (ef-ih-KUH-see) claims on the label. Efficacy is the ability to produce an effect. As applied to disinfectant claims, efficacy means the effectiveness with which a disinfecting solution kills microorganisms when used according to the label instructions.

Salons and cosmetologists must be aware of the types of disinfectants that are on the market and any new products that become available.

Salons pose a lower infection risk when compared to hospitals. For this reason, hospitals must meet much stricter infection control standards. Even though salons pose a lower risk of spreading certain types of infections, it is still very important to clean and then disinfect all tools, implements, surfaces, and equipment correctly before using on any client.

Proper Use of Disinfectants

Implements must be thoroughly cleaned of all visible matter or residue before being placed in disinfectant solution. This is because residue will interfere with the disinfectant and prevent proper disinfection. Properly cleaned implements and tools, free from all visible debris, must be completely immersed in disinfectant solution. Complete immersion means there is enough liquid in the container to cover all surfaces of the item being disinfected, including the handles, for 10 minutes or for the time recommended by the manufacturer (**figure 5-10**).

Disinfectant Tips

- Use only on pre-cleaned, hard, nonporous surfaces—not on single-use abrasive files or buffers.

- Always wear gloves and safety glasses when handling disinfectant solutions.

- Always dilute products according to the instructions on the product label.

- An item must remain submerged in the disinfectant for 10 minutes unless the product label specifies differently.

- To disinfect large surfaces such as tabletops, carefully apply the disinfectant onto the pre-cleaned surface, or use a disinfectant spray and allow it to remain wet for 10 minutes, unless the product label specifies differently.

- If the product label or your state rules require, "complete immersion," the entire implement must be completely immersed in the solution.

- Change the disinfectant according to the instructions on the label. If the liquid is not changed as instructed, it will no longer be effective and may begin to promote the growth of microbes.

- Proper disinfection of a whirlpool, pipeless or air-jet pedicure spa requires that the disinfecting solution circulate for 10 minutes, unless the product label specifies otherwise.

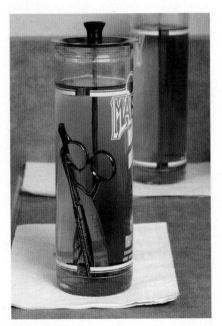

figure 5-10
Completely immerse tools in disinfectant.

After reading the next few sections, you will be able to:

LO **6**   List the types of disinfectants and the steps to using them properly.

? DID YOU KNOW?

Not all household bleaches are effective as disinfectants. To be effective, the bleach must have an EPA-registration number and contain at least 5 percent sodium hypochlorite and be diluted properly to a 10 percent solution—9 parts water to 1 part bleach.

Types of Disinfectants

Disinfectants are not all the same. Some are appropriate for use in the salon and some are not. You should be aware of the different types of disinfectants and the ones that are recommended for salon use.

Disinfectants Appropriate for Salon Use

Quaternary ammonium compounds (KWAT-ur-nayr-ree uh-MOH-neeum KAHM-powndz), also known as *quats* (KWATZ), are disinfectants that are very effective when used properly in the salon. The most advanced type of these formulations is called multiple quats. Multiple quats contain sophisticated blends of quats that work together to dramatically increase the effectiveness of these disinfectants. Quat solutions usually disinfect implements in 10 minutes. These formulas may contain anti-rust ingredients. They should be removed from the solution after the specified period, rinsed (if required), dried, and stored in a clean, covered container.

Phenolic disinfectants (fi-NOH-lik dis-in-FEK-tents) are powerful disinfectants, known as tuberculocidal. They are a form of formaldehyde, have a very high pH, and can damage the skin and eyes. Phenolic disinfectants can be harmful to the environment if put down the drain. They have been used reliably over the years to disinfect salon tools; however, they do have drawbacks. Phenol can damage plastic and rubber and can cause certain metals to rust. Phenolic disinfectants should never be used to disinfect pedicure tubs or equipment (unless required by state rules). Extra care should be taken to avoid skin contact with phenolic disinfectants. Phenolics are known carcinogens, and as such should only be used in states where required

Bleach

Household bleach, 5.25 percent **sodium hypochlorite** (SOH-dee-um hy-puh-KLOR-ite), is an effective disinfectant and has been used extensively as a disinfectant in the salon for large surface areas such as countertops and floors. Using too much bleach can damage some metals and plastics, so be sure to read the label for safe use. Bleach can be corrosive to metals and plastics and can cause skin irritation and eye damage. Bleach should not be used to disinfect salon and spa tools and implements such as shears, combs, and brushes.

To mix a bleach solution, always follow the manufacturer's directions. Store the bleach solution away from heat and light. A fresh bleach solution should be mixed every 24 hours or when the solution has been contaminated. After mixing the bleach solution, date the container to ensure that the solution is not saved from one day to the next, but disposed of daily similar to other disinfectants. Bleach can be irritating to the lungs, so be careful about inhaling the fumes.

Disinfectant Safety

Disinfectants are pesticides (a type of poison) and can cause serious skin and eye damage. Some disinfectants appear clear while others, especially phenolic disinfectants, are a little cloudy. Always use caution when handling disinfectants and follow the safety tips below.

Safety Tips for Disinfectants

Always

- Keep an SDS on hand for the disinfectant(s) you use.

- Wear gloves and safety glasses when mixing disinfectants (**figure 5-11**).

- Avoid skin and eye contact.

- Add disinfectant to water when diluting (rather than adding water to a disinfectant) to prevent foaming, which can result in an incorrect mixing ratio.

- Use tongs, gloves, or a draining basket to remove implements from disinfectants.

- Keep disinfectants out of reach of children.

- Carefully measure and use disinfectant products according to label instructions.

- Follow the manufacturer's instructions for mixing, using, and disposing of disinfectants.

- Carefully follow the manufacturer's directions for when to replace the disinfectant solution in order to ensure the healthiest conditions for you and your client. Replace the disinfectant solution every day—more often if the solution becomes soiled or contaminated.

Never

- Let quats, phenols, bleach, or any other disinfectant come in contact with your skin. If you do get disinfectants on your skin, immediately wash the area with liquid soap and warm water. Then rinse the area and dry the area thoroughly.

- Place any disinfectant or other product in an unmarked container. All containers should be labeled (**figure 5-12**).

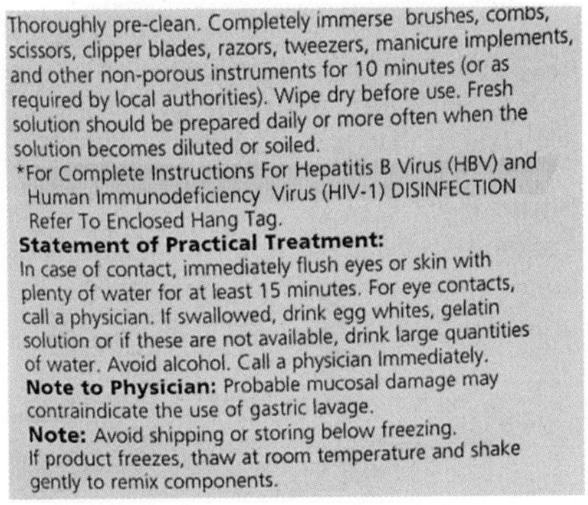

Jars or containers used to disinfect implements are often incorrectly called wet sanitizers. Disinfectant containers must be covered, but not airtight. Remember to clean the container every day and to wear gloves when you do. Always follow the manufacturer's label instructions for disinfecting products.

Disinfect or Dispose?

How can you tell which items in the salon can be disinfected and reused? There are two types of items used in salons: multiuse (reusable) items, and single-use (disposable) items.

- **Multiuse**, also known as *reusable*, items can be cleaned, disinfected, and used on more than one person even if the item is exposed to blood or body fluid. These items must have a hard, nonporous surface.

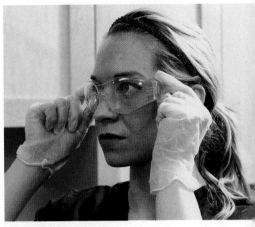

figure 5-11
Wear gloves and safety glasses while handling disinfectants.

Thoroughly pre-clean. Completely immerse brushes, combs, scissors, clipper blades, razors, tweezers, manicure implements, and other non-porous instruments for 10 minutes (or as required by local authorities). Wipe dry before use. Fresh solution should be prepared daily or more often when the solution becomes diluted or soiled.
*For Complete Instructions For Hepatitis B Virus (HBV) and Human Immunodeficiency Virus (HIV-1) DISINFECTION Refer To Enclosed Hang Tag.
Statement of Practical Treatment:
In case of contact, immediately flush eyes or skin with plenty of water for at least 15 minutes. For eye contacts, call a physician. If swallowed, drink egg whites, gelatin solution or if these are not available, drink large quantities of water. Avoid alcohol. Call a physician immediately.
Note to Physician: Probable mucosal damage may contraindicate the use of gastric lavage.
Note: Avoid shipping or storing below freezing. If product freezes, thaw at room temperature and shake gently to remix components.

figure 5-12
All containers should be labeled.

Examples of multiuse items are nippers, shears, combs, metal pushers, rollers, and permanent wave rods.

- **Single-use**, also known as *disposable*, items cannot be used more than once. These items are **porous**, items made or constructed of a material that has pores or openings and cannot be properly cleaned so that all visible residue is removed—such as pumice stones used for pedicures—or they are damaged or contaminated by cleaning and disinfecting. Examples of single-use items are wooden sticks, cotton balls, sponges, gauze, tissues, paper towels, nail files, and buffers. Single-use items must be thrown out after each use.

Keep a Logbook

Salons should always follow manufacturers' recommended schedules for cleaning and disinfecting tools and implements, disinfecting foot spas and basins, scheduling regular service visits for equipment, maintenance, and replacing parts when needed. Although your state may not require you to keep a logbook of all equipment usage, cleaning, disinfecting, testing, and maintenance, it may be advisable to keep one. Showing your logbook to clients provides them with peace of mind and confidence in your ability to protect them from infection and disease.

Disinfecting Nonelectrical Tools and Implements

State rules require that all multiuse tools and implements must be cleaned and disinfected before and after every service—even when they are used on the same person. Mix all disinfectants according to the manufacturer's directions, always adding the disinfectant to the water, not the water to the disinfectant (**figure 5-13**).

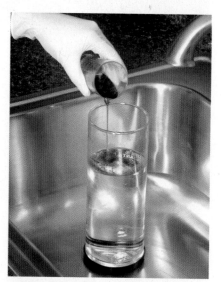

figure 5-13
Carefully pour disinfectant into the water when preparing disinfectant solution.

P 5-1 **Cleaning and Disinfecting Nonelectrical Tools and Implements**
See page 97

Disinfecting Electrical Tools and Equipment

Hair clippers, electrotherapy tools, nail drills, and other types of electrical equipment have parts that cannot be immersed in liquid. These items should be cleaned and disinfected using an EPA-registered disinfectant designed for use on these devices. Follow the procedures recommended by the disinfectant manufacturer for preparing the solution and follow the item's manufacturer directions for cleaning and disinfecting the device.

Disinfecting Work Surfaces

Before beginning every client service, all work surfaces must be cleaned and disinfected. Be sure to clean and disinfect tables, styling stations, shampoo sinks, chairs, arm rests, and any other surface that a customer's skin may have touched (**figure 5-14**). Clean doorknobs and handles daily to reduce transferring germs to your hands.

Cleaning Towels, Linens, and Capes

Clean towels, linens, and capes must be used for each client. After a towel, linen, or cape has been used on a client, it must not be used again

© Photo courtesy of King Research, Inc.

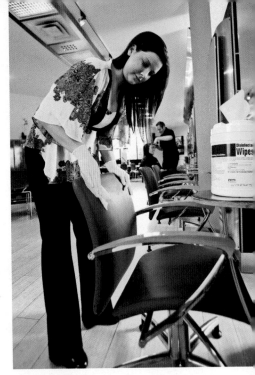

figure 5-14
Clean and disinfect styling stations regularly.

until it has been properly laundered. To clean towels, linens, and capes, launder according to the directions on the item's label. Be sure that towels, linens, and capes are thoroughly dried. Items that are not dry may grow mildew and bacteria. Store soiled linens and towels in covered or closed containers, away from clean linens and towels, even if your state regulatory agency does not require that you do so. Whenever possible, use disposable towels, especially in restrooms. Do not allow capes that are used for cutting, shampooing, and chemical services to touch the client's skin. Use disposable neck strips or towels. If a cape accidentally touches skin, do not use the cape again until it has been laundered.

Disinfecting Foot Spas and Pedicure Equipment

All equipment that contains water for pedicures (including whirlpool spas, pipeless units, foot baths, basins, tubs, sinks, and bowls) must be cleaned and disinfected after every pedicure, and the information must be entered into a logbook. Inspectors may issue fines if there is no logbook. Some state regulatory agencies allow single-use tub liners in pedicure equipment. Check with your state agency. If single-use liners are allowed in your state, be sure that you clean and disinfect all surfaces of the equipment that are not covered by the liner after every client.

Which Foot Spa Do I Have?

Many salons will refer to any of their pedicure chairs that circulate water as whirlpool spas, however this is a misconception. There are three types of foot spas that circulate water: whirlpool, air jet, and pipeless.

1. The *whirlpool foot spa* creates a massaging effect by re-circulating water through built in pipes and jets, similar to a Jacuzzi tub, and is often referred to as a piped foot spa. The whirlpool or piped foot spa has come under scrutiny because disease-causing microorganisms tend to grow inside the pipes despite the disinfecting process and therefore has been slowly discontinued in the industry.

2. The *air jet basin* uses a blower to force air through small holes in an air channel, creating an overall bubbling massage. Water does not circulate through these air channels.

3. The new standard in the industry is the *pipeless foot spa*. The pipeless foot spa uses impellers, the rotating blade of a pump, to circulate water. This type of foot spa is easily cleaned and disinfected.

All three foot spas have similar cleaning and disinfecting procedures.

4. The fourth type of foot spa is a *non-whirlpool foot basin* or *tub*. This type of tub does not circulate water. It can be connected to running water and a drain or be portable. If it is a portable tub, you will clean and disinfect it at the dispensary sink.

Ⓟ 5-2 **Cleaning and Disinfecting Whirlpool, Air-Jet, and Pipeless Foot Spas** *See page 99*

Ⓟ 5-3 **Cleaning and Disinfecting Basic Foot Basins or Tubs** *See page 103*

Soaps and Detergents

Chelating soaps (CHE-layt-ing SOHPS), also known as *chelating detergents*, work to break down stubborn films and remove the residue of pedicure products such as scrubs, salts, and masks. The chelating agents in these soaps work in all types of water, are low-sudsing, and are specially formulated to work in areas with hard tap water. Hard tap water reduces the effectiveness of cleaners and disinfectants. If your area has hard water, ask your local distributor for pedicure soaps that are effective in hard water. This information will be stated on the product's label.

Additives, Powders, and Tablets

There is no additive, powder, or tablet that eliminates the need for you to clean and disinfect. Products of this type cannot be used instead of EPA-registered liquid disinfectant solutions. You cannot replace proper cleaning and disinfection with a shortcut. Water sanitizers do not properly clean or disinfect equipment. They are designed for Jacuzzis and hydrotherapy tubs where no oils, lotions, or other enhancements are used. Therefore, water sanitizers do not work well in a salon environment. Never rely solely on water sanitizers to protect your clients from infection. Products that contain chloramine T, for example, are not effective disinfectants for equipment. These products only treat the water and have limited value in the salon. They do not replace proper cleaning and disinfection. Remember: There are no shortcuts!

Dispensary

The dispensary must be kept clean and orderly, with the contents of all containers clearly marked. Always store products according to the manufacturer's instructions and away from heat and out of direct sunlight. Keep the SDSs for all products used in the salon in a convenient, central location for the employees.

Hand Washing

Properly washing your hands is one of the most important actions you can take to prevent spreading germs from one person to another. Proper hand washing removes germs from the folds and grooves of the skin and from under the free edge of the nail plate by lifting and rinsing germs and contaminants from the surface.

You should wash your hands thoroughly before and after each service. Follow the hand washing procedure in this chapter. And, if you perform

❓ DID YOU KNOW?

Most pedicure spas hold five gallons of water; check with the manufacturer and be sure that you use the correct amount of disinfectant. Also, be sure that you are using a disinfectant that is appropriate for the pedicure spa.

Remember:

1 gallon = 128 ounces

5 gallons = 640 ounces

If you are working with a pedicure spa that holds five gallons of water, you will have to measure the correct amount of water needed to cover the jets and then add the correct amount of disinfectant.

nail services, your client should first wash his or her hands using a clean and disinfected nail brush before the service begins.

Antimicrobial and antibacterial soaps can dry the skin, and medical studies suggest that they are no more effective than regular soaps or detergents. The true benefit of hand washing comes from the friction created by the soap bubbles that can "pull" pathogens off the skin surface. Repeated hand washing can also dry the skin, so using a moisturizing hand lotion after washing is a good practice. Be sure the hand lotion is in a pump container, not a jar.

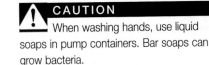

CAUTION
When washing hands, use liquid soaps in pump containers. Bar soaps can grow bacteria.

Ⓟ 5-4 **Proper Hand Washing** *See page 104*

Avoid using very hot water to wash your hands. Remember: You must wash your hands thoroughly before and after each service, so do all you can to reduce any irritation that may occur.

Waterless Hand Sanitizers

Antiseptics (ant-ih-SEP-tiks) are chemical germicides formulated for use on skin and are registered and regulated by the Food and Drug Administration (FDA). Antiseptics generally contain a high volume of alcohol, and these products are intended to reduce the numbers of microbes and slow growth on the skin. Neither type of antiseptic can clean the hands of dirt and debris; this can only be accomplished with liquid soap, a soft-bristle brush, and water. Use hand sanitizers only after properly cleaning your hands, or when hand washing is not an option. Never use an antiseptic to disinfect instruments or other surfaces. They are ineffective for that purpose.

After reading the next few sections, you will be able to:

LO❼ **Define Standard Precautions.**

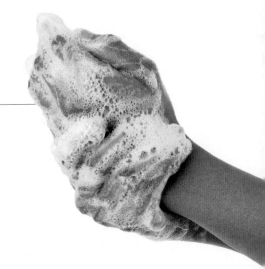

Follow Standard Precautions to Protect You and Your Clients

Standard Precautions are guidelines published by the Centers for Disease Control and Prevention (CDC) that require the employer and employee to assume that all human blood and body fluids are potentially infectious. Because it may not be possible to identify clients with infectious diseases, strict infection control practices should be used with all clients. In most instances, clients who are infected with the hepatitis B virus or other bloodborne pathogens are **asymptomatic**, which means that they show no symptoms or signs of infection. Bloodborne pathogens are more difficult to kill than germs that live outside the body.

© Samuel Borges Photography/Shutterstock.com

Occupational Health and Safety Administration and CDC set safety standards and precautions that protect employees in situations when they could be exposed to bloodborne pathogens. Precautions include proper hand washing, wearing gloves, and properly handling and disposing of sharp instruments and any other items that may have been contaminated by blood or other body fluids. It is important that specific procedures are followed if blood or body fluid is present.

Personal Protective Equipment (PPE)

Many chemicals used in the salon will bear labels that require the use of personal protective equipment such as gloves and safety glasses when working with their products. However, some equipment, such as gloves, offer protection from exposure to pathogens and should be worn whenever practical.

Gloves

The Occupational Safety and Health Act defines PPEs as "specialized clothing or equipment worn by an employee for protection against a hazard." The hazards this particular standard refers to are bloodborne pathogens, such as hepatitis and HIV.

Standard Precautions include guidelines for the use of gloves, masks, and eyewear when contact with blood or body secretions containing blood or blood elements is a possibility. The Standard Precautions standard within OSHA reads: "Standard Precautions shall be observed to prevent occupational exposure to blood or other potentially infectious materials. Occupational exposure includes any reasonably anticipated skin, eye, mucous membrane, or potential contact with blood or other potentially infectious materials that may result from the performance of an employee's duties[1]." It does not say "only wear gloves when there is exposure to a large amount of blood." Cosmetologists must prevent their occupational exposure to any amount of blood, no matter how miniscule, through the use of gloves, masks, and eye protection.

Gloves are single-use equipment; a new set is used for every client, and sometimes must be changed during the service, according to the protocol. Removal of gloves is performed by inverting the cuffs, pulling them off inside out, and then disposing of them into the trash (figure 5-15). The glove taken off first is held in the hand with a glove still on it and then that glove with the cuff inverted is pulled over the first glove inside out (figure 5-16). The first glove is then inside the second one, which has the service side now on the inside against the other glove, and they are disposed of together.

If a manicure and pedicure are being performed on the same client, a new set is to be worn for each service. If the services require moving from one place of service to another several times, several sets of gloves will need to be used. The technician is to perform hand washing after removing each set of gloves and before putting on a new set when two services are being performed together, or use antimicrobial gel cleanser between sets of gloves during the same appointment.

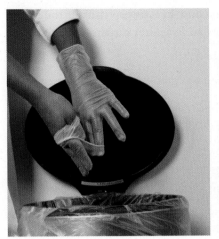

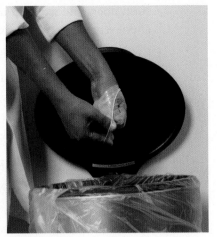

figure 5-15
Remove gloves by inverting the cuffs, pulling them off inside out.

figure 5-16
The glove with the cuff inverted is pulled over the first glove inside out and are disposed of together.

⚠ **CAUTION** Taking the time to conduct a thorough hair and scalp analysis will enable you to determine whether a client has any open wounds or abrasions. If the client does have an open wound or abrasion, do not perform services of any kind for the client.

An Exposure Incident: Contact with Blood or Body Fluid

You should never perform a service on any client who comes into the salon with an open wound or an abrasion. Sometimes accidents happen while a service is being performed in the salon, however.

An **exposure incident** is contact with nonintact (broken) skin, blood, body fluid, or other potentially infectious materials that is the result of the performance of an employee's duties. Should you or the client suffer a cut or abrasion that bleeds during a service, follow the steps outlined in Procedure 5-5.

🅟 5-5   **Handling an Exposure Incident** *See page 105*

DID YOU KNOW?
- It is your professional and legal responsibility to follow state and federal laws and rules.
- You must keep your license current and notify the licensing agency if you move or change your name.
- You must check your state's website weekly for any changes or updates to rules and regulations.

After reading the next few sections, you will be able to:

LO⑧   List your responsibilities as a salon professional.

List Your Professional Responsibilities

You have many responsibilities as a salon professional, but none is more important than protecting your clients' health and safety. Never take shortcuts for cleaning and disinfecting. You cannot afford to skip steps or save money when it comes to safety.

Infection control practices should be a part of the normal routine for you and your coworkers so that the salon and staff project a steadfast professional image. The following are some simple guidelines that will keep the salon looking its best.

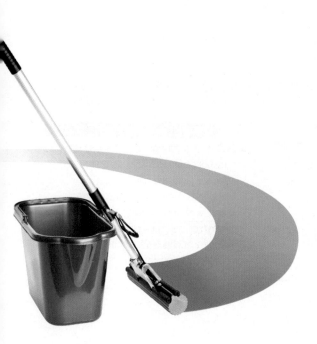

- Keep floors and workstations dust-free. Sweep hair off the floor after every client. Mop floors and vacuum carpets every day.

- Control dust, hair, and other debris.

- Keep trash in a covered waste receptacle to reduce chemical odors and fires.

- Clean fans, ventilation systems, and humidifiers at least once each week.

- Keep all work areas well-lit.

- Clean and disinfect restroom surfaces, including door handles.

- Provide toilet tissue, paper towels, liquid soap, properly disinfected soft-bristle nail brushes, and a container for used brushes in the restroom.

- Never place food in the same refrigerator used to store salon products.

- Prohibit eating, drinking, and smoking in areas where services are performed or where product mixing occurs (e.g., back bar area). Consider having a smoke-free salon. Even when you do not smoke in the service areas, the odor can flow into those areas.

- Empty waste receptacles regularly throughout the day.

- Make sure all containers are properly marked and properly stored.

- Never place any tools or implements in your mouth or pockets.

- Properly clean and disinfect all multiuse tools before reusing them.

- Store clean and disinfected tools in a clean, covered container. Clean drawers may be used for storage if only clean items are stored in the drawers. Always isolate used implements away from disinfected implements.

- Avoid touching your face, mouth, or eye areas during services.

- Clean and disinfect all work surfaces after every client.

- Have clean, disposable paper towels for each client.

- Always properly wash your hands before and after each service.

- Use clean linens and disposable towels on clients. Keep soiled linens separate from clean linens. Use single-use neck strips or clean towels to avoid skin contact with shampoo capes and cutting or chemical protection gowns. If a cape touches the client's skin, do not reuse that cape until it is properly laundered.

- Never provide a nail service to clients who have not properly washed their hands and carefully scrubbed under the free edge of their nails with a disinfected nail brush.

- Use effective exhaust systems in the salon. This will help ensure proper air quality in the salon.

CLEANING AND DISINFECTING NONELECTRICAL TOOLS AND IMPLEMENTS

Nonelectrical tools and implements include items such as combs, brushes, clips, hairpins, metal pushers, makeup brushes (synthetic only), tweezers, and nail clippers.

IMPLEMENTS & MATERIALS

You will need all of the following implements, materials, and supplies:

- ☐ Covered storage container
- ☐ Disinfectant container
- ☐ Disposable gloves
- ☐ Liquid disinfectant
- ☐ Liquid soap
- ☐ Safety glasses
- ☐ Scrub brush
- ☐ Timer
- ☐ Tongs
- ☐ Towels

PROCEDURE

1 It is important to wear safety glasses and gloves while disinfecting nonelectrical tools and implements to protect your eyes from unintentional splashes of disinfectant and to prevent possible contamination of the implements by your hands as well as to protect your hands from the powerful chemicals in the disinfectant solution.

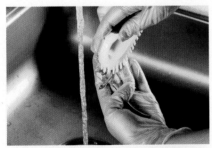

2 Rinse all implements with warm running water, and then scrub them thoroughly with soap or detergent, a properly disinfected nail brush, and warm water. Brush grooved items, if necessary, and open hinged implements to scrub the revealed area.

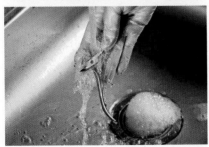

3 Rinse away all traces of soap from the implements with warm running water. The presence of soap in most disinfectants will cause them to become inactive. Soap is most easily rinsed off in warm, not hot, water. Hotter water is not more effective.

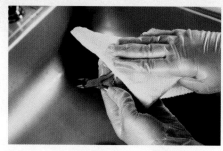

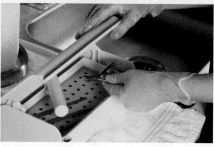

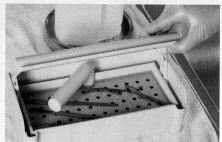

④ Dry implements thoroughly with a clean or disposable towel, or allow them to air dry on a clean towel. Your implements are now properly cleaned and ready to be disinfected.

⑤ If the disinfection solution is visibly dirty, or if the solution has been contaminated, it must be replaced. Completely immerse cleaned implements in an appropriate disinfection container holding an EPA-registered disinfectant for the required time (at least 10 minutes or according to the manufacturer's instructions). Set a timer. Remember to open hinged implements before immersing them in the disinfectant.

⑥ After the required disinfection time has passed, remove tools and implements from the disinfection solution with tongs or gloved hands, rinse the tools and implements well in warm running water, and pat them dry.

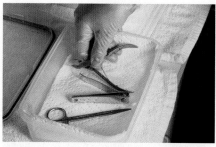

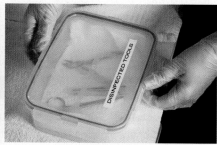

⑦ Store dry, disinfected tools and implements in a clean, covered container until needed.

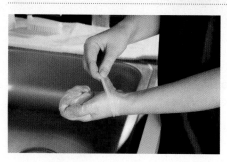

⑧ Remove gloves and thoroughly wash your hands with warm running water and liquid soap. Rinse and dry hands with a clean fabric or disposable towel.

CLEANING AND DISINFECTING WHIRLPOOL, AIR-JET, AND PIPELESS FOOT SPAS

IMPLEMENTS & MATERIALS

You will need all of the following implements, materials, and supplies:

- ☐ Chelating detergent
- ☐ Cleaning logbook
- ☐ Disposable gloves
- ☐ EPA–registered hospital liquid disinfectant
- ☐ Liquid soap
- ☐ Paper towels
- ☐ Safety glasses
- ☐ Scrub brush
- ☐ Timer

PROCEDURE

After every client:

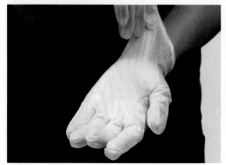

① Put on gloves and safety glasses.

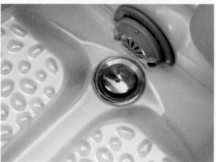

② Drain all water from the pedicure basin if it has not already been drained.

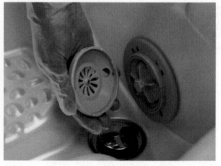

③ Remove the covers from the impellers and any other removable components according to the manufacturer's instructions. Most parts simply twist off.

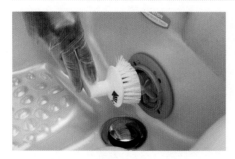

④ Thoroughly scrub all removable components, the impellers, and the areas behind each with liquid soap; a clean, disinfected brush; and clean, warm water to remove all visible residue. For whirlpool and air jet basins, this step is done at the end of each day.

5 Rinse and replace the properly cleaned screen and other removable parts.

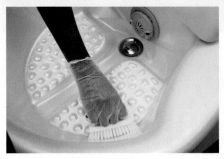

6 Scrub all visible residue from the inside walls of the basin with a clean, disinfected brush; liquid soap; and clean, warm water. Brushes must be cleaned and disinfected after each use; otherwise, they can transfer pathogens to other foot spas.

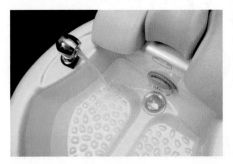

7 Rinse the basin with clean, warm water and drain.

8 Refill the basin with clean, warm water. If the basin has jets, be sure to put enough water in to cover the jets.

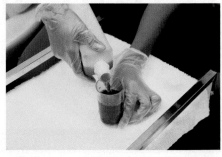

9 Measure the correct amount (read the product label for mixing instructions) of the EPA-registered hospital disinfectant, and add it to the water in the basin.

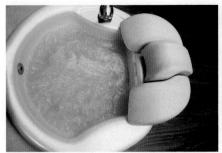

10 Circulate the disinfectant through the basin for 10 minutes or the length of time indicated on the product label. Set the timer to keep track of the time.

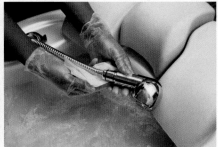

11 Clean and disinfect all external parts and surfaces.

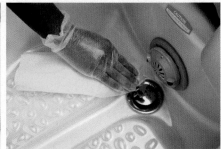

12 Drain; rinse with clean, warm water; and wipe the pedicure basin dry with a clean paper towel.

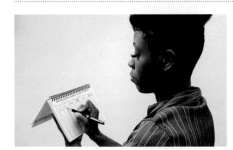

13 Record the disinfection information into the salon's logbook if required by state law or by salon policy.

In addition to the procedures performed after each client, you also need to circulate chelating detergent through the foot spas at the <u>end of every day</u>. Chelating soaps break down stubborn films and help remove pedicure product residues. Follow these steps:

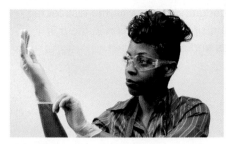

1 Put on gloves and safety glasses.

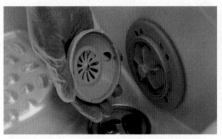

2 If your equipment includes removable parts, remove the screen and any other removable parts. (A screwdriver may be necessary.)

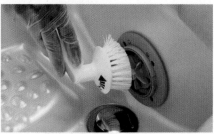

3 Clean the screen and other removable parts and the areas behind them with a clean, disinfected brush, liquid soap, and water to remove all visible residue. Replace the properly cleaned screen and other removable parts.

4 Fill the basin with warm water and chelating detergent (cleansers designed for use in hard water). *Important note: Please check whether chelating detergent is required for your type of the foot spa by your state or the manufacturer.*

5 Circulate the chelating detergent through the system for 5 to 10 minutes, following the manufacturer's instructions. If excessive foaming occurs, discontinue circulation and let it soak for the remainder of the time as instructed.

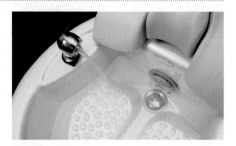

6 Drain the soapy solution, and rinse the basin with clean water.

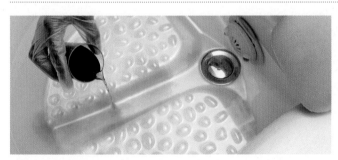

7 Refill the basin with clean water. Measure the correct amount (as indicated in the mixing instructions on the label) of the EPA-registered disinfectant and add it to the water in the basin. Circulate the disinfectant through the basin for 10 minutes or the length of time indicated on the disinfectant label. Set a timer to keep track of the time.

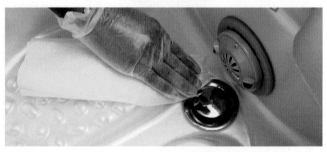

8 Drain, rinse with clean water, and wipe dry with a clean paper towel. Allow the basin to dry completely, unless you are performing the once-each-week disinfectant steps. Refer to those steps for additional information.

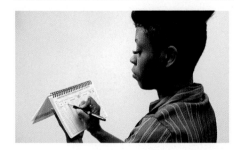

9 Record the disinfection information into the salon's logbook if required by state law or by salon policy.

In addition to the procedures performed after each client and at the end of each day, these steps are performed <u>at least once each week</u>:

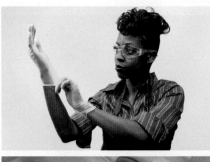

1 After your end-of-day cleaning procedure, *do not* drain the disinfectant solution. Turn the unit off and leave the disinfecting solution in the unit overnight. In the morning, put on gloves and safety glasses.

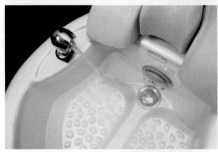

2 Drain all water from the basin and rinse the basin with clean water.

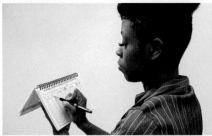

3 Refill the basin with clean water and flush the system.

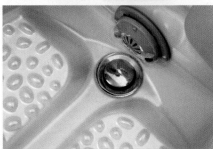

4 Record the disinfectant information into the salon's logbook if required by state law or by salon policy.

CLEANING AND DISINFECTING BASIC FOOT BASINS OR TUBS

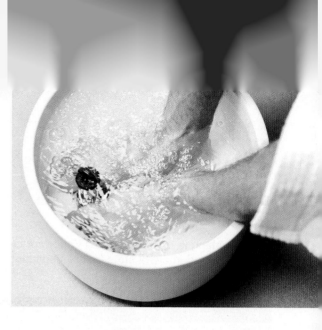

This procedure will demonstrate how to properly clean and disinfect non-whirlpool foot basins or tubs (also includes footbaths, sinks, and bowls). This type of tub does not circulate water. It can be connected to running water and a drain or be portable. If it is a portable tub, you will clean and disinfect it at the dispensary sink.

Any equipment that holds water for pedicures must be cleaned and disinfected after every pedicure.

IMPLEMENTS & MATERIALS

You will need all of the following implements, materials, and supplies:

- ☐ Cleaning logbook
- ☐ Disposable gloves
- ☐ EPA–registered hospital liquid disinfectant
- ☐ Liquid soap
- ☐ Paper towels
- ☐ Safety glasses
- ☐ Scrub brush
- ☐ Timer

PROCEDURE

1 Put on gloves and safety glasses. Drain all water from the foot basin or tub.

2 Scrub all inside surfaces of the foot basin or tub to remove all visible residue with a clean, disinfected brush, liquid soap, and clean water.

3 Rinse the basin or tub with clean water and drain.

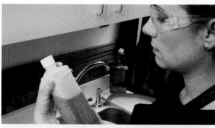

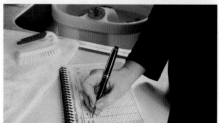

4 Refill the basin with clean water. Measure the correct amount of the EPA-registered hospital disinfectant (as indicated in mixing instructions on the label) and add it to the water in the basin. Set the timer, and leave this disinfectant solution in the basin for 10 minutes or the time recommended by the manufacturer.

5 Drain, rinse with clean water, and wipe dry with a clean paper towel.

6 Record the disinfection information into the salon's logbook if required by state law or by salon policy.

At the end of every day, perform the same procedure steps as after each client.

PROPER HAND WASHING

Hand washing is one of the most important procedures in your infection control efforts and is required in every state before beginning any service.

IMPLEMENTS & MATERIALS

You will need all of the following implements, materials, and supplies:

☐ Disposable paper towels ☐ Liquid soap in a pump container ☐ Nail brush

PROCEDURE

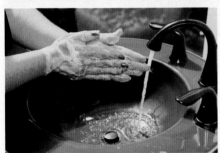

1 Turn the water on. The water should be warm, not hot. Wet your hands, and pump soap from a pump container onto the palm of your hand. Vigorously rub your hands together until a lather forms. Wash past your wrists. Continue for a minimum of 20 seconds.

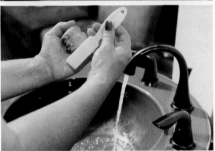

2 Wet and pump soap on a clean, disinfected nail brush. Brush your nails horizontally back and forth under the free edges. Change the direction of the brush to vertical and move the brush up and down along the nail folds of the fingernails. The process for brushing both hands should take about 60 seconds total. Rinse hands in running warm water.

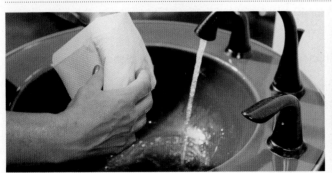

3 Use a clean cloth or a paper towel for drying your hands according to the salon policies or state rules/regulations.

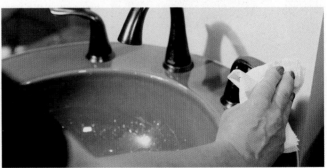

4 After drying your hands, use the towel to turn off the water and open the washroom door, and then dispose of the towel. Touching a doorknob with your bare fingers can re-contaminate your hands.

HANDLING AN EXPOSURE INCIDENT

IMPLEMENTS & MATERIALS

You will need all of the following implements, materials, and supplies:

- ☐ Antiseptic
- ☐ Bandages
- ☐ Biohazard sticker (optional depending on local/state laws)
- ☐ Cotton
- ☐ Disposable gloves
- ☐ Disposable paper towels
- ☐ EPA-registered hospital disinfectant
- ☐ Liquid soap
- ☐ Plastic bag
- ☐ Sharps box (optional depending on local/state laws)

PROCEDURE

Should you accidentally cut yourself, calmly take the following steps:

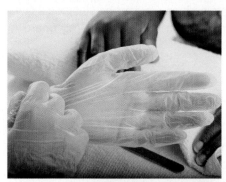

1 First, stop the service. Inform your client of what has happened and let the client know you are taking care of your cut, and the service will be interrupted for a couple of minutes. If the nature of your cut is severe, ask a salon employee to assist with the exposure incident.

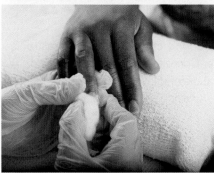

2 If receiving assistance, have the salon employee put on gloves. When appropriate, wash the injury with soap and water. Apply slight pressure to the wound with cotton to stop the bleeding, and then cleanse the area with an antiseptic.

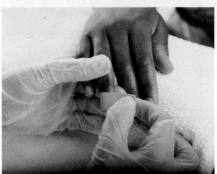

3 Apply an adhesive bandage to completely cover the wound.

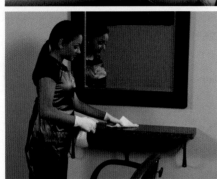

4 Now that your cut is properly cleaned and covered, put on gloves. Return to the service area, and remove any implements that may have been contaminated, placing them in your container for "dirty" items. If surfaces were contaminated, spray or wipe with approved disinfectant and allow to sit for the contact time listed on the product label.

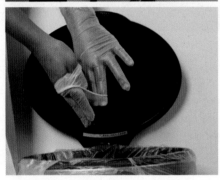

5 Discard all single-use, contaminated objects such as wipes, cotton balls, and your gloves in a plastic bag. Place the plastic bag in a closed trash container with a liner bag. Deposit sharp disposables in a sharps box. Dispose of trash items and sharps containers as required by state/local law. Information on these laws may be found on your local cosmetology board website or through the OSHA website.

6 Now that all disinfecting is complete, put on a new pair of gloves before you return to the service. Remember to dry any surfaces sprayed with disinfectant, and always use new implements to replace those that were contaminated.

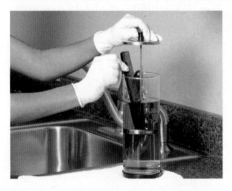

7 After the service has completed, thoroughly clean and disinfect all tools and implements used during the service. Completely immerse tools and implements in an EPA-registered hospital disinfectant solution for 10 minutes. See a physician if any signs of redness, swelling, pain, or irritation develop in the wounded area.

REVIEW QUESTIONS

1. What is the primary purpose of regulatory agencies?

2. What is an SDS? Where can you get these?

3. List the four types of microorganisms that are pertinent to cosmetology.

4. What is a contagious disease?

5. Is HIV a risk in the salon? Why or why not?

6. What is the difference between cleaning, disinfecting, and sterilizing?

7. What is complete immersion?

8. List at least six safety tips to follow when using disinfectants.

9. How do you know if an item can be disinfected?

10. Can porous items be disinfected?

11. What are Standard Precautions?

12. What is an exposure incident?

13. Describe the procedure for handling an exposure incident in the salon.

14. List the steps for cleaning and disinfecting whirlpool, air-jet, and pipeless foot spas after each client.

STUDY TOOLS

- **Reinforce what you just learned:** Complete the activities and exercises in your Theory or Practical Workbook, or your Study Guide.

- **Expand your knowledge:** Search for websites about the topics in this chapter and make a list of additional resources.

- **Study and prepare for your quiz:** Take the chapter test in your Exam Review or your Milady U: Online Licensing Prep.

- **Re-Test your knowledge:** Take the Chapter 5 *Quizzes!*

- **Learn even more:** Look up in a dictionary or search the internet for the definitions of any additional terms you want to learn about.

CHAPTER GLOSSARY

acquired immune deficiency syndrome (AIDS) uh-KWY-erd ih-MYOON di-FISH-en-see sin-drohm	p. 82	A disease that breaks down the body's immune system. AIDS is caused by the human immunodeficiency virus (HIV).
acquired immunity	p. 84	Immunity that the body develops after overcoming a disease, through inoculation (such as flu vaccinations) or through exposure to natural allergens such as pollen, cat dander, and ragweed.
allergy AL-ur-jee	p. 86	Reaction due to extreme sensitivity to certain foods, chemicals, or other normally harmless substances.
antiseptics ant-ih-SEP-tiks	p. 93	Chemical germicide formulated for use on skin; registered and regulated by the Food and Drug Administration (FDA).
asymptomatic	p. 93	Showing no symptoms or signs of infection.
bacilli bah-SIL-ee	p. 77	Singular: bacillus. Short, rod-shaped bacteria. They are the most common bacteria and produce diseases such as tetanus (lockjaw), typhoid fever, tuberculosis, and diphtheria.

bacteria bak-TEER-ee-ah	p. 76	One-celled microorganisms that have both plant and animal characteristics. Some are harmful; some are harmless.
bacterial spores	p. 79	Bacteria capable of producing a protective coating that allows them to withstand very harsh environments, and shed the coating when conditions become more favorable.
bactericidal back-teer-uh-SYD-ul	p. 76	Capable of destroying bacteria.
binary fission BY-nayr-ee FISH-un	p. 78	The division of bacteria cells into two new cells called daughter cells.
biofilms	p. 80	Colonies of bacteria that adhere together and adhere to environmental surfaces.
bloodborne pathogens	p. 82	Disease-causing microorganisms carried in the body by blood or body fluids, such as hepatitis and HIV.
chelating soaps CHE-layt-ing SOHPS	p. 92	Also known as *chelating detergents*; they break down stubborn films and remove the residue of pedicure products such as scrubs, salts, and masks.
clean (cleaning)	p. 76	A mechanical process (scrubbing) using soap and water or detergent and water to remove all visible dirt, debris, and many disease-causing germs. Cleaning also removes invisible debris that interfere with disinfection. Cleaning is what cosmetologists are required to do before disinfecting.
cocci KOK-sy	p. 77	Round-shaped bacteria that appear singly (alone) or in groups. The three types of cocci are staphylococci, streptococci, and diplococci.
contagious disease kon-TAY-jus dih-ZEEZ	p. 80	Also known as *communicable disease*; disease that is spread from one person to another person. Some of the more contagious diseases are the common cold, ringworm, conjunctivitis (pinkeye), viral infections, and natural nail or toe and foot infections.
contamination kuhn-tam-ih-NAY-shun	p. 81	The presence, or the reasonably anticipated presence, of blood or other potentially infectious materials on an item's surface or visible debris or residues such as dust, hair, and skin.
decontamination dee-kuhn-tam-ih-NAY-shun	p. 85	The removal of blood and all other potentially infectious materials on an item's surface, and the removal of visible debris or residue such as dust, hair, and skin.
diagnosis dy-ag-NOH-sis	p. 81	Determination of the nature of a disease from its symptoms and/or diagnostic tests. Federal regulations prohibit salon professionals from performing a diagnosis.
diplococci dip-lo-KOK-sy	p. 77	Spherical bacteria that grow in pairs and cause diseases such as pneumonia.
direct transmission	p. 78	Transmission of blood or body fluids through touching (including shaking hands), kissing, coughing, sneezing, and talking.
disease dih-ZEEZ	p. 74	An abnormal condition of all or part of the body, or its systems or organs, which makes the body incapable of carrying on normal function.
disinfectants dis-in-FEK-tents	p. 73	Chemical products approved by the EPA designed to destroy most bacteria (excluding spores), fungi, and viruses on surfaces.
disinfection (disinfecting) dis-in-FEK-shun	p. 76	A chemical process that destroys most, but not necessarily all, harmful organisms on environmental surfaces. The pathogens of concern in the cosmetology industry are effectively destroyed by the disinfection process, which is required in all states.

efficacy	p. 86	The ability to produce an effect.
ef-ih-KUH-see		
exposure incident	p. 95	Contact with non-intact (broken) skin, blood, body fluid, or other potentially infectious material that is the result of the performance of an employee's duties.
flagella	p. 78	Slender, hair-like extensions used by bacilli and spirilla for locomotion (moving about). May also be referred to as cilia.
fluh-JEL-uh		
folliculitis barbae	p. 83	Synonym *tinea barbae* (TIN-ee-uh BAR-bee). Also known as *barbers itch,* inflammation of the hair follicles caused by a bacterial infection from ingrown hairs. The cause is typically from ingrown hairs due to shaving or other epilation methods.
fah-lik-yuh-LY-tis BAR-bee		
fungi	p. 83	Single-cell organisms that grow in irregular masses that include molds, mildews, and yeasts; can produce contagious diseases such as ringworm.
FUN-jI		
fungicidal	p. 76	Capable of destroying fungi.
fun-jih-SYD-ul		
hepatitis	p. 82	A bloodborne virus that causes disease and can damage the liver.
hep-uh-TY-tus		
hospital disinfectants	p. 74	Disinfectants that are effective for cleaning blood and body fluids.
HOS-pih-tal dis-in-FEK-tents		
Human Immunodeficiency Virus	p. 82	Abbreviated HIV; virus that causes acquired immune deficiency syndrome (AIDS).
HYOO-mun ih-MYOO-noh-di-FISH-en-see VY-rus		
human papilloma virus	p. 82	Abbreviated HPV; a virus that causes warts in humans, but is also the cause of cervical cancer in women. When the virus infects the bottom of the foot and resembles small black dots, usually in clustered groups, it is also called plantar warts.
HYOO-mun pap-uh-LOW-ma VY-rus		
immunity	p. 84	The ability of the body to destroy and resist infection. Immunity against disease can be either natural or acquired, and is a sign of good health.
indirect transmission	p. 78	Transmission of blood or body fluids through contact with an intermediate contaminated object such as a razor, extractor, nipper, or an environmental surface.
infection	p. 75	The invasion of body tissues by disease-causing pathogens.
in-FEK-shun		
infection control	p. 75	Are the methods used to eliminate or reduce the transmission of infectious organisms.
infectious	p. 73	Caused by or capable of being transmitted by infection.
in-FEK-shus		
infectious disease	p. 75	Disease caused by pathogenic (harmful) microorganisms that enter the body. An infectious disease may be spread from one person to another person.
in-FEK-shus dih-ZEEZ		
inflammation	p. 79	A condition in which the body reacts to injury, irritation, or infection; characterized by redness, heat, pain, and swelling.
in-fluh-MAY-shun		
local infection	p. 79	An infection, such as a pimple or abscess, that is confined to a particular part of the body and appears as a lesion containing pus.
Material Safety Data Sheet	p. 72	Abbreviated MSDS; replaced by *Safety Data Sheet;* information compiled by the manufacturer about product safety, including the names of hazardous ingredients, safe handling and use procedures, precautions to reduce the risk of accidental harm or overexposure, and flammability warnings.

methicillin-resistant Staphylococcus aureus METH-eh-sill-en-ree-ZIST-ent staf-uh-loh-KOK-us OR-ee-us	p. 79	Abbreviated MRSA; a type of infectious bacteria that is highly resistant to conventional treatments due to incorrect doses or choice of antibiotic.
microorganism my-kroh-OR-gah-niz-um	p. 76	Any organism of microscopic or submicroscopic size.
mildew MIL-doo	p. 83	A type of fungus that affects plants or grows on inanimate objects, but does not cause human infections in the salon.
motility MOH-til-eh-tee	p. 77	Self-movement.
multiuse items	p. 89	Also known as *reusable items*; items that can be cleaned, disinfected, and used on more than one person, even if the item is accidentally exposed to blood or body fluid.
Mycobacterium fortuitum MY-koh-bak-TIR-ee-um for-TOO-i-tum	p. 73	A microscopic germ that normally exists in tap water in small numbers.
natural immunity	p. 84	Immunity that is partly inherited and partly developed through healthy living.
nonpathogenic non-path-uh-JEN-ik	p. 76	Harmless microorganisms that may perform useful functions and are safe to come in contact with since they do not cause disease or harm.
nonporous nahn-POHW-rus	p. 74	An item that is made or constructed of a material that has no pores or openings and cannot absorb liquids.
occupational disease	p. 81	Illness resulting from conditions associated with employment, such as prolonged and repeated overexposure to certain products or ingredients.
parasites	p. 84	Organisms that grow, feed, and shelter on or in another organism (referred to as the host), while contributing nothing to the survival of that organism. Parasites must have a host to survive.
parasitic disease	p. 81	Disease caused by parasites, such as lice and mites.
pathogenic path-uh-JEN-ik	p. 77	Harmful microorganisms that can cause disease or infection in humans when they invade the body.
pathogenic disease	p. 81	Disease produced by organisms, including bacteria, viruses, fungi, and parasites.
phenolic disinfectants fi-NOH-lik dis-in-FEK-tents	p. 88	Powerful tuberculocidal disinfectants. They are a form of formaldehyde, have a very high pH, and can damage the skin and eyes.
porous POHW-rus	p. 90	Made or constructed of a material that has pores or openings. Porous items are absorbent.
pus	p. 79	A fluid created by infection.
quaternary ammonium compounds KWAT-ur-nayr-ree uh-MOH-neeum KAHM-powndz	p. 88	Commonly known as "quats"; are products made of quaternary ammonium cations and are designed for disinfection on nonporous surfaces. They are appropriate for use in non-critical (non-invasive) environments and are effective against most pathogens of concern in the salon environment.
Safety Data Sheet	p. 72	Abbreviated SDS; required by law for all products sold. SDSs include safety information about products compiled by the manufacturer, including hazardous ingredients, safe use and handling procedures, proper disposal guidelines, precautions to reduce the risk of accidental harm or overexposure, and more.
sanitizing	p. 70	A chemical process for reducing the number of disease-causing germs on cleaned surfaces to a safe level.

scabies SKAY-beez	p. 84	A contagious skin disease that is caused by the itch mite, which burrows under the skin.
single-use items	p. 90	Also known as *disposable items*; items that cannot be used more than once. These items cannot be properly cleaned so that all visible residue is removed—such as pumice stones used for pedicures—or they are damaged or contaminated by cleaning and disinfecting.
sodium hypochlorite SOH-dee-um hy-puh-KLOR-ite	p. 88	Common household bleach; an effective disinfectant for the salon.
spirilla spy-RIL-ah	p. 77	Spiral or corkscrew-shaped bacteria that cause diseases such as syphilis and Lyme disease.
Standard Precautions	p. 93	Abbreviated SP; precautions such as wearing personal protective equipment to prevent skin and mucous membranes where contact with a client's blood, body fluids, secretions (except sweat), excretions, non-intact skin, and mucous membranes is likely. Workers must assume that all blood and body fluids are potential sources of infection, regardless of the perceived risk.
staphylococci staf-uh-loh-KOK-sy	p. 77	Pus-forming bacteria that grow in clusters like a bunch of grapes. They cause abscesses, pustules, and boils.
sterilization stayr-ih-luh-ZAY-shun	p. 84	The process that completely destroys all microbial life, including spores.
streptococci strep-toh-KOK-sy	p. 77	Pus-forming bacteria arranged in curved lines resembling a string of beads. They cause infections such as strep throat and blood poisoning.
systemic infection	p. 79	Infection that affects the body as a whole, often due to under-functioning or over-functioning of internal glands or organs. This disease is carried through the blood stream or the lymphatic system.
tinea barbae TIN-ee-uh BAR-bee	p. 83	A superficial fungal infection caused by a variety of dermatophytes that commonly affects the skin. It is primarily limited to the bearded areas of the face and neck or around the scalp. A person with this condition may have deep, inflamed or non-inflamed patches of skin on the face or the nape of the neck.
tinea capitis TIN-ee-uh KAP-ih-tis	p. 83	A fungal infection of the scalp characterized by red papules, or spots, at the opening of the hair follicles.
tinea pedis TIN-ee-uh PED-us	p. 83	A ringworm fungus of the foot.
toxins TAHK-sinz	p. 83	Various poisonous substances produced by some microorganisms (bacteria and viruses).
tuberculocidal disinfectants tuh-bur-kyoo-LOH-sy-dahl dis-in-FEK-tents	p. 74	Disinfectants that kill the bacteria that causes tuberculosis.
tuberculosis tuh-bur-kyoo-LOH-sus	p. 74	A disease caused by bacteria that are transmitted through coughing or sneezing.
virucidal vy-ru-SYD-ul	p. 76	Capable of destroying viruses.
virus VY-rus	p. 80	A parasitic submicroscopic particle that infects and resides in cells of biological organisms.

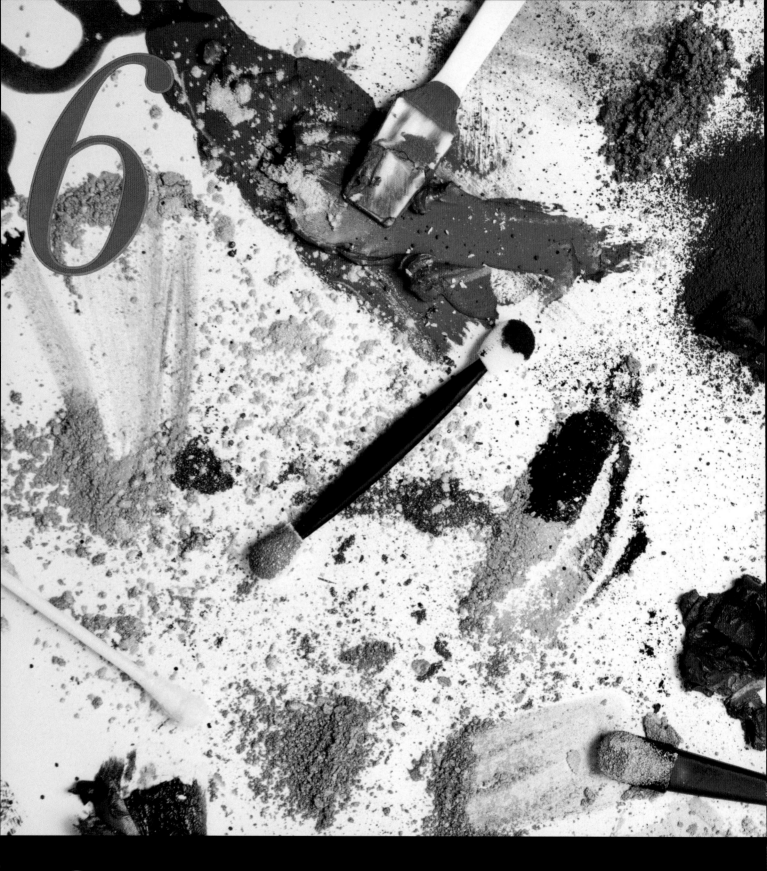

6

GENERAL ANATOMY & PHYSIOLOGY

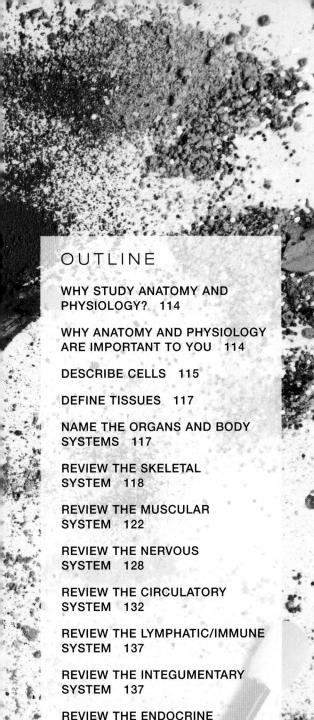

LEARNING OBJECTIVES

After completing this chapter, you will be able to:

LO❶
Define and explain the importance of anatomy and physiology to the cosmetology profession.

LO❷
Describe cells, their structure, and their reproduction.

LO❸
Define tissue and identify the four types of tissues found in the body.

LO❹
Name the 11 main body systems and explain their basic functions.

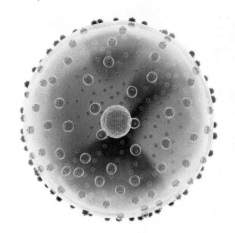

C osmetologists are licensed to touch and perform services on clients in ways that are not permitted in many other occupations. This is a very important responsibility and, as a cosmetologist, you should consider it an honor to be able to aid others in achieving a greater sense of well-being. How can you do this? You can begin by having a solid understanding of the anatomy and physiology of the human body.

© Sebastian Kaulitzki/Shutterstock.com

why study
ANATOMY AND PHYSIOLOGY?

Cosmetologists should study and have a thorough understanding of anatomy and physiology because:

> Understanding how the human body functions as an integrated whole is a key component to understanding how a client's hair, skin, and nails may react to various treatments and services.

> You will need to be able to recognize the difference between what is considered normal and what is considered abnormal for the body in order to determine whether specific treatments and services are appropriate and what should be referred to a physician.

> Understanding the bone and muscle structure of the human body will help you use the proper application of services and products for scalp manipulations and facials.

After reading the next few sections, you will be able to:

LO Define and explain the importance of anatomy and physiology to the cosmetology profession.

Why Anatomy and Physiology Are Important to You

While you should have an overall knowledge of human anatomy, cosmetology is primarily limited to the skin, muscles, nerves, circulatory system, and bones of the head, face, neck, shoulders, arms, hands, lower legs, and feet. Understanding the anatomy of these areas will help you develop techniques that can be used during scalp massage, facials, manicures, pedicures, and as part of a ritual at the shampoo station. In addition, knowing the bones of the skull and facial structure is important to designing flattering hairstyles that gracefully drape the head and for skillfully applying cosmetics. This chapter will provide you with the definitions and "map" of the human body as a point of reference to be used when you discuss specific services later in the text.

Anatomy (ah-NAT-ah-mee) is the study of the human body structures that can be seen with the naked eye and how the body parts are organized; it is the science of the structure of organisms or of their parts.

Physiology (fiz-ih-OL-oh-jee) is the study of the functions and activities performed by the body's structures. The ending **-ology** (AHL-O-jee) means *study of.*

After reading the next few sections, you will be able to:

LO❷ Describe cells, their structure, and their reproduction.

Describe Cells

Cells are the basic units of all living things—from bacteria to plants to animals, including human beings. Without cells, life does not exist. As a basic functional unit, the cell is responsible for carrying on all life processes.

Basic Structure of the Cell

The cells of all living things are composed of a substance called **protoplasm** (PROH-toh-plaz-um), a colorless jelly-like substance found inside cells in which food elements such as proteins, fats, carbohydrates, mineral salts, and water are present. You can visualize the protoplasm of a cell as being similar to raw egg white. In addition to protoplasm, most cells also include a nucleus, cytoplasm, and the cell membrane (**figure 6-1**).

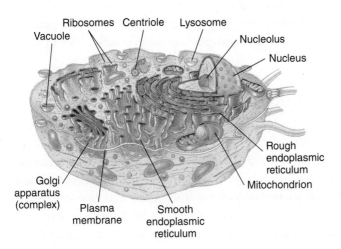

Ribosomes Centriole Lysosome
Vacuole
Nucleolus
Nucleus
Rough endoplasmic reticulum
Mitochondrion
Golgi apparatus (complex)
Plasma membrane
Smooth endoplasmic reticulum

figure 6-1
Basic structure of the cell

figure 6-2
Phases of mitosis

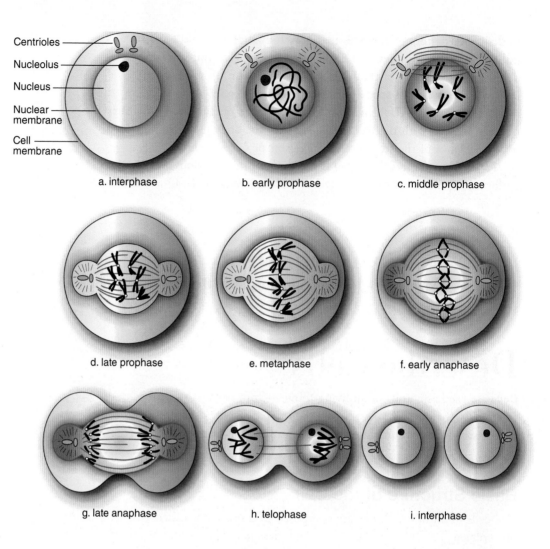

Centrioles
Nucleolus
Nucleus
Nuclear membrane
Cell membrane

a. interphase b. early prophase c. middle prophase

d. late prophase e. metaphase f. early anaphase

g. late anaphase h. telophase i. interphase

The **nucleus** (NOO-klee-us) is the dense, active protoplasm found in the center of the cell; it plays an important part in cell reproduction and metabolism. You can visualize the nucleus as the yolk in the middle of a raw egg.

The **cytoplasm** (sy-toh-PLAZ-um) is the watery fluid that surrounds the nucleus of the cell and is needed for growth, reproduction, and self-repair. It is the protoplasm of the cell.

The **cell membrane** (SELL MEM-brayn) is the cell part that encloses the protoplasm and permits soluble substances to enter and leave the cell.

Cell Reproduction and Division

Cells have the ability to reproduce, thus providing new cells for the growth and replacement of worn or injured ones. **Mitosis** (my-TOH-sis) is the usual process of cell reproduction of human tissues that occurs when the cell divides into two identical cells called daughter cells (**figure 6-2**). As long as conditions are favorable, the cell will grow and reproduce. Favorable conditions include an adequate supply of food, oxygen, and water; suitable temperatures; and the ability to eliminate waste products.

After reading the next few sections, you will be able to:

LO**3**   Define tissue and identify the four types of tissues found in the body.

Define Tissues

Tissue (TISH-oo) is a collection of similar cells that perform a particular function. Each kind of tissue has a specific function and can be recognized by its characteristic appearance. Body tissues are composed of large amounts of water, along with various other substances. There are four types of tissue in the body:

- **Connective tissue** is fibrous tissue that binds together, protects, and supports the various parts of the body. Examples of connective tissue are bone, cartilage, ligaments, tendons, blood, lymph, and **adipose tissue** (ADD-ih-pohz TISH-oo), a technical term for fat. Adipose tissue gives smoothness and contour to the body while protecting internal organs and insulating the body.

- **Epithelial tissue** (ep-ih-THEE-lee-ul TISH-oo) is a protective covering on body surfaces, such as skin, mucous membranes, the tissue inside the mouth, the lining of the heart, digestive and respiratory organs, and the glands.

- **Muscle tissue** contracts and moves various parts of the body.

- **Nerve tissue** (NURV TISH-oo) carries messages to and from the brain and controls and coordinates all bodily functions. Nerve tissue is composed of special cells known as neurons that make up the nerves, brain, and spinal cord.

After reading the next few sections, you will be able to:

LO**4**   Name the 11 main body systems and explain their basic functions.

Name the Organs and Body Systems

Organs are structures composed of specialized tissues designed to perform specific functions in plants and animals. During development of a fetus, tissues are "assigned" to specific functions in the body and they develop specifically for those functions. For example, lung tissue would not work as a part of the brain as it is designed to serve a specific function in the lungs. **Body systems** are groups of body organs acting together to perform one or more functions (**figure 6-3**). **Table 6-1** outlines

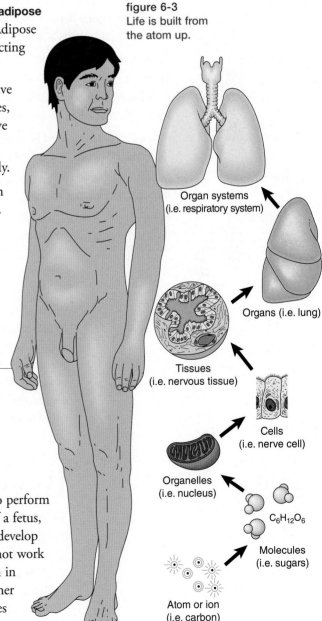

figure 6-3
Life is built from the atom up.

Organ systems
(i.e. respiratory system)

Organs (i.e. lung)

Tissues
(i.e. nervous tissue)

Cells
(i.e. nerve cell)

Organelles
(i.e. nucleus)

$C_6H_{12}O_6$

Molecules
(i.e. sugars)

Atom or ion
(i.e. carbon)

table 6-1

THE ELEVEN BODY SYSTEMS, THEIR FUNCTIONS, AND MAJOR ORGANS

Body Systems	Function	Major Organs
Circulatory	Controls movement of blood throughout the body	Heart, blood vessels
Digestive (gastrointestinal)	Breaks down food into nutrients or waste for nutrition or excretion	Stomach, intestines, salivary and gastric glands
Endocrine	Controls hormone levels within the body that determine growth, development, sexual function, and health of entire body	Endocrine glands, hormones
Excretory	Eliminates waste from the body reducing build up of toxins	Kidneys. liver, skin, large intestines, lungs
Integumentary	Provides protective covering and regulates body temperature	Skin, oil/sweat glands, hair, nails
Immune (lymphatic)	Protects the body from disease by developing immunities and destroying pathogens and toxins	Lymph, lymph nodes, thymus gland, spleen
Muscular	Covers, shapes and hold the skeletal in place. Muscles contract to allow for movement of body structures.	Muscles, connective tissues
Nervous	Coordinates all other body systems allowing them to work efficiently and react to the environment	Brain, spinal cord, nerves, eyes
Reproductive	Produces offspring and allows for transfer of genetic material. Differentiates between the sexes	Female: ovaries, uterus, vagina Male: testes, prostate, penis
Respiratory	Makes blood and oxygen available to body structures through respiration; eliminates carbon dioxide	Lungs, air passages
Skeletal	Forms the physical foundation of the body: 206 bones that are connected by moveable and immovable joints	Bones, joints

the body systems, indicating the functions of each system and the major organs that are associated with that system.

As a summary, understand that the basic structure and function is the *cell*. Cells are organized into layers or groups called *tissues*. Groups of tissues form complex structures that perform certain functions called *organs*. Organs are arranged in *body systems*. Body systems are arranged to form an *organism*, for example the human body.

Review the Skeletal System

The **skeletal system** forms the physical foundation of the body and is composed of 206 bones that vary in size and shape and are connected by movable and immovable joints.

Except for the tissue that forms the major part of the teeth, bone is the hardest tissue in the body. It is composed of connective tissue consisting of about one-third organic matter, such as cells and blood; and two-thirds minerals, mainly calcium carbonate and calcium phosphate.

The primary functions of the skeletal system are to:

- Give shape and support to the body.

- Protect various internal structures and organs.

- Serve as attachments for muscles and act as levers to produce body movement.

- Help produce both white and red blood cells (one of the functions of bone marrow).

- Store most of the body's calcium supply, as well as phosphorus, magnesium, and sodium.

A **joint** (JOYNT) is the connection between two or more bones of the skeleton. There are two types of joints: movable, such as elbows, knees, and hips; and immovable, such as the joints found in the pelvis and skull, which allow little or no movement. There are exceptions to this such as childbirth, where special hormones allow for flexibility of the pelvic joints.

Bones of the Skull

The **skull** is the skeleton of the head and is divided into two parts:

- **Cranium** (KRAY-nee-um). An oval, bony case that protects the brain.

- **Facial skeleton**. The framework of the face that is composed of 14 bones (figure 6-4).

Bones of the Cranium

The following are the cranium's eight bones:

- **Occipital bone** (ahk-SIP-ih-tul BOHN). Hindmost bone of the skull, below the parietal bones; forms the back of the skull above the nape.

- **Parietal bones** (puh-RY-uh-tul BOHNS). Bones that form the sides and top of the cranium. There are two parietal bones.

- **Frontal bone** (FRUNT-ul BOHN). Bone that forms the forehead.

- **Temporal bones** (TEM-puh-rul BOHNS). Bones that form the sides of the head in the ear region. There are two temporal bones.

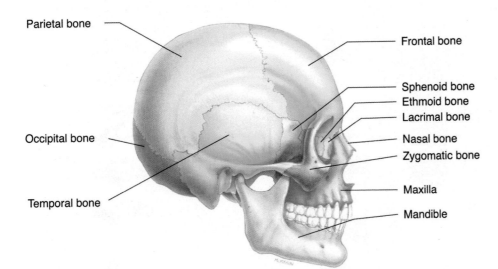

figure 6-4
Bones of the cranium and the face

- **Ethmoid bone** (ETH-moyd BOHN). Light spongy bone between the eye sockets; forms part of the nasal cavities.

- **Sphenoid bone** (SFEEN-oyd BOHN). Bone that joins all of the bones of the cranium together.

The ethmoid and sphenoid bones are not affected when performing services or giving a massage.

Bones of the Face

There are 14 bones of the face, but those listed below are most involved in the practice of cosmetology:

- **Nasal bones** (NAY-zul BOHNS). Bones that form the bridge of the nose. There are two nasal bones.

- **Lacrimal bones** (LAK-ruh-mul BOHNS). Small, thin bones located at the front inner wall of the orbits (eye sockets). There are two lacrimal bones.

- **Zygomatic bones** (zy-goh-MAT-ik BOHNS), also known as *malar bones* or *cheekbones*. Bones that form the prominence of the cheeks. There are two zygomatic bones.

- **Maxillae** (mak-SIL-ee) (singular: maxilla [mak-SIL-uh]). Bones of the upper jaw. There are two maxillae.

- **Mandible** (MAN-duh-bul). Lower jawbone; largest and strongest bone of the face.

Bones of the Neck

The main bones of the neck are the following:

- **Hyoid bone** (HY-oyd BOHN). U-shaped bone at the base of the tongue that supports the tongue and its muscles. It is the one and only bone of the throat.

- **Cervical vertebrae** (SUR-vih-kul VURT-uh-bray). The seven bones of the top part of the vertebral column, located in the neck region (**figure 6-5**).

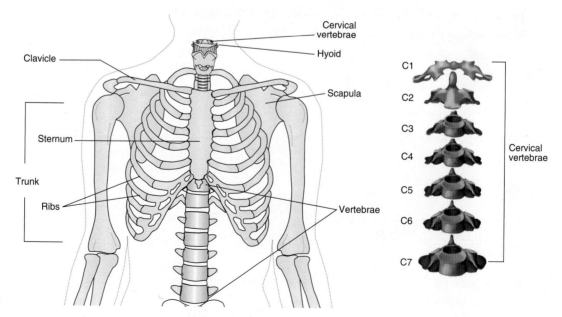

figure 6-5
Bones of the neck, shoulders, and back

Bones of the Chest, Shoulder, and Back

The bones of the trunk, or torso, are the following:

- **Thorax** (THOR-aks), also known as *chest* or *pulmonary trunk* (PUL-muh-nayr-ee TRUNK). Consists of the sternum, ribs, and thoracic vertebrae. It is an elastic, bony cage that serves as a protective framework for the heart, lungs, and other internal organs.

- **Ribs**. Twelve pairs of bones forming the wall of the thorax.

- **Scapula** (SKAP-yuh-luh), also known as *shoulder blade*. Large, flat, triangular bone of the shoulder. There are two scapulae.

- **Sternum** (STUR-num), also known as *breastbone*. Flat bone that forms the ventral (front) support of the ribs.

- **Clavicle** (KLAV-ih-kul), also known as *collarbone*. Bone that joins the sternum and scapula.

Bones of the Arms and Hands

The important bones of the arms and hands that you should know include the following:

- **Humerus** (HYOO-muh-rus). Uppermost and largest bone in the arm, extending from the elbow to the shoulder.

- **Ulna** (UL-nuh). Inner and larger bone in the forearm (lower arm), attached to the wrist and located on the side of the little finger.

- **Radius** (RAY-dee-us). Smaller bone in the forearm (lower arm) on the same side as the thumb (figure 6-6).

- **Carpus** (KAR-pus), also known as *wrist*. Flexible joint composed of a group of eight small, irregular bones (carpals) held together by ligaments.

- **Metacarpus** (met-uh-KAR-pus). Bones of the palm of the hand; parts of the hand containing five bones between the carpus and phalanges.

- **Phalanges** (fuh-LAN-jeez) (singular: phalanx [FAY-langks]). Also known as *digits*. Bones of the fingers or toes (figure 6-7). There are three phalanges in each finger and two in the thumb.

Bones of the Leg, Ankle, and Foot

The four bones of the leg are the following:

- **Femur** (FEE-mur). Heavy, long bone that forms the leg above the knee.
- **Tibia** (TIB-ee-ah). Larger of the two bones that form the leg below the knee. The tibia may be visualized as a bump on the big-toe side of the ankle.
- **Fibula** (FIB-ya-lah). Smaller of the two bones that form the leg below the knee. The fibula may be visualized as a bump on the little-toe side of the ankle.
- **Patella** (pah-TEL-lah). Also known as *accessory bone* or *kneecap*. Forms the kneecap joint (figure 6-8).

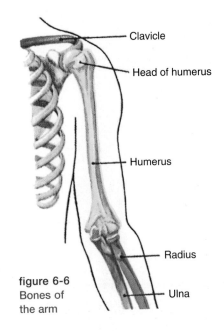

figure 6-6
Bones of the arm

Labels: Clavicle, Head of humerus, Humerus, Radius, Ulna

? DID YOU KNOW?

Fingernails provide protection for the delicate tips of the phalanges in the hand. If a phalange is accidentally broken, the finger loses much of its fine dexterity, and it becomes more difficult to pick up very small objects such as sewing needles or coins.

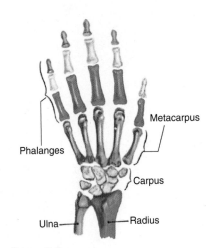

figure 6-7
Bones of the hand

Labels: Metacarpus, Phalanges, Carpus, Ulna, Radius

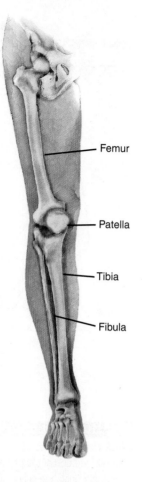

figure 6-8
Bones of
the leg

— Femur

— Patella

— Tibia

— Fibula

The ankle joint is composed of three bones:

- Tibia. Bone that comes down from the lower leg bone.

- Fibula. Bone that comes down from the lower leg bone.

- **Talus** (TA-lus), also known as *ankle bone*. Third bone of the ankle joint.

The foot is made up of 26 bones. These can be subdivided into three general categories:

- **Tarsal** (TAHR-sul). There are seven tarsal bones—talus, calcaneus (heel), navicular, three cuneiform bones, and the cuboid.

- **Metatarsal** (met-ah-TAHR-sul). Long and slender bones, similar to the metacarpal bones of the hand. There are five metatarsal bones.

- Phalanges. Fourteen bones that compose the toes. Toe phalanges are similar to the finger phalanges. There are three phalanges in each toe, except for the big toe, which has only two (figure 6-9).

Review the Muscular System

The **muscular system** (MUS-kuyh-lur SIS-tum) is the body system that covers, shapes, and holds the skeletal system in place; the muscular system contracts and moves various parts of the body.

Cosmetologists must be concerned with the voluntary muscles that control movements of the arms, hands, lower legs, and feet. It is important to know where these muscles are located and what they control. These muscles can become fatigued from excessive work or injury, and your clients will benefit greatly from the massaging techniques you incorporate into your services.

Muscles are fibrous tissues that have the ability to stretch and contract according to demands of the body's movements.

A muscle has three parts (figure 6-10):

- **Origin**. The part of the muscle that does not move and is attached closest to the skeleton.

- **Belly**. The middle part of the muscle.

- **Insertion**. The part of the muscle that moves and is farthest from the skeleton.

Pressure in massage is usually directed from the insertion to the origin.

Muscular tissue can be stimulated by:

- Massage (hand, electric vibrator, or water jets).

- Electrical therapy current. (See Chapter 13, Basics of Electricity, for additional information on types of electrical therapy current.)

- Infrared light.

figure 6-9
Bones of the
ankle and foot

— Tibia

Fibula —

— Talus

— Navicular   Tarsals

Calcaneus
(heel)

Cuboid —

— Cuneiforms (3)

Metatarsals (5)

V IV III II I

Phalanges (14)

- Dry heat (heating lamps or heating caps).
- Moist heat (steamers or moderately warm steam towels).
- Nerve impulses (through the nervous system).
- Chemicals (certain acids and salts).

Muscles of the Scalp

The four muscles of the scalp are the following:

- **Epicranius** (ep-ih-KRAY-nee-us), also known as *occipitofrontalis* (ahk-SIP-ih-toh frun-TAY-lus). Broad muscle that covers the top of the skull and consists of the occipitalis and frontalis.

- **Occipitalis** (ahk-SIP-i-tahl-is). Back (posterior) portion of the epicranius; the muscle that draws the scalp backward.

- **Frontalis** (frun-TAY-lus). Front (anterior) portion of the epicranius; the muscle of the scalp that raises the eyebrows, draws the scalp forward, and causes wrinkles across the forehead.

- **Epicranial aponeurosis** (ep-ih-KRAY-nee-al ap-uh-noo-ROH-sus). Tendon that connects the occipitalis and frontalis muscles (figure 6-11).

Muscles of the Neck

The muscles of the neck include the following:

- **Platysma muscle** (plah-TIZ-muh MUS-ul). Broad muscle extending from the chest and shoulder muscles to the side of the chin; responsible for lowering the lower jaw and lip.

- **Sternocleidomastoideus** (STUR-noh-KLEE-ih-doh-mas-TOYD-ee-us). Muscle of the neck that lowers and rotates the head.

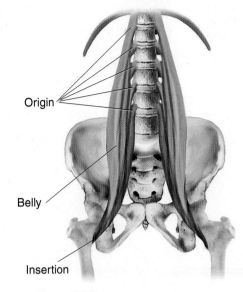

figure 6-10
Muscle origin and insertion

DID YOU KNOW?
About 40 to 50 percent of body weight is in muscles. And there are over 630 muscles that make your body move.

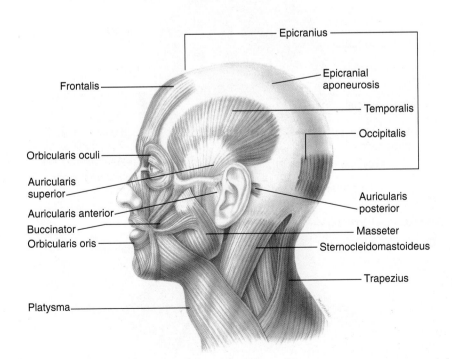

figure 6-11
Muscles of the head, face, and neck

Muscles of the Eye

The eye muscles include the following:

- **Orbicularis oculi muscle** (or-bik-yuh-LAIR-is AHK-yuh-lye MUS-ul). Ring muscle of the eye socket; enables you to close your eyes.

- **Corrugator muscle** (KOR-oo-gay-tohr MUS-ul). Muscle located beneath the frontalis and orbicularis oculi muscle that draws the eyebrow down and wrinkles the forehead vertically (**figure 6-12**).

- **Levator palpebrae superioris muscle** (lih-VAYT-ur [PAL-puh-bree] soo-peer-ee-OR-is MUS-ul). Thin muscle that controls the eyelid and can be easily damaged during makeup application.

Muscles of the Nose

The muscle of the nose that you should remember is the following:

- **Procerus muscle** (proh-SEE-rus MUS-ul). Covers the bridge of the nose, lowers the eyebrows, and causes wrinkles across the bridge of the nose.

There are other nasal muscles that contract and expand the openings of the nostrils, but they are not of major concern to cosmetologists.

Muscles of the Mouth

The important muscles of the mouth are the following:

- **Buccinator muscle** (BUK-sih-nay-tur MUS-ul). Thin, flat muscle of the cheek between the upper and lower jaw that compresses the cheeks and expels air between the lips.

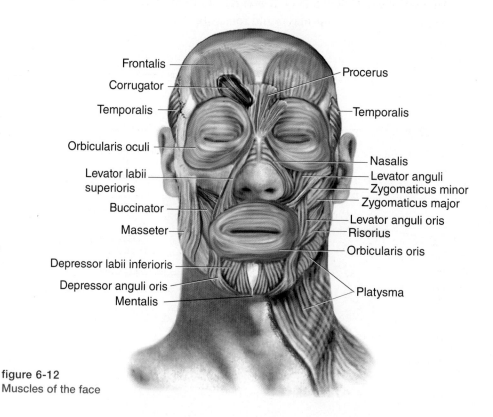

figure 6-12
Muscles of the face

- **Depressor labii inferioris muscle** (dee-PRES-ur LAY-bee-eye in-FEER-ee-or-us MUS-ul), also known as *quadratus labii inferioris muscle* (kwah-DRAY-tus LAY-bee-eye in-feer-ee-OR-is MUS-ul). Muscle surrounding the lower lip; lowers the lower lip and draws it to one side, as in expressing sarcasm.

- **Levator anguli oris muscle** (lih-VAYT-ur ANG-yoo-ly OH-ris MUS-ul), also known as *caninus muscle* (kay-NY-nus MUS-ul). Muscle that raises the angle of the mouth and draws it inward.

- **Levator labii superioris muscle** (lih-VAYT-ur LAY-bee-eye soo-peer-ee-OR-is MUS-ul), also known as *quadratus labii superioris muscle* (kwah-DRA-tus LAY-bee-eye soo-peer-ee-OR-is MUS-ul). Muscle surrounding the upper lip; elevates the upper lip and dilates the nostrils, as in expressing distaste.

- **Mentalis muscle** (men-TAY-lis MUS-ul). Muscle that elevates the lower lip and raises and wrinkles the skin of the chin.

- **Orbicularis oris muscle** (or-bik-yuh-LAIR-is OH-ris MUS-ul). Flat band of muscle around the upper and lower lips that compresses, contracts, puckers, and wrinkles the lips.

- **Risorius muscle** (rih-ZOR-ee-us MUS-ul). Muscle of the mouth that draws the corner of the mouth out and back, as in grinning.

- **Triangularis muscle** (try-ang-gyuh-LAY-rus MUS-ul). Muscle extending alongside the chin that pulls down the corners of the mouth.

- **Zygomaticus major muscles** (zy-goh-mat-ih-kus MAY-jor MUS-uls). Muscles on both sides of the face that extend from the zygomatic bone to the angle of the mouth. These muscles pull the mouth upward and backward, as when you are laughing or smiling.

- **Zygomaticus minor muscles** (zy-goh-mat-ih-kus MY-nor MUS-uls). Muscles on both sides of the face that extend from the zygomatic bone to the upper lips. These muscles pull the upper lip backward, upward, and outward, as when you are smiling (figures 6-11 and 6-12).

Muscles that Attach the Arms to the Body

The muscles that attach the arms to the body are the following:

- **Latissimus dorsi** (lah-TIS-ih-mus DOR-see). Large, flat, triangular muscle covering the lower back. It helps extend the arm away from the body and rotate the shoulder.

- **Pectoralis major** (pek-tor-AL-is MAY-jor) and **pectoralis minor** (pek-tor-AL-is MY-nur), located under the pectoralis major (not shown in figure 6-14). Muscles of the chest that assist the swinging movements of the arm.

- **Serratus anterior** (ser-RAT-us an-TEER-ee-or). Muscle of the chest that assists in breathing and in raising the arm.

- **Trapezius** (trah-PEE-zee-us). Muscle that covers the back of the neck and the upper and middle region of the back; rotates and controls swinging movements of the arm (figures 6-13 and 6-14).

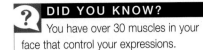

? DID YOU KNOW?
You have over 30 muscles in your face that control your expressions.

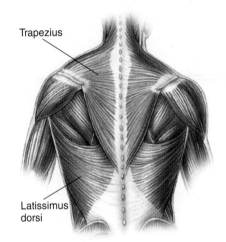

Trapezius

Latissimus dorsi

figure 6-13
Muscles of the back that attach the arms to the body

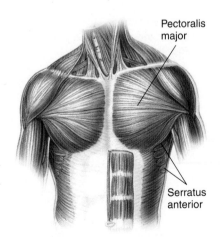

Pectoralis major

Serratus anterior

figure 6-14
Muscles of the chest that attach the arms to the body

Muscles of the Shoulder and Arm

There are three principal muscles of the shoulders and upper arms (figure 6-15):

- **Bicep** (BY-sep). Muscle that produces the contour of the front and inner side of the upper arm; lifts the forearm and flexes the elbow.

- **Deltoid** (DEL-toyd). Large, triangular muscle covering the shoulder joint that allows the arm to extend outward and to the side of the body.

- **Tricep** (TRY-sep). Large muscle that covers the entire back of the upper arm and extends the forearm.

The forearm is made up of a series of muscles and strong tendons (figure 6-15). As a cosmetologist, you will be concerned with the following muscles of the forearm:

- **Extensors** (ik-STEN-surs). Muscles that straighten the wrist, hand, and fingers to form a straight line.

- **Flexor** (FLEK-sur). Extensor muscle of the wrist involved in flexing the wrist.

- **Pronator** (proh-NAY-tohr). Muscle that turns the hand inward so that the palm faces downward.

- **Supinator** (SOO-puh-nayt-ur). Muscle of the forearm that rotates the radius outward and the palm upward.

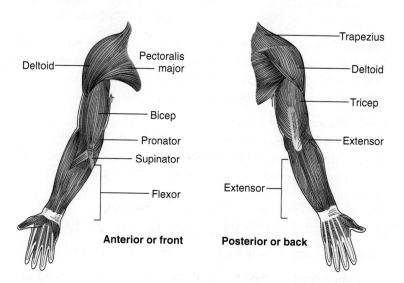

figure 6-15
Muscles of the anterior and posterior shoulder and arm

Muscles of the Hand

The hand is one of the most complex parts of the body, with many small muscles that overlap from joint to joint and provide the flexibility and strength to open and close the hand and fingers. Important muscles to know include the following:

- **Abductors** (ab-DUK-turz). Muscles that draw a body part, such as a finger, arm, or toe, away from the midline of the body or of an extremity. In the hand, abductors separate the fingers.

- **Adductors** (ah-DUK-turz). Muscles that draw a body part, such as a finger, arm, or toe, inward toward the median axis of the body or of an extremity. In the hand, adductors draw the fingers together (figure 6-16).

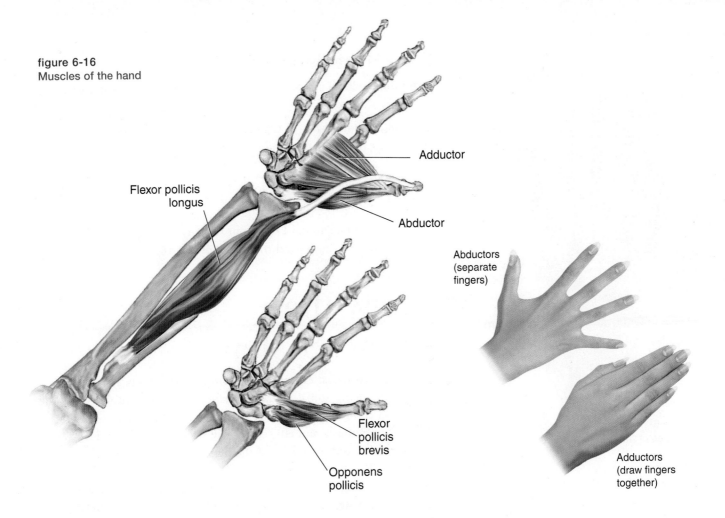

figure 6-16
Muscles of the hand

Flexor pollicis longus

Adductor

Abductor

Abductors (separate fingers)

Flexor pollicis brevis

Opponens pollicis

Adductors (draw fingers together)

Muscles of the Lower Leg and Foot

As a cosmetologist, you will use your knowledge of the muscles of the lower leg and foot during a pedicure. The muscles of the foot are small and provide proper support and cushioning for the foot and leg.

The muscles of the lower leg include the following:

- **Extensor digitorum longus** (ik-STEN-sur dij-it-TOHR-um LONG-us). Muscle that bends the foot up and extends the toes.

- **Extensor hallucis longus** (ik-STEN-sur ha-LU-sis LONG-us). Muscle that extends the big toe and flexes the foot.

- **Tibialis anterior** (tib-ee-AHL-is an-TEHR-ee-ohr). Muscle that covers the front of the shin. It bends the foot upward and inward.

- **Peroneus longus** (per-oh-NEE-us LONG-us). Muscle that covers the outer side of the calf. It inverts the foot and turns it outward.

- **Peroneus brevis** (per-oh-NEE-us BREV-us). Muscle that originates on the lower surface of the fibula. It bends the foot down and out.

- **Gastrocnemius** (gas-truc-NEEM-e-us). Muscle that is attached to the lower rear surface of the heel and pulls the foot down.

- **Soleus** (SO-lee-us). Muscle that originates at the upper portion of the fibula and bends the foot down (figure 6-17).

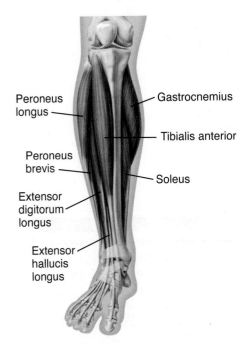

Peroneus longus

Gastrocnemius

Tibialis anterior

Peroneus brevis

Soleus

Extensor digitorum longus

Extensor hallucis longus

figure 6-17
Muscles of the lower leg

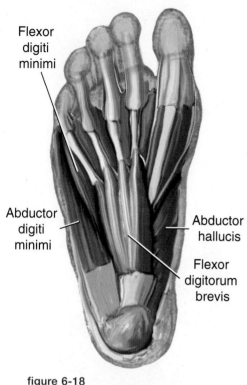

Flexor
digiti
minimi

Abductor
digiti
minimi

Abductor
hallucis

Flexor
digitorum
brevis

figure 6-18
Muscles of the foot (bottom)

The muscles of the feet include the following:

- **Flexor digiti minimi** (FLEK-sur dij-it-ty MIN-eh-mee). Muscle that moves the little toe.

- **Flexor digitorum brevis** (FLEK-sur dij-ut-TOHR-um BREV-us). Muscle that flexes the toes and helps maintain balance while walking and standing.

- **Abductor hallucis** (ab-DUK-tohr ha-LU-sis). Muscle that moves the big toe away from the other toes.

- **Abductor digiti minimi** (ab-DUK-tohr dij-it-ty MIN-eh-mee). Muscle that separates the fingers and the toes (**figure 6-18**).

Review the Nervous System

The **nervous system** is an exceptionally well-organized body system, composed of the brain, spinal cord, and nerves, that is responsible for controlling and coordinating all other systems of the body and makes them work harmoniously and efficiently. The scientific study of the structure, function, and pathology of the nervous system is known as **neurology** (nuh-RAHL-uh-jee).

An understanding of how nerves work will help you perform services in a more proficient manner when administering shampoos and massage techniques.

Divisions of the Nervous System

The nervous system can be divided into three main subdivisions:

- The **central nervous system (CNS)** consists of the brain, spinal cord, spinal nerves, and cranial nerves. It controls consciousness and many mental activities, functions of the five senses (sight, sound, taste, touch, and smell), and voluntary muscle actions, including all body movements and facial expressions.

- The **peripheral nervous system (PNS)** (puh-RIF-uh-rul NURV-vus SIS-tum) is a system of nerves that connects the peripheral (outer) parts of the body to the central nervous system; it has both sensory and motor nerves. Its function is to carry impulses, or messages, to and from the central nervous system.

- The **autonomic nervous system (ANS)** (aw-toh-NAHM-ik NURV-us SIS-tum) is the part of the nervous system that controls the involuntary muscles; it regulates the action of the smooth muscles, glands, blood vessels, heart, and breath (**figure 6-19**).

The Brain and Spinal Cord

The **brain** is the part of the central nervous system contained in the cranium. It is the largest and most complex organization of nerve tissue

? **DID YOU KNOW?**
Some sources divide the nervous system into two main divisions (central and peripheral), and then further divides the peripheral into autonomic and somatic subdivisions which represent the involuntary versus voluntary actions of the peripheral nervous system.

and it controls sensation, muscles, activity of glands, and the power to think, sense, and feel.

The **spinal cord** is the portion of the central nervous system that originates in the brain and extends down to the lower extremity of the trunk. It is protected by the spinal column. Thirty-one pairs of spinal nerves extending from the spinal cord are distributed to the muscles and skin of the trunk and limbs.

Nerves

Nerves are whitish cords made up of bundles of nerve fibers, held together by connective tissue, through which impulses are transmitted. Nerves have their origin in the brain and spinal cord and send their branches to all parts of the body (**figure 6-20**).

Types of Nerves

There are two types of nerves:

- **Sensory nerves**, also known as *afferent nerves* (AAF-eer-ent NURVS), carry impulses or messages from the sense organs to the brain, where sensations such as touch, cold, heat, sight, sound, taste, smell, pain, and pressure are experienced. Sensory nerve endings called receptors are located close to the surface of the skin. Impulses pass from the sensory nerves to the brain and back through the motor nerves to the muscles; the muscles move as a result of the completed circuit.

- **Motor nerves**, also known as *efferent nerves* (EF-uh-rent NURVS), carry impulses from the brain to the muscles or glands. These transmitted impulses produce movement.

The simplest form of nervous activity that includes a sensory and motor nerve is called a reflex. A **reflex** (REE-fleks) is an automatic reaction to a stimulus that involves the movement of an impulse from a sensory receptor along the sensory nerve to the spinal cord. A responsive impulse is sent along a motor neuron to a muscle, causing a reaction (for example, the quick removal of your hand from a hot object). Reflexes do not have to be learned; they are automatic.

Nerves of the Head, Face, and Neck

Cranial nerves connect the brain with the muscles of the head, face, and neck (**figure 6-21a**).

The largest of the cranial nerves is the **fifth cranial nerve**, also known as *trifacial nerve* (try-FAY-shul NURV) or *trigeminal nerve*

ACTIVITY

There are sensory nerve endings all over the body. Try gently pinching a small piece of the skin on your arm. You feel a slight pressure, right? That is the sensory nerve endings sending a message from your arm to your brain that something is happening to the arm.

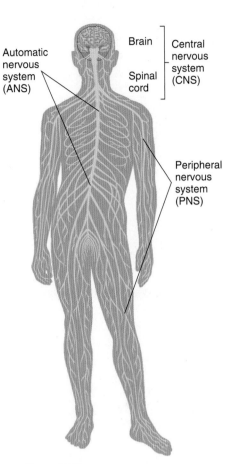

figure 6-19
Divisions of the nervous system

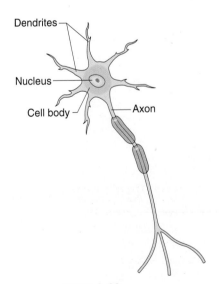

figure 6-20
A neuron or nerve cell

figure 6-21a
Nerves of the head, face, and neck

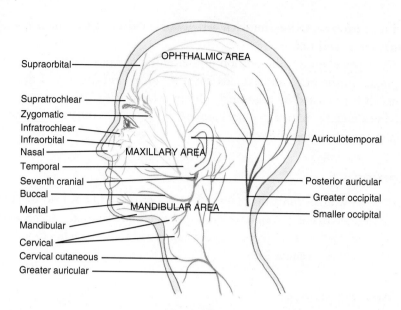

Supraorbital

Supratrochlear
Zygomatic
Infratrochlear
Infraorbital
Nasal
Temporal
Seventh cranial
Buccal
Mental
Mandibular

Cervical
Cervical cutaneous
Greater auricular

OPHTHALMIC AREA

MAXILLARY AREA

MANDIBULAR AREA

Auriculotemporal

Posterior auricular
Greater occipital
Smaller occipital

(try-JEM-un-ul NURV). It is the chief sensory nerve of the face and serves as the motor nerve of the muscles that control chewing (figure 6-21b). It consists of three branches:

- **Ophthalmic nerve** (ahf-THAL-mik NURV). Supplies impulses to the skin of the forehead, upper eyelids, and interior portion of the scalp, orbit, eyeball, and nasal passage.

- **Mandibular nerve** (man-DIB-yuh-lur NURV). Affects the muscles of the chin, lower lip, and external ear.

- **Maxillary nerve** (MAK-suh-lair-ee NURV). Supplies impulses to the upper part of the face.

The **seventh cranial nerve**, also known as the *facial nerve*, is the chief motor nerve of the face (figure 6-21c). Its divisions and their branches supply and control all the muscles of facial expression. It emerges near the lower part

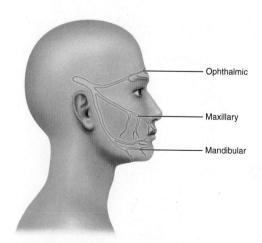

Ophthalmic

Maxillary

Mandibular

figure 6-21b
Fifth cranial nerve

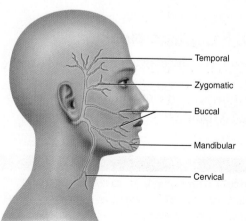

Temporal

Zygomatic

Buccal

Mandibular

Cervical

figure 6-21c
Seventh cranial nerve

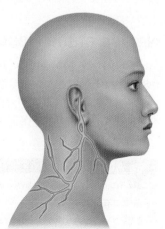

figure 6-21d
Eleventh cranial nerve

of the ear and extends to the muscles of the neck. The following are the most important branches of the facial nerve:

- **Posterior auricular nerve** (poh-STEER-ee-ur aw-RIK-yuh-lur NURV). Affects the muscles behind the ear at the base of the skull.

- **Temporal nerve** (TEM-poh-rul NURV). Affects the muscles of the temple, side of the forehead, eyebrow, eyelid, and upper part of the cheek.

- *Zygomatic nerve (upper and lower)*. Affects the muscles of the upper part of the cheek.

- **Buccal nerve** (BUK-ul NURV). Affects the muscles of the mouth.

- **Marginal mandibular nerve** (MAR-jin-ul man-DIB-yuh-lur NURV). Affects the muscles of the chin and lower lip.

- **Cervical nerves** (SUR-vih-kul NURVS). Affect the side of the neck and the platysma muscle.

The **eleventh cranial nerve**, also known as the *accessory nerve*, is a motor nerve that controls the motion of the neck and shoulder muscles (figure 6-21d). This nerve is important to cosmetologists because it is affected during facials, primarily when you are giving a massage to your client.

Nerves of the Arm and Hand

The principal nerves of the arm and hand are the following:

- **Digital nerve** (DIJ-ut-tul NURV). Sensory–motor nerve that, with its branches, supplies impulses to the fingers.

- **Radial nerve** (RAY-dee-ul NURV). Sensory–motor nerve that, with its branches, supplies the thumb side of the arm and back of the hand.

- **Median nerve** (MEE-dee-un NURV). Sensory–motor nerve that is smaller than the ulnar and radial nerves and that, with its branches, supplies the arm and hand.

- **Ulnar nerve** (UL-nur NURV). Sensory–motor nerve that, with its branches, affects the little-finger side of the arm and palm of the hand (figure 6-22).

Nerves of the Lower Leg and Foot

The nerves of the lower leg and foot are the following:

- **Sciatic nerve** (sy-AT-ik NURV). The largest and longest nerve in the body. It passes through the gluteal region into the thigh, where it branches into smaller nerves. Pain from injury or compression of the sciatic nerve can radiate throughout the abdomen and be sensed in the lower back, hip, or lower abdomen.

- **Tibial nerve** (TIB-ee-al NURV). Division of the sciatic nerve that passes behind the knee. It subdivides and supplies impulses to the knee, the muscles of the calf, the skin of the leg, and the sole, heel, and underside of the toes.

- **Common peroneal nerve** (KAHM-un per-oh-NEE-al NURV). Division of the sciatic nerve that extends from behind the knee to

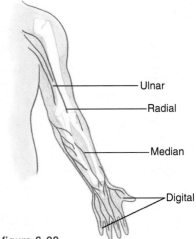

figure 6-22
Nerves of the arm and hand

DID YOU KNOW?

The ulnar nerve runs along the bottom of the elbow. This explains why leaning on the elbows for long periods can cause the little fingers to go numb. This is due to localized inflammation (irritation and swelling) around the nerve. This is also the nerve that is associated with the term "funny bone." It is the impulse of the ulnar nerve when you hit your elbow against an object that causes the sensation of "hitting your funny bone."

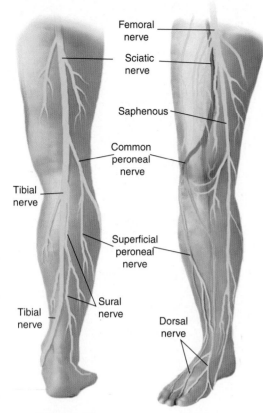

figure 6-23
Nerves of the lower leg and foot

wind around the head of the fibula to the front of the leg, where it divides into two branches.

- **Deep peroneal nerve** (DEEP pare-oh-NEE-uhl NURV), also known as *anterior tibial nerve*. Extends down the front of the leg, behind the muscles. It supplies impulses to these muscles and also to the muscles and skin on the top of the foot and adjacent sides of the first and second toes (not shown in **figure 6-23**).

- **Superficial peroneal nerve** (soo-pur-FISH-ul pare-oh-NEE-uhl NURV), also known as *musculocutaneous nerve* (MUS-kyoo-loh-kyoo-TAY-nee-us NURV). Extends down the leg, just under the skin, supplying impulses to the muscles and the skin of the leg, as well as to the skin and toes on the top of the foot, where it becomes the **dorsal nerve** (DOOR-sal NURV), also known as *dorsal cutaneous nerve*. The dorsal nerve extends up from the toes and foot, just under the skin, supplying impulses to the toes and foot, as well as the muscles and skin of the leg.

- **Saphenous nerve** (sa-FEEN-us NURV). Supplies impulses to the skin of the inner side of the leg and foot. The saphenous nerve begins in the thigh.

- **Sural nerve** (SUR-ul NURV). Supplies impulses to the skin on the outer side and back of the foot and leg (**figure 6-23**).

Review the Circulatory System

The **circulatory system**, also known as *cardiovascular system* (KAHRD-ee-oh-VAS-kyoo-lur SIS-tum) or *vascular system*, controls the steady circulation of the blood through the body by means of the heart and blood vessels. The circulatory system consists of the heart, arteries, veins, and capillaries that distribute blood throughout the body.

The Heart

The **heart** is a muscular, cone-shaped organ that keeps the blood moving within the circulatory system. It is often referred to as the body's pump.

The blood is in constant and continuous circulation from the time that it leaves the heart, is distributed throughout the body to deliver nutrients and oxygen, and then returns to the heart to be sent to the lungs and replenished with oxygen. Two systems are important to this circulation (**figure 6-24**):

- **Pulmonary circulation** (PUL-muh-nayr-ee sur-kyoo-LAY-shun). Takes deoxygenated blood to the lungs for oxygenation and waste removal and then returns that blood to the heart (left atrium) so oxygen-rich blood can be delivered to the body.

- **Systemic circulation** (sis-TEM-ik sur-kyoo-LAY-shun), also known as *general circulation*. Carries the oxygen-rich blood from the heart throughout the body and returns deoxygenated blood back to the heart.

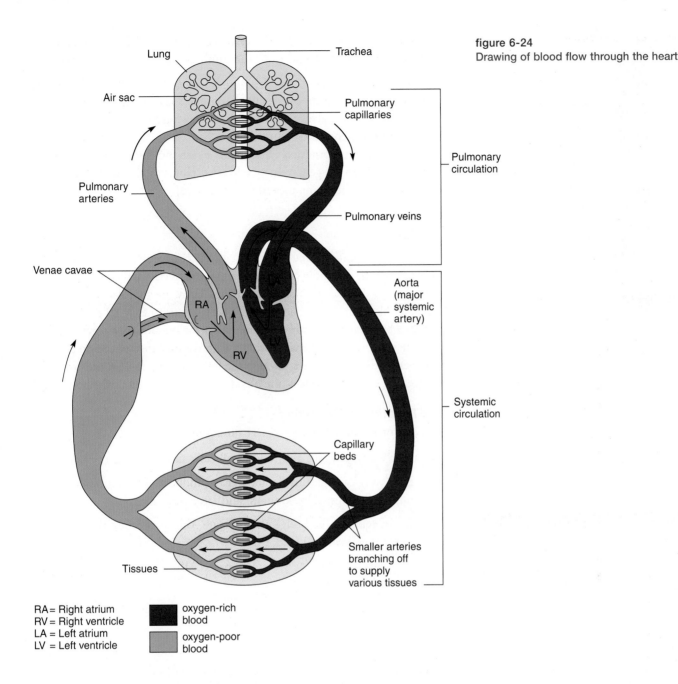

figure 6-24
Drawing of blood flow through the heart

Lung

Trachea

Air sac

Pulmonary capillaries

Pulmonary circulation

Pulmonary arteries

Pulmonary veins

Venae cavae

RA

Aorta (major systemic artery)

RV

LV

Systemic circulation

Capillary beds

Smaller arteries branching off to supply various tissues

Tissues

RA = Right atrium
RV = Right ventricle
LA = Left atrium
LV = Left ventricle

oxygen-rich blood

oxygen-poor blood

Blood Vessels

The **blood vessels** are tube-like structures that include the arteries, arterioles, capillaries, venules, and veins. The function of these vessels is to transport blood to and from the heart and then to various tissues of the body. The types of blood vessels important to a cosmetologist are:

- **Arteries** (AR-tuh-rees). Thick-walled, muscular, flexible tubes that carry oxygenated blood away from the heart to the arterioles. The largest artery in the body is the **aorta** (ay-ORT-uh).

- **Arterioles** (ar-TEER-ee-ohls). Small arteries that deliver blood to capillaries.

- **Capillaries** (KAP-ih-lair-eez). Tiny, thin-walled blood vessels that connect the smaller arteries to venules. Capillaries bring nutrients to the cells and carry away waste materials.

Blood flow toward the heart

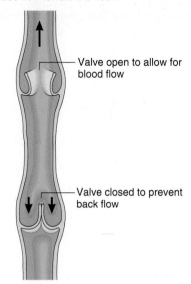

Valve open to allow for blood flow

Valve closed to prevent back flow

figure 6-25
Valves in the veins

- **Venules** (VEEN-yools). Small vessels that connect the capillaries to the veins. They collect blood from the capillaries and drain it into the veins.

- **Veins.** Thin-walled blood vessels that are less elastic than arteries; veins contain cup-like valves that keep blood flowing in one direction to the heart and prevent blood from flowing backward. Veins carry blood containing waste products back to the heart and lungs for cleaning and to pick up oxygen. Veins are located closer to the outer skin surface of the body than arteries (figure 6-25).

The Blood

Blood is a nutritive fluid circulating through the circulatory system (heart and blood vessels) to supply oxygen and nutrients to cells and tissues and to remove carbon dioxide and waste from them. There are approximately 8 to 10 pints of blood in the human body. Blood is approximately 80 percent water. It is bright red in the arteries (except for the pulmonary artery) and dark red in the veins. The color change occurs with the exchange of carbon dioxide for oxygen as the blood passes through the lungs, and again with the exchange of oxygen for carbon dioxide as the blood circulates throughout the body.

Chief Functions of the Blood

Blood performs the following critical functions:

- Carries water, oxygen, and food to all cells and tissues of the body.

- Carries away carbon dioxide and waste products to be eliminated through the lungs, skin, kidneys, and large intestines.

- Helps to equalize the body's temperature, thus protecting the body from extreme heat and cold.

- Works with the immune system to protect the body from harmful toxins and bacteria.

- Seals leaks found in injured blood vessels by forming clots, thus preventing further blood loss.

Arteries of the Head, Face, and Neck

The **common carotid arteries** (KAHM-un kuh-RAHT-ud ART-uh-rees) are the main arteries that supply blood to the head, face, and neck. They are located on both sides of the neck, and each artery is divided into an internal and external branch.

The **internal carotid artery** supplies blood to the brain, eyes, eyelids, forehead, nose, and internal ear. The **external carotid artery** supplies blood to the anterior (front) parts of the scalp, ear, face, neck, and sides of the head (figure 6-26).

Two branches of the internal carotid artery that are important to know are the following:

- **Supraorbital artery** (soo-pruh-OR-bih-tul AR-tuh-ree). Supplies blood to the upper eyelid and forehead.

- **Infraorbital artery** (in-frah-OR-bih-tul AR-tuh-ree). Supplies blood to the muscles of the eye.

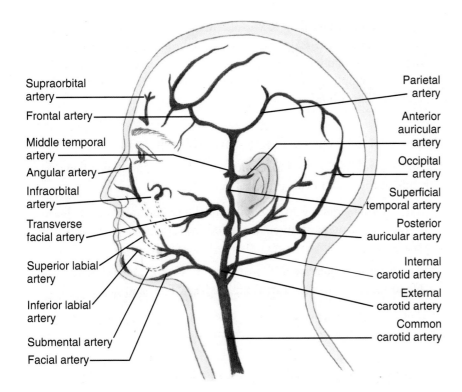

figure 6-26
Arteries of the head, face, and neck.

Supraorbital artery

Frontal artery

Middle temporal artery

Angular artery

Infraorbital artery

Transverse facial artery

Superior labial artery

Inferior labial artery

Submental artery

Facial artery

Parietal artery

Anterior auricular artery

Occipital artery

Superficial temporal artery

Posterior auricular artery

Internal carotid artery

External carotid artery

Common carotid artery

There are four branches of the external carotid artery—the facial artery, the superficial temporal artery, the occipital artery, and the posterior auricular artery.

The **facial artery**, also known as the *external maxillary artery* (eks-TUR-nul MAK-sah-lair-ee ART-uh-ree), supplies blood to the lower region of the face, mouth, and nose. Some of the important facial artery branches include:

- **Submental artery** (sub-MEN-tul ART-uh-ree). Supplies blood to the chin and lower lip.

- **Inferior labial artery** (in-FEER-ee-ur LAY-bee-ul ART-ur-ee). Supplies blood to the lower lip.

- **Angular artery** (ANG-gyoo-lur ART-ur-ee). Supplies blood to the side of the nose.

- **Superior labial artery** (soo-PEER-ee-ur LAY-bee-ul AR-tuh-ree). Supplies blood to the upper lip and region of the nose.

The **superficial temporal artery** (soo-pur-FISH-ul TEM-puh-rul AR-tuh-ree) is a continuation of the external carotid artery and supplies blood to the muscles of the front, side, and top of the head. Some of the important superficial temporal artery branches include:

- **Frontal artery**. Supplies blood to the forehead and upper eyelids.

- **Parietal artery** (puh-RY-ate-ul ART-uh-ree). Supplies blood to the side and crown of the head.

- **Transverse facial artery** (tranz-VURS FAY-shul ART-ur-ee). Supplies blood to the skin and masseter muscle (coordinates opening and closing of the mouth).

- **Middle temporal artery**. Supplies blood to the temples.

- **Anterior auricular artery** (an-TEER-ee-ur aw-RIK-yuh-lur ART-uh-ree). Supplies blood to the front part of the ear.

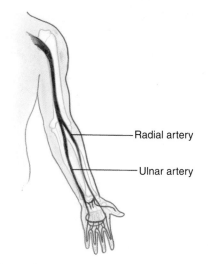

figure 6-27
Arteries of the arm and hand

The **occipital artery** (ahk-SIP-it-ul AR-tuh-ree) supplies blood to the skin and muscles of the scalp and back of the head up to the crown.

The **posterior auricular artery** (poh-STEER-ee-ur aw-RIK-yuh-lur ART-tuh-ree) supplies blood to the scalp, the area behind and above the ear, and the skin behind the ear.

Veins of the Head, Face, and Neck

The blood returning to the heart from the head, face, and neck flows on each side of the neck in two principal veins:

- The **internal jugular vein** (in-TUR-nul JUG-yuh-lur VAYN) is located at the side of the neck to collect blood from the brain and parts of the face and neck.

- The **external jugular vein** is located at the side of the neck and carries blood returning to the heart from the head, face, and neck.

The most important veins of the face and neck are parallel to the arteries and take the same names as the arteries.

Blood Supply to the Arm and Hand

The ulnar and radial arteries are the main blood supply of the arms and hands.

The **ulnar artery** (UL-nur AR-tuh-ree) and its numerous branches supply blood to the little-finger side of the arm and palm of the hand.

The **radial artery** (RAY-dee-ul AR-tur-ree) and its branches supply blood to the thumb side of the arm and the back of the hand; the radial artery also supplies blood to the muscles of the skin, hands, fingers, wrist, elbow, and forearm.

While the arteries are found deep in the tissues, the veins lie nearer to the surface of the arms and hands (figure 6-27).

Blood Supply to the Lower Leg and Foot

The major arteries that supply blood to the lower leg and foot are the popliteal artery and its branches and the dorsalis pedis artery.

The **popliteal artery** (pop-lih-TEE-ul ART-uh-ree), which supplies blood to the foot, divides into two separate arteries known as the anterior tibial artery and the posterior tibial artery.

- **Anterior tibial artery** (an-TEER-ee-ur TIB-ee-al ART-uh-ree). Supplies blood to the lower leg muscles and to the muscles and skin on the top of the foot and adjacent sides of the first and second toes. This artery continues to the foot, where it becomes the dorsalis pedis artery.

- **Posterior tibial artery** (poh-STEER-ee-ur TIB-ee-al ART-uh-ree). Supplies blood to the ankle and the back of the lower leg.

The **dorsalis pedis artery** (DOR-sul-is PEED-us ART-uh-ree) supplies blood to the foot.

As in the arms and hand, the important veins of the lower leg and foot are almost parallel with the arteries and take the same names (figure 6-28).

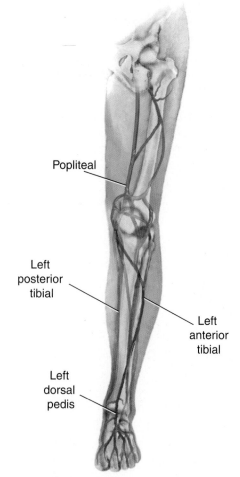

figure 6-28
Arteries of the lower leg and foot
(left leg view)

Review the Lymphatic/Immune System

The **lymphatic/immune system** (lim-FAT-ik ih-MYOON SIS-tum) is made up of lymph, lymph nodes, the thymus gland, the spleen, and lymph vessels. The lymphatic/immune system carries waste and impurities away from the cells and protects the body from disease by developing immunities and destroying disease-causing microorganisms. **Lymph** (LIMF) is a clear fluid that circulates in the lymph spaces (lymphatics) of the body. Lymph helps carry wastes and impurities away from the cells before it is routed back to the circulatory system. The lymphatic/immune system is closely connected to the cardiovascular system. They both transport streams of fluids, like rivers throughout the body. The difference is that the lymphatic/immune system transports lymph, which eventually returns to the blood where it originated.

Lymphatic vessels start as tubes that are closed at one end. They can occur individually or in clusters that are called **lymph capillaries**—blind-end tubes that are the origin of lymphatic vessels. **Lymph nodes** are gland-like structures found inside lymphatic vessels. Lymph nodes filter the lymphatic vessels, which helps fight infection.

The primary functions of the lymphatic/immune system are to:

- Carry nourishment from the blood to the body cells.

- Act as a defense against toxins and bacteria, and remove by-products of infection such as pus and dead tissue.

- Remove waste material from the body cells to the blood.

- Provide a suitable fluid environment for the cells.

Review the Integumentary System

The **integumentary system** (in-TEG-yuh-ment-uh-ree SIS-tum) consists of the skin and its accessory organs, such as the oil and sweat glands, sensory receptors, hair, and nails. It is a very complex system that serves as a protective covering and helps regulate the body's temperature (figure 6-29).

The word *integument* means a natural covering. So you can think of the skin as a protective overcoat for your body against the outside elements that you encounter every day, such as germs, chemicals, and sun exposure. Skin is also water-resistant.

Skin structure and growth are discussed in detail in Chapter 7, Skin Structure, Growth, and Nutrition.

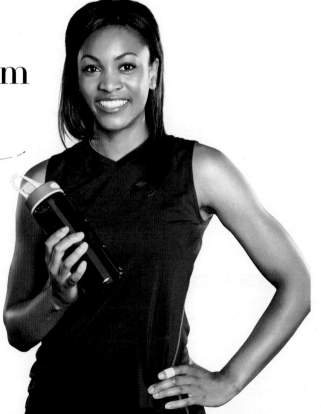

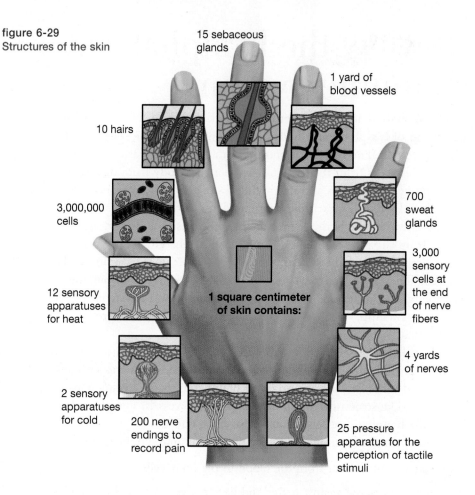

figure 6-29
Structures of the skin

15 sebaceous glands

1 yard of blood vessels

10 hairs

3,000,000 cells

700 sweat glands

3,000 sensory cells at the end of nerve fibers

12 sensory apparatuses for heat

1 square centimeter of skin contains:

4 yards of nerves

2 sensory apparatuses for cold

200 nerve endings to record pain

25 pressure apparatus for the perception of tactile stimuli

Review the Endocrine System

The **endocrine system** (EN-duh-krin SIS-tum) is a group of specialized glands that affect the growth, development, sexual functions, and health of the entire body. **Glands** are secretory organs that remove and release certain elements from the blood to convert them into new compounds.

There are two main types of glands:

- **Endocrine glands** (EN-duh-krin GLANDZ), also known as *ductless glands*, such as the thyroid and pituitary glands, release hormonal secretions directly into the bloodstream.

- **Exocrine glands** (EK-suh-krin GLANDZ), also known as *duct glands*, such as sweat and oil glands of the skin, produce a substance that travels through small, tube-like ducts.

The endocrine glands and the hormones they secrete have a tremendous influence on your body (figure 6-30). **Hormones** (HOR-mohnz) are secretions, such as insulin, adrenaline, and estrogen, that stimulate functional activity or other secretions in the body. Hormones influence the welfare of the entire body. They affect sleep, digestion, growth, sexual development, and many other important functions. You can see that endocrine glands are as important to us as our brain.

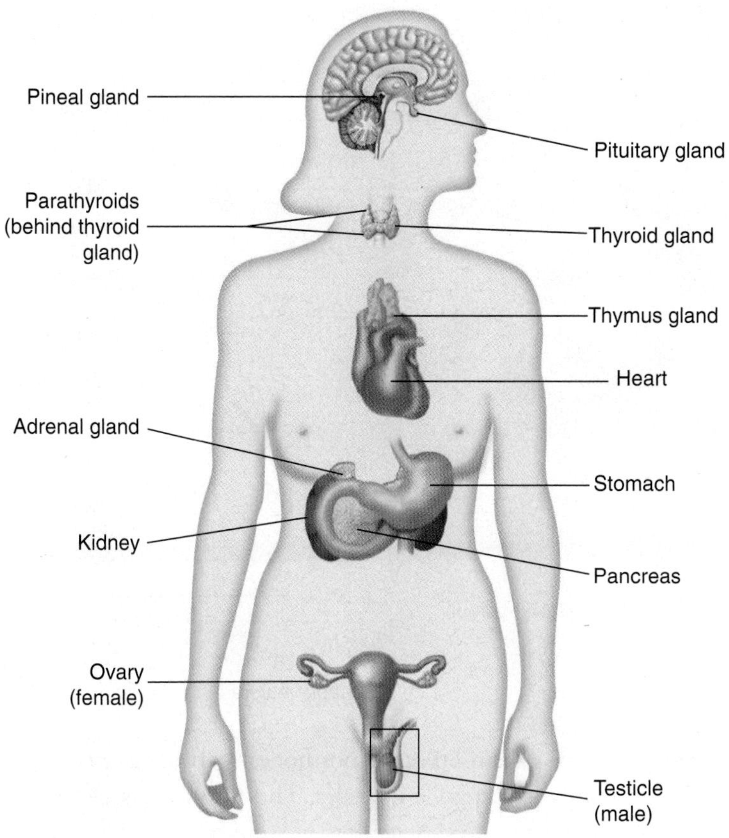

figure 6-30
Endocrine glands and other
body organs

Pineal gland

Pituitary gland

Parathyroids
(behind thyroid
gland)

Thyroid gland

Thymus gland

Heart

Adrenal gland

Stomach

Kidney

Pancreas

Ovary
(female)

Testicle
(male)

The endocrine glands and their functions are as follows:

- **Pineal gland** (PY-nee-ul GLAND). Plays a major role in sexual development, sleep, and metabolism.

- **Pituitary gland** (puh-TOO-uh-tair-ee GLAND). This gland affects almost every physiologic process of the body: growth, blood pressure, contractions during childbirth, breast-milk production, sexual organ functions in both women and men, thyroid gland function, and the conversion of food into energy (metabolism).

- **Thyroid gland** (THY-royd GLAND). Controls how quickly the body burns energy (metabolism), makes proteins, and how sensitive the body should be to other hormones. Thyroid malfunction is very common and sometimes can be seen by cosmetologist as a change in the growth rate of hair or nails or quality or texture of hair or nails that changes significantly.

Review the Reproductive System

The **reproductive system** (ree-proh-DUK-tiv SIS-tum) includes the ovaries, uterine tubes, uterus, and vagina in the female (**figure 6-31a**) and the testes, prostate gland, penis, and urethra in the male (**figure 6-31b**). This performs the function of producing offspring and passing on the genetic code from one generation to another.

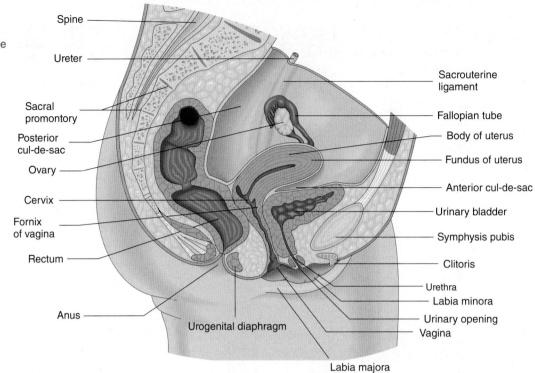

figure 6-31a
The female reproductive system

Spine

Ureter

Sacral promontory

Posterior cul-de-sac

Ovary

Cervix

Fornix of vagina

Rectum

Anus

Urogenital diaphragm

Sacrouterine ligament

Fallopian tube

Body of uterus

Fundus of uterus

Anterior cul-de-sac

Urinary bladder

Symphysis pubis

Clitoris

Urethra

Labia minora

Urinary opening

Vagina

Labia majora

The reproductive system produces hormones—primarily estrogen in females and primarily testosterone in males. These hormones affect and change the skin in several ways. Acne, loss of scalp hair, facial hair growth and color, and darker skin pigmentations are some of the results of changing or fluctuating hormones. Fortunately, cosmetologists have access to many products and treatments that can address unwanted changes of this nature and help clients feel more comfortable and confident about themselves. This is one more example of how important your role is in your clients' lives.

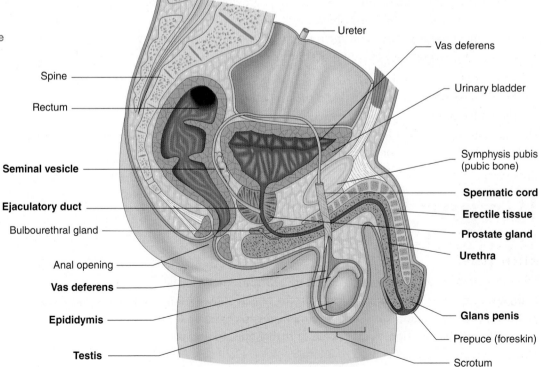

figure 6-31b
The male reproductive system

Spine

Rectum

Seminal vesicle

Ejaculatory duct

Bulbourethral gland

Anal opening

Vas deferens

Epididymis

Testis

Ureter

Vas deferens

Urinary bladder

Symphysis pubis (pubic bone)

Spermatic cord

Erectile tissue

Prostate gland

Urethra

Glans penis

Prepuce (foreskin)

Scrotum

REVIEW QUESTIONS

1. Why is the study of anatomy and physiology important to cosmetologists?

2. Define anatomy and physiology.

3. Name and describe the basic structures of a cell.

4. List and describe the functions of the four types of tissue found in the human body.

5. What are organs?

6. Name the 11 main body systems and their functions.

7. List the primary functions of the skeletal system.

8. Name and describe the two types of nerves found in the body and how they work.

9. Name and briefly describe the five types (venous and arterial) of blood vessels found in the body.

10. Name and discuss the two main types of glands found in the human body.

STUDY TOOLS

- **Reinforce what you just learned:** Complete the activities and exercises in your Theory or Practical Workbook, or your Study Guide.

- **Expand your knowledge:** Search for websites about the topics in this chapter and make a list of additional resources.

- **Study and prepare for your quiz:** Take the chapter test in your Exam Review or your Milady U: Online Licensing Prep.

- **Re-Test your knowledge:** Take the Chapter 6 Quizzes!

- **Learn even more:** Look up in a dictionary or search the internet for the definitions of any additional terms you want to learn about.

CHAPTER GLOSSARY

abductor digiti minimi ab-DUK-tohr dij-it-ty MIN-eh-mee	p. 128	Muscle that separates the fingers and the toes.
abductor hallucis ab-DUK-tohr ha-LU-sis	p. 128	Muscle that moves the big toe away from the other toes.
abductors ab-DUK-turz	p. 126	Muscles that draw a body part, such as a finger, arm, or toe, away from the midline of the body or of an extremity.
adductors ah-DUK-turz	p. 126	Muscles that draw a body part, such as a finger, arm, or toe, inward toward the median axis of the body or of an extremity.
adipose tissue ADD-ih-pohz TISH-oo	p. 117	The technical term for fat; it gives smoothness and contour to the body.
anatomy ah-NAT-ah-mee	p. 115	The study of human body structures that can be seen with the naked eye and how the body parts are organized; the science of the structure of organisms or of their parts.

angular artery ANG-gyoo-lur ART-ur-ee	p. 135	Branch of the facial artery that supplies blood to the side of the nose.
anterior auricular artery an-TEER-ee-ur aw-RIK-yuh-lur ART-uh-ree	p. 135	Branch of the superficial temporal artery that supplies blood to the front part of the ear.
anterior tibial artery an-TEER-ee-ur TIB-ee-al ART-uh-ree	p. 136	One of the popliteal arteries (the other is the posterior tibial artery) that supplies blood to the lower leg muscles and to the muscles and skin on the top of the foot and adjacent sides of the first and second toes. This artery continues to the foot where it becomes the dorsalis pedis artery.
aorta ay-ORT-uh	p. 133	The largest artery in the body.
arteries AR-tuh-rees	p. 133	Thick-walled, muscular, flexible tubes that carry oxygenated blood away from the heart to the arterioles.
arterioles ar-TEER-ee-ohls	p. 133	Small arteries that deliver blood to capillaries.
autonomic nervous system aw-toh-NAHM-ik NURV-us SIS-tum	p. 128	Abbreviated ANS; the part of the nervous system that controls the involuntary muscles; regulates the action of the smooth muscles, glands, blood vessels, heart, and breathing.
belly	p. 122	The middle part of the muscle.
bicep BY-sep	p. 126	Muscle that produces the contour of the front and inner side of the upper arm; lifts the forearm and flexes the elbow.
blood	p. 134	Nutritive fluid circulating through the circulatory system (heart and blood vessels) to supply oxygen and nutrients to cells and tissues and to remove carbon dioxide and waste from them.
blood vessels	p. 133	Tube-like structures that include arteries, arterioles, capillaries, venules, and veins.
body systems	p. 117	Also known as *systems*; groups of body organs acting together to perform one or more functions. The human body is composed of 11 major systems.
brain	p. 128	Part of the central nervous system contained in the cranium; it is the largest and most complex nerve tissue and controls sensation, muscles, activity of glands, and the power to think, sense, and feel.
buccal nerve BUK-ul NURV	p. 131	Branch of the seventh cranial nerve that affects the muscles of the mouth.
buccinator muscle BUK-sih-nay-tur MUS-ul	p. 124	Thin, flat muscle of the cheek between the upper and lower jaw that compresses the cheeks and expels air between the lips.
capillaries KAP-ih-lair-eez	p. 133	Tiny, thin-walled blood vessels that connect the smaller arteries to the venules. Capillaries bring nutrients to the cells and carry away waste materials.
carpus KAR-pus	p. 121	Also known as *wrist*; flexible joint composed of a group of eight small, irregular bones (carpals) held together by ligaments.
cell membrane SELL MEM-brayn	p. 116	A cell part that encloses the protoplasm and permits soluble substances to enter and leave the cell.

cells	p. 115	Basic units of all living things—from bacteria to plants to animals, including human beings.
central nervous system	p. 128	Abbreviated CNS; consists of the brain, spinal cord, spinal nerves, and cranial nerves.
cervical nerves SUR-vih-kul NURVS	p. 131	Branches of the seventh cranial nerve; originate at the spinal cord and affect the side of the neck and the platysma muscle.
cervical vertebrae SUR-vih-kul VURT-uh-bray	p. 120	The seven bones of the top part of the vertebral column, located in the neck region.
circulatory system	p. 132	Also known as *cardiovascular system* or *vascular system*; The body system that controls the steady circulation of the blood through the body by means of the heart and blood vessels.
clavicle KLAV-ih-kul	p. 121	Also known as *collarbone*; the bone that joins the sternum and scapula.
common carotid arteries KAHM-un kuh-RAHT-ud ART-uh-rees	p. 134	Main arteries that supply blood to the head, face, and neck.
common peroneal nerve KAHM-un per-oh-NEE-al NURV	p. 131	A division of the sciatic nerve that extends from behind the knee to wind around the head of the fibula to the front of the leg where it divides into two branches.
connective tissue	p. 117	Fibrous tissue that binds together, protects, and supports the various parts of the body. Examples of connective tissue are bone, cartilage, ligaments, tendons, blood, lymph, and fat (see *adipose tissue*).
corrugator muscle KOR-oo-gay-tohr MUS-ul	p. 124	Muscle located beneath the frontalis and orbicularis oculi muscles that draws the eyebrow down and wrinkles the forehead vertically.
cranium KRAY-nee-um	p. 119	An oval, bony case that protects the brain.
cytoplasm sy-toh-PLAZ-um	p. 116	The protoplasm of a cell; the watery fluid that surrounds the nucleus of the cell and is needed for growth, reproduction, and self-repair.
deep peroneal nerve DEEP pare-oh-NEE-uhl NURV	p. 132	Also known as *anterior tibial nerve*; it extends down the front of the leg, behind the muscles. It supplies impulses to these muscles and also to the muscles and skin on the top of the foot and adjacent sides of the first and second toes.
deltoid DEL-toyd	p. 126	Large, triangular muscle covering the shoulder joint that allows the arm to extend outward and to the side of the body.
depressor labii inferioris muscle dee-PRES-ur LAY-bee-eye in-FEER-ee-or-us MUS-ul	p. 125	Also known as *quadratus labii inferioris muscle*; muscle surrounding the lower lip; lowers the lower lip and draws it to one side, as in expressing sarcasm.
digestive system	p. 118	Also known as *gastrointestinal system*; the body system that is responsible for breaking down foods into nutrients and wastes; consists of the mouth, stomach, intestines, salivary and gastric glands, and other organs.
digital nerve DIJ-ut-tul NURV	p. 131	Sensory–motor nerve that, with its branches, supplies impulses to the fingers.

dorsal nerve DOOR-sal NURV	p. 132	Also known as *dorsal cutaneous nerve*; a nerve that extends up from the toes and foot, just under the skin, supplying impulses to toes and foot, as well as the muscles and skin of the leg, where it becomes the superficial peroneal nerve.
dorsalis pedis artery DOR-sul-is PEED-us ART-uh-ree	p. 136	Artery that supplies blood to the foot.
eleventh cranial nerve	p. 131	Also known as *accessory nerve*; a motor nerve that controls the motion of the neck and shoulder muscles.
endocrine glands EN-duh-krin GLANDZ	p. 138	Also known as *ductless glands*; glands such as the thyroid and pituitary gland that release hormonal secretions directly into the bloodstream.
endocrine system EN-duh-krin SIS-tum	p. 138	The body system consisting of a group of specialized glands that affect the growth, development, sexual functions, and health of the entire body.
epicranial aponeurosis ep-ih-KRAY-nee-al ap-uh-noo-ROH-sus	p. 123	Tendon that connects the occipitalis and frontalis muscles.
epicranius ep-ih-KRAY-nee-us	p. 123	Also known as *occipitofrontalis*; the broad muscle that covers the top of the skull and consists of the occipitalis and frontalis.
epithelial tissue ep-ih-THEE-lee-ul TISH-oo	p. 117	A protective covering on body surfaces, such as skin, mucous membranes, the tissue inside the mouth, the lining of the heart, digestive and respiratory organs, and the glands.
ethmoid bone ETH-moyd BOHN	p. 120	Light, spongy bone between the eye sockets; forms part of the nasal cavities.
exocrine glands EK-suh-krin GLANDZ	p. 138	Also known as *duct glands*; they produce a substance that travels through small, tube-like ducts. Sweat glands and oil glands of the skin belong to this group.
extensor digitorum longus ik-STEN-sur dij-it-TOHR-um LONG-us	p. 127	Muscle that bends the foot up and extends the toes.
extensor hallucis longus ik-STEN-sur ha-LU-sis LONG-us	p. 127	Muscle that extends the big toe and flexes the foot.
extensors ik-STEN-surs	p. 126	Muscles that straighten the wrist, hand, and fingers to form a straight line.
external carotid artery eks-TUR-nul kuh-RAHT-ud ART-uh-rees	p. 134	Artery that supplies blood to the anterior (front) parts of the scalp, ear, face, neck, and sides of the head.
external jugular vein	p. 136	Vein located at the side of the neck that carries blood returning to the heart from the head, face, and neck.
facial artery FAY-shul ART-ur-ee	p. 135	Also known as *external maxillary artery*; branch of the external carotid artery that supplies blood to the lower region of the face, mouth, and nose.
facial skeleton	p. 119	The framework of the face; composed of 14 bones.
femur FEE-mur	p. 121	Heavy, long bone that forms the leg above the knee.
fibula FIB-ya-lah	p. 121	Smaller of the two bones that form the leg below the knee. The fibula may be visualized as a bump on the little-toe side of the ankle.

fifth cranial nerve	p. 129	Also known as *trifacial nerve* or *trigeminal nerve*; the chief sensory nerve of the face that serves as the motor nerve of the muscles that control chewing.
flexor digiti minimi FLEK-sur dij-it-ty MIN-eh-mee	p. 128	Muscle that moves the little toe.
flexor digitorum brevis FLEK-sur dij-ut-TOHR-um BREV-us	p. 128	Muscle that flexes the toes and helps maintain balance while walking and standing.
flexor FLEK-sur	p. 126	Extensor muscle of the wrist involved in flexing the wrist.
frontal artery	p. 135	Branch of the superficial temporal artery that supplies blood to the forehead and upper eyelids.
frontal bone FRUNT-ul BOHN	p. 119	The bone that forms the forehead.
frontalis frun-TAY-lus	p. 123	Front (anterior) portion of the epicranius; muscle of the scalp that raises the eyebrows, draws the scalp forward, and causes wrinkles across the forehead.
gastrocnemius gas-truc-NEEM-e-us	p. 127	Muscle attached to the lower rear surface of the heel and pulls the foot down.
glands	p. 138	Organs that remove and release certain elements from the blood to convert them into new compounds.
heart	p. 132	Muscular, cone-shaped organ that keeps the blood moving within the circulatory system.
hormones HOR-mohnz	p. 138	Secretions, such as insulin, adrenaline, and estrogen, that stimulate functional activity or other secretions in the body. Hormones influence the welfare of the entire body.
humerus HYOO-muh-rus	p. 121	Uppermost and largest bone in the arm, extending from the elbow to the shoulder.
hyoid bone HY-oyd BOHN	p. 120	U-shaped bone at the base of the tongue that supports the tongue and its muscles.
inferior labial artery in-FEER-ee-ur LAY-bee-ul ART-ur-ee	p. 135	Branch of the facial artery that supplies blood to the lower lip.
infraorbital artery in-frah-OR-bih-tul AR-tuh-ree	p. 134	Branch of the internal carotid artery that supplies blood to the muscles of the eye.
insertion	p. 122	The movable part of the muscle that is farthest from the skeleton.
integumentary system in-TEG-yuh-ment-uh-ree SIS-tum	p. 137	The body system that consists of skin and its accessory organs, such as the oil and sweat glands, sensory receptors, hair, and nails; it serves as a protective covering and helps regulate the body's temperature.
internal carotid artery	p. 134	Artery that supplies blood to the brain, eyes, eyelids, forehead, nose, and internal ear.
internal jugular vein in-TUR-nul JUG-yuh-lur VAYN	p. 136	Vein located at the side of the neck to collect blood from the brain and parts of the face and neck.
joint JOYNT	p. 119	A connection between two or more bones of the skeleton.

lacrimal bones LAK-ruh-mul BOHNS	p. 120	Small, thin bones located at the front inner wall of the orbits (eye sockets).
latissimus dorsi lah-TIS-ih-mus DOR-see	p. 125	Large, flat, triangular muscle covering the lower back.
levator anguli oris muscle lih-VAYT-ur ANG-yoo-ly OH-ris MUS-ul	p. 125	Also known as *caninus muscle*; muscle that raises the angle of the mouth and draws it inward.
levator labii superioris muscle lih-VAYT-ur LAY-bee-eye soo-peer-ee-OR-is MUS-ul	p. 125	Also known as *quadratus labii superioris muscle*; muscle surrounding the upper lip. It elevates the upper lip and dilates the nostrils, as in expressing distaste.
levator palpebrae superioris muscle lih-VAYT-ur [insert palpebrae] soo-peer-ee-OR-is MUS-ul	p. 124	Thin muscle that controls the movement of the eyelid.
lymph LIMF	p. 137	Clear fluid that circulates in the lymph spaces (lymphatics) of the body. Lymph helps carry wastes and impurities away from the cells before it is routed back to the circulatory system.
lymph capillaries	p. 137	Blind-end tubes that are the origin of lymphatic vessels.
lymph nodes	p. 137	Gland-like structures found inside lymphatic vessels; filter the lymphatic vessels and help fight infection.
lymphatic/immune system lim-FAT-ik ih-MYOON SIS-tum	p. 137	The body system that consists of lymph, lymph nodes, the thymus gland, the spleen, and lymph vessels. It carries waste and impurities away from the cells and protects the body from disease by developing immunities and destroying disease-causing microorganisms.
mandible MAN-duh-bul	p. 120	Lower jawbone; largest and strongest bone of the face.
mandibular nerve man-DIB-yuh-lur NURV	p. 130	Affects the muscles of the chin, lower lip, and external ear.
marginal mandibular nerve MAR-jin-ul man-DIB-yuh-lur NURV	p. 131	Branch of the seventh cranial nerve that affects the muscles of the chin and lower lip.
maxillae mak-SIL-ee	p. 120	Singular: maxilla. Bones of the upper jaw.
maxillary nerve MAK-suh-lair-ee NURV	p. 130	Branch of the fifth cranial nerve that supplies impulses to the upper part of the face.
median nerve MEE-dee-un NURV	p. 131	Sensory–motor nerve that is smaller than the ulnar and radial nerves and that, with its branches, supplies the arm and hand.
mentalis muscle men-TAY-lis MUS-ul	p. 125	Muscle that elevates the lower lip and raises and wrinkles the skin of the chin.
metacarpus met-uh-KAR-pus	p. 121	Bones of the palm of the hand; parts of the hand containing five bones between the carpus and phalanges.
metatarsal met-ah-TAHR-sul	p. 122	One of three subdivisions of the foot; long and slender bones, similar to the metacarpal bones of the hand. The other two subdivisions are the tarsal and phalanges.
middle temporal artery TEM-puh-rul AR-tuh-ree	p. 135	Branch of the superficial temporal artery that supplies blood to the temples.

mitosis my-TOH-sis	p. 116	The usual process of cell reproduction of human tissues that occurs when the cell divides into two identical cells called daughter cells.
motor nerves	p. 129	Also known as *efferent nerves*; carry impulses from the brain to the muscles or glands.
muscle tissue	p. 117	Tissue that contracts and moves various parts of the body.
muscular system MUS-kuyh-lur SIS-tum	p. 122	The body system that covers, shapes, and holds the skeletal system in place; the muscular system contracts and moves various parts of the body.
nasal bones NAY-zul BOHNS	p. 120	Bones that form the bridge of the nose.
nerve tissue NURV TISH-oo	p. 117	Tissue that carries messages to and from the brain and controls and coordinates all bodily functions.
nerves	p. 129	Whitish cords made up of bundles of nerve fibers held together by connective tissue, through which impulses are transmitted.
nervous system	p. 128	Body system that consists of the brain, spinal cord, and nerves; controls and coordinates all other systems of the body and makes them work harmoniously and efficiently.
neurology nuh-RAHL-uh-jee	p. 128	Scientific study of the structure, function, and pathology of the nervous system.
nucleus NOO-klee-us	p. 116	Dense, active protoplasm found in the center of the cell; plays an important part in cell reproduction and metabolism.
occipital artery ahk-SIP-it-ul AR-tuh-ree	p. 136	Branch of the external carotid artery that supplies blood to the skin and muscles of the scalp and back of the head up to the crown.
occipital bone ahk-SIP-ih-tul BOHN	p. 119	The hindmost bone of the skull, below the parietal bones; forms the back of the skull above the nape.
occipitalis ahk-SIP-i-tahl-is	p. 123	Back (posterior) portion of the epicranius; muscle that draws the scalp backward.
-ology AHL-O-jee	p. 115	Word ending meaning *study of*.
ophthalmic nerve ahf-THAL-mik NURV	p. 130	Branch of the fifth cranial nerve that supplies impulses to the skin of the forehead, upper eyelids, and interior portion of the scalp, orbit, eyeball, and nasal passage.
orbicularis oculi muscle or-bik-yuh-LAIR-is AHK-yuh-lye MUS-ul	p. 124	Ring muscle of the eye socket; enables you to close your eyes.
orbicularis oris muscle or-bik-yuh-LAIR-is OH-ris MUS-ul	p. 125	Flat band of muscle around the upper and lower lips that compresses, contracts, puckers, and wrinkles the lips.
organs	p. 117	Structures composed of specialized tissues designed to perform specific functions in plants and animals.
origin	p. 122	The part of the muscle that does not move; attached closest to the skeleton.
parietal artery puh-RY-ate-ul ART-uh-ree	p. 135	Branch of the superficial temporal artery that supplies blood to the side and crown of the head.

parietal bones puh-RY-uh-tul BOHNS	p. 119	Bones that form the sides and top of the cranium.
patella pah-TEL-lah	p. 121	Also known as *accessory bone* or *kneecap*; forms the kneecap joint.
pectoralis major pek-tor-AL-is MAY-jor	p. 125	Muscles of the chest that assist the swinging movements of the arm.
pectoralis minor pek-tor-AL-is MY-nur	p. 125	Muscles of the chest that assist the swinging movements of the arm.
peripheral nervous system puh-RIF-uh-rul NURV-vus SIS-tum	p. 128	Abbreviated PNS; system of nerves that connects the peripheral (outer) parts of the body to the central nervous system; it has both sensory and motor nerves.
peroneus brevis per-oh-NEE-us BREV-us	p. 127	Muscle that originates on the lower surface of the fibula. It bends the foot down and out.
peroneus longus per-oh-NEE-us LONG-us	p. 127	Muscle that covers the outer side of the calf; inverts the foot and turns it outward.
phalanges fuh-LAN-jeez (singular: phalanx [FAY-langks])	p. 121	Singular: phalanx. Also known as *digits*; bones of the fingers or toes; one of the three subdivisions of the foot. The other two subdivisions are the tarsal and metatarsal.
physiology fiz-ih-OL-oh-jee	p. 115	The study of the functions and activities performed by the body's structures.
pineal gland PY-nee-ul GLAND	p. 139	Endocrine system gland that plays a major role in sexual development, sleep, and metabolism.
pituitary gland puh-TOO-uh-tair-ee GLAND	p. 139	The most complex organ of the endocrine system. This gland affects almost every physiologic process of the body: growth, blood pressure, contractions during childbirth, breast-milk production, sexual organ functions in both women and men, thyroid gland function, and the conversion of food into energy (metabolism).
platysma muscle plah-TIZ-muh MUS-ul	p. 123	Broad muscle extending from the chest and shoulder muscles to the side of the chin; responsible for lowering the lower jaw and lip.
popliteal artery pop-lih-TEE-ul ART-uh-ree	p. 136	Artery that supplies blood to the foot; divides into two separate arteries known as the anterior tibial artery and the posterior tibial artery.
posterior auricular artery poh-STEER-ee-ur aw-RIK-yuh-lur ART-tuh-ree	p. 136	Branch of the external carotid artery that supplies blood to the scalp, the area behind and above the ear, and the skin behind the ear.
posterior auricular nerve poh-STEER-ee-ur aw-RIK-yuh-lur NURV	p. 131	Branch of the seventh cranial nerve that affects the muscles behind the ear at the base of the skull.
posterior tibial artery poh-STEER-ee-ur TIB-ee-al ART-uh-ree	p. 136	One of the popliteal arteries (the other is the anterior tibial artery) that supplies blood to the ankle and the back of the lower leg.
procerus muscle proh-SEE-rus MUS-ul	p. 124	Muscle that covers the bridge of the nose, lowers the eyebrows, and causes wrinkles across the bridge of the nose.
pronator proh-NAY-tohr	p. 126	Muscle that turns the hand inward so that the palm faces downward.
protoplasm PROH-toh-plaz-um	p. 115	A colorless, jelly-like substance found inside cells in which food elements such as proteins, fats, carbohydrates, mineral salts, and water are present.

| **pulmonary circulation** | p. 132 | The system that takes deoxygenated blood from the heart to the lungs for oxygenation and waste removal and then returns that blood to the heart (left atrium) so oxygen-rich blood can be delivered to the body. |
| PUL-muh-nayr-ee sur-kyoo-LAY-shun | | |

| **radial artery** | p. 136 | Artery, along with numerous branches, that supplies blood to the thumb side of the arm and the back of the hand; supplies blood to the muscles of the skin, hands, fingers, wrist, elbow, and forearm. |
| RAY-dee-ul AR-tur-ree | | |

| **radial nerve** | p. 131 | Sensory–motor nerve that, with its branches, supplies the thumb side of the arm and back of the hand. |
| RAY-dee-ul NURV | | |

| **radius** | p. 121 | Smaller bone in the forearm (lower arm) on the same side as the thumb. |
| RAY-dee-us | | |

| **reflex** | p. 129 | Automatic reaction to a stimulus that involves the movement of an impulse from a sensory receptor along the sensory nerve to the spinal cord. |
| REE-fleks | | |

| **reproductive system** | p. 139 | The body system that includes the ovaries, uterine tubes, uterus, and vagina in the female and the testes, prostate gland, penis, and urethra in the male. This system performs the function of producing offspring and passing on the genetic code from one generation to another. |
| ree-proh-DUK-tiv SIS-tum | | |

| **respiratory system** | p. 118 | Body system consisting of the lungs and air passages; makes blood and oxygen available to body structures through respiration (breathing) and eliminating carbon dioxide. |
| RES-puh-rah-tor-ee SIS-tum | | |

| **ribs** | p. 121 | Twelve pairs of bones forming the wall of the thorax. |

| **risorius muscle** | p. 125 | Muscle of the mouth that draws the corner of the mouth out and back, as in grinning. |
| rih-ZOR-ee-us MUS-ul | | |

| **saphenous nerve** | p. 132 | Nerve of the leg that supplies impulses to the skin of the inner side of the leg and foot. |
| sa-FEEN-us NURV | | |

| **scapula** | p. 121 | Also known as *shoulder blade*; large, flat, triangular bone of the shoulder. There are two scapulae. |
| SKAP-yuh-luh | | |

| **sciatic nerve** | p. 131 | Largest and longest nerve in the body; it passes through the gluteal region into the thigh, where it branches into smaller nerves. Pain from injury or compression of the sciatic nerve can radiate throughout the abdomen and be sensed in the lower back, hip, or lower abdomen. |
| sy-AT-ik NURV | | |

| **sensory nerves** | p. 129 | Also known as *afferent nerves* (AAF-eer-ent NURVS); carry impulses or messages from the sense organs to the brain, where sensations of touch, cold, heat, sight, sound, taste, smell, pain, and pressure are experienced. |

| **serratus anterior** | p. 125 | Muscle of the chest that assists in breathing and in raising the arm. |
| ser-RAT-us an-TEER-ee-or | | |

| **seventh cranial nerve** | p. 130 | Also known as *facial nerve*; is the chief motor nerve of the face. Its divisions and their branches supply and control all the muscles of facial expression. It emerges near the lower part of the ear and extends to the muscles of the neck. |

| **skeletal system** | p. 118 | Forming the physical foundation of the body, it composed of 206 bones that vary in size and shape and are connected by movable and immovable joints. |

| **skull** | p. 119 | Skeleton of the head; divided into two parts: cranium and facial skeleton. |

soleus SO-lee-us	p. 127	Muscle that originates at the upper portion of the fibula and bends the foot down.
sphenoid bone SFEEN-oyd BOHN	p. 120	Bone that joins all of the bones of the cranium together.
spinal cord	p. 129	Portion of the central nervous system that originates in the brain and extends down to the lower extremity of the trunk. It is protected by the spinal column.
sternocleidomastoideus STUR-noh-KLEE-ih-doh-mas-TOYD-ee-us	p. 123	Muscle of the neck that lowers and rotates the head.
sternum STUR-num	p. 121	Also known as *breastbone*; flat bone that forms the ventral (front) support of the ribs.
submental artery sub-MEN-tul ART-uh-ree	p. 135	Branch of the facial artery that supplies blood to the chin and lower lip.
superficial peroneal nerve soo-pur-FISH-ul pare-oh-NEE-uhl NURV	p. 132	Also known as *musculocutaneous nerve* (MUS-kyoo-loh-kyoo-TAY-nee-us NURV); extends down the leg, just under the skin, supplying impulses to the muscles and the skin of the leg, as well as to the skin and toes on the top of the foot, where it becomes the dorsal nerve.
superficial temporal artery soo-pur-FISH-ul TEM-puh-rul AR-tuh-ree	p. 135	A continuation of the external carotid nerve artery; supplies blood to the muscles of the front, side, and top of the head.
superior labial artery soo-PEER-ee-ur LAY-bee-ul AR-tuh-ree	p. 135	Branch of the facial artery that supplies blood to the upper lip and region of the nose.
supinator SOO-puh-nayt-ur	p. 126	Muscle of the forearm that rotates the radius outward and the palm upward.
supraorbital artery soo-pruh-OR-bih-tul AR-tuh-ree	p. 134	Branch of the internal carotid artery that supplies blood to the upper eyelid and forehead.
sural nerve SUR-ul NURV	p. 132	Nerve of the lower leg that supplies impulses to the skin on the outer side and back of the foot and leg.
systemic circulation sis-TEM-ik sur-kyoo-LAY-shun	p. 132	Also known as *general circulation*; system that carries the oxygen-rich blood from the heart throughout the body and returns deoxygenated blood back to the heart.
talus TA-lus	p. 122	Also known as *ankle bone*; one of three bones that comprise the ankle joint. The other two bones are the tibia and fibula.
tarsal TAHR-sul	p. 122	One of three subdivisions of the foot. There are seven bones—talus, calcaneus, navicular, three cuneiform bones, and the cuboid. The other two subdivisions are the metatarsal and the phalanges.
temporal bones TEM-puh-rul BOHNS	p. 119	Bones that form the sides of the head in the ear region.
temporal nerve TEM-poh-rul NURV	p. 131	Branch of the seventh cranial nerve that affects the muscles of the temple, side of the forehead, eyebrow, eyelid, and upper part of the cheek.
thorax THOR-aks	p. 121	Also known as *chest* or *pulmonary trunk* (PUL-muh-nayr-ee TRUNK); consists of the sternum, ribs, and thoracic vertebrae; elastic, bony cage that serves as a protective framework for the heart, lungs, and other internal organs.

thyroid gland THY-royd GLAND	p. 139	Gland of the endocrine system that controls how quickly the body burns energy (metabolism), makes proteins, and how sensitive the body should be to other hormones.
tibia TIB-ee-ah	p. 121	Larger of the two bones that form the leg below the knee. The tibia may be visualized as a bump on the big-toe side of the ankle.
tibial nerve TIB-ee-al NURV	p. 131	A division of the sciatic nerve that passes behind the knee. It subdivides and supplies impulses to the knee, the muscles of the calf, the skin of the leg, and the sole, heel, and underside of the toes.
tibialis anterior tib-ee-AHL-is an-TEHR-ee-ohr	p. 127	Muscle that covers the front of the shin; bends the foot upward and inward.
tissue TISH-oo	p. 117	A collection of similar cells that perform a particular function.
transverse facial artery tranz-VURS FAY-shul ART-ur-ee	p. 135	Branch of the superficial temporal artery that supplies blood to the skin and masseter muscle.
trapezius trah-PEE-zee-us	p. 125	Muscle that covers the back of the neck and upper and middle region of the back; rotates and controls swinging movements of the arm.
triangularis muscle try-ang-gyuh-LAY-rus MUS-ul	p. 125	Muscle extending alongside the chin that pulls down the corners of the mouth.
tricep TRY-sep	p. 126	Large muscle that covers the entire back of the upper arm and extends the forearm.
ulna UL-nuh	p. 121	Inner and larger bone in the forearm (lower arm); attached to the wrist and located on the side of the little finger.
ulnar artery UL-nur AR-tuh-ree	p. 136	Artery, along with numerous branches, that supplies blood to the little-finger side of the arm and palm of the hand.
ulnar nerve UL-nur NURV	p. 131	Sensory–motor nerve that, with its branches, affects the little-finger side of the arm and palm of the hand.
veins	p. 134	Thin-walled blood vessels that are less elastic than arteries; veins contain cup-like valves that keep blood flowing in one direction to the heart and prevent blood from flowing backward.
venules VEEN-yools	p. 134	Small vessels that connect the capillaries to the veins. They collect blood from the capillaries and drain it into veins.
zygomatic bones zy-goh-MAT-ik BOHNS	p. 120	Also known as *malar bones* (MAY-lur BOHNS) or *cheekbones*; bones that form the prominence of the cheeks.
zygomaticus major muscles zy-goh-mat-ih-kus MAY-jor MUS-uls	p. 125	Muscles on both sides of the face that extend from the zygomatic bone to the angle of the mouth. These muscles pull the mouth backward, upward, and outward, as when you are laughing or smiling.
zygomaticus minor muscles zy-goh-mat-ih-kus MY-nor MUS-uls	p. 125	Muscles on both sides of the face that extend from the zygomatic bone to the upper lips. These muscles pull the upper lip backward, upward, and outward, as when you are smiling.

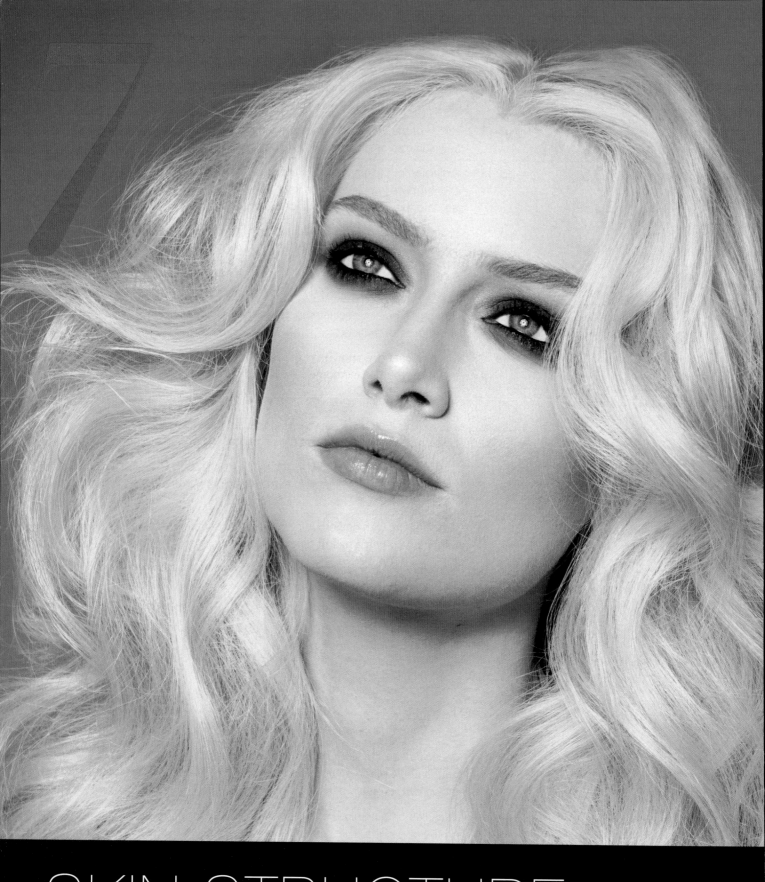

SKIN STRUCTURE, GROWTH, & NUTRITION

LEARNING OBJECTIVES

After completing this chapter, you will be able to:

LO❶
Describe the structure and composition of the skin.

LO❷
List the six functions of the skin.

LO❸
Name the classes of nutrients essential for good health.

LO❹
Identify the food groups and dietary guidelines recommended by the U.S. Department of Agriculture (USDA).

LO❺
List and describe the vitamins that can help the skin.

Clear, glowing skin is one of today's most important hallmarks of beauty. No matter how advanced the latest skin care technology may be, you still have to learn how to care for your client's skin and know what you should do to keep it healthy. That means you must study the structure of the skin, how skin grows, and why it is important to maintain a healthy diet.

why study

SKIN STRUCTURE, GROWTH, AND NUTRITION?

Cosmetologists should study and have a thorough understanding of skin structure, growth, and nutrition because:

> Knowing the skin's underlying structure and basic needs is crucial in order to provide excellent skin care for clients.

> You will need to recognize adverse conditions, including skin diseases, inflamed skin, and infectious skin disorders so that you can refer clients to medical professionals for treatment when necessary.

> Twenty-first century skin care has entered the realm of high technology, so you must learn about and understand the latest developments in ingredients and state-of-the-art delivery systems in order to help protect, nourish, and preserve the health and beauty of your clients' skin.

After reading the next few sections, you will be able to:

LO ❶ Describe the structure and composition of the skin.

Know the Anatomy of the Skin

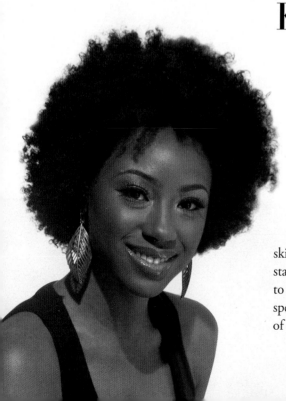

The medical branch of science that deals with the study of skin—its nature, structure, functions, diseases, and treatment—is called **dermatology** (dur-muh-TAHL-uh-jee). A **dermatologist** (dur-muh-TAHL-uh-jist) is a physician who specializes in diseases and disorders of the skin, hair, and nails. Dermatologists attend four years of college, four years of medical school, and about four years of specialty training in dermatology. Because some skin symptoms may be a sign of internal disease, many dermatologists have additional training in internal medicine.

Cosmetologists may be allowed to clean skin, preserve the health of skin, and beautify the skin, depending on the laws and regulations of their state. In some states, a cosmetologist must become an esthetician in order to perform certain services on the skin. An **esthetician** (es-thuh-TISH-un) specializes in the cleansing, beautification, and preservation of the health of skin on the entire body, including the face and neck.

Cosmetologists are not allowed to diagnose, prescribe, or provide any type of treatment for abnormal conditions, illnesses, or diseases. Cosmetologists refer clients with medical issues to dermatologists more than to any other type of physician.

The skin is the largest organ of the body. If the skin of an average adult were stretched out, it would cover over 3,000 square inches and weigh about six to nine pounds. Our skin protects the network of muscles, bones, nerves, blood vessels, and everything else inside our bodies. It is the only natural barrier between our bodies and the environment.

Healthy skin should be free of any visible signs of disease, infection, or injury. It is slightly moist, soft, and flexible. Ideally, healthy skin has a smooth, fine-grained texture (feel and appearance). The surface of healthy skin is slightly acidic, and its immune responses react quickly to organisms that touch or try to enter it. Appendages of the skin include hair, nails, and sudoriferous (sweat) and sebaceous (oil) glands.

Continued, repeated pressure on any part of the skin, especially the hands and feet, can cause it to thicken and develop into a **callus** (KAL-us), which is an important and needed protective layer that prevents damage to the underlying skin.

The skin of the scalp is constructed similarly to the skin elsewhere on the human body, but the scalp has larger and deeper hair follicles to accommodate the longer hair of the head.

The skin is composed of two main divisions: the epidermis and the dermis (figure 7-1).

? DID YOU KNOW?

A callus is nature's way of protecting the skin from damage and infection. Complete removal of a callus is a medical procedure that should not be performed in the salon.

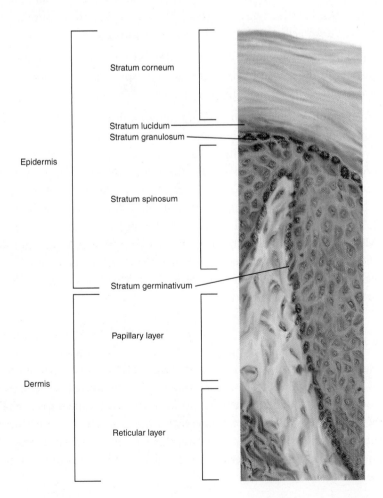

Epidermis
- Stratum corneum
- Stratum lucidum
- Stratum granulosum
- Stratum spinosum
- Stratum germinativum

Dermis
- Papillary layer
- Reticular layer

figure 7-1
Layers of the skin

The Epidermis

The **epidermis** (ep-uh-DUR-mis) is the outermost and thinnest layer of the skin. It contains no blood vessels, but has many small nerve endings. The epidermis is made up of five layers.

1. The **stratum corneum** (STRAT-um KOR-nee-um), also known as *horny layer* (HOR-nee LAY-ur), is the outer layer of the epidermis. The stratum corneum is the layer we see when we look at the skin and it is the layer cared for by salon products and services. Its scale-like cells are continually being shed and replaced by cells coming to the surface from underneath. These cells are made up of **keratin** (KAIR-uh-tin), a fibrous protein that is also the principal component of hair and nails. The cells combine with lipids (fats) produced by the skin to help make the stratum corneum a protective, water-resistant layer. The complex of lipids between the cells is known as the **barrier function** (BEAR-ee-ur FUNK-shun). The barrier function's purpose is to keep the skin moist by preventing water evaporation, and to guard against irritants penetrating the skin surface.

2. The **stratum lucidum** (STRAT-um LOO-sih-dum) is the clear, transparent layer under the stratum corneum; it consists of small cells through which light can pass. This layer is thicker on the palms of the hands and the soles of the feet.

3. The **stratum granulosum** (STRAT-um gran-yoo-LOH-sum), also known as *granular layer* (GRAN-yuh-lur LAY-ur), is the layer of the epidermis that is composed of cells that look like granules and are filled with keratin. The cells die as they are pushed to the surface to replace dead cells that are shed from the stratum corneum.

4. The **stratum spinosum** (STRAT-um spy-NOH-sum) is the spiny layer just above the stratum germinativum. The spiny layer is where the process of skin cell shedding begins.

5. The **stratum germinativum** (STRAT-um jer-mih-nah-TIV-um), more commonly called the *basal cell layer* (BAY zel CEL LAY-ur), is the deepest layer of the epidermis. This is the live layer of the epidermis that produces new epidermal skin cells and is responsible for the growth of the epidermis. It is composed of several layers of differently shaped cells. The basal cell layer also contains special cells called **melanocytes** (muh-LAN-uh-syts), which produce the dark skin pigment called melanin. Melanin protects the sensitive cells in the dermis (which is located below the epidermis) from the destructive effects of excessive ultraviolet (UV) light from the sun or from ultraviolet lamps. Melanin is discussed in greater detail later in this chapter.

The Dermis

The **dermis** (DUR-mis), also known as *derma* (DUR-muh), *corium* (KOH-ree-um), *cutis* (KYOO-tis), or *true skin*, is the underlying or inner layer of the skin. The dermis extends to form the subcutaneous tissue. The highly sensitive dermis layer of connective tissue is about 25 times thicker than the epidermis. Within its structure, there are numerous blood vessels, lymph vessels, nerves, sudoriferous (sweat) glands, sebaceous (oil) glands, and hair follicles, as well as arrector pili muscles. **Arrector pili muscles** (ah-REK-tohr PY-leh MUS-uls) are the small, involuntary muscles in the base of the hair follicle that cause goose flesh—or *goose bumps*, as many people call them—and papillae. The dermis is comprised of two layers: the papillary (superficial layer) and the reticular (deeper layer).

1. The **papillary layer** (PAP-uh-lair-ee LAY-ur) is the outer layer of the dermis, directly beneath the epidermis. Here you will find the **dermal papillae** (DUR-mul puh-PIL-eye) (singular: dermal papilla [DUR-mul puh-PIL-uh]), which are small, cone-shaped elevations at the base of the hair follicles. Some papillae contain looped capillaries, and others contain small epidermal structures called **tactile corpuscles** (TAK-tile KOR-pusuls), with nerve endings that are sensitive to touch and pressure. This layer also contains melanocytes, the pigment-producing cells. The top of the papillary layer where it joins the epidermis is called the **epidermal–dermal junction** (ep-ih-DUR-mul–DUR-mul JUNK-shun).

2. The **reticular layer** (ruh-TIK-yuh-lur LAY-ur) is the deeper layer of the dermis that supplies the skin with all of its oxygen and nutrients. It contains the following structures within its network:

   - Fat cells
   - Blood vessels
   - Lymph vessels
   - Sebaceous (oil) glands
   - Sudoriferous (sweat) glands
   - Hair follicles
   - Arrector pili muscles
   - Nerve endings

   Subcutaneous tissue (sub-kyoo-TAY-nee-us TISH-oo), also known as *adipose tissue* (AD-uh-pohs TISH-oo) or *subcutis tissue* (sub-KYOO-tis TISH-oo), is the fatty tissue found below the dermis. It gives smoothness and contour to the body, contains fats for use as energy, and also acts as a protective cushion for the skin. Subcutaneous tissue varies in thickness according to the age, gender, and general health of the individual (figure 7-2).

Fluids of the Skin

Blood and lymph vessels are located in the reticular dermis. Blood delivers nutrients and oxygen to the skin and takes away cellular waste products and carbon dioxide. Nutrients are molecules from food, such as protein, carbohydrates, and fats. These nutrients are necessary for cell life, repair, and growth. The skin cannot be nourished properly from the outside in with cosmetic products; it must have nourishment from foods that we eat.

Lymph, the clear fluids of the body that bathe the skin cells, remove toxins and cellular waste and have immune functions that help protect the skin and body against disease. Networks of blood arteries and lymph vessels in the subcutaneous tissue send their smaller branches to hair papillae, hair follicles, and skin glands.

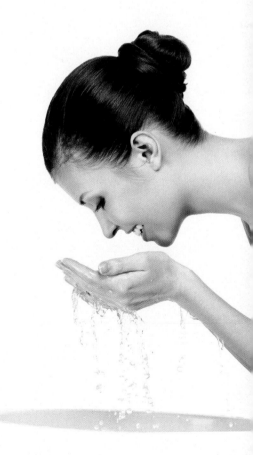

figure 7-2
Structures of the skin

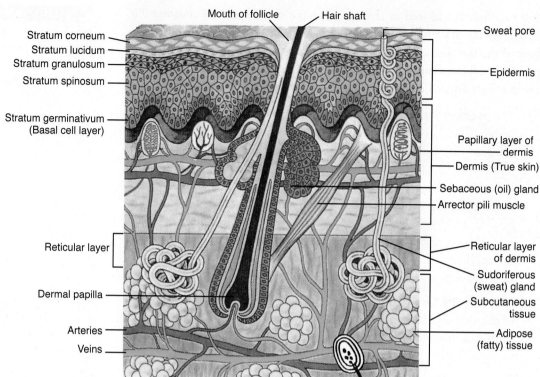

Mouth of follicle — Hair shaft

Sweat pore

Stratum corneum
Stratum lucidum
Stratum granulosum
Stratum spinosum

Epidermis

Stratum germinativum
(Basal cell layer)

Papillary layer of dermis
Dermis (True skin)
Sebaceous (oil) gland
Arrector pili muscle

Reticular layer

Reticular layer of dermis
Sudoriferous (sweat) gland
Subcutaneous tissue

Dermal papilla

Arteries

Veins

Adipose (fatty) tissue

Nerves of the Skin

The skin contains the surface endings of the following nerve fibers:

- **Motor nerve fibers** (MOH-tur NURV FY-burs) are distributed to the arrector pili muscles attached to the hair follicles. Motor nerves carry impulses from the brain to the muscles.

- **Sensory nerve fibers** (SEN-soh-ree NURV FY-burs) react to heat, cold, touch, pressure, and pain. These sensory receptors send messages to the brain.

- **Secretory nerve fibers** (seh-KREE-toh-ree NURV FY-burs) are distributed to the sudoriferous (sweat) and sebaceous (oil) glands of the skin. Secretory nerves, which are part of the autonomic nervous system, regulate the excretion of perspiration from the sudoriferous glands and control the flow of sebum (a fatty or oily secretion of the sebaceous glands) to the surface of the skin.

Sense of Touch

The papillary layer of the dermis houses the nerve endings that provide the body with the sense of touch, pain, heat, cold, and pressure. Nerve endings are most abundant in the fingertips. Complex sensations, such as vibrations, seem to depend on the sensitivity of a combination of these nerve endings.

Skin Color

The color of the skin—whether fair, medium, or dark—depends primarily on **melanin** (MEL-ah-nin), the tiny grains of pigment (coloring matter) that are produced by melanocytes and then deposited into cells in the basal layer of the epidermis and the papillary layers of the dermis. The color of the skin is a hereditary trait and varies among races and nationalities. Genes determine the amount and type of pigment produced in an individual.

The body produces two types of melanin: **pheomelanin** (fee-oh-MEL-uh-nin), which is red to yellow in color, and **eumelanin** (yoo-MEL-uh-nin), which is dark brown to black. People with light-colored skin mostly produce pheomelanin, while those with dark-colored skin mostly produce eumelanin. The size of melanin granules varies from one individual to another.

Melanin helps protect sensitive cells from the sun's UV light, but it does not provide enough protection to prevent skin damage. Daily use of a **broad spectrum sunscreen** with a sun protection factor (SPF) of 15 or higher can help the melanin protect the skin from burning, skin cancer, and premature aging (figure 7-3). *Broad spectrum* means that the sunscreen product has been shown to protect against both UV-A and UV-B radiation from the sun.

Strength and Flexibility of the Skin
The skin gets its strength, form, and flexibility from two specific structures found within the dermis: collagen and elastin. These two structures are composed of flexible protein fibers and they make up 70 percent of the dermis.

? DID YOU KNOW?
The word *collagen* comes from the Greek words *kolla*, meaning glue, and *gennan*, meaning to produce.

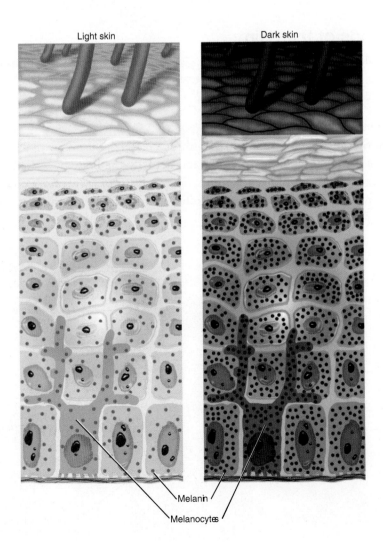

Light skin   Dark skin

Melanin
Melanocytes

figure 7-3
Melanocytes in the epidermis produce melanin.

Collagen (KAHL-uh-jen) is a fibrous protein that gives the skin form and strength. This fiber makes up a large percentage of the dermis and provides structural support by holding together all of the structures found in this layer. When collagen fibers are healthy, they allow the skin to stretch and contract as needed. If collagen fibers become weakened due to age, lack of moisture, environmental damage such as UV light, or frequent changes in weight, the skin will begin to lose its tone and suppleness. Wrinkles and sagging are often the result of collagen fibers losing their strength.

Elastin (ee-LAS-tin) is a protein base similar to collagen that forms elastic tissue. Elastin is interwoven with the collagen fibers. Elastin fiber gives the skin its flexibility and elasticity. It helps the skin regain its shape, even after being repeatedly stretched or expanded. Elastin can be weakened by the same factors that weaken collagen.

Both types of fibers are important to the overall health and appearance of the skin. As we age, gravity causes these fibers to weaken. In the end, a loss of elasticity results in sagging skin.

A majority of scientists now believe that most signs of skin aging are caused by sun exposure over a lifetime. Using a daily broad spectrum sunscreen with an SPF of 15 or higher, maintaining a moisturizing skin-care regimen, and keeping skin free of disease will slow the weakening of collagen and elastin fibers and help skin look young longer.

Glands of the Skin

The skin contains two types of duct glands that extract materials from the blood to form new substances. These are sudoriferous glands and sebaceous glands (figure 7-4).

Sudoriferous (Sweat) Glands

Sudoriferous glands (sood-uh-RIF-uhrus GLANZ), also known as **sweat glands**, excrete perspiration and detoxify the body by excreting excess salt and unwanted chemicals. They consist of a **secretory coil** (seh-KREET-toh-ree KOYL), the coiled base of the sudoriferous gland,

figure 7-4
Sudoriferous gland and sebaceous gland

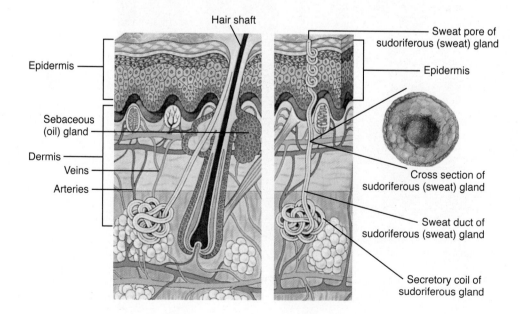

Hair shaft

Epidermis

Sebaceous (oil) gland

Dermis

Veins

Arteries

Sweat pore of sudoriferous (sweat) gland

Epidermis

Cross section of sudoriferous (sweat) gland

Sweat duct of sudoriferous (sweat) gland

Secretory coil of sudoriferous gland

and a tube-like sweat duct that ends at the surface of the skin to form the sweat pore. Practically all parts of the body are supplied with sudoriferous glands, which are more numerous on the palms of the hands, the soles of the feet, the forehead, and the underarm (armpit).

The sudoriferous glands regulate body temperature and help eliminate waste products from the body. The evaporation of sweat cools the skin's surface. The activity of sudoriferous glands is greatly increased by heat, exercise, emotions, and certain drugs.

The excretion of sweat is controlled by the nervous system. Normally, one to two pints of salt-containing liquids are eliminated daily through sweat pores in the skin.

Sebaceous (Oil) Glands

Sebaceous glands (sih-BAY-shus GLANZ), also known as *oil glands*, are connected to the hair follicles. They consist of little sacs with ducts that open into the follicles. These glands secrete **sebum** (SEE-bum), a fatty or oily substance that lubricates the skin and preserves the softness of the hair. With the exceptions of the palms of the hands and the soles of the feet, these glands are found in all parts of the body, particularly in the face and scalp where they are larger.

Ordinarily, sebum flows through the oil ducts leading to the mouths of the hair follicles. However, when the sebum hardens and the duct becomes clogged, a pore impaction called an **open comedo** (OH-pen KAHM-uh-doe) (plural: comedones [KAHM-uh-dohnz]), also known as *blackhead*, a hair follicle filled with dead keratinized cells and sebum, is formed.

A second type of comedo, called a **closed comedo** (closed KAHM-uh-doe), also known as a *whitehead*, is also filled with dead cells and sebum, but has a very small surface follicle opening and appears as a small white bump just under the skin surface (figure 7-5).

This type of lesion can lead to acne, a papule, or a pustule (figure 7-6).

Acne (AK-nee), also known as **acne vulgaris** (AK-nee vull-GAIR-us), is a skin disorder characterized by chronic inflammation of the sebaceous glands from retained secretions and bacteria known as **Propionibacterium acnes** (pro-PEE-ah-nee-back-tear-ee-um AK-nes), abbreviated P. acnes, the technical term for acne bacteria. A **papule** (PAP-yool), also known as **pimple**, is a small elevation on the skin that contains no fluid but may develop pus. A **pustule** (PUS-chool) is a raised, inflamed papule with a white or yellow center containing pus in the top of the lesion referred to as the "head" of the pimple.

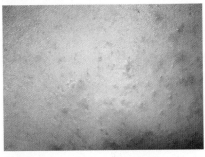
figure 7-5
Open and closed comedones

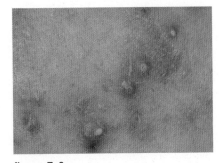
figure 7-6
Acne papules and pustules

After reading the next few sections, you will be able to:

LO❷ List the six functions of the skin.

Functions of the Skin

The six principal functions of the skin are protection, sensation, heat regulation, excretion, secretion, and absorption.

1. **Protection** The skin protects the body from injury and bacterial invasion. The outermost layer of the epidermis is rendered water-resistant

by a thin layer of sebum and fatty lipids. The fatty lipids, known as the barrier function, exist between the cells and are produced through the cell renewal process. This outermost layer is resistant to wide variations in temperature, minor injuries, chemically active substances, and many forms of bacteria.

2. **Sensation** By stimulating different sensory nerve endings, the skin responds to heat, cold, touch, pressure, and pain. When the nerve endings are stimulated, a message is sent to the brain. You respond by saying "Ouch" if you feel pain, by scratching if you have an itch, or by pulling away if you touch something hot. Some sensory nerve endings are located near hair follicles (figure 7-7).

3. **Heat regulation** The skin protects the body from the environment. A healthy body maintains a constant internal temperature of about 98.6 degrees Fahrenheit (37 degrees Celsius). As changes occur in the outside temperature, the blood and sudoriferous glands of the skin make necessary adjustments to allow the body to be cooled by the evaporation of sweat.

4. **Excretion** Perspiration from the sudoriferous glands is excreted through the skin. Water lost through perspiration takes salt and other chemicals with it.

5. **Secretion** Sebum is secreted by the sebaceous glands. This oil lubricates the skin, keeping it soft and pliable. Oil also keeps hair soft. Emotional stress and hormone imbalances can increase the flow of sebum.

6. **Absorption** Some ingredients can be absorbed by the outer layers of the skin, but very few ingredients can penetrate the epidermis. Small amounts of fatty materials, such as those used in many advanced skin care formulations, may be absorbed between the cells and through the hair follicles and sebaceous gland openings. However, cosmetic products are not formulated to penetrate the epidermis.

figure 7-7
Sensory nerve endings in the skin

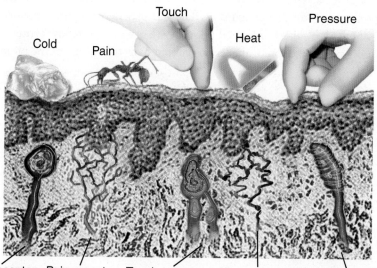

Cold receptor   Pain receptor   Touch receptor   Heat receptor   Pressure receptor

After reading the next few sections, you will be able to:

LO ③   Name the classes of nutrients essential for good health.

LO ④   Identify the food groups and dietary guidelines recommended by the U.S. Department of Agriculture (USDA).

LO ⑤   List and describe the vitamins that can help the skin.

Promote Nutrition and Skin Health

For your own benefit, as well as for the benefit of your clients, you should have a basic understanding of how to maintain healthy skin by making the right nutritional choices. You have heard people say, "You are what you eat." Mainly, that is very true. To keep the body healthy, people must ensure that what they eat helps regulate hydration (keeping a healthy level of water in the body), oil production, and overall function of the cells. Skin disorders, fatigue, stress, depression, and some diseases can be caused by an unhealthful diet or improper hydration.

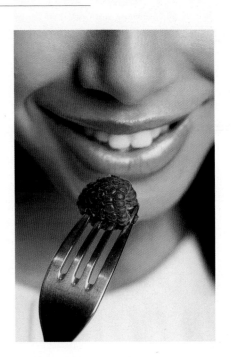

Essential Nutrients

There are six classes of nutrients that the body needs:

1. **Carbohydrates**—needed for energy to run every function within the body.

2. **Vitamins**—required for many body functions to occur.

3. **Fats**—needed for many body functions including hormones, sebum production, and absorption of fat soluble vitamins A, D, E, and K.

4. **Minerals**—used by cells to produce important biochemicals that have many body functions.

5. **Proteins**—important for building muscle and blood tissues, and for cell repair and replacement.

6. **Water**—makes up 50 to 70 percent of the body's weight and is necessary for virtually every function of the cells and body.

These essential nutrients are obtained through eating and drinking. The body cannot make nutrients in sufficient amounts to sustain itself properly.

The United States Department of Agriculture (USDA) developed a special program to help people determine the amounts of food they need to eat from the five basic food groups. It is called MyPlate and can be viewed at choosemyplate.gov. The food groups are:

- Grains

- Dairy

- Vegetables

- Protein foods (examples: meat, poultry, seafood, beans, and eggs)

- Fruits

? DID YOU KNOW?

If you want more information about nutrition, you can go to the USDA's special website at choosemyplate.gov. There many information sources on this easy-to-use page including daily nutrition advice, healthy recipes and meal planning, and weight loss information.

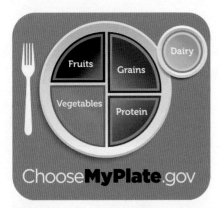

Courtesy of U.S. Department of Agriculture.

figure 7-8
MyPlate shows the five food groups and their appropriate proportions.

Eating the recommended amounts of foods from the five basic groups is the best way to support and maintain the health of the skin. See the recommended daily food amounts in **figure 7-8**.

In addition to following the recommendations included in the MyPlate program, the USDA and the United States Department of Health and Human Services have established dietary guidelines to assist people with a balanced diet. For much more information on necessary vitamins and minerals in the diet, check out the National Institute of Health's (NIH) page at nlm.nih.gov/medlineplus/ and search for "vitamins."

- Eat a variety of foods. Check out choosemyplate.gov for the right mix of foods.

- Select a diet that is high in fresh fruits, vegetables, and grain products and low in fats, saturated fat, and cholesterol.

- Eat moderate amounts of salt and sugar, including the sodium and modified sugars that are in prepared food products.

- Drink an appropriate amount of water. (See the formula in the Did You Know? sidebar to determine the appropriate amount of water based on your body weight.)

- Keep consumption of alcoholic beverages to a minimum.

- Balance your diet with the right amount of physical activity.

- Maintain or improve your weight.

Vitamins and Dietary Supplements

Vitamins play an important role in the skin's health, often aiding in healing and softening the skin and in fighting diseases. There 13 essential vitamins: A, C, D, E, K, and 8 B-complex vitamins. Vitamins A, D, E, and K are fat-soluble vitamins, found in fats in foods, and can be stored in the body. Vitamins C and B-complex are water-soluble, meaning the body uses and loses them quickly, so they must be replenished regularly.

Vitamins such as A, C, D, and E have been shown to have positive effects on the skin's health when taken by mouth. If a person's daily food consumption is lacking in nutrients, vitamin and mineral supplements

❓ DID YOU KNOW?

Do you want to know how much water you should drink every day? Here is an easy formula that will tell you the number of ounces of water you should be drinking each day:

Divide your body weight by two. The result is the number of ounces of water that you should drink every day. Example: 160 pounds ÷ 2 = 80 ounces of water.

Keep in mind that the average water bottle that most people carry with them holds just a bit over 16 ounces (1 pint). Therefore, a person who weighs 160 pounds should drink at least 5 bottles of water. (80 ounces ÷ 16 ounces = 5 bottles.)

People who are very active should drink even more water.

One of the best ways to follow a healthy diet is to read food labels. Food labels can help you select healthy foods. Food labels also contain nutrition facts about serving size, number of servings per container, calorie information, and the quantities of nutrients per serving. If you have any questions or concerns about the ingredients or nutritional value of a food product, contact the manufacturer by telephone or through a website to obtain supplemental information.

purchased through a health food store, vitamin store, or pharmacy can help provide some of the nutrients needed. Be sure to read the recommended daily allowance (RDA) for each vitamin and mineral supplement. These recommendations are listed on the supplement labels. Again, if you have any questions or concerns about the supplements, especially if the level of any nutrient is over 100 percent of the RDA, contact the manufacturer either by telephone or through a website. Remember that vitamins are nutritional supplements, not cosmetic ingredients. In fact, the law prohibits manufactures from claiming that any skin care product or cosmetic has nutritional value.

The following vitamins can help the skin in significant ways:

- **Vitamin A** supports the overall health of the skin and aids in the health, function, and repair of skin cells. It has been shown to improve the skin's elasticity and thickness.

- **Vitamin C** is an important substance needed for the proper repair of the skin and tissues. This vitamin aids in and accelerates the skin's healing processes. Vitamin C also is vitally important in fighting the aging process and promotes the production of collagen in the skin's dermal tissues, keeping the skin healthy and firm.

- **Vitamin D** enables the body to properly absorb and use calcium, the element needed for proper bone development and maintenance. Vitamin D also promotes rapid healing of the skin.

- **Vitamin E** helps protect the skin from the harmful effects of the sun's UV light. Some people claim that vitamin E helps to heal damage to the skin's tissues when taken by mouth.

Because the nutrients the body needs for proper functioning and survival must come primarily from what we eat and drink, you should not depend on supplements to make up for poor nutrition. If your daily food consumption is lacking in nutrients, you should strive to improve your diet rather than relying on vitamins and mineral supplements to provide nourishment.

Clients may occasionally ask you about nutrition and their skin. You can refer them to some of the informational websites listed within this chapter. If clients ask you detailed questions about nutrition, you should tell them to seek the advice of a physician or a registered dietician/nutritionist.

Water and the Skin

There is one element that no person can live without: water. To function properly, the body relies heavily on the benefits of water. This is especially true when it comes to the skin. Water composes 50 to 70 percent of body weight. The amount of water needed by an individual varies depending on body weight and the level of daily physical activity (figure 7-9).

Drinking pure water is essential to the health of the skin and body because it sustains the health of the cells, assists with the elimination of toxins and waste, helps regulate the body's temperature, and aids in proper digestion. All these functions, when performing properly, help keep the skin healthy, vital, and attractive.

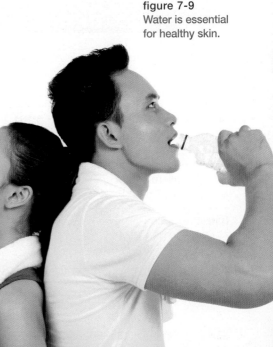

figure 7-9
Water is essential for healthy skin.

REVIEW QUESTIONS

1 Define *dermatology*.

2 Briefly describe healthy skin.

3 Name the main divisions of the skin and the layers within each division.

4 List the three types of nerve fibers found in the skin.

5 Name the two types of glands contained within the skin and describe their functions.

6 What are collagen and elastin?

7 Explain how collagen and elastin can be weakened.

8 What are the six important functions of the skin?

9 What are the six classes of nutrients that the body needs and how are they obtained?

10 What are the five basic food groups?

11 Can the skin be nourished with cosmetic products?

12 Name four vitamins that can help the skin and describe how they help.

13 What is the one essential item that no person can live without and why is it essential to the skin and body?

STUDY TOOLS

- **Reinforce what you just learned:** Complete the activities and exercises in your Theory or Practical Workbook, or your Study Guide.

- **Expand your knowledge:** Search for websites about the topics in this chapter and make a list of additional resources.

- **Study and prepare for your quiz:** Take the chapter test in your Exam Review or your Milady U: Online Licensing Prep.

- **Re-Test your knowledge:** Take the Chapter 7 *Quizzes*!

- **Learn even more:** Look up in a dictionary or search the internet for the definitions of any additional terms you want to learn about.

CHAPTER GLOSSARY

acne AK-nee	p.161	Also known as *acne vulgaris*; skin disorder characterized by chronic inflammation of the sebaceous glands from retained secretions and Propionibacterium acnes (P. acnes) bacteria.
acne vulgaris AK-nee vull-GAIR-us	p.161	Also known as *acne*; a skin disorder characterized by chronic inflammation of the sebaceous glands from retained secretions and bacteria known as Propionibacterium acnes (P. acnes) bacteria.
arrector pili muscles ah-REK-tohr PY-leh MUS-uls	p.157	Small, involuntary muscles in the base of the hair follicle that cause goose flesh, sometimes called *goose bumps*, and papillae.
barrier function BEAR-ee-ur FUNK-shun	p.156	The complex of lipids between the cells that keep the skin moist by preventing water evaporation, and to guard against irritants penetrating the skin surface.

broad spectrum sunscreen	p.159	Means that the sunscreen product has been shown to protect against both UV-A and UV-B radiation of the sun.
callus KAL-us	p.155	Thickening of the skin caused by continued, repeated pressure on any part of the skin, especially the hands and feet.
closed comedo closed KAHM-uh-doe	p.161	Plural: comedones (KAHM-uh-dohnz). Also known as *whitehead*; a follicle impacted with dead cells and solidified sebum, appearing as a small white bump just under the skin surface. Closed comedones have an extremely small surface opening.
collagen KAHL-uh-jen	p.160	Fibrous protein that gives the skin form and strength.
dermal papillae DUR-mul puh-PIL-eye	p.157	Singular: dermal papilla (DUR-mul puh-PIL-uh). Small, cone-shaped elevations at the base of the hair follicles that fit into the hair bulb.
dermatologist dur-muh-TAHL-uh-jist	p.154	Physician who specializes in diseases and disorders of the skin, hair, and nails.
dermatology dur-muh-TAHL-uh-jee	p.154	Medical branch of science that deals with the study of skin and its nature, structure, functions, diseases, and treatment.
dermis DUR-mis	p.156	Also known as *derma*, *corium*, *cutis*, or *true skin*; underlying or inner layer of the skin.
elastin ee-LAS-tin	p.160	Protein base similar to collagen that forms elastic tissue.
epidermal–dermal junction ep-ih-DUR-mul–DUR-mul JUNK-shun	p.157	The top of the papillary layer where it joins the epidermis.
epidermis ep-uh-DUR-mis	p.156	Outermost and thinnest layer of the skin; it is made up of five layers: stratum corneum, stratum lucidum, stratum granulosum, stratum spinosum, and stratum germinativum.
esthetician es-thuh-TISH-un	p.154	A specialist in the cleansing, beautification, and preservation of the health of skin on the entire body, including the face and neck.
eumelanin yoo-MEL-uh-nin	p.159	A type of melanin that is dark brown to black in color. People with dark-colored skin mostly produce eumelanin. There are two types of melanin; the other type is pheomelanin.
keratin KAIR-uh-tin	p.156	Fibrous protein of cells that is also the principal component of hair and nails.
melanin MEL-ah-nin	p.158	Tiny grains of pigment (coloring matter) that are produced by melanocytes and deposited into cells in the stratum germinativum layer of the epidermis and in the papillary layers of the dermis. There are two types of melanin: pheomelanin, which is red to yellow in color, and eumelanin, which is dark brown to black.
melanocytes muh-LAN-uh-syts	p.156	Cells that produce the dark skin pigment called melanin.
motor nerve fibers MOH-tur NURV FY-burs	p.158	Fibers of the motor nerves that are distributed to the arrector pili muscles attached to hair follicles. Motor nerves carry impulses from the brain to the muscles.

open comedo OH-pen KAHM-uh-doe	p.161	Plural: comedones (KAHM-uh-dohnz). Also known as *blackhead*; hair follicle filled with keratin and sebum.
papillary layer PAP-uh-lair-ee LAY-ur	p.157	Outer layer of the dermis, directly beneath the epidermis.
papule PAP-yool	p.161	Also known as *pimple*; small elevation on the skin that contains no fluid but may develop pus.
pheomelanin fee-oh-MEL-uh-nin	p.159	A type of melanin that is red to yellow in color. People with light-colored skin mostly produce pheomelanin. There are two types of melanin; the other type is eumelanin.
pimple	p.161	Also known as *papule*; small elevation on the skin that contains no fluid but may develop pus.
Propionibacterium acnes pro-PEE-ah-nee-back-tear-ee-um AK-nes	p.161	Abbreviated P. acnes; technical term for acne bacteria.
pustule PUS-chool	p.161	Raised, inflamed papule with a white or yellow center containing pus in the top of the lesion referred to as the "head" of the pimple.
reticular layer ruh-TIK-yuh-lur LAY-ur	p.157	Deeper layer of the dermis that supplies the skin with oxygen and nutrients; contains fat cells, blood vessels, sudoriferous (sweat) glands, hair follicles, lymph vessels, arrector pili muscles, sebaceous (oil) glands, and nerve endings.
sebaceous glands sih-BAY-shus GLANZ	p.161	Also known as *oil glands*; glands connected to hair follicles. Sebum is the fatty or oily secretion of the sebaceous glands.
sebum SEE-bum	p.161	A fatty or oily secretion that lubricates the skin and preserves the softness of the hair.
secretory coil seh-KREET-toh-ree KOYL	p.160	Coiled base of the sudoriferous (sweat) gland.
secretory nerve fibers seh-KREE-toh-ree NURV FY-burs	p.158	Fibers of the secretory nerve that are distributed to the sudoriferous glands and sebaceous glands. Secretory nerves, which are part of the autonomic nervous system (ANS), regulate the excretion of perspiration from the sweat glands and control the flow of sebum to the surface of the skin.
sensory nerve fibers SEN-soh-ree NURV FY-burs	p.158	Fibers of the sensory nerves that react to heat, cold, touch, pressure, and pain. These sensory receptors send messages to the brain.
stratum corneum STRAT-um KOR-nee-um	p.156	Also known as *horny layer*; outer layer of the epidermis.
stratum germinativum STRAT-um jer-mih-nah-TIV-um	p.156	More commonly called the basal cell layer; deepest, live layer of the epidermis that produces new epidermal skin cells and is responsible for growth.
stratum granulosum STRAT-um gran-yoo-LOH-sum	p.156	Also known as *granular layer*; layer of the epidermis composed of cells that look like granules and are filled with keratin; replaces cells shed from the stratum corneum.
stratum lucidum STRAT-um LOO-sih-dum	p.156	Clear, transparent layer of the epidermis under the stratum corneum.
stratum spinosum STRAT-um spy-NOH-sum	p.156	The spiny layer just above the stratum germinativum layer.

subcutaneous tissue sub-kyoo-TAY-nee-us TISH-oo	p.157	Also known as *adipose* or *subcutis tissue*; fatty tissue found below the dermis that gives smoothness and contour to the body, contains fat for use as energy, and also acts as a protective cushion for the outer skin.
sudoriferous glands sood-uh-RIF-uhrus GLANZ	p.160	Also known as *sweat glands*; excrete perspiration and detoxify the body by excreting excess salt and unwanted chemicals.
sweat glands	p.160	They excrete perspiration and detoxify the body by excreting excess salt and unwanted chemicals.
tactile corpuscles TAK-tile KOR-pusuls	p.157	Small epidermal structures with nerve endings that are sensitive to touch and pressure.
vitamin A	p.165	Supports the overall health of the skin; aids in the health, function, and repair of skin cells; has been shown to improve the skin's elasticity and thickness.
vitamin C	p.165	An important substance needed for proper repair of the skin and tissues; promotes the production of collagen in the skin's dermal tissues; aids in and promotes the skin's healing process.
vitamin D	p.165	Enables the body to properly absorb and use calcium, the element needed for proper bone development and maintenance. Vitamin D also promotes rapid healing of the skin.
vitamin E	p.165	Helps protect the skin from the harmful effects of the sun's UV light.

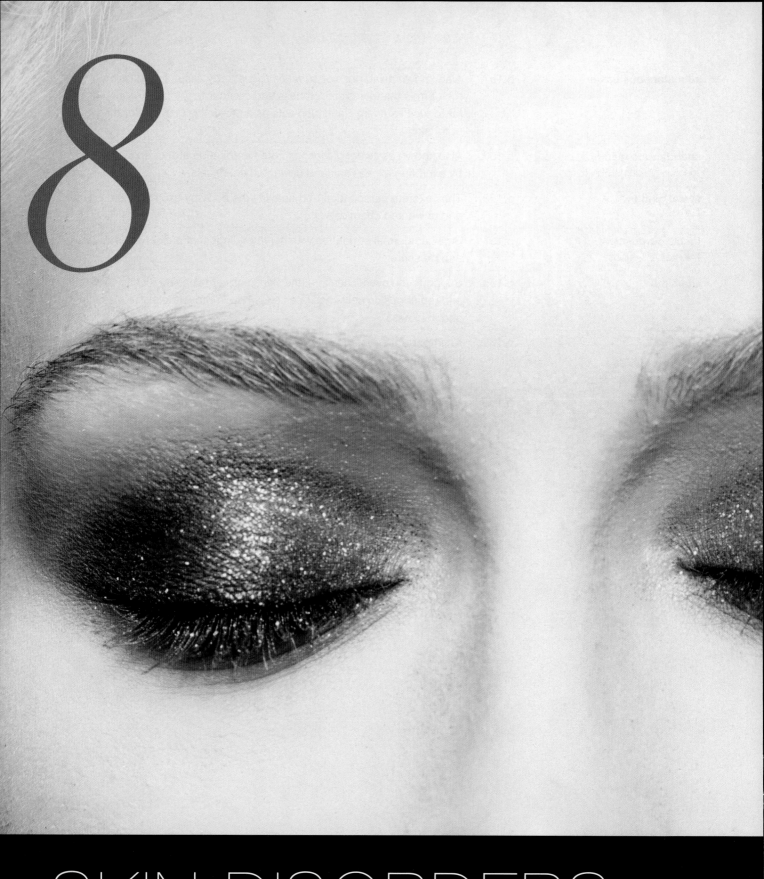

8

SKIN DISORDERS & DISEASES

LEARNING OBJECTIVES

After completing this chapter, you will be able to:

LO 1
Identify and describe common skin lesions, differentiating between primary and secondary lesions.

LO 2
List and describe common disorders of the sebaceous glands.

LO 3
List and describe common changes in skin pigmentation.

LO 4
Identify the forms of skin cancer including symptoms and mortality rates.

LO 5
Identify and describe the major causes of acne and current treatments.

LO 6
List the factors that contribute to the aging of the skin.

LO 7
Explain the effects of exposure to the sun on the skin.

LO 8
Describe contact dermatitis and prevention measures for cosmetologists.

Skin is the largest organ of the body and vital to our very existence! While it is designed to protect us, it is also the most visible organ of the body, and healthy skin is often associated with good health in general. Choosing a career in skin care to help people achieve maximum skin health and overcome or reduce the effects of skin disorders can be very rewarding.

Skin care specialists are in high demand in many salons and spas and earn excellent salaries. Some stylists find caring for the skin less arduous and physically demanding than styling hair and choose to balance their day by scheduling services in both areas. Whatever your reason, skin care is an area of rapid change and growth and a topic on most clients' minds. Knowing the basics of skin care and how the skin functions will allow you to advise clients on their skin care regimens when they seek your professional opinion.

why study
SKIN DISORDERS AND DISEASES?

Cosmetologists should study and have a thorough understanding of skin disorders and diseases for the following reasons:

> Providing even the most basic of skin care services requires an understanding of the underlying structure of the skin and common skin problems.

> The ability to recognize skin disorders and know when the client should be referred for medical treatment or when they can be treated by the cosmetologist is essential.

> Being fully qualified to offer skin care treatments adds another dimension of service for your clients.

Identify Disorders and Diseases of the Skin

Like any other organ of the body, the skin is susceptible to a variety of diseases, disorders, and ailments. In your work as a practitioner, you will often see skin and scalp disorders, so you must be prepared to recognize certain common skin conditions and know which you can help to treat and which must be referred to a physician. Occasionally, you may be asked to apply or use on a client a scalp treatment prescribed by a

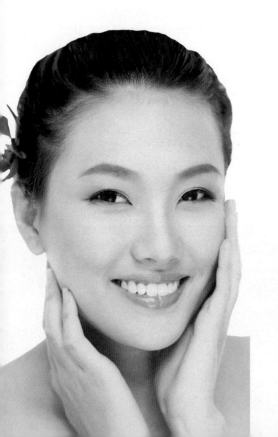

physician, which must be applied in accordance with a physician's directions.

A dermatologist is a physician who specializes in diseases and disorders of the skin, hair, and nails. Dermatologists attend four years of college, four years of medical school, and then complete specialty training in dermatology. When referring your client for medical evaluation, it may be helpful to explain the role of a dermatologist, although many clients will start first with their family doctor.

It is very important that a salon not serve a client who is suffering from an inflamed skin disorder, infectious or not, without a physician's note permitting the client to receive services. The cosmetologist should be able to recognize these conditions and sensitively suggest that proper measures be taken to prevent more serious consequences. One of the most visible signs of an issue with the skin is inflammation that may present as swelling and redness, often with no known cause. While some inflammation lasts for a very short period, such as a sunburn, and may leave a scar, long-term inflammation is the most concerning as it can cause permanent damage to the tissues. If your client has long-term inflammation of the skin, it is important to refer them to a physician to determine the cause and discuss possible treatments.

Numerous important terms relating to skin, scalp, and hair disorders that you should be familiar with are described in subsequent sections.

After reading the next few sections, you will be able to:

LO❶ Identify and describe common skin lesions, differentiating between primary and secondary lesions.

Lesions of the Skin

A **lesion** (LEE-zhun) is a mark on the skin that may indicate an injury or damage that changes the structure of tissues or organs. A lesion can be as simple as a freckle or as dangerous as a skin cancer. Lesions can indicate skin disorders or diseases and may be symptomatic of other internal diseases. Being familiar with the principal skin lesions will help you be able to distinguish between conditions that may and may not be treated in a salon or spa.

Primary Lesions of the Skin

Primary lesions (PRY-mayr-ee LEE-zhun) are lesions that are a different color than the color of the skin and/or lesions that are raised above the surface of the skin. They are often differentiated by size and layers of skin affected. These may require medical referral. Refer to **table 8-1** for a description of primary lesions and examples of each.

table 8-1

PRIMARY LESIONS

Primary lesions	Pronunciation	Image	Graphic	Description	Examples
Bulla	BULL-uh, (plural: bullae [BULL-ay])			Large blister containing a watery fluid; similar to a vesicle. Requires medical referral.	Contact dermatitis, large second degree burns, bulbous impetigo, perriphigus
Cyst and **tubercle**	SIST TOO-bur-kul	© Courtesy DermNet NZ		Closed, abnormally developed sac that contains pus, semifluid, or morbid matter, above or below the skin. A cyst can be drained of fluid and a tubercle cannot. Requires medical referral.	*Cyst*: Severe acne *Tubercle*: Lipoma, erythema nodosum
Macule	MAK-yool, (plural: maculae [MAK-yuh-ly])	© Aneese/Photos.com		Flat spot or discoloration on the skin.	Freckle or "liver" spot
Nodule	NOD-yool	© Sue McDonald /Shutterstock.com		A solid bump larger than 0.4 inches (1 cm) that can be easily felt. Requires medical referral.	Swollen lymph nodes, rheumatoid nodules
Papule	PAP-yool	© Ocskay Bence/Shutterstock.com		A small elevation on the skin that contains no fluid, but may develop pus.	Acne, warts, elevated nevi

Primary lesions	Pronunciation	Image	Graphic	Description	Examples
Pustule	PUS-chool	© Faiz Zaki/Shutterstock.com		Raised, inflamed, papule with a white or yellow center containing pus in the top of the lesion.	Acne, impetigo, folliculitis
Tumor	TOO-mur	© Courtesy DermNet NZ		Abnormal mass varying in size, shape, and color. Any type of abnormal mass, not always cancer. Requires medical referral.	Cancer
Vesicle	VES-ih-kel			Small blister or sac containing clear fluid, lying within or just beneath the epidermis. Requires medical referral if cause is unknown or untreatable with over-the-counter products.	Poison ivy, poison oak
Wheal	WHEEL	© Margoe Edwards/Shutterstock.com		An itchy, swollen lesion that can be caused by a blow, scratch, bite of an insect, or urticaria (skin allergy), or the sting of a nettle. Typically resolves on its own, but referral to a physician should be considered when the condition lasts more than three days.	Hives, mosquito bites

Secondary Lesions

Secondary skin lesions (SEK-un-deh-ree SKIN LEE-zhun) are characterized by piles of material on the skin surface, such as a crust or scab, or by depressions in the skin surface, such as an ulcer. Refer to table 8-2 for a description of secondary lesions and examples of each.

table 8-2

SECONDARY LESIONS

Secondary lesion	Pronunciation	Image	Graphic	Description	Examples
Crust	kruhst	© Pan Xunbin/Shutterstock.com		Dead cells that form over a wound or blemish while healing; accumulation of sebum and pus, sometimes mixed with epidermal cells.	Scab, sore
Excoriation	ek-skor-ee-AY-shun	R. Baran "The Nail in Differential Diagnosis" with permission of Informa (London).		Skin sore or abrasion produced by scratching or scraping.	Nail cuticle damage from nail biting
Fissure	FISH-ur	© librakv/Shutterstock.com		Crack in the skin that penetrates the dermis.	Severely cracked and/or chapped hands, lips, or feet
Keloid	KEE-loyd			A thick scar resulting from excessive growth of fibrous tissue. Keloids will form along any type of scar for people susceptible to them.	
Scale	skeyl	© librakv/Shutterstock.com		Thin, dry, or oily plate of epidermal flakes.	Excessive dandruff, psoriasis

Secondary lesion	Pronunciation	Image	Graphic	Description	Examples
Scar or **cicatrix**	Skahr OR SIK-uh-triks	© Geo-grafika/Shutterstock.com		Slightly raised or depressed area of the skin that forms as a result of the healing process related to an injury or lesion.	Post-operative repair
Ulcer	UL-sur	© Ilya Andriyanov/Shutterstock.com		Open lesion on the skin or mucous membrane of the body; accompanied by loss of skin depth and possibly weeping of fluids or pus. Requires medical referral, particularly in clients with underlying medical conditions such as diabetes.	Chicken pox, herpes

After reading the next few sections, you will be able to:

LO**2** List and describe common disorders of the sebaceous glands.

Identify Disorders of the Sebaceous (Oil) Glands

There are several common disorders of the sebaceous (oil) glands that the cosmetologist should be able to understand and identify.

An *open comedo*, also known as *blackhead*, is a hair follicle filled with keratin and sebum. Comedones appear most frequently on the face, especially in the T-zone—the center of the face (**figure 8-1**). When the sebum of the comedo is exposed to the environment, it oxidizes and turns black. When the follicle is closed and not exposed to the environment, the sebum remains a white or cream color and is a *closed comedo*, also known as *whitehead*, and appears as a small bump just under the skin surface.

figure 8-1
Comedones

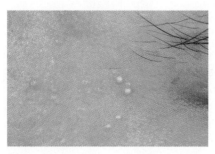

figure 8-2
Milia

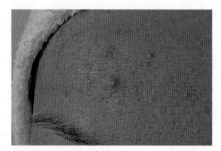

figure 8-3
Acne

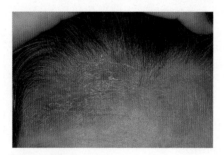

figure 8-4
Seborrheic dermatitis

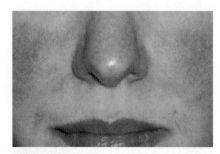

figure 8-5
Rosacea

Comedones can be removed by trained beauty professionals as long as proper procedures are employed and the procedure is performed in a clean environment using extraction implements that have been properly cleaned and disinfected.

Milia (MIL-ee-uh) are benign, keratin-filled cysts that appear just under the epidermis and have no visible opening. They resemble small sesame seeds and are almost always perfectly round. They are commonly associated with newborn babies, but can appear on the skin of people of all ages. They are usually found around the eyes, cheeks, and forehead, and they appear as small, firm whitish masses (figure 8-2). Milia is often mistakenly called whiteheads; however, whiteheads are soft in comparison. Depending on the state, milia can be treated in the salon or spa.

Acne, also known as *acne vulgaris*, is a skin disorder characterized by chronic inflammation of the sebaceous glands from retained secretions and bacteria known as propionibacterium acnes (P. acnes), the scientific term for acne bacteria. Acne will be discussed in further detail later in this chapter (figure 8-3).

A **sebaceous cyst** (sih-BAY-shus SIST) is a large, protruding pocket-like lesion filled with sebum. Sebaceous cysts are frequently seen on the scalp and the back and may be surgically removed by a dermatologist.

Seborrheic dermatitis (seb-oh-REE-ick derm-ah-TIE-tus) is a skin condition caused by an inflammation of the sebaceous glands, and is often characterized by redness, dry or oily scaling, crusting, and/or itchiness (figure 8-4). The red, flaky skin often appears in the eyebrows and beard, in the scalp and hairline, at the middle of the forehead, and along the sides of the nose. Mild flares of seborrheic dermatitis are sometimes treated with cortisone creams. Seborrheic dermatitis is a medical condition, but it can be helped in the salon with the application of non-fatty skin care products designed for sensitive skin. Severe cases should be referred to a dermatologist, who will often prescribe topical antifungal medications.

Rosacea (roh-ZAY-shuh), formerly called *acne rosacea*, is a chronic condition that appears primarily on the cheeks and nose. It is characterized by flushing (redness), **telangiectasis** (tee-lang-jek-tay-shuhz) distended or dilated surface blood vessels), and, in some cases, the formation of papules and pustules. The cause of rosacea is unknown, but the condition is thought to be genetic. Certain factors are known to aggravate the condition in some individuals. These include exposure to heat, sun, and very cold weather; ingestion of spicy foods, caffeine, and alcohol; and stress. Rosacea can be treated and kept under control by using medication prescribed by a physician, using proper skin care products designed for especially sensitive skin, and avoiding the aggravating flare factors listed above (figure 8-5).

Identify Disorders of the Sudoriferous (Sweat) Glands

Anhidrosis (an-hih-DROH-sis) is a deficiency in perspiration or the inability to sweat, often a result of damage to autonomic nerves. This condition can be life threatening and requires medical attention.

Bromhidrosis (broh-mih-DROH-sis) is foul-smelling perspiration, usually noticeable in the armpits or on the feet, that is generally caused by bacteria. There are several effective treatments that vary from over-the-counter preparations to Botox injections and the use of lasers on the sweat glands. Severe cases require medical referral.

Hyperhidrosis (hy-per-hy-DROH-sis) is excessive sweating, caused by heat or general body weakness. Requires medical referral.

Miliaria rubra (mil-ee-AIR-ee-ah ROOB-rah), also known as *prickly heat*, is an acute inflammatory disorder of the sweat glands, characterized by the eruption of small, red vesicles accompanied by burning, itching skin. It is caused by exposure to excessive heat and usually clears in a short time without treatment.

Recognize Inflammations and Common Infections of the Skin

Conjunctivitis (kuhn-juhngk-tuh-VAHY-tis), also known as *pinkeye*, is an infection of the eye(s) and may be caused by a bacteria or a virus. It is generally extremely contagious, and clients who have conjunctivitis or obviously irritated eyes should be politely rescheduled and referred to a physician immediately. Any product touching infected eyes must be thrown away and all implements properly cleaned and disinfected.

Dermatitis (der-mah-TY-tis) is a term broadly used to describe any inflammatory condition of the skin.

Eczema (EG-zuh-muh) is an inflammatory, uncomfortable, and often chronic disease of the skin. It is characterized by moderate to severe inflammation, scaling, and sometimes severe itching. There are several different types of eczema. The most common type is atopic eczema, which is an inherited genetic disorder. Eczema is not contagious. All cases of eczema should be referred to a physician for treatment, which is often topical cortisone (figure 8-6).

Herpes simplex I (HER-peez SIM-pleks) is a recurring viral infection that often presents as a fever blister or cold sore, although many people have no symptoms. It is characterized by the eruption of a single vesicle or group of vesicles on a red swollen base. The blisters usually appear on the lips, nostrils, or other part of the face, and the sores can last up to three weeks. Herpes simplex II is caused by the same virus and is designated as type II because it occurs below the waist. Herpes simplex is contagious (figure 8-7) and requires medical referral. Drugs are now available to control the symptoms, but the virus always remains in the body of infected persons.

Impetigo (im-pet-EYE-go) is a contagious bacterial skin infection characterized by weeping lesions and usually caused by a staphylococcus bacteria. Impetigo normally occurs on the face (especially around the nasal passages) and is most frequently seen in children, although it is possible at

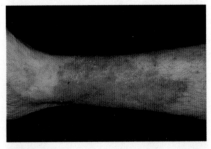

figure 8-6
Eczema

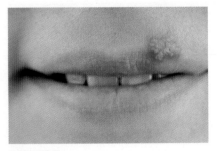

figure 8-7
Herpes simplex I

any age. Clients with any type of weeping, open facial lesions should be politely rescheduled and referred to a physician immediately.

Psoriasis (suh-RY-uh-sis) is a skin disease characterized by red patches covered with silver-white scales and is usually found on the scalp, elbows, knees, chest, and lower back. It is rarely found on the face. Psoriasis is caused by skin cells turning over faster than normal and when the condition is irritated, bleeding points can occur. Psoriasis is not contagious, but it requires medical referral. It is treatable, but it is not curable.

After reading the next few sections, you will be able to:

LO ③   List and describe common changes in skin pigmentation.

Recognize Pigment Disorders of the Skin

Pigment can be affected by internal factors such as heredity or hormonal fluctuations, or by external factors such as prolonged exposure to the sun. Abnormal colorations, known as **dyschromias** (dis-chrome-ee-uhs), accompany skin disorders and are symptoms of many systemic disorders. A change in pigmentation can also be observed when certain medications are being taken, such as photosensitivity related to use of certain antibiotics. The following disorders relate to changes in the pigmentation of the skin.

Hyperpigmentation (hy-pur-pig-men-TAY-shun) means darker than normal pigmentation, appearing as dark splotches. **Hypopigmentation** (hy-poh-pig-men-TAY-shun) is the absence of pigment, resulting in light or white splotches.

Albinism (AL-bi-niz-em) is congenital hypopigmentation, or absence of melanin pigment in the body, including the skin, hair, and eyes. Hair is silky white (**figure 8-8**). The skin is pinkish white and will not tan. The eyes are pink and the skin is sensitive to light and ages prematurely.

Chloasma (kloh-AZ-mah), also known as the *mask of pregnancy*, is a condition characterized by hyperpigmentation on the skin in spots that are not elevated. They are generally caused by cumulative sun exposure and can be helped by exfoliation or can be treated by a dermatologist.

Lentigines (len-TIJ-e-neez) (singular: lentigo [len-TY-goh]) is the technical term for freckles—small yellow-colored to brown-colored spots on skin exposed to sunlight and air. It is also commonly referred to as liver spots in older adults, although there is no relationship to the liver.

Leukoderma (loo-koh-DUR-mah) is a skin disorder characterized by light, abnormal patches (hypopigmentation); it is caused by a burn, scar, inflammation, or congenital disease that destroys the pigment-producing cells. Examples are vitiligo and albinism.

Nevus (NEE-vus), also known as *birthmark*, is a small or large malformation of the skin due to abnormal pigmentation or dilated capillaries.

Stain is an abnormal brown-colored or wine-colored skin discoloration with a circular or irregular shape (**figure 8-9**). Its permanent color is due to

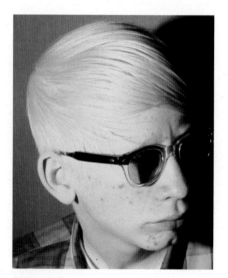

figure 8-8
Albinism

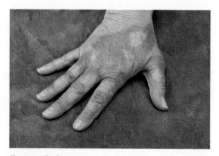

figure 8-9
Port wine stain

the presence of darker pigment. Stains can be present at birth, or they can appear during aging, after certain diseases, or after the disappearance of moles, freckles, and liver spots. The cause is often unknown.

Tan is the change in pigmentation of skin caused by exposure to the sun or ultraviolet light.

Vitiligo (vi-til-EYE-goh) is a hereditary condition that causes hypopigmented spots and splotches on the skin that often appear milky white. Recent research suggests that this disorder is part of an autoimmune disease (**figure 8-10**). Skin with vitiligo must be protected from overexposure to the sun.

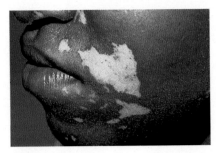

figure 8-10
Vitiligo

List Hypertrophies of the Skin

A **hypertrophy** (hy-PUR-truh-fee) of the skin is an abnormal growth of the skin. Many hypertrophies are benign, which means they are harmless.

A **keratoma** (kair-uh-TOH-mah) is an acquired, superficial, thickened patch of epidermis. A callus is a keratoma that is caused by continued, repeated pressure or friction on any part of the skin, especially the hands and feet. If the thickening grows inward, it is called a corn.

A **mole** is a small brownish spot or blemish on the skin, ranging in color from pale tan to brown or bluish black. Some moles are small and flat, resembling freckles; others are raised and darker in color. Large dark hairs often occur in moles. Any change in a mole requires medical attention.

A **skin tag** is a small brown-colored or flesh-colored outgrowth of the skin (**figure 8-11**). Skin tags occur most frequently on the neck and chest and can be easily removed by a dermatologist.

A **verruca** (vuh-ROO-kuh), also known as *wart*, is a hypertrophy of the papillae and epidermis. It is caused by a virus and is infectious. Verruca can spread from one location to another, particularly along a scratch in the skin. A dermatologist can be helpful in removing and reducing the recurrence of warts.

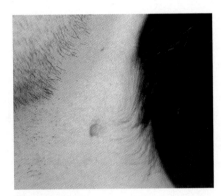

figure 8-11
Skin tags

After reading the next few sections, you will be able to:

LO❹ Identify the forms of skin cancer including symptoms and mortality rates.

Understand Skin Cancer

Skin cancer has become one of the most common cancers because of the large number of people diagnosed every year. It is also becoming one of the most common causes of cancer-related deaths because of general complacency about prevention and a lack of knowledge about the signs and real risks, particularly in young people. Cosmetologists should recognize the signs of potential skin cancer and always refer clients to see a physician. In this case, "better safe than sorry" is absolutely true! Do not let someone's young age or general good health stop you from being the one who saves someone's life through early diagnosis and treatment. There are three types of skin cancer (table 8-3).

Clients should be advised to regularly see a dermatologist for checkups of the skin, especially if any changes in coloration, size, or shape of a mole are detected, if the skin bleeds unexpectedly, or a lesion or scrape does not heal quickly.

Home self-examinations can also be an effective way to check for signs of potential skin cancer between scheduled doctor visits. When performing a self-care exam, clients should be advised to check for any changes in existing moles and pay attention to any new visible growths on the skin. Clients should also be advised to ask a spouse, friend, or loved one to check areas they cannot adequately see on a routine basis. This would include the back, scalp, and around the ears.

If detected early, anyone with these three forms of skin cancer has a good chance for survival. Cosmetologists serve a unique role by being able

table 8-3

TYPES OF SKIN CANCER

Moles	Description	Image
Normal Mole	Small brownish spot on the skin ranging in color from pale tan to brown or bluish black. *Note*: This is NOT a type of skin cancer.	
Basal Cell Carcinoma (BAY-zul SEL kar-sin-OH-mah)	Most common and least severe skin cancer; characterized by light or pearly nodules and has a 90 percent survival rate with early diagnosis and treatment.	
Squamous Cell Carcinoma (SKWAY-mus SEL kar-sin-OH-mah)	More serious than basal cell carcinoma; characterized by scaly red papules or nodules. It can spread to other parts of the body and survival rates depend on the stage at diagnosis.	
Malignant Melanoma (muh-LIG-nent mel-uh-NOH-mah)	Least common, but most dangerous, form of skin cancer; characterized by black or dark brown patches on the skin that may appear uneven in texture, jagged, or raised. Malignant melanoma is the least common, but is 100 percent fatal if left untreated—early detection and treatment can result in a 94 percent five-year survival rate, but that drops drastically (62 percent) once it reaches local lymph nodes.	

© D. Kucharski K. Kucharska/Shutterstock.com

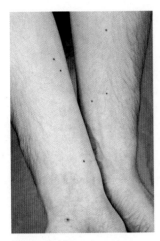

figure 8-12a
Normal mole

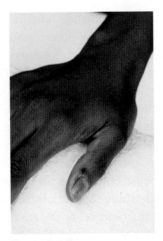

figure 8-12b
Normal mole

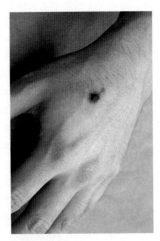

figure 8-12c
Moles with cancerous lesions

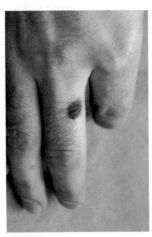

figure 8-12d
Moles with cancerous lesions

to recognize the appearance of serious skin disorders and referring the client to a dermatologist for diagnosis and treatment.

According to the American Cancer Society, professionals should use the ABCDE Cancer Checklist to spot signs of change in existing moles (figure 8-12 a–d):

When checking existing moles, look for changes in any of the following:

A. Asymmetry. One half of the mole does not match the other half.

B. Border irregularity. The edges of the mole are ragged or notched.

C. Color. The color of the mole is not the same all over. There may be shades of tan, brown, or black, and sometimes even patches of red, blue, or white.

D. Diameter. The mole is wider than about ¼" (although doctors are now finding melanomas that are smaller).

E. Evolution. The mole evolves or changes; it may include darkening or variations in color, it may itch or hurt; it may change in shape or growth.

For more information, contact the American Cancer Society at cancer.org or (800) ACS-2345.

After reading the next few sections, you will be able to:

LO ⑤ Identify and describe the major causes of acne and current treatments.

Examine Acne and Problem Skin

Common skin problems that affect clients' appearance, such as acne, can become a source of great concern, although most people have acne or another skin issue at some time in their lives. Acne is both a skin

> ⚠ **CAUTION**
> Do not treat moles or remove hair from moles. Removing a hair from a mole could irritate or cause a structural change to it. Only a physician should remove a hair from a mole.

disorder and an esthetic problem, and it is a major concern to anyone who suffers from it. Frequently misunderstood to be a teenage skin disorder, it can affect people at almost any age. Women often do not have acne problems until they reach their 20s, 30s, or beyond. Because acne affects the appearance, it is of interest to cosmetologists and estheticians, who are in a position to help their clients with treatment for minor cases or to provide dermatological referral for more severe acne.

A predisposition to acne is based on heredity and hormones. People with acne inherit the tendency to retain cells that gather on the walls of the follicle, eventually clumping and obstructing the follicle. Hormone levels directly affect the function of the sebaceous glands, increasing or decreasing the amount of sebum on the skin.

Retention hyperkeratosis (ree-TEN-shun HY-per-kera-toe-sis) is the hereditary tendency for acne-prone skin to retain dead cells in the follicle, forming an obstruction that clogs follicles and exacerbates inflammatory acne lesions such as papules and pustules.

The oiliness level of the skin is also hereditary. Overproduction of sebum by the sebaceous gland contributes to the development of acne by coating the dead cell buildup in the follicle with sebum, which hardens due to oxidation. This conglomeration of dead cells and solidified sebum obstruct the follicle.

Propionibacterium acne (P. acnes) is **anaerobic** (ann-air-ROH-bic), which means that these bacteria cannot survive in the presence of oxygen. When the follicles are obstructed, oxygen is blocked from the bottom of the follicles, allowing acne bacteria to multiply.

The main food source for acne bacteria is fatty acids, which are easily obtained from the abundance of sebum in the follicle. These bacteria flourish in this ideal environment, which has plenty of food (sebum) for the bacteria and is void of oxygen. The bacteria multiply, causing inflammation and swelling in the follicle, and eventually rupture the follicle wall. When the wall of the follicle ruptures, the immune system is alerted, causing blood to rush to the ruptured follicle, carrying white blood cells to fight the bacteria. Blood will surround and engulf the follicle, which is what causes the redness in pimples.

An acne papule is an inflammatory acne lesion resulting from this wall rupture and infusion of blood. A pustule forms from the papule when enough white blood cells accumulate to form pus, which is primarily composed of dead white blood cells.

Acne Treatment

Minor forms of acne can be treated without medical referral. The basics of acne treatment involve:

- Daily use of gentle cleansers formulated for a specific skin type. The use of harsh cleansers can make skin too dry and sebaceous glands will generate more sebum, creating an even bigger problem! These foamy, rinse-off products remove dirt, debris, and excess oil from the skin. Toners may be helpful for clients with excessively oily skin.

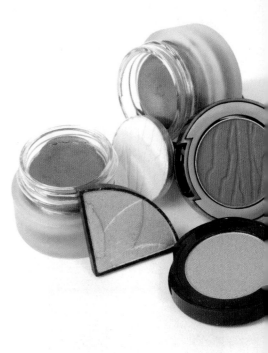

- Follicle exfoliants are leave-on products that help to remove cell buildup from the follicles, allowing oxygen to penetrate the follicles, killing bacteria. Commonly used ingredients in these products are alpha hydroxy acid, salicylic acid, and benzoyl peroxide. Benzoyl peroxide can be especially effective since it helps to shed cellular debris and also kill the acne bacteria. These are generally not used all over because of their drying properties, and are only used as a spot treatment.

- Avoidance of fatty skin care and cosmetic products is important because products that contain large amounts of fatty materials and oils can cause follicles to clog from the outside. Make sure all makeup and skin care products used on acne-prone skin are **noncomedogenic** (non-com-EE-doh-JENN-ic), which means the product has been designed and proven not to clog the follicles.

- Use of a light moisturizer to keep skin balanced and reduce the risk of excess sebum production can be helpful.

- Mild and moderate cases of acne are often treated by trained salon and spa professionals who have received specialized education in acne treatment.

After reading the next few sections, you will be able to:

LO ⑥　List the factors that contribute to the aging of the skin.

Analyze Aging Skin Issues

Aging of the skin is a concern of almost every client over 30 years of age, and has become a major area for new services and retail revenue within the salon and spa environment. There are two types of factors that influence aging of the skin: intrinsic factors and extrinsic factors.

Intrinsic Factors

Intrinsic factors (in-TRIN-zic FAK-torz) are skin-aging factors over which we have little control:

- Genetics and ethnicity play a significant role in how our skin will age. Our predisposition to skin disorders and our ability to tolerate sun exposure also play a role.

- Gravitational pull is the constant pulling downward on our skin and bodies and is a consistent factor for everyone.

- Facial expressions are the repeated movements of the face and result in the formation of expression lines, such as crow's-feet lines that form around the eyes; nasolabial folds that form from the corners of the nose to the corners of the mouth; and scowl lines that form between the eyes.

Extrinsic Factors

Extrinsic factors (ex-TRIN-zic FAK-torz) are primarily environmental factors that contribute to aging and the appearance of aging. Many scientists and dermatologists believe that these extrinsic factors are responsible for up to 85 percent of skin aging. Extrinsic factors include:

figure 8-13
Effects of aging and sun damage

Wrinkles of aging

Static lines

Dynamic lines

- Exposure to the sun. Tanning and sun bathing are significant offenders in the prevention of both aging and cancers of the skin and should always be discouraged by skin care professionals. However, the cumulative sun that we get in little doses every day also causes significant damage to the skin of most people and is the number one cause of the appearance of premature aging (figure 8-13). The key to preventing this prominent skin-aging factor is to use a broad-spectrum sunscreen every single day, and the easiest way to do this is to find a daily-use moisturizer with built-in sunscreen. As a cosmetologist, you can help your clients find the best sunscreen and moisturizer to use every day.

- Smoking is bad for more than just your lungs! It is bad for your body as a whole and does significant damage to the skin. Smoking produces tremendous numbers of **free radicals** (FREE RAD-ih-culs), unstable molecules that cause biochemical aging. These molecules, over time, can have a devastating effect on the body, causing wrinkling and sagging of the skin, particularly on the face and neck. Smoking also causes oxygen deprivation of the skin and body, which ultimately affects blood flow so the skin does not get adequate blood nutrients. This lack of blood flow causes the accumulation of cellular waste, often called toxins.

- Overuse of alcoholic beverages also has an overall effect on the body and the skin. Alcohol use inhibits the body from repairing itself and interferes with proper nutrition distribution to the skin and body tissues. Alcohol also dehydrates the skin by drawing essential water out of the tissues, which causes the skin to appear dull and dry.

- Individually, smoking and overuse of alcoholic beverages contribute to the aging process, but the combination of the two can be devastating to the tissues. The constant dilation and contraction that occur on the tiny capillaries and blood vessels, as well as the constant deprivation of oxygen and water to the tissues, quickly make the skin appear lifeless and dull. In these circumstances, it is very difficult for the skin to adjust and repair itself and the damage done by these lifestyle habits can be impossible to repair or diminish—often leaving people looking much older than they are.

- Stress plays a significant role in our overall health and contributes to premature aging of all organs, including the skin. Research now confirms that stress causes biochemical changes at the cellular level that can lead to the tissue damage that we call aging. Exercise, relaxation techniques, and a healthy state of mind can reduce stress levels, as can relaxing treatments like facials, aromatherapy, and massage.

- Poor nutrition deprives the skin of the proteins, fats, carbohydrates, vitamins, and minerals that are required to maintain, protect, and repair the skin, keeping it looking young and beautiful. Eating a well-balanced diet allows for all body systems to function at maximum performance and nourish the fragile tissues of the skin. One of the first signs of eating disorders is the dull complexion associated with repeated deprivation of needed nutrients.

- Exposure to pollution produces free radicals, interferes with proper oxygen consumption, and affects the lungs and other internal organs as well as the skin. The best defense against pollutants is the simplest one: Follow a good daily skin care routine. Routine washing and mild exfoliating (removing dead surface skin cells) help to remove the buildup of pollutants that have settled on the skin's surface throughout the day. The application of daily moisturizers, protective lotions, and even foundation products all help to protect the skin from airborne pollutants.

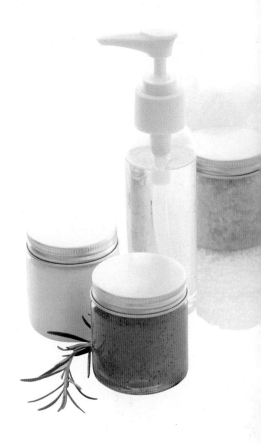

The appearance of aging skin can be greatly improved by practicing a good skin care program, especially at home. A professionally designed program for aging skin based on the client's needs, skin type, and condition severity involves a good hydrating sunscreen, an alpha or beta hydroxy acid exfoliating product, and products using state-of-the-art ingredients such as peptides and topical antioxidants designed specifically for aging skin.

© Khomulo Anna/Shutterstock.com

After reading the next few sections, you will be able to:

LO **7** Explain the effects of exposure to the sun on the skin.

Understand the Sun and Its Effects

The sun and its ultraviolet (UV) light have the greatest impact of all extrinsic factors on how skin ages. Approximately 80 to 85 percent of the symptoms of aging skin are caused by the accumulation of damaging rays from the sun. As we age, the collagen and elastin fibers of the skin naturally weaken, and this weakening happens at a much faster rate when the skin is frequently exposed to UV light without proper protection. When we call UV light a "UV ray" that is just a shorter way of saying that it is a form of radiation, and as such it can be damaging!

UVA rays, also known as *aging rays*, are deep-penetrating rays that can even go through a glass window. These rays weaken the collagen and elastin fibers, causing wrinkling and sagging of the tissues.

UVB rays, also known as *burning rays*, cause sunburns, tanning of the skin, and the majority of skin cancers. These are shorter rays that stop penetration at the base of the epidermis.

? DID YOU KNOW?
People used to believe light traveled in straight rays, but we now know that it oscillates in wave formations, called wavelengths. The word *ray* still remains, as UV rays, UVA and UVB rays or light rays, but it represents the term *radiation*.

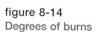

DID YOU KNOW?

You can actually get second-degree burns from sunburn (**figure 8-14**).

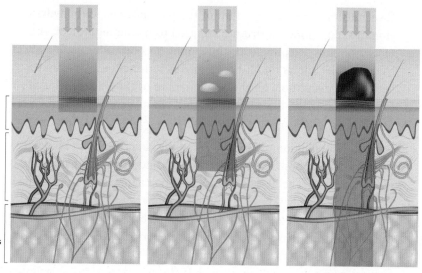

Epidermis

Dermis

Hypodermis - Subcutaneous fat

First degree burn   **Second degree burn**   **Third degree burn**

figure 8-14
Degrees of burns

© Alila Medical Media/Shutterstock.com

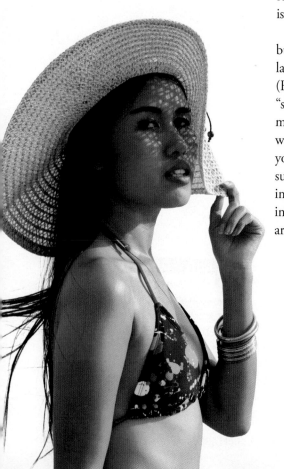

Protection from the Sun

The most common form of protection from the sun that most people think of is sunscreen, which is commonly applied to the face and body in anticipation of time in the sun. SPF stands for Sun Protection Factor and this number roughly designates the amount of time a person can be in the sun without burning when applied correctly. However, the actual amount of time that any specific SPF can offer protection is based on the time of day, altitude, skin type, and amount of sunscreen applied. The SPF only truly works when sunscreen is applied correctly. Clothing actually offers some barrier SPF, but it is minimal with hats offering an SPF of 5 and most cotton shirts an SPF of 6.

Two types of rays, UVA and UVB, are responsible for tanning and burning of the skin, so it is important to look for a sunscreen that is labeled as "broad spectrum," indicating it protects against UVA and UVB (FDA). Although some older sunscreen labels may read "waterproof" or "sweat proof," those claims are no longer allowed by the FDA. A sunscreen may only be labeled as "water resistant" and must indicate whether it is water resistant for 40 or 80 minutes. It is important that you talk with your clients about how to protect their skin from the damaging rays of the sun and the risks of skin cancer, offering them useful advice. It is also important that as a professional you stay up to date on the latest information and rules surrounding sun protection by reading current articles and visiting websites like FDA.gov.

- The number one way to prevent premature skin aging is to avoid deliberate sun exposure and to use a broad-spectrum sunscreen, which is one that filters both UVA and UVB rays and has an SPF (Sun Protection Factor) of at least 15, on a daily basis. Look for products that contain zinc oxide or titanium dioxide.

- Avoid prolonged exposure to the sun during peak hours, when UV exposure is highest. This is usually between 10 AM and 3 PM, and this time can be extended when at high altitudes or areas closer to the equator.

© Gina Smith/Shutterstock.com

- Sunscreen should be applied at least 30 minutes before sun exposure to allow time for absorption. Many people make the mistake of applying sunscreen after they have been exposed to the heat and sun for 30 minutes or more. The already inflamed skin is more likely to react to the sunscreen chemicals when the sunscreen is applied after sun exposure.

- Apply sunscreen liberally after swimming and after activities that result in heavy perspiration. If the skin is exposed to hours of sun, such as during a boat trip or day at the beach, sunscreen should be applied periodically throughout the day as a precaution.

- Avoid exposing children younger than six months of age to the sun.

- People who are prone to burning frequently and easily should wear a hat and protective clothing when participating in outdoor activities, in addition to using sunscreen. Redheads and blue-eyed blonds are particularly susceptible to sun damage.

After reading the next few sections, you will be able to:

LO ⑧ Describe contact dermatitis and prevention measures for cosmetologists.

Recognize Contact Dermatitis

Contact dermatitis is the most common work-related skin disorder for all cosmetology professionals. **Contact dermatitis** (KAHN-takt dur-mah-TYT-is) is an inflammation of the skin caused by having contact with certain chemicals or substances. Many of these substances are commonly used in cosmetology. There are two types of contact dermatitis: allergic contact dermatitis and irritant contact dermatitis.

Allergic Contact Dermatitis

Allergic contact dermatitis (AL-urg-jic KAHN-takt der-mah-TIT-tis), abbreviated ACD, occurs when a person (cosmetologist or client) develops an allergy to an ingredient or a chemical, usually caused by repeated skin contact with the chemical. **Sensitization** (sen-sih-TIZ-aye-shun) is an allergic reaction created by repeated exposure to a chemical or a substance. Monomer liquids, haircolor, and chemical texture solutions are all common causes of allergic reactions with repeated exposures.

Once an allergy to a product has been established, all services being done with the product must be discontinued until the allergic symptoms clear. The person affected by the allergy (cosmetologist or client) must stop using that particular product. In severe or chronic cases, affected people should see a dermatologist for allergy testing.

Common places for allergic contact dermatitis are listed below and include:

- On the fingers, palms, or on the back of the hand.
- On the face, especially the cheeks.
- On the scalp, hairline, forehead, or neckline.

If you examine the area where the problem occurs, you can usually determine the cause. For example, stylists often strand test haircolor with their bare fingers and hands, so it is no surprise when they find contact dermatitis on their fingers and hands.

Irritant Contact Dermatitis

Irritant contact dermatitis (IRH-ih-tent KAHN-takt der-mah-TIH-tus), abbreviated ICD, occurs when irritating substances temporarily damage the epidermis. Unlike allergic contact dermatitis, irritant contact dermatitis is not usually chronic if precautions are taken.

Corrosive substances or exfoliating agents are examples of products with irritant potential. Contact with irritant chemicals can cause damage to the epidermis because the irritant can enter the skin surface and cause possible inflammation, redness, swelling, itching, and burning and repeated exposure can worsen the condition.

The best way to prevent both types of occupational contact dermatitis is to use gloves or utensils when working with irritating chemicals. Cosmetologists should use gloves or utensils when applying chemicals such as haircolor, straighteners, or permanent wave solutions. Nail technicians should use gloves or utensils when applying nail products such as monomer liquids and polymer powders. Estheticians should use gloves or utensils when applying exfoliants such as peeling products and drying agents. All of these chemicals can irritate the skin of the hands and arms if precautions are not taken to avoid contact.

Frequent hand washing can result in dry hands, with cracks in the skin that can cause more irritation and that can allow penetration of irritant chemicals. Hand washing is important to prevent the spread of disease, but it should be followed by the frequent use of protective hand creams to keep the hands in good condition.

Protect Yourself

Taking the time to keep your implements, tools, equipment, and surfaces clean and disinfected is an important step in protecting yourself and avoiding a skin problem. Practice these suggestions with great diligence:

- Take extreme care to keep brush handles, containers, and table tops clean and free from product, dust, and residue. Repeatedly handling these items will cause overexposure if the items are not kept clean.
- Wear protective gloves whenever using products known to cause irritant or allergic contact dermatitis.
- Keep your hands clean and moisturized. Keeping the skin of the hands in excellent condition will help prevent irritant reactions.

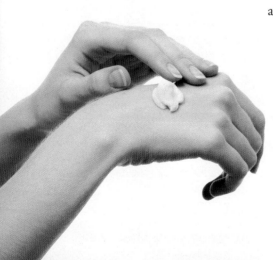

REVIEW QUESTIONS

1. Define a primary skin lesion and list three types.

2. Define a secondary skin lesion and list three types.

3. Name and describe at least five disorders of the sebaceous glands.

4. Name and describe at least five changes in skin pigmentation.

5. Name and describe the three forms of skin cancer.

6. What are the two major causes of acne and how should they be effectively treated?

7. What is the most significant factor in aging of the skin and increasing risk of all types of skin cancer?

8. Explain the effect of overexposure to the sun on the skin.

9. What is contact dermatitis and how it can be prevented?

STUDY TOOLS

- **Reinforce what you just learned:** Complete the activities and exercises in your Theory or Practical Workbook, or your Study Guide.

- **Expand your knowledge:** Search for websites about the topics in this chapter and make a list of additional resources.

- **Study and prepare for your quiz:** Take the chapter test in your Exam Review or your Milady U: Online Licensing Prep.

- **Re-Test your knowledge:** Take the Chapter 8 *Quizzes*!

- **Learn even more:** Look up in a dictionary or search the internet for the definitions of any additional terms you want to learn about.

CHAPTER GLOSSARY

acne	p. 178	A skin disorder characterized by chronic inflammation of the sebaceous glands from retained secretions and bacteria known as propionibacterium acnes (P. acnes), the scientific term for acne bacteria.
albinism AL-bi-niz-em	p. 180	Congenital hypopigmentation, or absence of melanin pigment of the body, including the skin, hair, and eyes.
allergic contact dermatitis AL-urg-jic KAHN-takt der-mah-TIT-tis	p. 189	Abbreviated ACD; an allergy to an ingredient or a chemical, usually caused by repeated skin contact with the chemical.
anaerobic ann-air-ROH-bic	p. 184	Cannot survive in the presence of oxygen.
anhidrosis an-hih-DROH-sis	p. 178	Deficiency in perspiration or the inability to sweat, often a result of damage to autonomic nerves.
basal cell carcinoma BAY-zul SEL kar-sin-OH-mah	p. 182	Most common and least severe type of skin cancer; often characterized by light or pearly nodules.

bromhidrosis broh-mih-DROH-sis	p. 179	Foul-smelling perspiration, usually noticeable in the armpits or on the feet, which is generally caused by bacteria.
bulla BULL-uh, (plural: BULL-ay)	p. 174	Plural: bullae. A large blister containing a watery fluid; similar to a vesicle, but larger.
chloasma kloh-AZ-mah	p. 180	Also known as *mask of pregnancy*; condition characterized by typically brown hyperpigmentation, generally on the face, which is not elevated.
cicatrix SIK-uh-triks	p. 177	Lightly raised mark on the skin formed after an injury or lesion of the skin has healed.
conjunctivitis kuhn-juhngk-tuh-VAHY-tis	p. 179	Also known as *pinkeye*; infection of the eye(s) that may be caused by a bacteria or a virus; generally extremely contagious.
contact dermatitis KAHN-takt der-mah-TYT-is	p. 189	An inflammation of the skin caused by having contact with certain chemicals or substances; many of these substances are used in cosmetology.
crust kruhst	p. 176	Dead cells that form over a wound or blemish while it is healing; an accumulation of sebum and pus, sometimes mixed with epidermal material.
cyst SIST	p. 174	Closed, abnormally developed sac that contains fluid, pus, semifluid, or morbid matter above or below the skin.
dermatitis der-mah-TY-tis	p. 179	Inflammatory condition of the skin.
dyschromias dis-chrome-ee-uhs	p. 180	Abnormal colorations of the skin that accompany skin disorders and are symptoms of many systemic disorders.
eczema EG-zuh-muh	p. 179	An inflammatory, uncomfortable, and often chronic disease of the skin; characterized by moderate to severe inflammation, scaling, and sometimes severe itching.
excoriation ek-skor-ee-AY-shun	p. 176	Skin sore or abrasion produced by scratching or scraping.
extrinsic factors ex-TRIN-zic FAK-torz	p. 186	Primarily environmental factors that contribute to aging and the appearance of aging.
fissure FISH-ur	p. 176	A crack in the skin that penetrates the dermis. Examples are severely cracked and/or chapped hands or lips.
free radicals FREE RAD-ih-culs	p. 186	Unstable molecules that cause biochemical aging, especially wrinkling and sagging of the skin.
herpes simplex I HER-peez SIM-pleks	p. 179	Recurring viral infection that often presents as a fever blister or cold sore.
hyperhidrosis hy-per-hy-DROH-sis	p. 179	Excessive sweating, caused by heat or general body weakness.
hyperpigmentation hy-pur-pig-men-TAY-shun	p. 180	Darker than normal pigmentation, appearing as dark splotches.
hypertrophy hy-PUR-truh-fee	p. 181	Abnormal growth of the skin.

hypopigmentation hy-poh-pig-men-TAY-shun	p. 180	Absence of pigment, resulting in light or white splotches.
impetigo im-pet-EYE-go	p. 179	Contagious bacterial skin infection characterized by weeping lesions; usually caused by a staphylococcus bacteria.
intrinsic factors in-TRIN-zic FAK-torz	p. 185	Skin-aging factors over which we have little control.
irritant contact dermatitis IRH-ih-tent KAHN-takt der-mah-TIH-tus	p. 190	Abbreviated ICD. Occurs when irritating substances temporarily damage the epidermis.
keloid KEE-loyd	p. 176	Thick scar resulting from excessive growth of fibrous tissue.
keratoma kair-uh-TOH-mah	p. 181	Acquired, superficial, thickened patch of epidermis. A callus is a keratoma caused by continued, repeated pressure or friction on any part of the skin, especially the hands and feet.
lentigines len-TIJ-e-neez (singular: len-TY-goh)	p. 180	Singular: lentigo. Technical term for freckles—small yellow-colored to brown-colored spots on skin exposed to sunlight and air.
lesion LEE-zhun	p. 173	A mark on the skin; may indicate an injury or damage that changes the structure of tissues or organs.
leukoderma loo-koh-DUR-mah	p. 180	Skin disorder characterized by light, abnormal patches (hypopigmentation); caused by a burn, scar, inflammation, or congenital disease that destroys the pigment-producing cells.
macule MAK-yool	p. 174	Plural: maculae (MAK-yuh-ly). Flat spot or discoloration on the skin, such as a freckle or a red spot left after a pimple has healed.
malignant melanoma muh-LIG-nent mel-uh-NOH-mah	p. 182	Most serious form of skin cancer; often characterized by black or dark brown patches on the skin that may appear uneven in texture, jagged, or raised.
milia MIL-ee-uh	p. 178	Benign, keratin-filled cysts that can appear just under the epidermis and have no visible opening.
miliaria rubra mil-ee-AIR-ee-ah ROOB-rah	p. 179	Also known as *prickly heat*; an acute inflammatory disorder of the sweat glands, characterized by the eruption of small, red vesicles and accompanied by burning, itching skin.
mole	p. 181	Small brownish spot or blemish on the skin, ranging in color from pale tan to brown or bluish black.
nevus NEE-vus	p. 180	Also known as *birthmark*; a small or large malformation of the skin due to abnormal pigmentation or dilated capillaries.
nodule NOD-yool	p. 174	A solid bump larger than 0.4 inches (1 centimeter) that can be easily felt.
noncomedogenic non-com-EE-doh-JENN-ic	p. 185	Product that has been designed and proven not to clog the follicles.
primary lesions PRY-mayr-ee LEE-zhuns	p. 173	Lesions that are a different color than the color of the skin, and/or lesions that are raised above the surface of the skin.

psoriasis suh-RY-uh-sis	p. 180	Skin disease characterized by red patches covered with silver-white scales; usually found on the scalp, elbows, knees, chest, and lower back. It is rarely found on the face.
retention hyperkeratosis ree-TEN-shun HY-per-kera-toe-sis	p. 184	The hereditary tendency for acne-prone skin to retain dead cells in the follicle, forming an obstruction that clogs follicles and exacerbates inflammatory acne lesions such as papules and pustules.
rosacea roh-ZAY-shuh	p. 178	Chronic condition that appears primarily on the cheeks and nose, and is characterized by flushing (redness), telangiectasis (distended or dilated surface blood vessels), and, in some cases, the formation of papules and pustules.
scale skeyl	p. 176	Any thin, dry, or oily plate of epidermal flakes. An example is abnormal or excessive dandruff.
scar Skahr	p. 177	Also known as *cicatrix*; a lightly raised mark on the skin formed after an injury or lesion of the skin has healed.
sebaceous cyst sih-BAY-shus SIST	p. 178	A large, protruding pocket-like lesion filled with sebum. Sebaceous cysts are frequently seen on the scalp and the back and may be surgically removed by a dermatologist.
seborrheic dermatitis seb-oh-REE-ick der-mah-TIE-tus	p. 178	Skin condition caused by an inflammation of the sebaceous glands. It is often characterized by redness, dry or oily scaling, crusting, and/or itchiness.
secondary skin lesions SEK-un-deh-ree SKIN LEE-uhns	p. 175	Characterized by piles of material on the skin surface, such as a crust or scab, or depressions in the skin surface, such as an ulcer.
sensitization sen-sih-TIZ-aye-shun	p. 189	Allergic reaction created by repeated exposure to a chemical or a substance.
skin tag	p. 181	A small brown-colored or flesh-colored outgrowth of the skin.
squamous cell carcinoma SKWAY-mus SEL kar-sin-OH-mah	p. 182	Type of skin cancer more serious than basal cell carcinoma; often characterized by scaly red papules or nodules.
stain	p. 180	Abnormal brown-colored or wine-colored skin discoloration with a circular and/or irregular shape.
tan	p. 181	Change in pigmentation of skin caused by exposure to the sun or ultraviolet light.
telangiectasis tee-lang-jek-tay-shuhz	p. 178	Distended or dilated surface blood vessels.
tubercle TOO-bur-kul	p. 174	Abnormal, rounded, solid lump above, within, or under the skin; larger than a papule.
tumor TOO-mur	p. 175	An abnormal mass varying in size, shape, and color.
ulcer UL-sur	p. 177	Open lesion on the skin or mucous membrane of the body; accompanied by pus and loss of skin depth and possibly weeping fluids or pus.

verruca vuh-ROO-kuh	p. 181	Also known as *wart*; hypertrophy of the papillae and epidermis.
vesicle VES-ih-kel	p. 175	Small blister or sac containing clear fluid, lying within or just beneath the epidermis.
vitiligo vi-til-EYE-goh	p. 181	Hereditary condition that causes hypopigmented spots and splotches on the skin that often appear milky white.
wheal WHEEL	p. 175	Itchy, swollen lesion that lasts only a few hours; caused by a blow or scratch, the bite of an insect, urticaria (skin allergy), or the sting of a nettle. Examples include hives and mosquito bites.

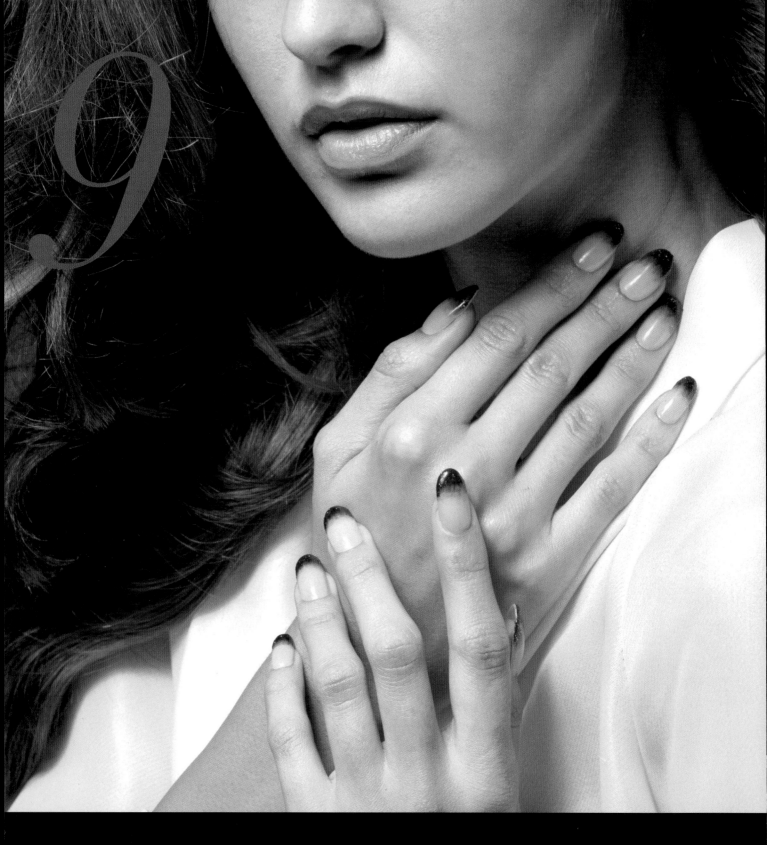

9

NAIL STRUCTURE
& GROWTH

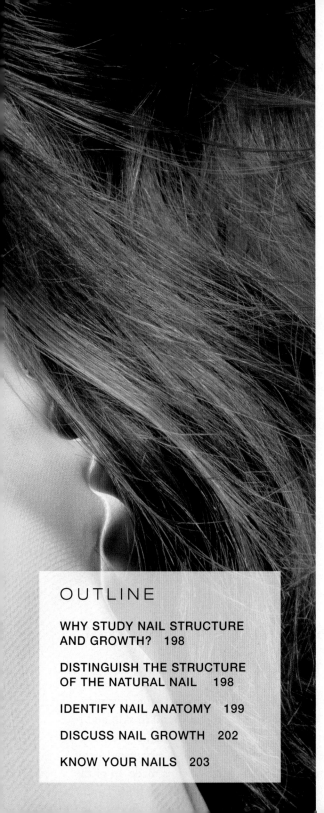

LEARNING OBJECTIVES

After completing this chapter, you will be able to:

LO❶
Describe the characteristics of normal, healthy nails.

LO❷
Describe the nine basic parts of the nail unit.

LO❸
Discuss how nails grow.

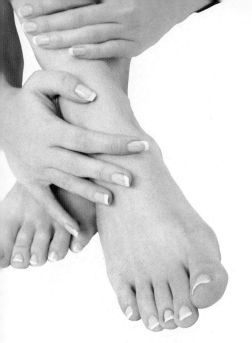

Y ou probably know that the natural nail has a cuticle. Do you know whether the cuticle is living or dead skin? And do you know where the plate and the bed are located in the natural nail? This chapter gives you the answers to these questions and more. So, read on, because you cannot perform professional nail services without understanding the structure and growth of the natural nail.

why study
NAIL STRUCTURE AND GROWTH?

Cosmetologists should study and have a thorough understanding of nail structure and growth because:

> Understanding the structure and growth of natural nails allows you to expertly groom, strengthen, and beautify nails.

> It is important to know the difference between the nail cuticle and the eponychium before performing nail services.

> Understanding the structure and growth cycles of the natural nail will prepare you for more advanced nail services.

After reading the next few sections, you will be able to:

LO **1**   Describe the characteristics of normal, healthy nails.

Distinguish the Structure of the Natural Nail

A **natural nail**, also known as *onyx* (AHN-iks), is the hard protective plate composed mainly of keratin, the fiber-shaped protein found in skin and hair. The keratin in natural nails is harder than the keratin in skin or hair. The natural nail is located at the end of the finger or toe. It is an appendage of the skin and is part of the integumentary system, which is made up of the skin and its various organs. Nail plates protect the tips of the fingers and toes, and their appearance can reflect the general health of the body.

A normal, healthy nail is firm but flexible. The surface is shiny, smooth, and unspotted with no wavy ridges, pits, or splits. A healthy nail also is whitish and translucent in appearance, with the pinkish color of the nail bed below showing through. In some races, the nail bed may have more yellow tones. The water content of the nail varies according to the relative humidity of the surrounding environment; in a humid environment, nails contain more water. A healthy nail may look dry and hard, but its water content is actually between 15 and 25 percent. The water content directly affects the nail's flexibility. The lower the water content, the more rigid the nail becomes. Using an oil-based nail conditioner or nail polish to coat the plate can reduce water loss or prevent excessive absorption and improve flexibility.

After reading the next few sections, you will be able to:

LO❷ Describe the nine basic parts of the nail unit.

Identify Nail Anatomy

The natural **nail unit** is composed of several major parts, including the nail plate, nail bed, matrix, cuticle, eponychium, perionychium, hyponychium, specialized ligaments, and nail folds (**figure 9-1**).

Nail Plate

The **nail plate** is a hardened keratin plate that sits on and covers the nail bed. It is the most visible and functional part of the nail unit. The nail plate is relatively porous and will allow water to pass through it much more easily than through normal skin of an equal thickness. As it grows, the nail plate slowly slides across the nail bed. The nail plate is formed by the matrix cells. The sole job of the matrix cells is to create nail plate cells. The nail plate may appear to be one solid piece, but is actually constructed of about 100 layers of nail cells. The **free edge** is the part of the nail plate that extends over the tip of the finger or toe.

Nail Bed

The **nail bed** is the portion of living skin that supports the nail plate as it grows toward the free edge. Because it is richly supplied with blood vessels, the nail bed has a pinkish appearance from the lunula to the area just before the free edge of the nail. The nail bed contains many nerves, and is attached to the nail plate by a thin layer of tissue called the **bed epithelium** (BED ep-ih-THEE-lee-um). The bed epithelium helps guide the nail plate along the nail bed as it grows. As a professional, you should understand the difference and use the proper names for the parts of the nail unit—for example, nail polish is applied to the nail "plate," not the nail "bed."

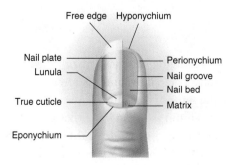

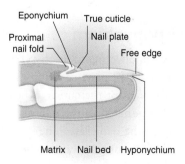

figure 9-1
Structure of the natural nail

Matrix

The **matrix** (MAY-trikz) is the area where the nail plate cells are formed. It is composed of matrix cells that produce the nail plate cells. The matrix area contains nerves, lymph, and blood vessels to nourish the matrix cells. As long as it is nourished and healthy, the matrix will continue to create new nail plate cells.

The matrix extends from under the nail fold at the base of the nail plate. The visible part of the matrix that extends from underneath the living skin is called the **lunula** (LOO-nuh-luh). It is the whitish, half-moon shape underneath the base of the nail. The whitish color is caused by the reflection of light off the surface of the visible part of the underlying matrix. The lighter color of the lunula shows the true color of the matrix. Every nail has a lunula, but some lunulas are short and remain hidden under the eponychium.

Growth and appearance of the nails can be affected if an individual is in poor health, if a nail disorder or disease is present, or if there has been an injury to the matrix.

Cuticle

The **cuticle** (KYOO-tih-kul) is the dead, colorless tissue attached to the natural nail plate. The cuticle comes from the underside of the skin that lies above the natural nail plate. This tissue sticks tight to the nail plate and can be difficult to remove. Its job is to seal the space between the natural nail plate and living skin above (the eponychium) to prevent entry of foreign material and microorganisms and to help avoid injury and infection.

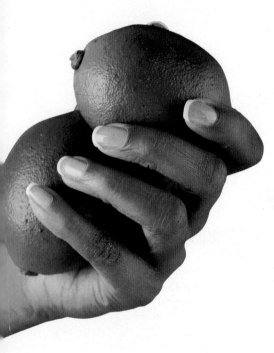

Sometimes the names used for professional nail products are confusing. To avoid this problem, know the proper names for the various parts of the nail unit and pay close attention to what the product is actually designed to do.

For example, look at products marketed as nail *cuticle moisturizers*, *softeners*, or *conditioners*. The cuticle is dead skin on the nail plate, so why are these products designed to moisturize, soften, and condition the cuticle? That does not make any sense! Cuticle moisturizers, softeners, and conditioners are *actually* designed for the eponychium, lateral sidewalls, and hyponychium—not for the cuticle!

Cuticle removers are properly named: they remove the dead cuticle. These professional products can quickly dissolve soft tissue and, when carefully applied to the nail plate, they speed up removal of stubborn cuticle tissue. Misunderstandings about the correct names for the parts of the nail cause a great deal of confusion, so make sure you learn these terms and use them properly.

Eponychium

The **eponychium** (ep-oh-NIK-ee-um) is the living skin at the base of the natural nail plate covering the matrix area. The eponychium is often mistaken for the cuticle. They are *not* the same. The cuticle is the *dead tissue* adhered to the nail plate; the eponychium is *living tissue* that grows up to the nail plate. The cuticle comes from the underside of this area where it completely detaches from the eponychium and strongly attaches to the new growth of nail plate. It pulls free to form a seal between the natural nail plate and the eponychium.

Many people cannot tell the difference between the nail cuticle and the eponychium, but it is easy when you use this simple checklist:

- Is the tissue adhering directly to the natural nail plate, but can be removed with gentle scraping?
- Is the tissue very thin and colorless, but easily visible under close inspection?
- Is the tissue nonliving and not directly attached to living skin?

If you answered yes to *any* of the questions above, then this tissue is called the *cuticle*.

- Is the tissue part of the skin that grows up to the base of the natural nail plate?
- Is the tissue any part of the skin that covers the nail matrix and lunula?
- If you cut deeply into this tissue, will it bleed?

If you answered yes to *any* of the questions above, this tissue is called the *eponychium*.

Cosmetologists are permitted to gently push back the eponychium, but are prohibited from cutting or trimming any part of the eponychium, since it is living skin. Cutting living skin is outside the scope of cosmetology and not allowed under any conditions or circumstances.

Perionychium

Perionychium (payr-eeuh-NIK-ee-um), as shown in figure 9-1, is the living skin bordering the root and sides of a fingernail or toenail.

Hyponychium

The **hyponychium** (hy-poh-NIK-ee-um) is the slightly thickened layer of skin under the nail that lies between the fingertip and the free edge of the nail plate. It forms a protective barrier that prevents microorganisms from invading and infecting the nail bed.

Specialized Ligaments

A **ligament** (LIG-uh-munt) is a tough band of fibrous tissue that connects bones or holds an organ in place. Specialized ligaments attach the nail bed and matrix bed to the underlying bone. These ligaments are located at the base of the matrix and around the edges of the nail bed.

Nail Folds

The **nail folds** are folds of normal skin that surround the nail plate. These folds form the **nail groove**, or furrow, on each side of the nail. The **sidewall**, also known as the *lateral nail fold* (LAT-ur-ul NAYL FOHLD), is the fold of skin overlapping the side of the nail.

ACTIVITY

Use a small magnifying glass to examine the hands of at least 10 friends or classmates. Look at the nail cuticle and eponychium on each finger. Observe how the thin cuticle tissue attaches to and rides on top of the nail plate as the cuticle emerges from under the eponychium at the base of the nail plate. Then examine the eponychium to see how these two differ in appearance from the cuticle. Identify which tissue can be removed and which tissue should never be cut.

Discuss Nail Growth

In Chapter 7, Skin Structure, Growth, and Nutrition, you learned that nutrition, exercise, and a person's general health affects the health of the skin. These factors affect the growth and health of the nail plate as well.

A normal nail grows forward from the matrix and extends over the tip of the finger. Normal, healthy nails can grow in a variety of shapes, depending on the shape of the matrix. The length, width, and curvature of the matrix determine the thickness, width, and curvature of the natural nail plate. For example, a longer matrix produces a thicker nail plate, and a highly curved matrix creates a highly curved free edge. No product or procedure can make the nail plate grow thicker because a thicker nail plate would require a larger matrix.

The average rate of nail plate growth in the normal adult is about ¹⁄₁₀" to ⅛" (2.5 mm to 3 mm) per month, but many factors affect this growth rate. Age, for example, affects nail growth. Compared with the nails of an average adult, children's nails grow more rapidly, while elderly adults' nails grow at a slower rate. Seasons also affect nail growth rate; nails grow faster in the summer than they do in the winter. Pregnancy dramatically affects nail growth because of hormonal changes in the body. Nail growth rates increase dramatically during the last trimester of pregnancy. The nail growth rate decreases quickly after delivery of the baby and returns to normal, as do hormone levels in the body. It is a myth that nail growth rate is increased by taking prenatal care vitamins; nail growth rates will accelerate whether or not a woman takes these vitamins. A nail's position on the body also affects its growth rate. Nail growth rate is fastest on the nail of the middle finger and slowest on the thumb, and toenails grow more slowly than fingernails. Although toenail plates grow more slowly than fingernail plates, they are thicker because the toenail matrix is longer than the matrix found on fingernails (figure 9-2).

figure 9-2
Various shapes of nails

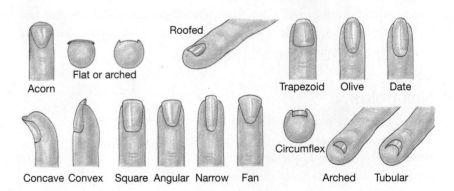

Acorn · Flat or arched · Roofed · Trapezoid · Olive · Date

Concave · Convex · Square · Angular · Narrow · Fan · Circumflex · Arched · Tubular

Nail Malformation

If the nail is abnormal in shape or form it is called **nail malformation**. This can be a temporary or permanent condition caused by disease, injury, or infection that has affected the matrix. In this case, it can change the shape or thickness of the nail plate and can appear altered or deformed. In fact, these conditions are generally the only reason a person will shed a nail. Healthy nails are not shed automatically or periodically in the way that healthy hair is shed. Ordinarily, replacement of a natural fingernail takes about four to six months. Toenails take about nine months to a year to be fully replaced.

The nail matrix is constantly creating new nail cells. Each time a new cell is created, it pushes the previously created cells upward and away from the matrix. This causes the plate to flow slowly toward the free edge, but only as quickly as new cells are produced. If a small portion of the matrix stops making new cells, the nail plate will become thinner and develop a narrow groove. As a person ages, parts of the nail matrix begin to permanently slow down production, causing the plate to develop a series of narrow grooves running down the length of the plate. This is considered to be a normal part of the aging process. Often these grooves are mistaken for "ridges." The matrix does not grow any ridges in the nail plate, only grooves, and filing away these so-called "ridges" only thins and weakens the entire nail plate.

Often after a disease, injury, or infection that has affected the nail's growth, the natural nail will return to its healthy growth as long as the matrix is healthy and undamaged. You will learn more about nail plate malformation and common disorders in the next chapter.

Know Your Nails

Many cosmetologists are interested in nails because of the creative opportunities they present. As with every other area of cosmetology, this creativity must be grounded in a full awareness of the structure and physiology of the nails and the surrounding tissue.

Working on strong, healthy nails can be a pleasure. Remember that as a licensed cosmetologist, you are allowed to work only on healthy nails and skin with no visible signs of disease or infection (figure 9-3).

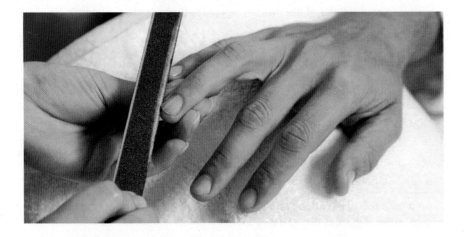

figure 9-3
Men's manicure

© bezikus/Shutterstock.com

REVIEW QUESTIONS

1. What is the technical term for the natural nail?

2. What is the major protein that makes up the natural nail?

3. Describe the appearance of a normal, healthy nail.

4. Name the basic parts of the nail unit.

5. Explain the difference between the nail plate and the nail bed.

6. What part of the nail unit contains the nerves, lymph, and blood vessels?

7. What is the difference between the cuticle and the eponychium?

8. Why are cosmetologists not allowed to cut the skin around the base of the nail plate, even if the client requests this during the service?

9. What can affect the growth of the nail plate?

STUDY TOOLS

- **Reinforce what you just learned:** Complete the activities and exercises in your Theory or Practical Workbook, or your Study Guide.

- **Expand your knowledge:** Search for websites about the topics in this chapter and make a list of additional resources.

- **Study and prepare for your quiz:** Take the chapter test in your Exam Review or your Milady U: Online Licensing Prep.

- **Re-Test your knowledge:** Take the Chapter 9 *Quizzes*!

- **Learn even more:** Look up in a dictionary or search the internet for the definitions of any additional terms you want to learn about.

CHAPTER GLOSSARY

bed epithelium BED ep-ih-THEE-lee-um	p. 199	Thin layer of tissue that attaches the nail plate and the nail bed.
cuticle KYOO-tih-kul	p. 200	Dead, colorless tissue attached to the natural nail plate.
eponychium ep-oh-NIK-ee-um	p. 200	Living skin at the base of the natural nail plate that covers the matrix area.
free edge	p. 199	Part of the nail plate that extends over the tip of the finger or toe.
hyponychium hy-poh-NIK-ee-um	p. 201	Slightly thickened layer of skin under the nail that lies between the fingertip and free edge of the natural nail plate.
ligament LIG-uh-munt	p. 201	Tough band of fibrous tissue that connects bones or holds an organ in place.
lunula LOO-nuh-luh	p. 200	Visible part of the matrix that extends from underneath the living skin; it is the whitish, half-moon shape at the base of the nail.
matrix MAY-trikz	p. 200	Area where the nail plate cells are formed; this area is composed of matrix cells that produce the nail plate.

nail bed	p. 199	Portion of the living skin that supports the nail plate as it grows toward the free edge.
nail folds	p. 201	Folds of normal skin that surround the natural nail plate.
nail groove	p. 201	Furrow on each side of the nail.
nail malformation	p. 203	When the nail is abnormal in shape or form.
nail plate	p. 199	Hardened keratin plate that sits on and covers the natural nail bed. It is the most visible and functional part of the natural nail unit.
nail unit	p. 199	Composed of several major parts of the fingernail including the nail plate, nail bed, matrix, cuticle, eponychium, hyponychium, specialized ligaments, and nail fold. Together, all of these parts form the nail unit.
natural nail	p. 198	Also known as *onyx*; the hard protective plate is composed mainly of keratin, the same fibrous protein found in skin and hair. The keratin in natural nails is harder than the keratin in skin or hair.
perionychium payr-eeuh-NIK-ee-um	p. 201	The tissue bordering the root and sides of a fingernail or toenail.
sidewall	p. 201	Also known as *lateral nail fold*; the fold of skin overlapping the side of the nail.

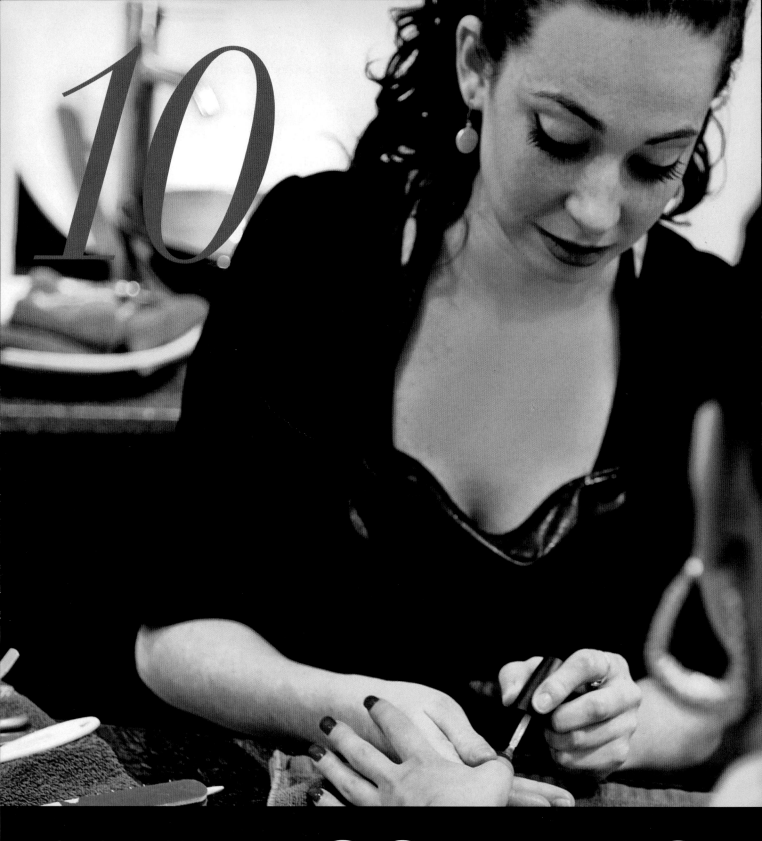

10

NAIL DISORDERS
& DISEASES

LEARNING OBJECTIVES

After completing this chapter, you will be able to:

LO❶
List and describe the various disorders and irregularities of nails.

LO❷
Recognize diseases of the nails that should not be treated in the salon.

LO❸
Perform a hand, nail, and skin analysis on a client.

OUTLINE

To perform professional and responsible service and care, you need to learn about the structure and growth of the nail, as you did in Chapter 9, Nail Structure and Growth. Now you must learn about the disorders and diseases of nails so that you will know when it is safe to work on a client. Nails are an interesting and surprising part of the human body. They are small mirrors into an individual's general health. Certain health conditions may first be revealed by a change in the nails, a visible disorder, or poor nail growth. Some conditions are easily treated in the salon—hangnails, for instance, or bruised nail beds that need camouflage—but some are infectious and cannot be treated by salon professionals. Carefully studying this chapter will vastly improve your knowledge and expertise in caring for nails.

why study
NAIL DISORDERS AND DISEASES?

Cosmetologists should study and have a thorough understanding of nail disorders and diseases because:

> You must be able to identify those conditions on a client's nails and determine if they should or should not be treated in the salon.

> You must acknowledge infectious conditions that may be present so you can take the appropriate steps to protect yourself and your clients from the spread of disease.

> You need to be able to recognize conditions that may signal mild to serious health problems that warrant the attention of a doctor.

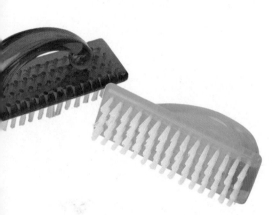

After reading the next few sections, you will be able to:

LO❶ List and describe the various disorders and irregularities of nails.

Pinpoint Common and Uncommon Nail Disorders

As you now know, a normal, healthy nail is firm but flexible. The surface is shiny, smooth, and unspotted with no wavy ridges, pits, or splits. A healthy nail also is whitish and translucent in appearance, with the pinkish color of the nail bed showing through. In some races, the nail bed may have more yellow tones. A **nail disorder** is a condition caused by injury,

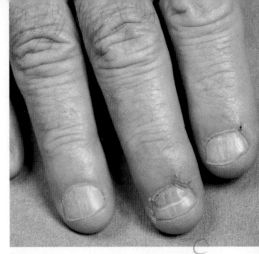

figure 10-1
Beau's lines

heredity, or previous disease of the nail unit. Most, if not all, of your clients have experienced a common nail disorder at some time in their lives. A cosmetologist should recognize common or normal disorders as well as abnormal nail conditions, understand what to do, and be able to help a client with a nail disorder in one of two ways:

- You can tell clients that they may have a disorder and refer them to a physician if required.

- You can cosmetically improve certain nail plate conditions if the problem is cosmetic and not a medical condition.

It is your professional responsibility and a requirement of your license to know which option to choose. A client whose nail or skin is infected, inflamed, broken, or swollen should not receive services and should be referred to a physician to determine the type of treatment that is required.

Common Nail Disorders

Beau's lines (BOWZ LYNEZ), sometimes called *furrows* (FUR-ohs) or *corrugations* (kor-uh-GAY-shuns), are visible depressions running across the width of the natural nail plate (figure 10-1). They usually result from major illness or injury that has traumatized the body, such as pneumonia, adverse drug reaction, surgery, heart failure, massive injury, or a long-lasting high fever. Beau's lines occur because the matrix slows down in producing nail cells for several weeks or a month. This causes the nail plate to grow thinner for a period of time. The nail plate thickness usually returns to normal after the illness or condition is resolved.

Blue fingernails, named for the nail bed color, is usually caused by a lack of circulating oxygen in the red blood cells. It may also represent a high level of an abnormal form of hemoglobin in the circulation. If normal color returns upon warming and/or massage, the cause is due to the fingers and nails not getting enough blood supply due to cold, constriction (of the tissues or the blood vessels that supply the tissues), or some other reason. If the fingernails remain blue, then there may be an underlying disease or structural abnormality interfering with the body's ability to deliver oxygenated red blood.

Bruised nail beds are a condition in which a blood clot forms under the nail plate, causing a dark purplish spot. These discolorations are usually due to small injuries to the nail bed. The dried blood absorbs into the nail bed epithelium tissue on the underside of the nail plate and grows out with it. Treat this injured nail gently and advise your clients to be more careful with their nails if they want to avoid this problem in the future. Advise them to treat their nails like jewels, not tools! This condition can usually be covered with nail polish or camouflaged with an opaque nail enhancement.

Discolored nails are nails that turn a variety of colors, which may indicate surface staining, a systemic disorder, or poor blood circulation. Although quite common, a discolored nail may be caused by several factors such as surface stains from nail polish, foods, dyes, or smoking. A discolored nail could also be caused by an internal discoloration of the nail plate due to biological, medical, or even pharmaceutical reasons.

DID YOU KNOW?
Clients cannot sign a waiver or verbally give a cosmetologist permission to disobey state or federal rules and regulations.

Eggshell nails are noticeably thin, white nail plates that are more flexible than normal. Eggshell nails are normally weaker and can curve over the free edge. The condition is usually caused by improper diet, hereditary factors, internal disease, or medication. Be very careful when manicuring these nails because they are fragile and can break easily. Use the fine side of an abrasive board (240 grit or higher) to file them gently, but only if needed. It is best not to file a nail plate of this type. A thin protective overlay of enhancement product can be helpful, but do not extend these nails beyond the free edge.

Hangnail is a condition in which the living skin around the nail plate splits and tears (figure 10-2). Dry skin or small cuts can result in hangnails. If there is no sign of infection or an open wound, advise the client that proper nail care, such as hot oil manicures, will aid in correcting the condition. Also, never cut the living skin around the natural nail plate, even if it is dry and rough looking. Other than to carefully remove the thin layer of dead cuticle tissue on the nail plate, you should not cut skin anywhere on the hands or feet. Hangnails can be carefully trimmed, as long as the living skin is not cut or torn in the process. It is against state board regulations to intentionally cut or tear the client's skin and can lead to serious infections for which you and the salon may be legally liable. If not properly cared for, a hangnail can become infected. Clients with symptoms of infections in their fingers should be referred to a physician. Signs of infection are redness, pain, swelling, or pus.

Koilonychia (koyal-oh-NICK-ee-uh) are soft spoon nails with a concave shape that appear scooped out. The depression is usually large enough to hold a drop of liquid. Often spoon nails are a sign of iron deficiency, anemia, or a liver condition known as hemochromatosis, in which your body absorbs too much iron from the food you eat. Spoon nails can also be associated with heart disease and hypothyroidism or other long-term illness.

Leukonychia spots (loo-koh-NIK-ee-ah SPATS), also known as *white spots*, are whitish discolorations of the nails, usually caused by minor injury to the nail matrix. It is a myth that these are caused by a vitamin or mineral deficiency (e.g., calcium or zinc). They appear frequently in the nails but do not indicate disease. As the nail continues to grow, the white spots eventually grow off and disappear (figure 10-3).

Melanonychia (mel-uh-nuh-NIK-ee-uh) is darkening of the fingernails or toenails. It may be seen as a black band within the nail plate extending from the base to the free edge (figure 10-4). In some cases, it may affect the

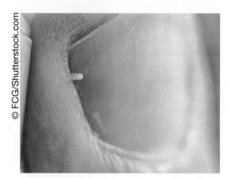

figure 10-2
Hangnail

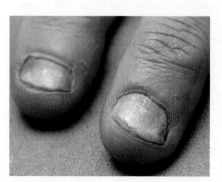

figure 10-3
Leukonychia spots

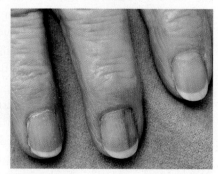

figure 10-4
Melanonychia

entire nail plate. A localized area of increased pigment cells (melanocytes), usually within the matrix, is responsible for this condition. As matrix cells form the nail plate, melanin is laid down within the plate by the melanocytes. This is a fairly common occurrence and considered normal in people of color, but could be indicative of a disease condition in Caucasians.

Onychophagy (ahn-ih-koh-FAY-jee), also known as *bitten nails*, is the result of a habit of chewing the nail or the hardened, damaged skin surrounding the nail plate (figure 10-5). Advise clients that frequent manicures and care of the hardened eponychium can often help them overcome this habit, at the same time improving the health and appearance of the hands. Sometimes the application of nail enhancements can beautify deformed nails and discourage the client from biting the nails. However, the bitten, damaged skin should not be treated by a cosmetologist. If the skin is broken or infected, no services can be provided until the area is healed.

Onychorrhexis (ahn-ih-koh-REK-sis) refers to split or brittle nails that have a series of lengthwise ridges giving a rough appearance to the surface of the nail plate (figure 10-6). This condition is usually caused by injury to the matrix, excessive use of cuticle removers, harsh cleaning agents, aggressive filing techniques, or heredity. Nail services can be performed only if the nail is not split, exposing the nail bed. Nail enhancement product should never be applied if the nail bed is exposed. This condition may be corrected by softening the nails with a conditioning treatment and discontinuing the use of harsh detergents, cleaners, or improper filing. These nail plates often lack sufficient moisture, so twice-daily treatments with a high quality, penetrating nail oil can be very beneficial. Nail hardeners should always be avoided on brittle nails, since these products will increase brittleness.

Plicatured nail (plik-a-CHOORD NAYL), also known as *folded nail*, is a type of highly curved nail plate usually caused by injury to the matrix, but it may be inherited. This condition often leads to ingrown nails (figure 10-7).

Ridges are vertical lines running down the length of the natural nail plate that are caused by uneven growth of the nails, usually the result of normal aging. Older clients are more likely to have these ridges, and unless the ridges become very deep and weaken the nail plate, they are perfectly normal. When manicuring a client with this condition, carefully buff the nail plate to minimize the appearance of these ridges. This helps to remove or minimize the ridges, but great care must be taken not to overly thin the nail plate, which

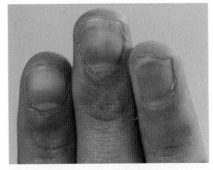
figure 10-5
Onychophagy or bitten nails

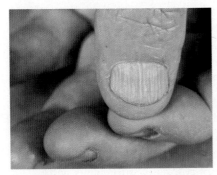
figure 10-6
Onychorrhexis

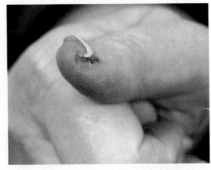
figure 10-7
Plicatured nail

could lead to nail plate weakness and additional damage. Ridge filler is less damaging to the natural nail plate and can be used with colored polish to give a smooth appearance while keeping the nail plate strong and healthy.

A **splinter hemorrhage** (SPLIN-tohr HEM-err-aje) is caused by physical trauma or injury to the nail bed that damages the capillaries and allows small amounts of blood flow. As a result, the blood stains the bed epithelium tissue that forms rails to guide the nail plate along the nail bed during growth. This blood oxidizes and turns brown or black, giving the appearance of a small splinter underneath the nail plate. Splinter hemorrhages will always be positioned lengthwise in the direction of growth (pointing toward the front and back of the nail plate) because this is how the bed epithelium rails grow. Splinter hemorrhages are normal and usually associated with some type of hard impact or other physical trauma to the fingernail or toenail.

Uncommon or Abnormal Nail Disorders

Onychauxis (ahn-ih-KAHK-sis) refers to the thickening of nails. It is usually observed in both the toenails and the fingernails and may present in a number of different ways. Its treatment is to trim or bring the nails down to size, but if the nails are ingrown it is advisable to ask a doctor for assistance. **Onychogryposis** (ahn-ih-koh-gry-POH-sis), also known as *ram's horn* or *claw nails*, is an enlargement of the fingernails or toenails accompanied by increased thickening and curvature. This condition is usually found on the great toes.

Nail pterygium (NAYL teh-RIJ-ee-um) is an abnormal condition that occurs when the skin is stretched by the nail plate. This disorder is usually caused by serious injury, such as burns, or an adverse skin reaction to chemical nail enhancement products. The terms *cuticle* and *pterygium* do not designate the same thing and they should never be used interchangeably. Nail pterygium is abnormal and is caused by damage to the eponychium or hyponychium.

Do not treat nail pterygium and never push the extension of skin back with an instrument. Doing so will cause more injury to the tissues and will make the condition worse. The gentle massage of conditioning oils or creams into the affected area may be beneficial. If this condition becomes irritated, painful, or shows signs of infection, recommend that the client see a physician for examination and proper treatment.

Nail plates with a deep or sharp curvature at the free edge have this shape because of the matrix; the greater the curvature of the matrix, the greater the curvature of the free edge. Increased curvature can range from mild to severe pinching of the soft tissue at the free edge. In some cases, the free edge pinches the sidewalls into a deep curve. This is known as **pincer nail** (PIN-sir NAYL), also known as *trumpet nail*. The nail can also curl in on itself (figure 10-8), may be deformed only on one sidewall, or the edges of the nail plate may curl around to form the shape of a trumpet or sharp cone at the free edge. In each of these cases, the natural nail plate should be carefully trimmed and filed. Extreme or unusual cases should be referred to a qualified medical doctor or podiatrist.

A brief summary of nail disorders is found in table 10-1.

You should never provide any type of nail services to clients with a nail bacterial or fungal infection.

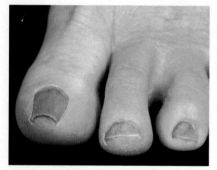

figure 10-8
Pincer or trumpet nail

table 10-1

OVERVIEW OF NAIL DISORDERS

Disorder	Signs or Symptoms
Beau's Lines (BOWZ LYNEZ)	Visible depressions running across the width of the natural nail plate; usually a result of major illness or injury that has traumatized the body.
Blue Fingernails	Blue or purple nail bed, usually from poor circulation.
Bruised Nail Beds	Dark purplish spots, usually due to physical injury.
Discolored Nails	Nails turn a variety of colors; may indicate surface staining, a systemic disorder, or poor blood circulation.
Eggshell Nails	Noticeably thin, white nail plates that are more flexible than normal and can curve over the free edge; usually caused by improper diet, hereditary factors, internal disease, or medication.
Hangnail	Living skin around the nail plate (often the eponychium) that becomes split or torn.
Koilonychia (koyal-oh-NICK-ee-uh)	Also known as *spoon nails*; inverted or concave nails.
Leukonychia Spots (loo-koh-NIK-ee-ah SPATS)	Also known as *white spots*; whitish discolorations of the nail usually caused by minor injury to the nail matrix. Not related to the body's health or vitamin deficiencies.
Melanonychia (mel-uh-nuh-NIK-ee-uh)	Darkening of the fingernails or toenails; may be seen as a black band within the nail plate extending from the base to the free edge.
Nail Pterygium (NAYL teh-RIJ-ee-um)	Abnormal stretching of skin around the nail plate; usually caused by serious injury, such as burns, or an adverse skin reaction to chemical nail enhancement products or an allergic skin reaction.
Onychauxis (ahn-ih-KAHK-sis)	Thickening of the fingernails or toenails.
Onychogryposis (ahn-ih-koh-gry-POH-sis	Also known as *ram's horn* or *claw nails;* an enlargement of the fingernails or toenails accompanied by increased thickening and curvature.
Onychophagy (ahn-ih-koh-FAY-jee)	Also known as *bitten nails*; chewed nails or chewed hardened skin surrounding the nail plate.
Onychorrhexis (ahn-ih-koh-REK-sis)	Split or brittle nails that have a series of lengthwise ridges giving a rough appearance to the surface of the nail plate.
Pincer Nail (PIN-sir NAYL)	Also known as *trumpet nail;* increased crosswise curvature throughout the nail plate caused by an increased curvature of the matrix; the edges of the nail plate may curl around to form the shape of a trumpet or sharp cone at the free edge.
Plicatured Nail (plik-a-CHOORD NAYL)	Also known as *folded nail;* a type of highly curved nail plate, usually caused by injury to the matrix, but it may be inherited.
Ridges	Vertical lines running the length of the natural nail plate that are caused by uneven growth of the nails, usually the result of normal aging.
Splinter Hemorrhage (SPLIN-tohr HEM-err-aje)	Physical trauma or injury to the nail bed that damages the capillaries and allows a small amount of blood flow.

After reading the next few sections, you will be able to:

LO❷ Recognize diseases of the nails that should not be treated in the salon.

Recognize Nail Diseases

Many disorders are caused by disease. **Onychosis** (ahn-ih-KOH-sis) is any deformity or disease of the natural nail. Since there are several nail diseases that you may come across, it is important to know if they are infectious and cannot be serviced, or if it is noninfectious and can receive a partial or specialized service.

A brief overview of nail diseases is found in **table 10-2.**

table 10-2

OVERVIEW OF NAIL DISEASES

Disease	Signs or Symptoms
Nail Psoriasis (NAYL suh-RY-uh-sis)	Tiny pits or severe roughness on the surface of the nail plate.
Onychia (uh-NIK-ee-uh)	Inflammation of the nail matrix followed by shedding of the nail.
Onychocryptosis (ahn-ih-koh-krip-TOH-sis)	Also known as *ingrown nails;* nail grows into the sides of the tissue around the nail.
Onycholysis (ahn-ih-KAHL-ih-sis)	Lifting of the nail plate from the nail bed, without shedding, usually beginning at the free edge and continuing toward the lunula area.
Onychomadesis (ahn-ih-koh-muh-DEE-sis)	Separation and falling off of a nail plate from the nail bed; can affect fingernails and toenails.
Onychomycosis (ahn-ih-koh-my-KOH-sis)	Fungal infection of the natural nail plate.
Paronychia (payr-uh-NIK-ee-uh)	Bacterial inflammation of the tissues surrounding the nail. Redness, pus, and swelling are usually seen in the skin fold adjacent to the nail plate.
Pseudomonas Aeruginosa (SUE-duh-MOAN-us aye-ru-jin-oh-sa)	Common bacteria that can lead to a bacterial infection that appears as a green, yellow, or black discoloration on the nail bed.
Pyogenic Granuloma (py-oh-JEN-ik gran-yoo-LOH-muh)	Severe inflammation of the nail in which a lump of red tissue grows up from the nail bed to the nail plate.
Tinea Pedis (TIN-ee-uh PED-us)	Also known as *athlete's foot;* red, itchy rash on the skin on the bottom of feet and/or between the toes, usually between the fourth or fifth toe.

Go to a library or use the Internet to research the term *scope of practice* for medical doctors, dermatologists, and podiatrists. You should be familiar with what these professionals do as well as the strict limitations placed on cosmetologists' *scope of practice* so that you'll better understand what you cannot do.

Product manufacturers can always provide you with additional information and guidance. Call them whenever you have any questions related to safe handling and proper use.

Infectious Nail Diseases

Any nail disease that shows signs of infection or inflammation (redness, pain, swelling, or pus) should not be diagnosed or treated in the salon. Medical examination is required for all nail diseases and treatment will be determined by the physician.

A person's occupation can cause a variety of nail infections. For instance, infections develop more readily in people who regularly place their hands in harsh cleaning solutions. Natural oils are removed from the skin by frequent exposure to soaps, solvents, and many other types of substances.

Onychia (uh-NIK-ee-uh) is an inflammation of the nail matrix followed by shedding of the natural nail plate. Any break in the skin surrounding the nail plate can allow pathogens to infect the matrix. Be careful to avoid injuring sensitive tissue and make sure that all implements are properly cleaned and disinfected. Improperly cleaned and disinfected nail implements can cause this and other diseases if an accidental injury occurs.

Onychomycosis (ahn-ih-koh-my-KOH-sis) is a fungal infection of the natural nail plate (figure 10-9). When the infection begins at the cuticle it is called *proximal subungual onychomycosis*. A common form is whitish patches that can be scraped off the surface of the nail. Another common form of this infection shows long whitish or pale yellowish streaks within the nail plate. These types of infection often begin with a small separation between the end of the nail and the nail bed. Many fungal infections start as an innocent bang and separation. Soft yellow material gradually builds up in the separation and the nail will thicken and yellow. Untreated, the disease will progress toward the matrix resulting in a partially destroyed nail. It is very important to keep this clean and dry. Do not poke things under your nail to clean it. You should not apply product to a fungal nail until it is healed.

As you learned in Chapter 5, Infection Control: Principles and Practices, fungi are parasites that may cause infections of the feet and hands. Nail fungi are of concern to the salon because they are contagious and can be transmitted through contaminated implements. Fungi can spread from nail to nail on the client's feet, but it is much less likely that these pathogens will cause fingernail infections. Fungal infections prefer to grow in conditions where the skin is warm, moist, and dark, that is, on feet inside shoes.

It is extremely unlikely that a cosmetologist could become infected from a client, but it is possible to transmit fungal infections from one client's foot or toe to another client. With proper cleaning and disinfection practices, the transmission of fungal infections can be easily avoided. Clients with suspected nail fungal infection must be referred to a physician.

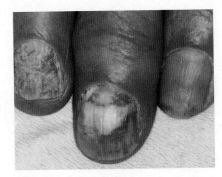

figure 10-9
Onychomycosis

© Courtesy of Robert Baran, MD (France)

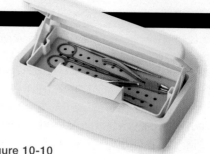

figure 10-10
Always practice strict rules regarding cleaning and disinfecting when working with nails.

Paronychia (payr-uh-NIK-ee-uh) is a bacterial inflammation of the tissues surrounding the nail. Redness, pus, and swelling are usually seen in the skin fold adjacent to the nail plate. Individuals who work with their hands in water, such as dishwashers and bartenders, or who must wash their hands continually, such as health-care workers and food processors, are more susceptible to paronychia because their hands are often very dry or chapped from excessive exposure to water, detergents, and harsh soaps. This makes them much more likely to develop infections.

Toenails, because they spend a lot of time in a warm, moist environment, are often more susceptible to paronychia infections as well. Use moisturizing hand lotions to keep skin healthy, and keep feet clean and dry.

The green, yellow, or black discoloration on a nail bed is usually a bacterial infection such as ***Pseudomonas aeruginosa*** (SUE-duh-MOAN-us aye-ru-jin-oh-sa), one of several common bacteria that can cause a nail infection, or Staphylococcus aureus. These naturally occurring skin bacteria can grow rapidly to cause an infection if conditions are correct for growth (figure 10-11). In the past, discolorations of the nail plate (especially those between the plate and nail enhancements) were generally referred to as *molds*, which is a type of fungus. This term should not be used when referring to infections of the fingernails or toenails. A typical pseudomonal bacterial infection on the nail plate can be identified in the early stages as a light-green spot that becomes darker in its advanced stages. Clients with these symptoms should be immediately referred to a physician for treatment. It is illegal for a cosmetologist to diagnose or treat a nail infection. Do not remove the nail enhancement unless directed to do so by the client's treating physician.

Bacterial or fungal infections can be caused by the use of implements that are contaminated with large numbers of these bacteria. Water does not cause infections but can support bacterial and fungal growth. Infections are caused by large numbers of bacteria or fungal organisms on a surface. This is why proper cleaning and preparation of the natural nail plate, as well as cleaning, disinfection, and/or sterilization of implements, are so important. If these pathogens are not present, infections cannot occur.

Pyogenic granuloma (py-oh-JEN-ik gran-yoo-LOH-muh) is a severe inflammation of the nail in which a lump of red tissue grows up from the nail bed to the nail plate.

Tinea pedis (TIN-ee-uh PED-us), also known as *athlete's foot*, is the medical term for fungal infections of the feet. These infections can occur

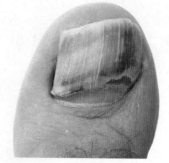

figure 10-11
Pseudomonas aeruginosa

© murat5234/Shutterstock.com

on the bottoms of the feet and often appear as a red itchy rash in the spaces between the toes, most often between the fourth and fifth toe. There is sometimes a small degree of scaling of the skin. Clients with this condition should be advised to wash their feet every day and dry them completely. This will make it difficult for the infection to live or grow. Advise clients to wear cotton socks and change them at least twice per day. They should also avoid wearing the same pair of shoes each day, since shoes can take up to 24 hours to dry completely. Over-the-counter antifungal powders can help keep feet dry and may help speed healing (figure 10-12).

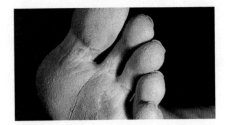
figure 10-12
Tinea pedis

Noninfectious Nail Diseases

Nail psoriasis (NAYL suh-RY-uh-sis) is a noninfectious condition that affects the surface of the natural nail plate causing tiny pits or severe roughness on the surface of the nail plate. Sometimes these pits occur randomly and sometimes they appear in evenly spaced rows. Nail psoriasis can also cause the surface of the plate to look like it has been filed with a coarse abrasive, can cause a ragged free edge, or can cause both (figure 10–13). People with skin psoriasis often experience this nail disorder. Neither skin nor nail psoriasis are infectious diseases. Nail psoriasis can also affect the nail bed, causing it to develop yellowish to reddish spots underneath the nail plate, called *salmon patches*. When all of these symptoms are present on the nail unit at the same time, nail psoriasis becomes a likely cause of the client's problem nails and they should be referred to a physician for diagnoses and treatment, if needed.

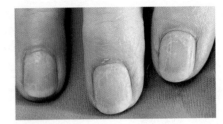
figure 10-13
Nail psoriasis

Onychocryptosis (ahn-ih-koh-krip-TOH-sis), also known as *ingrown nails*, can affect either the fingers or toes (figure 10-14). In this condition, the nail grows into the sides of the living tissue around the nail. The movements of walking can press the soft tissues up against the nail plate, contributing to the problem. If the tissue around the nail plate is not infected, or if the nail is not imbedded in the flesh, you can carefully trim the corner of the nail in a curved shape to relieve the pressure on the nail groove. However, if there is any redness, pain, swelling, or irritation, you may not provide any services. Cosmetologists are not allowed to service ingrown nails. Refer the client to a physician.

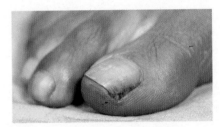
figure 10-14
Onychocryptosis

Onycholysis (ahn-ih-KAHL-ih-sis) is the lifting of the nail plate from the bed without shedding, usually beginning at the free edge and continuing toward the lunula area (figure 10-15). This is usually the result of physical injury, trauma, or allergic reaction of the nail bed and less often related to a health disorder. It often occurs on natural nails when they are filed too aggressively, on nail enhancements when they are improperly removed, or on toenails when clients wear shoes without sufficient room for the toes. If there is no indication of an infection or open sores, a basic manicure or pedicure may be given. The nail plate should be short to avoid further injury, and the area underneath the nail plate should be kept clean and dry. If the trauma that caused the onycholysis is removed, the area will begin to slowly heal itself. Eventually the nail plate will grow off the free edge and the hyponychium will reform the seal that provides a natural barrier against infection (figure 10-16).

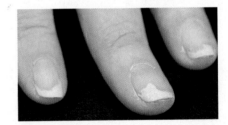
figure 10-15
Onycholysis

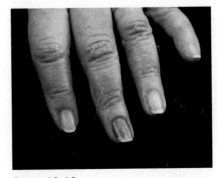
figure 10-16
Onycholosis caused by trauma

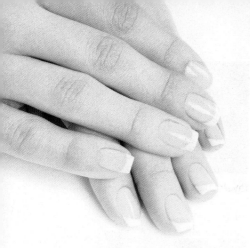

Onychomadesis (ahn-ih-koh-muh-DEE-sis) is the separation and falling off of a nail plate from the nail bed. It can affect fingernails and toenails. In most cases, the cause can be traced to a localized infection, injuries to the matrix, or a severe systemic illness. Drastic medical procedures, such as chemotherapy, may also be the cause.

Whatever the reason, once the problem is resolved, a new nail plate will eventually grow again. If onychomadesis is present, do not apply enhancements to the nail plate. If there is no indication of an infection or open sores, a basic manicure or pedicure service may be given.

After reading the next few sections, you will be able to:

LO❸ Perform a hand, nail, and skin analysis on a client.

Perform Hand, Nail, and Skin Analysis

It is very important to perform a hand and nail analysis on every client before beginning a nail service. This examination will allow a cosmetologist to identify disease, disorders, and conditions including signs of infection which may be identified through pain, redness, swelling, throbbing, and pus. A proper analysis will help to determine not only the needed service, but also if a service should not be performed.

Use these simple steps to perform a hand, nail, and skin analysis:

- Always begin a hand, skin, and nail analysis by cleaning the hands of both the cosmetologist and the client.

- Using the senses of sight and touch, observe the following:

  1. The moisture level of the skin. It should be soft and supple. There should be no signs of dehydration or flaking skin.

  2. The temperature of the skin. Cold skin may indicate poor circulation. Warm skin may indicate infection.

  3. The condition of the skin. Redness may indicate inflammation or infection. It should be free of any disease or disorder.

  4. Tenderness to the touch of the skin. Feel the client's hands and ask if they have any pain. If they have pain, it may require caution or special techniques during massage.

  5. Examine the condition and length of the nails including the shape of the free edge and cuticle and the thickness of the nail plate. Know when to refer the client to a physician—this is why cosmetologists need to study nail disease, disorders, and conditions.

After performing the nail examination, share your findings with your client:

1. Identify any form of onychosis—disease, disorder, or condition.

2. Note the apparent cause—systemic, environmental, etc.

3. Suggest the proper service or refer to a physician.

4. Discuss home maintenance and a future service plan.

1. In what situation should a nail service not be performed?

2. Name at least eight common nail disorders and describe their appearance.

3. What conditions do fungal organisms favor for growth?

4. What is *Pseudomonas aeruginosa*? Why is it important to learn about it?

5. What is the most effective way to avoid transferring infections among your clients?

6. Can a cosmetologist offer treatment advice for a client who has developed a nail infection?

7. Can a cosmetologist treat an ingrown toenail if there is no sign of pus or discharge? Why?

8. Name two common causes of onycholysis.

STUDY TOOLS

- **Reinforce what you just learned:** Complete the activities and exercises in your Theory or Practical Workbook, or your Study Guide.

- **Expand your knowledge:** Search for websites about the topics in this chapter and make a list of additional resources.

- **Study and prepare for your quiz:** Take the chapter test in your Exam Review or your Milady U: Online Licensing Prep.

- **Re-Test your knowledge:** Take the Chapter 10 *Quizzes*!

- **Learn even more:** Look up in a dictionary or search the internet for the definitions of any additional terms you want to learn about.

CHAPTER GLOSSARY

Beau's lines BOWZ LYNEZ	p. 209	Sometimes called *furrows* (FUR-ohs) or *corrugations* (kor-uh-GAY-shuns); visible depressions running across the width of the natural nail plate; usually a result of major illness or injury that has traumatized the body.
blue fingernails	p. 209	Named for the nail bed color; is usually caused by a lack of circulating oxygen in the red blood cells.
bruised nail beds	p. 209	Condition in which a blood clot forms under the nail plate, causing a dark purplish spot. These discolorations are usually due to small injuries to the nail bed.
discolored nails	p. 209	Nails turn a variety of colors; may indicate surface staining, a systemic disorder, or poor blood circulation.
eggshell nails	p. 210	Noticeably thin, white nail plates that are more flexible than normal and can curve over the free edge.
hangnail	p. 210	A condition in which the living tissue surrounding the nail plate splits or tears.

koilonychia koyal-oh-NICK-ee-uh	p. 210	Soft spoon nails with a concave shape that appear scooped out.
leukonychia spots loo-koh-NIK-ee-ah SPATS	p. 210	Also known as *white spots*; whitish discolorations of the nails, usually caused by injury to the matrix area; not related to the body's health or vitamin deficiencies.
melanonychia mel-uh-nuh-NIK-ee-uh	p. 210	Darkening of the fingernails or toenails; may be seen as a black band within the nail plate, extending from the base to the free edge.
nail disorder	p. 208	Condition caused by an injury or disease of the nail unit.
nail psoriasis NAYL suh-RY-uh-sis	p. 217	A noninfectious condition that affects the surface of the natural nail plate causing tiny pits or severe roughness on the surface of the nail plate.
nail pterygium NAYL teh-RIJ-ee-um	p. 212	Abnormal condition that occurs when the skin is stretched by the nail plate; usually caused by serious injury, such as burns, or an adverse skin reaction to chemical nail enhancement products.
onychauxis ahn-ih-KAHK-sis	p. 212	Thickening of nails.
onychia uh-NIK-ee-uh	p. 215	Inflammation of the nail matrix followed by shedding of the natural nail.
onychocryptosis ahn-ih-koh-krip-TOH-sis	p. 217	Also known as *ingrown nails*; nail grows into the sides of the tissue around the nail.
onychogryposis ahn-ih-koh-gry-POH-sis	p. 212	Also known as *ram's horn* or *claw nails*; an enlargement of the fingernails or toenails accompanied by increased thickening and curvature.
onycholysis ahn-ih-KAHL-ih-sis	p. 217	Lifting of the nail plate from the nail bed without shedding, usually beginning at the free edge and continuing toward the lunula area.
onychomadesis ahn-ih-koh-muh-DEE-sis	p. 218	The separation and falling off of a nail plate from the nail bed; affects fingernails and toenails.
onychomycosis ahn-ih-koh-my-KOH-sis	p. 215	Fungal infection of the natural nail plate.
onychophagy ahn-ih-koh-FAY-jee	p. 211	Also known as *bitten nails*; result of a habit of chewing the nail or chewing the hardened skin surrounding the nail plate.
onychorrhexis ahn-ih-koh-REK-sis	p. 211	Split or brittle nails that have a series of lengthwise ridges giving a rough appearance to the surface of the nail plate.
onychosis ahn-ih-KOH-sis	p. 214	Any deformity or disease of the natural nails.
paronychia payr-uh-NIK-ee-uh	p. 216	Bacterial inflammation of the tissues surrounding the nail. Redness, pus, and swelling are usually seen in the skin fold adjacent to the nail plate.
pincer nail PIN-sir NAYL	p. 212	Also known as *trumpet nail*; increased crosswise curvature throughout the nail plate caused by an increased curvature of the matrix. The edges of the nail plate may curl around to form the shape of a trumpet or sharp cone at the free edge.
plicatured nail plik-a-CHOORD NAYL	p. 211	Also known as *folded nail*; a type of highly curved nail usually caused by injury to the matrix, but may be inherited.

Pseudomonas aeruginosa SUE-duh-MOAN-us aye-ru-jin-oh-sa	p. 216	Common bacteria that can lead to a bacterial infection that appears as a green, yellow, or black discoloration on the nail bed.
pyogenic granuloma py-oh-JEN-ik gran-yoo-LOH-muh	p. 216	Severe inflammation of the nail in which a lump of red tissue grows up from the nail bed to the nail plate.
ridges	p. 211	Vertical lines running through the length of the natural nail plate that are caused by uneven growth of the nails, usually the result of normal aging.
splinter hemorrhage SPLIN-tohr HEM-err-aje	p. 212	Hemorrhage caused by trauma or injury to the nail bed that damages the capillaries and allow small amounts of blood flow.
tinea pedis TIN-ee-uh PED-us	p. 216	Also known as *athlete's foot*; medical term for fungal infections of the feet; red, itchy rash of the skin on the bottom of the feet and/or in between the toes, usually found between the fourth and fifth toe.

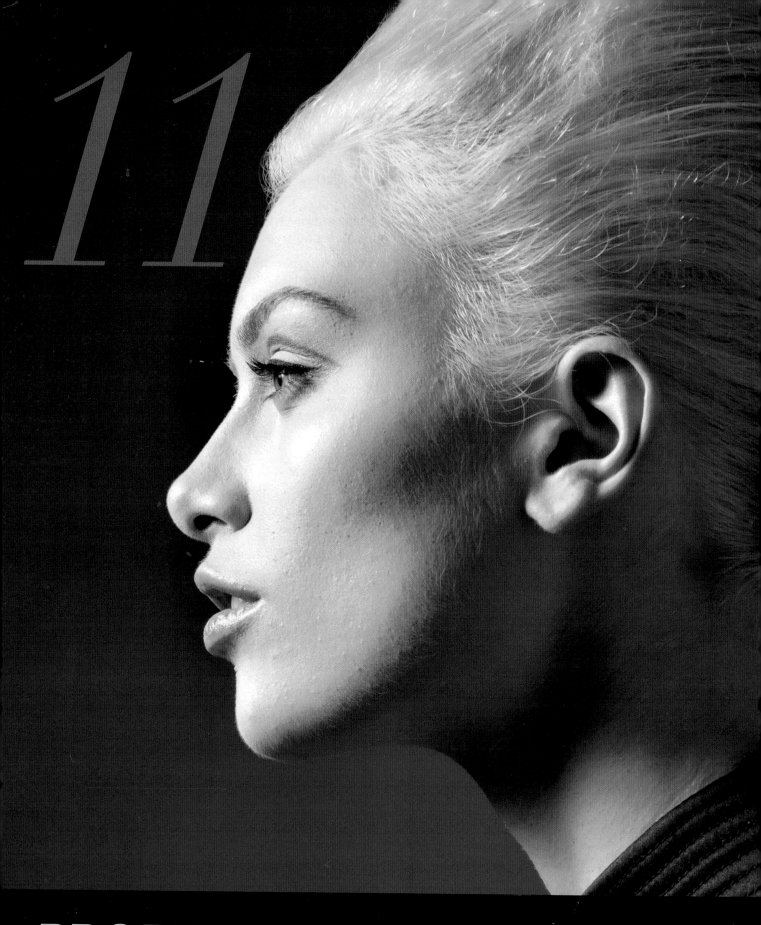

11

PROPERTIES OF THE HAIR AND SCALP

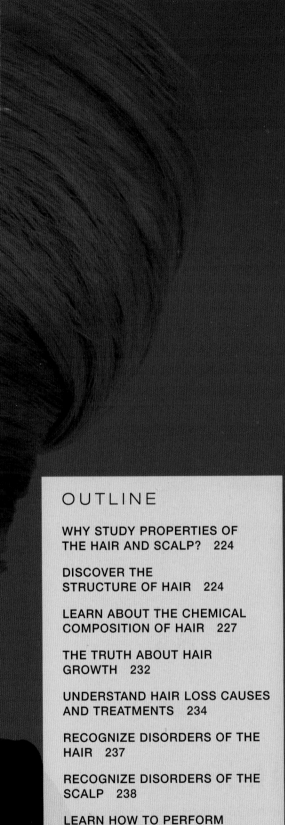

LEARNING OBJECTIVES

After completing this chapter, you will be able to:

LO❶
Identify and distinguish the different structures of the hair root.

LO❷
Point out and differentiate the differences among the three main layers of the hair shaft.

LO❸
Identify and explain the three types of side bonds in the cortex.

LO❹
Name and compare the differences among the three cycles of hair growth.

LO❺
Give examples of the common types of hair loss and explain what can cause hair loss.

LO❻
Identify and explain at least three options for hair loss treatment.

LO❼
Learn to identify the most common hair and scalp disorders seen in the salon and school, and then name which ones a physician should treat.

LO❽
Compare and describe the different factors that should be considered during a hair and scalp analysis.

From Lady Godiva's infamous horseback ride to the sought-after celebrity styles that make headlines every day, hair has been one of humanity's most enduring obsessions. The term *crowning glory* aptly describes the importance placed on hair, how good we feel when our hair looks great, and just how distressing a bad hair day really can be. This is why hairstylists play such an important role in many people's lives. All professional hair services must be based on a thorough understanding of the growth, structure, and composition of hair.

why study
PROPERTIES OF THE HAIR AND SCALP?

Cosmetologists should study and have a thorough understanding of the properties of the hair and scalp because:

> You need to know how and why hair grows and how and why it falls out in order to be able to differentiate between normal and abnormal hair loss.

> Knowing what creates natural color and texture is a vital part of being able to offer a variety of chemical services to clients.

> Spotting an unhealthy scalp condition that could be harboring a communicable disease or even be causing permanent hair loss is a way to aid your client in caring for their scalp and their hair's well-being.

After reading the next few sections, you will be able to:

LO **1**   Identify and distinguish the different structures of the hair root.

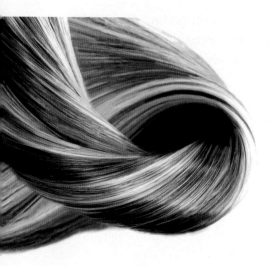

Discover the Structure of Hair

The scientific study of hair and its diseases and care is called **trichology** (trih-KAHL-uh-jee), which comes from the Greek words *trichos* (hair) and *ology* (the study of). The hair, skin, nails, and glands are part of the integumentary system. Although we no longer need hair for warmth and protection, hair still has an enormous impact on our psychology.

A mature strand of human hair is divided into two parts: the hair root and the hair shaft. The **hair root** is the part of the hair located below the surface of the epidermis (outer layer of the skin). The **hair shaft** is the portion of the hair that projects above the epidermis (figure 11-1).

Structures of the Hair Root

The five main structures of the hair root include the hair follicle, hair bulb, dermal papilla, arrector pili muscle, and sebaceous (oil) glands.

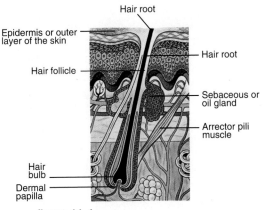

figure 11-1
Structures of the hair

- The **hair follicle** (HAYR FAWL-ih-kul) is the tube-like depression or pocket in the skin or scalp that contains the hair root. Hair follicles are distributed all over the body, with the exceptions of the palms of the hands and the soles of the feet. The follicle extends downward from the epidermis into the dermis (the inner layer of skin), where it surrounds the dermal papilla. Sometimes more than one hair will grow from a single follicle.

- The **hair bulb** (HAYR BULB) is the lowest part of a hair strand. It is the thickened, club-shaped structure that forms the lower part of the hair root. The lower part of the hair bulb fits over and covers the dermal papilla.

- The **dermal papilla** (DERMAL puh-PIL-uh) (plural: dermal papillae) is a small, cone-shaped elevation located at the base of the hair follicle that fits into the hair bulb. The dermal papilla contains the blood and nerve supply that provides the nutrients needed for hair growth. Some people refer to the dermal papilla as the "mother" of the hair because it contains the blood and nerve supply that provides the nutrients needed for hair growth.

- The **arrector pili muscle** is the small, involuntary muscle in the base of the hair follicle. Strong emotions or a cold sensation cause it to contract, which makes the hair stand up straight and results in what we call *goose bumps*.

- **Sebaceous glands** are the oil glands in the skin that are connected to the hair follicles. The sebaceous glands secrete a fatty or an oily substance called **sebum**. Sebum lubricates the skin.

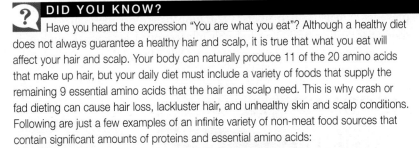

? DID YOU KNOW?

Have you heard the expression "You are what you eat"? Although a healthy diet does not always guarantee a healthy hair and scalp, it is true that what you eat will affect your hair and scalp. Your body can naturally produce 11 of the 20 amino acids that make up hair, but your daily diet must include a variety of foods that supply the remaining 9 essential amino acids that the hair and scalp need. This is why crash or fad dieting can cause hair loss, lackluster hair, and unhealthy skin and scalp conditions. Following are just a few examples of an infinite variety of non-meat food sources that contain significant amounts of proteins and essential amino acids:

- Proteins in plant-based foods such as nuts, soy, and whole (unrefined) wheat and grains
- Nitrogen-fixing, seed-bearing plants, such as peas and all varieties of legumes (beans), are very good sources of proteins and amino acids.

Food combinations such as the following are also examples of non-meat food sources that contain plenty of proteins and amino acids:

- Whole wheat (or other whole grain) pasta and mushrooms, and fruits such as tomato, eggplant, and zucchini
- Peanut butter and whole grain or whole wheat bread
- Whole grain rice and beans
- Beans and corn

Structures of the Hair Shaft

The three main layers of the hair shaft are the hair cuticle, cortex, and medulla (figure 11-2).

- The **hair cuticle** (HAYR KYOO-ti-kul) is the outermost layer of the hair. It consists of a single overlapping layer of transparent, scale-like cells that look like shingles on a roof. The cuticle layer provides a barrier that protects the inner structure of the hair as it lies tightly against the cortex. It is responsible for creating the shine and the smooth, silky feel of healthy hair.

   To feel the cuticle, pinch a single healthy strand of hair between your thumb and forefinger. Starting near the scalp, pull upward on the strand. The strand should feel sleek and smooth. Next, hold the end of the hair strand with one hand, and then pinch the strand with the thumb and forefingers of your other hand. Move your fingers down the hair shaft. In this direction, the hair feels rougher because you are going against the natural growth of the cuticle layer. A healthy, compact cuticle layer is the hair's primary defense against damage. A lengthwise cross-section of hair shows that although the hair cuticle scales overlap, each individual cuticle scale is attached to the cortex (figure 11-3). These overlapping scales make up the cuticle layer. Swelling the hair by applying substances such as haircolor raises the cuticle layer and opens the space between the scales, which allows liquids to penetrate into the cortex.

   A healthy hair cuticle layer protects the hair from penetration and prevents damage to hair fibers. Oxidation haircolors, permanent waving solutions, and chemical hair relaxers must have an alkaline pH to penetrate the cuticle layer because a high pH swells the cuticle and causes it to lift and expose the cortex.

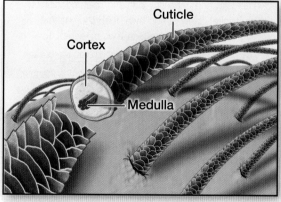

figure 11-2
Cross-section of hair cuticle

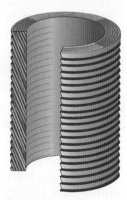

figure 11-3
Hair cuticle layer

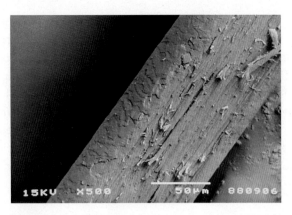

figure 11-4
Hair shaft with part of the hair cuticle
stripped off, exposing the cortex

- The **cortex** (KOR-teks) is the middle layer of the hair. It is a fibrous protein core formed by elongated cells containing melanin pigment. About 90 percent of the total weight of hair comes from the cortex. The elasticity of the hair and its natural color are the result of the unique protein structures located within the cortex. The changes involved in oxidation haircoloring, wet setting, thermal styling, permanent waving, and chemical hair relaxing take place within the cortex (**figure 11-4**).

- The **medulla** (muh-DUL-uh) is the innermost layer of the hair and is composed of round cells. It is quite common for very fine and naturally blond hair to entirely lack a medulla. Generally, only thick, coarse hair contains a medulla. All male beard hair contains a medulla. The medulla is not involved in salon services.

Learn About the Chemical Composition of Hair

Hair is composed of protein that grows from cells originating within the hair follicle. This is where the hair begins. As soon as these living cells form, they begin their journey upward through the hair follicle. They mature in a process called **keratinization** (kair-uh-ti-ni-ZAY-shun). As these newly formed cells mature, they fill up with a fibrous protein called **keratin**. After they have filled with keratin, the cells move upward, lose their nucleus, and die. By the time the hair shaft emerges from the scalp, the cells of the hair are completely keratinized and are no longer living. The hair shaft that emerges is a nonliving fiber composed of keratinized protein.

Hair is approximately 90 percent protein. The protein is made up of long chains of amino acids, which, in turn, are made up of elements. The major elements that make up human hair are carbon, oxygen, hydrogen, nitrogen, and sulfur and are often referred to as the **COHNS elements** (KOH-nz EL-uh-ments). These five elements are also found in skin and nails. Table 11-1 shows the percentages of each element in a typical strand of hair.

table 11-1

THE COHNS ELEMENTS

Element	Percentage in Normal Hair
Carbon	51%
Oxygen	21%
Hydrogen	6%
Nitrogen	17%
Sulfur	5%

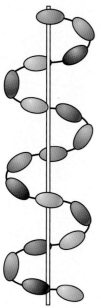

figure 11-5
Polypeptide chains intertwine in a spiral shape called a helix

Proteins are made of long chains of **amino acids** (uh-MEE-noh AS-udz), units that are joined together end-to-end like pop beads. The strong, chemical bond that joins amino acids is a **peptide bond** (PEP-tyd BAHND), also known as end bond. A long chain of amino acids linked by peptide bonds is called a **polypeptide chain** (pahl-ee-PEP-tyd CHAYN). **Proteins** (PROH-teenz) are long, coiled complex polypeptides made of amino acids. The spiral shape of a coiled protein is called a **helix** (HEE-licks), which is created when the polypeptide chains intertwine with each other (**figure 11-5**).

After reading the next few sections, you will be able to:

LO❸ Identify and explain the three types of side bonds in the cortex.

Side Bonds of the Cortex

The cortex is made up of millions of polypeptide chains. Polypeptide chains are cross-linked like the rungs on a ladder by three different types of **side bonds** that link the polypeptide chains together and are responsible for the extreme strength and elasticity of human hair. They are essential to services such as wet setting, thermal styling, permanent waving, and chemical hair relaxing (see Chapter 20, Chemical Texture Services). The three types of side bonds are hydrogen, salt, and disulfide bonds (**figure 11-6**).

- A **hydrogen bond** is a weak, physical, cross-link side bond that is easily broken by water or heat. Although individual hydrogen bonds are very weak, there are so many of them that they account for about one-third of the hair's overall strength. Hydrogen bonds are broken by wetting the hair with water (**figure 11-7**). That allows the hair to be stretched and wrapped around rollers. The hydrogen bonds reform when the hair dries.

- A **salt bond** is also a weak, physical, cross-link side bond between adjacent polypeptide chains. Salt bonds depend on pH, so they are easily broken by strong alkaline or acidic solutions (**figure 11-8**). Even though they are weak bonds, there are so many of them that they account for about one-third of the hair's overall strength.

- A **disulfide bond** (dy-SUL-fyd BAHND) is a strong, chemical, side bond that is very different from the physical side bond of a hydrogen bond or salt bond. The disulfide bond joins the sulfur atoms of two neighboring **cysteine** (SIS-ti-een) amino acids to create one **cystine** (SIS-teen). The cystine joins together two polypeptide strands. Although there are far fewer disulfide bonds than hydrogen or salt bonds, disulfide bonds are so much stronger that they also account for about one-third of the hair's overall strength.

Disulfide bonds are not broken by water. They are broken by permanent waves and chemical hair relaxers that alter the shape of hair

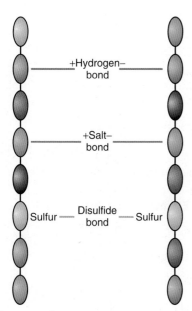

figure 11-6
Side bonds between polypeptide chains

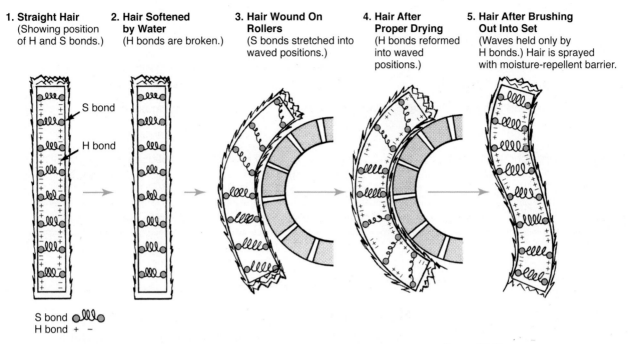

1. **Straight Hair**
(Showing position of H and S bonds.)

2. **Hair Softened by Water**
(H bonds are broken.)

3. **Hair Wound On Rollers**
(S bonds stretched into waved positions.)

4. **Hair After Proper Drying**
(H bonds reformed into waved positions.)

5. **Hair After Brushing Out Into Set**
(Waves held only by H bonds.) Hair is sprayed with moisture-repellent barrier.

S bond
H bond

S bond ⬭⬭
H bond + −

figure 11-7
Changes in hair cortex during wet setting

(**table 11-2**). Additionally, normal amounts of heat, such as the heat used in conventional thermal styling, do not break disulfide bonds. The bonds can be broken by extreme heat produced by boiling water and some high-temperature thermal styling tools such as straightening or flat irons.

Thio permanent waves break disulfide bonds and reform the bonds with thio neutralizers. Hydroxide chemical hair relaxers break disulfide bonds and then convert them to **lanthionine bonds** (lan-THY-oh-neen BAHNDZ) when the relaxer is rinsed from the hair. The disulfide bonds that are treated with hydroxide relaxers are broken permanently and can never be reformed (see Chapter 20, Chemical Texture Services).

figure 11-8
Changes in hair cortex during permanent waving

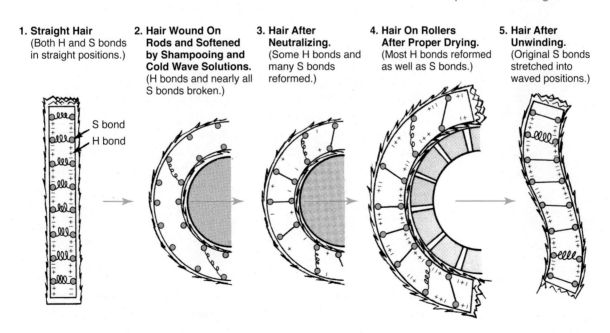

1. **Straight Hair**
(Both H and S bonds in straight positions.)

2. **Hair Wound On Rods and Softened by Shampooing and Cold Wave Solutions.**
(H bonds and nearly all S bonds broken.)

3. **Hair After Neutralizing.**
(Some H bonds and many S bonds reformed.)

4. **Hair On Rollers After Proper Drying.**
(Most H bonds reformed as well as S bonds.)

5. **Hair After Unwinding.**
(Original S bonds stretched into waved positions.)

S bond
H bond

table 11-2

BONDS OF THE HAIR

Bond	Type	Strength	Broken By	Reformed By
Hydrogen	Side bond	Weak, physical	Water or heat	Drying or cooling
Salt	Side bond	Weak, physical	Changes in pH	Normalizing pH
Disulfide	Side bond	Strong, chemical	1. Thio perms and thio relaxers 2. Hydroxide relaxers 3. Extreme heat	1. Oxidation with neutralizer 2. Converted to lanthionine bonds
Peptide	End bond	Strong, chemical	Chemical depilatories	Not reformed; hair dissolves

Hair Pigment

All natural hair color is the result of the pigment located within the cortex. **Melanin** are the tiny grains of pigment in the cortex that give natural color to the hair. The two types of melanin are eumelanin and pheomelanin.

- **Eumelanin** provides natural dark brown to black color to the hair and is the dark pigment predominant in black and brunette hair.

- **Pheomelanin** is the lighter pigment that provides natural colors ranging from red and ginger to yellow and blond tones.

Natural hair color in a person's hair is due to the presence of the mixture of these pigments. More eumelanin gives darker hair and the amount can vary from person to person and also across a person's head. When we look at a hair under the microscope, the eumelanin pigment granules are oval (elliptical) in shape and the pheomelanin pigments are partly oval and partly rod-shaped. Gray hair contains only a few scattered melanin granules and white hair does not contain any melanin.

Wave Pattern

The **wave pattern** of hair refers to the shape of the hair strand. It is described as straight, wavy, curly, or extremely curly (figure 11-9).

Natural wave patterns are the result of genetics. Although there are many exceptions, as a general rule, Asians and Native Americans tend to have extremely straight hair, Caucasians tend to have straight, wavy, or curly hair, and African Americans tend to have extremely curly hair. But straight, wavy, curly, and extremely curly hair occur in all races—anyone of any race, or mixed race, can have hair with varying degrees of curl from straight to extremely curly. The wave pattern may also vary from strand to strand on the same person's head. It is not uncommon for an individual to have different amounts of curl in different areas of the head. Individuals with curly hair often have straighter hair in the crown and tighter curl in other areas. Straight blond hair is round with more pheomelanin, straight black hair is round with mostly eumelanin, and straight gray hair lack melanin. Curly hair is oval in shape (figure 11-10).

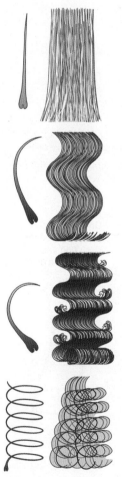

figure 11-9
Straight, wavy, curly, and extremely curly hair strands

Basis of Hair Color and Texture

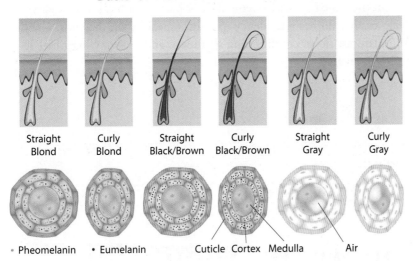

Straight Blond · Curly Blond · Straight Black/Brown · Curly Black/Brown · Straight Gray · Curly Gray

· Pheomelanin · Eumelanin Cuticle Cortex Medulla Air

Alila Medical Media/Shutterstock.com

figure 11-10
Individuals with curly hair often have straighter hair in the crown and tighter curl in other areas.

Several theories attempt to explain the cause of natural curly hair, but there is no single, definite answer that explains why some hair grows straight and other hair grows curly. The most popular theory claims that the shape of the hair's cross-section determines the amount of curl. This theory claims that hair with a round cross-section is straight, hair with an oval to flattened oval cross-section is wavy or curly, and hair with a flattened to flattened oval cross-section is extremely curly (table 11–3).

Extremely Curly Hair

Extremely curly hair grows in long twisted spirals. Cross-sections appear flattened and vary in shape and thickness along their length. Compared to straight or wavy hair, which tends to possess a fairly regular and uniform diameter along a single strand, extremely curly hair is fairly irregular, showing varying diameters along a single strand. Some extremely curly hair has a natural tendency to form a coil like a telephone cord. Coiled hair

> **? DID YOU KNOW?**
> The term *hair color* (two words) refers to the color of hair created by nature. *Haircolor* (one word) is the term used in the beauty industry to refer to artificial haircoloring products. Gray hair is caused by the absence of melanin. Gray hair grows from the hair bulb in exactly the same way that pigmented hair grows. It has the same structure, but without the melanin pigment.

table 11-3
WAVE PATTERN AND CROSS-SECTIONS

	Wave Pattern	Shape of Cross-Section
	Straight Hair	Round cross-section
	Wavy or Curly Hair	Oval to round cross-section
	Extremely Curly Hair	Elliptical cross-section

usually has a fine texture, with many individual strands winding together to form the coiled locks. Extremely curly hair often has low elasticity, breaks easily, and has a tendency to knot, especially on the ends. Gentle scalp manipulations, conditioning shampoo, and a detangling rinse help minimize tangles.

After reading the next few sections, you will be able to:

LO ④ Name and compare the differences among the three cycles of hair growth.

The Truth About Hair Growth

The two main types of hair found on the body are vellus hair and terminal hair (figure 11-11).

Vellus hair (VEL-us HAYR), also known as *lanugo hair* (luh-NOO-goh HAYR), is short, fine, unpigmented, and downy hair that appears on the body. Vellus hair almost never has a medulla. It is commonly found on infants and can be present on children until puberty. On adults, vellus hair is usually found in places that are normally considered hairless (forehead, eyelids, and bald scalp), as well as nearly all other areas of the body except the palms of the hands and the soles of the feet. The follicles that produce vellus hairs do not have sebaceous glands. Women normally retain 55 percent more vellus hair than men. Vellus hair helps with the evaporation of perspiration.

Terminal hair (TUR-mih-nul HAYR) is the long, coarse, pigmented hair found on the scalp, legs, arms, and bodies of males and females. Terminal hair is coarser than vellus hair, and, with the exception of gray hair, it is pigmented. It usually has a medulla.

Hormonal changes during puberty cause some areas of fine vellus hair to be replaced with thicker terminal hair. All hair follicles are capable of producing either vellus or terminal hair, depending on genetics, age, and hormones.

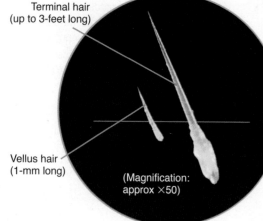

figure 11-11
Vellus hair and terminal hair

Terminal hair
(up to 3-feet long)

Vellus hair
(1-mm long)

(Magnification:
approx ×50)

Pfizer Inc.

Growth Cycles of Hair

Hair growth occurs in cycles. Each complete cycle has three phases that are repeated over and over again throughout life. The three phases are anagen, catagen, and telogen.

1. During the **anagen phase** (AN-uh-jen FAYZ), also known as *growth phase*, new hair is produced. New cells are actively manufactured in the hair follicle. During this phase, hair cells are produced faster than any other normal cell in the human body. The average growth of

healthy scalp hair is about ½ (0.5) inch (1.25 centimeters) per month. The rate of growth varies on different parts of the body, between sexes, and with age. Scalp hair grows faster on women than on men. Scalp hair grows rapidly between the ages of 15 and 30, but slows down sharply after the age of 50.

About 90 percent of scalp hair is growing in the anagen phase at any time. The anagen phase generally lasts from three to five years, but in some cases, it can last as long as 10 years. The longer the anagen cycle is, the longer the hair is able to grow. This is why some people can only grow their hair down to their shoulders, while others can grow it down to the floor!

2. The **catagen phase** (KAT-uh-jen FAYZ) is the brief transition period between the growth and resting phases of a hair follicle. It signals the end of the anagen phase. During the catagen phase, the follicle canal shrinks and detaches from the dermal papilla. The hair bulb disappears and the shrunken root end forms a rounded club. Less than one percent of scalp hair is in the catagen phase at any time. The catagen phase is very short, lasting from one to two weeks.

3. The **telogen phase** (TEL-uh-jen FAYZ), also known as resting phase, is the final phase in the hair cycle and lasts until the fully grown hair is shed. The hair is either shed during the telogen phase or remains in place until the next anagen phase, when the new hair growing in pushes it out. A little less than 10 percent of scalp hair is in the telogen phase at any one time.

The telogen phase lasts for approximately three to six months. As soon as the telogen phase ends, the hair returns to the anagen phase and begins the entire cycle again. On average, the entire growth cycle repeats itself once every 4 to 5 years.

Myths and Facts about Hair Growth

As a stylist, you may hear opinions about hair growth from your clients or from other stylists. Here are some myths and facts about hair growth:

Myth. Shaving, clipping, and cutting the hair on the head makes it grow back faster, darker, and coarser.

Fact. Shaving or cutting the hair on the head has no effect on hair growth. When hair is blunt cut to the same length, it grows back more evenly. Although it may seem to grow back faster, darker, and coarser, shaving or cutting hair on the head has no effect on hair growth.

Myth. Scalp massage increases hair growth.

Fact. Scalp massages are very stimulating to the scalp and can increase blood circulation, relax the nerves in the scalp, and tighten the scalp muscles. However, it has not been scientifically proven that any type of stimulation or scalp massage increases hair growth. Minoxidil and finasteride are the only treatments that have been scientifically proven to increase hair growth and are approved for that purpose by the Food and Drug Administration (FDA). Products that claim to increase hair growth are regulated as drugs and are not cosmetics.

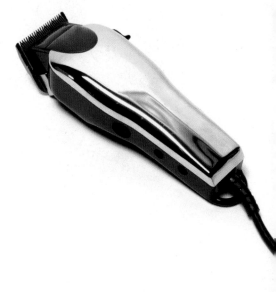

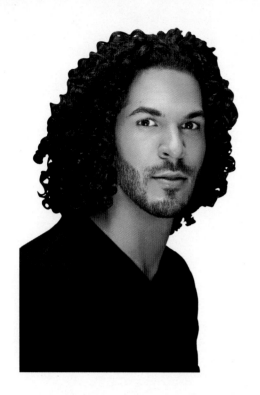

Myth. Gray hair is coarser and more resistant than pigmented hair.
Fact. Other than the lack of pigment, gray hair is exactly the same as pigmented hair. Although gray hair may be resistant, it is not resistant simply because it is gray. Pigmented hair on the same person's head is just as resistant as the gray hair. Gray hair is simply more noticeable than pigmented hair.
Myth. The amount of natural curl is always determined by racial background.
Fact. Anyone of any race, or mixed race, can have hair from straight to extremely curly. It is also true that within races individuals have hair with varying degrees of curl in different areas of the head.
Myth. Hair with a round cross-section is straight, hair with an oval cross-section is wavy, and hair with a flattened cross-section is curly.
Fact. In general, cross-sections of straight hair are often round, cross-sections of wavy and curly hair tend to be more oval to flattened oval, and cross-sections of extremely curly hair have a flattened cross-section. However, cross-sections of hair can be almost any shape, and the shape of the cross-section does not always relate to the amount of curl or the shape of the follicle.

After reading the next few sections, you will be able to:

LO⑤ Give examples of the common types of hair loss and what can cause hair loss.

Understand Hair Loss Causes and Treatments

Under normal circumstances, we all lose some hair every day. Normal, daily hair loss is the natural result of the anagen, catagen, and telogen phases of the hair's growth cycle that were explained earlier in this chapter.

The growth cycle provides for the continuous growth, fall, and replacement of individual hair strands. A hair that is shed in the telogen phase is replaced by a new hair, in that same follicle, in the next anagen phase. This natural shedding of hair accounts for normal daily hair loss. Although estimates of the rate of hair loss have long been quoted at 100 to 150 hairs per day, recent measurements indicate that the average rate of hair loss is closer to 35 to 40 hairs per day.

The Emotional Impact of Hair Loss

Although the medical community does not always recognize hair loss as a medical condition, the anguish felt by many of those who suffer from abnormal hair loss is very real and all too often overlooked. Results from a study that investigated perceptions of bald and balding men showed that compared to men who had hair, bald men were perceived as:

- Less physically attractive (by both sexes).

- Less assertive.

- Less successful.

- Less personally likable.

- Older (by about 5 years).

A study of how bald men perceive themselves showed that greater hair loss had a more significant impact than moderate hair loss. Men with more severe hair loss:

- Experience significantly more negative social and emotional effects.

- Are more preoccupied with their baldness.

- Make some effort to conceal or compensate for their hair loss.

Abnormal hair loss is not as common in women as it is in men, but it can be very traumatic and devastating for women who experience it because, as studies indicate, women have a greater emotional investment in their appearance. Many women with abnormal hair loss feel anxious, helpless, and less attractive. They may think that they are the only ones who have the problem. They also tend to worry that their hair loss is a symptom of a serious illness and sometimes try to disguise it from everyone, even their doctors, which is usually a mistake.

Over 63 million people in the United States suffer from abnormal hair loss. As a professional hairstylist, it is likely that you will be the first person that a hair loss sufferer will confide in, so it is important that you have a basic understanding of the different types of hair loss and the products and services that are available.

Types of Abnormal Hair Loss

Abnormal hair loss is called **alopecia** (al-oh-PEE-shah). The three most common types of abnormal hair loss are androgenic alopecia, alopecia areata, and postpartum alopecia.

Androgenic alopecia (an-druh-JEN-ik al-oh-PEE-shah), also known as *androgenetic alopecia* (an-druh-je-NET-ik al-oh-PEE-shah), is hair loss that is characterized by miniaturization of terminal hair that is converted into vellus hair. It is usually the result of genetics, age, or hormonal changes that cause terminal hair to miniaturize (**figure 11-12**).

Androgenic alopecia can begin as early as the teens and is frequently seen by the age of 40. By age 35, almost 40 percent of both men and women, show some degree of hair loss.

In men, androgenic alopecia is known as male pattern baldness and usually progresses to the familiar horseshoe-shaped fringe of hair. In women, it shows up as generalized thinning over the entire crown area. Androgenic alopecia affects millions of men and women in the United States.

Alopecia areata (al-oh-PEE-shah air-ee-AH-tah) is an autoimmune disorder that causes the affected hair follicles to be mistakenly attacked by a person's own immune system. White blood cells stop the hair growth during the anagen phase. It is a highly unpredictable skin disease that affects an estimated 5 million people in the United States

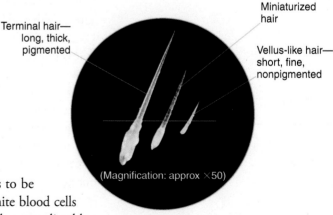

Terminal hair—
long, thick,
pigmented

Miniaturized
hair

Vellus-like hair—
short, fine,
nonpigmented

(Magnification: approx ×50)

figure 11-12
Miniaturization of the hair follicle

Pfizer Inc.

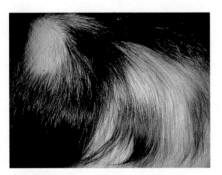

figure 11-13
Alopecia areata

alone. This hair disorder usually begins with one or more small, round, smooth bald patches on the scalp and can progress to total scalp hair loss, known as **alopecia totalis** (al-oh-PEE-shah toh-TAHL-us), or complete body hair loss, called **alopecia universalis** (al-oh-PEE-shah yoo-nih-vur-SAA-lis).

Alopecia areata occurs in males and females of all ages, races, and ethnic backgrounds and most often begins in childhood. The scalp usually shows no obvious signs of inflammation, skin disorder, or disease (figure 11-13).

Postpartum alopecia (POHST-pahr-tum al-oh-PEE-shah) is temporary hair loss experienced at the end of a pregnancy. For some women, pregnancy seems to disrupt the normal growth cycle of hair. There is very little normal hair loss during pregnancy, but then there is sudden and excessive shedding towards the end and sometimes up to 12 months after the pregnancy. Although this is usually very traumatic to the new mother, the growth cycle generally returns to normal within one year after the baby is delivered.

After reading the next few sections, you will be able to:

LO⑥ Identify and explain at least three options for hair loss treatment.

Hair Loss Treatments

Of all treatments that are said to counter hair loss, there are only two products—minoxidil and finasteride—that have been proven to stimulate hair growth and are approved by the FDA for sale in the United States.

Minoxidil is a topical (applied to the surface of the body) medication that is put on the scalp twice a day and has been proven to stimulate hair growth. It is sold over the counter (OTC) as a nonprescription drug. Minoxidil is available for both men and women and comes in two different strengths: 2 percent regular-strength solution and 5 percent extra-strength solution. It is not known to have any serious negative side effects. The most well-known minoxidil product on the market is Rogaine®.

Finasteride is an oral prescription medication for men only. Although finasteride is more effective and convenient than minoxidil, possible side effects include weight gain and loss of sexual function. Women may not use this treatment, and pregnant women or those who might become pregnant are cautioned not to even touch finasteride tablets because of the

Courtesy of Robert A. Silverman, M.D., Clinical Associate Professor, Department of Pediatrics, Georgetown University.

strong potential for birth defects. These over-the-counter medications slow the rate of hair loss and, in some cases, grow new hair. But once you stop using it, hair loss returns. In addition to the treatments described above, there are also several surgical options available to treat alopecia. A hair transplant is the most common permanent hair replacement technique. This process consists of removing small sections of hair, including the follicle, papilla, and hair bulb, from an area where there is a lot of hair (usually in the back) and transplanting them into the bald area. These sections grow normally in the new location. Only licensed surgeons may perform this procedure, and several surgeries are usually necessary to achieve the desired results. The cost of each surgery can range from $8,000 to over $20,000.

Hairstylists can offer a number of nonmedical options to counter hair loss. Some salons specialize in nonsurgical hair replacement systems such as wigs, toupees, hair weavings, and hair extensions. With proper training, you can learn to fit, color, cut, and style wigs and toupees. Hair weavings and hair extensions allow you to enhance a client's natural hair and create a look that boosts self-esteem (see Chapter 19, Wigs and Hair Additions).

After reading the next few sections, you will be able to:

LO **7** Learn to identify the most common hair and scalp disorders seen in the salon and school, and then name which ones a physician should treat.

Recognize Disorders of the Hair

The following disorders of the hair range from those that are commonplace and not particularly troublesome to those that are far more unusual or distressing:

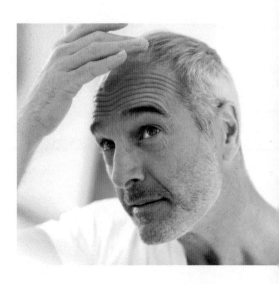

- **Canities** (kah-NIT-eez) is the technical term for gray hair. Canities results from the loss of the hair's natural melanin pigment. Other than the absence of pigment, gray hair is exactly the same as pigmented hair. The two types of canities are congenital and acquired.

- Congenital canities exists at or before birth. It occurs in albinos, who are born without pigment in the skin, hair, and eyes, and occasionally in individuals with normal hair. A patchy type of congenital canities may develop either slowly or rapidly, depending on the cause of the condition.

- Acquired canities develops with age and is the result of genetics. Although genetics is also responsible for premature canities, acquired canities may develop due to prolonged anxiety or illness.

- **Ringed hair** is a variety of canities, characterized by alternating bands of gray and pigmented hair throughout the length of the hair strand.

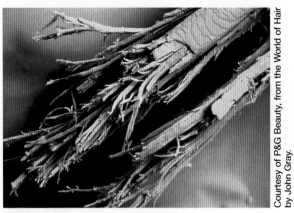

figure 11-14
Trichoptilosis

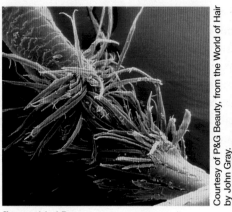

Courtesy of P&G Beauty, from the World of Hair by John Gray.

figure 11-15
Trichorrhexis nodosa

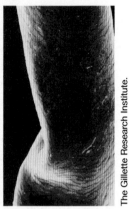

The Gillette Research Institute.

figure 11-16
Monilethrix

- **Hypertrichosis** (hi-pur-trih-KOH-sis), also known as *hirsuties* (hur-SOO-shee-eez), is a condition of abnormal growth of hair. It is characterized by the growth of terminal hair in areas of the body that normally grow only vellus hair. Mustaches or light beards on women are examples of hypertrichosis.

  Treatments for hypertrichosis include electrolysis, photoepilation, laser hair removal, shaving, tweezing, electronic tweezers, depilatories, epilators, threading, and sugaring (see Chapter 22, Hair Removal).

- **Trichoptilosis** (trih-kahp-tih-LOH-sus) is the technical term for split ends (figure 11-14). Hair conditioning treatments will soften and lubricate dry ends but will not repair split ends. The only way to remove split ends is by cutting them.

- **Trichorrhexis nodosa** (trik-uh-REK-sis nuh-DOH-suh) is the technical term for knotted hair (figure 11-15). It is characterized by brittleness and the formation of nodular swellings along the hair shaft. The hair breaks easily, and the broken fibers spread out like a brush along the hair shaft. Treatments include softening the hair with conditioners and moisturizers.

- **Monilethrix** (mah-NIL-ee-thriks) is the technical term for beaded hair (figure 11-16). The hair breaks easily between the beads or nodes. Treatments include hair and scalp conditioning.

- **Fragilitas crinium** (fruh-JIL-ih-tus KRI-nee-um) is the technical term for brittle hair. The hairs may split at any part of their length. Treatments include hair and scalp conditioning and haircutting above the split to prevent further damage.

Recognize Disorders of the Scalp

The skin is in a constant state of renewal. The outer layer of skin that covers your body is constantly being shed and replaced by new cells from below. The average person sheds about nine pounds of dead skin each year.

The skin cells of a normal, healthy scalp fall off naturally as small, dry flakes, without being noticed.

Dandruff can be easily mistaken for dry scalp because the symptoms of both conditions are a flaky, irritated scalp, but there is a difference. Dandruff commonly produces an oily scalp, but—just as the name indicates—the scalp is dry with the condition of dry scalp. The flakes from a dry scalp are much smaller and less noticeable than the larger flakes seen with dandruff. Dry scalp can result from contact dermatitis, sunburn, or extreme age, and is usually made worse by a cold, dry climate.

Dandruff

Pityriasis (pit-ih-RY-uh-sus) is the technical term for dandruff, which is characterized by the excessive production and accumulation of skin cells. Instead of the normal, one-at-a-time shedding of tiny individual skin cells, dandruff is the shedding of an accumulation of large, visible clumps of skin cells (figure 11-17).

Although the cause of dandruff has been debated for many years, current research confirms that dandruff is the result of a fungus called malassezia (mal-uh-SEEZ-ee-uh). **Malassezia** is a naturally occurring fungus that is present on all human skin but causes the symptoms of dandruff when it grows out of control. Some individuals are also more susceptible to malassezia's irritating effects. Factors such as stress, age, hormones, and poor hygiene can cause the fungus to multiply and dandruff symptoms to worsen.

Modern antidandruff shampoos contain the antifungal agents pyrithione zinc, selenium sulfide, or ketoconazole that control dandruff by suppressing the growth of malassezia. Antidandruff shampoos that contain pyrithione zinc are available in a variety of formulas for all hair types and are gentle enough to be used every day, even on color-treated hair. Frequent use of an antidandruff shampoo is essential for controlling dandruff. And although good personal hygiene and proper cleaning and disinfecting are important, dandruff is not contagious.

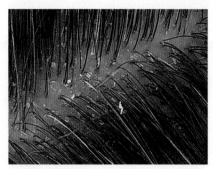

figure 11-17
Pityriasis, more commonly known as dandruff

⚠ **CAUTION**

You may find it difficult to speak with your client about a scalp disorder. After all, it is not easy to tell a client that you cannot perform a scheduled service because there may be something wrong with their scalp. If you feel that you cannot perform the service on your client and need help speaking with them about it, seek guidance from your instructor or salon manager.

If you encounter such a situation and feel you are ready to discuss the situation with your client, try this approach.

"Mrs. Smith, I noticed that your scalp looks different today. I am not licensed to diagnose any scalp disorders, but I am concerned and think you should see a physician about it as soon as possible. For your safety, I should not continue with the service you have scheduled."

Do not let your client try to talk you into performing the service. It could put you, your other clients, and the salon at risk of spreading the scalp disorder.

There are two principal types of dandruff:

- **Pityriasis capitis simplex** (pit-ih-RY-uh-sus KAP-ih-tis SIM-pleks) is the technical term for classic dandruff that is characterized by scalp irritation, large flakes, and an itchy scalp. The scales may attach to the scalp in masses, scatter loosely in the hair, or fall to the shoulders. Regular use of antidandruff shampoos, conditioners, and topical lotions are the best treatment.

- **Pityriasis steatoides** (pit-ih-RY-uh-sus stee-uh-TOY-deez) is a more severe case of dandruff characterized by an accumulation of greasy or waxy scales, mixed with sebum, that stick to the scalp in crusts. As explained in Chapter 8, Skin Disorders and Diseases, when this condition is accompanied by redness and inflammation, it is called seborrheic dermatitis. Seborrheic dermatitis also can be found in the eyebrows or beard. You should not perform a service on anyone who has dandruff, as the scalp is irritated and itchy. Antidandruff shampoo can be recommended to a client with mild conditions, but anyone with severe conditions must be referred to a physician.

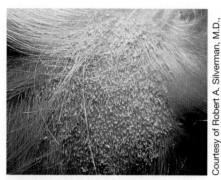

figure 11-18
Tinea capitis

Fungal Infections (Tinea)

Tinea (TIN-ee-uh) is the technical term for ringworm. It is characterized by itching, scales, and, sometimes, painful circular lesions. Several patches may be present at one time. Tinea is caused by a fungal organism and not a parasite, as the old-fashioned term *ringworm* seems to suggest. Tinea infections are named for the part or location of the body they infect.

All forms of tinea are contagious and can be easily transmitted from one person to another. Infected skin scales or hairs that contain the fungi are known to spread the disease. Bathtubs, swimming pools, and unclean personal articles are also sources of transmission. Practicing approved cleaning and disinfection procedures will help prevent the spread of this disease in the salon.

As you read in Chapter 5, Infection Control: Principals and Practices, *tinea capitis,* sometimes called "ringworm of the scalp," is another type of fungal infection characterized by red papules, or spots, at the opening of the hair follicles. The patches spread and the hair becomes brittle. Hair often breaks off leaving only a stump or the hair may be shed from the enlarged open follicle (**figure 11-18**). Tinea barbae is a superficial fungal infection caused by a variety of dermatophytes that commonly affects the skin. It is primarily limited to the bearded areas of the face and neck or around the scalp (**figure 11-19**). It is similar to tinea capitis in appearance. You should not perform a service on anyone who has or who you suspect may have tinea barbae. A client with this condition must be referred to a physician for medical treatment.

Tinea favosa (TIN-ee-uh fah-VOH-suh), also known as *tinea favus* (TIN-ee-uh FAH-vus), is characterized by dry, sulfur-yellow, cuplike crusts on the scalp called **scutula** (SKUCH-ul-uh). Scutula has a distinctive odor. Scars from tinea favosa are bald patches that may be pink or white and shiny (**figure 11-20**).

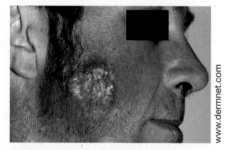

figure 11-19
Folliculitis barbae or tinea (ringworm) barbae

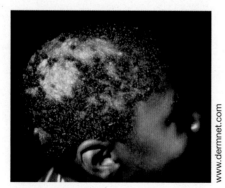

figure 11-20
Tinea favosa, also known as tinea favus

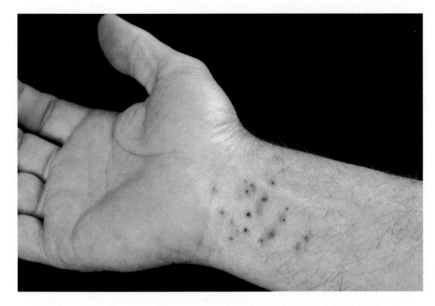

figure 11-21
Scabies infestation on wrist and arm

Remember: You should never perform a service on anyone who has or you suspect may have a fungal infection. If you are not certain about whether the condition is a fungal infection, be safe and refer your client to a physician.

Parasitic Infections

Scabies is a highly contagious skin disease caused by a parasite called a mite that burrows under the skin. Vesicles (blisters) and pustules (inflamed pimples with pus) usually form on the scalp from the irritation caused by this parasite. Excessive itching accompanies this condition and scratching the infected areas makes the affected area worse. Practicing approved cleaning and disinfection procedures is very important to prevent the spread of this disease (figure 11-21).

You should not perform a service on anyone who has scabies. A client with this condition must be referred to a physician for medical treatment.

Pediculosis capitis (puh-dik-yuh-LOH-sis KAP-ih-tis) is the infestation of the hair and scalp with head lice (figures 11-22 and 11-23). As these parasites feed on the scalp, it begins to itch. If the scalp is scratched, it can cause an infection. Head lice are transmitted from one person to another by contact with infested hats, combs, brushes, and other personal articles. You can distinguish head lice from dandruff flakes by looking closely at the scalp with a magnifying glass.

Properly practicing state board-approved cleaning and disinfection procedures will prevent the spread of this infestation. Several nonprescription medications are available.

You should not perform a service on anyone who has head lice. A client with this condition must be referred to a physician or a pharmacist.

Bacterial Infections

Bacterial infections of the scalp are caused by two strains of bacteria known as staphylococci and streptococci. Most common types of staphylococci infections are furuncles, carbuncles, and folliculitis.

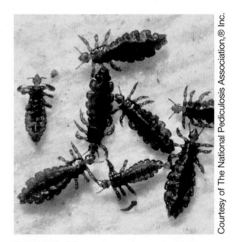

figure 11-22
Head lice

Courtesy of The National Pediculosis Association,® Inc.

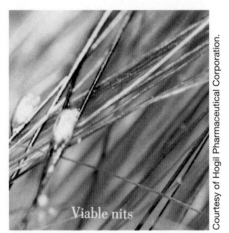

figure 11-23
Nits (lice eggs)

Viable nits

Courtesy of Hogil Pharmaceutical Corporation.

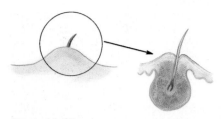

figure 11-24a
Furuncle (boil)

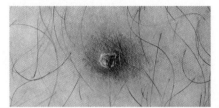

figure 11-24b

HERE'S A TIP
Remember to re-schedule the appointment if you refer a client to a physician. Follow up with a call two to three days before the appointment.

- A **furuncle** (FYOO-rung-kul) is the technical term for a boil, an acute, localized bacterial infection of the hair follicle that produces constant pain (**figures 11-24a** and **11-24b**). It is limited to a specific area and produces a pustule perforated by a hair.

- A **carbuncle** (KAHR-bung-kul) is an inflammation of the subcutaneous tissue caused by staphylococci. It is similar to a furuncle but is larger.

- Folliculitis is an infection of the hair follicles frequently caused by staphylococcus or other bacteria. Infections are seen as small, white-headed pimples around one or more follicles. Mild folliculitis may heal by itself in few days but deep or recurring ones need medical attention. One common example seen in hair salons is folliculitis barbae, also known as *pseudofolliculitis barbae*. It is an inflammation of hair follicles caused by a bacterial infection often caused by Staphylococcus aureus. Outside of healthcare, this is regularly referred to as *barber's itch* or *hot tub folliculitis*.

Properly practicing state board-approved cleaning and disinfection procedures will prevent the spread of these infections.

You should not perform a service on anyone who has a boil, carbuncle, or folliculitis. A client with any of these conditions must be referred to a physician for medical treatment.

After reading the next few sections, you will be able to:

LO⑧ Compare and describe the different factors that should be considered during a hair and scalp analysis.

Learn How To Perform a Thorough Hair and Scalp Analysis

All successful salon services must begin with a thorough analysis of the condition of the client's scalp and client's hair type. Knowing the client's scalp condition and the client's hair type allows you to prepare and make decisions about the results that can be expected from the service.

Because different types of hair react differently to the same service, it is essential that a thorough analysis be performed before all salon services. Hair analysis is performed by observation using the senses of sight, touch, sound, and smell. The four most important factors to consider in hair analysis are texture, density, porosity, and elasticity. Other factors that you should also be aware of are growth pattern and dryness versus oiliness.

Texture

Hair texture is the thickness or diameter of the individual hair strand. Hair texture can be classified as coarse, medium, or fine (**figures 11-25, 11-26,**

© Inxti/Shutterstock.com

242   PART 2 | GENERAL SCIENCES

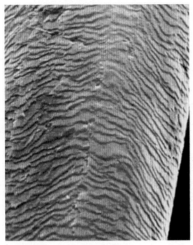

figure 11-25
Coarse hair

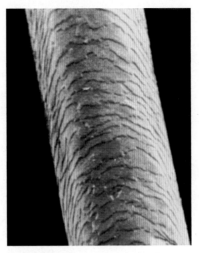

figure 11-26
Medium hair

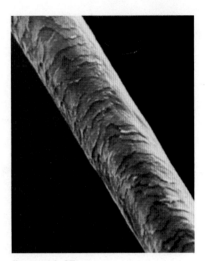

figure 11-27
Fine hair

and 11-27) and can vary from strand to strand on the same person's head. It is not uncommon for hair from different areas of the head to have different textures. Hair on the nape (back of the neck), crown, temples, and front hairline of the same person may have different textures.

Coarse hair texture has the largest diameter. It is stronger than fine hair for the same reason that a thick rope is stronger than a thin rope. It is often more resistant to processing than medium or fine hair, so it usually requires more processing when you are applying products such as hair lighteners, haircolors, permanent waving solutions, and chemical hair relaxers.

Medium hair texture is the most common texture and is the standard to which other hair is compared. Medium hair does not pose any special problems or concerns.

Fine hair has the smallest diameter and is more fragile, easier to process, and more susceptible to damage from chemical services than coarse or medium hair.

As with hair cuticle analysis, hair texture can be determined by feeling a single dry strand between the fingers. Take an individual strand from four different areas of the head—front hairline, temple, crown, and nape—and hold each strand securely with one hand while feeling it with the thumb and forefinger of the other hand. With a little practice, you will be able to feel the difference between coarse, medium, and fine hair diameters (figure 11-28).

FOCUS ON

Selling retail products increases client retention. A client who takes home a retail product is more than twice as likely to return for services. Recommending products for home use is an important part of a successful career as a hairstylist. Your client needs to know what products to use and how to use them.

A complete hair analysis will enable you to recommend the right products for your client with confidence. It is your job to know more about your client's specific needs than anyone else and to recommend the right products to satisfy those needs. Your clients consider you to be their expert in hair care, so do not be shy about analyzing their needs and making recommendations to them since they genuinely benefit from your advice.

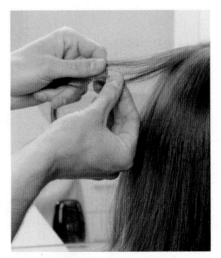

figure 11-28
Testing for hair texture

table 11-4

AVERAGE NUMBER OF HAIRS ON THE HEAD BY HAIR COLOR

Hair Color	Average Number of Hairs on Head
Blond	140,000
Brown	110,000
Black	108,000
Red	80,000

Density

Hair density measures the number of individual hair strands on one square inch (2.5 square centimeters) of scalp. It indicates how many hairs there are on a person's head. Hair density can be classified as low, medium, or high (also known as thin, medium, or thick/dense). Hair density is different from hair texture—individuals with the same hair texture can have different densities.

Some individuals may have coarse hair texture (each hair has a large diameter), but low hair density (a low number of hairs on the head). Others may have fine hair texture (each hair has a small diameter), but high hair density (a high number of hairs on the head).

The average hair density is about 2,200 hairs per one square inch. Hair with high density (thick or dense hair) has more hairs per one square inch, and hair with low density (thin hair) has fewer hairs per one square inch. The average head of hair contains about 100,000 individual hair strands. The number of hairs on the head generally varies with the color of the hair. Blonds usually have the highest density, and people with red hair tend to have the lowest. **Table 11-4** shows hair density by hair color.

Porosity

Hair porosity is the ability of the hair to absorb moisture. The degree of porosity is directly related to the condition of the cuticle layer. Healthy hair with a compact cuticle layer is naturally resistant to being penetrated by moisture and is referred to as **hydrophobic** (hy-druh-FOHB-ik). Porous hair has a raised cuticle layer that easily absorbs moisture and is called **hydrophilic** (hy-druh-FIL-ik).

Hair with average porosity is considered to be normal hair (**figure 11-29**). Chemical services performed on this type of hair will usually process as expected, according to the texture.

Hair with low porosity is considered resistant (**figure 11-30**). Chemical services performed on hair with low porosity require a more alkaline solution than those on hair with high porosity. Alkaline solutions raise the cuticle and permit uniform saturation and processing on resistant hair.

Hair with high porosity is considered overly porous hair and is often the result of previous overprocessing (**figure 11-31**). Overly porous hair is

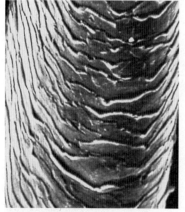

figure 11-29
Average porosity (normal hair)

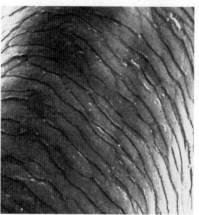

figure 11-30
Low porosity (resistant hair)

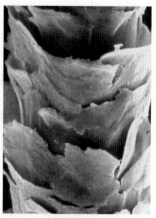

figure 11-31
High porosity (overly porous hair)

The Gillette Research Institute.

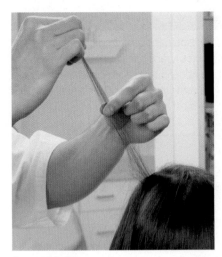

figure 11-32
Testing for hair porosity

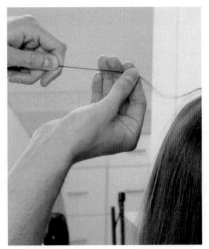

figure 11-33
Testing for hair elasticity

damaged, dry, fragile, and brittle. Chemical services performed on overly porous hair require less alkaline solutions with a lower pH, which help prevent additional overprocessing and damage.

The texture of the hair can be an indication of its porosity, but it is only a general rule of thumb. Different degrees of porosity can be found in all hair textures. Although coarse hair normally has a low porosity and is resistant to chemical services, in some cases coarse hair will have high porosity, perhaps as the result of previous chemical services.

You can check porosity on dry hair by taking a strand of several hairs from four different areas of the head (front hairline, temple, crown, and nape). Hold the strand securely with one hand while sliding the thumb and forefinger of the other hand from the end to the scalp. If the hair feels smooth and the cuticle is compact, dense, and hard, it is considered resistant. If you can feel a slight roughness, it is considered porous. If the hair feels very rough, dry, or breaks, it is considered highly porous and may have been overprocessed (figure 11-32).

Elasticity

Hair elasticity is the ability of the hair to stretch and return to its original length without breaking. Hair elasticity is an indication of the strength of the side bonds that hold the hair's individual fibers in place. Wet hair with normal elasticity will stretch up to 50 percent of its original length and return to that same length without breaking. Dry hair stretches about 20 percent of its length.

Hair with low elasticity is brittle and breaks easily. It may not be able to hold the curl from wet setting, thermal styling, or permanent waving. Hair with low elasticity is the result of weak side bonds that usually are a result of overprocessing. Chemical services performed on hair with low elasticity require a milder solution with a lower pH to minimize further damage and prevent additional overprocessing.

Check elasticity on wet hair by taking an individual strand from four different areas of the head (front hairline, temple, crown, and nape). Hold a single strand of wet hair securely and try to pull it apart (figure 11-33).

If the hair stretches and returns to its original length without breaking, it has normal elasticity. If the hair breaks easily or fails to return to its original length, it has low elasticity.

Hair Growth Patterns

Hair growth patterns are important to identify and consider, especially when preparing to shape and style the hair. During your hair analysis, you should identify any and all hair growth patterns and take them into consideration when creating the overall look, haircut, or hairstyle the client wants to achieve.

Hair follicles that grow out of the head at a perpendicular, 90-degree angle or in a straight direction from the head may cause the following growth patterns to result:

- A **hair stream** is hair flowing in the same direction, resulting from follicles sloping in the same direction. Two streams flowing in opposite directions from the head form a natural part in the hair.

- A **whorl** (WHORL) occurs when hair leaves the follicles at an angle; the hair will lie in a particular direction forming patterns or streams on the head. Often the streams spiral outward from a central point. Usually they run in a clockwise direction and sometimes more than one whorl can be seen in certain individuals (figure 11-34).

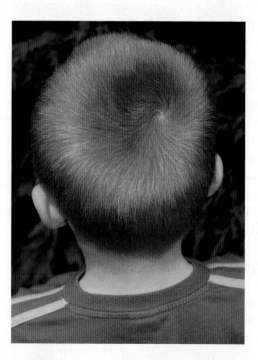

figure 11-34
Example of a whorl

© iStockphoto/RMAX

• A **cowlick** (KOW-lik) is due to a particular pattern of hair stream on the forehead. Cowlicks are usually more noticeable at the front hairline in people with short, thick hair but they may be located anywhere on the head (figure 11-35).

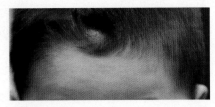

figure 11-35
Example of a cowlick

Dry Hair and Scalp

Dry hair and scalp can be caused by inactive sebaceous glands. These conditions are aggravated by excessive shampooing or by a dry climate. The lack of natural oils (sebum) leads to hair that appears dull, dry, and lifeless. Dry hair and scalp should be treated with products that contain moisturizers and emollients.

People with dry hair and scalp should avoid frequent shampooing along with the use of strong soaps, detergents, or products with a high alcohol content because these products could aggravate existing conditions. Dry hair should not be confused with overly porous hair that has been damaged by thermal styling, chemical services, or environmental conditions.

Oily Hair and Scalp

Oily hair and scalp, characterized by a greasy buildup on the scalp and an oily coating on the hair, are caused by improper shampooing or overactive sebaceous glands. Oily hair and scalp can be treated by properly washing with a normalizing shampoo. A well-balanced diet, exercise, regular shampooing, and good personal hygiene are essential to controlling oily hair and scalp.

Healthy Hair, Happy Clients

The more you learn about the structure of hair and how to keep it healthy, the more you will understand how salon services affect different hair types. This is the key to consistent results with your services and happy clients who recommend you to their friends.

REVIEW QUESTIONS

1. Name and describe the five main structures of the hair root.

2. Name and describe the three layers of the hair shaft.

3. Explain the process of keratinization.

4. What are polypeptide chains?

5. List and describe the three types of side bonds. Indicate whether they are strong or weak and why.

6. Name and describe the two types of melanin responsible for natural hair color.

7. Name and describe the two types of hair and their locations on the body.

8. What are the three phases of the hair growth cycle? What occurs during each phase?

9. What is the reason for normal daily hair loss?

10. What are the most common types of abnormal hair loss?

11. What are the only two approved hair loss treatments?

12. Name the two main types of dandruff. Can either one be treated in the salon?

13. Which hair and scalp disorders cannot be treated in the salon?

14. What four factors about the hair should be considered in a hair analysis?

STUDY TOOLS

- **Reinforce what you just learned:** Complete the activities and exercises in your Theory or Practical Workbook, or your Study Guide.

- **Expand your knowledge:** Search for websites about the topics in this chapter and make a list of additional resources.

- **Study and prepare for your quiz:** Take the chapter test in your Exam Review or your Milady U: Online Licensing Prep.

- **Re-Test your knowledge:** Take the Chapter 11 *Quizzes*!

- **Learn even more:** Look up in a dictionary or search the internet for the definitions of any additional terms you want to learn about.

CHAPTER GLOSSARY

alopecia al-oh-PEE-shah	p. 235	Abnormal hair loss.
alopecia areata al-oh-PEE-shah air-ee-AH-tah	p. 235	Autoimmune disorder that causes the affected hair follicles to be mistakenly attacked by a person's own immune system; usually begins with one or more small, round, smooth bald patches on the scalp.
alopecia totalis al-oh-PEE-shah toh-TAHL-us	p. 236	Total loss of scalp hair.
alopecia universalis al-oh-PEE-shah yoo-nih-vur-SAA-lis	p. 236	Complete loss of body hair.
amino acids uh-MEE-noh AS-udz	p. 228	Units that are joined together end-to-end like pop beads by strong, chemical peptide bonds (end bonds) to form the polypeptide chains that comprise proteins.

anagen phase AN-uh-jen FAYZ	p. 232	Also known as *growth phase*; phase during which new hair is produced.
androgenic alopecia an-druh-JEN-ik al-oh-PEE-shah	p. 235	Also known as *androgenetic alopecia* (an-druh-je-NET-ik al-oh-PEE-shah); hair loss characterized by miniaturization of terminal hair that is converted to vellus hair; in men, it is known as male pattern baldness.
arrector pili muscle	p. 225	The small, involuntary muscle in the base of the hair follicle.
canities kah-NIT-eez	p. 237	Technical term for gray hair; results from the loss of the hair's natural melanin pigment.
carbuncle KAHR-bung-kul	p. 242	Inflammation of the subcutaneous tissue caused by staphylococci; similar to a furuncle but larger.
catagen phase KAT-uh-jen FAYZ	p. 233	The brief transition period between the growth and resting phases of a hair follicle. It signals the end of the growth phase.
COHNS elements KOH-nz EL-uh-ments	p. 227	The five elements—carbon, oxygen, hydrogen, nitrogen, and sulfur—that make up human hair, skin, tissue, and nails.
cortex KOR-teks	p. 227	Middle layer of the hair; a fibrous protein core formed by elongated cells containing melanin pigment.
cowlick KOW-lik	p. 247	Tuft of hair that stands straight up.
cysteine SIS-ti-een	p. 228	An amino acid with a sulfur atom (S) that joins together two peptide strands.
cystine SIS-teen	p. 228	An amino acid formed when 2 cysteine amino acids (with single sulfur) are joined by their sulfur groups or disulfide bond.
dermal papilla DERMAL puh-PIL-uh	p. 225	Plural: dermal papillae. A small, cone-shaped elevation located at the base of the hair follicle that fits into the hair bulb.
disulfide bond dy-SUL-fyd BAHND	p. 228	Strong chemical side bond that joins the sulfur atoms of two neighboring cysteine amino acids to create one cystine, which joins together two polypeptide strands like rungs on a ladder.
eumelanin you-mell-ee-non	p. 230	Provides natural dark brown to black color to the hair and is the dark pigment predominant in black and brunette hair.
fragilitas crinium fruh-JIL-ih-tus KRI-nee-um	p. 238	Technical term for brittle hair.
furuncle FYOO-rung-kul	p. 242	Boil; acute, localized bacterial infection of the hair follicle that produces constant pain.
hair bulb	p. 225	Lowest part of a hair strand; the thickened, club-shaped structure that forms the lower part of the hair root.
hair cuticle HAYR KYOO-ti-kul	p. 226	Outermost layer of hair; consisting of a single, overlapping layer of transparent, scale-like cells that look like shingles on a roof.
hair density	p. 244	The number of individual hair strands on 1 square inch (2.5 square centimeters) of scalp.
hair elasticity HAYR ee-las-TIS-ut-ee	p. 245	Ability of the hair to stretch and return to its original length without breaking.
hair follicle HAYR FAWL-ih-kul	p. 225	The tube-like depression or pocket in the skin or scalp that contains the hair root.
hair porosity HAYR puh-RAHS-ut-ee	p. 244	Ability of the hair to absorb moisture.

hair root	p. 224	The part of the hair located below the surface of the epidermis.
hair shaft	p. 224	The portion of hair that projects above the epidermis.
hair stream	p. 246	Hair flowing in the same direction, resulting from follicles sloping in the same direction.
hair texture	p. 242	Thickness or diameter of the individual hair strand.
helix HEE-licks	p. 228	Spiral shape of a coiled protein created by polypeptide chains that intertwine with each other.
hydrogen bond HY-druh-jun BAHND	p. 228	A weak, physical, cross-link side bond that is easily broken by water or heat.
hydrophilic hy-druh-FIL-ik	p. 244	Easily absorbs moisture; in chemistry terms, capable of combining with or attracting water (water-loving).
hydrophobic hy-druh-FOHB-ik	p. 244	Naturally resistant to being penetrated by moisture.
hypertrichosis hi-pur-trih-KOH-sis	p. 238	Also known as *hirsuties* (hur-SOO-shee-eez); condition of abnormal growth of hair, characterized by the growth of terminal hair in areas of the body that normally grow only vellus hair.
keratin	p. 227	A fibrous protein that grows from cells originating within the hair follicle.
keratinization kair-uh-ti-ni-ZAY-shun	p. 227	Process by which newly formed cells in the hair bulb mature, fill with keratin, move upward, lose their nucleus, and die.
lanthionine bonds lan-THY-oh-neen BAHNDZ	p. 229	The bonds created when disulfide bonds are broken by hydroxide chemical hair relaxers after the relaxer is rinsed from the hair.
malassezia mal-uh-SEEZ-ee-uh	p. 239	Naturally occurring fungus that is present on all human skin, but is responsible for dandruff when it grows out of control.
medulla muh-DUL-uh	p. 227	Innermost layer of the hair that is composed of round cells; often absent in fine and naturally blond hair.
melanin	p. 230	The tiny grains of pigment in the cortex that give natural color to the hair.
monilethrix mah-NIL-ee-thriks	p. 238	Technical term for beaded hair.
pediculosis capitis puh-dik-yuh-LOH-sis KAP-ih-tis	p. 241	Infestation of the hair and scalp with head lice.
peptide bond PEP-tyd BAHND	p. 228	Also known as an *end bond*; chemical bond that joins amino acids to each other, end-to-end, to form a polypeptide chain.
pheomelanin	p. 230	The lighter pigment that provides natural colors ranging from red and ginger to yellow and blond tones.
pityriasis pit-ih-RY-uh-sus	p. 239	Technical term for dandruff; characterized by excessive production and accumulation of skin cells.
pityriasis capitis simplex pit-ih-RY-uh-sus KAP-ih-tis SIM-pleks	p. 240	Technical term for classic dandruff; characterized by scalp irritation, large flakes, and itchy scalp.
pityriasis steatoides pit-ih-RY-uh-sus stee-uh-TOY-deez	p. 240	Severe case of dandruff characterized by an accumulation of greasy or waxy scales mixed with sebum that stick to the scalp in crusts.
polypeptide chain pahl-ee-PEP-tyd CHAYN	p. 228	A long chain of amino acids linked by peptide bonds.
postpartum alopecia POHST-pahr-tum al-oh-PEE-shah	p. 236	Temporary hair loss experienced towards the end and after the pregnancy.

proteins PROH-teenz	p. 228	Long, coiled complex polypeptides made of amino acids.
ringed hair	p. 237	Variety of canities characterized by alternating bands of gray and pigmented hair throughout the length of the hair strand.
salt bond	p. 228	A weak, physical, cross-link side bond between adjacent polypeptide chains.
scutula SKUCH-ul-uh	p. 240	Dry, sulfur-yellow, cuplike crusts on the scalp in tinea favosa or tinea favus.
sebaceous glands	p. 225	The oil glands in the skin that are connected to the hair follicles.
sebum	p. 225	A fatty or oily substance secreted by the sebaceous glands that lubricates the skin.
side bonds	p. 228	Bonds that cross-link the polypeptide chains together and are responsible for the extreme strength and elasticity of human hair.
telogen phase TEL-uh-jen FAYZ	p. 233	Also known as *resting phase*; the final phase in the hair cycle that lasts until the fully grown hair is shed.
terminal hair TUR-mih-nul HAYR	p. 240	Long, coarse, pigmented hair found on the scalp, legs, arms, and bodies of males and females.
tinea TIN-ee-uh	p. 240	Technical term for ringworm—a contagious condition caused by fungal infection and not a parasite; characterized by itching, scales, and, sometimes, painful lesions.
tinea favosa TIN-ee-uh fah-VOH-suh	p. 240	Also known as *tinea favus*; fungal infection characterized by dry, sulfur-yellow, cuplike crusts on the scalp called scutula.
trichology trih-KAHL-uh-jee	p. 224	Scientific study of hair and its diseases and care.
trichoptilosis trih-kahp-tih-LOH-sus	p. 238	Technical term for split ends.
trichorrhexis nodosa trik-uh-REK-sis nuh-DOH-suh	p. 238	Technical term for knotted hair; it is characterized by brittleness and the formation of nodular swellings along the hair shaft.
vellus hair VEL-us HAYR	p. 232	Also known as *lanugo hair*; short, fine, unpigmented, and downy hair that appears on the body, with the exception of the palms of the hands and the soles of the feet.
wave pattern	p. 230	The shape of the hair strands; described as straight, wavy, curly, and extremely curly.
whorl WHORL	p. 246	Hair that forms in a circular pattern on the crown of the head.

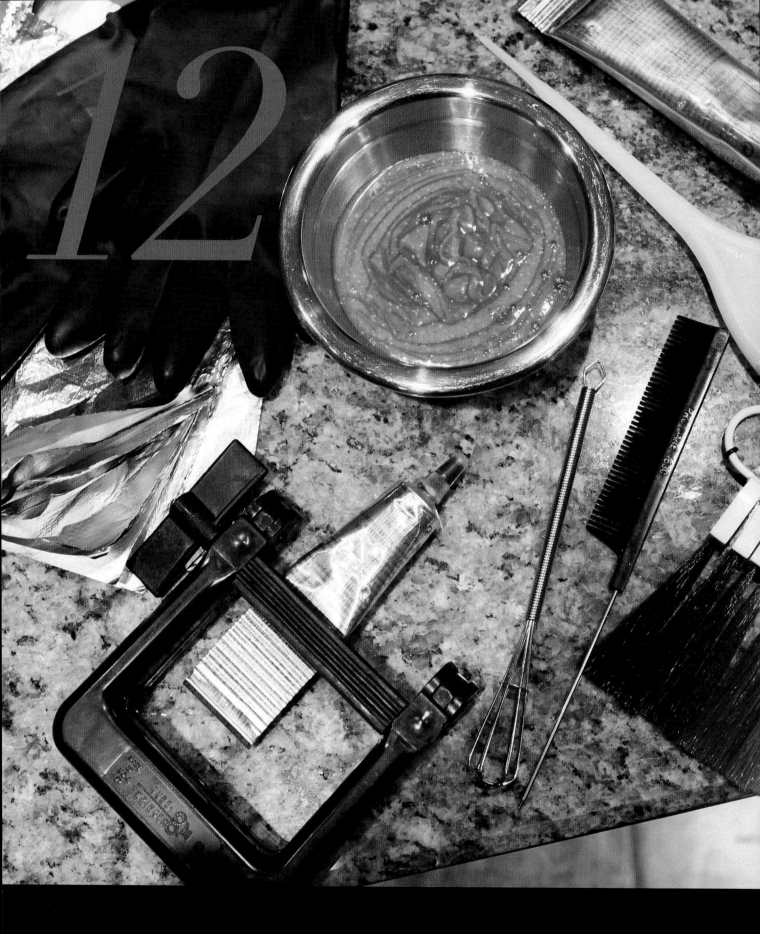

12

BASICS OF CHEMISTRY

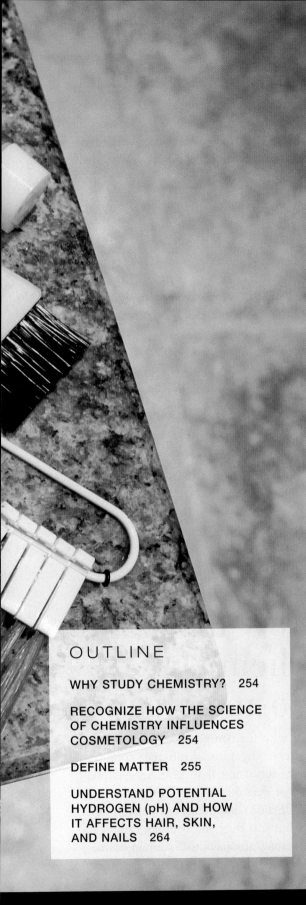

LEARNING OBJECTIVES

After completing this chapter, you will be able to:

LO❶
List the difference between organic and inorganic chemistry.

LO❷
Categorize and give examples of different substances for each of the different states of matter: solid, liquid, and gas.

LO❸
Summarize, in your own words, oxidation–reduction (redox) reactions.

LO❹
Define the differences between pure substances and physical mixtures.

LO❺
Evaluate the differences among solutions, suspensions, and emulsions.

LO❻
Explain what pH is and how the pH scale works.

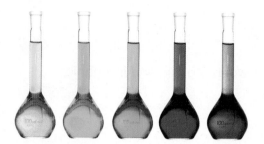

What do you think about when someone mentions the word *chemistry*? Beakers of mixtures bubbling in a lab? Test tubes filled with strange-looking liquids? Petri dishes growing fuzzy things? Most cosmetology services depend on the use of chemicals. So, studying the basics of chemistry means that you will have the knowledge you need to understand the products that you are using in the salon to give your clients the professional services they deserve.

why study
CHEMISTRY?

Cosmetologists should study and have a thorough understanding of chemistry because:

> Without an understanding of basic chemistry, you would not be able to use professional products effectively and safely.

> Every product used in the salon and in cosmetology services contains some type of chemical.

> With an understanding of chemistry, you will be able to troubleshoot and solve common problems you may encounter with chemical services.

After reading the next few sections, you will be able to:

LO ❶ **List the difference between organic and inorganic chemistry.**

Recognize How the Science of Chemistry Influences Cosmetology

Chemistry is the science that deals with the composition, structures, and properties of matter and how matter changes under different conditions.

Organic chemistry is the study of substances that contain the element carbon. All living things or things that were once alive, whether they are plants or animals, contain carbon. Organic compounds can contain other elements like nitrogen and oxygen, but it is the bond between carbon and hydrogen that makes it organic. Organic substances that contain both carbon and hydrogen can burn. Although the term *organic* is often used to mean safe or natural because of its association with living things such as foods or food ingredients, not all organic substances are natural, healthy, or safe.

You may be surprised to learn that gasoline, motor oil, plastics, synthetic fabrics, pesticides, and fertilizers are all organic substances.

All hair color products, chemical texturizers, shampoos, conditioners, styling aids, nail enhancements, and skin care products are organic chemicals. So remember, the word *organic*, as applied to chemistry, does not mean natural or healthy; it means that the material contains both carbon and hydrogen from either natural or synthetic sources.

Inorganic chemistry is the study of substances that do not contain the element carbon but may contain the element hydrogen. Most inorganic substances do not burn because they do not contain carbon. Inorganic substances are not, and never were, alive. Metals, minerals, glass, water, and air are inorganic substances. Pure water and oxygen are inorganic, yet they are essential to life. Hydrogen peroxide, hydroxide hair relaxers, titanium dioxide, and zinc oxide in sun protection creams are inorganic substances.

Define Matter

Matter is any substance that occupies space and has mass (weight). All matter has physical and chemical properties and exists in the form of a solid, liquid, or gas. Since matter is made from chemicals, everything made out of matter is a chemical.

Matter has physical properties that we can touch, taste, smell, or see. In fact, everything you can touch and everything you can see—with the exception of light and electricity—is matter. All matter is made up of chemicals. You can see visible light and light that electrical sparks create, but these are not made of matter. Light and electricity are forms of energy and energy is not matter. Everything known to exist in the universe is either made of matter or energy. There are no exceptions to this rule.

Energy does not occupy space or have mass. Energy is discussed further in Chapter 13, Basics of Electricity. This chapter is dedicated to matter.

Elements

An **element** is the simplest form of chemical matter. It cannot be broken down into a simpler substance without a loss of identity. There are 118 known elements today and of these 98 occur naturally and the rest are produced by synthetic methods from nuclear reactions. All matter in the universe is made up of these elements and they have their own distinct physical and chemical

---

? DID YOU KNOW?

Using the word *chemical* to describe something does not mean it is dangerous or harmful. Water and air are 100 percent chemicals. Even your body is completely composed of chemicals.

The vast majority of chemicals you come in contact with every day are safe and harmless. When chemicals do have the potential to cause harm, manufacturers are required to describe that potential harm on the packaging or label. There is no such thing as a chemical-free product, so do not be fooled by misleading marketing claims.

properties. Each element is identified by a letter symbol, such as *O* for oxygen, *C* for carbon, *H* for hydrogen, *N* for nitrogen, and *S* for sulfur. Symbols for all elements can be found in the Periodic Table of Elements in chemistry textbooks or by searching the Internet.

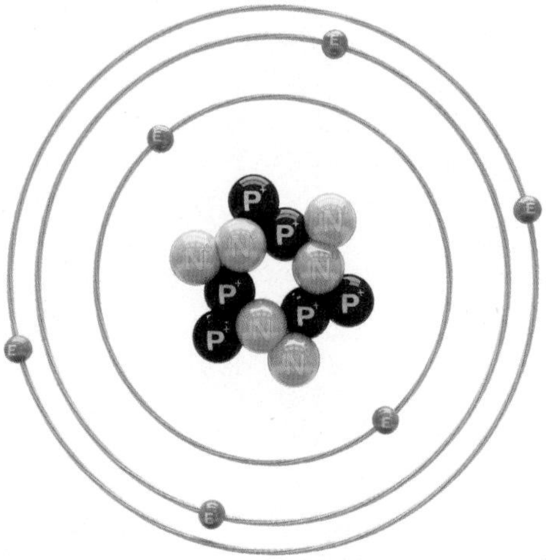

Atom

An **atom** is the basic unit of matter with a nucleus at the center surrounded by negatively charged **electrons** (E) that move around the nucleus in orbits. The nucleus consists of **protons** (P) (subatomic particles with a positive charge) and **neutrons** (N) (subatomic particles with no charge) and the number of protons determines the element. Atoms cannot be divided into simpler substances by ordinary chemical means. Figure 12-1 shows the atomic structure of carbon with six protons and six neutrons at the nucleus and six electrons in the orbit.

Molecules

Just as words are made by combining letters, molecules are made by combining atoms. A **molecule** (MAHL-uh-kyool) is a chemical combination of two or more atoms in definite (fixed) proportions. For example, water is made from hydrogen atoms and oxygen atoms. Carbon dioxide is made from carbon atoms and oxygen atoms.

Atmospheric oxygen and other chemical substances, such as nitrogen and water vapor, make up the air you breathe. This type of oxygen is called an **elemental molecule** (EL-uh-men-tul MAHL-uh-kyool), a molecule containing two or more atoms of the same element (in this case, oxygen) in definite (fixed) proportions. It is written as O_2. Ozone is another elemental molecule made up of oxygen. Ozone is a major component of smog and can be very dangerous. It contains three atoms of the element oxygen and is written as O_3 (figure 12-2).

Compound molecules (KAHM-pownd MAHL-uh-kyools), also known as *compounds*, are a chemical combination of two or more atoms of different elements in definite (fixed) proportions (figure 12-3). Sodium chloride (NaCl), common table salt, is an example of compound molecules. Each sodium chloride molecule contains one atom of the element sodium (Na) and one atom of the element chlorine (Cl).

figure 12-1
Atomic structure of carbon with six protons, six neutrons, and six electrons

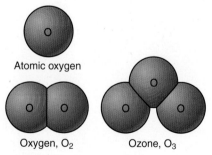

figure 12-2
Elemental molecules contain two or more atoms of the same element in definite (fixed) proportions.

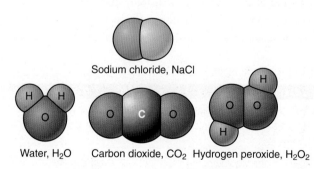

figure 12-3
Compound molecules contain two or more atoms of different elements in definite (fixed) proportions.

LO ❷   Describe and give examples of different substances for each of the different states of matter: solid, liquid, and gas.

States of Matter

All matter exists in one of three different physical forms:

- Solid
- Liquid
- Gas

These three forms are called the **states of matter**. Matter (table 12-1) becomes one of these states, depending on its temperature (figure 12-4).

Like many other substances, water (H_2O) can exist in all three states of matter, depending on its temperature. For example, water changes according to how the temperature changes, but it is still water. When water freezes, it turns to ice. When ice melts, it turns back into water. When water boils, it turns to steam. When the steam cools, it turns back into water. The water stays the same chemical, but it becomes a different physical form. When one chemical changes its state of matter, the change is called a physical change. (See Physical and Chemical Changes in this chapter.)

Vapor is a liquid that has evaporated into a gas-like state. Vapors can return to being a liquid when they cool to room temperature, unlike a gas. Steam is an example of a vapor. Vapors are not a unique state of matter; they are liquids that have undergone a physical change.

Physical and Chemical Properties of Matter

Every substance has unique properties that allow us to identify it. The two types of properties are physical and chemical.

Physical properties are characteristics that can be determined without a chemical reaction and that do not involve a chemical change in the substance.

Solid

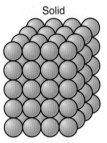

Liquid

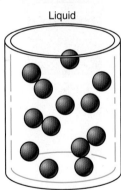

Gas

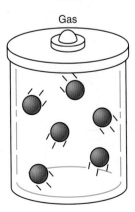

figure 12-4
Solid, liquid, and gas states of matter

table 12-1

STATES OF MATTER

State	Description	Examples
Solid	Rigid; has a fixed shape and volume.	Brush, roller, wooden nail pusher, ice
Liquid	Definite volume but takes the shape of its container.	Bleach, shampoo, haircolor, water
Gas	No fixed volume or shape; takes the shape and volume of its container. Can never be liquid at normal temperatures or pressures.	Propellant in hairspray, mousse, propane

Physical properties include color, solubility, odor, density, melting point, boiling point, hardness, and glossiness. (As described above, the state of matter that a substance becomes is an example of a physical property.)

Chemical properties are characteristics that can only be determined by a chemical reaction and a chemical change in the substance. Examples of chemical properties include the ability of iron to rust, wood to burn, or hair to change color through the use of haircolor and hydrogen peroxide.

After reading the next few sections, you will be able to:

LO ③   Summarize, in your own words, oxidation–reduction (redox) reactions.

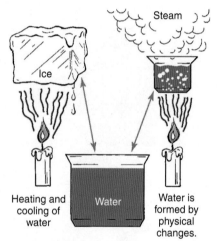

figure 12-5
Physical changes

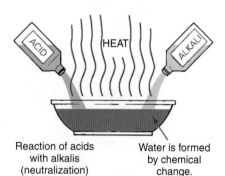

figure 12-6
Chemical changes

Physical and Chemical Changes

Matter can be changed in two different ways. Physical forces cause physical changes and chemical reactions cause chemical changes.

A **physical change** is a change in the form or physical properties of a substance, without a chemical reaction or the creation of a new substance. No chemical reactions are involved in physical change and no new chemicals are formed. Solid ice undergoes a physical change when it melts into water and then converts into steam when heat is applied (figure 12-5). A physical change occurs when nail polish is applied onto nails and the solvent evaporates, forming a layer or film on the nail.

A **chemical change** is a change in the chemical composition or make-up of a substance. This change is caused by chemical reactions that create new chemical substances, usually by combining or subtracting certain elements. Those new substances have different chemical and physical properties (figure 12-6). An example of a chemical change is the **oxidation** (ahk-sih-DAY-shun) of hair color. The term *oxidation* refers to a chemical reaction that combines a substance with oxygen to produce an oxide. Another example is the oxidation of melanin pigments in hair by hydrogen peroxide in lightening processes.

Oxidation–reduction, also known as *redox* (ree-DOCS), is a chemical reaction in which oxidation and reduction take place at the same time. When oxygen is chemically combined with a substance, the substance is oxidized. When oxygen is chemically removed from a substance, the substance is reduced.

> **? DID YOU KNOW?**
> Depilatory products are designed to help people to remove unwanted hair. The primary active ingredient in these types of cosmetics is some version of thioglycolic acid. The acid reacts with the cystine amino acids in hair and breaks down the S-S linkages. The hair is reduced to a jelly-like mass that can then be wiped away. This is an example of a chemical reaction.

An **oxidizing agent** is a substance that releases oxygen. Hydrogen peroxide (H_2O_2), which can be thought of as water with an extra atom of oxygen, is an example of an oxidizing agent. A **reducing agent** is a substance that adds hydrogen to a chemical compound or subtracts oxygen from the compound. When hydrogen peroxide is mixed with an oxidation haircolor, oxygen is subtracted from the hydrogen peroxide and the hydrogen peroxide is reduced. At the same time, oxygen is added to the haircolor and the haircolor is oxidized. In this example, haircolor is the reducing agent.

So far, we have considered oxidation only as the addition of oxygen and reduction only as loss of oxygen. Although the first known oxidation reactions involved oxygen, many oxidation reactions do not involve oxygen. Oxidation also results from loss of hydrogen and reduction also results from addition of hydrogen (figure 12-7). Redox reactions are also responsible for the chemical changes created by haircolors, hair lighteners, permanent wave solutions, and thioglycolic acid neutralizers. These chemical services would not be possible without oxidation–reduction (redox) reactions.

Under certain circumstances, chemical reactions can release a significant amount of heat. These types of chemical reactions are called **exothermic reactions** (ek-soh-THUR-mik ree-AK-shunz). In fact, all oxidation reactions are exothermic reactions. An example of an exothermic reaction is a nail product that hardens (polymerizes) to create nail enhancements. Exothermic reactions occur but usually clients cannot feel the heat being released.

Combustion (kum-BUS-chun) is the rapid oxidation of a substance accompanied by the production of heat and light. Lighting a match is an example of rapid oxidation. Oxidation requires the presence of oxygen; this is the reason that there cannot be a fire without air.

OXIDATION	REDUCTION
+ Oxygen	− Oxygen
− Hydrogen	+ Hydrogen

figure 12-7
Chart of oxidation and reduction reactions

After reading the next few sections, you will be able to:

LO④ Explain the differences between pure substances and physical mixtures.

Pure Substances and Physical Mixtures

All matter can be classified as either a pure substance or a physical mixture (blend).

A **pure substance** is a chemical combination of matter in definite (fixed) proportions. Pure substances have unique properties. Aluminum foil is an example of a pure substance. It has only atoms of the element aluminum. Most substances do not exist in a pure state. Air contains many substances, including nitrogen, carbon dioxide, and water vapor. This is an example of a physical mixture. A **physical mixture** is a physical combination of matter in any proportion. The properties of a physical mixture are the combined properties of the substances in the mixture. Salt water is a physical mixture of salt and water in any proportion. The properties of salt water are the properties contained in salt and in water: Salt water is salty and wet. Most of the products cosmetologists and nail technicians use are physical mixtures (figure 12-8).

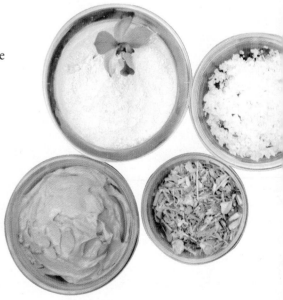

figure 12-8

Examples of pure substances
and physical mixtures

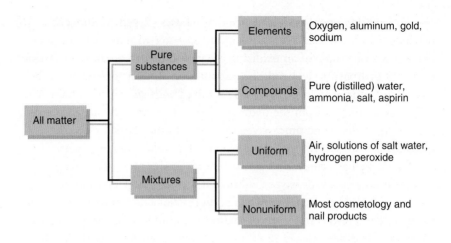

Table 12-2 summarizes the differences between pure substances and physical mixtures.

After reading the next few sections, you will be able to:

LO⑤ **Explain the differences among solutions, suspensions, and emulsions.**

Solutions, Suspensions, and Emulsions

Solutions, suspensions, and emulsions are all physical mixtures. The differences among solutions, suspensions, and emulsions are determined by the types of substances, the size of the particles, and the solubility of the substances.

- A **solution** is a stable physical mixture of two or more substances in a solvent. The **solute** (SAHL-yoot) is the substance that is dissolved into solution. The **solvent** (SAHL-vent) is the substance that dissolves the solute and makes the solution. For example, when salt is dissolved in water, salt is the solute and water is the solvent. Water is known as a universal solvent because it has the ability to dissolve more substances than any other solvent.

table 12-2

DIFFERENCES BETWEEN PURE SUBSTANCES AND PHYSICAL MIXTURES

Pure Substances	Physical Mixtures
United chemically	United physically
Definite (fixed) proportions	Any proportions
Unique chemical and physical properties	Combined chemical and physical properties
Salt and pure (distilled) water are examples of pure substances.	Salt water is a physical mixture.

ACTIVITY

Pour an ounce of a clear hair styling spay into a cup. Cover it loosely with a paper towel and set it aside for a week. What happens when the liquid evaporates? What does the residue look like? Touch and feel the residue. What is it made from? When styling compounds or polymers are dissolved in alcohol/water mixture, is it a physical or chemical change?

All liquids are either miscible or immiscible. **Miscible** (MIS-uh-bul) liquids are mutually soluble, meaning that they can be mixed together to form clear solutions. Water and alcohol are examples of miscible liquids as in a nail polish remover. When these substances are mixed together, they will stay mixed, forming a solution. Solutions contain small particles that are invisible to the naked eye. Solutions are usually transparent, although they may be colored. They do not separate when left still. Again, salt water is an example of a solution with a solid dissolved in a liquid. Water is the solvent that dissolves the salt (solute) and holds it in solution.

Immiscible (im-IS-uh-bul) liquids are not capable of being mixed together to form stable solutions. Water and oil are examples of immiscible liquids. These substances can be mixed together, but they will separate when left sitting still. When immiscible liquids are combined, they form suspensions.

- **Suspensions** (sus-PEN-shunz) are unstable physical mixtures of undissolved particles in a liquid. Compared with solutions, suspensions contain larger and fewer miscible particles. The particles are generally visible to the naked eye but are not large enough to settle quickly to the bottom. Suspensions are not usually transparent and may be colored. They are unstable and separate over time, which is why some lotions and creams can separate in the bottle and need to be shaken before they are used. Another example of a suspension is the glitter in nail polish that can separate from the polish.

  The suspension will separate when left sitting still and must be shaken before using. Calamine lotion and nail polish are other examples of suspensions.

- An **emulsion** (ee-MUL-shun) is an unstable physical mixture of two or more immiscible substances (substances that normally will not stay blended) plus a special ingredient called an emulsifier. An **emulsifier** (ee-MUL-suh-fy-ur) is an ingredient that brings two normally incompatible materials together and binds them into a uniform and fairly stable blend. Emulsions are considered to be a special type of suspension because they can separate, but the separation usually happens very slowly over a long period of time. An example of an emulsion is hand lotion. A properly formulated emulsion, stored under ideal conditions, can be stable up to three years. Since conditions are rarely ideal, all cosmetic emulsions should be used within one year of purchase. Always refer to the product's instructions and cautions for specific details.

DID YOU KNOW?

Soaps were the first synthetic surfactants. People began making soaps about 4,500 years ago by boiling oil or animal fat with wood ashes. Modern soaps are made from animal fats or vegetable oils. Traditional bar soaps are highly alkaline and combine with the minerals in hard water to form an insoluble film that coats skin and can cause hands to feel dry, itchy, and irritated. Cosmetologists who are performing nail services should be aware that soaps can leave a film on the nail plate, which could contribute to lifting of the nail enhancement. Modern synthetic surfactants have overcome these disadvantages and are superior to soaps; many are milder on the skin than soaps used in the past.

table 12-3

DIFFERENCES AMONG SOLUTIONS, SUSPENSIONS, AND EMULSIONS

Solutions	Suspensions	Emulsions
Miscible	Slightly miscible	Immiscible
No surfactant	No surfactant	Surfactant
Small particles	Larger particles	Largest particles
Stable mixture	Unstable, temporary mixture	Limited stability through an emulsifier
Usually clear	Usually cloudy	Usually a solid color
Solution of nail primer	Nail polish, glitter in nail polish	Shampoos, conditioners, hand lotions

Table 12-3 offers a summary of the differences among solutions, suspensions, and emulsions.

Surfactants (sur-FAK-tants) are substances that allow oil and water to mix, or emulsify. They are one type of emulsifier. The term *surfactant* is a contraction for surface active agents—substances that allow oil and water to mix, or emulsify. A surfactant molecule has two distinct parts (**figure 12-9**): The head of the surfactant molecule is hydrophilic (hy-drah-FIL-ik), capable of combining with or attracting water (water-loving), and the tail is **lipophilic** (ly-puh-FIL-ik), having an affinity for or an attraction to fat and oils (oil-loving). Following the like-dissolves-like rule, the hydrophilic head dissolves in water and the lipophilic tail dissolves in oil. So a surfactant molecule mixes with and dissolves in both oil and water and temporarily joins them together to form an emulsion.

In an **oil-in-water (O/W) emulsion**, oil droplets are emulsified in water. The droplets of oil are surrounded by surfactant molecules with their lipophilic tails pointing in and their hydrophilic heads pointing out. Tiny oil droplets form the internal portion of each O/W emulsion because the oil is completely surrounded by water (**figure 12-10**). Oil-in-water emulsions do not feel as greasy as water-in-oil emulsions because the oil is hidden and water forms the external portion of the emulsion.

In a **water-in-oil (W/O) emulsion**, water droplets are emulsified in oil. The droplets of water are surrounded by surfactants with their hydrophilic heads pointing in and their lipophilic tails pointing out (**figure 12-11**).

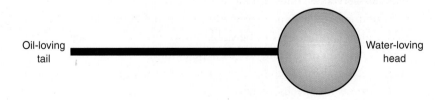

Oil-loving tail | Water-loving head

figure 12-9
A surfactant molecule

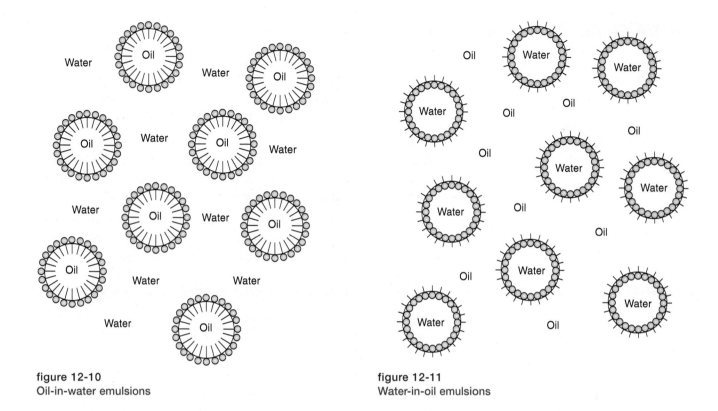

figure 12-10
Oil-in-water emulsions

figure 12-11
Water-in-oil emulsions

Tiny droplets of water form the internal portion of a W/O emulsion because the water is completely surrounded by oil. Water-in-oil emulsions feel greasier than oil-in-water emulsions because the water is hidden and oil forms the external portion of the emulsion. Styling creams, cold creams, and foot balms are examples.

Other Physical Mixtures

Ointments, pastes, pomades, and styling waxes are semisolid mixtures made with any combination of petrolatum (petroleum jelly), oil, and wax.

Powders are a physical mixture of one or more types of solids. Off-the-scalp, powdered hair lighteners are physical mixtures. These mixtures may separate during shipping and storage and should be thoroughly mixed by shaking the container before each use.

Common Chemical Product Ingredients

Cosmetologists use many chemical products when performing client services. Following are some of the most common chemical ingredients used in salon products.

- **Volatile alcohols** (VAHL-uh-tul AL-kuh-hawlz) are those that evaporate easily, such as isopropyl alcohol (rubbing alcohol) and ethyl alcohol (hairspray and alcoholic beverages). These chemicals are familiar to most people but there are many other types of alcohols, from free-flowing liquids to hard, waxy solids. Fatty alcohols, such as cetyl alcohol and cetearyl alcohol, are nonvolatile alcohol waxes that are used as skin conditioners.

- **Alkanolamines** (al-kan-oh-LAH-mynz) are alkaline substances used to neutralize acids or raise the pH of many hair products. They are often used in place of ammonia because they produce less odor.

- **Ammonia** (uh-MOH-nee-uh) is a colorless gas with a pungent odor that is composed of hydrogen and nitrogen. It is used to raise the pH in hair products to allow the solution to penetrate the hair shaft. Ammonium hydroxide and ammonium thioglycolate are examples of ammonia compounds that are used to perform chemical services in a salon.

- **Glycerin** (GLIS-ur-in) is a sweet, colorless, oily substance. It is used as a solvent and as a moisturizer in skin and body creams.

- **Silicones** (SIL-ih-kohnz) are a special type of oil used in hair conditioners, water-resistant lubricants for the skin, and nail polish dryers. Silicones are less greasy than other oils and form a breathable film that does not cause comedones (blackheads). Silicones also give skin a silky, smooth feeling and great shine to hair. Certain silicone resins (silicone gums) can withstand high pH environments and can be incorporated into relaxers and permanent wave formulations[i].

- **Volatile organic compounds (VOCs)** are compounds that contain carbon (organic) and evaporate very easily (volatile). For example, a common VOC used in hairspray is SD alcohol (ethyl alcohol). Volatile organic solvents such as ethyl acetate and isopropyl alcohol are used in nail polish, base and top coats, and polish removers.

After reading the next few sections, you will be able to:

LO**6** Explain what pH is and how the pH scale works.

Understand Potential Hydrogen (pH) and How It Affects Hair, Skin, and Nails

Although **pH**, the abbreviation used for *potential hydrogen*, is often mentioned when talking about salon products, it is one of the least understood chemical properties. Notice that *pH* is written with a small *p* (which represents a quantity) and a capital *H* (which represents the hydrogen ion). The term *pH* represents the quantity of hydrogen ions. Understanding pH and how it affects the hair, skin, and nails is essential to understanding all salon services. For more information about the pH of products used in salon services, see Chapter 15, Scalp Care, Shampooing, and Conditioning, and Chapter 20, Chemical Texture Services.

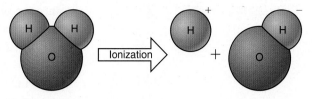

figure 12-12
The ionization of water

Water and pH

Before you can understand pH, you need to learn about ions. An **ion** (EYE-on) is an atom or molecule that carries an electrical charge. **Ionization** (eye-on-ih-ZAY-shun) is the separation of an atom or molecule into positive and negative ions. An ion with a negative electrical charge is an **anion** (AN-eye-on). An ion with a positive electrical charge is a **cation** (KAT-eye-on).

In water, some of the water (H_2O) molecules naturally ionize into hydrogen ions and hydroxide ions. The pH scale measures these ions. The hydrogen ion (H^+) is acidic. The more hydrogen ions there are in a substance, the more acidic it will be. The hydroxide ion (OH-) is alkaline. The more hydroxide ions there are in a substance, the more alkaline it will be. pH is only possible because of this ionization of water. Only products that contain water can have a pH.

In pure (distilled) water, each water molecule that ionizes produces one hydrogen ion and one hydroxide ion (**figure 12-12**). Pure water has a neutral pH because it contains the same number of hydrogen ions as hydroxide ions. It is an equal balance of 50 percent acidic and 50 percent alkaline. The pH of any substance is always a balance of both acidity and alkalinity. As acidity increases, alkalinity decreases. The opposite is also true; as alkalinity increases, acidity decreases. Even the strongest acid also contains some alkalinity.

The pH Scale

A **pH scale** is a measure of the acidity and alkalinity of a substance. It has a range of 0 to 14. A pH of 7 is a neutral solution, a pH below 7 indicates an **acidic solution**, and a pH above 7 indicates an **alkaline solution** (figure 12-13). The term **logarithm** (LOG-ah-rhythm) means multiples of 10.

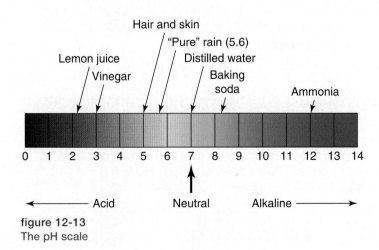

figure 12-13
The pH scale

Since the pH scale is a logarithmic scale, a change of one whole number represents a tenfold change in pH. This means, for example, that a pH of 8 is 10 times more alkaline than a pH of 7. A change of two whole numbers represents a change of 10 times 10, or a 100-fold change. So a pH of 9 is 100 times more alkaline than a pH of 7. Even a small change on the pH scale represents a large change in the pH.

pH is always a balance of both acidity and alkalinity. Pure water has a pH of 7, which is an equal balance of acid and alkaline. Although a pH of 7 is neutral on the pH scale, it is not neutral compared to the hair and skin, which have an average pH of 5. Pure (distilled) water, with a pH of 7, is 100 times more alkaline than a pH of 5, so pure water is 100 times more alkaline than your hair and skin. This difference in pH is the reason pure water can cause the hair to swell as much as 20 percent and the reason that water is drying to the skin.

Acids and Alkalis

All acids owe their chemical reactivity to the hydrogen ion. Acids have a pH below 7.0.

Alpha hydroxy acids (AHAs) (al-FAH HY-drok-see AS-udz), derived from plants (mostly fruit), are examples of acids often used in salons to exfoliate the skin and to help adjust the pH of a lotion, conditioner, or cream. Acids contract and close the hair cuticle. One such acid is **thioglycolic acid** (thy-oh-GLY-kuh-lik AS-ud), a colorless liquid or white crystals with a strong unpleasant odor that is used in permanent waving solutions. **Glycolic acid** is an alpha hydroxy acid used in exfoliation and to lower the pH of products.

All **alkalis** (AL-kuh-lyz), also known as *bases*, owe their chemical reactivity to the hydroxide ion. Alkalis are compounds that react with acids to form salts. Alkalis have a pH above 7.0. They feel slippery and soapy on the skin. Alkalis soften and swell hair, skin, the cuticle on the nail plate, and calloused skin.

Sodium hydroxide, commonly known as lye, is a very strong alkali used in chemical hair relaxers, callous softeners, and drain cleaners. These products must be used according to manufacturers' instructions, and it is very important that you do not let the products touch or sit on the skin as they may cause injury to or a burning sensation on the skin. Sodium hydroxide products may be especially dangerous if they get into the eyes, so always wear safety glasses to avoid eye contact. Consult the product's SDS for more specific information on safe use.

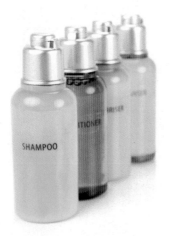

ACTIVITY

For a product to have a pH, it must contain water. Shampoos, conditioners, haircolor, permanent waves, relaxers, lotions, and creams have a pH. Divide into groups and research these products online to find their pH. If the information is not available online, contact the manufacturers. Make a chart and compare your findings with what your classmates found. How will the pH of these products affect the hair?

Here is a hint to save you some time: Oils, waxes, and nail polish have no pH because they contain no water.

Acid-Alkali Neutralization Reactions

The same reaction that naturally ionizes water into hydrogen ions and hydroxide ions also runs in reverse. When acids and alkalis are mixed together in equal proportions, they neutralize each other to form water (figure 12-14). Neutralizing shampoos and normalizing lotions used to neutralize hair relaxers work by creating an acid-alkali neutralization reaction. Liquid soaps are usually slightly acidic and can neutralize alkaline callous softener residues left on the skin after rinsing.

Chemistry Will Help You in the Salon

Whether you are studying the pH of products, redox reactions, suspensions, solutions, or emulsions, there is a lot to learn about how chemistry affects the products you use in the salon. Having a basic understanding of chemistry will help you use professional products effectively and safely in the salon.

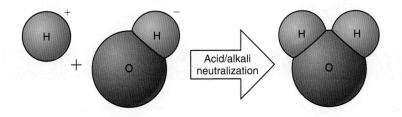

figure 12-14
Acid and alkali neutralization reaction

REVIEW QUESTIONS

1. What is chemistry?

2. Why is a basic understanding of chemistry important to a cosmetologist?

3. What are the differences among between organic and inorganic chemistry?

4. What is matter?

5. What is an element?

6. What are atoms?

7. Explain the difference between elemental molecules and compound molecules. Give examples.

8. Name and describe the three states of matter.

9. What are the physical and chemical properties of matter? Give examples.

10. What is the difference between physical and chemical change? Give examples.

11. Explain oxidation–reduction (redox).

12. Explain pure substances and physical mixtures. Give examples.

13. What are the differences among solutions, suspensions, and emulsions? Give examples.

14. Define pH and the pH scale.

STUDY TOOLS

- **Reinforce what you just learned:** Complete the activities and exercises in your Theory or Practical Workbook, or your Study Guide.

- **Expand your knowledge:** Search for websites about the topics in this chapter and make a list of additional resources.

- **Study and prepare for your quiz:** Take the chapter test in your Exam Review or your Milady U: Online Licensing Prep.

- **Re-Test your knowledge:** Take the Chapter 12 *Quizzes*!

- **Learn even more:** Look up in a dictionary or search the internet for the definitions of any additional terms you want to learn about.

CHAPTER GLOSSARY

acidic solution	p. 265	A solution that has a pH below 7.0 (neutral).
alkaline solution	p. 265	A solution that has a pH above 7.0 (neutral).
alkalis AL-kuh-lyz	p. 266	Also known as *bases*; compounds that react with acids to form salts.
alkanolamines al-kan-oh-LAH-mynz	p. 264	Alkaline substances used to neutralize acids or raise the pH of many hair products.
alpha hydroxy acids al-FAH HY-drok-see AS-udz	p. 266	Abbreviated AHAs; acids derived from plants (mostly fruit) that are often used to exfoliate the skin.
ammonia uh-MOH-nee-uh	p. 264	Colorless gas with a pungent odor that is composed of hydrogen and nitrogen.

anion AN-eye-on	p. 265	An ion with a negative electrical charge.
atoms	p. 256	The smallest chemical components (often called particles) of an element; structures that make up the element and have the same properties of the element.
cation KAT-eye-on	p. 265	An ion with a positive electrical charge.
chemical change	p. 258	A change in the chemical composition or make-up of a substance.
chemical properties	p. 258	Characteristics that can only be determined by a chemical reaction and a chemical change in the substance.
chemistry	p. 254	Science that deals with the composition, structures, and properties of matter and how matter changes under different conditions.
combustion kum-BUS-chun	p. 259	Rapid oxidation of a substance accompanied by the production of heat and light.
compound molecules KAHM-pownd MAHL-uh-kyools	p. 256	Also known as compounds; a chemical combination of two or more atoms of different elements in definite (fixed) proportions.
electrons	p. 256	Subatomic particles with a negative charge.
element	p. 255	The simplest form of chemical matter; an element cannot be broken down into a simpler substance without a loss of identity.
elemental molecule EL-uh-men-tul MAHL-uh-kyool	p. 256	Molecule containing two or more atoms of the same element in definite (fixed) proportions.
emulsifier ee-MUL-suh-fy-ur	p. 261	An ingredient that brings two normally incompatible materials together and binds them into a uniform and fairly stable blend.
emulsion ee-MUL-shun	p. 261	An unstable physical mixture of two or more immiscible substances (substances that normally will not stay blended) plus a special ingredient called an emulsifier.
exothermic reactions ek-soh-THUR-mik ree-AK-shunz	p. 259	Chemical reactions that release a significant amount of heat.
glycerin GLIS-ur-in	p. 264	Sweet, colorless, oily substance used as a solvent and as a moisturizer in skin and body creams.
glycolic acid	p. 266	An alpha hydroxy acid used in exfoliation and to lower the pH of products.
immiscible im-IS-uh-bul	p. 261	Liquids that are not capable of being mixed together to form stable solutions.
inorganic chemistry	p. 255	The study of substances that do not contain the element carbon, but may contain the element hydrogen.
ion EYE-on	p. 265	An atom or molecule that carries an electrical charge.
ionization eye-on-ih-ZAY-shun	p. 265	The separation of an atom or molecule into positive and negative ions.
lipophilic ly-puh-FIL-ik	p. 262	Having an affinity for or an attraction to fat and oils (oil-loving).

logarithm	p. 265	Multiples of 10.
LOG-ah-rhythm		
matter	p. 255	Any substance that occupies space and has mass (weight).
miscible	p. 261	Liquids that are mutually soluble, meaning that they can be mixed together to form stable solutions.
MIS-uh-bul		
molecule	p. 256	A chemical combination of two or more atoms in definite (fixed) proportions.
MAHL-uh-kyool		
neutrons	p. 256	Subatomic particles with no charge.
oil-in-water emulsion	p. 262	Abbreviated O/W emulsion; oil droplets emulsified in water.
organic chemistry	p. 254	The study of substances that contain the element carbon.
oxidation	p. 258	A chemical reaction that combines a substance with oxygen to produce an oxide.
ahk-sih-DAY-shun		
oxidation–reduction	p. 258	Also known as *redox* (ree-DOCS); a chemical reaction in which the oxidizing agent is reduced (by losing oxygen) and the reducing agent is oxidized (by gaining oxygen).
oxidizing agent	p. 259	Substance that releases oxygen.
pH	p. 264	The abbreviation used for potential hydrogen. pH represents the quantity of hydrogen ions.
pH scale	p. 265	A measure of the acidity and alkalinity of a substance; the pH scale has a range of 0 to 14, with 7 being neutral. A pH below 7 is an acidic solution; a pH above 7 is an alkaline solution.
physical change	p. 258	A change in the form or physical properties of a substance without a chemical reaction or the creation of a new substance.
physical mixture	p. 259	A physical combination of matter in any proportion.
physical properties	p. 257	Characteristics that can be determined without a chemical reaction and that do not cause a chemical change in the substance.
protons	p. 256	Subatomic particles with a positive charge.
pure substance	p. 259	A chemical combination of matter in definite (fixed) proportions.
reducing agent	p. 259	A substance that adds hydrogen to a chemical compound or subtracts oxygen from the compound.
silicones	p. 264	Special type of oil used in hair conditioners, water-resistant lubricants for the skin, and nail polish dryers.
SIL-ih-kohnz		
solute	p. 260	The substance that is dissolved in a solution.
SAHL-yoot		
solution	p. 260	A stable physical mixture of two or more substances.
solvent	p. 260	The substance that dissolves the solute and makes a solution.
states of matter	p. 257	The three different physical forms of matter: solid, liquid, and gas.
surfactants	p. 262	A contraction of surface active agents; substances that allow oil and water to mix, or emulsify.
sur-FAK-tants		
suspensions	p. 261	Unstable physical mixtures of undissolved particles in a liquid.

thioglycolic acid thy-oh-GLY-kuh-lik AS-ud	p. 266	A colorless liquid or white crystals with a strong unpleasant odor that is used in permanent waving solutions
volatile alcohols	p. 264	Alcohols that evaporate easily.
volatile organic compounds	p. 264	Abbreviated VOCs; compounds that contain carbon (organic) and evaporate very easily (volatile).
water-in-oil emulsion	p. 262	Abbreviated W/O emulsion; water droplets emulsified in oil.

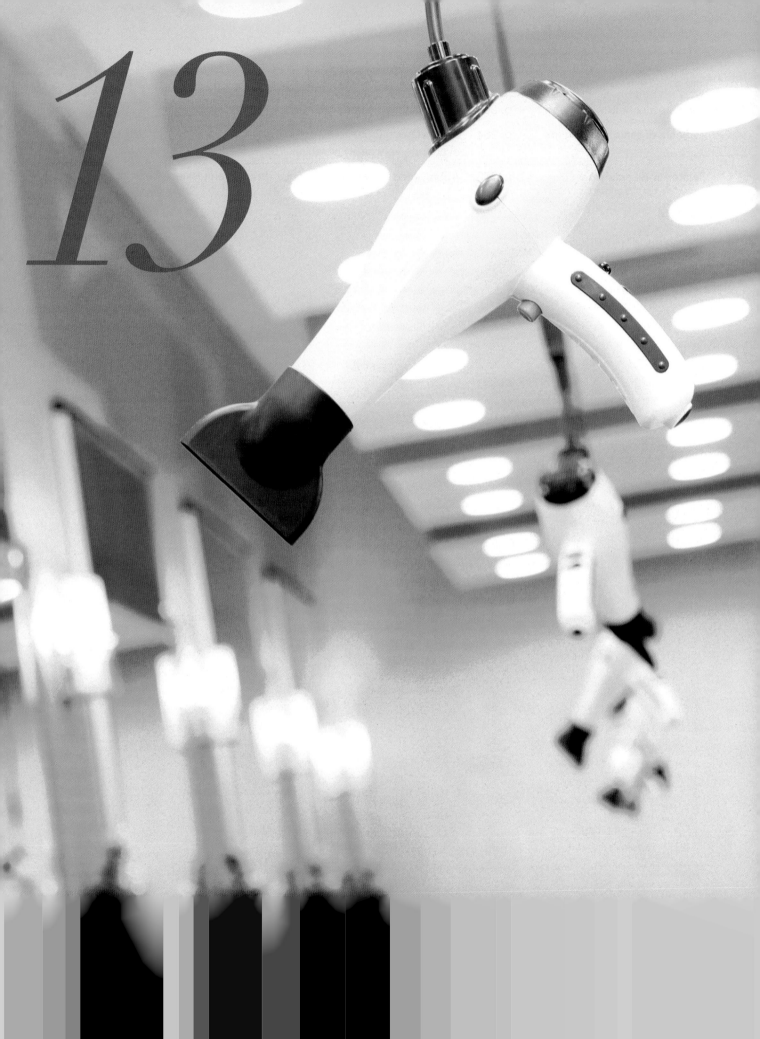

13

LEARNING OBJECTIVES

After completing this chapter, you will be able to:

LO ❶
Identify the nature of electricity and the two types of electric current.

LO ❷
List electrical measurements.

LO ❸
Understand the principles of electrical equipment safety.

LO ❹
Examine the main electric modalities used in cosmetology.

LO ❺
Outline other types of electrical equipment that cosmetologists use and describe how to use them.

LO ❻
Explain the electromagnetic spectrum, visible spectrum of light, and invisible light.

LO ❼
Compare the types of light therapy and their benefits.

OUTLINE

You decided to enter this field because you love cosmetology and all of the services it offers to clients: hairstyling, haircoloring, perms, facials, mani-pedis. How many of these services could you offer without using electricity? As you study this chapter, you will learn how important it is for cosmetology professionals to have a basic working knowledge of electricity.

why study
BASICS OF ELECTRICITY?

Cosmetologists should study and have a thorough understanding of the basics of electricity because:

> Cosmetologists use and rely upon a variety of electrical appliances. Knowing what electricity is and how it works will allow you to use it wisely and safely.

> A basic understanding of electricity will enable you to properly use and care for your equipment and tools.

> Electricity and its use impact other aspects of the salon environment, such as lighting and the temperature of styling irons. Therefore, it impacts the services you offer your clients.

After reading the next few sections, you will be able to:

LO❶   Identify the nature of electricity and the two types of electric current.

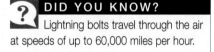

Understand Electricity

If you look at lightning on a stormy night, what you will see are the effects of electricity. If you plug a poorly wired appliance into a socket and sparks fly out of the socket, you will also see the effects of electricity. You are not really seeing electricity, however; instead, you are seeing its *visual* effects on the surrounding air. Electricity does not occupy space or have mass (weight), so it is not matter. If it is not matter, then what is it? **Electricity** (ee-lek-TRIS-ih-tee) is the movement of electrons from one atom to another along a conductor. Electricity is a form of energy that, when in motion, exhibits magnetic, chemical, or thermal effects.

An **electric current** (ee-LEK-trik KUR-unt) is the flow of electricity along a conductor. All materials can be classified as conductors or nonconductors (insulators) depending on the ease with which an electric current can be transmitted through them.

A **conductor** (kahn-DUK-tur) is any material that conducts electricity. Most metals are good conductors. This means that electricity will pass through the material easily. Copper is a particularly good conductor and is used in electric wiring and electric motors. Pure (distilled) water is a poor conductor, but the ions usually found in ordinary water, such as tap water or a river or a lake, make it a good conductor. This explains why you should not swim in a lake during an electrical storm.

A **nonconductor**, (nahn-kun-DUK-tur), also known as *insulator* (IN-suh-layt-ur), is a material that does not transmit electricity. Rubber, silk, wood, glass, and cement are good insulators. Electric wires are composed of twisted metal threads (the conductor) covered with a rubber or plastic coating (the nonconductor or insulator). A **complete electric circuit** (kahm-PLEET ee-LEK-trik SUR-kit) is the path of negative and positive electric currents moving from the generating source through the conductors and back to the generating source.

Types of Electric Current

There are two types of electric current:

- **Direct current** (dy-REKT KUR-unt), abbreviated DC, is a constant, even-flowing current that travels in one direction only and is produced by chemical means. Flashlights, mobile telephones, and cordless hairstyling tools use the direct current produced by batteries. The battery in your car stores electric energy. Without it, your car would not start. An **inverter** (in-VUR-tur) is an apparatus that changes direct current to alternating current. Inverters usually have a plug and a cord. They allow you to use appliances outside of the salon or your home that normally would have to be plugged into an electric wall outlet. The mobile phone charger in a car is an example of an inverter (**figure 13-1**).

- **Alternating current** (AWL-tur-nayt-ing KUR-rent), abbreviated AC, is a rapid and interrupted current, flowing first in one direction and then in the opposite direction; it is produced by mechanical means and changes directions 60 times per second. Corded hair dryers, curling irons, electric files, and table lamps that plug into a wall outlet use alternating current. A **rectifier** (REK-ti-fy-ur) is an apparatus that changes alternating current (AC) to direct current (DC). Cordless electric clippers and mobile phone chargers use a rectifier to change the AC from an electric wall outlet to the DC needed to recharge their batteries.

Table 13-1 outlines the differences between direct current and alternating current.

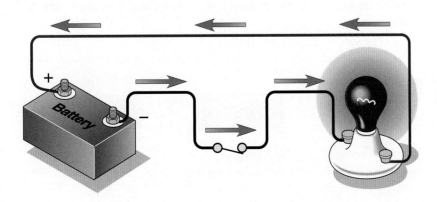

figure 13-1
A complete direct current (DC) electric circuit

table 13-1

DIRECT CURRENT (DC) AND ALTERNATING CURRENT (AC)

Direct Current	Alternating Current
Constant, even flow	Rapid and interrupted flow
Travels in one direction	Travels in two directions
Produced by chemical means	Produced by mechanical means

After reading the next few sections, you will be able to:

LO **2** **List electrical measurements.**

Electrical Measurements

The flow of an electric current can be compared to water flowing through a hose on a shampoo sink in the salon. Without pressure, neither water nor electricity would flow.

- A **volt** (VOLT), abbreviated V and also known as *voltage* (VOL-tij), is the unit that measures the pressure or force that pushes electric current forward through a conductor (**figure 13-2**). Car batteries are 12 volts. Normal electric wall sockets that power your hair dryer and curling iron are 120 volts. Most air conditioners and clothes dryers run on 240 volts. A higher voltage indicates more power. Nominal system voltage is 240, minimum service voltage requirement is 220.

- An **ampere** (AM-peer), abbreviated A and also known as *amp* (AMP), is the unit that measures the strength of an electric current. Just as the sink hose must be large enough to carry the amount of water flowing through it, a wire also must be large enough to carry the amount of electricity (amps) flowing through it. A hair dryer rated at 12 amps must have a cord that is twice as thick as one rated at 6 amps; otherwise, the cord might overheat and start a fire. A higher amp rating indicates a greater number of electrons and a stronger current (**figure 13-3**).

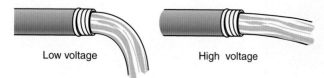

Low voltage   High voltage

figure 13-2
Volts measure the pressure or force that pushes the electric current forward through a conductor.

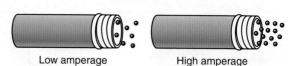

Low amperage   High amperage

figure 13-3
Amps measure the strength of the electric current.

- A **milliampere** (mil-ee-AM-peer), abbreviated mA, is ¹⁄₁,₀₀₀ of an ampere. The current used for facial and scalp treatments is measured in milliamperes; an ampere current would be much too strong. If used for facials and scalp treatments, an ampere current would damage the skin or body.

- An **ohm** (OHM), abbreviated O, is a unit that measures the resistance of an electric current. Current will not flow through a conductor unless the force (volts) is stronger than the resistance (ohms).

- A **watt** (WAHT), abbreviated W, is a unit that measures how much electric energy is being used in one second. A 40-watt light bulb uses 40 watts of energy per second.

- A **kilowatt** (KIL-uh-waht), abbreviated kw, is 1,000 watts. The electricity in your house is measured in kilowatts per hour (kwh). A 1,000-watt (1-kilowatt) hair dryer uses 1,000 watts of energy per second.

After reading the next few sections, you will be able to:

LO ❸ Understand the principles of electrical equipment safety.

Practice Electrical Equipment Safety

When working with electricity, you must always be concerned with your own safety, as well as the safety of your clients. All electrical equipment should be inspected regularly to determine whether it is in safe working order. Careless electrical connections and overloaded circuits can result in an electrical shock, a burn, or even a serious fire.

Safety Devices

A wire that is not large enough to carry the electrical current passing through it will overheat. The heating element in your hair dryer or curling iron heats up because it is not large enough to carry the electric current. Heating elements are designed to overheat and are safe when used properly, but when the electrical wires in a wall overheat, they can cause a fire. If excessive current passes through a circuit or a fuse, the circuit breaker turns off the circuit to prevent overheating.

© Vasilius/Shutterstock.com

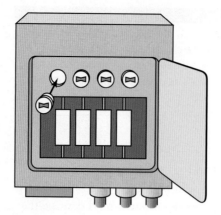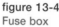

figure 13-4
Fuse box

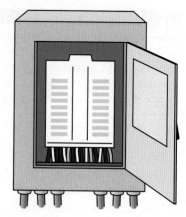

figure 13-5
Circuit breakers

These are the electrical safety devices that you may encounter when working in a salon:

- A **fuse** (FYOOZ) prevents excessive current from passing through a circuit. It is designed to blow out or melt when the wire becomes too hot from overloading the circuit with too much current, such as when too many appliances or faulty equipment is connected to an electric source. To re-establish the circuit, disconnect the appliance, check all connections and insulation, insert a new fuse, then reconnect the appliance. Fuses are often found in older buildings that have not been renovated or modernized (**figure 13-4**).

- A **circuit breaker** (SUR-kit BRAYK-ar) is a switch that automatically interrupts or shuts off an electric circuit at the first indication of an overload. Circuit breakers have replaced fuses in modern electric circuits. They have all the safety features of fuses but do not require replacement and can simply be reset by switching the circuit breaker back on. Your hair dryer has a circuit breaker located in the electric plug that is designed to protect you and your client in case of an overload or short circuit. When a circuit breaker shuts off, you should disconnect the appliance and check all connections and insulation before resetting it (**figure 13-5**).

Grounding

Grounding (GROWND-ing) completes an electric circuit and carries the current safely away. It is another important way to promote electrical safety. All electrical appliances must have at least two rectangular electrical connections, or prongs, on the plug. This is called a two-prong plug. The two prongs supply electric current to the circuit. If you look closely at the two prongs, you will see that one is slightly larger than the other. This guarantees that the plug can be inserted into an outlet only one way and protects you and your client from an electric shock in the event of a short circuit.

For added protection, some appliances (especially the ones with metal casing) have a third circular electric connection that is a grounding pin. This is called a three-prong plug. The grounding pin is designed to guarantee a safe path of electricity and protect the user from electrical shock even if a wire comes loose. Appliances with a third circular grounding pin offer the most protection for you and your clients (**figure 13-6**).

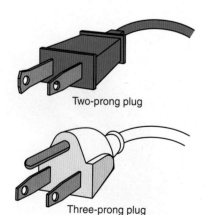

Two-prong plug

Three-prong plug

figure 13-6
Two-prong and three-prong plugs

Ground Fault Interrupter (GFI)

Ground fault interrupters are designed to protect from electrical shock by interrupting a household circuit when there is a leak in the circuit. GFI's are required by the electrical code for receptacles in bathrooms, kitchens, and some outside receptacles. GFI is designed to detect currents of few milliamperes and trip a breaker at the receptacle or at the breaker panel to remove shock hazard. When it is working properly it has a green light and when it trips the light turns red. Once the appliance is removed from the socket it can be reset with a "reset" button on the panel (figure 13-7).

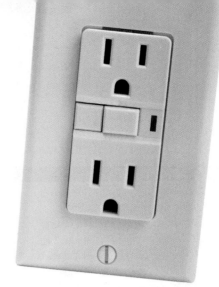

figure 13-7
GFI outlet

Guidelines for Safe Use of Electrical Equipment

Salon fires are often caused by electrical problems such as shorts in the wiring of the building or improper use of items such as appliances, extension cords, and plugs. Careful attention to electrical safety involves following recommended UL guidelines, manufacturer's directions, and the safety instructions and policies of your salon. The guidelines below will help you use electricity and electrical equipment safely.

- All the electrical appliances you use should be UL certified (figure 13-8).

- Read all instructions carefully before using any piece of electrical equipment.

- Disconnect all appliances when not in use; pull on the plug, not the cord, to disconnect.

- Inspect all electrical equipment regularly.

- Keep all wires, plugs, and electrical equipment in good repair.

- Use only one plug in each outlet; overloading may cause the circuit breaker to pop. If more than one plug is needed in an area, use a power strip with a surge protector (figure 13-9).

- Avoid contact, for both you and your client, with water and metal surfaces when using electricity and do not handle electrical equipment with wet hands.

- Keep electrical cords off the floor and away from everyone's feet; getting tangled in a cord could cause you or your client to trip.

- Do not leave your client unattended while the client is connected to an electrical device.

- Do not attempt to clean around electric outlets while equipment is plugged in.

- Do not touch two metal objects at the same time if either is connected to an electric current.

- Do not step on or place objects on electrical cords.

- Do not allow electrical cords to become twisted; this can cause a short circuit.

- Do not attempt to repair electrical appliances. If you have a problem with electric wiring or an electrical device or appliance, tell your supervisor immediately, take the device to a repair store, or call a certified electrician or repair representative to resolve the issue.

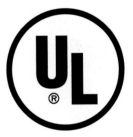

figure 13-8
UL symbol, as it appears on electrical devices

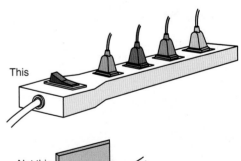

This

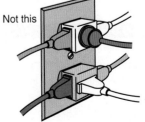

Not this

figure 13-9
Use only one plug per outlet on a power strip or on the wall.

Understand Electrotherapy

The use of electrical currents to treat the skin is commonly referred to as electrotherapy (ee-lek-troh-thair-uh-pee). Currents used in electrical facial and scalp treatments are called **modalities** (MOH-dal-ih-tees). Each modality produces a different effect on the skin.

An **electrode** (ee-LEK-trohd), also known as *probe*, is an applicator for directing electric current from an electrotherapy device to the client's skin. It is usually made of carbon, glass, or metal. Each modality requires two electrodes—one negative and one positive—to conduct the flow of electricity through the body. The only exception to this rule is the Tesla high-frequency current, which is covered in more depth later in this chapter.

Polarity

Polarity (poh-LAYR-ut-tee) is the negative or positive pole of an electric current. The electrodes on many electrotherapy devices have one negatively charged pole and one positively charged pole. The positive electrode is called an **anode** (AN-ohd); the anode is usually red and is marked with a *P* or a plus (+) sign. The negative electrode is called a **cathode** (KATH-ohd); it is usually black and is marked with an *N* or a minus (–) sign (**figure 13-10**). The negatively charged electrons from cathode flows to positively charged anode. If the electrodes are not marked, ask your instructor, salon manager, or supervisor to help you determine the positive and negative poles.

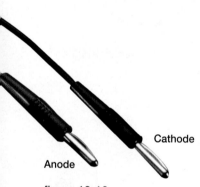

Cathode

Anode

figure 13-10
Anode and cathode

Modalities

The main modalities used in cosmetology are galvanic current, microcurrent, and Tesla high-frequency current.

Galvanic Current

Galvanic current (gal-VAN-ik KUR-unt) is a constant and direct current, having a positive and negative pole, that produces chemical changes when it passes through the tissues and fluids of the body.

Two different chemical reactions are possible with galvanic current, depending on the polarity (positive or negative) that is used (**table 13-2**). The **active electrode** (AK-tiv ee-LEK-trohd) is the electrode used on the area to be treated. The **inactive electrode** (in-AK-tiv ee-LEK-trohd) is the opposite pole from the active electrode. The effects produced by the positive pole are the exact opposite of those produced by the negative pole. Galvanic current is used to infuse water soluble products into unbroken skin and the scientific term for that process is called phoresis.

Iontophoresis (eye-ahn-toh-foh-REE-sus) is the process of infusing water-soluble products into the skin with the use of electric current, such as the use of the positive and negative poles of a galvanic machine.

table 13-2

EFFECTS OF GALVANIC CURRENT

Positive Pole (Anode) Cataphoresis	Negative Pole (Cathode) Anaphoresis
Produces acidic reactions	Produces alkaline reactions
Closes the pores	Opens the pores
Soothes nerves	Stimulates and irritates the nerves
Decreases blood supply	Increases blood supply
Contracts blood vessels	Expands blood vessels
Hardens and firms tissues	Softens tissues

Cataphoresis (kat-uh-foh-REE-sus) infuses an acidic (positive) product into deeper tissues using galvanic current from the positive pole toward the negative pole.

Anaphoresis (an-uh-foh-REE-sus) infuses an alkaline (negative) product into the tissues from the negative pole toward the positive pole. **Desincrustation** (des-inkrus-TAY-shun) is a form of anaphoresis and is a process used to soften and emulsify grease deposits (oil) and blackheads in the hair follicles. Desincrustation is frequently used to treat acne, milia (small, white cyst-like pimples), and comedones (blackheads and whiteheads).

Microcurrent

Microcurrent (MY-kroh-kur-unt) is an extremely low level of electricity that mirrors the body's natural electrical impulses. Microcurrent can be used for iontophoresis, firming, toning, and soothing skin. It also can help heal inflamed tissue such as acne.

Newer microcurrent devices have negative and positive polarity in one probe, not two probes. This allows the client to relax rather than to have to hold on to one of the probes during the service or treatment (**figure 13-11**).

Microcurrent does not travel throughout the entire body; it serves only the specific area being treated.

Microcurrent can be effective in the following ways:

- Improves blood and lymph circulation
- Produces acidic and alkaline reactions
- Opens and closes hair follicles and pores
- Increases muscle tone
- Restores elasticity
- Reduces redness and inflammation
- Minimizes healing time for acne lesions
- Improves the natural protective barrier of the skin
- Increases metabolism

When microcurrent is used during aging-skin treatments, it may give your client's skin a softer, firmer, more hydrated appearance.

⚠ **CAUTION**

Do not use negative galvanic current on skin with broken capillaries or pustular acne conditions or on clients with high blood pressure or metal implants.

⚠ **CAUTION**

As with all electric current devices, microcurrent should not be used on clients with pacemakers, epilepsy, cancer, pregnancy, phlebitis, or thrombosis. It also should not be used on anyone under a physician's care for a condition that may exclude them from using certain ingredients or products or from having treatments. If you are unsure about whether it is appropriate to treat clients, ask them to obtain physician consent for the service.

? **DID YOU KNOW?**

The Tesla high-frequency current is named after an electrical engineer named Nikola Tesla who was born in 1856 in Croatia. He moved to the United States in 1884, where he did the majority of the work on alternating current. Tesla died in New York City in 1943.

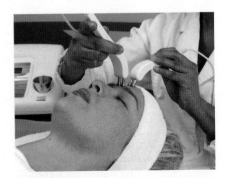

figure 13-11
A microcurrent treatment

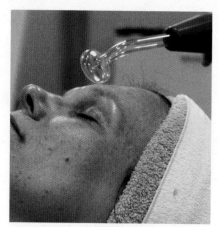

figure 13-12
Applying Tesla high-frequency current with a facial electrode

Tesla High-Frequency Current

The **Tesla high-frequency current** (TES-luh HY-FREE-kwen-see KUR-ent), also known as *violet ray*, is a thermal or heat-producing current with a high rate of oscillation or vibration that is commonly used for scalp and facial treatments. Tesla current does not produce muscle contractions, and the effects can be either stimulating or soothing, depending on the method of application. The electrodes are made from either glass or metal and only one electrode is used to perform a service (**figure 13-12**).

The benefits of the Tesla high-frequency current are:

- Stimulates blood circulation

- Increases elimination and absorption

- Increases skin metabolism

- Improves germicidal action

- Relieves skin congestion

As you learn more about facials and treatments, you will become familiar with the term *contraindication*, a condition that requires avoiding certain treatments, procedures, or products to prevent undesirable side effects.

After reading the next few sections, you will be able to:

LO**5** Outline other types of electrical equipment that cosmetologists use and describe how to use them.

⚠ CAUTION
Tesla high-frequency current should not be used on clients who are pregnant or who have epilepsy (seizures), asthma, high blood pressure, a sinus blockage, a pacemaker, or metal implants. The client also should avoid contact with metal, such as chair arms, jewelry, and metal bobby pins during the treatment. A burn may occur if contact is made.

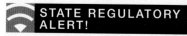
STATE REGULATORY ALERT!
Always be certain that you are in compliance with your state's regulations for licensing and use of electric current devices.

Identify Other Electrical Equipment

As a cosmetologist, you will be using many types of electrical equipment and tools. Here are a few of the most common electrical tools you may encounter, along with some information regarding their use:

- Conventional hood hair dryers or heat lamps are sources of dry heat that can be used to shorten chemical processing time. Since dry heat causes evaporation, the hair must be covered with a plastic cap to avoid drying the hair during a chemical process.

- Ionic hair dryers with the crystalline mineral tourmaline and styling irons are effective at combating static electricity and flyaway hair. When tourmaline is heated, it produces positive and negative ions that cancel the electric charges in the hair that cause static electricity. Claims that ionic dryers dry hair faster or condition hair have not been proven.

- Electric curling and flat irons are available in many types and sizes. They have built-in heating elements and plug directly into a wall outlet. Thermal styling tools now have the capacity to get extremely hot (up to 410 degrees Fahrenheit, or higher, on some styling tools). This extreme heat causes the water within the hair to boil and can severely damage hair.

- Heating caps provide a uniform source of heat and can be used with hair and scalp conditioning treatments.

- Haircolor processing machines, or accelerating machines, shorten the time it takes to process chemical hair services. These processors usually look similar to a hood dryer and dispense a hot water vapor inside the hood. A haircolor service processed with a machine at 90 degrees Fahrenheit (32 degrees Celsius) will process twice as fast as it would at a normal room temperature of 72 degrees Fahrenheit (22 degrees Celsius).

- A steamer or vaporizer produces moist, uniform heat that can be applied to the head or face. Steamers warm and cleanse the skin by increasing the flow of both oil and sweat. Some steamers also may be used for hair and scalp conditioning treatments. Estheticians often add essential oils to a facial steamer as part of a skin therapy and to enhance a client's general well-being.

- Light therapy equipment includes lasers, light-emitting diode (LED), and intense pulse light. These types of equipment are medical devices and should be used only by licensed professionals. Light therapy is described in the next section.

After reading the next few sections, you will be able to:

LO⑥ Explain the electromagnetic spectrum, visible spectrum of light, and invisible light.

Explain Light Energy and Light Therapy

The **electromagnetic spectrum** (ee-lek-troh-MAG-ne-tik SPEK-trum), also known as *electromagnetic spectrum of radiation*, is the name given to all of the forms of energy (or radiation) that exist. The forms of energy in the electromagnetic spectrum are radio waves (used by radios and televisions), microwaves (used in microwave ovens), light waves (infrared light, visible light, and ultraviolet light used for light therapy services), X-rays (used by physicians and dentists), and gamma rays (used for nuclear power plants) (**figure 13-13**).

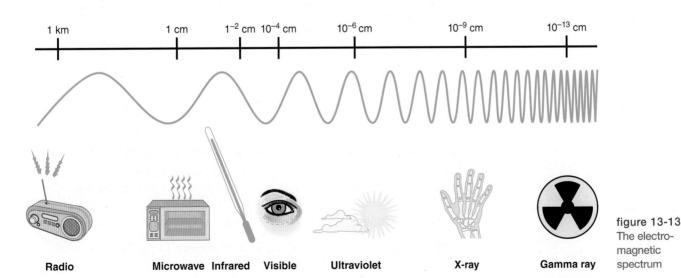

figure 13-13
The electromagnetic spectrum

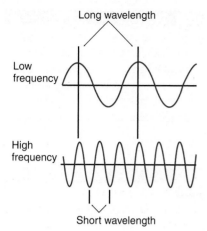

figure 13-14
Waveform patterns of long and short wavelengths

Energy moves through space on waves. These waves are similar to the waves caused when a stone is dropped on the surface of water. Each type of energy has its own **wavelength**, the distance between successive peaks of electromagnetic waves. A **waveform** is the measurement of the distance between two wavelengths. Some wavelengths are long and some are short (table 13-3). Long wavelengths have low frequency, meaning that the number of waves is less frequent (fewer waves) within a waveform pattern. Short wavelengths have higher frequency because the number of waves is more frequent (more waves) within a waveform pattern (figure 13-14).

Visible Spectrum of Light

The **visible spectrum of light** is the part of the electromagnetic spectrum that can be seen. Visible light makes up only 35 percent of natural sunlight. Within the visible spectrum of light, violet has the shortest wavelength and red has the longest. The wavelength of infrared light is just below that of red light and the wavelength of ultraviolet light is just above that of violet light.

Although they are referred to as *light*, infrared light and ultraviolet light are not really light. Ultraviolet light and infrared light, which are covered in more depth later in this chapter, are also forms of electromagnetic energy but they are invisible because their wavelengths are beyond the visible spectrum of light. Invisible light makes up 65 percent of natural sunlight (figure 13-15).

table 13-3

LONG WAVELENGTHS COMPARED WITH SHORT WAVELENGTHS

Long Wavelengths	Short Wavelengths
Low frequency	High frequency
Deeper penetration	Less penetration
Less energy	More energy

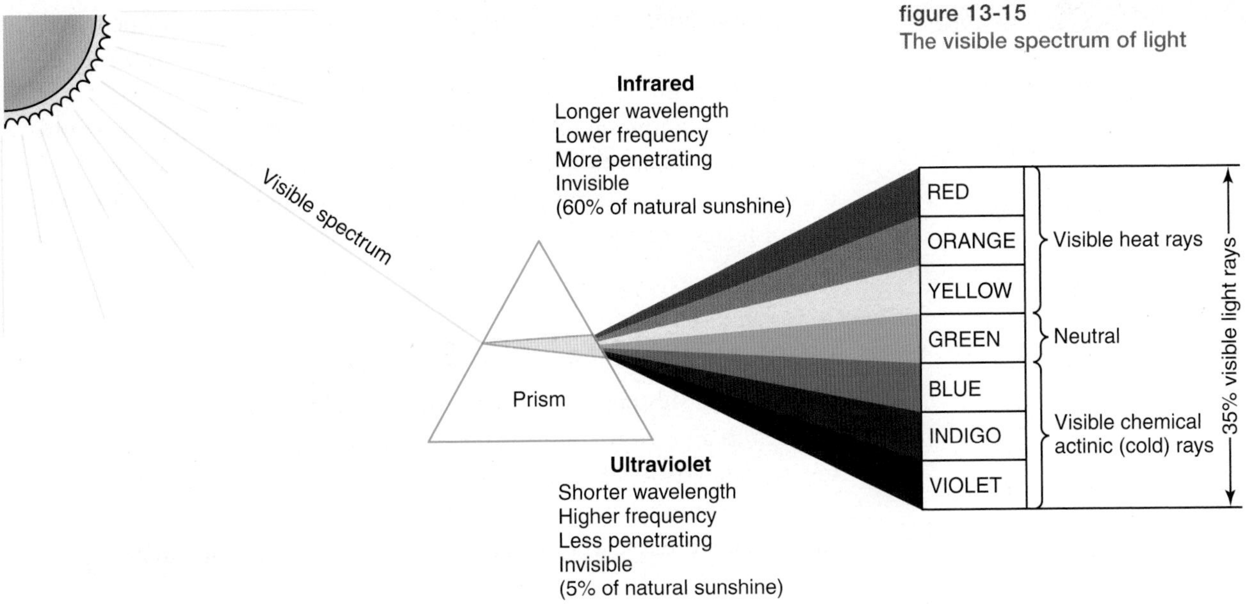

figure 13-15
The visible spectrum of light

Infrared
Longer wavelength
Lower frequency
More penetrating
Invisible
(60% of natural sunshine)

Visible spectrum

Prism

Ultraviolet
Shorter wavelength
Higher frequency
Less penetrating
Invisible
(5% of natural sunshine)

RED	
ORANGE	} Visible heat rays
YELLOW	
GREEN	} Neutral
BLUE	
INDIGO	} Visible chemical actinic (cold) rays
VIOLET	

35% visible light rays

Invisible Light

Invisible light is the light at either end of the visible spectrum of light that is invisible to the naked eye. Before the visible violet light of the spectrum is ultraviolet light; it is the shortest and least-penetrating light of the spectrum. Beyond the visible red light of the spectrum is infrared light, which produces heat.

Ultraviolet light (ul-truh-VY-uh-let LYT), abbreviated UV light and also known as *cold light* or *actinic light* (ak-TIN-ik LYT), is invisible light that has a short wavelength (giving it higher energy), is less penetrating than visible light, causes chemical reactions to happen more quickly than visible light, produces less heat than visible light, and kills some germs.

UV light prompts the skin to produce vitamin D, a fat-soluble vitamin that is good for bone growth and health. We need sunlight to survive on the planet but overexposure to UV light can cause premature aging of the skin and skin cancer. Incidence of skin cancer has reached a near-epidemic level, with over one million new cases being diagnosed each year. It is estimated that one in five Americans will develop skin cancer and that 90 percent of those cancers will be the result of exposure to UV radiation from natural sunlight, sun lamps, and tanning beds.

There are three types of UV light:

• **Ultraviolet A (UVA).** Ultraviolet A light has the longest wavelength of the UV light spectrum and penetrates directly into the dermis of the skin, damaging the collagen and elastin. UVA light is the light that is often used in tanning beds.

• **Ultraviolet B (UVB).** Ultraviolet B light is often called the burning light because it is most associated with sunburns. Excessive use of both UVA and UVB light can cause skin cancers.

• **Ultraviolet C (UVC).** Ultraviolet C light is blocked by the ozone layer. If the Earth loses the protective layer of the ozone, life will no longer exist as we know it. We do not want to deplete the ozone layer because it protects us from UVC radiation.

? DID YOU KNOW?
If light from the sun is passed through a glass prism (usually a glass or plastic prism resembles a pyramid shape after it is cut), it will appear in seven different colors, known as the rainbow, displayed in the following manner: violet (the shortest wavelength), indigo, blue, green, yellow, orange, and red (the longest wavelength). These colors, which are visible to the eye, constitute visible light.

? DID YOU KNOW?
Some animals can see parts of the visible spectrum that humans cannot. For example, many insects can see ultraviolet light.

⚠ CAUTION
Although the application of UV light can be beneficial, it must be done with the utmost care in a proper manner by a qualified professional because overexposure can lead to skin damage and skin cancer. It has been used to kill bacteria on the skin and to help the body produce vitamin D. Dermatologists use UV therapy in addition to drugs for the treatment of psoriasis.

Infrared light (in-fruh-RED LYT) has longer wavelengths, penetrates more deeply, has less energy, and produces more heat than visible light. Infrared light makes up 60 percent of natural sunlight.

Infrared lamps are used mainly during hair conditioning treatments and to process haircolor. They are also used in spas and saunas for relaxation and for warming up muscles. Infrared light has been used to diminish signs of aging such as wrinkles, to heal wounds, and to increase circulation.

Light Versus Heat and Energy

Catalysts are substances that speed up chemical reactions. Some catalysts use heat as an energy source while others use light. Whatever the energy source, catalysts absorb energy like a battery. At the appropriate time, they pass this energy to the initiator and the reaction begins. Like other chemicals, a catalyst will not get consumed in a chemical reaction.

After reading the next few sections, you will be able to:

LO **7** Compare the types of light therapy and their benefits.

Light Therapy

Light therapy, also known as *phototherapy*, is the application of light rays to the skin for the treatment of wrinkles, capillaries, pigmentation, or hair removal. Lasers and light therapy devices have been used for decades, but some of the original techniques are still valid today. Lasers are designed to focus all of the light power to a specific depth and in one direction within the skin, using the same color of light. In contrast, other light therapies have multiple depths, colors, and wavelengths and the light may be scattered. The most important point to remember about light therapy is that the equipment you use is selected based on the skin type and condition you are treating.

Lasers

Laser is an acronym for *light amplification stimulation emission of radiation*; it is a medical device that uses electromagnetic radiation for hair removal and skin treatments. There are many types of lasers used to treat a variety of skin conditions. All lasers work by selective **photothermolysis** (FOTO-ther-moll-ih-sis), a process that turns the light from the laser device into heat. Depending on the intended use and type, lasers can remove blood vessels, disable hair follicles, remove tattoos, or eliminate some wrinkles without destroying surrounding tissue. Lasers have been used for decades in a variety of surgical procedures. In laser hair removal the light is converted to heat as it passes through the skin. The heat is absorbed by melanin in the follicles and the follicles are damaged, inhibiting hair growth. **Figure 13-16** shows removing facial hair with a laser.

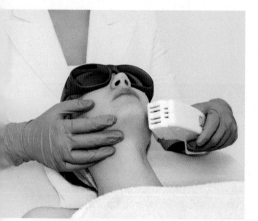

figure 13-16
Removing facial hair with laser

© carol.anne/Shutterstock.com

Lasers work by means of a medium (solid, liquid or gas, or semi-conductor) that emits light when stimulated by a power source. The medium is placed in a specifically designed chamber with mirrors located inside both ends. That chamber is stimulated by an energy source, such as electric current, which, in turn, stimulates the particles. The mirrors create light that becomes trapped and goes back and forth through the medium, gaining energy with each pass. The medium determines the wavelength of the laser and its use.

Most lasers are classified as a Level II medical device or above, which means that estheticians must be working under the supervision of a qualified physician to operate the laser.

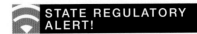
Light-Emitting Diode (LED)

A **light-emitting diode**, abbreviated LED, is a medical device used to reduce acne, increase blood circulation, and improve the collagen content in the skin. The LED works by releasing light onto the skin to stimulate specific responses at precise depths of the skin tissue. Each color of light corresponds to a different depth—measured in one billionths of a meter, which are called nanometers—in the tissue. The LED light color seeks a color in the skin tissue known as a **chromophore**, a color component within the skin such as blood or melanin. The term chromophore is derived from the Greek term *chroma,* meaning color. When the colored light reaches a specific depth in the tissue, it triggers a reaction, such as stimulating circulation or reducing bacteria. Depending on the type of equipment used, the LED can be blue, red, yellow, or green. Blue light LED reduces acne. Red light increases circulation and improves the collagen and elastin production in the skin. Yellow light reduces swelling and inflammation and green light reduces hyperpigmentation (**table 13-4**). Blue light LED also can be used in medical procedures performed by physicians for precancerous lesions (**figure 13-17**).

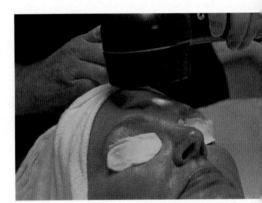

figure 13-17
LED treatment reduces redness and improves the collagen content in the skin.

Courtesy of Revitalight

table 13-4

BENEFICIAL EFFECTS OF LED THERAPY

Color nm (nanometers)	Beneficial Effects
Blue light 570 nm	Reduces acne and reduces bacteria
Red light 640 nm	Increases circulation Improves collagen and elastin production Stimulates wound healing
Yellow light 590 nm	Reduces swelling and inflammation Improves lymphatic flow Detoxifies and increases circulation
Green light 525 nm	Reduces hyperpigmentation Reduces redness Calms and soothes

figure 13-18
Acne before and after treatment

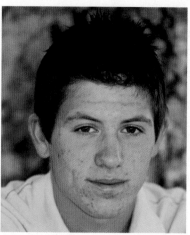

© iStock.com/jtyler

Figure 13-18 shows the result from before and after treatment with Blue light LED therapy in reducing acne. A remarkable decrease in wrinkle reduction is illustrated in (figure 13-19) with LED red light.

As with all light therapies, it is important to be certain that you have viewed the client consultation form for any contraindications. Light therapy should not be performed on anyone who has light sensitivities (photosensitivities), phototoxic reactions, is taking antibiotics, has cancer or epilepsy, is pregnant, or is under a physician's care. If you are not sure whether you should treat certain clients, refer them to their physicians.

Intense Pulse Light

Intense pulse light is a medical device that uses multiple colors and wavelengths (broad spectrum) of focused light to treat spider veins, hyperpigmentation, rosacea and redness, wrinkles, enlarged hair follicles and pores, and excessive hair. As with most devices, multiple treatments are required. These treatments are provided only under the supervision of a qualified physician.

From dermatologists using UV therapy for treating psoriasis to estheticians using blue light therapy for acne to surgeons using lasers for advanced surgical procedures, the power of light therapy is here to stay.

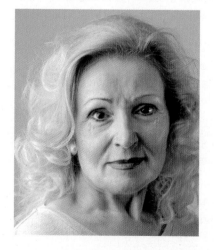
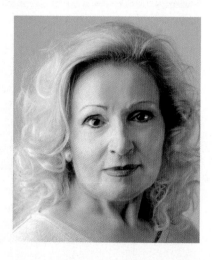

© ollyy/Shutterstock.com

figure 13-19
Before and after anti-wrinkle treatment

REVIEW QUESTIONS

1. Define electric current.

2. Explain the difference between a conductor and a nonconductor (insulator).

3. Describe the two types of electric current and give examples of each.

4. Explain the difference between a volt and an amp.

5. Define ohm.

6. Define watt and kilowatt.

7. Explain the function of a fuse.

8. What is the purpose of a circuit breaker?

9. What is the purpose of grounding?

10. List at least five steps to take for electrical safety.

11. List and describe the two main electric modalities (currents) used in cosmetology.

12. What are electromagnetic radiation, visible light, and invisible light?

13. List and describe the two main types of light therapy.

14. What are the benefits of LED therapies?

15. Identify the colors of LED lights and their wavelengths (nm)?

16. Name two important precautions to observe when using light therapy.

STUDY TOOLS

- **Reinforce what you just learned:** Complete the activities and exercises in your Theory or Practical Workbook, or your Study Guide.

- **Expand your knowledge:** Search for websites about the topics in this chapter and make a list of additional resources.

- **Study and prepare for your quiz:** Take the chapter test in your Exam Review or your Milady U: Online Licensing Prep.

- **Re-Test your knowledge:** Take the Chapter 12 *Quizzes!*

- **Learn even more:** Look up in a dictionary or search the internet for the definitions of any additional terms you want to learn about.

CHAPTER GLOSSARY

active electrode AK-tiv ee-LEK-trohd	p. 280	Electrode of an electrotherapy device that is used on the area to be treated.
alternating current AWL-tur-nayt-ing KUR-rent	p. 275	Abbreviated AC; rapid and interrupted current, flowing first in one direction and then in the opposite direction; produced by mechanical means and changes directions 60 times per second.
ampere AM-peer	p. 276	Abbreviated A and also known as *amp* (AMP); unit that measures the strength of an electric current.
anaphoresis an-uh-foh-REE-sus	p. 281	Process of infusing an alkaline (negative) product into the tissues from the negative pole toward the positive pole.
anode AN-ohd	p. 280	Positive electrode of an electrotherapy device; the anode is usually red and is marked with a *P* or a plus (+) sign.

CHAPTER 13 | BASICS OF ELECTRICITY   289

catalysts	p. 286	Substances that speed up chemical reactions.
cataphoresis kat-uh-foh-REE-sus	p. 281	Process of fusing an acidic (positive) product into deeper tissues using galvanic current from the positive pole toward the negative pole.
cathode KATH-ohd	p. 280	Negative electrode of an electrotherapy device; the cathode is usually black and is marked with an *N* or a minus (–) sign.
chromophore	p. 287	A color component within the skin such as blood or melanin.
circuit breaker SUR-kit BRAYK-ar	p. 278	Switch that automatically interrupts or shuts off an electric circuit at the first indication of overload.
complete electric circuit kahm-PLEET ee-LEK-trik SUR-kit	p. 275	The path of negative and positive electric currents moving from the generating source through the conductors and back to the generating source.
conductor kahn-DUK-tur	p. 274	Any material that conducts electricity.
desincrustation des-inkrus-TAY-shun	p. 281	A form of anaphoresis; process used to soften and emulsify grease deposits (oil) and blackheads in the hair follicles.
direct current dy-REKT KUR-unt	p. 275	Abbreviated DC; constant, even-flowing current that travels in one direction only and is produced by chemical means.
electric current ee-LEK-trik KUR-unt	p. 274	Flow of electricity along a conductor.
electricity ee-lek-TRIS-ih-tee	p. 274	The movement of electrons from one atom to another along a conductor.
electrode ee-LEK-trohd	p. 280	Also known as *probe*; applicator for directing electric current from an electrotherapy device to the client's skin.
electromagnetic spectrum ee-lek-troh-MAG-ne-tik SPEK-trum	p. 283	Also known as *electromagnetic spectrum of radiation*; name given to all of the forms of energy (or radiation) that exist.
fuse FYOOZ	p. 278	Prevents excessive current from passing through a circuit.
galvanic current gal-VAN-ik KUR-unt	p. 280	Constant and direct current, having a positive and negative pole, that produces chemical changes when it passes through the tissues and fluids of the body.
grounding GROWND-ing	p. 278	Completes an electric circuit and carries the current safely away.
inactive electrode in-AK-tiv ee-LEK-trohd	p. 280	Opposite pole from the active electrode.
infrared light in-fruh-RED LYT	p. 286	Infrared light has longer wavelengths, penetrates more deeply, has less energy, and produces more heat than visible light; it makes up 60 percent of natural sunlight.
intense pulse light	p. 288	A medical device that uses multiple colors and wavelengths (broad spectrum) of focused light to treat spider veins, hyperpigmentation, rosacea and redness, wrinkles, enlarged hair follicles and pores, and excessive hair.
inverter in-VUR-tur	p. 275	Apparatus that changes direct current to alternating current.
invisible light	p. 285	Light at either end of the visible spectrum of light that is invisible to the naked eye.

iontophoresis eye-ahn-toh-foh-REE-sus	p. 280	Process of infusing water-soluble products into the skin with the use of electric current, such as the use of the positive and negative poles of a galvanic machine.
kilowatt KIL-uh-waht	p. 277	Abbreviated kw; 1,000 watts.
laser	p. 286	Acronym for light amplification stimulation emission of radiation; a medical device that uses electromagnetic radiation for hair removal and skin treatments.
light-emitting diode	p. 287	Abbreviated LED; a medical device used to reduce acne, increase blood circulation, and improve the collagen content in the skin.
light therapy	p. 286	Also known as *phototherapy*; the application of light rays to the skin for the treatment of wrinkles, capillaries, pigmentation, or hair removal.
microcurrent MY-kroh-kur-unt	p. 281	An extremely low level of electricity that mirrors the body's natural electrical impulses.
milliampere mil-ee-AM-peer	p. 277	Abbreviated mA; $\frac{1}{1,000}$ of an ampere.
modalities MOH-dal-ih-tees	p. 280	Currents used in electrical facial and scalp treatments.
nonconductor nahn-kun-DUK-tur	p. 275	Also known as *insulator* (IN-suh-layt-ur); a material that does not transmit electricity.
ohm OHM	p. 277	Abbreviated O; unit that measures the resistance of an electric current.
photothermolysis FOTO-ther-moll-ih-sis	p. 286	Process that turns the light from a laser device into heat.
polarity poh-LAYR-ut-tee	p. 280	Negative pole or positive pole of an electric current.
rectifier REK-ti-fy-ur	p. 275	Apparatus that changes alternating current (AC) to direct current (DC).
Tesla high-frequency current TES-luh HY-FREE-kwen-see KUR-ent	p. 282	Also known as *violet ray*; thermal or heat-producing current with a high rate of oscillation or vibration that is commonly used for scalp and facial treatments.
ultraviolet light ul-truh-VY-uh-let LYT	p. 285	Abbreviated UV light and also known as *cold* light or *actinic* light (ak-TIN-ik LYT); invisible light that has a short wavelength (giving it higher energy), is less penetrating than visible light, causes chemical reactions to happen more quickly than visible light, produces less heat than visible light, and kills germs.
visible spectrum of light	p. 284	The part of the electromagnetic spectrum that can be seen. Visible light makes up only 35 percent of natural sunlight.
volt (VOLT)	p. 276	Abbreviated V and also known as *voltage*; unit that measures the pressure or force that pushes electric current forward through a conductor.
watt (WAHT)	p. 277	Abbreviated W; unit that measures how much electric energy is being used in one second.
waveform	p. 284	Measurement of the distance between two wavelengths.
wavelength	p. 284	Distance between successive peaks of electromagnetic waves.

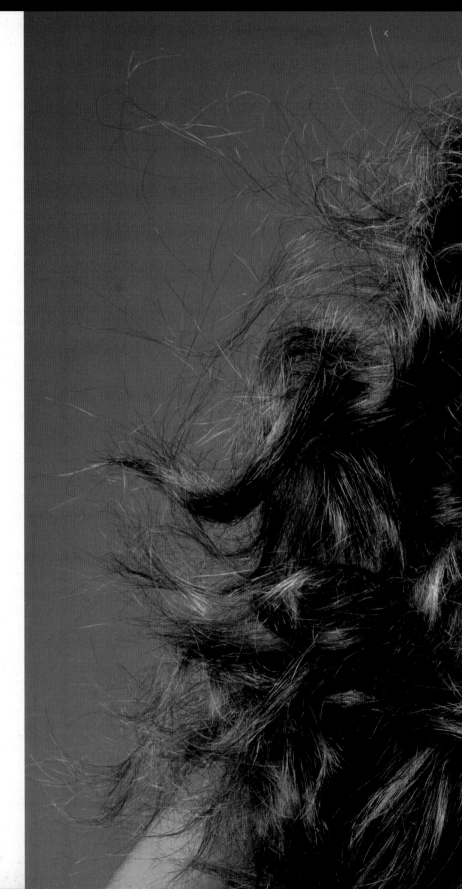

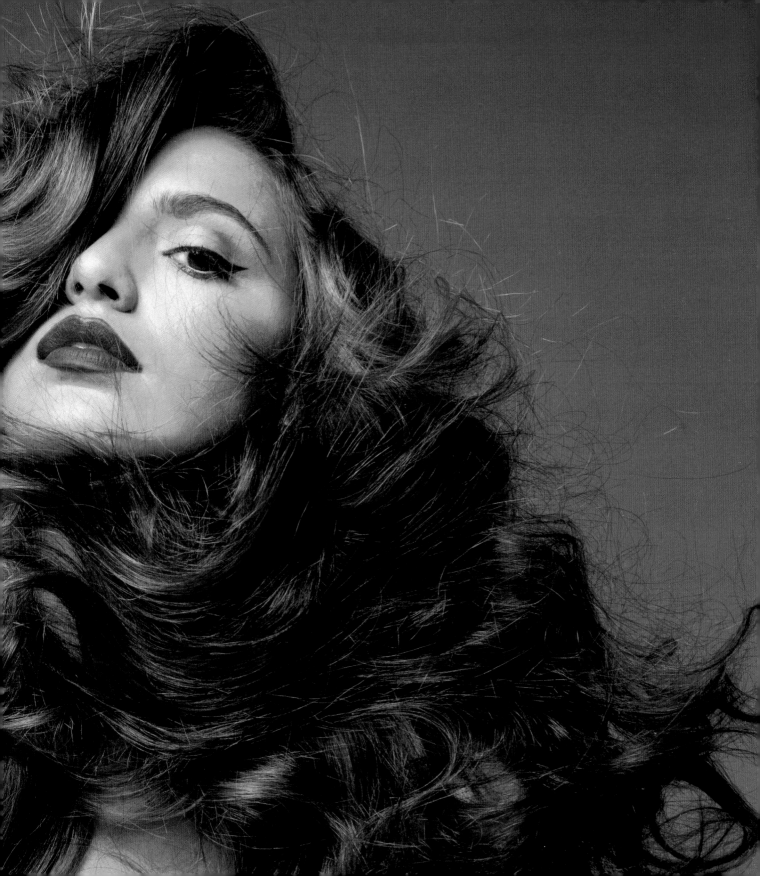

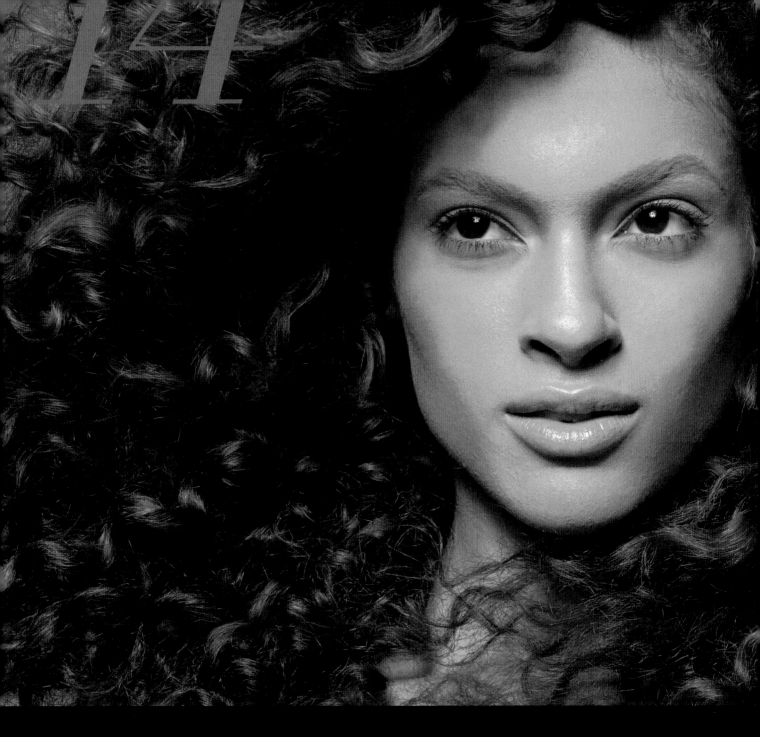

14

PRINCIPLES OF HAIR DESIGN

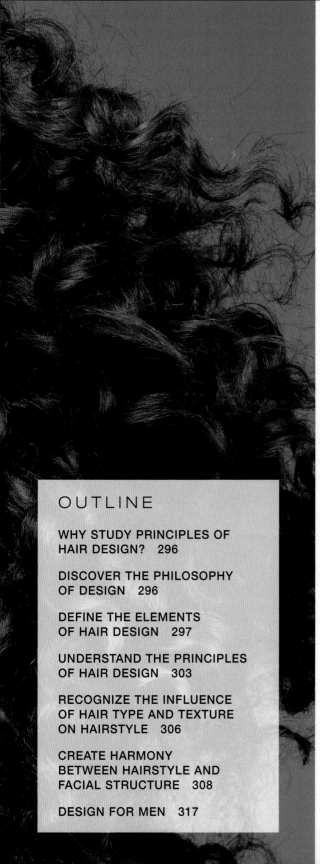

LEARNING OBJECTIVES

After completing this chapter, you will be able to:

LO❶
Describe sources of hair design inspiration.

LO❷
List the five elements of hair design and how they relate to hairstyling.

LO❸
Explain the five principles of hair design and recognize their specific contribution to a hairstyle.

LO❹
Understand the influence of hair type and texture on design.

LO❺
Identify the seven different facial shapes and design a beneficial hairstyle for each.

LO❻
Explain two design considerations for men.

Design is the foundation of all artistic applications. All artists—architects, fashion designers, and interior designers, among many others—have a strong visual eye. The odds are that you do too, since you have chosen to pursue a career in the beauty industry.

Do you want to be known as a good stylist or a great one? To add value to your career as a stylist, take the time to learn how to design the best hairstyle for your client. That process begins with analyzing the entire person by using the elements and principles of design to enhance positive features and minimize more challenging ones. An understanding of design and art principles will help you develop the artistic skill and judgment needed to create the best possible design for your client.

why study
PRINCIPLES OF HAIR DESIGN?

As a cosmetologist, you should study and have a thorough understanding of the principles of hair design because:

> You will be better able to understand why a particular hairstyle will or will not be the best choice for a client.

> The principles of design will serve as helpful guidelines to assist you in achieving your styling vision.

> You will be able to create haircuts and styles designed to help clients camouflage areas of concern while emphasizing their most attractive areas.

After reading the next few sections, you will be able to:

LO **Describe sources of hair design inspiration.**

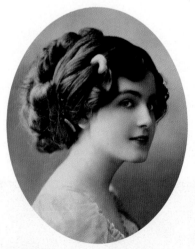

figure 14-1
Soft beauty from 1910

Discover the Philosophy of Design

Have a vision. Inspiration can emerge from many sources: movies, TV, magazines, videos, even a person on the street—anything, anywhere—can spark the creative process. One of the best sources of inspiration can be found in nature. The rhythm and movement of ocean waves have inspired painters, poets, composers, and hairstylists. Historical and contemporary art forms provide a great source for visual creativity. At times, you may find yourself looking to the past for inspiration. A hairstyle from an earlier era might inspire you to reinvent it in a way that works for today (figures 14-1 and 14-2). Modern inspiration in fashion often starts as individual expression then moves to the streets as a phenomenon or trend.

© Michaela Stejskalova/Shutterstock.com

Follow a plan. A good designer always envisions the end result before beginning. For example, when an architect designs a building, he or she first visualizes the final product. Then the architect completes drawings and takes the necessary steps to create the design in a model. In hair design, the stylist first envisions changes in texture, form, and direction, and then creatively plans the end result.

Work at the plan. Once inspired, you will need to decide which tools and techniques are needed to achieve your design. Organize your thoughts so that the tools and products needed are available and ready for use. When working out the details and planning of a design, practice your technique and intended plan on a mannequin first. There is always the chance that your original concept will turn into something entirely different as you work through your design concept. There are no failures if the experience is a lesson learned. If you are open to change, the creative process will be exciting and satisfying.

Try and try again. As a designer, you will need to develop a visual understanding of which hairstyles work best on different face shapes and body types. It takes time and experience to train your eye to recognize the best design decision. Along with learning through study of the chapters in this text, it is best to practice over and over until you gain a working knowledge of the process. Don't get frustrated. The more you practice, the better you will become. All good stylists have made a significant number of design mistakes in the past—great stylists learn and grow from each experience. Having a strong design foundation will help make you a great stylist. Once you have these skills, your creative juices will kick in and you can move beyond the basics.

Take calculated risks. Having a strong foundation in technique along with practicing personal skills will allow you to take calculated risks. It is important in this field to take those risks and build your creativity. Often stylists limit positive risks and confine themselves to their current comfort zone. Sometimes comfort zones can translate into "dated and uninspiring." Always explore new possibilities and customize your design to each client's individual needs and lifestyle. Great hairstylists find inspiration everywhere by keeping an eye out for what is new in the beauty industry and by dedicating themselves to their continuing education. You can keep growing by having your eyes and mind always open to learning.

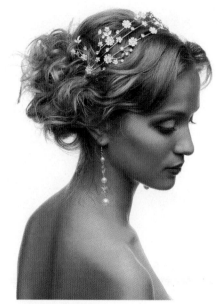

figure 14-2
Updated version of soft beauty

After reading the next few sections, you will be able to:

LO❷ List the five elements of hair design and how they relate to hairstyling.

Define the Elements of Hair Design

To begin to understand the creative process involved in hairstyling, it is critical to learn the five basic elements of three-dimensional design. These elements are line, form, space, design texture, and color.

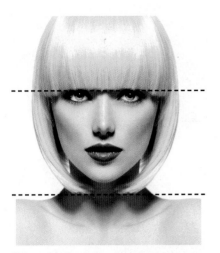

figure 14-3
Horizontal lines create width
in a hairstyle.

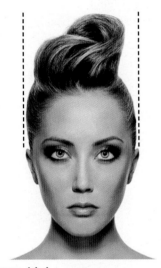

figure 14-4
Vertical lines in a hairstyle

Line

Line defines form and space. The presence of one line nearly always means that there are others involved. Lines create the shape, design, and movement of a hairstyle. Horizontal, vertical, diagonal, and curved lines can all interrelate and create illusions. The eye follows the lines in a design. They can be straight or curved. Lines are impactful in styling, but they also are obvious in haircutting and haircoloring. If understood correctly, they can effectively be used to promote the focal point of a style. There are four basic types of lines:

- **Horizontal lines** create width in hair design. They extend in the same direction and maintain a constant distance apart and are parallel from the floor and relative to the horizon (figure 14-3).

- **Vertical lines** create length and height in hair design. They make a hairstyle appear longer and narrower as the eye follows the lines up and down (figure 14-4).

- **Diagonal lines** are positioned between horizontal and vertical lines. They are often used to emphasize or minimize facial features. Diagonal lines are also used to create interest in hair design (figure 14-5).

- **Curved lines**, lines moving in a circular or semi-circular direction, soften a design. They can be large or small, a full circle, or just part of a circle (figure 14-6). Curved lines may move in a clockwise or counter-clockwise direction to create the illusion of movement. They can be placed horizontally, vertically, or diagonally. Curved lines repeating in opposite directions create a wave (figure 14-7).

Designing with Lines

Hairstyles are created by the types of line, direction, or combination you choose. The overall look of the hair design can be established through various line placements.

- **Single lines** are used in the one-length hairstyle. These hairstyles are best for clients requiring the lowest maintenance when styling their hair (figure 14-8).

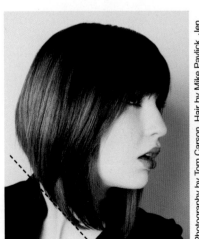

figure 14-5
Diagonal lines can create
interest in a hairstyle.

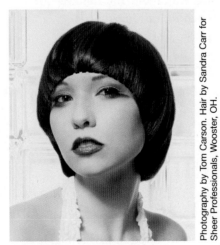

figure 14-6
Curved lines can soften a hairstyle.

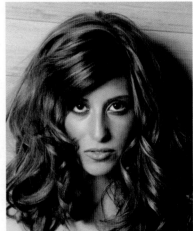

figure 14-7
Wave

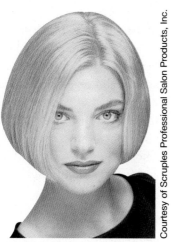

figure 14-8
Single-line hairstyle

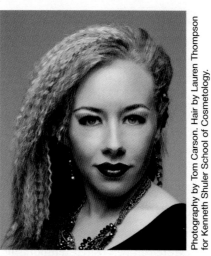

figure 14-9
Repeating lines in a hairstyle

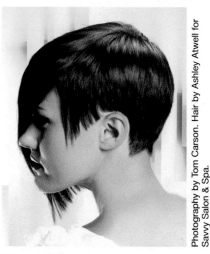

figure 14-10
Contrasting lines

- **Parallel lines** are repeating lines in a hairstyle. The lines can be straight or curved. The repetition of lines creates more interest in the design. Crimping hair or crinkle-wave is an example of a style using curved, parallel lines (figure 14-9).

- **Contrasting lines** are horizontal and vertical lines that meet at a 90-degree angle. These lines create a hard edge. Contrasting lines in a design usually create distinct looks and work best for clients able to carry off a strong style (figure 14-10).

- **Transitional lines** are usually curved lines that are used to blend and soften horizontal or vertical lines. These lines are used frequently when texturizing a haircut along with hair color placement and color blending (figure 14-11).

- **Directional lines** are lines with a definite forward or backward movement.

Form

Form is the mass or general outline of a hairstyle. It is three-dimensional and has length, width, and depth. Form may also be referred to as volume. Solid, smoother forms with minimal texture most often give a slimming appearance to the outline of the style, where more textured forms can add weight. The hair form should be in proportion to the shape of the head and face, the length and width of the neck, and the shoulder line (figure 14-12).

Space

Space is the area surrounding the form or the area the hairstyle occupies. We are more aware of the (positive) form than the (negative) spaces. In hair design, with every movement the relationship of the form and space changes. A hairstylist must keep every angle in mind—not only of the forms being created, but of the spaces surrounding the forms as well. The space may contain curls, curves, waves, straight hair, or any combination.

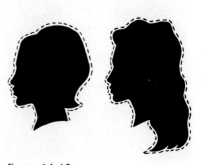

figure 14-11
Transitional lines

figure 14-12
The outline of the hairstyle is the form.

Design Texture

Design texture refers to the directional wave patterns or illusion of motion in the hair. The design texture must be taken into consideration when creating a style for your client. All hair, whether straight, wavy, curly, or excessively curly has a unique directional pattern and its own movement. For example, straight hair reflects light better than other patterns; it also reflects the most light when it is cut to a single length (figure 14-13). Wavy hair can be combed directionally to create horizontal lines (figure 14-14). Curly hair is more coiled and often grows more compact together. Curly hair will reflect less light and can create a larger form than straight or wavy hair (figure 14-15).

Creating Design Texture with Styling Tools

Texture can be created temporarily with the use of heat and/or wet styling techniques. Curling irons, hot rollers, or even flat irons can be used to create a wave or curl. Curly hair can be straightened using a flat brush, round brush, and the heat of a blow dryer or flat iron (figure 14-16).

Crimping irons are used to create interesting and unusual wave patterns, like zigzags. Hair can also be wet-set with rollers, wrapped with bobby pins or pincurled to create curls and waves. Finger waves, braids, and locs are other ways of creating temporary textured pattern changes (figures 14-17 and 14-18). You will learn more about styling techniques in subsequent chapters.

Changing Design Texture with Chemicals

Chemically infused services that make changes in the natural texture, curl, or wave pattern in the hair are considered permanent and will never revert back to the original pattern. (figure 14-19). As the hair grows long enough to alter the texture or pattern, a re-touch chemical process will need to be done on the new growth to make the design pattern uniform. Curly hair can be straightened with relaxers, and straight hair can be curled with permanent waves.

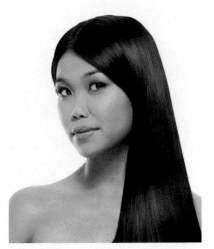
figure 14-13
Straight hair

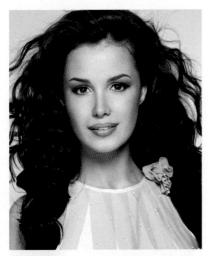
figure 14-14
Wavy hair

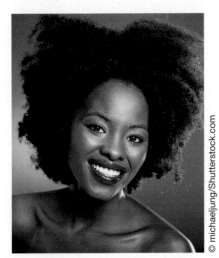
figure 14-15
Very curly hair

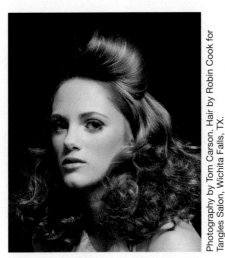
figure 14-16
Wave patterns can be altered temporarily.

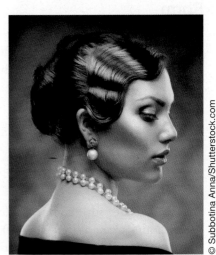
figure 14-17
Finger waves and curls

© Alliance/Shutterstock.com

© Valua Vitaly/Shutterstock.com

© michaeljung/Shutterstock.com

Photography by Tom Carson. Hair by Robin Cook for Tangles Salon, Wichita Falls, TX.

© Subbotina Anna/Shutterstock.com

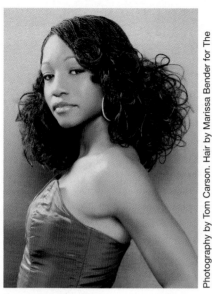

figure 14-18
Fine braids create temporary waves.

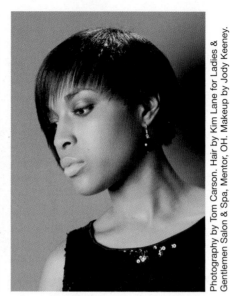

figure 14-19
Chemically altered hairstyle

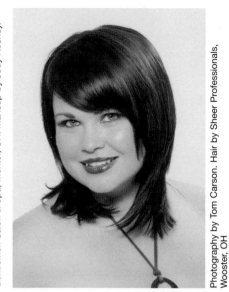

figure 14-20
Straight wave patterns are flattering on a round face.

Keratin based chemical treatments used for smoothing or straightening the hair are also available in today's market. This process, however, is not completely permanent. Depending on the manufacturer, strength, timing, and application, the product results last 120 days on average. These techniques are covered in detail in Chapter 20, Chemical Texture Services.

Tips for Designing with Directional Wave Patterns

- Use creative discretion when using multiple directional wave pattern combinations together in one design. This design is ideal for a client who wants to achieve a trendy multi-textured look with volume and unconstructed lines; however, may be less appropriate for more conservative professionals who wish for a smoother finished design.

- Smooth patterns accent the face and are particularly useful when you wish to narrow a round head shape (figure 14-20).

- Curly patterns take attention away from the face and can be used to soften square or rectangular features (figure 14-21).

Haircolor

Haircolor plays an important role in hair design, both visually and psychologically. It can be used to help define texture and line in a design. Haircolor can work to your advantage in many ways, from covering gray to changing the all-over color of a client's hair. Color can make all or part of the design appear larger or smaller by adding or subtracting volume. Depending on placement, color can accent or de-emphasize a particular part of a style or client feature. Color is also known to have a positive impact on one's mood and or attitude, if done well. In Chapter 21, Haircoloring, you will learn more about enhancing hair design by using haircolor as an important element.

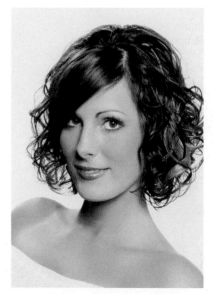

figure 14-21
Curly wave patterns soften angular faces.

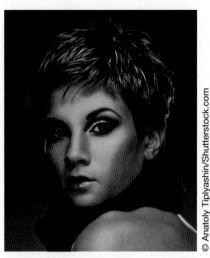

figure 14-22
Light colors appear closer
to the surface.

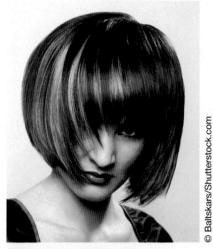

figure 14-23
Creating dimension with color

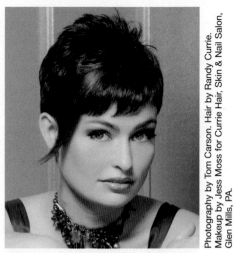

figure 14-24
Contrasting color accents the line.

figure 14-25
Strong color contrast

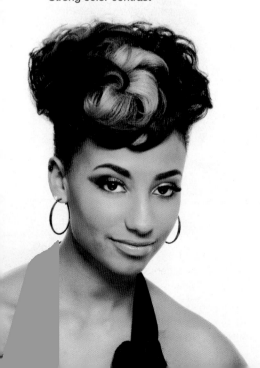

Dimension with Color

The look of the hair design can change depending on the chosen colors, along with the pattern and placement. Light and warm colors create the illusion of volume. Dark, cool colors recede or move in toward the head, creating the illusion of less volume. The illusion of dimension, or depth, is created when lighter and warmer colors alternate with those that are darker and cooler (figures 14-22 and 14-23).

Lines with Color

Color acts as an illusion and helps to create lines of attention. Because the eye is drawn to the lightest color present, you can use a light color to draw a line in a hairstyle in the direction you want the eye to travel, as with highlights around the fringe or facial area. A single line of color, or a series of repeated lines of color, can create a bold, dramatic accent or work to enhance blunt lines around the perimeter of a style (figure 14-24).

How Color Selection Can Influence a Design

When choosing a color, it is important to map out and understand your design plan. Create a visual plan for placement and patterns of your color choices. With the colors selected to include in the design, consider how they weigh with the other variables. Consult with your client about their color objectives and/or what look or impact he or she is trying to achieve. For instance, if a client has a gold tone to her skin, warm haircolors are more flattering than cool haircolors. For a more conservative or natural look when using two or more colors, choose colors with similar tones within two levels of each other. When using high contrast colors in most salon situations, you should use one color sparingly. A strong contrast can create an attention-grabbing look and should only be used on clients who are trendy and can carry off a bold look (figure 14-25). These are all important factors when considering color and will give you more leverage to more predictable results.

You will learn more about haircolor and the proper tools for color selection in Chapter 21, Haircoloring.

After reading the next few sections, you will be able to:

LO❸ Explain the five principles of hair design and recognize their specific contribution to a hairstyle.

Understand the Principles of Hair Design

Five important principles in art and design—proportion, balance, rhythm, emphasis, and harmony—are also the basis of hair design. The better you understand these principles, the more confident you will feel about creating styles that are pleasing to the eye.

Proportion

Proportion is the comparative relationship of one thing to another. For example, a 60-inch television set might be considered out of proportion or scale in a very small bedroom. Understanding facial and head proportion is important. A person with a very small chin and a very wide forehead might be said to have a head shape that is not in proportion. A well-chosen hairstyle could create the illusion of better proportion for such a client.

Body Proportion

It is essential when designing a hairstyle that you take into account the client's body shape and size. As a cosmetologist, you will have the opportunity to assist in developing the total image of a client. It is important to gain a brief understanding of body proportion to create styles that best fit each individual client.

Challenges in body proportion become more obvious if the hair form is too small or too large. Though there are subtle differences between individuals, there is a fairly standard range of proportion between the head and the body. The measurement of the head is the distance from the top of the head to the chin. This unit of measurement is most often used to establish the proportions of the entire body A general guide for classic proportion is that the hair should not be wider than the center of the shoulders, regardless of the body structure. Keep in mind that the best hairstyles are those that create harmony between the client's height and weight. Cropped to above shoulder-length styles with gentle wave patterns are usually best for shorter smaller frames, while taller fuller proportions should aim for a medium-length style, with softer curves. When choosing a style for a woman with large hips or broad shoulders, for instance, you would normally create a style with more volume (**figure 14-26**). But the same large hairstyle would appear out of proportion on a petite woman (**figure 14-27**).

Balance

Balance is establishing equal or appropriate proportions to create symmetry. In hairstyling, it can be the proportion of height to width.

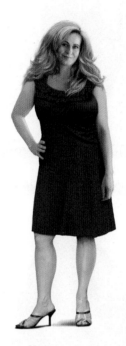
figure 14-26
A large hairstyle balances a large body structure.

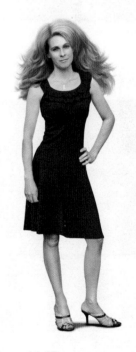
figure 14-27
A large hairstyle makes a petite woman look smaller.

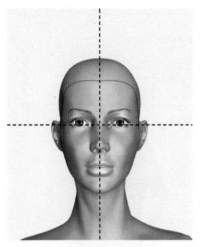

figure 14-28
Measuring symmetry of the head

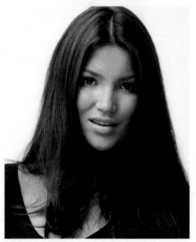

figure 14-29
Both sides equidistant from center

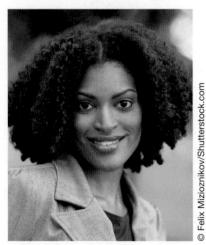

figure 14-30
Symmetry with different shapes, same volume

Balance can be symmetrical or asymmetrical. Often when you are dissatisfied with a finished hair design, it is because the style is out of balance.

To measure symmetry, divide the face into four equal parts. The lines cross at the central axis, the reference point for judging the balance of the hair design. You can then decide if the hairstyle looks pleasing to the eye and is in correct balance (figure 14-28).

Symmetrical balance (sih-MET-rih-kal BAL-antz) occurs when an imaginary line is drawn through the center of the face and the two resulting halves form a mirror image of one another. Both sides of the hairstyle are the same distance from the center, the same length, and have the same volume when viewed from the front (figures 14-29 and 14-30).

Asymmetrical balance (A-sym-et-rical BAL-antz) is established when the two imaginary halves of a hairstyle have an equal visual weight, but are positioned unevenly. Opposite sides of the hairstyle are different lengths or have a different volume. Asymmetry can be horizontal or diagonal (figures 14-31 and 14-32).

Rhythm

Rhythm is a regular pulsation or recurrent pattern of movement in a design. In music or dance, rhythm can be fast or slow. In hair design, a fast rhythm moves quickly; tight curls are an example. A slow rhythm can be seen in larger shapes or long waves (figures 14-33 and 14-34).

Emphasis

The **emphasis**, also known as *focus*, in a design is what draws the eye first, before it travels to the rest of the design. A hairstyle may be well balanced, with good rhythm and harmony, and yet still be boring. Create interest with an area of emphasis or focus by using the following:

- Wave patterns (figure 14-35)
- Color (figure 14-36)

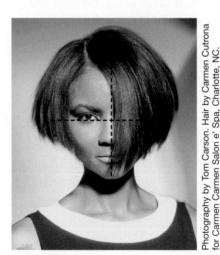

figure 14-31
Horizontal asymmetry

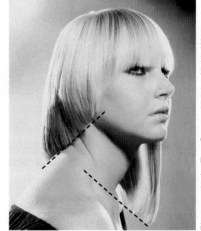

figure 14-32
Diagonal asymmetry

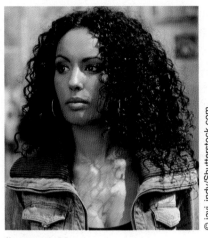

figure 14-33
Fast rhythm

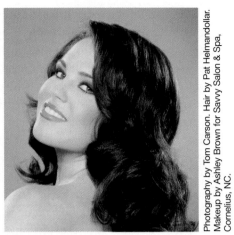

figure 14-34
Slow rhythm

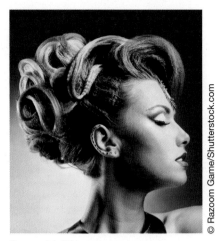

figure 14-35
Creating emphasis with various
wave patterns

- Change in form (figure 14-37)
- Ornamentation (figure 14-38)

Choose an area of the head or face that you want to emphasize. Keep the design simple so that it is easy for the eye to follow from the point of emphasis through to the rest of the style. You can have multiple points of emphasis as long as you do not use too many and as long as they are decreasing in size and importance. Remember, less is more.

Harmony

Harmony is the creation of unity in a design and is the most important of the art principles. Harmony holds all the elements of the design together. When a hairstyle is harmonious it has the following elements:

- A form with interesting lines
- A pleasing color or combination of colors and textures
- A balance and rhythm that together strengthen the design

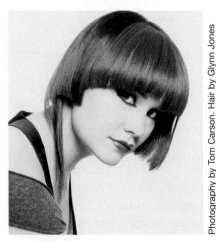

figure 14-36
Creating emphasis with color

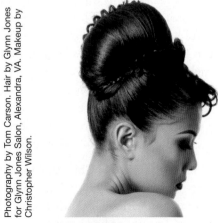

figure 14-37
Creating emphasis with form and
texture changes

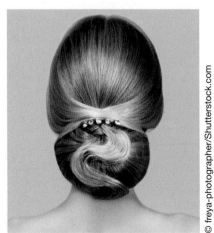

figure 14-38
Ornament as focal point

A harmonious design is never too busy and it is in proportion to the client's facial and body structure. A successful harmonious design includes an area of emphasis from which the eyes move to the rest of the style.

The principles of design may be used in modern hairstyling to guide you as you decide how best to achieve a beautiful appearance for your client. The best results are obtained when each of your client's facial features and profile is properly analyzed for its strengths and weaknesses. Your job is to accentuate a client's best features and to downplay features that do not add to the person's appearance. Every hairstyle you create for every client should be properly proportioned to body type and correctly balanced to the person's head, length of neck, and facial features. The hairstyle should attractively frame the client's face. An artistic and suitable hairstyle will take into account physical characteristics such as the following:

- Shape of the head, including the front view (face shape), profile, and back view
- Length of neck
- Facial features (perfect as well as imperfect features)
- Body shape and posture

milady pro™ **LEARN MORE!**

Optional info on **Hair Design** topics and tutorials can be found at miladypro.com Keyword: *FutureCosPro*

After reading the next few sections, you will be able to:

LO❹   Understand the influence of hair type and texture on design.

Recognize the Influence of Hair Type and Texture on Hairstyle

Your client's hair type is a major consideration in the selection of a hairstyle. Hair type is categorized by two defining characteristics: directional patterns and hair texture.

All hair has natural directional patterns, such as waves that must be taken into consideration when designing a style. These patterns are straight, wavy, curly, and extremely curly. Hair texture, density, and the relationship between the two are also important factors in choosing a style. The basic hair textures are: fine, medium, and coarse. Hair density, or hair per square inch, ranges from very thin to very thick.

Keep in mind the following guidelines for different types of hair:

- **Straight, fine hair.** This combination usually hugs the head shape due to the lack of body or volume, and marginal elasticity. The silhouette is small and narrow. If this is not appropriate for the client based on the facial features or body structure, think about what styling aids or chemical services can be recommended to achieve the most flattering style. Left natural, this hair type may not support many styling options.

- **Straight, medium hair.** This type of hair offers more versatility in styling. It responds well to blow drying with various sized brushes and has a good amount of movement. It will also respond well to rollers and thermal styling.

- **Straight, coarse hair.** This hair is hard to curl and carries more volume than the previous two types. It casts a slightly wider silhouette and responds well to thermal styling with flat tools. Take note that round brushing may increase the unwanted volume in this hair type. The hair is still quite resistant with a more compact cuticle, therefore chemical services may take a little longer to process.

- **Wavy, fine hair.** This type of hair can appear fuller when diffused with heat and the appropriate haircut and style. The cuticle is a bit more raised than straighter hair types, so subsequently may be prone to minimal frizz and may be considered a bit fragile. With layering, it can look fuller, and respond well to blow drying and chemical services appropriate for smoothing and straightening.

- **Wavy, medium hair.** This type of hair offers the most versatility in styling as it has the most uniformity of pattern. It responds well to heat and is easily diffused when dried from its natural state to look curly, or be easily straightened by blow drying.

- **Wavy, coarse hair.** This hair type can produce a silhouette that is very voluminous if it is not shaped properly. Although blow drying can be effective with this hair type, the process is often much easier for the stylist than for the client. Clients with this hair often feel that their hair is too wavy when straight, and not curly enough for a curly style. A soft perm could easily bring the client to a wash-and-wear curly style. A chemical relaxer or keratin-based chemical treatment used for smoothing or straightening may be a good alternative if the client prefers a straighter look. Perhaps simply removing some weight from the interior with texture shears would be a great option.

- **Curly, fine hair.** When this hair type is worn long, it often separates, revealing the client's scalp unless the hair is very dense. This hair type responds well to mild relaxers, keratin-based chemical treatments used for smoothing/straightening, and color services. Blow drying the hair straight may require a bit more attention, as it sometimes tends to tangle easily. Using a thermal protecting detangle product before blow drying could alleviate some of the work.

- **Curly, medium hair.** This hair type creates a silhouette with subliminal volume. When left natural, this type of hair gives a soft, romantic look. The silhouette should be in proportion to the client's body shape and not overwhelm it. When shaping the hair, keep in mind where the weight line of the haircut will fall. This hair responds well to relaxers, keratin-based chemical treatment, and color.

- **Curly, coarse hair.** This hair type usually represents a mixture of coiled to extremely coiled hair strands. It is usually very compacted and offers little to no movement. Because of its many twists and turns, this hair is prone to tangles and dryness. Products containing moisture should be a focus when servicing clients with this hair type. Remember while cutting this hair type that the hair will shrink considerably when dry, making it appear much shorter; therefore it is suggested to cut dry.

- **Very curly, fine hair.** The most flattering shape for the client must be determined before you begin styling. For ease of styling, this hair type is generally best cut short. If the hair is long, the silhouette will be horizontally full and extremely voluminous. Chemical services and chemical smoothing services take well, but ensure that you follow all manufactures directions and recommended timing so that the hair's integrity is not compromised. Smoothing the hair using a blow dryer and thermal flat iron is also a great option. Remember to always use a protecting product when using any thermal appliance or tool.

- **Extremely curly, medium hair.** This silhouette can promote horizontal lines of volume, as it tends to widen as it grows longer because of the amount of curls. Chemical relaxers and chemical smoothers work very well to make the shape narrower. Pressing and thermal straighteners are also good options. If the hair is left in its natural state, cropping it close to the head in a flattering shape is great for ease of styling and low maintenance. This hair type offers versatility of styles that incorporate twists and braids, keeping the hair moisturized during styling for healthy looking results!

- **Extremely curly, coarse hair.** This silhouette will be extremely wide. Chemical relaxing is often recommended to make it more manageable and offer additional styling options. This hair type often appears quite dense and offers limited flexibility. If left in its natural state without chemicals, this hair type responds well to short, cropped layers along with braided, loc, or twisted styles which make the silhouette look more narrow while defining the curl pattern.

After reading the next few sections, you will be able to:

LO ⑤ Identify the seven different facial shapes and design a beneficial hairstyle for each.

Create Harmony between Hairstyle and Facial Structure

Perhaps one of the most challenging opportunities you will face as a stylist is speaking to your client about styles that will best accent their facial shape. Not every look that a client wants will work with their given facial shape. A client's facial shape is determined by the position and prominence of the facial bones. A good way to determine facial shape and to have the client understand what is possible is to pull all of the client's hair completely off the face using a towel or hair band to better observe just the client's face. There are seven basic facial shapes: oval, round, square, triangle (pear-shaped), oblong, diamond, and inverted triangle (heart-shaped). To recognize each facial shape and to be able to style the hair in the most flattering design with that facial shape in mind, you should be acquainted with the characteristics of each. Remember, when designing a style for your client's facial type, you generally are trying to create the illusion of an oval shaped face. Incorporate this process into your consultation by sharing this information with the client and show him or her pictures of hairstyles that are best suited for each shape and also share reasons why certain facial shapes do not do well with some styles. To determine a facial shape, divide the face into three zones: forehead to eyebrows, eyebrows to end of nose, and end of nose to bottom of chin.

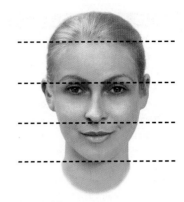

figure 14-39
Ideal facial proportions

Oval Facial Type

The contour and proportions of the oval face shape form the basis and ideals for evaluating and modifying all other facial types (figure 14-39).

Facial contour: The oval face is about one and a half times longer than its width across the brow. The forehead is slightly wider than the chin (figure 14-40). It visibly has no areas that dominate the others. A person with an oval face can wear any hairstyle unless there are other considerations, such as eyeglasses, length and shape of nose, or profile. (See the Special Considerations section later in this chapter.)

Round Facial Type

Facial contour: Round hairline and round chin line; wide face.
Objective: To create the illusion of length to the face, since this will make the face appear slimmer.
Styling choice: A hairstyle that has height or volume on top and closeness or no volume at the sides (figures 14-41a and b).

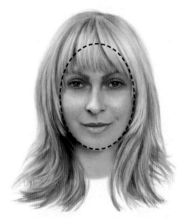

figure 14-40
The oval face shape is considered ideal and works with any hairstyle.

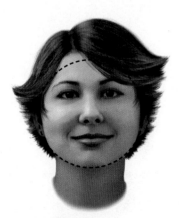

figure 14-41a
The round face shape is widest at the center of the face. A style like this one accentuates the width at the center of the face, so it is not a good choice.

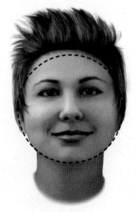

figure 14-41b
This style helps the round face shape appear longer and more oval by using additional volume at the top of the head and decreasing volume at the temple.

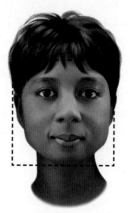

figure 14-42a
The square face shape is accentuated with this hairstyle because the style has little volume and does not help to soften the squared edges of the face shape.

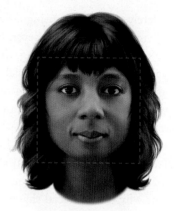

figure 14-42b
With its soft waves, close-to-the-head bangs, and curls at the chin, this hairstyle has volume at the temple area. It is very flattering for the square face shape.

Square Facial Type

Facial contour: Wide at the temples, narrow at the middle third of the face, and squared off at the jaw.

Objective: To offset or round out the square features.

Styling choice: Soften the hair around the temples and jaw by bringing the shape or silhouette close to the head form. Create volume in the area between the temples and jaw by adding width around the ear area (figures 14-42a and b).

Triangular (Pear-Shaped) Facial Type

Facial contour: Narrow forehead, wide jaw and chin line.

Objective: To create the illusion of width in the forehead.

Styling choice: A hairstyle that has volume at the temples and some height at the top. You can disguise the narrowness of the forehead with a soft bang or fringe (figures 14-43a and b).

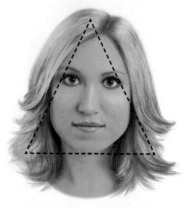

figure 14-43a
This style—long, flat-on-top, and curly length—does nothing to soften the angles of a triangular face.

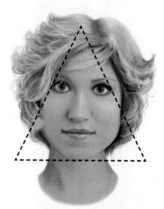

figure 14-43b
A much more flattering look for the triangular face shape. This style adds fullness to the top half of the head balancing the chin area and making the overall look more proportionate.

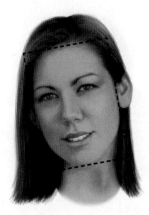

figure 14-44a
With no width at the center of the hairstyle, the oblong face shape is quite obvious.

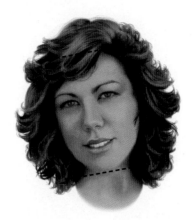

figure 14-44b
Adding volume to the temple and side areas creates the appearance of width and balance for this oblong face shape.

ACTIVITY

Partner up with a classmate. Using a standard tape measure, take turns measuring facial features.

1. Measure the forehead (across the forehead and above the eyebrows). Write down the number.
2. Using the middle of the ear as a guide, measure across the face from one ear to the other. Write down the number.
3. The last measurement should be from one side of the lower jaw bone to the other. Write down the number.

Check to see what proportions your measurements indicate and follow what you learned to determine your partner's facial shape and what hairstyle would work best on them. Discuss why this style would work best.

Oblong Facial Type

Facial contour: Long, narrow face with hollow cheeks.
Objective: To make the face appear shorter and wider.
Styling choice: Keep the hair fairly close to the top of the head. Add volume on the sides to create the illusion of width. The hair should not be too long, as this will elongate the oblong shape of the face. Chin-length styles are most effective for this facial type (**figures 14-44a and b**).

Diamond Facial Type

Facial contour: Narrow forehead, extreme width through the cheekbones, and narrow chin.
Objective: To reduce the width across the cheekbone line.
Styling choice: Increase the fullness across the jaw line and forehead while keeping the hair close to the head at the cheekbone line. Avoid hairstyles that lift away from the cheeks or move back from the hairline on the sides near the ear area (**figures 14-45a and b**).

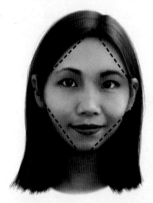

figure 14-45a
This hairstyle accentuates the diamond face shape by being close to the head and exposing the forehead, adding to the width of the face.

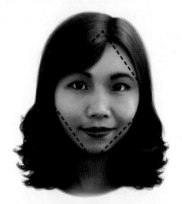

figure 14-45b
To create the illusion of balance for a diamond face shape, keep the sides closer to the face and create volume at the top and chin area.

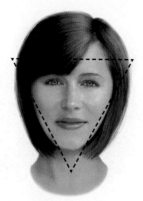

figure 14-46a
The inverted triangle-shaped face, also called the heart-shaped face, is not flattered by a hairstyle whose lines mimic the face shape.

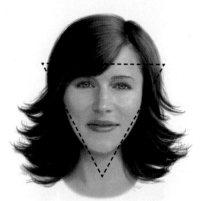

figure 14-46b
The inverted triangle-shaped face looks best in a hairstyle that has curl and volume in the lower half of the face.

Inverted Triangle (Heart-Shaped) Facial Type

Facial contour: Wide forehead and narrow chin line.

Objective: To decrease the width of the forehead and increase the width in the lower part of the face.

Styling choice: Style the hair close to the head with no volume. A bang or fringe is recommended. Gradually increase the width of the silhouette as you style the middle third of the shape in the cheekbone area and near the ears, and keep the silhouette at its widest at the jaw and neck area (figures 14-46a and b).

Profiles

The **profile** is the outline of the face, head, or figure seen in a side view. There are three basic profiles: straight, convex, and concave.

The **straight profile** is considered the ideal. The face when viewed in profile is neither convex (curving outward) nor concave (curving inward); although even a straight profile has a very slight curvature. Generally, all hairstyles are flattering to the straight or ideal profile (figure 14-47).

The **convex profile** (kahn-VEKS PRO-fyl) has a receding forehead and chin. It calls for an arrangement of curls or bangs over the forehead. Keep the style close to the head at the nape and move hair forward in the chin area (figures 14-48 and 14-49).

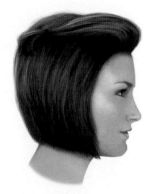

figure 14-47
Straight profile

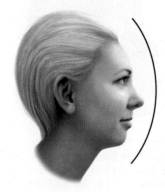

figure 14-48
Convex profile

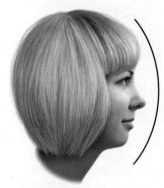

figure 14-49
Styling for a convex profile

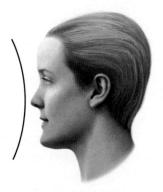

figure 14-50
Concave profile

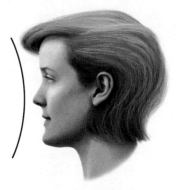

figure 14-51
Styling for a concave profile

The **concave profile** (kahn-KAYV PRO-fyl) has a prominent forehead and chin, with other features receding inward. It should be accommodated by softly styling the hair at the nape with an upward movement. Do not build hair onto the forehead (figures 14-50 and 14-51).

Special Considerations

An understanding of facial features and proportions will make it easier for you to analyze each client's face. You can then apply the design principles you have learned to help balance facial structural challenges. Dividing the face into three sections is one way to do this analysis.

Top Third of the Face

- **Wide forehead:** Direct hair forward over the sides of the forehead (figure 14-52).

- **Narrow forehead:** Direct hair away from the face at the forehead. Lighter highlights may be used at the temples to create the illusion of width (figure 14-53).

- **Receding forehead:** Direct the bangs over the forehead with an outwardly directed volume (figure 14-54).

- **Large forehead:** Use bangs with little or no volume to cover the forehead (figure 14-55).

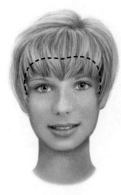

figure 14-52
Wide forehead

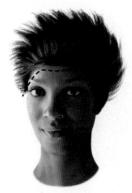

figure 14-53
Narrow forehead

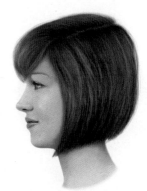

figure 14-54
Receding forehead

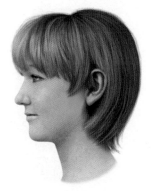

figure 14-55
Large forehead

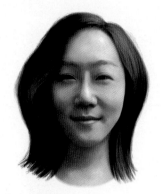
figure 14-56
Close-set eyes

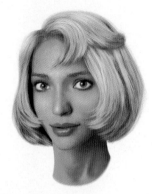
figure 14-57
Wide-set eyes

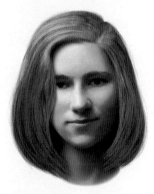
figure 14-58
Crooked nose

Middle Third of the Face

- **Close-set eyes:** Usually found on long, narrow faces. Direct hair back and away from the face at the temples. A side movement from a diagonal back part with some height is advisable. A slight lightening of the hair at the corner of the eyes will give the illusion of width (figure 14-56).

- **Wide-set eyes:** Usually found on round or square faces. Use a higher half bang to create length in the face. This will give the face the illusion of being larger and will make the eyes appear more proportional. The hair should be slightly darker at the sides than the top (figure 14-57).

- **Crooked nose:** Asymmetrical, off-center styles are best, as they attract the eye away from the nose. Symmetrical styles will accentuate the fact that the face is not even (figure 14-58).

- **Wide, flat nose:** Draw the hair away from the face and use a center part to help elongate and narrow the nose (figure 14-59).

- **Long, narrow nose:** Stay away from styles that are tapered close to the head on the sides, with height on top. Middle parts or too much hair directed toward the face are also poor choices. These will only accentuate any long, narrow features on the face. Instead, select a style where the hair moves away from the face, creating the illusion of wider facial features (figure 14-60).

- **Small nose:** A small nose often gives a child-like look; therefore, it is best to design an age-appropriate hairstyle that would not be associated with children. Hair should be swept off the face, creating a line from nose to ear. The top hair should be moved off the forehead to give the illusion of length to the nose (figure 14-61).

- **Prominent nose:** To draw attention away from the nose, bring hair forward at the forehead with softness around the face (figure 14-62).

Lower Third of the Face

- **Round jaw:** Use straight lines at the jaw line (figure 14-63).
- **Square jaw:** Use curved lines at the jaw line (figure 14-64).

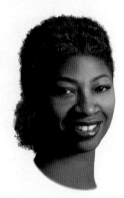
figure 14-59
Wide, flat nose

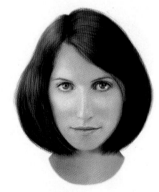
figure 14-60
Long, narrow nose

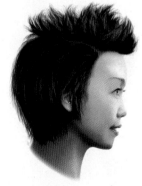
figure 14-61
Small nose

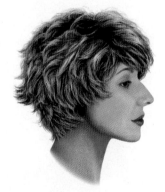
figure 14-62
Prominent nose

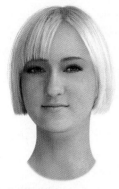

figure 14-63
Round jaw

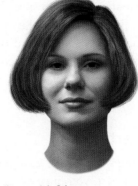

figure 14-64
Square jaw

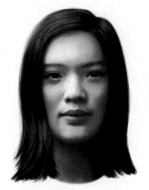

figure 14-65
Long jaw

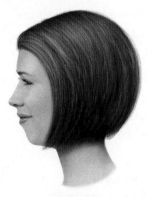

figure 14-66
Receding chin

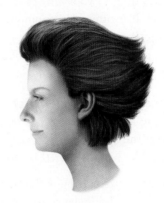

figure 14-67
Small chin

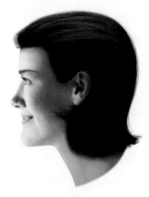

figure 14-68
Large chin

- **Long jaw:** Hair should be full and fall below the jaw to direct attention away from it (figure 14-65).
- **Receding chin:** Hair should be directed forward in the chin area (figure 14-66).
- **Small chin:** Move the hair up and away from the face along the chin line (figure 14-67).
- **Large chin:** The hair should be either longer or shorter than the chin line so as to avoid drawing attention to the chin (figure 14-68).

Head Shape

Not all head shapes are round. It is important to evaluate the head shape before deciding on a hairstyle. Design the style with volume in areas that are flat or small while reducing the volume of the hair in areas that are large or prominent (figure 14-69).

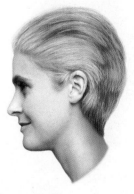

figure 14-69
Perfect oval

Styling for People Who Wear Glasses

Eyeglasses have become a fashion accessory and many people change their eyewear as often as their clothes. It is important for you to know whether your clients ever wear glasses so you can take that into account when designing the appropriate hairstyle. Keep in mind that when clients put on their glasses, the arms of the glasses (the part that rests on the ear) can push the hair at the ear and cause it to stick out.

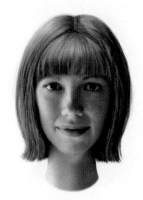

figure 14-70
Triangular part

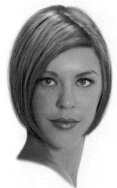

figure 14-71
Diagonal part in bangs

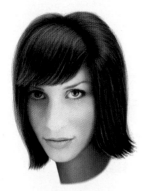

figure 14-72
Curved part

If you are choosing a short haircut, you may want to reconsider the length of the hair around the ear, opting to either leave it a little longer or cut the hair above and around the ear. For styling purposes, choose a style in which there is enough hair covering the ear (fine hair may pop out at the ear), or direct the hair away from the face, so that the arms of the glasses are not an issue.

Hair Partings

Hair partings can be the focal point of a hairstyle. Because the eye is drawn to a part, you must be careful in the placement. When possible, it is usually best to use a natural parting. You may, however, want to create a part according to your client's head shape or facial features, or for a desired hairstyle. It is often challenging to create a hairstyle working against the natural crown parting. For best results, you might try to incorporate the natural part into the finished style. The following are suggestions for hair partings that suit the various facial types.

Partings for the Bang (Fringe)

The **bang area**, also known as *fringe area*, is the triangular section that begins at the apex, or high point of the head, and ends at the front corners. The bang is parted in three basic ways:

- A triangular parting is the basic parting for bang sections and gives a symmetrical balance to the features on the face (figure 14-70).

- A diagonal parting gives height to a round or square face and width to a long, thin face (figure 14-71).

- A curved part is used for a receding hairline or high forehead (figure 14-72).

Style Partings

There are four other partings that can be used to highlight facial features:

- Center partings are classic. They are used for an oval face, but also give an oval illusion to wide and round faces. (figure 14-73).

- Side partings are used to direct hair across the top of the head. They help develop height on top and make thin hair appear fuller (figure 14-74).

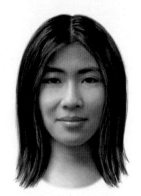

figure 14-73
Center part

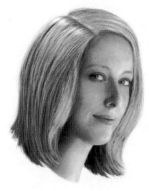

figure 14-74
Side part

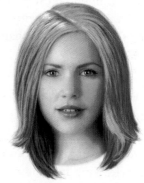

figure 14-75
Diagonal part

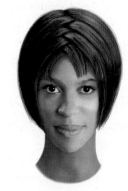

figure 14-76
Zigzag part

- Diagonal back partings are used to create the illusion of width or height in a hairstyle (figure 14-75).
- Zigzag partings create a dramatic effect (figure 14-76).

After reading the next few sections, you will be able to:

LO **6** Explain two design considerations for men.

Design for Men

All the design principles and elements you have just read about work for men's hairstyles as well as for women's. Men's styles have become more individualized since the early 1960s, when the Beatles hit the music and fashion scene and greatly revolutionized men's hairstyling. As trends continue, men's hairstyles are typically a bit longer, more tousled, and more disheveled than in past years. Men are also choosing layered texture for design and movement in their style. All hair lengths and forms such as spikes, mohawks, twists, and locs are now acceptable for men, giving them more choices than ever before (figure 14-77). Bald head options are also becoming more popular to promote a man's individual style.

As a professional, you should be able to recommend styles that are both flattering and appropriate for the client's lifestyle, career, and hair type. Men are concerned about their hair and grooming it properly, therefore you should also be able to suggest products that will work well with the style and be able to provide maintenance tips to use at home.

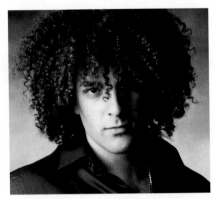

figure 14-77
Twist style on naturally curly hair

Choosing Facial Hair Design

Mustaches, beards, and sideburns can be a great way for a male client to show his individual style. They can also be used to camouflage facial flaws. For example, if a man does not have a prominent chin when you look at his profile, a neatly trimmed full beard and mustache can be a good solution (figure 14-78). If a man has a wide face and full cheeks, a fairly close-trimmed or even faded beard and mustache would be very thinning to the overall appearance while also creating a more youthful and trendy look.

A man who is balding with closely trimmed hair could also look very good in a closely groomed beard and mustache. Sideburns, mustaches, and beard shapes are largely dictated by current trends and fashions. No matter what the trend is, it is important that the shapes appear well groomed and are flattering to the client. Facial hair can be groomed using a facial trimmer or a straight razor for closer more precise linings. It is suggested to always use a shaving cream product to ensure that the tool glides smoothly across the face, limiting the potential for skin punctures.

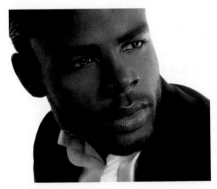

figure 14-78
Full beard and mustache with faded design line

© Coka/Shutterstock.com

© holbox/Shutterstock.com

1. What are possible sources a hair designer might use for inspiration?

2. List the five elements of hair design and give a brief definition of each.

3. List the five principles of hair design and describe one form that uses each principle.

4. What influence does hair type and texture have on hairstyle?

5. List and describe the seven facial shapes and explain how hair design can be used to highlight or camouflage facial features.

6. How do the elements and principles of hair design apply to men?

STUDY TOOLS

- **Reinforce what you just learned:** Complete the activities and exercises in your Theory or Practical Workbook, or your Study Guide.

- **Expand your knowledge:** Search for websites about the topics in this chapter and make a list of additional resources.

- **Study and prepare for your quiz:** Take the chapter test in your Exam Review or your Milady U: Online Licensing Prep.

- **Re-Test your knowledge:** Take the Chapter 14 *Quizzes*!

- **Learn even more:** Look up in a dictionary or search the internet for the definitions of any additional terms you want to learn about.

CHAPTER GLOSSARY

asymmetrical balance A-sym-et-rical BAL-antz	p. 304	Is established when two imaginary halves of a hairstyle have an equal visual weight, but the two halves are positioned unevenly. Opposite sides of the hairstyle are different lengths or have a different volume. Asymmetry can be horizontal or diagonal.
balance	p. 303	Establishing equal or appropriate proportions to create symmetry. In hairstyling, it is the relationship of height to width.
bang area	p. 316	Also known as *fringe area*; triangular section that begins at the apex, or high point of the head, and ends at the front corners.
concave profile kahn-KAYV PRO-fyl	p. 313	Curving inward; prominent forehead and chin, with other features receded inward.
contrasting lines	p. 299	Horizontal and vertical lines that meet at a 90-degree angle and create a hard edge.
convex profile kahn-VEKS PRO-fyl	p. 312	Curving outward; receding forehead and chin.
curved lines	p. 298	Lines moving in a circular or semi-circular direction; used to soften a design.

design texture	p. 300	Wave patterns that must be taken into consideration when designing a style.
diagonal lines	p. 298	Lines positioned between horizontal and vertical lines. They are often used to emphasize or minimize facial features.
directional lines	p. 299	Lines with a definite forward or backward movement.
emphasis	p. 304	Also known as *focus*; the place in a hairstyle where the eye is drawn first before traveling to the rest of the design.
form	p. 299	The mass or general outline of a hairstyle. It is three-dimensional and has length, width, and depth.
harmony	p. 305	The creation of unity in a design; the most important of the art principles. Holds all the elements of the design together.
horizontal lines	p. 298	Lines parallel to the floor and relative to the horizon; create width in hair design.
parallel lines	p. 299	Repeating lines in a hairstyle; may be straight or curved.
profile	p. 312	Outline of the face, head, or figure seen in a side view.
proportion	p. 303	The comparative relationship of one thing to another; the harmonious relationship among parts or things.
rhythm	p. 304	A regular pulsation or recurrent pattern of movement in a design.
single lines	p. 298	A hairstyle with only one line, such as the one-length hairstyle.
space	p. 299	The area surrounding the form or the area the hairstyle occupies.
straight profile	p. 312	Neither convex nor concave; considered the ideal.
symmetrical balance Sym-et-rical BAL-antz	p. 304	Two halves of a style; form a mirror image of one another.
transitional lines	p. 299	Usually curved lines that are used to blend and soften horizontal or vertical lines.
vertical lines	p. 298	Lines that are straight up and down; create length and height in hair design.

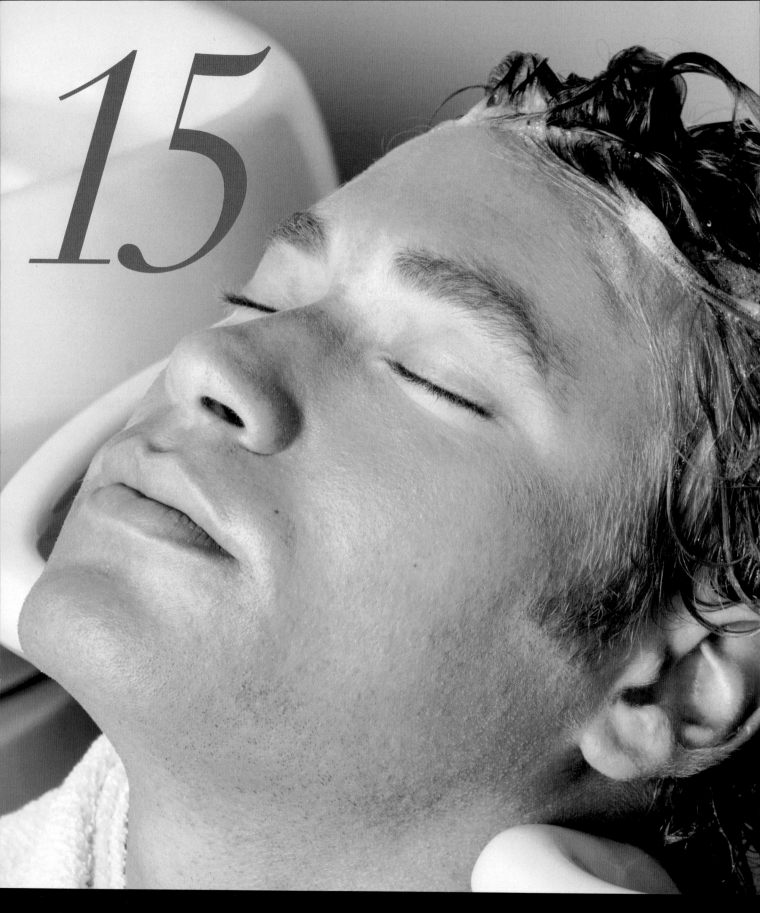

15

SCALP CARE, SHAMPOOING, AND CONDITIONING

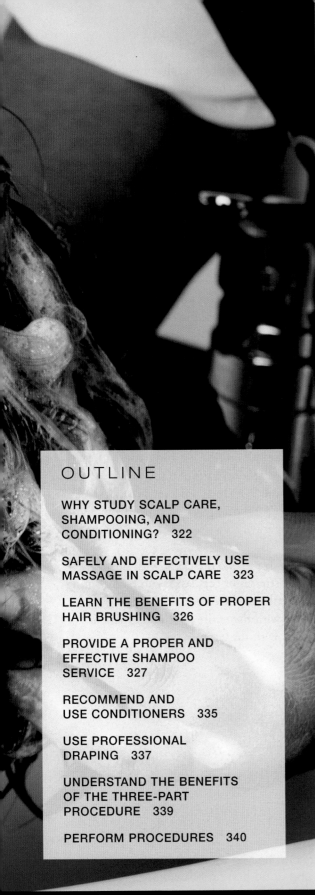

LEARNING OBJECTIVES

After completing this chapter, you will be able to:

LO ❶
Identify the two most basic requirements for scalp care.

LO ❷
Demonstrate a scalp massage during a shampoo service.

LO ❸
Examine the differences and similarities of treating scalp and hair that are dry, oily, and/or affected by dandruff.

LO ❹
Describe how hair brushing contributes to a healthy scalp.

LO ❺
Evaluate the uses and benefits of the various types of shampoo.

LO ❻
Evaluate the uses and benefits of the various types of conditioners.

LO ❼
Demonstrate appropriate draping for a basic shampooing and conditioning, and draping for a chemical service.

LO ❽
Identify the three-part procedure of a hair care service and explain why it is useful.

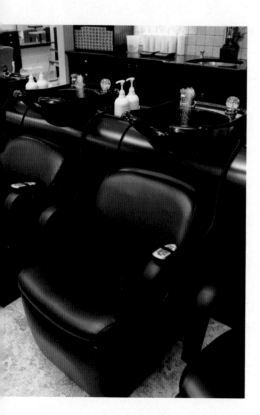

When clients visit a salon for the first time, they immediately begin making judgments about the surroundings. How does the salon look? What kind of music is playing? Does the receptionist greet them with a smile and call them by name? While all of these factors are part of a good salon experience, it is what happens when the client moves into the service area that can assist in the professional promotion of you and your salon business.

When you arrive at your salon, take a good look around. Ensure that you have done everything you can to prepare your client for a positive experience:

- Make sure you are dressed for success and present a happy and professional posture and healthy hygiene.
- Make sure your working station and back bar area are clean and organized and prepared with the tools needed for the business day.
- Adjust the temperature for client comfort and create an atmosphere of relaxation with soft music if possible.

Remember the old adage—*You only get one chance to make a good first impression.* Take the opportunity to stack the odds in your favor!

One of the most important experiences that a stylist provides is the shampoo. Making this a pleasurable and memorable experience can have a great impact on building your reputation as a stylist and building loyalty and repeat business for your salon. Often called simply "the shampoo," this first step of the service actually encompasses three different processes: scalp care and massage, shampooing, and conditioning. The shampoo can and should be a soothing, pleasurable experience that sets the mood for the entire visit.

The shampoo is an opportunity to provide the client with quality relaxation time that is free from the stresses of the day. It can be nurturing and, when done well, add great benefits to the hair for styling.

Remember: If clients are happy with the entire shampoo experience, they are far more likely to be happy with the entire service.

why study
SCALP CARE, SHAMPOOING, AND CONDITIONING?

Cosmetologists should study and have a thorough understanding of scalp care, shampooing, and conditioning because:

> The shampoo service is the first opportunity to reinforce your position as a professional who attends to the specific, individual needs of your client.

> You will be able to examine, identify, and address hair and scalp conditions that do not require a physician's care and be able to refer clients to a physician if a more serious issue is identified.

> A general knowledge of product category choices will assist you in determining the best preparation for other services to be performed.

> A successful home-care regimen recommendation will keep your work looking its best for all to see.

After reading the next few sections, you will be able to:

LO❶ Identify the two most basic requirements for scalp care.

LO❷ Demonstrate a scalp massage during a shampoo service.

LO❸ Examine the differences and similarities of treating scalp and hair that are dry, oily, and/or affected by dandruff.

Safely and Effectively Use Massage in Scalp Care

The two basic requirements for a healthy scalp are cleanliness and stimulation. Since similar manipulations are given with all scalp treatments, scalp massage is a procedure you will perform often and one that you should learn to do well. Remember all safety practices when servicing clients in your salon. The comfort and protection of the client's skin, hair, and clothing are all part of your responsibility as a stylist and important to their satisfaction with your service.

Proper maintenance of the hair and scalp begins with the hygiene practice of shampooing. The hair should be shampooed as often as necessary to remove dirt, oils and product build-up. If the hair and scalp is improperly addressed and cleansed, there is potential to promote unhealthy disorders of the scalp due to the buildup of dirt, product and oils.

Most often, one of the most memorable services in the salon is the shampoo coupled with a great scalp massage. The massage is a method of manipulating the scalp by rubbing, tapping, kneading, or stroking it with the hands. It can provide beneficial qualities such as increasing blood circulation and calming tenseness. Usually done once after the hair has been cleansed, massage techniques are initiated along with the conditioning service. The conditioner is applied and the massage manipulations begin, allowing the conditioning product to penetrate more evenly, offering the nourishing benefits in a tension-reducing atmosphere. Follow the recommended instructions and timing for the conditioning service and apply gentle pressure during the massage as not to irritate the client's scalp from over-manipulation.

When performing a scalp massage, remember to keep the client's head supported and maintain contact with the head at all times. Use slow, deliberate motions and a soft touch. It is also important for you as the stylist to be relaxed. Your hands, fingers, and shoulders should be free of stiff, mechanical movements. Utilize proper body positioning to maintain your balance and rhythm control.

Before performing a shampoo service that includes a scalp massage, complete a client intake or health screening form. During the consultation, acknowledge and discuss any medical condition your client listed that may produce undesirable side effects for a scalp massage. Ask the client if they have discussed massage with their physician and, if applicable, encourage them to seek their physician's advice as to whether or not a scalp massage is advisable before performing the service.

Many clients who have high blood pressure (hypertension), diabetes, or circulatory conditions may still have massage without concern, especially if their condition is being treated and carefully looked after to monitored by a physician. Massage is, however, not recommended for clients with severe, uncontrolled hypertension. If your client expresses a concern about having a scalp massage, or if there is any concern on your part, be conservative and do not proceed with the service. Create a relaxing environment for massage. Soft music and limited dialogue enhances the massage experience.

Procedure 15-7, Scalp Massage, explains the protocol and massage manipulations that are used in scalp massage. There are massage techniques that are designed for relaxation and those that are done in conjunction with a treatment. The main difference between the two are the products you use. For simple relaxation, most any conditioner can be used to create a very enjoyable experience for your client. Treatment massages are generally suggested to address conditions of the scalp such as dryness, minimal flaking, and to temporarily soothe a tight scalp. The manipulations would mirror those of a relaxation massage but would include the pre application of appropriate products. Be sure to follow all of the manufacturer's directions whenever a special scalp treatment product is used.

Scalp massage offers the opportunity to elevate your expertise and deliver a great salon experience. This can lead to profitable client retentions and a foundation for ongoing business referrals.

Basic massage manipulations will be further discussed and detailed in Chapter 23, Facials. These techniques are universal in theory and can be adapted and applied to the scalp as well. In addition, understanding the muscles, the location of blood vessels, and the nerve points of the scalp and neck will help guide you to those areas most likely to benefit from massage movements. For details on this information, see Chapter 6, General Anatomy and Physiology.

Ⓟ 15-7 **Scalp Massage** *See page 352*

Normal Hair and Scalp Treatment

The purpose of a general scalp treatment is to maintain the scalp and hair in a clean and healthy condition. A hair or scalp treatment should be recommended only after a hair and scalp examination. Educate the client about any potential scalp and/or hair concerns and involve her in understanding the overall hair benefits of a professional scalp treatment. Encourage the service, however if the client does not wish an immediate treatment, recommend scheduling the treatment for an alternate time. If the client agrees to the treatment, follow all manufacturer's directions prior to proceeding with the service.

Dry Hair and Scalp Treatment

A dry hair and scalp treatment should be used when there is a deficiency of natural oil on the scalp and hair. Dry scalp can derive from many sources. The elements such as sun, water, and wind can add dryness to the scalp and hair. Chemicals, harsh soaps, and topical products can also contribute to dryness. To address this concern, select scalp preparations containing moisturizing and emollient ingredients. Avoid the use of high-detergent based cleansers, preparations containing a mineral- or oil base, greasy preparations, or lotions with high alcohol content. During a dry hair and scalp treatment, a scalp steamer, which resembles a hooded dryer, can be used to help resolve the moisture balance in the hair. Through the use of steam, water and treatment are delivered into the cuticle layer of the hair and scalp. (figure 15-1).

Oily Hair and Scalp Treatment

Excessive oiliness is caused by overactive sebaceous glands. These glands are sometimes active due to genetics but can also be aggravated by over-exertion, misuse and layering of heavy products, and physical changes in the body. During this type of massage, manipulate the scalp using a kneading technique to increase blood circulation to the surface. This will reduce any hardened sebum that has been collected in the pores of the scalp and can be removed with gentle pressing or squeezing. To normalize the function of these glands and discourage further build-up, excess sebum should be flushed out or rinsed with each treatment.

figure 15-1
Scalp steamers can be used with hair and scalp treatments to help infuse moisture.

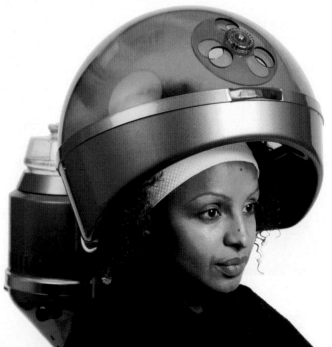

Antidandruff Treatment

As you may remember from Chapter 11, Dandruff is the visible shedding of skin cells and the result of a fungus called malassezia (māl-SĒ-zē-). The dandruff can sit on the scalp and create dryness, itchiness, and discomfort. Modern antidandruff shampoos, conditioners, and topical lotions contain antifungal agents that control dandruff by suppressing the growth of malassezia. Moisturizing salon treatments also soften and loosen scalp scales that stick to the scalp in crusts. Because of the ability of fungus to resist treatment, additional salon treatments and the frequent use of antidandruff home care should be recommended. The use of an infrared lamp used with massage could help to penetrate the product into the hair shaft and scalp while keeping the scalp warm and moist enough to loosen and lift the agitated cells that should be removed from the scalp during the rinsing process and potentially after the shampoo.

After reading the next few sections, you will be able to:

LO④ Describe how hair brushing contributes to a healthy scalp.

Learn the Benefits of Proper Hair Brushing

Correct hair brushing stimulates blood circulation to the scalp; brushing helps remove dust, dirt, and hairspray buildup from the hair and gives hair added shine. You should include a thorough hair brushing prior to the beginning of every shampoo (figure 15-2). When performing a scalp treatment, pay attention to the pressure used in brushing. Brush gently to remove debris and buildup while not allowing the brush to over-stimulate or prick the scalp area. You should always begin brushing the hair from the ends first and then work up towards the scalp. You can then freely brush the hair to rid of all tangles. This allows a proper detangling procedure without after additional friction or stress to the hair. Combing the hair with a wide-toothed comb is generally suggested for wet hair detangling post the shampoo process.

There are certain times, however, when brushing, massaging, or shampooing the scalp is not recommended. Check the list below for some of the situations when brushing should be avoided:

- If the scalp is irritated.
- Prior to a chemical service (follow manufacturer's directions).
- Prior to or after haircolor service (semi-permanent or permanent).
- Prior to or after bleach lightening or highlighting services (follow manufacturer's directions).

If shampooing is recommended by the manufacturer prior to a service, shampoo gently to avoid scalp irritation.

There are many brushes on the market; the most highly recommended hairbrushes are those made from natural bristles. Natural bristles have many tiny overlapping layers or scales, which clean and add luster to the hair. Hairbrushes with nylon bristles are shiny and smooth and are more suitable for hairstyling. Paddle brushes with rubber interior bristles and plastic vent brushes are also widely used especially when detangling wet hair.

figure 15-2
Include a thorough hair brushing as part of every shampoo and scalp treatment.

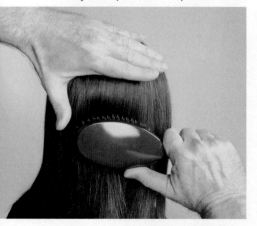

Ⓟ 15-3 **Hair Brushing** *See page 345*

After reading the next few sections, you will be able to:

LO⑤   Evaluate the uses and benefits of the various types of shampoo.

Provide a Proper and Effective Shampoo Service

The shampoo service provides a good opportunity to make sure that the hair and scalp are properly cleansed and nourished, providing a great canvas for styling and ongoing hair care. Prior to any service, analyze the client's hair and scalp. Always check the scalp and hair for any of the following conditions because they may alter your product choices or even your professional ability to perform the service:

- Dry, dehydrated hair
- Excessive shedding of the hair
- Thinning of the hair
- Dry, tight scalp
- Oily scalp
- Abnormal flaking on the scalp
- Open wounds or scalp irritations
- Scalp disorders or diseases
- Tick or lice infestation

If there are any open wounds, reddened scalp irritations, abnormal scalp flaking, or apparent diseases or infestations, immediately direct the client to a physician and do not continue with the service.

In salons where shampoos are performed by salon assistants, these assistants should always alert the stylist about any hair or scalp conditions, including suspected diseases or disorders. A client with an infectious disease is never to be treated in the salon and should be referred to a physician.

The primary purpose of a shampoo is to cleanse the hair and scalp prior to a service. This is also the best time to educate your client about the importance of home hair care and to suggest the best hair care products to use at home.

To be effective, a shampoo must remove all dirt, oils, cosmetics, and skin debris without adversely affecting either the scalp or hair. The scalp and hair need to be cleansed regularly to combat the accumulation of oils and perspiration that mix with the natural scales and dirt to create a breeding ground for disease-producing bacteria. Hair should only be shampooed as often as necessary. Excessive shampooing strips the hair of its protective oil (sebum) that, in small amounts, seals and protects the hair's cuticle. As a general rule, oily hair needs to be shampooed more often than normal or dry hair.

Always maintain good posture to protect against muscle aches, back strain, discomfort, fatigue, and other physical problems that can result from the action of performing a shampoo. The most important rule regarding posture is to always keep your shoulders back while performing a shampoo. Avoid slumping over the client or placing your torso, arms, and back into an unnatural position this will help avoid injury. Remember, too, to hold your abdomen and core in, thereby lifting your upper body. Free-standing shampoo bowls allow for healthier body alignment and help reduce strain on the back and shoulders.

Let's take a moment to look at the composition of a basic shampoo product.

Ⓟ 15-6   **Basic Shampooing and Conditioning** *See page 348*

Selecting the Proper Shampoo

There are many types of shampoo available on the market. As a professional cosmetologist, you should become skilled at selecting shampoos that support the health of the hair, whether the hair is natural or chemically altered. There are numerous products on the market that target the hair's specific needs. There are shampoos for color-treated hair, color toning, and some that even protect the fading of haircolor. There are shampoo choices for chemically relaxed hair, hair processed with keratin-based products that are used for smoothing or straightening, as well as cleansers for hair treated with cold wave products. Manufacturer's also produce shampoo products to meet the needs of the hair type and texture. Formulas have been developed to remedy fine and limp hair, coarse and dense hair, and some can enhance volume, remove frizz, and provide additional strength to the hair. For any situation you can imagine, there is a shampoo formulated to answer that market need. Most shampoo products contain water combined with various percentages of surfactants, lathering agents, and other ingredients that assist in maintaining or balancing the pH levels. Always read labels and accompanying literature carefully so that you can make informed decisions about the use of various shampoos. A thorough knowledge of your products will help you choose the right product and additionally recommend them as home-care items for purchase by your clients.

Select a shampoo according to the condition of the client's hair and scalp. Hair can usually be characterized as oily, dry, normal, or chemically treated. Keep in mind that some clients have multiple hair conditions and may need products to address various concerns. It is not uncommon to find shampoo products marketed to help many concerns or to neutralize conditions.

For example, chemically treated hair (hair that has been lightened, colored, permed, chemically relaxed, or processed with a keratin straightener) may require a product, such as a sulfate-free shampoo, that is less harsh and more conditioning. In addition, hair that has been abused by the use of harsh shampoos or damaged by improper care and exposure to the elements such as wind, sun, cold, and heat may also need to be treated with more conditioning agents.

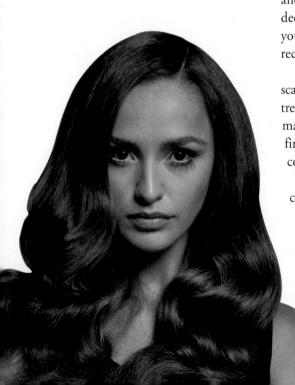

Using the right home-care products can make all the difference in how your clients' hair looks, feels, and behaves. It is your job to recommend and educate clients about which products they should be using, as well as how and why. Otherwise, they will make their own uninformed decisions, perhaps buying inferior products at the drugstore or supermarket. The wrong product choice can make a good haircut look bad, can negatively affect the client's opinion of your work, and can affect the outcome of a chemical service. Remember: You want your clients to look their best so that they become good advertising for you.

The pH Scale

Chapter 12, Basics of Chemistry, provides you with an overview of important chemistry basics, including pH and surfactants. Refer to that chapter as necessary. The following is a brief review of pH as it applies to shampoo.

Understanding pH levels will help you select the proper shampoo for your client. The amount of hydrogen in a solution, which determines whether it is alkaline or acidic, is measured on a pH scale that has a range from 0 to 14. The pH of a neutral solution, one which is neither acidic nor alkaline, is 7. A shampoo that is acidic will have a pH ranging from 0 to 6.9; a shampoo that is alkaline will have a pH 7.1 or higher. The more alkaline the shampoo, the stronger and harsher it is. A high-pH shampoo can leave the hair dry, brittle, and porous. A high-pH shampoo can cause fading in color-treated hair. A slightly acidic shampoo more closely matches the ideal pH of hair.

The Chemistry of Water

Water is the most abundant and important element on Earth. It is classified as a universal solvent because it is capable of dissolving more substances than any other solvent known to science.

Fresh water from lakes and streams is purified by sedimentation (matter sinking to the bottom) and filtration (water passing through a

---

FOCUS ON

Seven Ways to Make a Good Shampoo Experience Great!

1. The scalp is always massaged according to the preference of the client. Some clients have a sensitive scalp and want a very light massage, while others want a firm massage. In order to service every client to the best of your ability, ask about massage preferences before beginning the procedure.

2. Always ask the client if the water feels too warm, too cool, or just right; adjust the temperature accordingly.

3. Do not allow the water or your hands to touch the client's face during the shampoo. Allowing the face to get wet may cause irritation or remove makeup and can potentially turn an otherwise great shampoo into an unpleasant experience.

4. It is easy to miss the nape of the neck when shampooing and rinsing, so you should always double-check this area before escorting the client to your station.

5. Throughout the shampoo, be very careful not to drench the towel that is draped around the client's neck. If the towel becomes damp, replace it with a clean, dry towel before leaving the shampoo area.

6. When blotting the hair after the shampoo, be careful once again not to touch the face. If you remove part of your client's makeup, she may feel self-conscious during the entire visit.

7. As you learn to give a great shampoo, you should also learn how to give a great relaxation massage. You may hear your clients say, "Don't stop, you can do that for hours," every time they come to you. Even though you may hear this five times a day, it is always satisfying to know that you are making your clients feel good!

porous substance, such as a filter paper or charcoal) to remove suspended clay, sand, and organic material. Before the water enters public water pipelines, small amounts of chlorine are added to kill bacteria. Boiling water at a temperature of 212 degrees Fahrenheit (100 degrees Celsius) will also destroy most microbes. Water can be further treated by distillation, a process of heating water so that it becomes a vapor, and then condensing the purified vapor so that it collects as a liquid. Distillation is often used in the manufacturing of cosmetics.

Water is of crucial importance in the cosmetology industry because it is used for shampooing, mixing solutions, and many other functions. Depending on the kinds and amounts of minerals present in water, water can be classified as either hard or soft. You will be able to make a more professional shampoo selection if you know whether the water in your salon and area is hard or soft. Most water-softener companies can supply you with a water-testing kit to determine how hard or soft your water is (soft, slightly hard, moderately hard, hard, or extremely hard).

Soft water is rainwater or chemically softened water that contains only small amounts of minerals and, therefore, allows soap and shampoo to lather freely. For this reason, it is preferred for shampooing. **Hard water** is often found in well water and contains minerals that reduce the ability of soap or shampoo to lather. Hard water may also change the results of the haircoloring service. However, a water treatment process can soften hard water.

Always remember to monitor the temperature and pressure of the water before and during the professional service. Warmer, tepid water is adequate for rinsing shampoo and chemical product and cooler water works well to close the cuticle post-service, helping to add shine and vibrancy to the hair.

The Chemistry of Shampoo

To determine which shampoo will leave your client's hair in the best condition for the intended service, you need to understand the chemical and botanical ingredients regularly found in shampoos. Many shampoos have ingredients in common. It is often the small differences in formulation that make one shampoo better than another for a particular hair texture or condition.

Water is the main ingredient in most shampoos. Generally it is not just plain water, but purified or **deionized water** (DEE-eye-on-ized WAH-ter), water that has had impurities, such as calcium and magnesium and other metal ions that would make a product unstable, removed. Water is usually the first ingredient listed, which indicates that the shampoo contains more water than anything else. From there on, ingredients are listed in descending order, according to the percentage of each ingredient in the shampoo.

Surfactants

The second ingredient that most shampoos have in common is the primary surfactant (or base detergent). Surfactants are cleansing or surface active agents. A surfactant molecule has two ends: a hydrophilic or water-attracting head and a lipophilic or oil-attracting tail. During

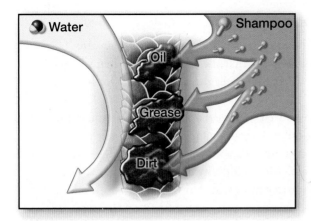

figure 15-3
The tail of the shampoo molecule is attracted to oil and dirt.

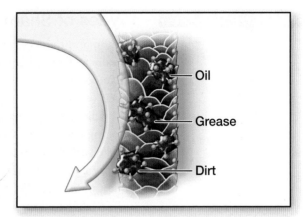

figure 15-4
Shampoo causes oils to roll up into small globules.

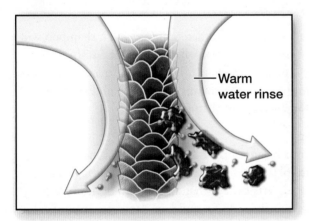

figure 15-5
The heads of the shampoo molecules attach to water molecules.

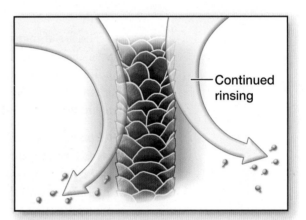

figure 15-6
Thorough rinsing washes away debris and excess shampoo.

the shampooing process, the hydrophilic head attracts water and the lipophilic tail attracts oil. This creates a push/pull process that causes the oils, dirt, and deposits to roll up into little balls that can be lifted off in the water and rinsed from the hair. Even shampoos that are marketed as surfactant-free have gentle cleansing agents added to the base (figures 15-3 through 15-6).

Other ingredients are added to the base surfactants to create a wide variety of shampoo formulas. **Moisturizer**, which is a product formulated to add moisture to dry hair or promote the retention of moisture, is a common additive along with oil, protein, preservative, foam enhancer, and perfume.

ACTIVITY

List all the hair products used in your school, along with the hair types appropriate for each. Analyze the hair of one or two classmates and recommend a particular shampoo and conditioner. List the benefits of each product for that particular "client." With your instructor's guidance, you might even try using your recommended choices on your classmates. Keep a record of what products you use, how the hair feels and behaves afterward, and your classmates' own opinions about the products.

Types of Shampoo

Shampoo products are the most widely purchased of all hair care products. Consumer studies show that the fastest growth items in the shampoo market are products that meet the specific needs of hair and scalp concerns.

Clients are increasingly well informed about beauty products from reading about them in beauty magazines and other consumer reports. Make sure that you are current with your product knowledge and technical theory for proper hair care. Your credibility as a professional will be in question if your client is better informed than you are.

Many good shampoos exist for every type of hair and/or scalp condition. There are shampoos for dry, oily, fine, coarse, limp, lightened, permed, relaxed, or color-treated and chemically treated hair. There are shampoos that deposit a slight amount of color to color-treated hair and those that cleanse hair of styling product buildup, mineral deposits, and so forth.

The list of ingredients is your key to determining which shampoo will leave a client's hair shiny and manageable, which will treat a scalp or hair condition, and which will prepare the hair for a chemical treatment. Now that you are familiar with pH and the chemistry of water and shampoo, here are some of the different types of shampoos.

pH-Balanced Shampoo

A **pH-balanced shampoo** is balanced to the pH of skin and hair (4.5 to 5.5). Many shampoos are pH balanced by the addition of citric, lactic, or phosphoric acid. Most experts believe that an acid pH of 4.5 to 5.5 is essential to preventing excessive dryness and hair damage during the cleansing process. Shampoos that are pH balanced help to close the hair cuticle and are recommended for hair that has been color-treated or lightened.

Conditioning Shampoo

Conditioning shampoo, also known as *moisturizing shampoo*, is designed to make the hair appear smooth and shiny and to improve the manageability of the hair. Protein and biotin are just two examples of conditioning agents that boost shampoos so that they can meet current grooming needs. These conditioning agents restore moisture and elasticity, strengthen the hair shaft, and add volume. They also are **nonstripping**, meaning that they do not remove artificial color from the hair.

Medicated Shampoo

Medicated shampoo contains special ingredients that are very effective in reducing dandruff or relieving other scalp conditions. Some medicated shampoos have to be prescribed by a physician. They can be quite strong and could affect the color of color-treated or lightened hair. In some cases, the shampoo must remain on the scalp for a longer period of time than other shampoos in order for the active ingredient to work. Always read and follow the manufacturer's instructions carefully.

Clarifying Shampoo

Clarifying shampoo contains an active chelating agent that binds to metals (such as iron and copper) and removes them from the hair, as well as an

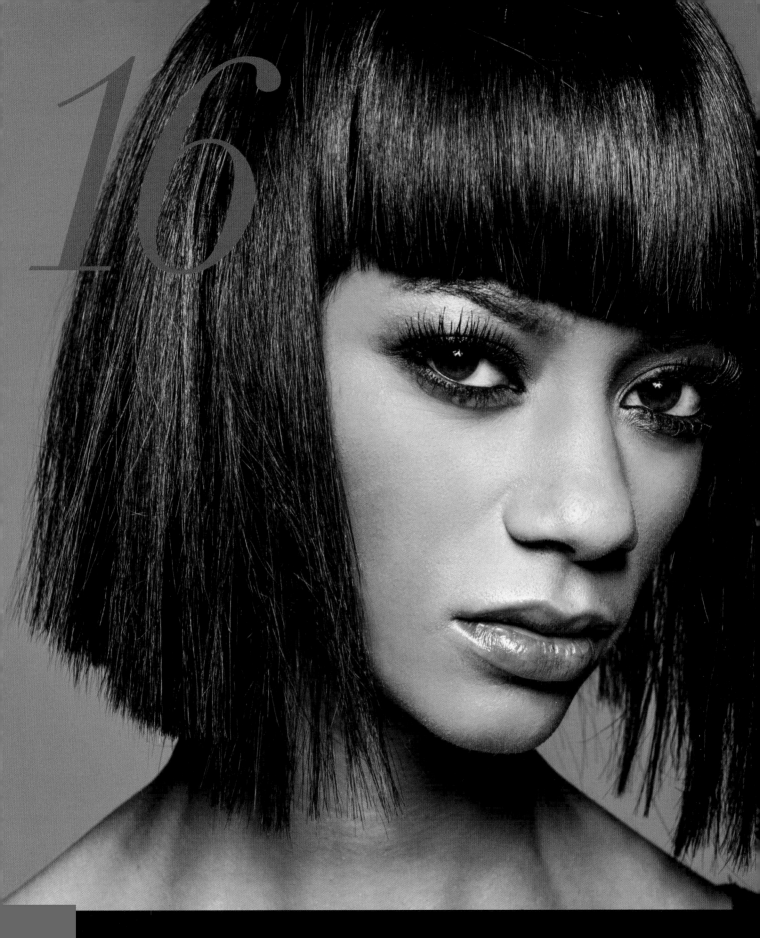

16

LEARNING OBJECTIVES

After completing this chapter, you will be able to:

LO❶
Identify the reference points on the head and understand their role in haircutting.

LO❷
Define lines, sections, elevations, and guidelines.

LO❸
List the factors involved in a successful client consultation.

LO❹
Explain the uses of the various tools of haircutting.

LO❺
Name three things you can do to ensure good posture and body position while cutting hair.

LO❻
Perform the four basic haircuts.

LO❼
List the multiple ways to section and cut the bang (fringe) area.

LO❽
Discuss and explain three different texturizing techniques performed with shears.

LO❾
Explain a clipper cut.

LO❿
Identify the uses of a trimmer.

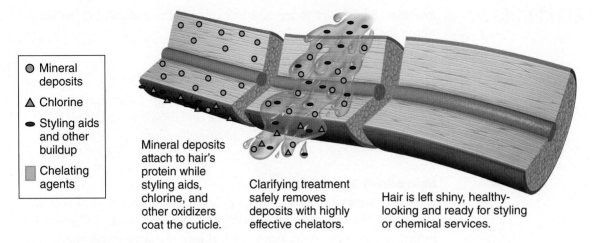

- ○ Mineral deposits
- △ Chlorine
- ● Styling aids and other buildup
- ▧ Chelating agents

Mineral deposits attach to hair's protein while styling aids, chlorine, and other oxidizers coat the cuticle.

Clarifying treatment safely removes deposits with highly effective chelators.

Hair is left shiny, healthy-looking and ready for styling or chemical services.

figure 15-7
Clarifying shampoos should be used when a buildup is evident, after swimming, and prior to all chemical services.

equalizing agent that enriches hair, helps retain moisture, and makes hair more manageable. Clarifying shampoo should be used when a buildup is evident, after swimming, and prior to all chemical services (**figure 15-7**).

Balancing Shampoo

For oily hair and scalp, **balancing shampoo** will wash away excess oiliness, while preventing the hair from drying out.

Strengthening Shampoo

Strengthening shampoo contains a variety of strengthening and nourishing ingredients and is designed to repair damaged and brittle hair.

Dry Shampoo

Sometimes, the state of a client's health makes a wet shampoo uncomfortable or hard to manage. For instance, an elderly client may experience some discomfort at the shampoo bowl due to pressure on the back of the neck. In such a case, it is advisable to use a **dry shampoo**, also known as *powder shampoo*, which cleanses the hair without the use of soap and water. The powder picks up dirt and oils as you brush or comb it through the hair. It also adds volume to the hair. Dry shampoo can also be used between shampoos to rid of excess oils and extend the life of a style. The elimination of oils promotes the luster of the hair and allows volume to return to the hairstyle. Follow the manufacturer's instructions. Never give a dry shampoo before performing a chemical service.

A dry shampoo can be applied at the stylist's station, with the client draped as for a chemical service. Follow the manufacturer's directions, as they will vary. For the most part, you will be applying the powder directly to the hair from scalp to the ends, and then brushing through with a natural-bristle brush to remove oil and dirt (**figure 15-8**).

Sulfate-Free Shampoo

Sulfate-free shampoo, sometimes called soap-free shampoos, are formulated with little to no alkaline soap base. They are manufactured as wetting agents to be compatible with hair and soft water sources and generally are

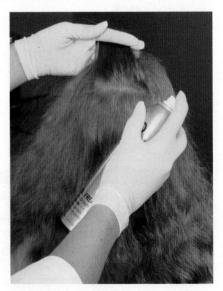

figure 15-8
Apply the dry shampoo directly onto the scalp and out to the hair ends, then brush through with a natural-bristle brush to remove oil and dirt.

known to be sensitive to artificial hair color and to maintaining the natural oils in the hair.

Shampoos for Thinning Hair

Shampoos marketed for thinning hair are usually formulated to be gentler and have a lighter molecular weight that encourages a clean environment for healthy hair growth. These shampoos contain volume-boosting ingredients that give the illusion of additional volume and density to the hair.

Neutralizing Shampoo

A **neutralizing shampoo** is designed to re-balance the pH level of your hair by neutralizing any alkali and unwanted residues in the hair. It works to help return the hair to the average pH of hair after a chemical interaction. A neutralizing or balancing shampoo is most often used as part of the chemical relaxing process.

Color-Enhancing Shampoo

Color-enhancing shampoo is created by combining the surfactant base with basic color pigment. It is similar to a temporary color rinse because it is attracted to porous hair and results in only slight color changes that are removed with plain shampooing. Color-enhancing shampoos are used to brighten, to add a slight hint of color, and to eliminate unwanted color tones, such as gold or brassiness and overly cool strands.

Shampoos with Keratin Protein Added

A shampoo with keratin protein added is designed to help strengthen the hair as it cleanses. It is manufactured with artificial protein molecules added to the shampoo base to cling to the natural protein in the hair.

Shampoo for Hairpieces and Wigs

Prepared wig-cleaning solution is available for these hair enhancements (for more information on wigs and their care, see Chapter 19, Wigs and Hair Additions).

Shampooing Clients with Special Needs

Clients with disabilities or those who are wheelchair bound will usually tell you how they prefer to be shampooed. Some clients in wheelchairs will allow you to shampoo their hair while they remain seated in their

FOCUS ON

Suggest Products to Take Home

You can begin to establish your professional relationship during the shampoo by giving clients information about what you are doing and why. Clients are definitely becoming more product and ingredient savvy with hair care products. They also seek information on the basic details of their services. Let clients know what shampoo and conditioner you are using and why you have selected those products especially for their hair. Mention that these products are available for purchase, and emphasize their

benefits. Making the products available in the salon enables the client the opportunity to purchase products that will enable them to re-create the styling service performed in the salon. They will often make a purchase based on your advice and will thank you for your professional recommendation.

You will often find that the stylist with the highest client retention also has the highest retail/home-care sales in the salon. This stylist has gained the clients' trust and professional respect.

wheelchair, facing the shampoo bowl and bending forward, with a towel to protect their face. If the wheelchair is the correct height in relation to the shampoo bowl, shampoo as normal while the client remains in the wheelchair.

Sometimes a client will arrive in the salon with their hair freshly shampooed from home and other times a dry shampoo is appropriate. The same goes for clients with other special needs. Always ask about their preferences and make their comfort and safety a priority.

After reading the next few sections, you will be able to:

LO**6**   Evaluate the uses and benefits of the various types of conditioner.

Recommend and Use Conditioners

Conditioner is a special chemical agent applied to the hair to deposit protein or moisturizer to help restore the hair's strength, infuse moisture, give hair body, and protect hair against possible breakage. Conditioners are a temporary remedy or cosmetic fix for hair that feels dry or appears damaged. They can only repair hair to a certain extent; conditioners cannot improve the quality of new hair growth.

Conditioning treatments can restore luster, shine, manageability, and strength while the damaged hair grows long enough to be cut off and replaced by new, healthier hair. Because of frequent shampooing, the use of thermal styling tools, and chemical services, conditioning is a must for clients who care about their hair.

Conditioners are available in the following basic types:

- **Cleansing conditioner.** Cleansing conditioners offer gentle cleansing while providing extra nourishment for your hair. They are usually free of harmful detergents and contain less irritating surfactants. This type of cleanser doesn't typically remove all of the natural oils and cleans hair without feeling stripped.

- **Rinse-out conditioner.** Finishing rinses or cream rinses that are rinsed out after they are worked through the hair for detangling.

- **Treatment or repair conditioner.** Deep, penetrating conditioners that restore protein and moisture and sometimes require longer processing time or the application of heat.

- **Leave-in conditioner.** Applied to the hair and not rinsed out.

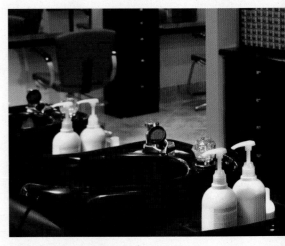

Most conditioners contain silicone along with moisture-binding **humectants** (hew-MECK-tents), substances that absorb moisture or promote the retention of moisture. Silicone reflects light and makes the hair appear shiny. Other ingredients reduce frizz or bulk up the hair. Most treatments and leave-ins contain proteins, which penetrate the cortex and reinforce the hair shaft from within.

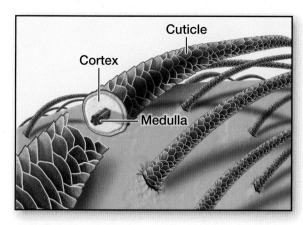

figure 15-9
Moisturizing conditioners contain humectants that attract moisture from the air and are absorbed into the cortex.

Since the hair's cuticle is made up of overlapping scales, a healthy cuticle lies down smoothly and reflects light, giving the appearance of shiny hair. Conditioners, detangling rinses, and cream rinses smooth the cuticle and coat the hair shaft to achieve healthier looking hair.

The cortex makes up 90 percent of the hair strand. The cortex can be penetrated with **protein conditioner**, products designed to penetrate the cortex and reinforce the hair shaft from within to temporarily reconstruct the hair. Moisturizing conditioners also contain humectants that attract moisture from the air and are absorbed into the cortex (**Figure 15-9**).

Other Conditioning Agents

Other conditioning agents that you need to be familiar with include the following:

- **Spray-on thermal protector** is applied to hair prior to any thermal service to protect the hair from the harmful effects of blowdrying, thermal irons, or electric rollers.

- **Scalp conditioner**, usually found in a cream base, is used to soften and improve the health of the scalp. It contains moisturizing and emollient (ee-MAHL-yunt) ingredients.

- **Medicated scalp lotion** is a conditioner that promotes healing of the scalp.

- **Scalp astringent lotion** (SKALP-UH-STRA-in_jent LOW-shun) removes oil accumulation from the scalp and is used after a scalp treatment and before styling.

Table 15-1 lists the types of products suitable for various hair types.

table 15-1

MATCHING PRODUCTS TO HAIR TYPES

Hair type	Fine	Medium	Coarse
Straight	• volumizing shampoo • detangler, if necessary • protein treatments	• pH/acid-balanced shampoo • finishing rinse • protein treatments	• moisturizing shampoo • leave-in conditioner • moisturizing treatments
Wave, curly, extremely curly	• fine hair shampoo • light leave-in conditioner • protein • spray-on thermal protectors treatments	• pH/acid-balanced shampoo • leave-in conditioner • moisturizing treatment	• moisturizing shampoo • leave-in conditioner • protein and moisturizing treatments
Dry and damaged (perms, color, relaxers, blowdrying, sun, hot irons)	• gentle cleansing shampoo or cleansing conditioner • light leave-in conditioner • protein and moisturizing repair treatments • spray-on thermal protection	• shampoo for chemically treated hair • moisturizing conditioner • protein and moisturizing repair treatments	• deep-moisturizing shampoo for damaged hair • leave-in conditioner • deep-conditioning treatments and hair masks

Deep-Conditioning Treatment

Deep-conditioning treatment, also known as *hair mask* or *conditioning pack*, is a chemical mixture of concentrated protein and intensive moisturizer. It penetrates the cuticle layer and is the chosen therapy when a moisturizing and/or protein treatment is desired. These conditioners come in the forms of creams, lotions, and sometimes in a serum form.

After reading the next few sections, you will be able to:

LO Demonstrate appropriate draping for a basic shampooing and conditioning, and draping for a chemical service.

Use Professional Draping

After the client consultation and before any professional cosmetology service can begin, the client must be appropriately draped for the service or services they are to receive. Client draping is an important aspect of every overall service because it contributes to the client's safety and comfort.

Have you ever been in a salon for a haircut and had your clothing get wet during a shampoo because you weren't properly draped? Or worse yet, have you ever had a haircolor service and then, once the service was over, realized that the haircolor was all over the collar of your shirt or somewhere else on your clothing, because the stylist didn't protect your clothing properly? Not only are these incidences annoying to the client, they are completely avoidable when the stylist takes the time to ensure a professional draping. Prior to draping, request that the client remove all jewelry. The client should be responsible for securing all of her personal items. If the salon has a safe locker service, offer that service to the client to secure his or her valuables.

Before the draping service, make sure that proper sanitary practices are used and that each cape has been laundered in a disinfecting solution prior to use. Always use a protective neck strip and/or towel between the neck of the client and the band of the cape to ensure protection for the client.

There are two types of draping that are used in the salon. They are:

1. Shampoo draping

2. Chemical service draping

A shampoo draping, sometimes called a wet draping, is a draping used when a client is in the salon for a shampoo and styling or a shampoo and haircutting service. Turn client's collar inward if applicable. Two terry cloth towels are used to protect the client from getting wet: one under the plastic shampoo cape and one over the cape. When shampooing, make sure to position the cape on the outside of the shampoo chair. Once the shampoo service is completed and before the haircutting or hairstyling service begins, the terry cloth towels are removed and replaced with a paper neck strip, and the plastic cape is replaced with a haircutting or styling cape. The neck strip is less bulky and will allow a natural fall to the

hair for more precision while cutting. The dry haircutting cape is more comfortable for the client and will allow the hair to move more freely.

Ⓟ 15-4 **Draping for a Basic Shampooing and Conditioning** *See page 346*

A chemical draping is used for clients who will have a chemical service or treatment, such as a haircoloring, permanent wave, or chemical hair relaxing.

In a chemical drape, turn client's inward if applicable or offer a smock as not to damage clothing.

The client is draped with two terry towels, one under the cape and one over the cape, the same as you learned for a wet set. The towels and cape however, remain as a part of the drape until the service is completed and are regularly checked for dryness and replaced by the stylist if needed to ensure the comfort of the client.

Ⓟ 15-5 **Draping for a Chemical Service** *See page 347*

Be sure to read and follow the manufacturer's directions regarding whether or not a shampoo is required before using a particular chemical product such as haircolor. If the manufacturer requires that the client be shampooed before the color product is applied, then follow the procedure

---

ACTIVITY

Role playing is a good way to practice recommending retail products to clients. Pair off with a classmate. One student should take the role of the stylist and the other should play a client. Your scene might go like this:

Stylist: Have you encountered any problems with your scalp or hair since your last salon visit, Mrs. Benson?

Mrs. Benson: Actually, I have been noticing some flaking and dryness at the top of my head.

Stylist: I noticed that as well during my hair analysis today. I'm going to use this shampoo for color-treated hair and finish with this moisturizing conditioner. [Show shampoo and conditioner bottles to the client and place them in her hands.] After your hair has gone through a chemical service such as haircoloring, we need to make sure that we are replenishing the hair with the necessary moisture lost during the process. The hair and scalp need a balance of moisture and protein to stay healthy.

Mrs. Benson: That sounds good. But won't the conditioner make my hair feel limp?

Stylist: Not at all, I'll be using a light-weight conditioner. It will infuse moisture where needed and the residue will simply rinse off. It will leave your hair silky and shiny and not weigh it down. If you like it, you can purchase some before you leave. You know, using the right shampoo and conditioner will help keep your hair healthy between visits to the salon.

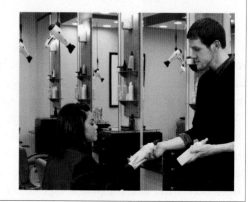

Mrs. Benson: Great! Let's do it!

for shampoo draping, shampoo the client gently, and, before the chemical service is to begin, re-drape the client for a chemical service.

After reading the next few sections, you will be able to:

LO**8** Identify the three-part procedure of a hair care service and explain why it is useful.

Understand the Benefits of the Three-Part Procedure

It is easier to keep track of what you are doing, to remain organized, and to give consistent service if you break your hair-care procedures into three individual parts. The Three-Part Procedure consists of: 1) pre-service, 2) actual service, and 3) post-service.

Part One: Pre-Service Procedure

The pre-service procedure is an organized, step-by-step plan for the cleaning and disinfecting of your tools, implements, and materials; for setting up your station; and for meeting, greeting, and escorting your client to your service area.

ℙ 15-1   **Pre-Service Procedure** *See page 340*

Part Two: Service Procedure

The service procedure is an organized, step-by-step plan for accomplishing the actual service the client has requested such as a shampoo, haircut, haircoloring, or chemical service.

Part Three: Post-Service Procedure

The post-service procedure is an organized, step-by-step plan for caring for your client after the procedure has been completed. It details helping your client through the scheduling and payment process of the salon and provides information for you on how to prepare for the next client.

ℙ 15-2   **Post-Service Procedure** *See page 343*

PRE-SERVICE PROCEDURE

A. CLEANING AND DISINFECTING

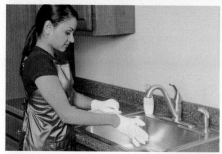

1️⃣ Put on a fresh pair of gloves while performing this pre-service to prevent possible contamination of the implements by your hands and to protect your hands from the powerful chemicals in the disinfectant solution.

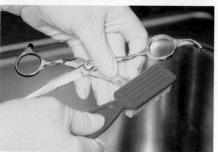

2️⃣ Clean all tools and implements such as combs, brushes, rollers, clips, scissors, and any other reusable, nonelectrical items by first rinsing them in warm running water and then thoroughly washing them with soap, a small nylon brush, and warm water. Brush grooved items, if necessary, and open hinged tools to scrub the revealed area.

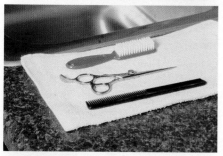

3️⃣ Rinse away all traces of soap with warm running water. The presence of soap in most disinfectants can cause them to become inactive. Dry the items thoroughly with a clean fabric or disposable towel or allow them to air dry on a clean towel. Your implements are now properly cleaned and ready to be disinfected.

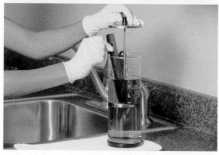

4️⃣ Immerse cleaned implements in an appropriate disinfection container holding an EPA-registered disinfectant for the required time (usually 10 minutes). Remember to open hinged implements before immersing them in disinfectant solution. If the disinfectant solution is visibly dirty, the solution has been contaminated and must be replaced.

5️⃣ Remove implements, avoiding skin contact, and rinse and dry tools thoroughly.

6️⃣ Store disinfected implements in a clean, dry, sterile container until needed.

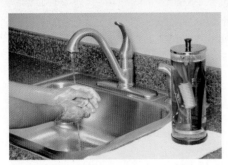

7 Remove gloves and thoroughly wash your hands with liquid soap. Then rinse and dry them with a clean fabric or disposable towel.

B. BASIC STATION SETUP

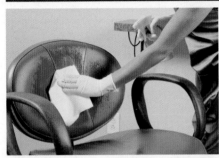

8 Put on a fresh pair of gloves and clean and disinfect your station and client chair with an approved disinfectant cleaner.

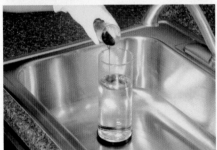

9 Each day, ensure that the disinfection container is filled with clean disinfectant solution at least 20 minutes before your first service. Use a disinfectant approved by your states board regulations, and follow the manufacturer's directions for use. Change the disinfectant every day or when the solution is visibly contaminated with debris.

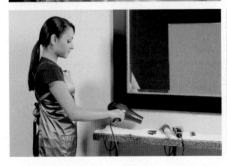
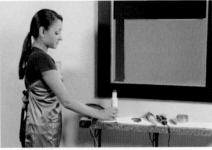

10 Collect all implements and professional products that you will use during the service, along with any electrical equipment such as a blow dryer or clippers, and bring them to your station.

C. STYLIST PREPARATION

11 Review your appointment schedule for the day and resolve any potential time conflicts or challenges you perceive.

12 Retrieve the client's intake form and service record card and review them. If the appointment is for a new client, be sure to either have a blank or digital consultation form at your station or ensure that the receptionist enters intake form information into the system when the client is checked in (so it is available digitally to review).

13 Organize yourself by taking care of your personal needs before the client arrives—use the restroom, get a drink of water, return a personal call—complete whatever you need to so that when your client arrives, your full attention is focused on his or her needs.

14 Turn off your cell phone. Be sure that you eliminate anything that can distract you from your client while they are in the salon.

15 Take a moment to clear your head of all personal concerns and issues. Take a couple of deep breaths and remind yourself that you are committed to providing your client with fantastic service and your full attention.

16 Wash your hands thoroughly before going to greet your client.

D. GREET CLIENT

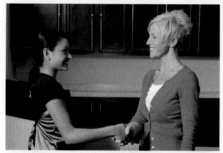

17 Greet the client in the reception area with a warm smile and in a professional manner. Introduce yourself if you have never met and shake hands. If the client is new, ask her for the intake form she filled out in the reception area.

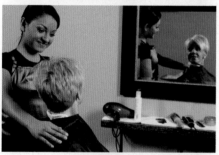

18 Escort the client to your station and invite them to take a seat. Make sure your client is comfortable before beginning the service. Remember, the client is a person with whom you want to build an ongoing relationship. By showing a client respect, you lay the foundation that establishes trust in you as a professional.

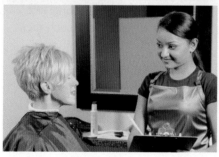

19 Perform a consultation before beginning the service. Discuss the information on the intake form, note any changes on the service record, and determine a course of action for the service.

POST-SERVICE PROCEDURE

A. ADVISE CLIENT AND PROMOTE PRODUCTS

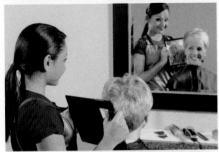

1 Before your client leaves your styling chair, determine if he or she is satisfied. Be receptive and not defensive. Listen to any questions or concerns. If necessary, make any adjustments or give an explanation as to what adjustments are achievable. Determine a plan for future visits.

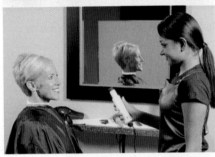

2 Advise the client about proper at-home maintenance and explain the benefits of using professional products at home. This is the time to discuss your retail product recommendations. Explain why the recommended products are important and how to use them.

B. SCHEDULE NEXT APPOINTMENT AND THANK CLIENT

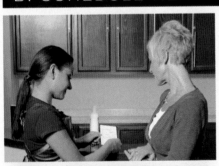

3 Escort the client to the reception desk, write up a service ticket that describes the service provided, and recommended home-care products. Place all the recommended professional retail home-care products on the counter for the client. Review the service ticket and the product recommendations with your client.

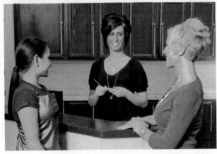

4 After the client has paid for their service and take-home products, ask him or her if you can schedule the next appointment. Set up the date, time, and services for this next appointment. Write the information on your business card and give it to the client.

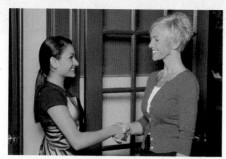

5 Thank the client for the opportunity and invite her or him to return for additional services. Encourage the client to contact you should he or she have any questions or concerns about the service provided. Genuinely wish the client well, shake their hand, and wish him or her a great day.

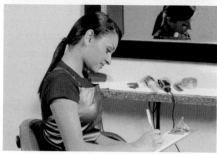

6 Return to your station and record all service information, observations, and product recommendations on the intake form and service record card. Be sure you return the intake form and service record card to the proper place for filing.

C. PREPARE WORK AREA AND IMPLEMENTS FOR NEXT CLIENT

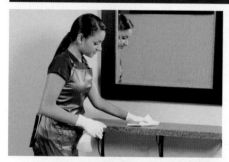

7 Put on a fresh pair of gloves and clean, then disinfect and reorganize your station, sweep and dispose of hair properly in a covered trash receptacle. Place all used towels and capes in the laundry. Close and remove any styling products or aids you used.

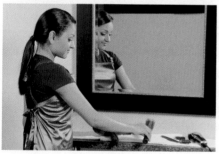

8 Clean and then disinfect all used tools and implements. Follow all steps for disinfecting implements described in the pre-service procedure.

9 Reset your station with disinfected tools and the proper styling products and prepare to greet your next client.

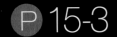

P 15-3

HAIR BRUSHING

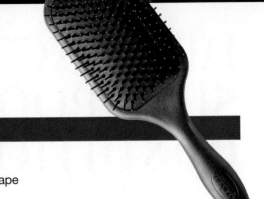

IMPLEMENTS & MATERIALS

You will need all of the following implements, materials, and supplies:

□ Comb   □ Neck strip   □ Shampoo cape
□ Two terry cloth towels □ Hairbrush

PREPARATION

Perform:

P 15-1 **Pre-Service Procedure** *See page 340*

PROCEDURE

1 Show your client to the shampoo chair and assist him or her in becoming comfortable.

2 Drape your client for a shampoo. (**See Procedure 15-4, Draping for a Basic Shampooing and Conditioning.**)

3 Ask the client to remove all hair ornaments, jewelry, and glasses and put them in a secure place.

4 Examine the condition of scalp to be sure there are no abrasions. If the scalp has open abrasions, do not continue with the service. Have client consult a physician.

5 Part the hair using a half-head parting.

6 Further subsection the hair 1 inch (2.5 centimeters) from the front hairline to crown.

7 Hold the hair in your non-dominant hand between thumb and fingers.

8 Lay brush (held in dominant hand) with bristles down on the hair, close to the scalp.

9 Rotate the brush by turning your wrist slightly and sweeping bristles the full length of the hair shaft.

10 Repeat brushing three times on each strand.

11 Continue brushing until the entire head has been brushed.

12 Now move on to the next portion of the service.

POST-SERVICE

Complete:

P 15-2 **Post-Service Procedure** *See page 343*

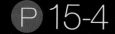 15-4

DRAPING FOR A BASIC SHAMPOOING AND CONDITIONING

IMPLEMENTS & MATERIALS

You will need all of the following implements, materials, and supplies:

☐ Shampoo cape   ☐ Two terry cloth towels   ☐ Neck strip

PROCEDURE

1 Once the client is comfortably seated in the shampoo chair, turn their collar to the inside of their shirt, if needed.

2 Place a terry cloth towel, folded lengthwise and diagonally, across the client's shoulders and cross the ends under the client's chin.

3 Place a shampoo cape over the towel and fasten it in the back securely, making sure it does not touch the client's skin.

4 Place another terry cloth towel over the cape and secure it in the front.

5 Proceed with the shampoo procedure. **(See Procedure 15-6, Basic Shampooing and Conditioning.)**

6 Once the shampoo is completed, escort the client back to your work station.

7 Help the client to get comfortably seated and, using towel two of the original draping, completely towel dry the hair. Once towel dried, pin long hair up and out of the way.

8 Remove the shampoo cape and towel one. Dispose of towels one and two properly.

9 Secure a neck strip around the client's neck. Place and fasten a cutting or styling cape over the neck strip. Fold the neck strip down over the cape so that no part of the cape touches the client's skin.

10 Proceed with the scheduled service.

DRAPING FOR A CHEMICAL SERVICE

IMPLEMENTS & MATERIALS

You will need all of the following implements, materials, and supplies:

☐ Chemical Service cape   ☐ Two terry cloth towels

PROCEDURE

1 Once the client is comfortably seated in the shampoo or styling chair, turn their collar to the inside of their shirt, if needed.

2 Place a terry cloth towel, folded lengthwise and diagonally, across the client's shoulders and cross the ends under the client's chin.

3 Place a chemical service cape over the towel and fasten it in the back securely, making sure it does not touch the client's skin.

4 Place another terry cloth towel over the cape and secure it in the front.

5 Proceed with the chemical service. Be sure to check both towels used in the draping. If either towel becomes wet or soiled with chemicals or other product, replace it promptly.

BASIC SHAMPOOING AND CONDITIONING

IMPLEMENTS & MATERIALS

You will need all of the following implements, materials, and supplies:

- □ Conditioner
- □ Hairbrush
- □ Hooded dryer
- □ Plastic cap
- □ Shampoo
- □ Shampoo cape
- □ Three towels
- □ Wide tooth comb

PREPARATION | PROCEDURE

Perform:

ⓟ 15-1 **Pre-Service Procedure** *See page 340*

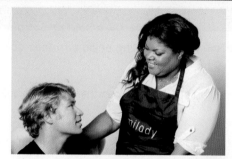

1 Show your client to the shampoo chair and assist him or her in becoming comfortable.

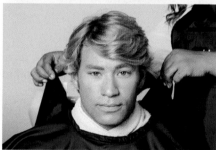

2 Drape your client for a shampoo. (**See Procedure 15-4, Draping for a Basic Shampooing and Conditioning.**)

3 Ask the client to remove all hair ornaments, jewelry, and glasses and put them in a secure place.

4 Examine the condition of the scalp to be sure there are no abrasions. If scalp has open abrasions, do not continue with the service. Have the client consult a physician.

5 Brush hair thoroughly. (**See Procedure 15-3, Hair Brushing.**)

6 Assist the client in leaning back into the shampoo bowl, making sure that his or her neck fits properly into the neck rest.

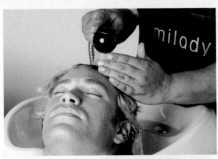

7 Turn on the water and adjust volume and temperature of water spray. Test the water temperature on your inner wrist; monitor by keeping your fingers under spray. Saturate the hair with warm water. Lift the hair and work it with your free hand; protect the client's face, ears, and neck from the spray.

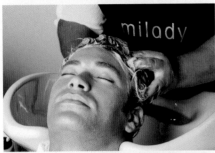

8 Apply a small amount of shampoo. Begin at the hairline and work back and into lather using the cushions (pads) of fingertips.

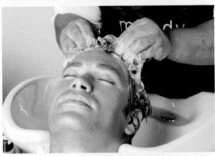

9 Begin at front hairline and work in back and forth movements until the top of the head is reached.

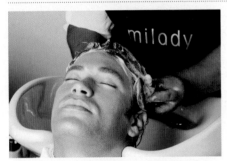

10 Continue to back of head, shifting fingers back about one inch at a time.

11 Lift the head with either hand, depending on whether you are right- or left-handed; with the non-dominant hand, start at the top of the right ear, using back and forth movement, and work to back of the head.

12 Drop your fingers down about one inch and repeat the process until right side of the head has been shampooed.

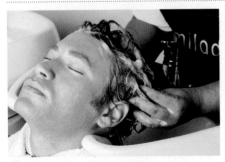

13 Beginning at the left ear, repeat the prior two steps on the left side of the head.

14 Allow the client's head to relax and work around the hairline with your thumbs in a rotary movement.

15 Repeat all steps until the scalp has been thoroughly shampooed. Remove excess lather by squeezing the hair gently.

16 Rinse the hair thoroughly, using a strong spray of water.

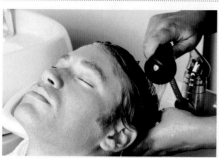 **17** Lift the hair at crown and back to permit the spray to rinse the hair until the water runs clear.

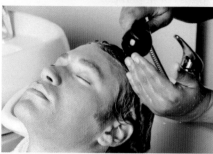 **18** Cup your hand and pat the hair, forcing the spray against the base scalp area.

19 Shampoo and rinse again if needed.

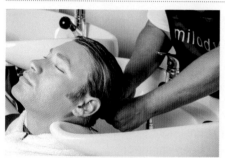 **20** Gently squeeze excess water from the hair.

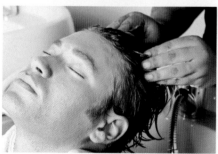 **21** Apply conditioner throughout the hair.

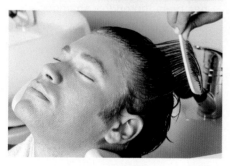 **22** Gently comb conditioner through, distributing it with a wide-tooth comb.

㉓ Massage scalp, if applicable. **(See Procedure 15-7, Scalp Massage.)**

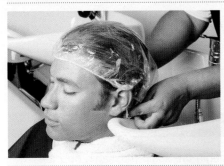

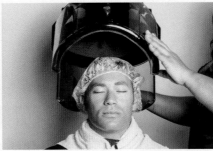

㉔ If conditioner is to remain on the hair more than 1 minute, as in a deep-conditioning treatment, place a plastic cap on the client's head and sit the client upright for the recommended time. If heat is required, follow manufacturer's directions.

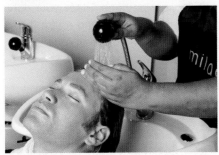

㉖ Remove excess moisture from the hair at the shampoo bowl, before the client sits up, by partially towel drying the hair and wiping excess moisture from around the client's face and ears with the ends of towel.

㉗ Lift the towel and drape it over the client's head by placing your hands on top of the towel and massaging until the hair is partially dry. Ask the client to sit up.

㉕ Rinse the hair thoroughly.

㉘ Clean out the shampoo bowl, removing any loose hair, and wipe out bowl.

㉙ Escort the client back to your work station.

㉚ Once the client is comfortably seated, completely towel dry the hair and, if needed, pin it up and out of the way. Change the drape to keep the client's clothing dry and then comb the client's hair, beginning with the ends at the nape of the neck.

㉛ Now you are ready to proceed with the rest of the service.

POST-SERVICE

Complete:

Ⓟ 15-2 **Post-Service Procedure** See page 343

SCALP MASSAGE

PREPARATION	PROCEDURE

Perform:

P 15-1 **Pre-Service Procedure** *See page 340*

P 15-6 **Basic Shampooing and Conditioning** *See page 348* **Perform through step 23.**

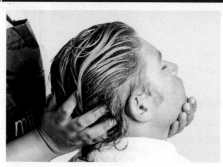

1 To begin the scalp massage, cup the client's chin in your left hand. Place your right hand at the base of the skull and rotate the head gently. Reverse the position of your hands and repeat.

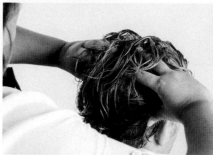

2 Place your fingertips on each side of the client's head; slide your hands firmly upward, spreading the fingertips until they meet at the top of the head. Repeat four times.

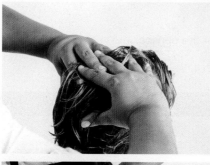

3 Place your fingertips again on each side of the client's head, this time 1 inch (2.5 centimeters) back from where you placed your fingertips in step 2. Slide your hands firmly upward, spreading the fingertips until they meet at the top of the head, rotate and move the client's scalp. Repeat four times.

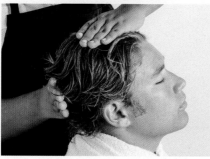

4 Hold the back of the client's head with your left hand. Place your stretched thumb and the fingers of your right hand on the client's forehead. Move your hand slowly and firmly upward to 1 inch (2.5 centimeters) past the hairline. Repeat four times.

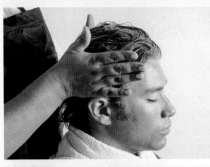

5 Place the palms of your hands firmly against the client's scalp. Lift the scalp in a rotary movement, first with your hands placed above the client's ears and second with your hands placed at the front and back of the client's head.

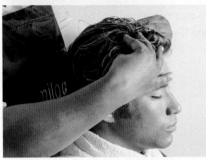

6 Place the fingers of both hands at the client's forehead. Massage around the hairline by lifting and rotating.

7 Repeat the preceding movement over the entire head moving back towards the nape.

8 Resume Basic Shampooing Service with step 24.

POST-SERVICE

Complete:

 15-2 **Post-Service Procedure** *See page 343*

See page 343

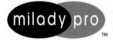 **Check out miladypro.com for additional resources and training to enhance your technical skills.   Keyword:** *FutureCosPro*

REVIEW QUESTIONS

1. What are two important requirements for a healthy scalp?

2. How should scalp and hair that are dry, oily, or have dandruff be treated?

3. What are the benefits of scalp massage?

4. Why is hair brushing important to maintaining a healthy scalp and hair?

5. What shampoo is recommended most to address dandruff? on product buildup? on hair that is damaged?

6. What is the action of conditioner on the hair?

7. List and describe two types of professional draping? At what point in the service do you remove or replace the towels and cape used for each.

8. Describe the benefits of using the Three-Part Procedure and list the parts.

STUDY TOOLS

- **Reinforce what you just learned:** Complete the activities and exercises in your Theory or Practical Workbook, or your Study Guide.

- **Expand your knowledge:** Search for websites about the topics in this chapter and make a list of additional resources.

- **Study and prepare for your quiz:** Take the chapter test in your Exam Review or your Milady U: Online Licensing Prep.

- **Re-Test your knowledge:** Take the Chapter 15 *Quizzes!*

- **Learn even more:** Look up in a dictionary or search the internet for the definitions for any additional terms you want to learn about.

CHAPTER GLOSSARY

balancing shampoo	p. 333	Shampoo designed to wash away excess oiliness while preventing the hair from drying out.
clarifying shampoo	p. 332	Shampoo containing an active chelating agent that binds to metals (such as iron and copper) and removes them from the hair; contains an equalizing agent that enriches hair, helps retain moisture, and makes hair more manageable.
color-enhancing shampoo	p. 334	Shampoo created by combining the surfactant base with basic color pigments that help to extend the vibrancy of the haircolor while adding hydration for hue intensity.
conditioner	p. 335	Special chemical agent applied to the hair to deposit protein or moisturizer to help restore hair strength, infuse moisture, give hair body, or to protect hair against possible breakage.

conditioning shampoo	p. 332	Also known as *moisturizing shampoo*; shampoo designed to make the hair appear smooth and shiny and to improve the manageability of the hair.
deep-conditioning treatment	p. 337	Also known as *hair mask* or *conditioning pack*; chemical mixture of concentrated protein and intensive moisturizer.
deionized water DEE-eye-on-ized WAH-ter	p. 330	Water that has had impurities (such as calcium and magnesium and other metal ions that would make a product unstable) removed.
dry shampoo	p. 333	Also known as *powder shampoo*; shampoo that cleanses the hair without the use of soap and water.
hard water	p. 330	Water that contains minerals that reduce the ability of soap or shampoo to lather.
humectants hew-MECK-tents	p. 335	Substances that absorb moisture or promote the retention of moisture.
medicated scalp lotion	p. 336	Conditioner that promotes healing of the scalp.
medicated shampoo	p. 332	Shampoo containing special chemicals or drugs that are very effective in reducing dandruff or relieving other scalp conditions.
moisturizer	p. 331	Product formulated to add moisture to dry hair or promote the retention of moisture.
neutralizing shampoo	p. 334	Shampoo used for chemically processed or relaxed hair that is designed to re-balance the pH level of the hair by neutralizing any alkali and unwanted residues in the hair; after a chemical interaction, it works to help return the hair to the average pH.
nonstripping	p. 332	Product that does not remove artificial color from the hair.
pH-balanced shampoo	p. 332	Shampoo that is balanced to the pH of skin and hair (4.5 to 5.5).
protein conditioner	p. 336	Product designed to penetrate the cortex and reinforce the hair shaft from within.
scalp astringent lotion SKALP-UH-STRA-in_jent LOW-shun	p. 336	Product used to remove oil accumulation from the scalp; used after a scalp treatment and before styling.
scalp conditioner	p. 336	Product, usually in a cream base, used to soften and improve the health of the scalp.
sulfate-free shampoo	p. 333	Shampoo that does not contain harsh soap detergents. They are formulated with little to no alkaline soap base; manufactured as wetting agents to be compatible with hair and soft water sources, and generally are known to be sensitive to artificial hair color and to maintaining the natural oils in the hair.
soft water	p. 330	Rainwater or chemically softened water that contains only small amounts of minerals and, therefore, allows soap and shampoo to lather freely.
spray-on thermal protector	p. 336	Product applied to hair prior to any thermal service to protect the hair from the harmful effects of blowdrying, thermal irons, or electric rollers.
strengthening shampoo	p. 333	Shampoo that contains a variety of strengthening and nourishing ingredients and is designed to repair damaged and brittle hair.

As you embark on your career, you will find haircutting to be an exciting art form. The stylist is given the opportunity to shape, design, and cut hair into endless designs. Cutting hair with confidence has the potential to bring great success to every stylist. Gaining knowledge through experience with well-developed techniques will solidify your foundation as well as your confidence. The best way to develop the foundational skills needed is being educated in the principles of haircutting and precision haircutting methods. Precision haircutting is not just the art of being precise in your haircut; it is the application of a systematic plan. When combined with the principles of haircutting, you will have a better understanding of how to approach any haircut. However, first you must know the rules before you break them. You will need to have an understanding of the techniques and tools of cutting.

why study
HAIRCUTTING?

Cosmetologists should study and have a thorough understanding of haircutting because:

> Haircutting is the basic foundational skill upon which all other hair design is built.

> Being able to rely on your haircutting skills and techniques when creating a haircut is what will build confidence, trust, and loyalty between a cosmetologist and his or her clients.

> The ability to duplicate an existing haircut or create a new haircut from a photo will build a stronger professional relationship between stylist and client.

> A good haircut that is easy to style and maintain will make clients happy with their experience and will build repeat services.

> Studying the fundamentals will allow you to understand advanced haircutting techniques.

> Specializing in haircutting will increase your career opportunities and profits as a hairstylist.

After reading the next few sections, you will be able to:

 Identify the reference points on the head and understand their role in haircutting.

Understand the Basic Principles of Haircutting

Good haircuts begin with an understanding of the shape of the head, referred to as the **head form**, also known as *head shape*. Hair responds differently on various areas of the head depending on the length and the cutting

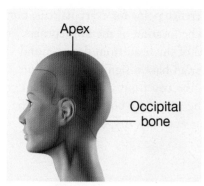

figure 16-1
Reference points

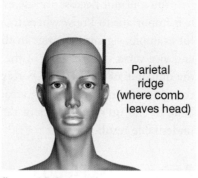

figure 16-2
The parietal ridge

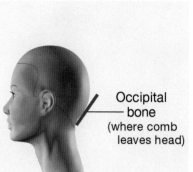

figure 16-3
The occipital bone

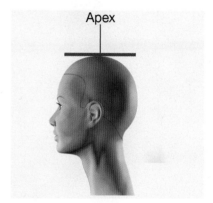

figure 16-4
The apex

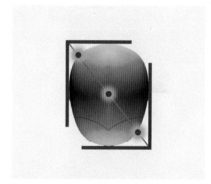

figure 16-5
Locating the four corners

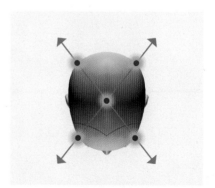

figure 16-6
Another way to locate the four corners

technique used. Being aware of where the head form curves, turns, and changes will help you achieve the look that you and your client are seeking.

Reference Points

Reference points on the head mark where the surface of the head changes, such as the ears, jawline, occipital bone, or apex. These points are used to establish design lines (**figure 16-1**).

An understanding of head shape and reference points will help you in the following ways:

- Finding balance within the design, so that both sides of the haircut turn out the same.

- Developing the ability to create the same haircut consistently.

- Showing where and when it is necessary to change technique to make up for irregularities (such as a flat crown) in the head form.

Standard reference points are defined below:

- **Parietal ridge** (puh-RY-ate-ul RIJ). This is the widest area of the head, starting at the temples and ending at the bottom of the crown. This area is easily found by placing a comb flat on the side of the head: The parietal ridge is found where the head starts to curve away from the comb. The parietal ridge is also referred to as the *crest area* (**figure 16-2**).

- **Occipital bone** (ahk-SIP-ih-tul BOHN). The bone that protrudes at the base of the skull is the occipital bone. To find the occipital bone, simply feel the back of the skull or place a comb flat against the nape and find where the comb leaves the head (**figure 16-3**).

- **Apex** (AY-peks). This is the highest point on the top of the head. This area is easily located by placing a comb flat on the top of the head. The comb will rest on that highest point (**figure 16-4**).

- **Four corners.** These may be located in one of two ways. One is by placing two combs flat against the side and back, and then locating the back corner at the point where the two combs meet (**figure 16-5**). The second is by making two diagonal lines crossing the apex of the head, which then point directly to the front and back corners (**figure 16-6**).

You will not necessarily use every reference point for every haircut, but it is important to know where they are. The location of the four corners, for example, signals a change in the shape of the head from flat to round and vice versa. This change in the surface can have a significant effect on the outcome of the haircut. For example, the two front corners represent the widest points in the bang area. Cutting past these points can cause the bang to end up on the sides of the haircut once it is dry, creating an undesirable result.

Areas of the Head

The areas of the head are described below (figure 16-7):

- **Top.** By locating the parietal ridge, you can find the hair that grows on the top of the head. This hair lies on the head shape. Hair that grows below the parietal ridge, or crest, hangs because of gravity. You can locate the top by parting the hair at the parietal ridge, and continuing all the way around the head.

- **Front.** By making a parting, or drawing a line from the apex to the back of the ear, you can separate the hair that naturally falls in front of the ear from the hair behind the ear. Everything that falls in front of the ear is considered the front.

- **Sides.** The sides are easy to locate. They include all hair from the back of the ear forward, below the parietal ridge.

- **Crown.** The crown is the area between the apex and the back of the parietal ridge. On many people, the crown is flat and is the site of cowlicks or whorls. Because of this, it is extremely important to pay special attention to this area when haircutting.

- **Nape.** The nape is the area at the back part of the neck and consists of the hair below the occipital bone. The nape can be located by taking a horizontal parting, or by making a horizontal line across the back of the head at the occipital bone.

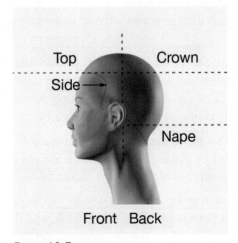

figure 16-7
The areas of the head

- **Back.** By making a parting or drawing a line from the apex to the back of the ear, you can locate the back of the head, which consists of all the hair that falls naturally behind the ear. When you have identified the front, you have also identified the back.

- **Bang area.** also known as *fringe area*. The bang area is a triangular section that begins at the apex and ends at the front corners (**figure 16-8**). This area can be located by placing a comb on top of the head so that the middle of the comb is balanced on the apex. The spot where the comb leaves the head in front of the apex is where the bang area begins. Note that the bang area, when combed into a natural falling position, falls no farther than the outer corners of the eyes.

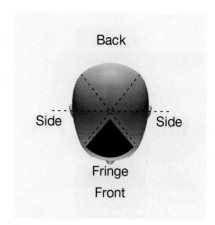

figure 16-8
The bang (fringe) area

After reading the next few sections, you will be able to:

LO❷ Define lines, sections, elevations, and guidelines.

Lines, Sections, and Angles

All haircuts are made up of lines, sections, and angles. A **line** is a thin, continuous mark used as a guide. A **section** is the working area that the hair is separated into prior to cutting. The two basic lines used in haircutting are straight and curved. The head itself is made up of curved and straight lines. When you cut lines in a haircut, the hair will fall into a shape. An **angle** is created when the space between two lines or surfaces intersects at a given point. The angle in which you cut the line is what gives the hair direction and shape. Angles are important elements in creating a strong foundation and consistency in haircutting because this is how shapes are created (**figure 16-9**). There are three types of straight lines in haircutting: horizontal, vertical, and diagonal (**figure 16-10**).

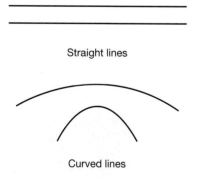

figure 16-9
Types of lines

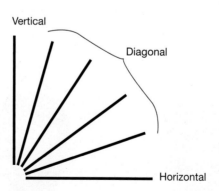

figure 16-10
The types of straight lines in a haircut are horizontal, vertical, and diagonal lines.

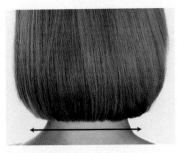

figure 16-11
Horizontal line on a haircut

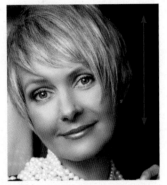

figure 16-12
Vertical lines on a haircut

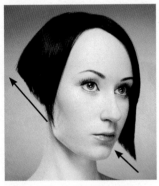

figure 16-13
Diagonal lines on a haircut

- **Horizontal lines.** These are parallel from the floor and relative to the horizon. Horizontal lines direct the eye from one side to the other. Horizontal lines build weight. They are used to create one-length and low-elevation haircuts and to add weight (figure 16-11).

- **Vertical lines.** These are usually described in terms of up and down and are perpendicular to the horizon; they are the opposite of horizontal. Vertical lines remove weight to create graduated or layered haircuts and are used with higher elevations (figure 16-12).

- **Diagonal lines.** These are between horizontal and vertical and they have a slanting or sloping direction (figure 16-13). **Beveling** and *stacking* are techniques using diagonal lines to create angles by cutting the ends of the hair with a slight increase or decrease in length. Beveling also can be accomplished by rolling the hair around the index and middle finger to flip the hair up or under and then cut.

  There are two types of diagonal lines:
  - **Diagonal forward.** Creates movement toward the face.
  - **Diagonal back.** Creates movement away from the face.

For control during haircutting, the hair is parted into working areas called **sections**. Each section may be divided into smaller areas called **subsections**. A **part** or **parting** is the line dividing the hair at the scalp, separating one section of hair from another, creating subsections. Sections are made up of the combination of two basic line types, curved and straight. Sections are used to subdivide sometimes many areas of the head into smaller segments that will be included in the haircut design. There are four types of sections used in haircutting: horseshoe, pivoting, profile, and radial.

- **Horseshoe section.** Taken from recession to recession, separates the head at the parietal ridge to below the crown allowing you to have control when layering or graduating the hair (figures 16-14a through 16-14c).

- **Pivoting section.** Also referred to as *pie shape sections;* rotates from a central point and used in layering and graduation. (figures 16-14d and 16-14e).

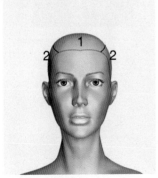

figure 16-14a
Horseshoe section, front of head

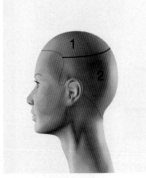

figure 16-14b
Horseshoe section, side of head

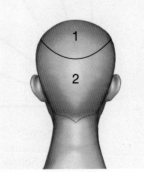

figure 16-14c
Horseshoe section, back of head

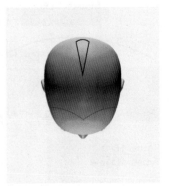

figure 16-14d
Pivoting section, top of head

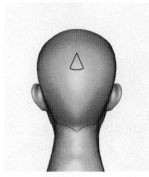

figure 16-14e
Pivoting section, back of head

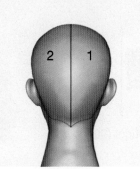

figure 16-14f
Profile section, back of head

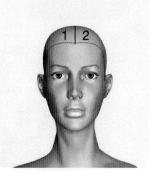

figure 16-14g
Profile section, front of head

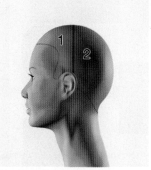

figure 16-14h
Radial section, side of head

- **Profile section.** Center forehead to center nape. Divides the head in two sections (a right and left profile) and allowing subsectioning to take place (**figures 16-14f** and **16-14g**).
- **Radial section.** A section that is taken from ear to ear and divides the head from front to back starting behind the apex in the crown (**figure 16-14h**).

Elevation

Elevation, also known as *projection* or *lifting*, is the degree at which a subsection of hair is held, or elevated, from the head when cutting. Elevation creates **graduation** and layers, and is usually described in degrees (**figure 16-15**). In a blunt or one-length haircut, there is no elevation (0 degrees). Elevation occurs when you lift any section of hair above 0 degrees. If a haircut is not a single length, you can be sure that elevation was used.

When a client brings in a picture of a haircut she would like, you should be able to look at the picture and determine what elevations were used. Once you understand the effects of elevation, you can create any shape you desire. The most commonly used elevations are 45 and 90 degrees. The more you elevate the hair, the more graduation and layering you create. When the hair is elevated below 90 degrees, you are building weight. When you elevate the hair at 90 degrees or higher you are removing weight, or layering the hair. The length of the hair also affects the end result. The weight of longer hair often makes it appear heavier or less layered. You will usually need to use less elevation on curly hair than on straighter textures, or leave the hair a bit longer because of **shrinkage**, which is when hair contracts or lifts through the action of moisture loss/drying.

Cutting Line or Finger Angle

The **cutting line** is the angle at which the fingers are held when cutting the line that creates the end shape. It is also known as *cutting position, cutting angle* (using degrees), *finger angle,* and *finger position.* The cutting line can

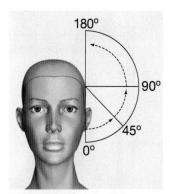

figure 16-15
Hair that falls at 0 degrees in natural fall elevated up to 180 degrees relative to head form.

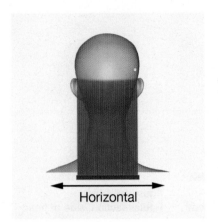

figure 16-16
Horizontal cutting line

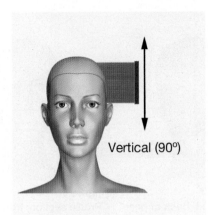

figure 16-17
Vertical cutting line

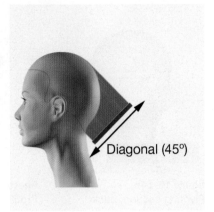

figure 16-18
Diagonal cutting line

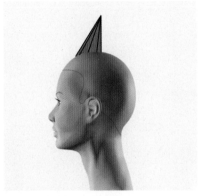

figure 16-19
Stationary guideline

be described as horizontal, vertical, diagonal, or by using degrees in relation to the angle to the head (**figures 16-16** through **16-18**).

Guidelines

A **guideline**, also known as *guide*, is a subsection of hair that determines the length the hair will be cut. Guidelines are located either at the **perimeter**, the outer line, or the **interior** inner or internal line, of the cut. The guideline is usually the first section cut when creating a shape. The two types of guidelines in haircutting are stationary and traveling.

A **stationary guideline** does not move (**figure 16-19**). All other sections are combed to the stationary guideline and cut at the same angle and length. Stationary guidelines are used in blunt (one-length) haircuts (**figure 16-20**) or in haircuts that use overdirection to create a length or weight increase (**figure 16-21**).

A **traveling guideline**, also known as *movable guideline*, moves as the haircut progresses (**figure 16-22**). Traveling guidelines are used when

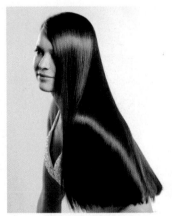

figure 16-20
Blunt (one-length) haircut

© Bairachnyi Dmitry/Shutterstock.com

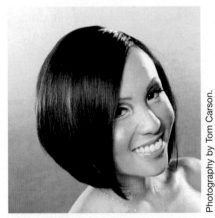

figure 16-21
Graduated haircut, that uses overdirection to create a length increase

Photography by Tom Carson.

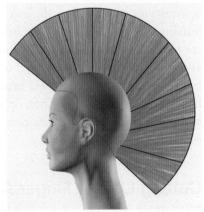

figure 16-22
Traveling guidelines

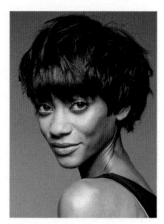

figure 16-23
Uniform-layered haircut

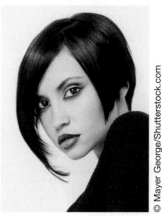

figure 16-24
Graduated haircut

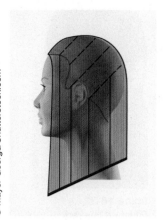

figure 16-25
Blunt haircut variation:
diagonal cutting line

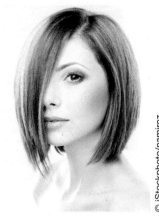

figure 16-26
Finished blunt haircut
variation

creating layered or graduated haircuts (**figure 16-23** and **figure 16-24**). The guideline travels with you as you work through the haircut. When you use a traveling guide, you take a small slice of the previous subsection and move it to the next position, or subsection, where it becomes your new guideline.

The following are just a few of the shapes that can be created by using different elevations, cutting lines, and either stationary or traveling guidelines. Keep in mind the varying amounts of weight that result from these combinations.

Figures 16-25 and **16-26** show a blunt (one-length) haircut with no elevation, a diagonal cutting line, and a stationary guideline. To achieve the layered shape in **figures 16-27** and **16-28**, a 90-degree elevation was used with a vertical cutting line and a traveling guideline. The shape shown in **figures 16-29** and **16-30** was cut using a 45-degree elevation throughout the sides and back, creating a stacked effect with a diagonal (45-degree) cutting line. The top was cut using a 90-degree elevation (layered), and the entire shape was created using a traveling guideline.

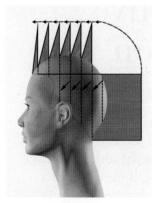

figure 16-27
Layered haircut variation:
vertical cutting line

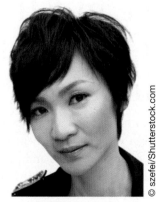

figure 16-28
Finished layered haircut
variation

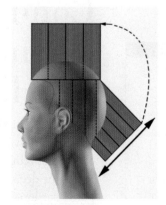

figure 16-29
Graduated haircut variation:
stacked effect

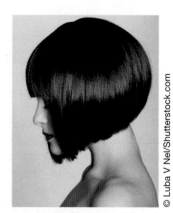

figure 16-30
Finished graduated haircut
variation

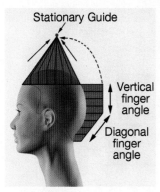

figure 16-31
Overdirection in layered
haircut

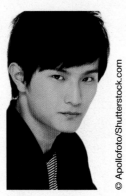

figure 16-32
Finished layered
haircut

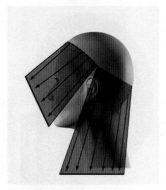

figure 16-33
Overdirection in long-
layered haircut

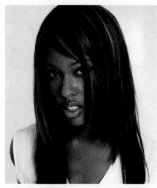

figure 16-34
Finished long-layered haircut

Overdirection

Overdirection is best understood by comparing it to elevation. Whereas elevation is simply the degree to which you lift a section away from the head, overdirection occurs when you comb the hair away from its natural falling position, rather than straight out from the head. Overdirection is used mostly in graduated and layered haircuts and where you want to create a length increase in the design.

For example, you are working on a layered haircut and want the hair to be longer toward the front. You can overdirect the sections to a stationary guideline at the back of the ear (**figures 16-31** and **16-32**). Or, if you are creating a haircut with shorter layers around the face and longer layers in the back, you can overdirect sections to a stationary guideline at the front (**figures 16-33** and **16-34**).

After reading the next few sections, you will be able to:

LO❸   **List the factors involved in a successful client consultation.**

Conduct an Effective Client Consultation for Haircutting

A great haircut always begins with a great consultation. A consultation is a conversation between you and your client when you find out what the client is looking for, offer suggestions and professional advice, and come to a joint decision about the most suitable haircut. If the client has a particular look in mind, you can discuss whether that look is a good choice for the client.

It can be difficult when a client asks for something that you know will not be the best look for him or her. This is when you will want to use gentle persuasion and positive reinforcement to offer alternative suggestions that will work with the client's hair texture, face shape, and lifestyle.

A great place to begin the consultation is to analyze the client's freshly cleansed and unstyled hair for its natural behavior. Ask the client if there is anything he or she would like to discuss with you about their hair. Sometimes the client may ask you for your suggestions. Before recommending anything, you should consider the client's lifestyle and hair type. What is his or her lifestyle? How much time is he or she willing to spend on his or her hair every day? Does the client want something that is classic or trendy? Problems may arise, for example, when a client with naturally curly hair is asking for a haircut that is really designed for straight hair. Will the client be willing to take the time to blowdry it straight every day? You will need to analyze hair density and texture, growth patterns, and hairline. If the client has hair that grows straight up at the nape and is requesting a short haircut that is soft and wispy at the nape, you should suggest other haircuts that will work with their hairline.

Face Shape

Another part of the consultation is analyzing the face shape. To analyze the shape of a client's face, pull all the hair away with a clip or wrap the hair in a towel. Look for the widest areas, the narrowest areas, and the balance of the features. A quick way to analyze a face shape is to determine if it is wide or long. Look for the features that you want to bring out and those you want to de-emphasize. See Chapter 14, Principles of Hair Design, for examples of face shapes.

By analyzing the face shape, you can begin to make decisions about the best haircut for the client. An important thing to remember is that weight and volume draw attention to a specific area. For example, if a client has a wide face, a hairstyle with fuller sides makes the face appear wider, whereas a narrower style will give length to the face. If the client has a long face, a hairstyle with fullness on the sides will add width. If a client has a narrow forehead, on the other hand, you can add visual width by increasing volume or weight in that area. In order to balance out face shapes or draw the eye away from certain features, you need to add or remove weight or volume in other areas. **Figures 16-35** and **16-36** illustrate two face shapes and haircuts that help create balance.

Another important point to consider is the client's profile, or how she or he looks from the side. Turn the chair so you can see your client's profile. Pull the hair away from the face and up and away from the neck. What do you see? Look for features to emphasize, such as a nice jawline or lovely neck. Look also for features to de-emphasize, such as a prominent or receding chin, a double chin, or an overly large nose. The haircut you choose should flatter the client by emphasizing good features and taking attention away from features that are not as flattering. For example, if a client has a prominent chin, you will want to balance the shape by adding volume or weight above or below the chin line (**figure 16-37**). If the client has a prominent nose, you can balance the shape of the profile by adding weight and fullness to the back of the head and bang area (**figure 16-38**).

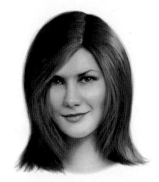
figure 16-35
Wide face with suitable hairstyle

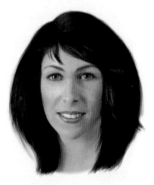
figure 16-36
Narrow face with suitable hairstyle

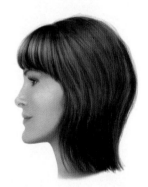
figure 16-37
Flattering style for client with prominent chin

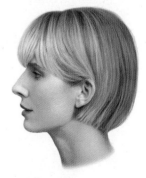
figure 16-38
Flattering style for client with prominent nose

The consultation is also the time to decide on the type of part the client will wear. Will you be working with a natural parting, a center parting, or a side parting?

During the consultation, it is helpful to use parts of the face and body as points of reference when describing the length of the haircut. For example, you could ask, "Would you like your hair to fall chin length or shoulder length?"

Hair shrinks when it dries. Once you and the client have decided on the length, keep in mind that the hair will shrink ¼ inch (0.6 centimeters) to ½ inch (1.25 centimeters) as it dries. In other words, you need to cut wet hair ¼ to ½ inch longer than the desired length. If the hair is curly, it will shrink ½ to 2 inches (1.25-5 centimeters) or more. Be sure to check with your instructor when deciding on cutting length for curly-haired clients.

Hair Analysis

As discussed in more detail in Chapter 11, Properties of the Hair and Scalp, there are four characteristics that determine the behavior of the hair:

- Growth patterns
- Texture
- Density
- Elasticity

Hairlines and Growth Patterns

Both the hairline and growth patterns are important to examine. The **hairline** is the hair that grows at the outermost perimeter along the face, around the ears, and on the neck. The **growth pattern** is the direction in which the hair grows from the scalp, also referred to as *natural fall* or *natural falling position*. Cowlicks, whorls, and other growth patterns affect where the hair ends up once it is dry. You may need to use less tension when cutting these areas to compensate for hair being pushed up when it dries, especially in the nape, or to avoid getting a *hole* around the ear in a one-length haircut. Another crucial area is the crown.

Hair Density

Hair density is the number of individual hair strands on 1 square inch (2.5 cm²) of scalp. It is usually described as thin, medium, or thick.

The density of the hair will determine the size and number of the subsections needed to complete a cut. If there is too much hair in one subsection, it becomes difficult to see your guideline and to control the hair, because the hair is pushed away as you close the shears, producing an uneven line.

Hair Texture

Hair texture is based on the thickness or diameter of each hair strand, usually classified as coarse, medium, and fine.

Density and texture are important because the different hair textures respond differently to the same type of cutting. Some hair textures need more layers, and some need more weight. For example, coarse hair tends to stick out more, especially if it is cut too short; fine hair, though, can be

table 16-1

DENSITY AND TEXTURE

Texture	Density		
	Thin	Medium	Thick
Fine	Limp, needs weight.	Great for many cuts, especially blunt and low elevation. Razor cuts are good.	Usually needs more texturizing. Suitable for many haircuts.
Medium	Needs weight. Graduated shapes work well.	Great for most cuts. Hair can handle texturizing.	Many shapes are suitable. Texturizing usually necessary.
Coarse	Maintain some weight. Razor cuts not recommended.	Great for many shapes. Razor cuts appropriate if hair is in good condition.	Very short cuts do not work. Razors may frizz and *expand* hair. Maintain some length to weigh hair down.

cut to very short lengths and still lies flat. However, if a client has fine (texture) and thin (density) hair, cutting too short can result in the scalp showing through (**table 16-1**).

Wave Pattern

The wave pattern, or the amount of movement in the hair strand, varies from client to client, as well as within the same head of hair. A client may have completely straight hair (no wave), wavy hair, curly hair, extremely curly hair, or anything in between.

Imagine the same haircut cut at the same length on different types of hair: fine, thin hair (**figure 16-39**); thick, coarse hair (**figure 16-40**); and medium, curly hair (**figure 16-41**).

After reading the next few sections, you will be able to:

LO❹ **Explain the uses of the various tools of haircutting.**

Show Proper Use of Haircutting Tools

How do you choose and use the right tools for the job? To find the answer, you will need to understand the function and characteristics of your tools, how to use them in a way that is safe for both you and your client, and how to position your body so that your energy and effectiveness are maximized and protected.

There are several tools that you will need for haircutting. Understanding these implements and the results you can achieve with them is necessary for creating a great haircut. To do your best work, buy and use only high-quality professional implements from a reliable

figure 16-39
Uniform-layered haircut on fine thin hair

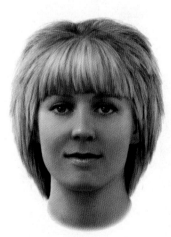

figure 16-40
Uniform-layered haircut on thick, coarse hair

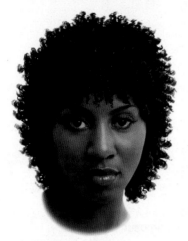

figure 16-41
Uniform-layered haircut on medium, curly hair

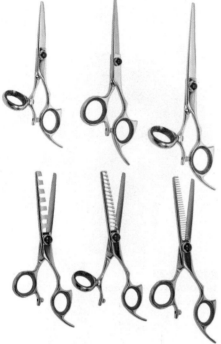

figure 16-42
Haircutting and texturizing shears

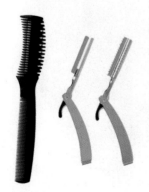

figure 16-43
Razors

manufacturer, use them properly, and take good care of them. Follow these simple suggestions, and your tools can last a lifetime.

- **Haircutting shears.** These shears, also known as *scissors*, are mainly used to cut blunt or straight lines in hair. They may also be used to slide cut, point cut, or to implement other texturizing techniques (discussed later in this chapter).

- **Texturizing shears.** Texturizing shears are mainly used to remove bulk from the hair. They are sometimes referred to as *thinning shears*, *tapering shears*, or *notching shears*. Many types of texturizing shears are used today, with varying amounts of teeth in the blades. A general rule of thumb is that the more teeth in the shear, the less hair is removed per cut. Notching shears are usually designed to remove more hair, with larger teeth set farther apart (**figure 16-42**).

- **Razors.** Straight razors or feather blades are mainly used when a softer effect on the ends of the hair is desired. Razors can be used to create an entire haircut, to thin hair out, or to texturize in certain areas. They come in different shapes and sizes, and with or without guards (**figures 16-43** and **16-44**).

- **Clippers.** These are mainly used when creating short haircuts, short tapers, fades, and flat tops. Clippers may be used without a guard to shave hair right to the scalp, with cutting guards of various lengths, and for the clipper-over-comb technique (**figure 16-45**).

- **Trimmers.** These are a smaller version of clippers and are also known as *edgers*. They are mainly used to remove excess or unwanted hair at the neckline and around the ears and to create crisp outlines. Trimmers are generally used on men's haircuts and very short haircuts for women.

- **Sectioning clips.** These come in a variety of shapes, styles, and sizes and can be made of plastic or metal. In general, two types are used: jaw or butterfly clips and duckbill clips. Both come in large and small sizes.

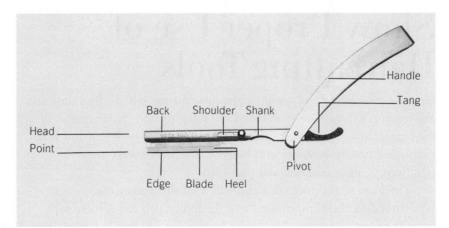

figure 16-44
Parts of a razor

- **Wide-tooth comb.** This comb is mainly used to detangle hair. The wide-tooth comb is rarely used when performing a haircut.
- **Tail comb.** This tool is mainly used to section and subsection the hair.
- **Barber comb.** This comb is mainly used for close tapers on the nape and sides when using the scissor-over-comb technique. The narrow end of the comb allows the shears to get very close to the head.
- **Styling or cutting comb.** Also referred to as an *all-purpose comb*, this tool is used for most haircutting procedures. It can be 6 to 8 inches (15–20cm) long and has fine teeth at one end and wider teeth at the other (figure 16-46).

All About Shears

Your haircutting shears will be one of the most important tools in your career as a professional cosmetologist. Having the right type, size, and make of shear for you—one that fits you well and is comfortable to use—is vital if you are to build a career in the salon.

Steel

All professional haircutting shears are made of steel. Three countries are primarily responsible for manufacturing the steel used to make professional shears: Japan, Germany, and the United States.

It is important for a stylist to know how to gauge the hardness of the metal a shear is made from because this is how you will determine if the shear can hold a sharp edge for an extended period of time. If the metal is too soft, the shear will not hold a sharp edge and will need to be sharpened more often than a shear made with a harder metal. The gauge is called the Rockwell hardness.

Generally, a shear with a Rockwell hardness of at least 56 or 57 is ideal. A shear with a Rockwell hardness that is higher than 63 can make the shear too hard and brittle to work with; the shear could even break if dropped.

There are many different grades of steel available on the market. As the strength or hardness of the steel increases, so does the shear's ability to retain a sharp edge, which means less frequent sharpening and maintenance.

Forged versus Cast Shears

Professional shears are made in one of two ways; they are either cast or forged.

Cast shears are made by a process whereby molten steel is poured into a mold. Once the metal is cooled, it takes on the shape of the mold.

One disadvantage of a cast shear is that sometimes the casting process can create tiny pinhole bubbles that create holes or voids. If a shear with a void is dropped, it could shatter. Also, if a cast shear is bent, it cannot be bent back into shape without the risk of breaking it because cast shears are often brittle.

Cast shears are less expensive to produce than forged shears, and they are usually less expensive to purchase.

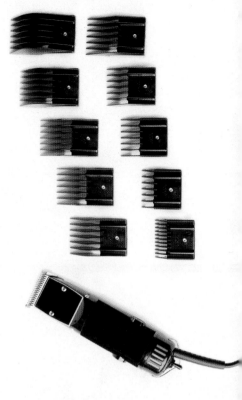

figure 16-45
Clippers and guards

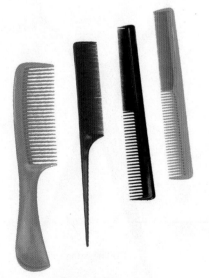

figure 16-46
From left to right: wide-tooth comb, tail comb, barber comb, and styling comb

A **forged** (FORJed) shear is made by a process of working metal to a finished shape by hammering or pressing. The metal is heated to temperatures between 2,100 degrees Fahrenheit and 2,300 degrees Fahrenheit (1,150 and 1,260°C), which expands the molecular structure of the steel so that when it is struck by a heavy object, the molecules move. After the hammering or pressing is completed, the metal is cooled in water, causing the molecules to compress. The process is repeated until the desired structure of the metal is achieved, thus making the metal much denser and harder than metal that goes through the casting process.

The forging process creates a more durable shear than the casting process. Forged shears are easier to repair if dropped or bent. With new technology in the manufacturing process, a forged shear is similar in price to a cast shear but is of much higher quality and durability. Forged shears last significantly longer than cast shears.

Some forged shears have handles that are welded to the blades. These shears undergo the same forging process, but usually the blades are made with a harder metal than the handles. The benefit of this construction is that the shears can be repaired and adjusted easily by a certified technician if they are dropped or become dull.

Parts of a Shear

You are going to be working with a pair or pairs of haircutting shears every day and will rely on them to enable you to create great haircuts that satisfy your clients and keep them coming into the salon for your services. Therefore, you should know and understand all of the parts of a typical haircutting shear (**figure 16-47**).

The cutting edge is the part of the blade that actually does the cutting. The pivot and the adjustment area are the parts that make your shears cut. (Your hand only directs where the shear travels.) The adjustment knob, when tightened, pulls the blades together at just the correct tension so that the hair does not fall or slide between the blades and it also allows the hair to rest on top of the blades so that when they are closed the hair is cut on the desired line.

The finger tang gives your pinky an additional contact point so the nerves and tendons in the pinky and hand are less stressed and pressure is relieved, allowing you to relax your grip so you can hold the shear more comfortably. The finger tang also allows you to have more control over the shear.

The ring-finger hole is where you place your ring finger. Do not use your middle finger when cutting, only your ring finger should be placed in the ring-finger hole.

The thumb hole is the bottom hole and, when properly fitted, should only go to, or slightly over, the cuticle.

Shear Maintenance

To keep your shears in excellent shape and reliable, given the demanding schedule you will keep, it is important to clean and maintain your shears on a regular basis. Get into the habit of caring for your shears and they will never let you down. You should use the following maintenance schedule, beginning now.

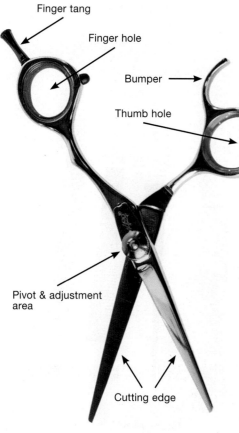

Finger tang

Finger hole

Bumper

Thumb hole

Pivot & adjustment area

Cutting edge

figure 16-47
Parts of a shear

- **Daily cleaning and lubrication.** Use a soft cloth or towel saturated with scissor oil, and thoroughly wipe the inside of the blades of your shear after every client. This will remove your previous client's hair, reduce buildup of chemicals and debris, and keep the blades lubricated to reduce friction caused by metal-to-metal contact. Proper lubrication and blade tension will extend the life of the blades and reduce the frequency with which your shear will need to be sharpened. If you own a swivel shear, lubricate the swivel joint as needed.

- **Daily tension adjustment and balancing.** Adjusting blade tension is an important task to make sure your shears are functioning correctly and to ensure that you get the best results from your shears. If the tension is too loose, it will allow your shears to fold the hair. If it is too tight, it will cause the shears to bind and cause unnecessary wear and user fatigue. To test for tension, hold the shears with the adjustment knob facing you and the thumb handle in your left hand. With the shear perfectly straight (and the blades pointed to the left for a right-handed shear or to the right for a left-handed shear), lift up on the ring finger to open the blades halfway. Then, let the ring-finger handle go. The blades should close ⅔ of the way, or, at the end of the shear, you should have about a 1- to 2-inch (2.5–5 cm) gap at the tips.

  If your shears need to be adjusted, you can tighten the tension by turning the adjustment knob to the right; you can loosen the tension by turning the adjustment knob to the left.

- **Weekly cleaning and lubrication.** Once a week, carefully open shears to a 90-degree angle and loosen the adjustment knob enough so that the blades allow a paper towel to fit between the pivot point, and then push out any hair particles or debris (be careful not to over loosen the adjustment knob or your shears could fall apart). After the area between the blades is cleaned, put one or two drops of top-quality scissor oil into the space between the blades. This removes dirt and debris from between the blades. Be careful not to put scissor oil directly under the adjustment knob because over lubrication may cause loss of blade tension, resulting in folding and bending of the hair when cutting.

- **Disinfecting shears.** You must disinfect your shears after each client by first thoroughly cleaning the shear with soap and water and then completely immersing in an EPA-registered disinfectant for the amount of time indicated on the disinfectant label. Be sure to thoroughly dry the shears; however, it is not recommended that you take the shears apart by loosening the screw to dry the area. You must relubricate your blades after disinfecting them because the oil will be removed from the blades during this process.

- **Sharpening shears.** You should only sharpen your shears as needed. Do not fall into the habit of automatically having them sharpened on a three- to six-month cycle, whenever the sharpening technician comes to the salon.

Remember, the better you care for your shears, the longer the edges will last between sharpening. On average, you should be able to go one year or longer between sharpening if you follow the oiling and adjustment

DID YOU KNOW?

The only difference between a titanium shear and any other shear is its color. Titanium is simply the finish that has been applied to the surface of the steel to change the appearance of the shear. Although claims may be made that titanium makes a shear better, sharper, stronger, or harder, it actually has no bearing or benefit on the shear except to coat it in color (**figure 16-48**).

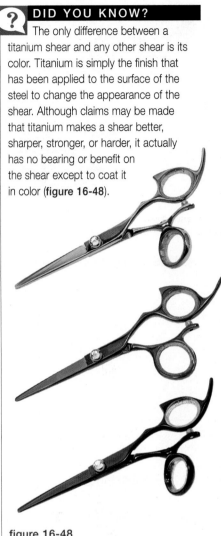

figure 16-48
Titanium shears

DID YOU KNOW?

- Shears with shorter blades are great for point cutting and cutting hair close to the head—like around the ears!
- Shears with longer blades are great for cutting long straight lines into the hair—like for blunt cuts!

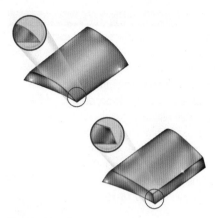

figure 16-49
Convex edge; beveled edge

directions described above. When you do need to have your shears sharpened, it is best to have a factory-certified technician sharpen your shears or to send them to the manufacturer for service.

Left-Handed versus Right-Handed Shears

There is a difference between a right-handed and a left-handed shear. Simply taking a right-handed shear and turning it over does not make it appropriate for a left-handed cutter because the blades of the shear need to be reversed.

It is important that you always use the correct shear for your dominant hand.

Purchasing Shears

You will purchase shears several times throughout your career and the purchase will very likely require a substantial expenditure. Keep in mind that buying a high-quality shear is an investment in your career. Here are some things to look for in a shear you are considering for purchase:

- **Know how the shear was manufactured.** Remember that forged shears are of higher quality than cast shears. Even though forged shears may cost a little more, they are more structurally sound and generally last longer.

- **Ask about the steel quality.** Be sure that you know the quality of the steel that the shear is made from and the Rockwell hardness. You will want at least a *440-A* steel or higher. As you go up the scale from *440-A* to *440-C* the steel gets harder, which means that the edges will last longer.

- **Decide on the right blade edge.** A full convex edge will give you the smoothest cut and is the sharpest edge possible (**figure 16-49**). See **table 16–2** for the differences in blade edges.

- **Decide on the best handle design for you.** Shears will have one of three types of handle grips and you will need to decide which one is best for you (**figure 16-50**). Shears with an *opposing grip* force the

Opposing grip

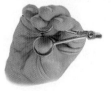

Offest grip

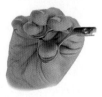

Crane grip

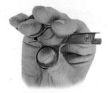

figure 16-50
Opposing grip, offset grip, crane or full offset grip

table 16-2

DIFFERENT BLADE EDGES

Convex Edge	Beveled Edge
Very sharp edge	Dull edge style
Smooth and quiet	Not smooth and can be noisy
Glides through the hair easily	Normally found on lower-quality shears
Best overall edge for the professional stylist	Not recommended for the professional stylist
Great for all kinds of cutting techniques, including slide cutting	Not recommended for professional salon use

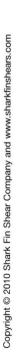

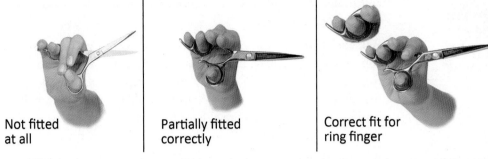

| Not fitted at all | Partially fitted correctly | Correct fit for ring finger |

figure 16-51
Finger-fitting system for the ring finger

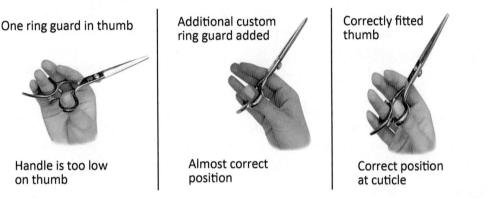

| One ring guard in thumb | Additional custom ring guard added | Correctly fitted thumb |
| Handle is too low on thumb | Almost correct position | Correct position at cuticle |

figure 16-52
Finger-fitting system for the thumb

thumb underneath the ring finger and can create stress and pressure on the nerves and tendons of the hand. An *offset grip* moves the thumb forward, so it is resting below the ring and middle finger. A *full offset* or *crane grip* is the most anatomically correct handle design because it positions the thumb grip under the index finger, which is how your hand is when relaxed. This position releases the pressure and stress put on the nerves and tendons of the hand and thumb.

- **Be sure the shears fit properly.** Since you will be working with your shears almost constantly, consider purchasing a shear that comes with a finger-fitting system so that the shear can be custom fitted to the exact size of your ring finger (figure 16-51) and thumb diameter (figure 16-52). A proper fit will ensure maximum performance, comfort, and control.

- **Hold the shears in your hands.** Since purchasing a shear is a very personal thing, you need to feel shears in your hand before you buy them. When you are ready to purchase your shears, select a vendor that has plenty of shear samples for you to try and a representative who will allow you all the time you need to make the right choice. Make sure the shear manufacturer offers a 30-day trial period, so that if you are not satisfied with the performance of the shears, you can exchange or return them for a full refund.

- **Swivel thumb shears.** Decide if you would like to use a swivel thumb shear. A popular option, the swivel shear provides great comfort and control. The swivel shear allows you to lower your shoulder and elbow

HERE'S A TIP

Ask yourself these simple questions when preparing to purchase a new pair of shears:

- Do these shears fit me correctly, and do they feel comfortable?
- Do these shears feel too loose or too big? Do I feel like I have complete control of these shears?
- Do these shears come with a set of ring guards to custom fit the shear to my exact ring finger and thumb diameter (figure 16-51a)?

Regardless of what anyone else says about their experience with a shear, you need to feel comfortable and satisfied with your purchase. Don't let anyone else's advice sway your choice in a shear.

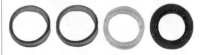

figure 16-51a
Custom finger-fitting system

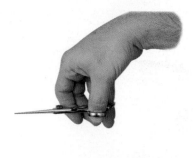

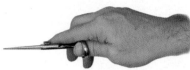

figure 16-53
Non-swivel shear (top).
Swivel shear (bottom).

HERE'S A TIP

Every type of shear has a distinct design and reason for its size, shape, and length (**table 16-3**). For example, when first starting out, you might want to use a 28-tooth thinning shear or 40-tooth blending shear. These are both safe starting shears for a new cutter because they render less dramatic cuts and are appropriate for many types of haircuts.

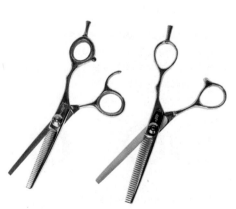

figure 16-54
Types of texture shears

and straighten the wrist while cutting, for a more relaxed working posture (**figure 16-53**).

- **Ask about the service agreement.** Regardless of the type of shears you decide to purchase, be sure that the company you buy your shears from can service them in a timely and convenient manner. Be sure that they have a person who is certified to sharpen their shears in your area. Otherwise, you may have to send your shears away to be sharpened, leaving you without them for a period of time.

- **Ask about the warranty.** Since every company offers a different warranty for their shears, make sure you know what the warranty period is and exactly what the warranty covers before you buy the shears. Should you have an issue with your shears, make sure you are satisfied with that company's warranty policy before you decide to make a purchase.

- **Analyze the cost of the shears.** A pair of shears that is made from high-quality steel, is forged instead of cast, and has the kind of warranty you will need as a new cosmetologist should cost between $250 and $350. If you are buying a cast shear, you should not pay more than $200. If the price of a cast shear is higher than $200, keep looking. Better-quality forged shears are available on the market for only slightly more.

- **Determine how many pairs of shears you need.** A good rule of thumb is to have two cutting shears and one thinning or blending shear available at all times. Your second shear is necessary so if anything happens to your main cutting shear, you can continue to service your clients while the damaged shear is being repaired.

Custom-Fitted Shears

Over the course of your career, you are likely to perform thousands of haircuts! Using shears that are properly fitted to your hand allows the

table 16-3

TYPES OF TEXTURE SHEARS

Types of Texture Shears (figure 16-54)	Uses
Chunking shear (5–9 teeth)	Great for taking out big sections (the wider the space between the blades, the more pronounced the cutting will be)
Texturizing shear (14–19 teeth)	Adds increased blending
Thinning shear (26–30 teeth)	Most universally used; consistent reduction of bulk (the closer together the teeth, the more blended the cut)
Blending shear (38–50 teeth)	Great for scissor-over-comb cutting

muscles and tendons of your hand and wrist to be as relaxed as possible and will help to protect you from long-term repetitive motion injuries such as carpal tunnel syndrome and other musculoskeletal (MUS-kyuh-lo-SKEL-uh-tul) disorders.

Prevention is the key to avoiding these problems, and a keen awareness of good work habits along with the proper tools and equipment will enhance your health and comfort. Remember, your hand's main job is to steer the shear—correct blade tension does the cutting.

Buying and using ergonomically correct and custom-fitted shears can help dramatically by:

- Allowing you to relax your grip, reducing thumb pressure while cutting, so the blades are not being forced together. This will also keep your blades sharper longer.

- Reducing the amount of pressure on the nerves and tendons in your hand. Too much pressure of this type can result in nerve damage; carpal tunnel syndrome; or wrist, shoulder, elbow, neck, and back pain.

- Allowing the shear to do the cutting work when properly adjusted and fitted to your hand.

Fitting the Shear Correctly

Fitting the shear correctly to your hand entails four components:

1. **Fitting the ring finger.** A properly fitted shear has a ring-finger hole that rests between the first and second knuckle—far enough back on the ring finger so that your pinky is resting comfortably on the finger tang. Once you have the shear in that position, there should be only a slight bit of extra space around your finger and the finger hole. A properly fitted ring finger will be centered in the middle of the finger hole.

2. **Fitting the thumb.** When your shear is properly fitted, the thumb hole will rest at or slightly over the cuticle area of your thumb, but not up to or over the knuckle. Once you have the shear at that location on your thumb, there can be a little extra space around your thumb and the thumb hole. A proper fit will have your cuticle centered underneath the center of the thumb ring guard.

3. **Relaxing your grip.** A relaxed grip allows to you to cut without any thumb pressure, so the blades are not being forced together. It reduces the amount of pressure on the nerves and tendons in your hand, which can result in damage, and it allows the shear to do the work of cutting.

4. **Correct finger position and alignment.** Correct nerve and tendon alignment while cutting hair is crucial to having a healthy career as a professional cosmetologist. Correct finger position allows your finger to stay properly aligned, which not only gives you correct nerve and tendon alignment in your hand, but also reduces the likelihood of developing hand health issues caused by improperly fitted shears. Look for a handle design that cradles your middle finger. This guarantees correct finger placement on the shear (**figure 16-56**).

DID YOU KNOW?

The correct way to measure the length of a shear is to start at the tip of the blades and measure to where the finger rest/tang connects to the back of the ring-finger opening. Do not include the length of the tang (**figure 16-55**).

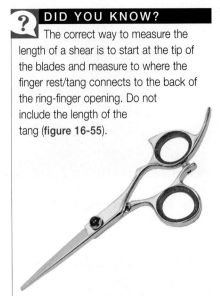

figure 16-55
How to measure shears

DID YOU KNOW?

You should never lend your shears to another stylist. Everyone cuts hair using a certain amount of hand pressure. Allowing someone else—someone who uses a different level of pressure than you use—to borrow your shears can recondition the blades. The result? Your shears may not cut correctly for you.

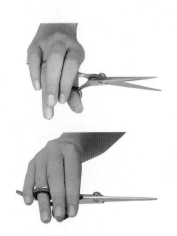

figure 16-56
Correct finger position and alignment

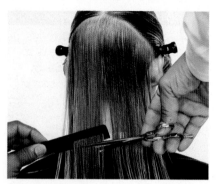
figure 16-57
Proper placement of ring finger
and little finger

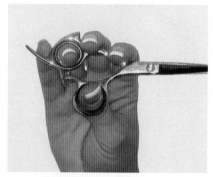
figure 16-58
Proper placement of thumb

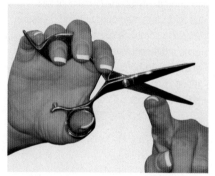
figure 16-59
Still and moving blades

Holding Your Tools

There are two important reasons to hold your tools properly:

- A proper hold gives you the most control and the best results when cutting hair.

- A proper hold helps you avoid muscle strain in your hands, arms, neck, and back.

Holding Your Shears

1. Open your right hand (left hand if you are left-handed), and place the ring finger in the finger grip of the still blade and the little finger on the finger tang (brace) (figure 16-57).

2. Place the thumb in the finger grip (thumb grip) of the moving blade (figure 16-58).

3. Practice opening and closing the shears. Concentrate on moving only your thumb. A great way to get the feel of this movement is to lay the still blade against the palm or forefinger of your other hand to hold it steady, while you move the other blade with your thumb (figure 16-59).

Holding the Shears and Comb

During the haircutting process, you will be holding the comb and shears at the same time. You may be tempted to put the comb down while cutting, but doing so will waste a lot of time. It is best to learn—from the start—to hold both tools during the entire haircut. In general, your cutting hand (dominant hand) does most of the work. It holds the shears, parts the hair, combs the hair, and cuts the hair. Your holding hand does just that: It holds the sections of hair and the comb while cutting. The holding hand helps you maintain control.

- **Palming the shears.** Remove your thumb from the thumb grip, leaving your ring and little fingers in the grip and finger rest. Curl your fingers in to palm the shears, which keeps them closed while you comb or part the hair (figure 16-60). This allows you to hold the comb and the shears at the same time. While palming the shears, hold the comb between thumb, index, and middle fingers (figure 16-61).

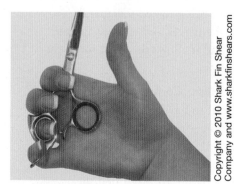
figure 16-60
Palming the shears

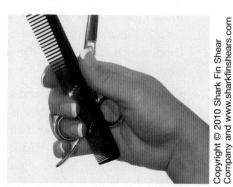
figure 16-61
Holding a comb and shears

- **Transferring the comb.** After you have combed a subsection into position, you will need to free up your cutting hand. Once your fingers are in place at the correct cutting position, transfer the comb by placing it between the thumb and index finger of your holding hand (the hand holding the subsection) (**figure 16-62**). You are now ready to cut the subsection.

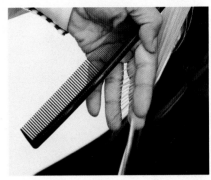

figure 16-62
Transferring the comb

Holding the Razor

The straight razor, or feather blade, is a versatile tool that can be used for an entire haircut or just for detailing and texturizing. Holding and working with a razor feels very different from holding and working with shears. The more you practice holding and palming the razor, the more comfortable you will become with this tool. There are two methods for holding the razor for cutting:

Method A

1. Open the razor so that the handle is higher than the shank. Place the thumb on the thumb grip, and the index, middle, and ring fingers on the shank.

2. Place the little finger in the tang, underneath the handle (**figure 16-63**).

3. When cutting a subsection, position the razor on top of the subsection, the part facing you, for maximum control (**figure 16-64**).

Method B

1. Open the razor until the handle and shank form a straight line.

2. Place the thumb on the grip and wrap the fingers around the handle (**figure 16-65**).

Just as you need to be able to hold the comb and the shears in your cutting hand while working, you also need to palm the razor so that you can comb and section hair during a haircut. Curl your ring finger and little finger to palm the razor. Hold the comb between your thumb and the index and middle fingers (**figure 16-66**). Most accidents with razors happen when combing the hair, not when cutting the hair, because of a

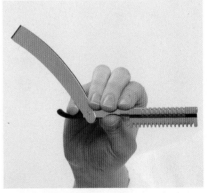

figure 16-63
Holding a razor properly

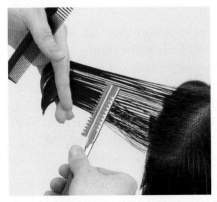

figure 16-64
Holding a razor for cutting

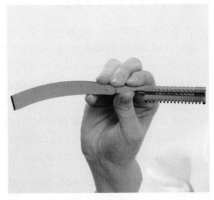

figure 16-65
Alternate method of holding a razor

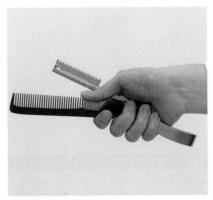

figure 16-66
Palming the razor

loose grip when palming. Be sure to practice keeping a firm grip on the razor with the ring and little fingers, which keeps the open blade from sliding and cutting your hand while you comb the hair.

Handling the Comb

Both the wide and fine teeth of the comb are regularly used when cutting hair. The wide teeth are used for combing and parting hair, while the finer teeth comb the section before cutting. The finer teeth provide more tension and are useful when cutting around the ears, when dealing with difficult hairlines, and when cutting curly hair. You should plan on spending some time practicing how to turn the comb in your hand while palming the shears.

Tension

Tension in haircutting is the amount of pressure applied when combing and holding a subsection. Tension is created by stretching or pulling the subsection.

Tension ranges from minimum to maximum. You control tension with your fingers when you hold the subsection of hair between them. Consistent tension is important for constant, even results in a haircut. Use maximum tension on straight hair when you want precise lines. With curly or wavy hair, less tension is better because a lot of tension will result in the hair shrinking even more than usual as it dries. Minimum or no tension should be used around the ears and on hairlines with strong growth patterns.

After reading the next few sections, you will be able to:

LO**5** Name three things you can do to ensure good posture and body position while cutting hair.

Understand Proper Posture and Body Position

It is important to be aware of your habits of posture (how you stand and sit) and body position (how you hold your body when cutting hair). As a working cosmetologist, you will be spending many hours on your feet and you may want to consider using a cutting stool and wearing proper footwear as preventive measures. Good posture and body position will help you avoid future back problems and ensure better haircutting results. The correct body position will help you move more efficiently during the haircut and help you maintain more control over the process.

- **Position the client.** Not only is your body position important, but so is your client's. Make sure that your client is sitting up straight and that his or her legs are not crossed. Gentle reminders as the haircut

⚠ **CAUTION**
Back and wrist strain may result if correct body posture and hand position are not maintained while cutting.

progresses may be necessary. Remember, you can move the client by turning the chair or raising/lowering the chair—whichever gives you the option of keeping your body in the same place—or by angling the client's chair so you can see what you are doing in the mirror.

- **Center your weight.** When working, keep your body weight centered and firm. When standing, keep your knees slightly bent rather than locked. Instead of bending at the waist, try bending one knee if you need to lean slightly one way or the other. When sitting, keep both feet on the floor.

- **Work in front of your section.** When cutting hair, a general rule of thumb is to stand or sit directly in front of the area you are cutting. By doing this, you keep your body weight centered and you will automatically find yourself moving around the head during a haircut. If you want to sit or stand in the same place, or be able to view what you are doing in the mirror, you need to move the client's chair. As much as possible, keep to the general rule of always standing in front of the area you are working on and positioning your hands according to the cutting line.

Hand Positions for Different Cutting Angles

- **Cutting over your fingers.** There are some situations in which you will be cutting over your fingers or on top of your knuckles. This hand position is used most often when cutting uniform or increasing layers (figure 16–67).

- **Cutting below the fingers.** When cutting a blunt haircut or a heavier graduated haircut, it is customary to use a horizontal cutting line. In this case, you will be cutting below your fingers or on the insides of your knuckles (figure 16-68).

- **Cutting palm-to-palm.** When cutting with a vertical or diagonal cutting line, cutting palm-to-palm is the best way to maintain control of the subsection, especially with regard to elevation and overdirection. Cutting palm-to-palm means that the palms of both hands are facing each other while cutting. This is different from cutting on the tops of your fingers or knuckles. Cutting palm-to-palm also helps to prevent strain on your back as you work (figures 16-69 and 16-70).

Learning how to control your shears is important because many techniques, such as scissor-over-comb and point cutting, are difficult to learn and perform if you hold the shears improperly.

Maintain Safety in Haircutting

It is absolutely essential for you to keep in mind that when you are cutting hair, accidents can happen. You will be handling sharp tools and instruments, and you must always protect yourself and your client by following the proper precautions.

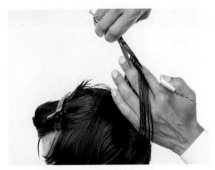
figure 16-67
Cutting over the fingers

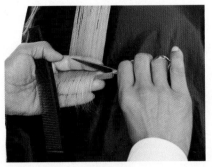
figure 16-68
Cutting below the fingers

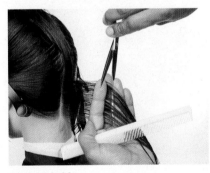
figure 16-69
Cutting palm-to-palm, vertical cutting line

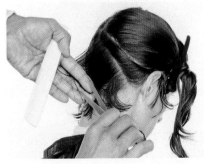
figure 16-70
Cutting palm-to-palm, diagonal cutting line

miladypro LEARN MORE!

Optional info on **Haircutting** topics and tutorials can be found at miladypro.com Keyword: *FutureCosPro*

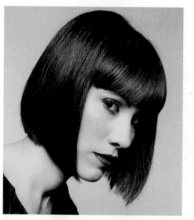

Always palm the shears and the razor when combing or parting the hair. This keeps the points of the shears closed and pointed away from the client while combing and prevents you from cutting yourself or the client. Palming the shears also reduces strain on the index finger and thumb while combing the hair.

Do not cut past the second knuckle when cutting below your fingers, or when cutting palm-to-palm. The skin is soft and fleshy past the second knuckle and is easy to cut.

When cutting around the ears, take extra care not to accidentally cut the ear. Cuts on the ears can produce large amounts of blood!

When working with a razor, learn with a guard. You should never practice holding, palming, or cutting with the razor without a guard unless directed and supervised by your instructor. Take extra care when removing and disposing of the razor blade. Discard used blades in a puncture-proof container.

After reading the next few sections, you will be able to:

LO6 Perform the four basic haircuts.

Cut Hair Using Basic Haircutting Techniques

The art of haircutting is made up of variations on four basic haircuts: blunt, graduated, layered, and long-layered. An understanding of these basic haircuts is essential before you can begin experimenting with other cuts and effects.

In a **blunt haircut**, also known as a *one-length haircut*, all the hair comes to a single hanging level, forming a weight line. The **weight line** is a visual line in the haircut where the ends of the hair hang together. The blunt cut is also referred to as a zero-elevation cut or no-elevation cut because it has no elevation or overdirection. It is cut with a stationary guide. The cutting line can be horizontal, diagonal, or rounded. Blunt haircuts are excellent for finer and thinner hair types because all the hair is cut to one length, therefore making it appear thicker (**figure 16-71**).

figure 16-71
Blunt haircut

Photography by Tom Carson. Hair by Laura Dorelli for Vanis Salon and Day Spa, Scheveville IN. Makeup by Amy Malone and Gretchen Wilson.

A **graduated haircut** is a slow or immediate build up of weight; this is caused by cutting the hair with tension, low to medium elevation, or overdirection. The most common elevation is 45 degrees. In a graduated haircut, there is a visual buildup of weight in a given area. The ends of the hair appear to be stacked. There are many variations and effects you can create with graduation simply by adjusting the degree of elevation, the amount of overdirection, or your cutting line (**figure 16-72**).

figure 16-72
Graduated haircut

Photography by Tom Carson. Hair by Antonio Morosi, hair stylist for Above and Beyond Salon, Vermillion, Ohio. Laura Hall, Color for Above and Beyond Salon,

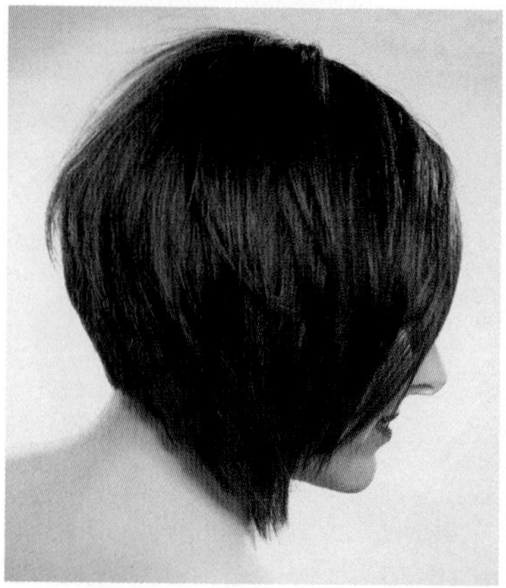

A **layered haircut** is an effect achieved by cutting the hair with elevation or overdirection. The hair is cut at higher elevations, usually 90 degrees. Layered haircuts generally have less weight than graduated haircuts. In a graduated haircut, the ends of the hair appear closer

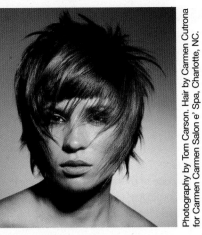

figure 16-73
Layered haircut

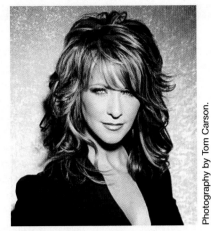

figure 16-74
Long-layered haircut

together. In a layered haircut, the ends appear farther apart. **Layers** create movement and volume in the hair by releasing weight. A layered haircut can be created with a traveling guide, a stationary guide, or both (**figure 16-73**).

Another basic haircut is the **long-layered haircut.** The hair is cut at a 90-degree elevation and then overdirected to maintain length and weight at the perimeter. This results in the length and weight of the hair, being elevated from 0 degrees (in natural fall) to 180 degrees when overdirected. This technique gives more volume to hairstyles and can be combined with other basic haircuts. The resulting shape will have shorter layers at the top and increasingly longer layers toward the perimeter. A long-layered haircut can be modified depending on the texture and density. For example, fine hair requires more weight in the interior. In this case you will use a stationary guide at the center profile and overdirect into the center section with a high elevation and overdirection (as demonstrated in Procedure 16-04 long-layered haircut); on thicker hair you can release more weight by using a traveling guide from your center profile section. (**figure 16-74**)

By using these four basic concepts, you can create any haircut you want. Every haircut is made up of one, two, or three of these basic techniques. Add a little texturizing, slide cutting, or scissor-over-comb, and you have advanced haircutting. Advanced haircutting is simply learning the basics and then applying them in any combination to create unlimited shapes and effects.

The Blunt Haircut

The blunt haircut—also known as a *bob, one-length, one-level,* or *pageboy haircut*—is an all-time classic. Although the line of the cut appears to be simple, the success of the cut relies on precision, which can be anything but simple when working with a variety of hair types, growth patterns, and animated clients.

The client's head should be slightly tilted when cutting the back sections and moved slowly upright and straight forward as you incorporate the sides and complete the remainder of the cut. For a blunt haircut, you

- Always make consistent and clean partings, which will give an even amount of hair to each subsection and produce more precise results.
- Make sure your lines and sections are clean and balanced.
- Take extra care when working in the crown and neckline, which sometimes have very strong growth patterns. These areas are potential danger zones.
- Another danger zone is the hair that grows around the ear or hangs over the ear in a finished haircut. Allow for the protrusion of the ear by either keeping more weight in this area or cutting with minimal tension.
- Always use consistent tension. Tension may range from maximum to minimum. You can maintain light tension by using the wide teeth of the comb and by not pulling the subsection too tightly. Use consistent tension for the entire section of hair.
- Pay attention to head position. If the head is not upright or in the position dictated by the haircut, it may alter the amount of elevation and overdirection.
- Maintain an even amount of moisture in the hair. Dry hair responds to cutting differently than wet hair and may give you uneven results in the finished haircut.
- Always work with your guideline. If you cannot see the guide, subsection before cutting. Using a subsection that is too big can result in a mistake that may be too big to fix. If a mistake is made while using a smaller subsection, the mistake is also smaller and therefore easier to correct.
- Always cross-check the haircut. **Cross-checking** is parting the haircut in the opposite way that you cut it, at the same elevation, to check for precision of line and shape. For example, if you use vertical partings in a haircut, cross-check the lengths with horizontal partings (**figure 16-75**).
- Use the mirror to see your elevation. You can also turn the client sideways so that you can see one side in the mirror while working on the opposite side. This helps create even lines and maintains visual balance while working.
- Check both sides. Always check that both sides are even by standing in front of your client.
- When cutting a stationary guide or overdirecting, stand in front of your section and always overdirect towards your body, your stationary guide, or a predetermined point. This will insure balance and control.
- Cutting curly hair: Remember that curly hair shrinks more than straight hair, anywhere from ½ to 2 inches or more (1.25 to 5 centimeters). Always leave the length longer than the desired end result.

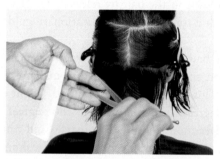

figure 16-75
Cross-checking

want to cut the hair in its natural position. If you cut a blunt haircut with the head forward, you will make two discoveries: (1) The line will not fall as you cut it, and (2) you will have created some graduation where you did not intend to. Blunt haircuts may be performed by either holding the sections between the fingers or using the comb to hold the hair with little or no tension. If the hair length is past the shoulders, sections need to be held between the fingers with minimal tension. For very long hair, it is often useful to have the client stand while you sit on a cutting stool as you work.

When cutting a blunt cut, be aware of the crown area, sometimes called the danger zone, because this is where irregular growth patterns are most often found. The crown can be challenging when you are doing blunt haircuts. Look at the scalp to see the natural growth pattern. You may want to cut this area at the very end of the haircut or cut it slightly longer than the guideline. Once the hair is dry, you can see where it falls and then match the length to the guideline.

Another danger zone is around the ears. Because ears do not lie flat against the head, you need to take special steps to keep an even cutting line. Always work with very little tension or no tension around the ears, unless you are working with shorter layers.

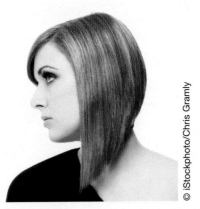

figure 16-76
A-line haircut

© iStockphoto/Chris Gramly

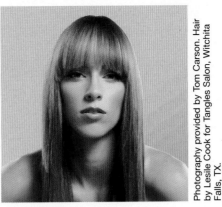

figure 16-77
Longer blunt haircut with
one-length fringe

Photography provided by Tom Carson. Hair by Lesile Cook for Tangles Salon, Witchita Falls, TX.

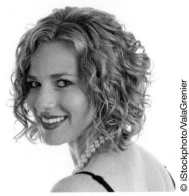

figure 16-78
Blunt haircut on curly hair

© iStockphoto/ValaGrenier

Used with the permission of the authors, Martin Gannon and Richard Thompson, as featured in their book, *Mahogany: Steps to Cutting, Colouring, and Finishing Hair.* © Martin Gannon and Richard Thompson, 1997.

Blunt cuts can be designed with or without bangs (fringe); on straight or curly hair; and with a short, medium, or long length.

 16-1   Blunt Haircut *See page 407*

Other Blunt Haircuts

The blunt haircut is the basis for many other classic cuts.

In a classic A-line bob, a diagonal forward cutting line (finger angle) is used (**figure 16-76**).

In this longer blunt haircut (**figure 16-77**), the bang has been left long and was cut with a horizontal finger angle. When blunt cutting longer hair, hold the hair between the fingers with very little tension.

Figure 16-78 illustrates a blunt haircut on curly hair. Note how the hair naturally graduates itself when it dries.

In a classic pageboy, the perimeter is curved, using a combination of horizontal and curved diagonal back lines (**figure 16-79**).

The Graduated Haircut

In this basic haircut, you will be utilizing vertical, horizontal, and diagonal cutting lines with a 45-degree elevation at the back, one finger's depth on the sides, and 90 degree elevation for the layers. Although you will use a side part, keep in mind that this haircut can also work with a center part or a bang. You will be using a stationary guideline and a traveling guideline.

FOCUS ON

Tips for Blunt Haircuts

- Always cut with minimal or no tension.
- Work with the natural growth patterns of the hair, keeping the client's head upright.
- Always comb the section twice before cutting to ensure that you have combed the hair clean from the parting to the ends. If using the wide teeth of the comb while cutting, always comb the section first with the fine teeth, then turn the comb around and re-comb with the wide teeth.
- Always maintain an even amount of moisture in the hair.
- Pay close attention to growth patterns in the crown and hairline.
- To avoid creating a hole in your line, take precaution to allow for the protrusion of the ears.

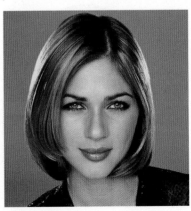

figure 16-79
Classic blunt haircut

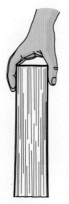

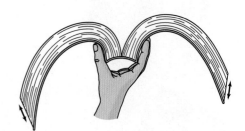

figure 16-80
Straight or blunt hanging line

figure 16-81
Beveled or graduated hanging line

Remember, a stationary guideline is a guideline that does not move. All other sections are combed toward the guideline and are cut to match it. A traveling guideline moves with you as you work through the haircut.

Here's a great way to understand what a graduated haircut looks like: Hold a telephone book by the spine with the pages hanging down. The edges of the pages make a straight line, just like a blunt haircut (**figure 16-80**). Now turn the book the other way, open it in the middle, and let the pages flop down on either side. The edges of the pages make a beveled line, just like a graduated haircut (**figure 16-81**).

Here is another type of graduated haircut, created with different cutting angles. In the classic graduated bob made popular by Vidal Sassoon, diagonal sections and finger angles are used to create a rounded or beveled effect. This haircut begins in the back, using a 45-degree elevation throughout, and gradually incorporates the sides and top (**figures 16-82** and **figure 16-83**).

In the examples in **figures 16-84, 16-85,** and **16-86,** you can see a shorter shape that has rounded weight. This haircut is created using diagonal partings that connect at the back of the ear. In front of the ear,

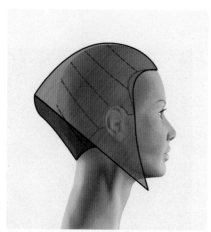

figure 16-82
Graduated design

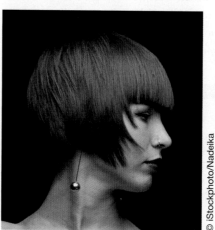

© iStockphoto/Nadeika

figure 16-83
Finished graduated design

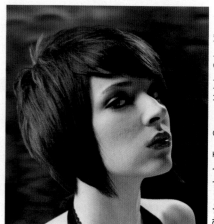

Photography by Tom Carson. Hair by Salon Visage, Knoxville, TN

figure 16-84
Finished graduated haircut: side view

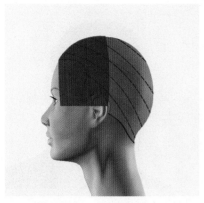

figure 16-85
Classic (round) graduated
haircut: design

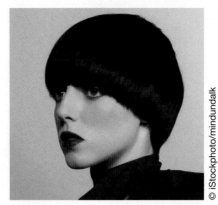

figure 16-86
Finished classic (round)
graduated haircut

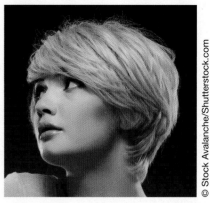

figure 16-87
A uniform-layered haircut

© iStockphoto/mindundalk

© Stock Avalanche/Shutterstock.com

the diagonal forward partings point down toward the face. Behind the ear, the diagonal back partings point down toward the back. The sides are elevated and overdirected to the back of the ear, producing more length toward the face. The back is cut using a traveling guideline, with each section overdirected to the previous section.

 16-2   Graduated Haircut *See page 414*

The Uniform-Layered Haircut

The third basic haircut is the layered haircut created with **uniform layers**. All the hair is elevated to 90 degrees from the scalp and cut at the same length. Your guide for this haircut is an interior traveling guideline. An **interior guideline** is inside the haircut rather than on the perimeter. The resulting shape will appear soft and rounded, with no built-up weight or corners. The perimeter of the hair will fall softly, because the vertical sections in the interior reduce weight (**figure 16-87**). This cut can be established on a variety of lengths and textures.

 16-3   Uniform-Layered Haircut *See page 418*

FOCUS ON

Tips for Graduated Haircuts

- Heavier graduated haircuts (those cut with lower elevations) work well on hair that tends to expand when dry. Coarse textures and curly hair will appear to graduate more than straight hair. Keep your elevation low below 45 degrees when working on these hair types.
- Fine hair is great for graduation. Because graduation builds weight, you can make thin or fine hair appear thicker and fuller. However, if hair is both fine and thin, avoid creating heavy weight lines. Softer graduation, using diagonal partings, will create a softer weight line. If hair has medium density but is fine in texture,

it is safe to elevate more because there is enough density to support it.
- Check the neckline carefully before cutting the nape short. If the hairline grows straight up, you may want to leave the length longer and the graduation lower, so that it falls below the hairline. You can also blend in a tricky hairline by using the scissor-over-comb technique, which is explained later in this chapter.
- Use the fine teeth of the comb and maintain even tension to ensure a precise line.

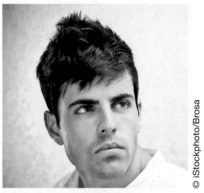

figure 16-88
Short-crop, men's haircut

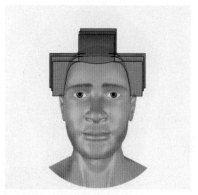

figure 16-89
Basic men's haircut design

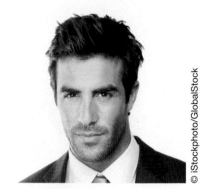

figure 16-90
Basic men's haircut

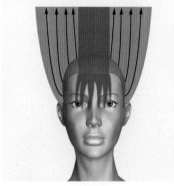

figure 16-91
Long-layered design

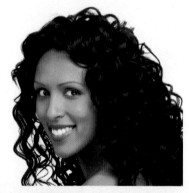

figure 16-92
Long-layered haircut on curly hair

Other Examples of Layered Haircuts

There are many variations on the basic layered haircut.

If you follow the uniform-layering technique but cut the hair much shorter, to 1 inch (2.5 centimeters) or so, you will create a *pixie*, *crop*, or *Caesar* haircut. This hairstyle is flattering on both men and women (figure 16-88).

If you follow the same method but keep the corners by holding your fingers vertically and not following the head form, you can create a square shape, which is common in a man's basic haircut (figures 16–89 and 16–90).

You can create a layered haircut with longer perimeter lengths, otherwise known as a *shag*, by cutting the top area the same as you do for uniform layers and then elevating the side and back sections straight up, overdirecting and blending them into the top length that is cut at 90 degrees (figures 16-91).

In the long-layered haircut, you will begin by cutting your perimeter line. After the perimeter is complete, you will begin creating layers using a 45-degree elevation along the front hairline and sides, in front of the ear. Your guide for the interior layers and top will be a center profile section elevated to 90 degrees extending from the occipital bone to the front hairline. This profile section will serve as your guide for the interior layers, which will be overdirected to match the guide which is cut at 90 degrees (figure 16-92).

Ⓟ 16-4 **Long-Layered Haircut** *See page 430*

Ⓟ 16-4 **Long-Layered Haircut** *See page 430*

FOCUS ON

Tips for Layered Haircuts

- When layering short hair, you will achieve the best results on medium to thicker densities. Cutting thin hair too short can expose the scalp.
- Coarse hair tends to stick out if cut shorter than 3 inches (8 cm). This hair texture needs the extra length to hold it down.
- When working on longer layered shapes in which you want to maintain thickness at the bottom, remember to keep the top

sections longer. Cutting the top layers too short will take too much hair away from the rest of the haircut and may leave you with a collapsed shape that is stringy at the bottom.

- If the client has hair past the shoulder blades, use slide cutting (explained later in this chapter) to connect the top sections to the lengths. This will maintain maximum length and weight at the perimeter of the haircut.

Understand Other Cutting Techniques

To go beyond the basic haircut, there are many techniques you can use to create different effects in hair. You can make wild hairlines calm down. You can make thick hair behave like thinner hair or make fine hair appear to be fuller. You can create more movement and add or reduce volume. You can also compensate for various growth patterns that exist on the same head of hair.

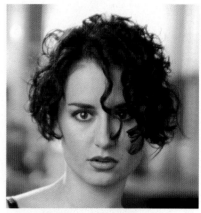

figure 16-93
Blunt haircut on curly hair

Cutting Curly Hair

Curly hair can be a challenge to cut. Once you gain confidence, curly hair can be a lot of fun to style. However, it is important to understand how curly hair behaves after it has been cut and dried. Although you can apply any cutting technique to curly hair, you will get very different results than you get when cutting straight hair. Curl patterns can range from slightly wavy to extremely curly, and curly-haired clients may have fine, medium, or coarse textures with a density ranging from thin to thick.

Examples of Basic Haircuts on Curly Hair

Let us take a look at some basic haircuts and how they work on wavy and curly hair. In figure 16-93, note how the hair appears stacked, even though it was cut with a blunt technique. Although the hair was not elevated, it appears graduated. Note how the volume in the graduated haircut (figure 16-94) is above the ears. The hair shrinks as it dries, resulting in a weight line that has graduated itself even higher. In the next example (figure 16-95), note the round shape. This is a uniform-layered cut on curly hair.

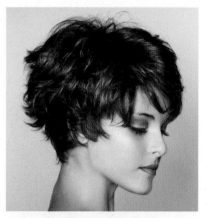

figure 16-94
Graduated haircut on wavy hair

FOCUS ON

Tips for Cutting Curly Hair

- Curly hair can appear shorter after it dries because of a shrinking effect. The curlier the hair, the more it will shrink. For every ¼ inch (0.6 centimeters) you cut when the hair is wet, it will shrink up to 1 inch (2.5 centimeters) when dry. Always keep this in mind when consulting with your client.
- So as not to cut curly hair shorter than desired, use minimal tension and/or the wide teeth of your comb when cutting and be sure not to stretch the hair as you cut it.
- Maintain a consistent dampness of the hair while cutting.
- Curly hair naturally graduates itself. If the shape you want to create has strong angles, you need to elevate less than when working with straight hair.
- Curly hair when dry has more volume than straight hair. This means that you will generally need to leave lengths longer, which ultimately helps weigh the hair down and keeps the shape from ending up too short.
- In general, a razor should not be used on curly hair. Doing so weakens the cuticle and causes the hair to frizz.
- Choose your texturizing techniques carefully. Avoid using the razor and work mostly with point cutting and free-hand notching to remove bulk and weight (these techniques are discussed later in this chapter).

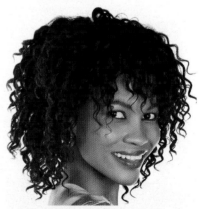

figure 16-95
Uniform-layered haircut on curly hair

After reading the next few sections, you will be able to:

LO **7** List the multiple ways to section and cut the bang (fringe) area.

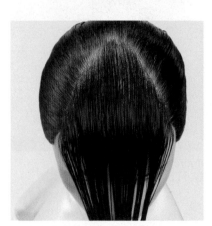

figure 16-96
Bang area

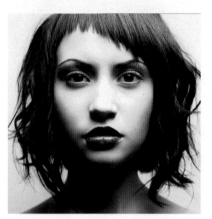

figure 16-97
asymmetric" to match text

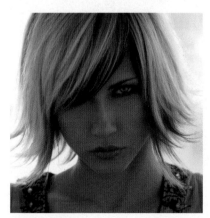

figure 16-98
Side swept bang

Cutting the Bangs (Fringe)

Because much of our haircutting history comes from England, you will sometimes hear the word *fringe* used instead of *bangs*. The two words mean the same thing. The bang or fringe area includes the hair that lies between the two front corners, or approximately between the outer corners of the eyes (figure 16-96). When cutting the bangs or fringe, be sure the hair is either damp or completely dry. Also, when combing and preparing to cut bangs and or fringe do not use tension, allow for the natural lift of the hair.

It is important to work with the natural **distribution**, where and how hair is moved over the head, when locating the bang area. Every head is different and you need to make sure that you cut only the hair that falls in that area. Otherwise, you can end up with short pieces falling where they don't belong, ruining the lines of the haircut. When creating bangs (fringe), you do not always cut all of the hair in this area, but you only cut more if you are blending into the sides or the top. Avoid cutting bangs on clients with strong cowlicks or low facial hairlines. A cowlick, when cut, is prone to stand straight up and not blend. A low facial hairline shortens the length of the forehead. By introducing bangs, the forehead length will shorten further. Always take into consideration suitability, texture, and face shape.

The bang (fringe) area is the focal point of a haircut and can compliment many hairstyles. It's also a perfect choice for the client looking for change without sacrificing length.

Practice cutting these five basic types of bangs (fringes).

Asymmetric Bang (Fringe). Designed for all hair lengths; this bang style makes a statement and can vary from subtle to bold. (figure 16-97). Use shears.

1. Start by placing an offset triangular section of hair at each corner of the eye.

2. Take a ½ inch (1.25 centimeters) subsection at the narrowest part of the offset triangle, elevate at 90 degrees, and cut 2–3 inches (5–7.5 centimeters) (or longer) in length—this will become a stationary guide.

3. Continue taking ½ inch (1.25 centimeters) subsections, elevate to 90 degrees, and overdirect to the stationary guide or, for thick hair, overdirect to the previously cut section.

4. Finish by blowdrying with a flat brush or comb. Using your comb for precision and angle, cut to desired length.

Side Swept Bang (Fringe). Most commonly used on mid-length to long hair, this bang is worn on the side and works great for the client with a natural side part (figure 16-98). Use shears or razor.

1. Find the natural side part and take a subsection from the side part to the opposite corner of the hairline, forming an offset triangle.

2. Starting at the side part (corner of the offset triangle), take a vertical section, elevate at 90 degrees, and blunt or point cut 3–4 inches in length (7.5–10 centimeters)—this will become a stationary guide. (The longer the guide, the longer the bang.)

3. Take a ½-inch (1.25 centimeters) pie-shape subsection and overdirect to the stationary guide. Continue taking ½ inch pie-shape subsections and overdirecting to the stationary guide.

4. Finish by cutting the perimeter at a 45-degree elevation from the face and cut on an angle, combing perpendicular to your section.

5. Blowdry and remove weight by slicing or with texturizing shears. This will encourage the hair to sweep to the side.

Versatile Bang (Fringe). Designed for all hair lengths, this type of bang can be worn on either side (**figure 16-99**). Use shears or razor.

1. Start by taking a (standard bang) triangle section at the top of the head.

2. Take a ½ inch (1.25 centimeters) central vertical section, elevate at 90 degrees, and blunt or point cut 4–5 inches (10–12.5 centimeters) in length—this will become a stationary guide. (The longer the guide, the longer the bang.)

3. Take a ½ inch (1.25 centimeters) subsection, elevate to 90 degrees, and overdirect to the center stationary guide. Continue taking ½ inch subsections and overdirecting to the center guide. Repeat on the opposite side.

4. Finish by cutting the perimeter into a slight "V" shape.

5. Blowdry and remove weight by slicing or with texturizing shears. Move from side to side and look for balance of weight.

Short Textured Bang (Fringe). Most commonly used on short hair. Use shears or razor (**figure 16-100**).

1. Once you've completed your short haircut, start by taking a 1-inch (2.5 centimeters) horizontal section at the front hairline from recession to recession, elevate to 90 degrees, and point cut 2–3 inches (5–7.5 centimeters) in length.

2. Blowdry the hair and detail the bang area visually. Using your cutting comb, elevate the hair and texturize with irregular deep point cutting. You may also use a razor to create a textured feel.

3. Use your mirror and always make sure you achieve balance; the density of the hair will dictate how much texturizing is needed. Use the carving technique for separation and detail.

Square Bang (Fringe). Designed for all hair lengths, this bang can be worn heavy or soft (**figure 16-101**). Use shears.

1. Start by taking a (standard bang) triangle section at the top of the head.

2. Take a ½-inch (1.25 centimeters) subsection in the front hairline, comb to natural fall (with minimal tension), and elevate two-fingers

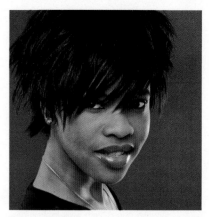
figure 16-99
Versatile bang

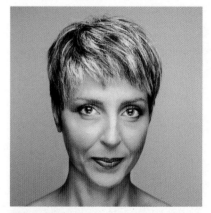
figure 16-100
Short textured bang

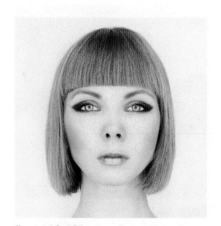
figure 16-101
Square bang

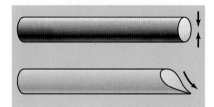

figure 16-102
Shear-cut and razor-cut strands

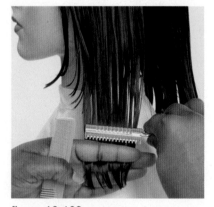

figure 16-103
Razor cutting parallel to subsection

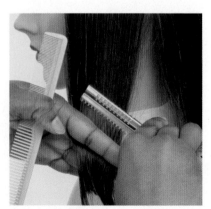

figure 16-104
Razor cutting at 45-degree angle

depth. Starting at the bridge of the nose, cut a square line and continue cutting until the corner of the eye. Repeat on the opposite side.

3. Continue taking ½-inch subsections, elevate to 1-finger depth, and cut square following the guide from the previously cut section.

4. For a heavy fringe, leave one length; for a softer fringe, layer using technique from the Versatile Bang (Fringe) (steps 2 and 3).

5. Finish by blowdrying with a flat brush or comb. For heavy bangs, use your comb (for precision) and detail to desired length. For a softer fringe, remove weight by deep point cutting or with texturizing shears.

Razor Cutting

A razor cut gives a totally different result than other haircutting technique. For instance, a razor cut gives a softer appearance than a shear cut. The razor is a great option when working with medium to fine hair textures. When you work with shears, the ends of the hair are cut blunt. When working with a razor, the ends are cut at an angle and the line is not blunt. This produces softer shapes with more visible separation, or a feathered effect, on the ends. With the razor, there is only one blade cutting the hair and it is a much finer blade than the shears. With shears, there are two blades that close on the hair, creating blunt ends (**figure 16-102**).

Any haircut you can create with shears can also be done with the razor. You can cut horizontal, vertical, and diagonal lines. The main difference is that the guide is above your fingers, whereas with shears the guide is usually below your fingers. Razor cutting is an entirely different technique from cutting with shears. The best way to become comfortable with the razor is to practice. Before cutting with a razor, review how to properly hold the razor in the Haircutting Tools section of this chapter.

There are two commonly used methods for cutting with a razor. In the first method, the razor is kept parallel to the subsection (**figure 16-103**). This technique is used to thin the ends of the hair and the entire length of the blade is used. The other approach is to come into the subsection with the blade at an angle (about 45 degrees). Here, you are using about one-third of the blade to make small strokes as you work through the subsection (**figure 16-104**). If the blade is not entering the hair at an angle

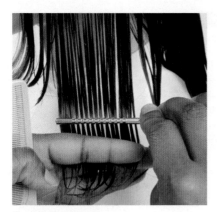

figure 16-105
Incorrect razor angle

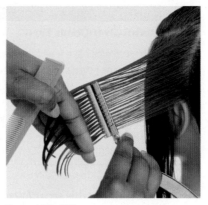

figure 16-106
Hand position in vertical section

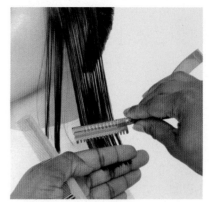

figure 16-107
Hand position on
horizontal section

and you attempt to push the razor through the hair, you place added stress on the hair and risk losing control of the hair (figure 16-105). Always remember that the blade needs to be at an angle when entering the hair.

When cutting a section, you move from top to bottom or side to side, depending on the section and finger angle. Examples of razor techniques and hand positions on a vertical and horizontal subsection, respectively, are found in figures 16-106 and 16-107.

Slide Cutting

Slide cutting is a method of cutting or layering the hair in which the fingers and shears glide along the edge of the hair to remove length. It is useful for removing length, blending shorter lengths to longer lengths, and it's a perfect way to layer very long hair and keep weight at the perimeter. Rather than opening and closing the shears, you keep them partially open as you slide along the edge of the section. This technique should only be performed on wet hair with very sharp shears.

There are two methods of holding the subsection when slide cutting. It is important to visualize the line you wish to cut before you begin (figure 16-108). In one method, you hold the subsection with tension beyond the cutting line (figure 16-109). In the other method, you place your shears on top of your knuckles and then use both hands to move simultaneously out the length to the ends. Practice this technique by cutting the section in front of your fingers. Once you've mastered this technique, and feel like you have control of your shears, you can then use both methods.

Scissor-Over-Comb

Scissor-over-comb, also known as *shear-over-comb*, is a barbering technique that has crossed over into cosmetology. In this technique, you hold the hair in place with the comb while using the tips of the shears to remove length. Scissor-over-comb is used to create very short tapers and allows you to cut from an extremely short length to longer lengths. In most cases, you start at the hairline and work your way up to the longer lengths.

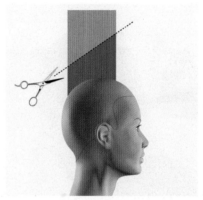

figure 16-108
Visualize your cutting line first.

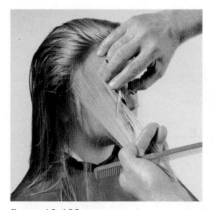

figure 16-109
Slide cutting

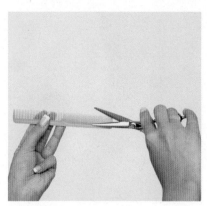

figure 16-110
Scissor-over-comb technique

It is best to use this technique on dry hair because then you can see exactly how much hair you are cutting and that helps you maintain control.

Lift (elevate) the hair away from the head using the comb, and allow the comb to act as your guide. Do not hold the hair between your fingers. Let the shear and comb move simultaneously up the head. It is important that one blade stays still and remains parallel to the spine of the comb as you move the thumb blade to close the shears. Try to cut with an even rhythm. Stopping the motion may cause steps or visible weight lines in the hair. Practice moving the comb and shears simultaneously, keeping the bottom blade still and opening and closing the shears with your thumb (**figure 16-110**).

The basic steps when working with the scissor-over-comb technique are summarized below:

1. Stand or sit directly in front of the section you are working on. The area that you are cutting should be at eye level.

2. Place the comb, teeth first, into the hairline and turn the comb so that the teeth are angled away from the head (**figure 16-111**).

3. With the still blade of the shears parallel to the spine of the comb, begin moving the comb up the head, continually opening and closing the thumb blade smoothly and quickly.

4. Angle the comb farther away from the head as you reach the area you are blending to avoid cutting into the length (weight) (**figure 16-112**).

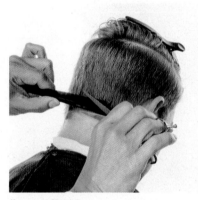

figure 16-111
Comb position

After reading the next few sections, you will be able to:

LO ⑧ Discuss and explain three different texturizing techniques performed with shears.

Texturizing

Texturizing is a technique often used in today's haircuts. **Texturizing** is the process of removing excess bulk without shortening the length. It can also be used to cut for effect within the hair length, causing wispy or spiky results. The term *texturize* should not be confused with *hair texture*, which is the diameter of the hair strand itself.

Texturizing techniques can be used to add or remove volume, to make hair move, and to blend one area into another. They can also be used to compensate for different densities that exist on the same head of hair. Texturizing can be done with cutting shears, thinning shears, or a razor.

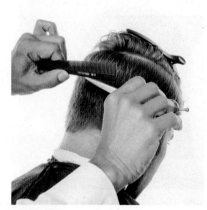

figure 16-112
Reaching the weight line

There are many texturizing techniques and a number of them will be explained in this section. You will need to practice all the techniques so that you can use them to create specific effects as needed.

Texturizing with Shears

- **Point cutting** is a technique performed on the ends of the hair using the tips, or points, of the shears to create a broken edge. This can be done on wet hair to remove length and on dry hair to soften the line, remove weight, and create a seamless effect. It is very easy to do on dry hair because the hair stands up and away from your fingers (figure 16-113). On wet hair (to remove length), hold the hair 1 to 2 inches (2.5 to 5 centimeters) from the ends. Turn your wrist so that the tips of the shears are pointing into the ends of the hair. Open and close the shears by moving your thumb as you work across the section. As you close the shears, move them away from your fingers to avoid cutting yourself. Move them back in toward your fingers as you open them. The more diagonal the angle of the shears, the more hair is taken away and the chunkier the effect (figure 16-114). Basically, you are cutting points in the hair.

  On dry hair, a more vertical (parallel) approach of the shear softens the edge, removes weight, creates a seamless effect, and removes less hair (figure 16-115).

- **Notching** is another version of point cutting. Notching is more aggressive and creates a chunkier effect. Notching is done toward the ends. Hold the section about 3 inches (7.5 centimeters) from the ends. Place the tips of your shears about 2 inches (5 centimeters) from the ends. Close your shears as you quickly move them out toward the ends. If you are working on very thick hair, you can repeat the motion every ⅛ inch (0.3 centimeters). On medium to fine hair, place your notches farther apart. This technique can be done on wet or dry hair (figure 16-116).

- **Free-hand notching** also uses the tips of the shears. Do not slide the shears, but simply snip out pieces of hair at random intervals. This technique is generally used on the interior of the section rather than at the ends. It works well on curly hair, where you do not want to add too many layers but instead want to release the curl and remove some density (figure 16-117).

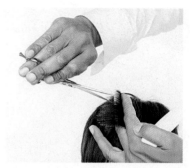
figure 16-113
Point cutting

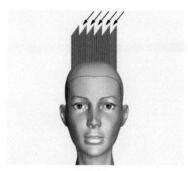
figure 16-114
Point cutting with diagonal angle of shears

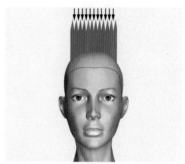
figure 16-115
Point cutting with vertical angle of shears

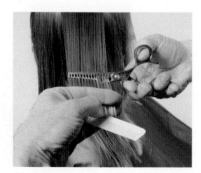
figure 16-116
Notching with notching shears

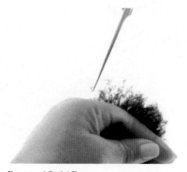
figure 16-117
Free-hand notching with cutting shears

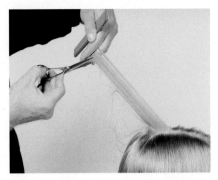
figure 16-118
Effilating

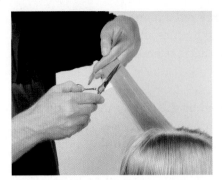
figure 16-119
Ideal open position

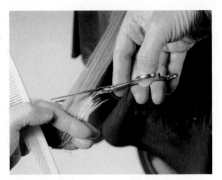
figure 16-120
Slicing with shears

- **Effilating**, also known as *slithering*, is the process of thinning the hair to graduated lengths with shears. In this technique, the hair strand is cut by a sliding movement of the shears with the blades kept partially opened (figure 16-118). Slithering reduces volume and creates movement.

- **Slicing** is a technique that removes weight and adds movement through the lengths of the hair. When slicing, fan out the section of hair to be cut and never completely close the shears. Use only the portion of the blades near the pivot. This prevents removing large pieces of hair (figures 16-119 and 16-120). This technique can be performed within a subsection or on the surface of the hair with haircutting or texturizing shears (figures 16-121 and 16-122). To slice an elevated subsection, work with either wet or dry hair. When slicing to remove weight or on the surface of the haircut, it is best to work on dry hair because you can see exactly how much hair you are taking away.

- **Carving** is a version of slicing that creates a visual separation in the hair. It works best on short hair (1½ to 3 inches or 3.75 to 7.5 centimeters in length). This technique is done by placing the still blade into the hair and resting it on the scalp. Move the shears through the hair, gently opening and partially closing them as you move, thus carving out areas (figure 16-123). The more horizontal your

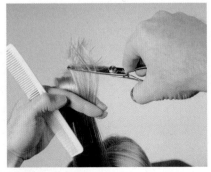
figure 16-121
Slicing through a subsection with texturizing shears

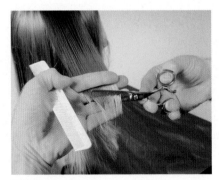
figure 16-122
Slicing through the surface with texturizing shears

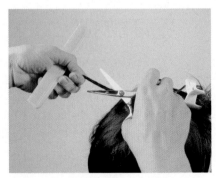
figure 16-123
Carving a twisted section of hair to remove the bulk

shears, the more hair you remove; the more vertical, the less hair you remove.

When carving the ends, you can add texture and separation to the perimeter of a haircut by holding the ends of a small strand of hair between your thumb and index finger and carving on the surface of that strand. Begin carving about 3 (8 cm) inches from the ends toward your fingers.

Texturizing with the Razor

- **Removing weight to taper the ends.** You can use the razor to remove weight to taper the hair. On damp hair, hold the section out from the head with your fingers at the ends. Place the razor flat to the hair, 2 to 3 inches (5 to 7.5 centimeters) away from your fingers. Gently stroke the razor, removing a thin sheet of hair from the area (**figure 16-124**). This tapers the ends of the section. This technique can be used on any area of the haircut where this effect is desired.

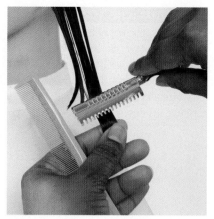
figure 16-124
Tapering the hair with a razor

- **Free-hand slicing at midshaft.** This technique can be used throughout the section or at the ends and should be done on wet hair. When working on the midshaft of the subsection, comb the hair out from the head and hold it with your fingers close to the ends. With the tip of the razor, slice out pieces of hair. The more vertical the movement, the less hair you remove; the more horizontal the movement, the more hair you remove. This technique releases weight from the subsection, allowing it to move more freely (**figure 16-125**).

Texturizing with Thinning Shears and Razor

- **Removing bulk (thinning).** Thinning shears were originally created for the purpose of thinning hair and blending. Many clients are afraid of the word *thinning*. A better choice of words would be *removing bulk* or *removing weight*. When using the thinning shears for this purpose, it is best to follow the same sectioning as used in the haircut. Comb the subsection out from the head and cut it with the thinning shears at least 4 to 5 inches (10 to 12.5 centimeters) from the scalp. On longer lengths, you may need to repeat the process again as you move out toward the ends. On coarse hair textures, stay farther away from the scalp, as sometimes the shorter hairs will poke through the haircut. On blunt haircuts, avoid thinning the top surfaces because you may see lines where the hair is cut with the thinning shears. When working on curly hair, it is best to use the free-hand notching technique rather than thinning shears.

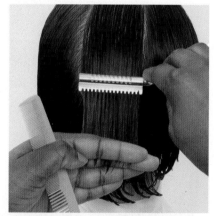
figure 16-125
Free hand-slicing at the midshaft to remove weight.

- **Removing weight from the ends.** You can also use thinning shears to remove bulk from the ends. This process works well on many hair textures. It can be used on both thin and thick hair, and it helps taper the perimeter of both graduated and blunt haircuts. Elevating each subsection out from the head, place the thinning shears into the hair at an angle and close the shears a few times as you work out toward the ends (**figure 16-126**).

- **Scissor-over-comb with thinning shears.** Practice is the best way to master this technique. This technique is useful for blending weight

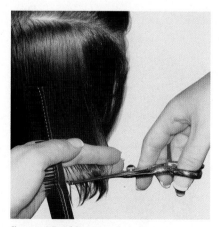
figure 16-126
Thinning out the ends with texturizing shears

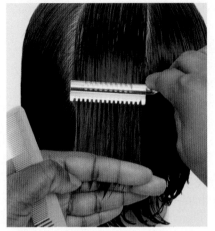

figure 16-127
Free hand-slicing on the ends to create separation throughout shape

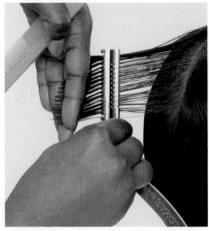

figure 16-128
Free hand-slicing on the ends to create a soft perimeter

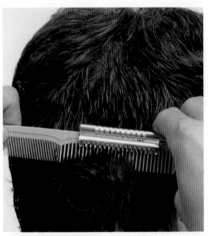

figure 16-129
Razor-over-comb technique

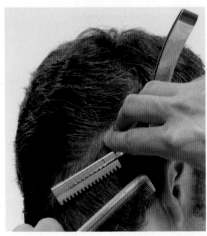

figure 16-130
Razor rotation

lines on fine textured hair and can also be used on thick and coarse textured hair that is cut very short, especially at the sides and the nape. This technique will help the hair lie closer to the head.

- **Other thinning shear techniques.** Any texturizing technique that can be performed with regular haircutting shears may also be performed with the thinning shears. When working on very fine or thin hair, try using the thinning shears for carving, point cutting, and slicing. This will help avoid over texturizing and removing too much weight.

- **Free-hand slicing with razor on the ends.** You can also use free-hand slicing on the ends of the hair to produce a softer perimeter or to create separation throughout the shape (figure 16-127). To create a soft perimeter, hold the ends of a small piece of hair in your fingertips. Beginning about 3 (8 cm) inches from your fingers, slice down one side of the piece toward your fingers (figure 16-128).

- **Razor-over-comb.** In this technique, the comb and the razor are used on the surface of the hair. Using the razor on the surface softens weight lines and causes the hair to lie closer to the head. This technique is used mainly on shorter haircuts. To perform this technique, place the comb into the hair with the teeth pointing down, a few 3 inches (8 cm) above the area on which you will be working. Make small, gentle strokes on the surface of the hair with the razor. Move the comb down as you move the razor down (figure 16-129). This is a great technique for tapering in the nape area or softening weight lines.

- **Razor rotation** is very similar to razor-over-comb. The difference is that with razor rotation you make small circular motions. Begin by combing the hair in the direction you will be moving in. Place the razor on the surface of the hair. Then allow the comb to follow the razor through the area just cut. Then comb back into the section or onto a new section. This helps soften the texture of the area and gives direction to the haircut (figure 16-130).

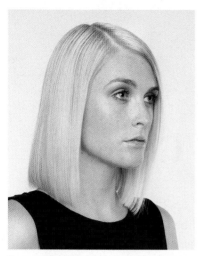

figure 16-131
Blunt haircut before texturizing

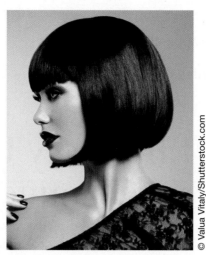

figure 16-132
Texturized blunt haircut

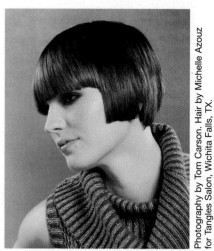

figure 16-133
Graduated haircut before texturizing

Basic Haircuts Enhanced with Texturizing Techniques

Examine these three basic haircuts and see how texturizing techniques have changed the appearance of each haircut.

- Figure 16-131 shows a diagonal forward blunt haircut before free-hand razor slicing, and figure 16-132 shows a different model with the same type of haircut after free-hand razor slicing and the addition of fringe.

- Figure 16-133 shows a graduated haircut before free-hand razor slicing, and figure 16-134 shows the same haircut after free-hand razor slicing.

- Figure 16-135 shows a uniform–layered haircut before texturizing and figure 16-136 shows the same haircut after notching on the ends and free-hand notching on the interior.

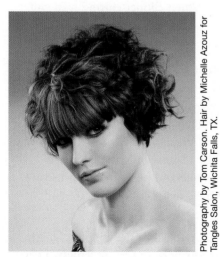

figure 16-134
Texturized graduated haircut

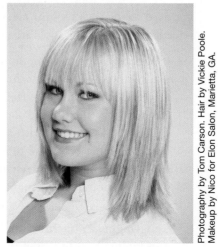

figure 16-135
Uniform-layered haircut before texturizing

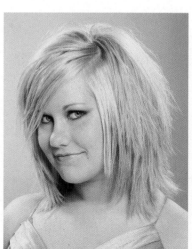

figure 16-136
Texturized uniform-layered haircut

Effectively Use Clippers and Trimmers

Other types of tools that all stylists should be familiar with are clippers and trimmers, which offer solutions for many haircutting challenges.

Clippers are electric or battery-operated tools that cut the hair by using two moving blades held in place by a metal plate with teeth. The blade action is faster than the eye can see. Clippers are mainly used for cutting shorter haircuts and can be used to create a **taper**, hair that is cut very short and close to the hairline and that gradually gets longer as you move up the head. While men have been getting clipper cuts for many years, today clippers are being used more and more in women's haircutting. Clippers can be used as follows:

- Without length guards, to remove hair completely (great for cleaning up necklines and around the ears).

- Without length guards, to taper hairlines from extremely short lengths into longer lengths, using the **clipper-over-comb** technique (this technique is very similar to scissor-over-comb, except that the clippers move side to side across the comb rather than bottom to top).

- With length guards, attachments that fit over the blade plate and vary in size from ⅛ inch to 1 inch (0.3 to 2.5 cm) for short, layered cuts.

Tools for Clipper Cutting

There are several tools to have on hand. When clipper cutting, you will not need to use each tool for every haircut but it is still important to understand when these tools are needed.

- **Clippers.** Clippers come in different shapes and sizes. They can be used with or without attachments. Trimmers, also called *edgers*, are usually cordless, smaller-sized clippers. They are mainly used to clean the necklines and around the ears (**figure 16-137**). Clean your clippers and trimmers with a clipper brush after each use. Apply one drop of clipper oil to the tops of the blades while the clipper is running. Disinfect the detachable blade and heel after each use as well. Always follow the manufacturer's instructions for care and cleaning.

- **Length guard attachments.** When attached to the clippers, length guards allow you to cut all the hair evenly to that exact length. They range from ⅛- to 1-inch (0.3 to 2.5 centimeters) wide and can be used in different combinations to create different lengths.

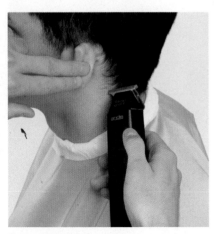

figure 16-137
Trimmer cutting around the ear

- **Haircutting shears.** Used mainly for removing length and detailing the haircut.

- **Thinning shears.** Also called *blending* or *tapering scissors*, these are great for removing excess bulk and for blending one area with another.

- **Combs.** With a regular cutting comb, the wider-spaced teeth are intended for combing and cutting. The finer-spaced teeth are used for detailing, scissor-over-comb, and clipper-over-comb techniques.

The classic barbering comb is often used in the nape, at the sides, and around the ears, and allows you to cut the hair very short and close to the head. The wide-tooth comb is used when cutting thicker and longer lengths where detailing is not required.

Basic Clipper Techniques

Basic techniques with clippers include clipper-over-comb and clipper cutting with length guard attachments.

Clipper-Over-Comb

The clipper-over-comb technique allows you to cut the hair very close to the scalp and create a flat top or square shape. The way you use the comb is the same as when you are working with scissor-over-comb. The main difference is that the clippers move across the comb, which requires that you keep the comb in position as you cut. The angle at which you hold the comb determines the amount of hair that is removed.

Clippers are more accurate when used on dry to slightly damp hair. Use the lever switch on the clipper or a numbered attachment to vary the distance that the clipper is held from the head.

Tips for working with the clipper-over-comb technique follow. This technique will be illustrated in the procedure for the men's basic clipper cut later in this chapter.

1. Stand directly in front of the section on which you are working. The area you are cutting should be at eye level.

2. Place the comb, teeth first, into the hairline, and turn the comb so that the teeth are angled slightly away from the head. Always work against the growth patterns of the hair to ensure that you are lifting the hair away from the head and cutting evenly.

3. Hold the comb stationary and cut the length against the comb, moving the clippers from right to left. (If you are left-handed, you will move the clippers left to right.)

4. Although your movements should be fluid, remember to stop momentarily to cut the section. Remove the comb from the hair and begin the motion again, using the previously cut section underneath as your guideline. Continue working up the head toward the weight or length.

Clipper Cutting with Attachments

Using the length guard attachments is a quick and easy way to create short haircuts. With practice, clipper cutting with attachments allows you to create many different shapes. For example, you can use the ¼-inch (6 mm) guard on the nape and sides. Then you can switch to the ½-inch (13 mm) guard as you reach the parietal area. This will maintain more length at the parietal area. This technique produces a square shape.

Men's Basic Clipper Cut

In this cut, the hair is cropped close along the bottom and sides and becomes longer as you travel up the head. The distance between the comb and the scalp determines the amount of hair to be cut. The clipper can be positioned horizontally, vertically, or diagonally.

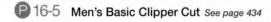

P 16-5   Men's Basic Clipper Cut *See page 434*

Using Trimmers

- **Using trimmers around the ears.** When cutting a clean line around the ears, use both hands to hold the edger sideways. Using just the outer edge on the skin, arc the edger up and around the ear (figure 16-138). As you reach the area behind the ear, use the comb to hold the hair in place, and continue with the arcing motion (figure 16-139).

- **Using trimmers at the neckline.** Clean up the hair on the neck that grows below the design line (figure 16-140). Trimmers also help create more defined lines at the perimeter (figure 16-141).

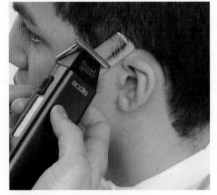

figure 16-138
Arcing trimmer at front of the ear

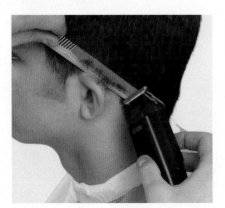

figure 16-139
Arcing trimmer at back of the ear with comb

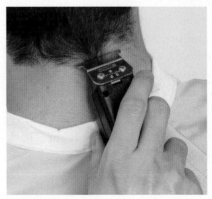

figure 16-140
Cleaning up neck hair

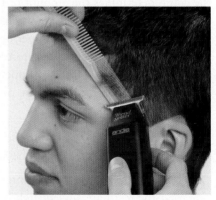

figure 16-141
Edging line at side perimeter

• **Using tattoo trimmers.** This is a great tool to use for those hard to reach areas because of its slender design. This trimmer is great for outlining, trimming beards and mustaches, and creating elaborate designs with ease. The thin blade allows a professional stylist to trim a precise cut without irritation to the skin or scalp.

Trimming Facial Hair

Clippers and trimmers can be used to trim beards and mustaches as well. The technique is very similar to scissor-over-comb and clipper-over-comb. When removing length, use the comb to control the hair and always cut against the comb (figure 16-142). You can also use the length guard attachments to trim a beard to the desired length (figure 16-143). If you choose to use haircutting shears to trim facial hair, you may want to keep a less expensive pair for this purpose because facial hair is very coarse and may dull your haircutting shears.

Some male clients have long eyebrows or excess hair in or on their ears. When performing a haircut or trimming facial hair, always check the ears and eyebrows, then ask the client if he would like you to remove any excess hair you may find. Carefully snip away the hair with your shears or trimmers, using complete focus.

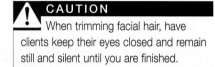

⚠ CAUTION
When trimming facial hair, have clients keep their eyes closed and remain still and silent until you are finished.

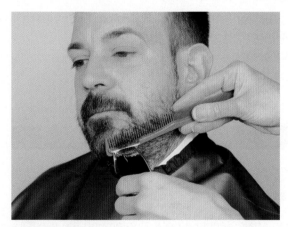

figure 16-142
Trimming beard with trimmer-over-comb

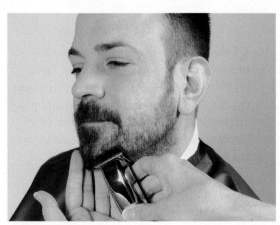

figure 16-143
Trimming beard with trimmer and guard

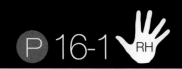

P 16-1 RH

BLUNT HAIRCUT

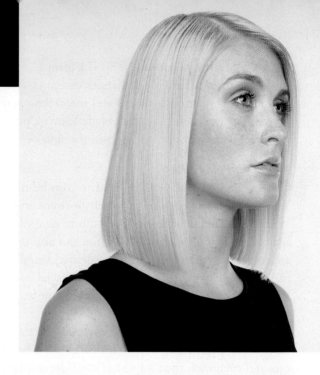

IMPLEMENTS & MATERIALS

You will need all of the following implements, materials, and supplies:

- ☐ Blowdryer
- ☐ Classic styling brush
- ☐ Cutting cape
- ☐ Cutting comb

- ☐ Haircutting shears
- ☐ Neck strip
- ☐ Sectioning clips

- ☐ Shampoo and conditioner
- ☐ Shampoo cape
- ☐ Spray bottle with water

- ☐ Styling product for finish
- ☐ Towels
- ☐ Wide-tooth comb

PREPARATION

Perform

P 15-1 **Pre-Service Procedure** *See page 340*

PROCEDURE

1 Drape your client for a shampoo.

2 Shampoo and condition the hair as necessary.

3 Escort the client back to the styling chair. Secure a neck strip around the client's neck. Place a cape over the neck strip and fasten in the back. Fold the neck strip down over the cape so that no part of the cape touches the client's skin.

4 Detangle the hair with the wide-tooth comb.

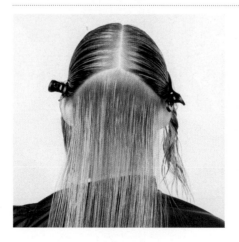

5 Part the hair in the center, from the front hairline through to the nape. Next create two diagonal forward partings from the occipital to behind the ear creating a 1/2 inch (1.3 cm) wide subsection. (The depth of the section may vary due to hair density.)

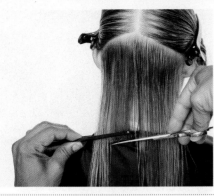
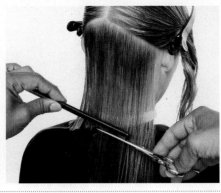

6 Angle the head forward slightly. Begin in the center and using the fine teeth, comb the hair to its natural fall. Parallel to the diagonal forward parting, at 0 degrees elevation, cut your first line. Repeat on the opposite side, starting the cut from the outer corner to the center creating a slight arc-shape line. Check balance.

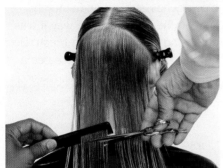

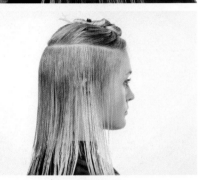

7 Now, from the top of the occipital to the top of each ear, create another set of diagonal forward partings. The head position will move up slightly, but the natural fall distribution and 0-degree elevation remain consistent. Cut parallel to your diagonal forward parting and follow the length of your guide.

8 Position the client's head upright. Beginning just below the crown and extending to the front hairline, create a horseshoe section. Starting in the rear of the horseshoe section, using the wide teeth, comb the hair over the previously cut hair to its natural fall (0-degree elevation). Following your guide beneath, cut the line along the comb until you reach the side, just below the ear.

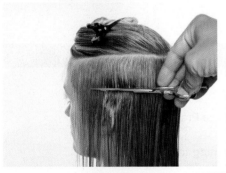

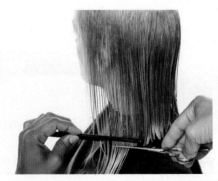

9 On the sides just behind the ear, continue to comb the hair to natural fall (cutting at 0 degrees), cutting the hair parallel to the horseshoe parting. Pay close attention to the protrusion of the ear and tap the hair above the comb before you cut to release any tension.

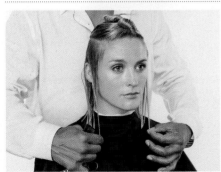

10 Repeat on the opposite side. Before moving on, stand behind the client and check the lengths on both sides while looking in the mirror. Make any needed adjustments.

11 Take another subsection from the horseshoe above the crown to the front hairline. Starting at the back, comb the hair to natural fall and cut at 0 degrees following your guide. When you reach the sides, continue the same technique as step 9.

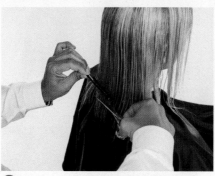 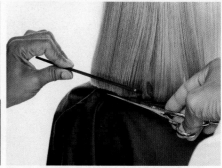

12 Release the remaining hair in the section and comb to natural fall. Be sure to notice any cowlicks or movement at the crown. From the back, continue combing the hair to natural fall. Follow your guide and cut at 0 degrees elevation.

13 To check the line for accuracy, blowdry hair straight and smooth section the hair the same way it was cut, using a classic styling brush. Do not use a round brush—it creates a bend in the ends of the hair, making it difficult to check the line.

14 Once the hair is dry, check the line in the mirror. You should see an even, horizontal line all the way around the head. Using the wide teeth, comb the hair to natural fall and clean up your bob line. (Avoid cutting your line shorter.)

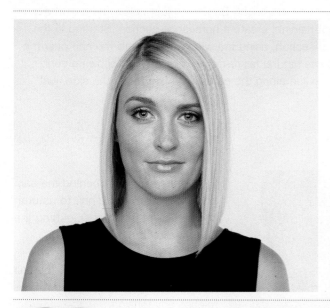

15 Finished look.

POST-SERVICE

Complete

P 15-2   **Post-Service Procedure** *See page 343*

milady pro Check out miladypro.com for additional resources and training to enhance your technical skills.   Keyword: *FutureCosPro*

BLUNT HAIRCUT

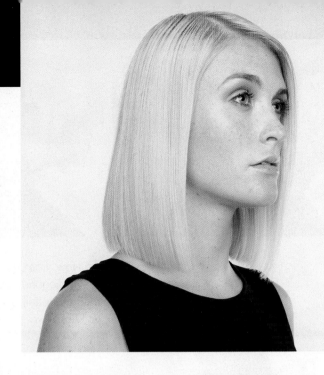

IMPLEMENTS & MATERIALS

You will need all of the following implements, materials, and supplies:

- Blowdryer
- Classic styling brush
- Cutting cape
- Cutting comb
- Haircutting shears
- Neck strip
- Sectioning clips
- Shampoo and conditioner
- Shampoo cape
- Spray bottle with water
- Styling product for finish
- Towels
- Wide-tooth comb

PREPARATION

Perform

P 16-1 **Blunt Haircut**
See page 404

PROCEDURE

1 Drape your client for a shampoo.

2 Shampoo and condition the hair as necessary.

3 Escort the client back to the styling chair. Secure a neck strip around the client's neck. Place a cape over the neck strip and fasten in the back. Fold the neck strip down over the cape so that no part of the cape touches the client's skin.

4 Detangle the hair with the wide-tooth comb.

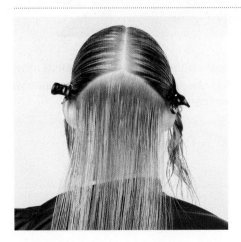

5 Part the hair in the center, from the front hairline through to the nape. Next create two diagonal forward partings from the occipital to behind the ear creating a 1/2 inch (1.3 cm) wide subsection. (The depth of the section may vary due to hair density.)

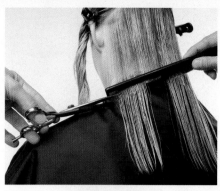

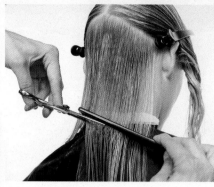

6 Angle the head forward slightly. Begin in the center and using the fine teeth, comb the hair to its natural fall. Parallel to the diagonal forward parting, at 0 degrees elevation, cut your first line. Repeat on the opposite side, starting cut from the center to the outer corner creating a slight arc-shape line. Check balance.

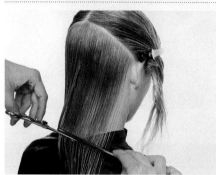

7 Now, from the top of the occipital to the top of each ear, create another set of diagonal forward partings. The head position will move up slightly, but the natural fall distribution and 0-degree elevation remain consistent. Cut parallel to your diagonal forward parting and follow the length of your guide.

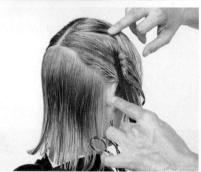

8 Position the client's head upright. Beginning just below the crown and extending to the front hairline, create a horseshoe section. Starting in the rear of your horseshoe section, using the wide teeth, comb the hair over the previously cut hair to its natural fall (0-degree elevation). Following your guide beneath, cut the line along the comb until you reach the side, just below the ear.

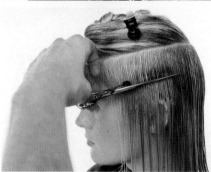

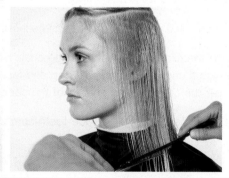

9 On the sides just behind the ear, continue to comb the hair to natural fall (cutting at 0 degrees), cutting the hair parallel to the horseshoe parting. Pay close attention to the protrusion of the ear and tap the hair above the comb before you cut to release any tension.

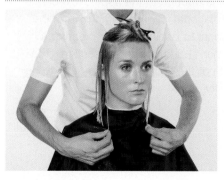

10 Repeat on the opposite side. Before moving on, stand behind the client and check the lengths on both sides while looking in the mirror. Make any needed adjustments.

11 Take another subsection from the horseshoe from above the crown to the front hairline. Starting at the back, comb the hair to natural fall and cut at 0 degrees following your guide. When you reach the sides continue the same technique as step 9.

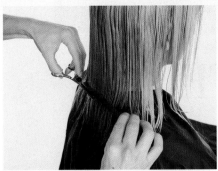

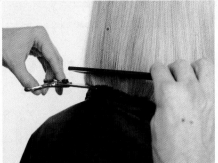

12 Release the remaining hair in the section and comb to natural fall. Be sure to notice any cowlicks or movement at the crown. From the back, continue combing the hair to natural fall. Follow your guide and cut at 0 degrees elevation.

13 To check the line for accuracy, blowdry the hair straight and smooth section the hair the same way it was cut, using a classic styling brush. Do not use a round brush—it creates a bend in the ends of the hair, making it difficult to check the line.

14 Once the hair is dry, check the line in the mirror. You should see an even, horizontal line all the way around the head. Using the wide teeth, comb the hair to natural fall and clean up your bob line. (Avoid cutting you line shorter.)

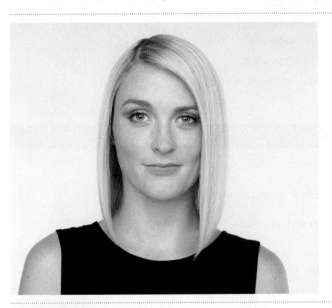

15 Finished look.

POST-SERVICE

Complete

P 15-2 **Post-Service Procedure** *See page 343*

milady pro Check out miladypro.com for additional resources and training to enhance your technical skills. Keyword: *FutureCosPro*

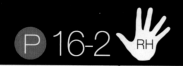

GRADUATED HAIRCUT

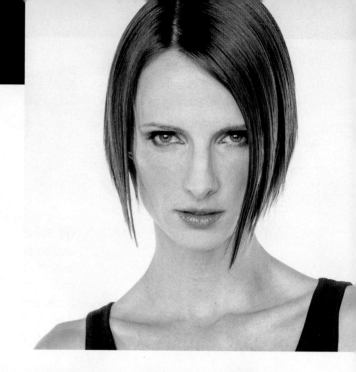

IMPLEMENTS & MATERIALS

You will need all of the following implements, materials, and supplies:

- ☐ Blowdryer
- ☐ Cutting cape
- ☐ Cutting or styling comb
- ☐ Haircutting shears
- ☐ Neck strip
- ☐ Sectioning clips
- ☐ Shampoo and conditioner
- ☐ Shampoo cape
- ☐ Spray bottle with water
- ☐ Styling product for finish
- ☐ Towels
- ☐ Wide-tooth comb

PREPARATION

Perform

P 15-1 **Pre-Service Procedure** *See page 340*

PROCEDURE

① Drape your client for a shampoo.

② Shampoo and condition the hair as necessary.

③ Escort the client back to the styling chair.

④ Secure a neck strip around the client's neck. Place a cape over the neck strip and fasten in the back. Fold the neck strip down over the cape so that no part of the cape touches the client's skin.

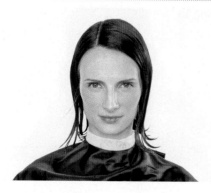

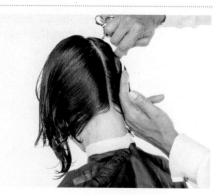

⑤ Begin your first section by taking the parting from the client's natural side part back to the crown. Then take a central parting from the crown to the nape.

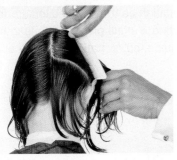
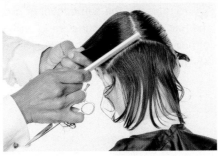

6 At the occipital bone, take a diagonal forward parting from the central parting to the middle of each ear. Then take a pivoting diagonal forward 1/2 inch (1.3 cm) wide subsection and elevate it to 45 degrees and cut parallel to your parting. Both your finger angle and elevation should be at 45 degrees.

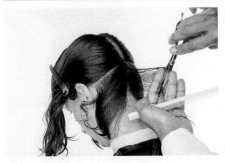
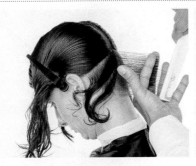
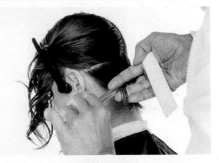

7 Make sure that your section is no longer than 2–3 inches (5–7.5 centimeters) in length or your graduation will sit too low. This will serve as your traveling guide.

8 Continue taking pivoting diagonal forward subsections, using the previously cut subsection as a traveling guide. Both your elevation and finger angle are held at 45 degrees. Elevate and cut parallel to your parting.

9 Once you've reached your last subsection, you should be parallel to your diagonal forward parting; continue to elevate at 45 degrees following your traveling guide.

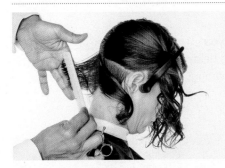
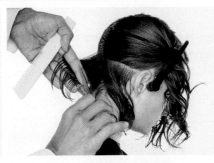
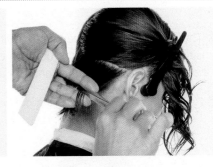

10 Repeat the same steps and technique on the opposite side. (Note the change in hand position. The tips of your fingers will now be palm up, pointing down.) Once completed, cross-check the balance from the outer edges on both sides.

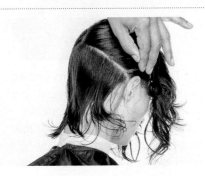

11 To begin the next section, take a diagonal forward parting from above the occipital bone extending to the top of each ear. Each side is then subsectioned and cut as before, using pivoting diagonal forward subsections to work your way through the section.

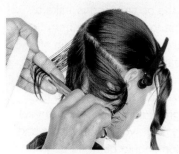

12 To maintain the same level of graduation as the first section, comb the hair parallel to your parting and, using a small piece of the length of hair cut from the first section as a guide, cut a stationary guide at a 45-degree elevation.

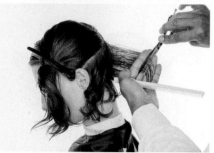
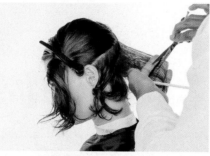

13 Repeat the same steps on the opposite side. Once completed, check for visual balance.

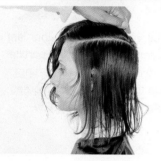
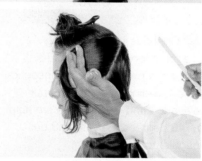

14 The next section will be a horseshoe section taken from just below the crown to the recession area on both sides. This section will be subdivided and cut using traveling diagonal forward subsections combed to natural fall and then elevated to 45 degrees and cut parallel to the horseshoe parting.

15 The elevation will decrease to one-finger's depth just behind the ear where you transition to the sides and the bob line begins. From the ear forward, the hair is held in the comb to release tension and cut at 0 degrees parallel to the horseshoe parting.

16 Repeat the same steps on the opposite side.

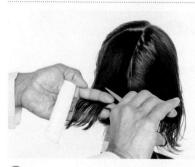
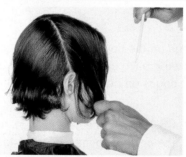
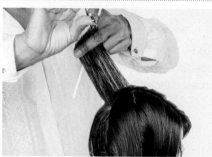

17 Continue taking sections from the horseshoe until the natural side part is reached and all remaining hair has been cut following your guide.

18 In preparation for layering, create a radial section by taking a radial parting from the crown to the top of each ear. Take a ½-inch wide (1.25 centimeters) central vertical subsection from the crown to the occipital.

19 The hair in this section is elevated to 90 degrees and overdirected back. Your guide will be taken from the perimeter of the graduation for the length. You will point cut following the head shape. (Do not cut below occipital or you will cut into your graduation.)

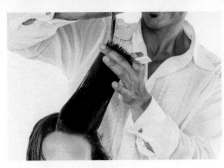

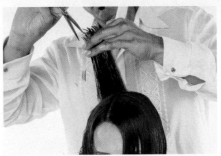

22 In the front, length is maintained by overdirecting back to a stationary guide at the radial section. Repeat the same steps on the opposite side.

20 Pivoting subsections are combed to 90 degrees, overdirected back, and, using a traveling guide, cut parallel to the head. When you've completed the radial section, repeat on the opposite side.

21 When you reach the sides, take a horizontal subsection from the natural side part, elevate to 90 degrees, overdirect back, and point cut following your guide from the radial section. (Make sure to keep your elbows up to avoid cutting into the perimeter.) Remember to begin at the natural side part and overdirect the section back to a stationary guide at the radial section.

23 Once the hair is dry, detail the perimeter: Starting at the nape, use the points of your shears for softness or blunt cut for a stronger line. At the sides, clean up your line at the perimeter. (Avoid cutting too much hair, remember that you are just detailing.)"

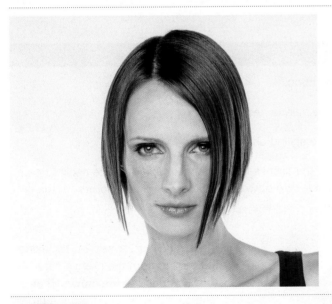

24 Finished look.

POST-SERVICE

Complete

P 15-2 **Post-Service Procedure** *See page 343*

milady pro   Check out miladypro.com for additional resources and training to enhance your technical skills.   Keyword: *FutureCosPro*

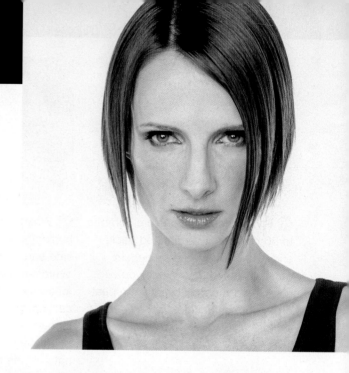

GRADUATED HAIRCUT

IMPLEMENTS & MATERIALS

You will need all of the following implements, materials, and supplies:

☐ Blowdryer

☐ Cutting cape

☐ Cutting or styling comb

☐ Haircutting shears

☐ Neck strip

☐ Sectioning clips

☐ Shampoo and conditioner

☐ Shampoo cape

☐ Spray bottle with water

☐ Styling product for finish

☐ Towels

☐ Wide-tooth comb

PREPARATION

Perform

P 15-1 **Pre-Service Procedure** *See page 340*

PROCEDURE

1. Drape your client for a shampoo.

2. Shampoo and condition the hair as necessary.

3. Escort the client back to the styling chair.

4. Secure a neck strip around the client's neck. Place a cape over the neck strip and fasten in the back. Fold the neck strip down over the cape so that no part of the cape touches the client's skin.

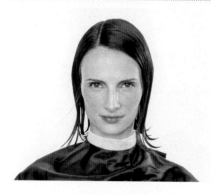

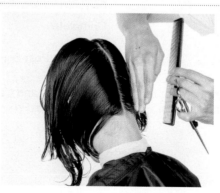

5. Begin your fist section by taking the parting from the client's natural side part back to the crown. Then take a central parting from the crown to the nape.

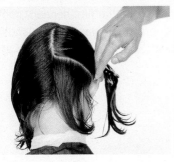

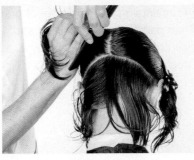

6 At the occipital bone, take a diagonal forward parting from the central parting to the middle of each ear. Then take a pivoting diagonal forward 1/2 inch (1.3 cm) wide subsection and elevate it to 45 degrees and cut parallel to your parting. Both your finger angle and elevation should be at 45 degrees.

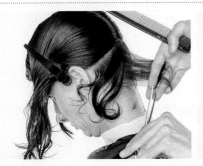

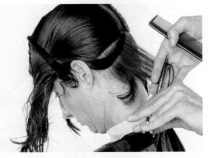

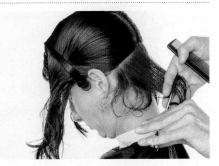

7 Make sure that your section is no longer than 2–3 inches (5–7.5 centimeters) in length or your graduation will sit too low. This will serve as your traveling guide.

8 Continue taking pivoting diagonal forward subsections, using the previously cut subsection as a traveling guide. Both your elevation and finger angle are held at 45 degrees. Elevate and cut parallel to your parting.

9 Once you've reached your last subsection, you should be parallel to your diagonal forward parting, continue to elevate at 45 degrees following your traveling guide.

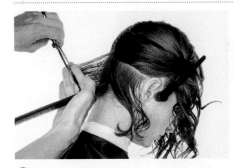

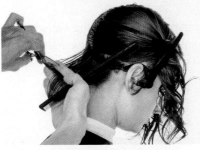

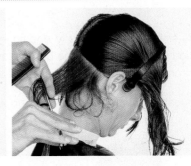

10 Repeat the same steps and technique on the opposite side. (Note the change in hand position. The tips of your fingers will now be palm up, fingers pointing up.) Once completed, cross-check the balance from the outer edges on both sides.

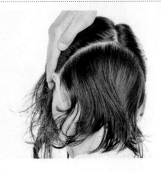

11 To begin the next section, take a diagonal forward parting from above the occipital bone extending to the top of each ear. Each side is then subsectioned and cut as before, using pivoting diagonal forward subsections to work your way through the section.

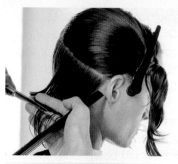

12 To maintain the same level of graduation as the first section, comb the hair parallel to your parting and, using a small piece of the length of hair cut from the first section as a guide, cut a stationary guide at a 45-degree elevation.

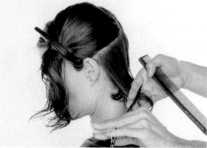

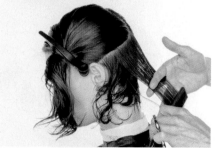

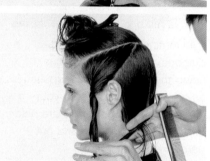

13 Repeat the same steps on the opposite side. Once completed, check for visual balance.

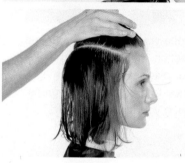

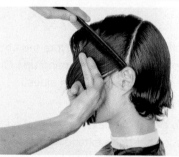

14 The next section will be a horseshoe section taken from just below the crown to the recession area on both sides. This section will be subdivided and cut using traveling diagonal forward subsections, combed to natural fall, and then elevated to 45 degrees and cut parallel to the horseshoe parting.

15 The elevation decreases to one finger's depth just behind the ear where you transition to the sides and the bob line begins. From the ear forward, the hair is held in the comb to release tension and cut at 0 degrees parallel to the horseshoe parting.

16 Repeat the same steps on the opposite side.

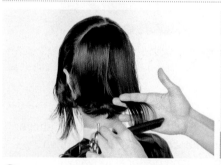

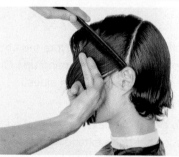

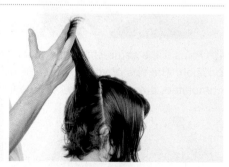

17 Continue taking sections from the horseshoe until the natural side part is reached and all remaining hair has been cut following your guide.

18 In preparation for layering, create a radial section by taking a radial parting from the crown to the top of each ear. Take a ½-inch wide (1.25 centimeters) central vertical subsection from the crown to the occipital.

19 The hair in this section is elevated to 90 degrees and overdirected back. Your guide will be taken from the perimeter of the graduation for the length. You will point cut following the head shape. (Do not cut below occipital or you will cut into your graduation.)

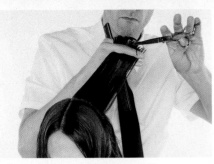

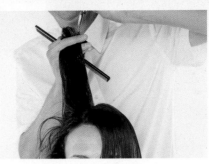

22 In the front, length is maintained by overdirecting back to a stationary guide at the radial section. Repeat the same steps on the opposite side.

20 Pivoting subsections are combed to 90 degrees overdirected back and, using a traveling guide, cut parallel to the head. When you've completed the radial section, repeat on the opposite side.

21 When you reach the sides, take a horizontal subsection from the natural side part, elevate to 90 degrees, overdirect up, and point cut following your guide from the radial section. (Make sure to keep your elbows up to avoid cutting into the perimeter.) Remember to begin at the natural side part and overdirect the section back to a stationary guide at the radial section.

23 Once the hair is dry, detail the perimeter: Starting at the nape, use the points of your shears for softness or blunt cut for a stronger line. At the sides, clean up your line at the perimeter. (Avoid cutting too much hair, remember that you are just detailing.)

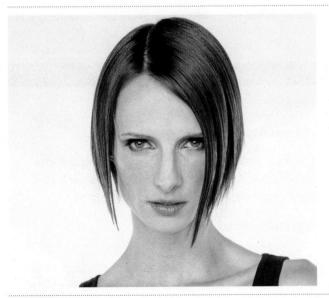

24 Finished look.

POST-SERVICE

Complete

P 15-2 **Post-Service Procedure** *See page 343*

milady pro Check out miladypro.com for additional resources and training to enhance your technical skills. Keyword: *FutureCosPro*

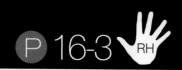

UNIFORM-LAYERED HAIRCUT

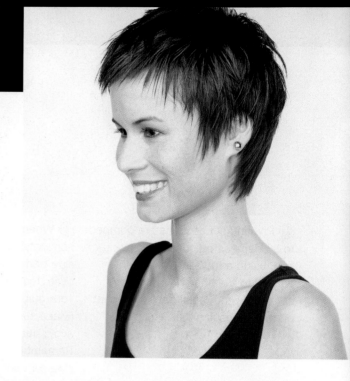

IMPLEMENTS & MATERIALS

You will need all of the following implements, materials, and supplies:

- ☐ Blowdryer
- ☐ Cutting cape
- ☐ Cutting or styling comb
- ☐ Haircutting shears
- ☐ Neck strip
- ☐ Paddle Brush
- ☐ Sectioning clips
- ☐ Shampoo and conditioner
- ☐ Shampoo cape
- ☐ Spray bottle with water
- ☐ Styling product for finish
- ☐ Towels
- ☐ Wide-tooth comb

PREPARATION

Perform

P 15-1 **Pre-Service Procedure** *See page 340*

PROCEDURE

1 Drape your client for a shampoo.

2 Shampoo and condition the hair as necessary.

3 Escort the client back to the styling chair. Secure a neck strip around the client's neck. Place a cape over the neck strip and fasten in the back. Fold the neck strip down over the cape so that no part of the cape touches the client's skin.

4 Detangle the hair with the wide-tooth comb.

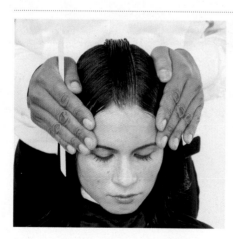

5 To create a guide, take a ½-inch wide (1.25 centimeters) profile section from the front hairline to the nape. Cut palm-to-palm until you've reached the apex, then switch hand position.

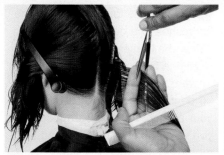 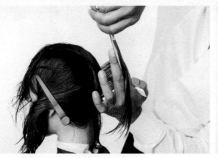 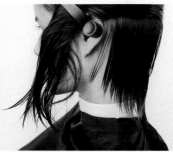

6 Starting at the nape, elevate the hair to 90 degrees and cut 3 inches (7.5 centimeters) in length working in small increments following the head shape.

7 Above occipital, switch hand position and cut to the second knuckle to avoid corners forming on the line. Follow the guide to the front hairline. Once you've cut the center guide, check the length for balance and remove any corners.

8 After completing the guide, make a horseshoe section from recession to recession and below the crown. Make sure your section is clean and balanced at both sides of the recession.

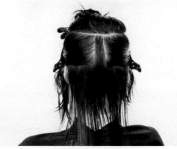

9 Take a horizontal parting from the occipital to the back of each ear and clip the section above your horizontal line. At the back, take a center section from the occipital to the nape dividing your first profile section guide in half.

10 Starting at the center back, take a slight diagonal forward parting through to the nape, incorporating your guide from the profile section.

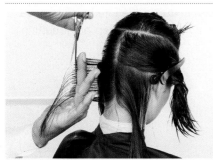 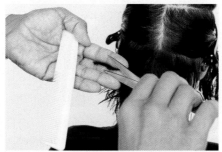 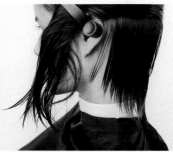

11 Elevate the hair to 90 degrees and cut parallel to the parting for your subsection following the guide. If you can't see your guide, take a smaller subsection. (Hand position is palm-to-palm when cutting the left side.)

12 Cross-check horizontally on every fourth section (any overdirection should be corrected section by section). The line should be round because you're following the head shape.

13 Continue taking slight diagonal forward subsections, elevating at 90 degrees, and cutting parallel to your parting for your subsection until you've reached back of the ear. Switch hand position and repeat on the opposite side.

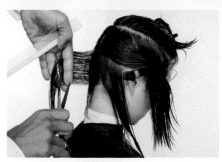

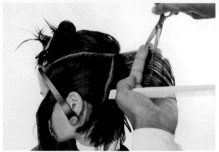

14 Release the lower portion of the horseshoe and cut palm-to-palm below the horseshoe on both sides. Continue taking slight diagonal forward subsections, elevating at 90 degrees, and cutting parallel to your parting. Follow your guide until you've completed the side and then repeat on the opposite side.

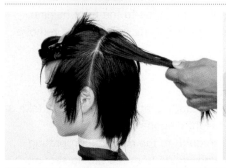

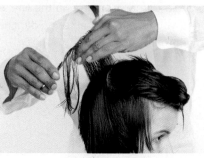

15 Release the horseshoe section. Then take a radial section from above the crown to the top of each ear separating the hair from front to back. Switch hand position and cut above your fingers for the remainder of the haircut.

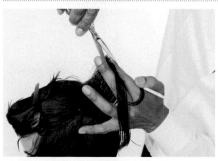

16 Pivoting pie shape sections are taken from below your radial section. Following your guide, elevate the hair at 90 degrees and cut until you have completed both sides. (Remember to cross-check.)

17 At this point, you should have a guide from the top, sides, and behind the radial section, allowing you to stay consistent and follow the head shape.

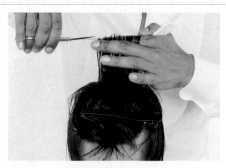

18 Continue taking horizontal subsections, elevating at 90 degrees, and cutting with the traveling guide until you've reached the front hairline. Repeat the same technique on the opposite side.

19 Dry the hair with your hands or a paddle brush. Once the haircut is dry, texturize the interior to remove weight by using deep point cutting.

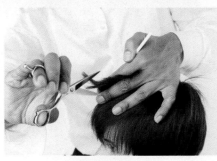
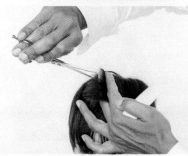

20 Hold the section 2 inches (5 centimeters) from the ends and enter the section parallel so you don't remove any length, work in 1-inch (2.5 centimeters) panels. (Do not angle your shears and close the blade on the way out to avoid cutting your fingers.)

21 Use your mirror and look at the balance. Detail the bang area (utilize the short textured bangs technique) and perimeter with point cutting and carving.

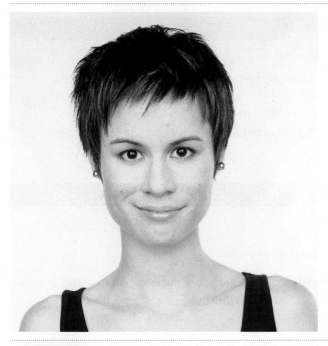

22 Finished look.

POST-SERVICE

Complete

 15-2 **Post-Service Procedure** *See page 343*

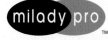 Check out miladypro.com for additional resources and training to enhance your technical skills.   Keyword: *FutureCosPro*

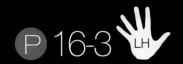
UNIFORM-LAYERED HAIRCUT

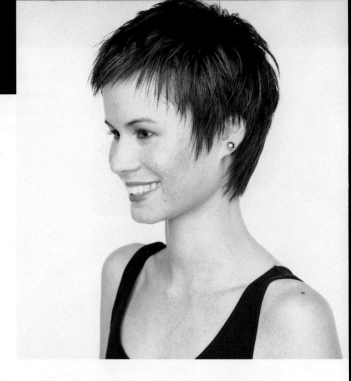

IMPLEMENTS & MATERIALS

You will need all of the following implements, materials, and supplies:

- ☐ Blowdryer
- ☐ Cutting cape
- ☐ Cutting or styling comb
- ☐ Haircutting shears
- ☐ Neck strip
- ☐ Paddle Brush
- ☐ Sectioning clips
- ☐ Shampoo and conditioner
- ☐ Shampoo cape
- ☐ Spray bottle with water
- ☐ Styling product for finish
- ☐ Towels
- ☐ Wide-tooth comb

PREPARATION

Perform

P 15-1 **Pre-Service Procedure** *See page 340*

PROCEDURE

1 Drape your client for a shampoo.

2 Shampoo and condition the hair as necessary.

3 Escort the client back to the styling chair. Secure a neck strip around the client's neck. Place a cape over the neck strip and fasten in the back. Fold the neck strip down over the cape so that no part of the cape touches the client's skin.

4 Detangle the hair with the wide-tooth comb.

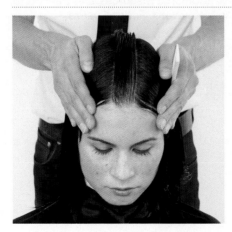

5 To create a guide, take a ½-inch wide (1.25 centimeters) profile section from the front hairline to the nape. Cut palm-to-palm until you've reached the apex, then switch hand position.

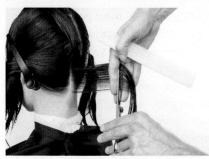

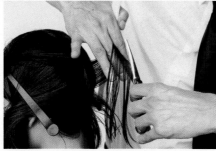

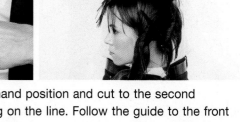

6 Starting at the nape, elevate the hair to 90 degrees and cut 3 inches (7.5 centimeters) in length working in small increments following the head shape.

7 Above the occipital, switch hand position and cut to the second knuckle to avoid corners forming on the line. Follow the guide to the front hairline. Once you've cut the center guide, check the length for balance and remove any corners.

8 After completing the guide, make a horseshoe section from recession to recession and below the crown. Make sure your section is clean and balanced at both sides of the recession.

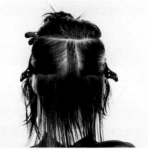

9 Take a horizontal parting from the occipital to the back of each ear and clip the section above your horizontal line. At the back, take a center section from the occipital to the nape dividing your first profile section guide in half.

10 Starting at the center back, take a slight diagonal forward parting through to the nape incorporating your guide from the profile section.

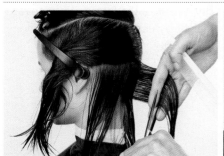

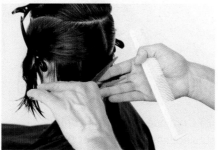

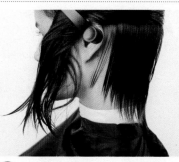

11 Elevate the hair to 90 degrees and cut parallel to the parting for your subsection following the guide. If you can't see your guide, take a smaller subsection. (Hand position is palm-to-palm when cutting the left side.)

12 Cross-check horizontally on every fourth section. (Any overdirection should be corrected section by section.) The line should be round because you are following the head shape.

13 Continue taking slight diagonal forward subsections, elevating at 90 degrees, and cutting parallel to your parting for your subsection until you've reached the back of the ear. Switch hand position and repeat on the opposite side.

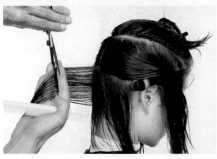

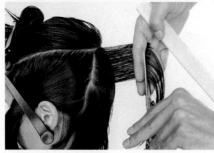

14 Release the lower portion of the horseshoe section and cut palm-to-palm below the horseshoe on both sides. Continue taking slight diagonal forward subsections, elevating at 90 degrees, and cutting parallel to your parting following your guide until you've completed the side and then repeat on the opposite side.

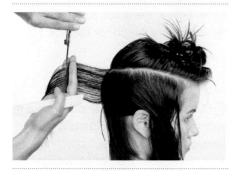

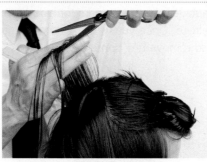

15 Release the horseshoe section. Then take a radial section from above the crown to the top of each ear, separating the hair from front to back. Switch hand position and cut above your fingers for the remainder of the haircut.

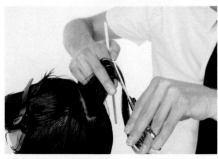

16 Pivoting pie shape sections are taken from below your radial section. Following your guide, elevate the hair at 90 degrees and cut until you have completed both sides. (Remember to cross-check.)

17 At this point, you should have a guide from the top, sides, and behind the radial section, allowing you to stay consistent and follow the head shape.

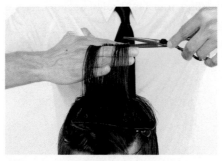

18 Continue taking horizontal subsections, elevating at 90 degrees, and cutting with the traveling guide until you've reached the front hairline. Repeat the same technique on the opposite side.

19 Dry the hair with your hands or a paddle brush. Once the haircut is dry, texturize the interior to remove weight by using deep point cutting.

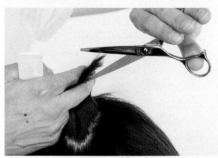

20 Hold the section 2 inches (5 centimeters) from the ends and enter the section parallel so you don't remove any length, work in 1-inch (2.5 centimeters) panels. (Do not angle you shears and close the blade on the way out to avoid cutting your fingers.)

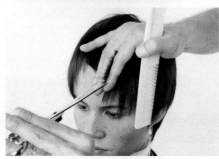

21 Use your mirror and look at the balance. Detail the bang area (utilize the short textured bangs technique) and perimeter with point cutting and carving.

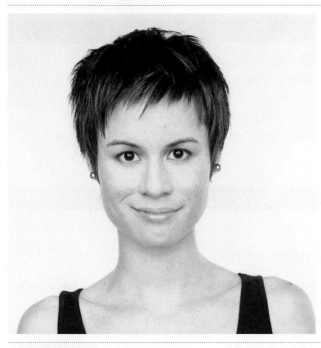

22 Finished look.

POST-SERVICE

Complete

 15-2 **Post-Service Procedure** *See page 343*

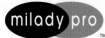 Check out miladypro.com for additional resources and training to enhance your technical skills.   Keyword: *FutureCosPro*

LONG-LAYERED HAIRCUT

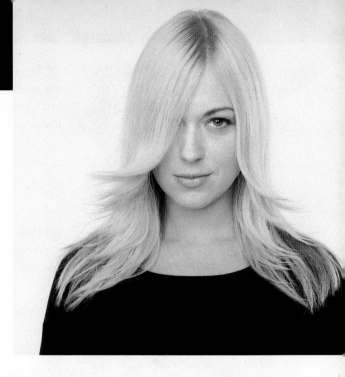

IMPLEMENTS & MATERIALS

You will need all of the following implements, materials, and supplies:

☐ Blowdryer

☐ Cutting cape

☐ Cutting or styling comb

☐ Haircutting shears

☐ Neck strip

☐ Round Brush (large)

☐ Sectioning clips

☐ Shampoo and conditioner

☐ Shampoo cape

☐ Spray bottle with water

☐ Styling product for finish

☐ Towels

☐ Wide-tooth comb

PREPARATION

Perform

P 15-1 **Pre-Service Procedure** *See page 340*

PROCEDURE

1 Drape your client for a shampoo.

2 Shampoo and condition the hair as necessary.

3 Escort the client back to the styling chair. Secure a neck strip around the client's neck. Place a cape over the neck strip and fasten in the back. Fold the neck strip down over the cape so that no part of the cape touches the client's skin.

4 Detangle the hair with the wide-tooth comb.

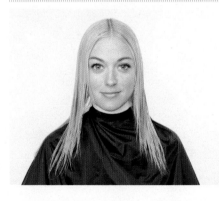

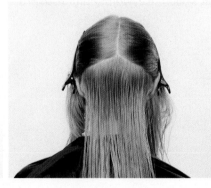

5 Begin by taking a central profile parting from the front hairline through to the nape. Then take two slight diagonal forward subsections ½-inch (1.25 centimeters) wide from the occipital to behind the ear. (The depth of the section may vary due to hair density.)

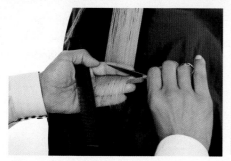 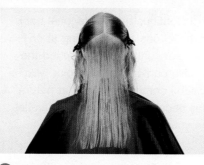 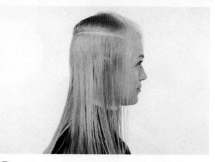

6 Tilt the head slightly forward. Starting in the center back, comb the hair to natural fall at 0 degrees. Cut (length) the line parallel to the parting. This will serve as your guide for the perimeter. The perimeter guide can be cut by either holding it with your fingers or a comb.

7 Take another ½-inch (1.25 cm) wide set of slight diagonal forward subsections from the top of the occipital to the top of each ear. The head position will move up slightly, but the natural fall distribution and 0-degree elevation will remain. Cut parallel to the parting and following the length of your guide.

8 With the client's head upright, take a horseshoe section from below the crown to the front hairline. Starting at the back of the head, comb the hair to natural fall and 0-degree elevation and cut the line following your guide.

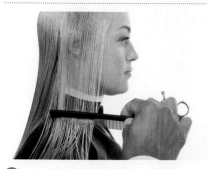 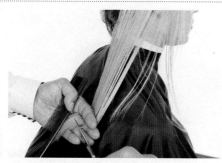 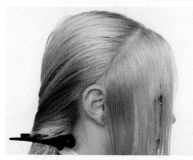

9 On the sides, comb the hair to natural fall and overdirect to behind the shoulder. Cut the line square to your guide. To do this, you will stand to the side to comb the hair into natural fall. Then step to the back and cut the line square.

10 Repeat the same technique on the opposite side. Continue cutting the hair in the horseshoe until you've reached the profile part (at the apex of the head) or run out of hair to cut.

11 On the sides, take a diagonal back parting from the profile part to the top of each ear.

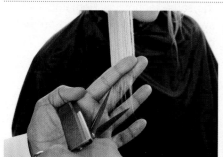 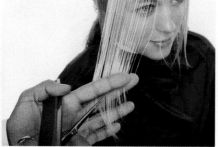

12 Standing to the front side of your client, comb the hair parallel to your diagonal back parting, elevate to a 45 degree, angle from the face. Starting at the bottom corner, cut the hair in small increments to the length of the chin.

13 To keep the length on the sides from front to back, avoid cutting your corner at the sideburn area or just in front of the ear. Clients with long hair want to see their length at the front and back.

14 Take another diagonal back subsection. This time, extend to behind the ear (incorporating the hair from your first diagonal back subsection). Comb the hair parallel to the parting, elevate at 45 degrees, and follow your guide.

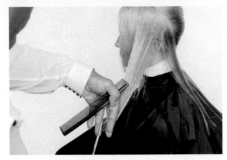

15 Although you're sectioning out and taking hair from behind the ear, this hair will not be cut. You will only be cutting hair from your corner, not what's behind the ear. Avoid overdirecting any hair beyond that point.

16 Continue taking diagonal back subsections and elevating at 45 degrees, until you've reached the profile parting. At that point, you will be combing the hair at natural fall because you're cutting parallel to your line.

17 Repeat the same technique on the opposite side, paying close attention to body position, balance, and your corner.

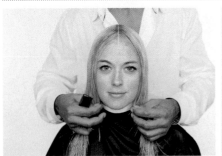

18 Once the sides are completed and you've checked your balance, take two diagonal forward partings at the top of the occipital to the back of each ear. The hair below your diagonal partings will be sectioned out of the way.

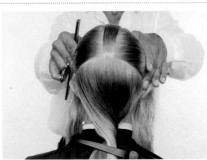

19 Starting at the front hairline take a ½-inch (1.25 centimeters) profile section to the occipital bone using your length from the chin as a guide.

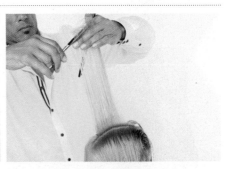

20 Elevate profile section to 90 degrees and, as you work toward the occipital, you will be overdirecting with your finger angle the length from the back at the occipital. The layered profile section will serve as a stationary guide for your interior layers.

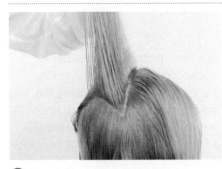

21 Below the crown and above the occipital, take a diagonal back subsection, elevate at 90 degrees, and overdirect to your center stationary guide. You should stand in front of the guide and overdirect the sections to your body, keeping your elbows up.

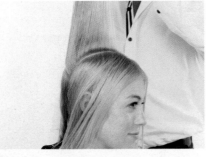

22 Continue taking diagonal back subsection, elevate up at 90 degrees, and overdirect to the stationary center guide. Continue until you've reached the front hairline section. Make sure you're combing the hair diagonally back and up into the center.

23 Repeat on the opposite side with the same technique. Remember to switch body position. Stand on the opposite side and in front of your guide.

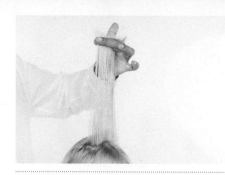

24 Crosscheck the haircut by taking a horizontal section at the top and looking for an increase in length. Remember when the hair travels to a stationary guide it increases in length. The line should still be consistent, a short to long angle.

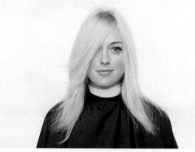

26 Once the hair is dry, detail the interior and perimeter using deep point cutting. Hold the section 3 inches (7.5 centimeters) from the ends and enter the hair parallel (use the entire length of the blade) so you don't remove any length.

27 Work in 1-inch (2.5 centimeters) panels. (Do not angle your shears and close the blade on the way out to avoid cutting your fingers.)

25 Section the hair the same manner it was cut and blowdry using a large round brush.

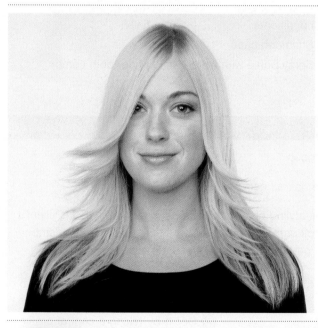

28 Finished look.

POST-SERVICE

Complete

P 15-2 **Post-Service Procedure** *See page 343*

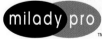

Check out miladypro.com for additional resources and training to enhance your technical skills.   Keyword: *FutureCosPro*

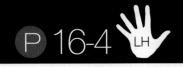

LONG-LAYERED HAIRCUT

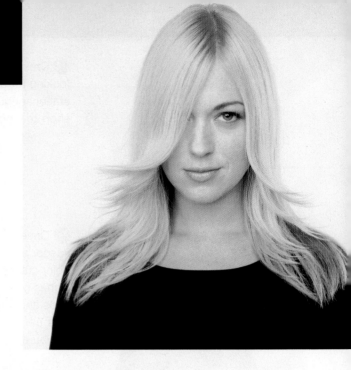

IMPLEMENTS & MATERIALS

You will need all of the following implements, materials, and supplies:

- ☐ Blowdryer
- ☐ Cutting cape
- ☐ Cutting or styling comb
- ☐ Haircutting shears
- ☐ Neck strip
- ☐ Round Brush (large)
- ☐ Sectioning clips
- ☐ Shampoo and conditioner
- ☐ Shampoo cape
- ☐ Spray bottle with water
- ☐ Styling product for finish
- ☐ Towels
- ☐ Wide-tooth comb

PREPARATION

Perform

P 15-1 **Pre-Service Procedure** *See page 340*

PROCEDURE

1️⃣ Drape your client for a shampoo.

2️⃣ Shampoo and condition the hair as necessary.

3️⃣ Escort the client back to the styling chair. Secure a neck strip around the client's neck. Place a cape over the neck strip and fasten in the back. Fold the neck strip down over the cape so that no part of the cape touches the client's skin.

4️⃣ Detangle the hair with the wide-tooth comb.

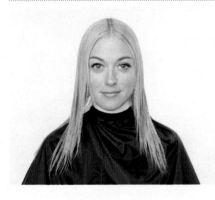

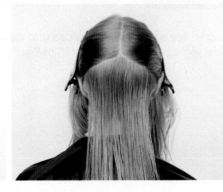

5️⃣ Begin by taking a central profile parting from the front hairline through to the nape. Then take two slight diagonal forward subsections ½-inch (1.25 centimeters) wide from the occipital to behind the ear. (The depth of the section may vary do to hair density.)

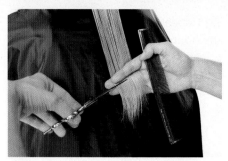

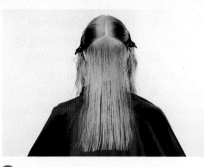

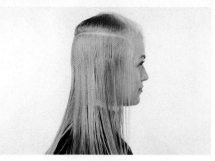

6 Tilt the head slightly forward. Starting in the center back, comb the hair to natural fall at 0 degrees. Cut (length) the line parallel to the parting. This will serve as your guide for the perimeter. The perimeter guide can be cut by either holding it with your fingers or a comb.

7 Take another ½-inch (1.25 cm) wide set of slight diagonal forward subsections from the top of the occipital to the top of each ear. The head position will move up slightly, but the natural fall distribution and 0-degree elevation will remain. Cut parallel to the parting and following the length of your guide.

8 With the client's head upright, take a horseshoe section from below the crown to the front hairline. Starting at the back of the head, comb the hair to natural fall and 0-degree elevation, and cut the line following your guide.

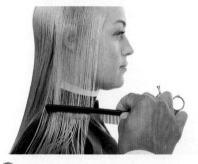

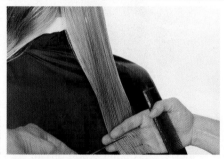

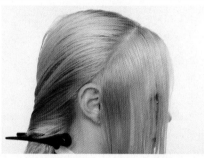

9 On the sides, comb the hair to natural fall and overdirect to behind the shoulder and cut the line square to your guide. To do this, you will stand to the side to comb the hair into natural fall. Then step to the back and cut the line square.

10 Repeat the same technique on the opposite side. Continue cutting the hair in the horseshoe until you've reached the profile part (at the apex of the head) or run out of hair to cut.

11 On the sides, take a diagonal back parting from the profile part to the top of each ear.

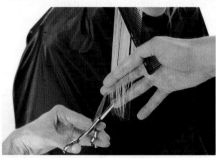

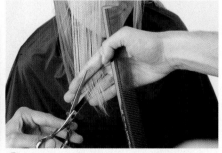

12 Standing to the front side of your client, comb the hair parallel to your diagonal back parting, elevate to a 45-degree angle from the face. Starting at the bottom corner, cut the hair in small increments to the length of the chin.

13 To keep the length on the sides from front to back, avoid cutting your corner at the sideburn area or just in front of the ear. Clients with long hair want to see their length at the front and back.

14 Take another diagonal back subsection. This time, extend to behind the ear (incorporating the hair from your first diagonal back subsection). Comb the hair parallel to the parting, elevate at 45 degrees, and follow your guide.

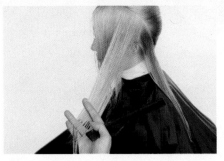

15 Although you're sectioning out and taking hair from behind the ear, this hair will not be cut. You will only be cutting hair from your corner, not what's behind the ear. Avoid overdirecting any hair beyond that point.

16 Continue the taking diagonal back subsections, and elevating at 45 degrees, until you've reached the profile parting. At that point, you will be combing the hair at natural fall because you're cutting parallel to your line.

17 Repeat the same technique on the opposite side, paying close attention to body position, balance, and your corner.

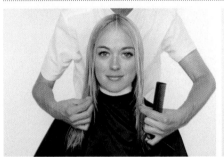

18 Once the sides are completed and you've checked your balance, take two diagonal forward partings at the top of the occipital to the back of each ear. The hair below your diagonal parting will be sectioned away.

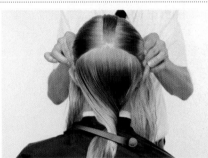

19 Starting at the front hairline take a ½-inch (1.25 centimeters) profile section to the occipital using your length from the chin as a guide.

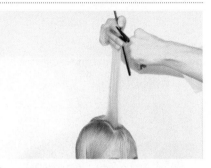

20 Elevate profile section to 90 degrees and, as you work toward the occipital, you will be overdirecting with your finger angle the length from the back at the occipital. The layered profile section will serve as a stationary guide for your interior layers.

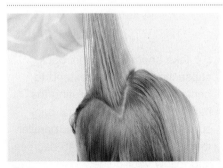

21 Below the crown and above the occipital, take a diagonal back subsection, elevate at 90 degrees, and overdirect to your center stationary guide. You should stand in front of the guide and overdirect the sections to your body, keeping your elbows up.

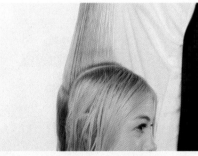

22 Continue taking diagonal back subsections, elevate up at 90 degrees, and overdirecting to the stationary center guide. Continue until you've reached the front hairline section. Make sure you're combing the hair diagonally back and up into the center.

23 Repeat on the opposite side with the same technique. Remember to switch body position. Stand on the opposite side and in front of your guide.

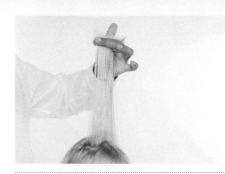

24 Cross-check the haircut by taking a horizontal section at the top and looking for an increase in length. Remember, when the hair travels to a stationary guide it increases in length. The line should still be consistent; a short to long angle.

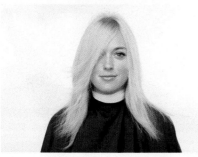

26 Once the hair is dry, detail the interior and perimeter using deep point cutting. Hold the section 3 inches (7.5 centimeters) from the ends and enter the hair parallel (use the entire length of the blade) so you don't remove any length.

27 Work in 1-inch (2.5 centimeters) panels. (Do not angle your shears and close the blade on the way out to avoid cutting your fingers.)

25 Section the hair the same manner it was cut and blowdry using a large round brush.

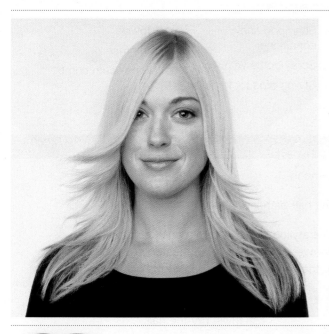

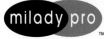

28 Finished look.

POST-SERVICE

Complete

 15-2 **Post-Service Procedure** *See page 343*

Check out miladypro.com for additional resources and training to enhance your technical skills.   Keyword: *FutureCosPro*

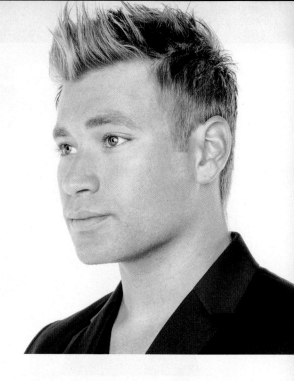

MEN'S BASIC CLIPPER CUT

IMPLEMENTS & MATERIALS

You will need all of the following implements, materials, and supplies:

☐ Blowdryer

☐ Clipper

☐ Cutting cape

☐ Haircutting comb

☐ Haircutting shears

☐ ¼-inch clipper guard (optional)

☐ Neck strip

☐ Shampoo and conditioner

☐ Spray bottle with water

☐ Styling product for finish

☐ Towels

☐ Trimmer

☐ Wide-tooth comb

PREPARATION

Perform

P 15-1 **Pre-Service Procedure** *See page 340*

PROCEDURE

1 Drape your client for a shampoo.

2 Shampoo and condition the hair as necessary.

3 Escort the client back to the styling chair. Secure a neck strip around the client's neck. Place a cape over the neck strip and fasten in the back. Fold the neck strip down over the cape so that no part of the cape touches the client's skin.

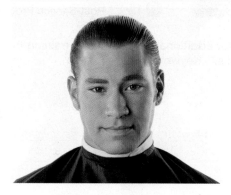

4 Towel dry the hair.

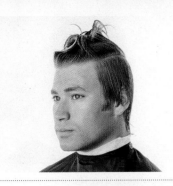
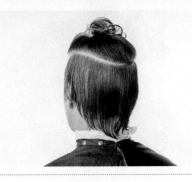

5 Begin the horseshoe section by taking a parting from recession to recession to create a section below the crown, dividing the top from the bottom. Make sure your section is clean and balanced.

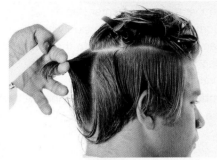

6 Starting at the back, elevate the hair up parallel to the horseshoe section and elevate at 90 degrees. You will be holding the section horizontally. With shears, cut the section 1½-inch (3.75 centimeters) in length on the inside of your fingers.

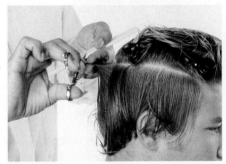
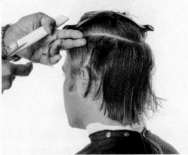

8 The section that you've cut around the horseshoe will serve as a guide.

7 Follow that same guide and technique around the horseshoe section. You should end up with a 1-inch (2.5 centimeters) section parallel to the horseshoe that follows the head shape. Cross-check the sides to eliminate any corners in your design line. When complete, blowdry the section below the horseshoe with a comb in a downward motion until dry.

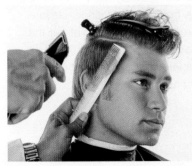
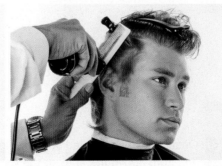
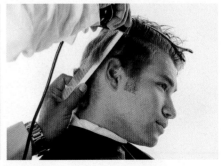

9 Using clippers, starting on the side of the front hairline, hold your comb in a slight diagonal back angle against the scalp. Elevate the hair out at 90 degrees to expose your guide. Place your clippers against the comb and cut the section up to your guide.

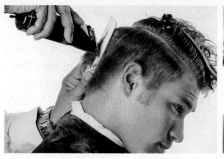 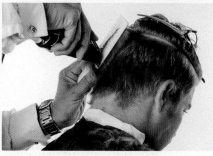 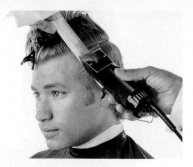

🔟 Tilt the comb at a 45-degree angle and cut short to long. The longest point will be your guide below the horseshoe. (For a tapered, uniform look, place the comb at the scalp and avoid tilting the comb.)

1️⃣1️⃣ The subsection cut will be no wider than the width of the comb. Use steady uniformed strokes and glide the clippers up the comb to the guide. Continue to comb the hair in a slight diagonal back fashion, elevating it at 90 degrees, and cutting to your guide.

1️⃣2️⃣ Continue this technique until you've reach the center back. Complete the opposite side with the same technique cutting to the center back and cross-check horizontally. Once you've completed the underneath, blowdry the hair below the horseshoe.

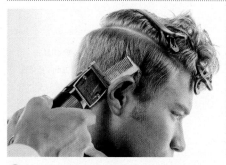 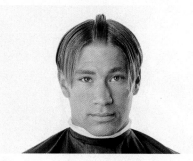

1️⃣3️⃣ Using the clipper and a ¼-inch (0.6 centimeters) guard, shorten and shape the hair around ears. Then blend or outline the perimeter of the haircut; you may use a clipper or trimmer.

1️⃣4️⃣ Using a water bottle, re-wet the top section. Switch back to cutting shears and create a ½-inch center profile section from the front hairline to your guide below the crown.

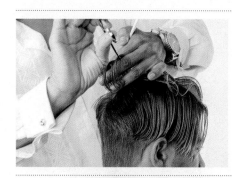 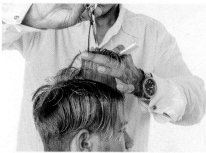

1️⃣5️⃣ Starting at the center back, using the 1½-inch (3.75 centimeters) guide from the horseshoe, elevate guide to 90 degrees. Point cut the guide following the head shape. Complete your profile section to the front hairline.

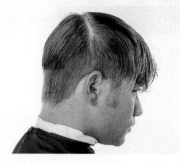

1️⃣6️⃣ Once you've completed your profile section, you will then take a radial section from above the apex to the parietal ridge.

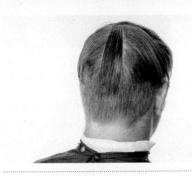

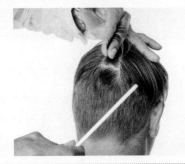

17 Here you will take pivoting pie-shape sections from below your radial section. Following your guideline, elevating the hair at 90 degrees, and point cutting until you've completed the radial section on both sides. (Remember to cross-check.)

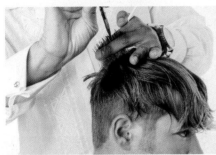

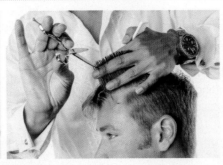

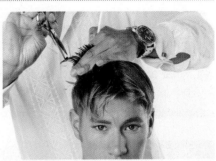

18 When you reach the top of the section, you will switch to making horizontal subsections, elevating at 90 degrees. These subsections will be point cut following your guide from the center and behind the radial section. When you reach the parietal ridge, elevate the hair at 90 degrees, and point cut the corners to blend with the sides. (Remember to cross-check.)

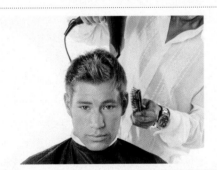

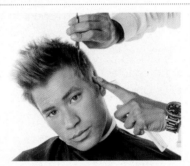

19 Blowdry with a vent brush and then detail the bangs with point cutting. Texturize with slicing and carving for a disheveled look.

20 Finished look.

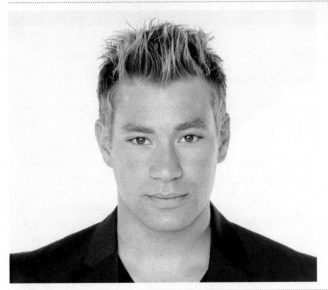

POST-SERVICE

Complete

P 15-2 **Post-Service Procedure** See page 343

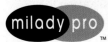

Check out miladypro.com for additional resources and training to enhance your technical skills. Keyword: *FutureCosPro*

REVIEW QUESTIONS

1. What are reference points and what is their function?

2. What are lines, sections, elevations, and guidelines?

3. What are important considerations to discuss with a client during a haircutting consultation?

4. What are a razor, haircutting shears, styling or cutting comb, and texturizing shears used for?

5. What are three things you can do to ensure good posture and body position while cutting hair?

6. Name and describe the four basic types of haircuts.

7. What is another name for *bangs*? When should you avoid cutting bangs? Name 5 basic types of bangs.

8. Name and describe three or more different texturizing techniques performed with shears.

9. What is a clipper cut?

10. How is a trimmer used?

STUDY TOOLS

- **Reinforce what you just learned:** Complete the activities and exercises in your Theory or Practical Workbook, or your Study Guide.

- **Expand your knowledge:** Search for websites about the topics in this chapter and make a list of additional resources.

- **Study and prepare for your quiz:** Take the chapter test in your Exam Review or your Milady U: Online Licensing Prep.

- **Re-Test your knowledge:** Take the Chapter 16 *Quizzes*!

- **Learn even more:** Look up in a dictionary or search the internet for the definitions for any additional terms you want to learn about.

CHAPTER GLOSSARY

angle	p. 361	Space between two lines or surfaces that intersect at a given point.
apex AY-peks	p. 359	Highest point on the top of the head.
beveling	p. 362	Haircutting technique using diagonal lines by cutting hair ends with a slight increase or decrease in length.
blunt haircut	p. 382	Also known as a *one-length haircut*; haircut in which all the hair comes to one hanging level, forming a weight line or area; hair is cut with no elevation or overdirection.
carving	p. 396	Haircutting technique done by placing the still blade into the hair, resting it on the scalp, and then moving the shears through the hair while opening and partially closing the shears.
cast	p. 371	Method of manufacturing shears; a metal-forming process whereby molten steel is poured into a mold and, once the metal is cooled, takes on the shape of the mold.

clipper-over-comb	p. 400	Haircutting technique similar to scissor-over-comb, except that the clippers move side to side across the comb rather than bottom to top.
cross-checking	p. 384	Parting the haircut in the opposite way from which you cut it in order to check for precision of line and shape.
crown	p. 360	Area of the head between the apex and back of the parietal ridge.
cutting line	p. 363	Angle at which the fingers are held when cutting, and, ultimately, the line that is cut; also known as *finger angle*, *finger position*, *cutting position*, or *cutting angle*.
diagonal back	p. 362	A type of diagonal line that creates movement away from the face.
diagonal forward	p. 362	A type of diagonal line that creates movement toward the face.
distribution	p. 390	Where and how hair is moved over the head.
effilating	p. 396	Also known as *slithering*; process of thinning the hair to graduated lengths with shears; cutting the hair with a sliding movement of the shears while keeping the blades partially opened.
elevation	p. 363	Also known as *projection* or *lifting*; the degree at which a subsection of hair is held, or lifted, from the head when cutting.
forged FORJed	p. 372	Process of working metal to a finished shape by hammering or pressing.
four corners	p. 359	Points on the head that signal a change in the shape of the head, from flat to round or vice versa.
free-hand notching	p. 395	Haircutting technique in which pieces of hair are snipped out at random intervals.
free-hand slicing	p. 397	Haircutting technique used to release weight from the subsection, allowing the hair to move more freely.
graduated haircut	p. 382	Slow or immediate buildup of weight; an effect or haircut that results from cutting the hair with tension, low to medium elevation, or overdirection.
graduation	p. 363	Elevation that occurs when a section is lifted above 0 degrees.
growth pattern	p. 368	Direction in which the hair grows from the scalp; also referred to as *natural fall* or *natural falling* position.
guideline	p. 364	Also known as *guide*; section of hair, located either at the perimeter or the interior of the cut, which determines the length the hair will be cut. Usually the first section that is cut to create a shape.
hairline	p. 368	Hair that grows at the outermost perimeter along the face, around the ears, and on the neck.
head form	p. 358	Also known as *head shape*; the shape of the head, which greatly affects the way the hair falls and behaves.
Interior	p. 364	Inner or internal part.
interior guideline	p. 387	Guideline that is inside the haircut rather than on the perimeter.
layered haircut	p. 382	Effect achieved by cutting the hair with elevation or overdirection; the hair is cut at higher elevations, usually 90 degrees or above, which removes weight.
layers	p. 383	Create movement and volume in the hair by releasing weight.

line	p. 361	Thin, continuous mark used as a guide; can be straight or curved, horizontal, vertical, or diagonal.
long-layered haircut	p. 383	Haircut in which the hair is cut at a 90-degree elevation and then overdirected to maintain length and weight at the perimeter.
nape	p. 360	Back part of the neck; the hair below the occipital bone.
notching	p. 395	Haircutting technique, a version of point cutting, in which the tips of the shears are moved toward the hair ends rather than into them; creates a chunkier effect.
occipital bone ahk-SIP-ih-tul BOHN	p. 359	Bone that protrudes at the base of the skull.
overdirection	p. 366	Combing a section away from its natural falling position, rather than straight out from the head, toward a guideline; used to create increasing lengths in the interior or perimeter.
palm-to-palm	p. 381	Cutting position in which the palms of both hands are facing each other.
parietal ridge puh-RY-ate-ul RIJ	p. 359	Widest area of the head, usually starting at the temples and ending at the bottom of the crown.
part/parting	p. 362	Line dividing the hair at the scalp, separating one section of hair from another, creating subsections.
perimeter	p. 364	Outer line of a hairstyle.
pivoting	p. 362	Rotates from a central point; also referred to as *pie shape sections*, used for layering and graduating.
point cutting	p. 395	Haircutting technique in which the tips of the shears are used to cut *points* into the ends of the hair.
razor-over-comb	p. 398	Texturizing technique in which the comb and the razor are used on the surface of the hair.
razor rotation	p. 398	Texturizing technique similar to razor-over-comb, done with small circular motions.
reference points	p. 359	Points on the head that mark where the surface of the head changes or the behavior of the hair changes, such as ears, jawline, occipital bone, apex, and so on; used to establish design lines that are proportionate.
scissor-over-comb	p. 393	Also known as *shear-over-comb*; haircutting technique in which the hair is held in place with the comb while the tips of the shears are used to remove length.
section	p. 361	To divide the hair by parting into uniform working areas for control. During haircutting, the working areas of the hair. Working in smaller sections gives better control.
shrinkage	p. 363	When hair contracts or lifts through the action of moisture loss or drying.
slicing	p. 396	Haircutting technique that removes weight and adds movement through the lengths of the hair; the shears are not completely closed, and only the portion of the blades near the pivot is used.
slide cutting	p. 393	Method of cutting or layering the hair in which the fingers and shears glide along the edge of the hair to remove length.

stationary guideline	p. 364	Guideline that does not move.
subsections	p. 362	Smaller sections within a larger section of hair, used to maintain control of the hair while cutting.
taper	p. 400	Haircutting effect in which there is an even blend from very short at the hairline to longer lengths as you move up the head; *to taper* is to narrow progressively at one end.
tension	p. 380	Amount of pressure applied when combing and holding a section, created by stretching or pulling the section.
texturizing	p. 394	Haircutting technique designed to remove excess bulk without shortening the length; changing the appearance or behavior of the hair through specific haircutting techniques using shears, thinning shears, or a razor.
traveling guideline	p. 364	Also known as *movable guideline*; guideline that moves as the haircutting progresses, used often when creating layers or graduation.
uniform layers	p. 387	Hair is elevated to 90 degrees from the scalp and cut at the same length.
weight line	p. 382	Visual line in the haircut where the ends of the hair hang together.

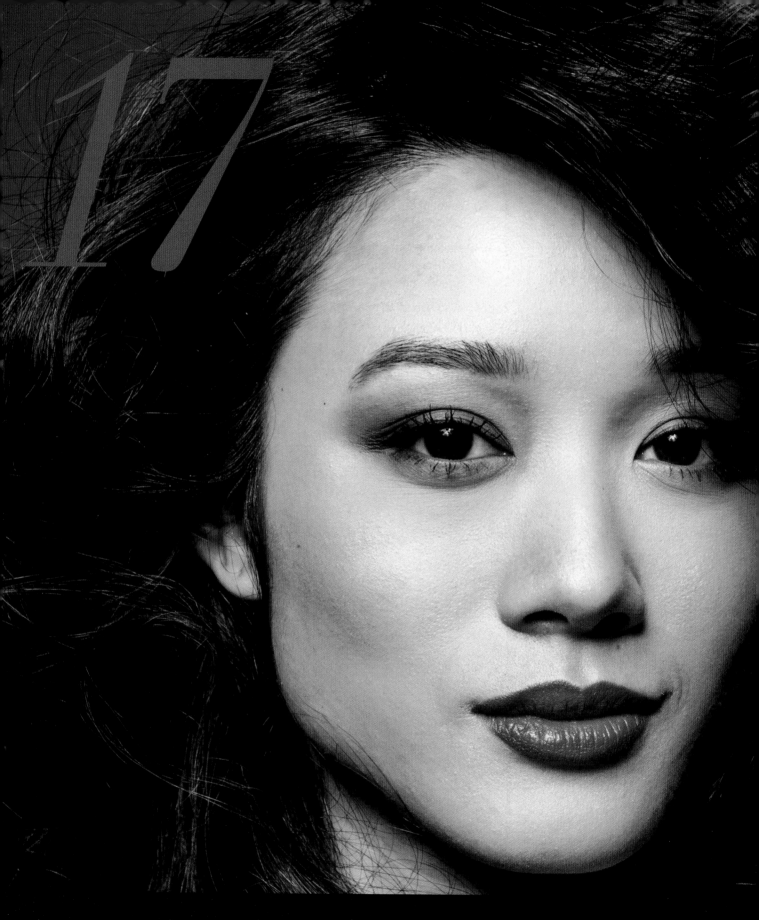

17

HAIRSTYLING

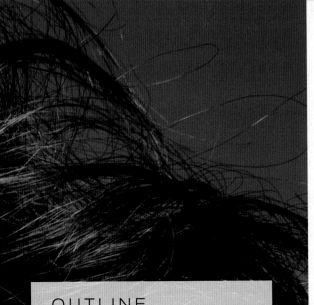

LEARNING OBJECTIVES

After completing this chapter, you will be able to:

LO❶
Execute finger waving, pin curling, roller setting, and hair wrapping.

LO❷
Perform various blowdry styling techniques and learn the proper use of blowdrying tools.

LO❸
Demonstrate the proper use of thermal irons.

LO❹
Demonstrate the proper use of a flat iron and show an understanding of heat settings.

LO❺
Demonstrate various thermal iron manipulations and explain how they are used.

LO❻
Perform the four basic curl patterns and explain the end result.

LO❼
Describe the three types of hair pressing.

LO❽
Understand the importance of preparation, sectioning, pinning, and balance with regard to updos.

LO❾
Create the two foundational updos for styling long hair.

The art of hairstyling or dressing the hair has always changed in direct relation to the fashion, art, and life of the times. When you compare the ornate hair fantasies of Marie Antoinette and her court prior to the French Revolution to the sleek bobs with finger waves and pin curls of flappers during the 1920s and 1930s, when streamline modern or art deco was the rage, you can see how a person's hairstyle reflects the period in which they live (figure 17-1).

The necessity of learning long hair and styling techniques is two-fold when becoming a cosmetologist. We can't call ourselves hairdressers if we only concentrate on one area of our craft. A hairdresser is a professional with well-rounded skills that can adapt to the individual needs of the client. By mastering "hair-dressing" we will not only learn discipline but finger dexterity or the manipulation of our hands. The basic long hair and styling techniques shown in this chapter can easily be adapted for salon work and also enable you to offer more options to your client. Focus on understanding these basic principles and over time you will build consistency, quality, and the confidence to approach any hairstyle.

why study
HAIRSTYLING?

Cosmetologists should study and have a thorough understanding of hairstyling because:

> Hairstyling is an important, foundational skill that allows the professional to articulate creativity and deliver a specific outcome desired by the client.

> Clients rely on you to teach them about their hair and how to style it so they can have a variety of options based on their lifestyle and fashion needs. You are the expert!

> The client looks to you for that special style desired for that special day.

> Hairstyling skills will enable you to help clients to be as contemporary as they would like to be, allowing them to keep up with the trends.

> This knowledge helps make you a well-rounded hairdresser, and it also creates discipline and cleanliness in your work.

> If one of your goals is to work on photo shoots or do editorial work for fashion, you must first master the basic techniques.

figure 17-1
Today, many women wear beautiful and dramatic finger wave styles for special occasions.

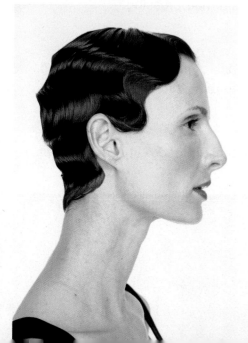

Start with a Client Consultation

The client consultation is always the first step in the hairstyling process. Have your client look through magazines to find styles that she likes, or better yet, show her your portfolio of hairstyles. A picture is worth a thousand words. When deciding the best hairstyle, take into consideration all that you have learned in Chapter 14, Principles of Hair Design, regarding face shape, hair type, and lifestyle.

Often, you will be called upon as a creative problem solver. What if, on the client's last visit to another salon, she asked for a hairstyle that was not right for her hair? Because the stylist did not suggest something more appropriate, the outcome was disastrous. Now you are being asked to fix the problem. If you can come up with an alternative style, one that is both flattering and easy to manage, she may become one of your most loyal clients.

Learn the Basics of Wet Hairstyling

Wet hairstyling tools include the following items:

- Combs
- Brushes
- Rollers (plastic)
- Pins (bobby pins and hairpins)
- Clips (duckbill, sectioning, double prong, and single prong)
- Clamps (sectioning clamps) (**figure 17-2**)

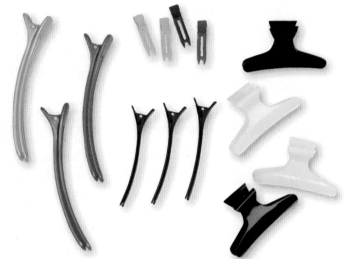

figure 17-2
Clips (left to right: duckbill, sectioning, double prong, and sectioning clamps)

After reading the next few sections, you will be able to:

LO **1** Execute finger waving, pin curling, roller setting, and hair wrapping.

Perform Finger Waving

Finger waving is the process of shaping and directing the hair into an S pattern through the use of the fingers, combs, and finger-waving lotion. Finger waving was all the rage in the 1920s and 1930s, which may have you wondering why you are being asked to learn this technique today. The answer is that many women today are influenced by the movie stars and celebrities they see wearing gorgeous, dramatic finger waves!

From Madonna to Tyra Banks, well-known celebrities have embraced the elegance of the finger-wave style for the red carpet and other special, highly televised and photographed events. Clients will ask you for the very same look for their own special occasions, and you need to be prepared! In addition to its use in today's fashions, finger waving teaches you the technique of moving and directing hair. It also provides valuable training in molding hair to the curved surface of the head and is an excellent introduction to hairstyling.

Finger-Waving Lotion

Finger-waving lotion also known as *liquid gel*, is a type of hair gel that makes the hair pliable enough to keep it in place during the finger-waving procedure. It is traditionally made from karaya (kuh-Ry-uh) gum, taken from trees found in Africa and India. Karaya gum is diluted for use on fine hair, or it can be used in a more concentrated consistency on medium or coarse hair. A good finger-waving lotion is harmless to the hair and does not flake when it dries. Be sure not to use too much of it at any one time. You will know if you have used too much because the hair will be too wet and the waving lotion will drip. Liquid styling gels are also commonly used in conjunction with finger waving and in many cases they have replaced traditional karaya gum products.

Other Methods of Finger Waving

Instead of completing one side before beginning the other, you may want to complete the first ridge on one side of the head and then move to the other side. After joining the two, you can repeat the process in this manner until you are finished with the entire head.

In vertical finger waving, the ridges and waves run up and down the head. Horizontal finger waves are sideways and parallel around the head. The procedure is the same for both.

P 17-1   **Preparing Hair for Wet Styling** *See page 475*

P 17-2   **Horizontal Finger Waving** *See page 481*

Form Pin Curls

Pin curls serve as the basis for patterns, lines, waves, curls, and rolls that are used in a wide range of hairstyles. You can use them on all types of hair, including straight, permanent waved, or naturally curly hair. Pin curls work best when the hair is layered and smoothly wound. This style makes springy and long-lasting curls with good direction and definition.

Parts of a Curl

Pin curls are made up of three principal parts: base, stem, and circle (**figure 17-3**).

The **base** is the stationary (non-moving) foundation of the curl, which is the area closest to the scalp; the panel of hair on which the pin curl is placed.

The **stem** is the section of the pin curl between the base and first arc (turn) of the circle that gives the curl its direction and movement; the hair between the scalp and the first turn of the pin curl.

The **circle** is the part of the curl that forms a complete circle and ultimately the wave. The size of the circle determines the width of the wave and its strength.

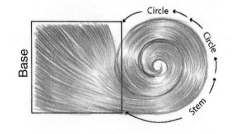

figure 17-3
Parts of a curl

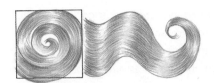

figure 17-4
No-stem curl unwound

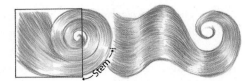

figure 17-5
Half-stem curl opened out

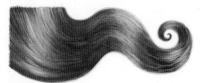

figure 17-6
Full-stem curl opened out

Mobility of a Curl

The stem determines the amount of mobility, or movement, in a section of hair. Curl mobility is classified as no stem, half stem, and full stem.

- The **no-stem curl** is placed directly on the base of the curl. It produces a tight, firm, long-lasting curl and allows minimum mobility (figure 17-4).

- The **half-stem curl** permits medium movement; the curl (circle) is placed half off the base. It gives good control to the hair (figure 17-5).

- The **full-stem curl** allows for the greatest mobility. The curl is placed completely off the base. The base may be a square, triangular, half-moon, or rectangular section, depending on the area of the head in which the full-stem curls are used. It gives as much freedom as the length of the stem will permit. If it is exaggerated, the hair near the scalp will be flat and almost straight. It is used to give the hair a strong, definite direction (figure 17-6).

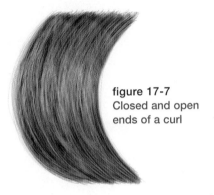

figure 17-7
Closed and open ends of a curl

Shaping for Pin Curl Placements

A **shaping** is a section of hair that is molded in a circular movement in preparation for the formation of curls. Shapings are either open- or closed-end. Always begin a pin curl at the open end, or convex side, of a shaping (figures 17-7 and 17-8).

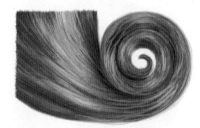

figure 17-8
Curl in the shaping

Open- and Closed-Center Curls

Open-center curls produce even, smooth waves and uniform curls. **Closed-center curls** produce waves that get smaller toward the ends. They are good for fine hair or if a fluffy curl is desired. Note the difference in the waves produced by pin curls with open centers and those with closed centers. The width of the curl determines the size of the wave. If you make pin curls with the ends outside the curl, the resulting wave will be narrower near the scalp and wider toward the ends (figures 17-9 and 17-10).

Curl and Stem Direction

Curls may be turned toward the face, away from the face, upward, downward, or diagonally. The finished result will be determined by the stem's direction.

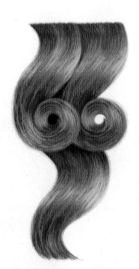

figure 17-9
Curl with open center

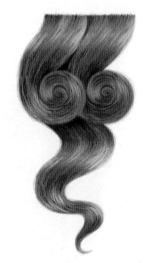

figure 17-10
Curl with closed center

The terms *clockwise curls* and *counterclockwise curls* are used to describe the direction of pin curls. Curls formed in the same direction as the movement of the hands of a clock are known as *clockwise curls*.

Curls formed in the opposite direction are known as *counterclockwise curls*.

Pin Curl Bases or Foundations

Before you begin to make pin curls, divide the wet hair into sections or panels. Then subdivide each section into the type of base required for the various curls. The most commonly shaped base is the arc base (half-moon or C-shaped). Others are rectangular, triangular, or square.

To avoid splits in the finished hairstyle, you must use care when selecting and forming the curl base. When the sections of hair are as close to equal as possible, you will get curls that are similar to one another. Each curl must lie flat and smooth on its base. If it is too far off the base, the curl will lie loose away from the scalp. The shape of the base, however, does not affect the finished curl.

- Rectangular base pin curls are usually recommended at the side front hairline for a smooth, upswept effect (**figure 17-11**). To avoid splits in the comb out, the pin curls must overlap.

- Triangular base pin curls are recommended along the front or facial hairline to prevent breaks or splits in the finished hairstyle. The triangular base allows a portion of the hair from each curl to overlap the next and this style can be combed into a wave without splits (**figure 17-12**).

- Arc base pin curls, also known as *half-moon* or *C-shaped base curls*, are carved out of a shaping. Arc base pin curls give good direction and may be used at the hairline or in the nape (**figure 17-13**).

- Square base pin curls are suitable for curly hairstyles without much volume or lift. They can be used on any part of the head and will comb out with lasting results. To avoid splits in the comb out, stagger the sectioning as shown in the illustration (square base, brick-lay fashion) (**figure 17-14**).

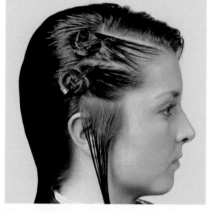
figure 17-11
Rectangular base pin curls

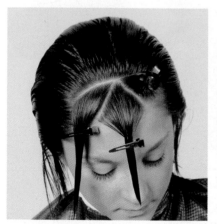
figure 17-12
Triangular base pin curls

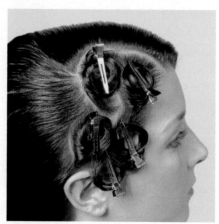
figure 17-13
Arc base pin curls

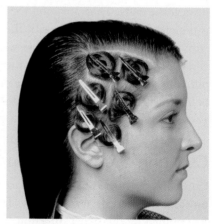
figure 17-14
Square base pin curls

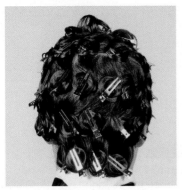

figure 17-15
Setting pattern for a wave.

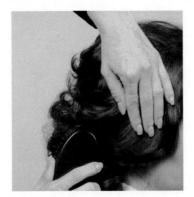

figure 17-16
Comb out of wave setting.

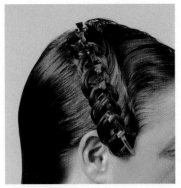

figure 17-17
Setting pattern for ridge curl

Pin Curl Techniques

Various methods are used to make pin curls. We will illustrate several methods below, but your instructor might demonstrate other methods that are equally effective.

One important technique to learn is called **ribboning** (RIB-un-ing), which involves forcing the hair between the thumb and the back of the comb to create tension. You can also ribbon hair by pulling the strands while applying pressure between your thumb and index finger out toward the ends of the strands.

Carved or Sculptured Curls

Pin curls sliced from a shaping and formed without lifting the hair from the head are referred to as **carved curls**, also known as *sculptured curls*.

Designing with Pin Curls

- To create a wave, use two rows of pin curls. Set one row clockwise and the second row counterclockwise (**figures 17-15** and **17-16**).

- **Ridge curls** are pin curls placed immediately behind or below a ridge to form a wave (**figures 17-17** and **17-18**).

- **Skip waves** are two rows of ridge curls, usually on the side of the head. Skip waves create a strong wave pattern with well-defined lines between the waves. This technique represents a combination of finger waving and pin curls (**figures 17-19** and **17-20**).

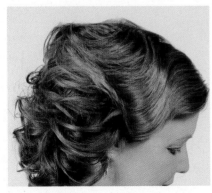

figure 17-18
Comb out for ridge curl

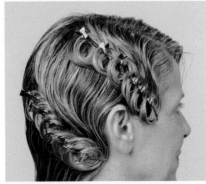

figure 17-19
Setting pattern for skip wave

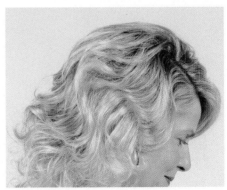

figure 17-20
Comb out of skip wave setting

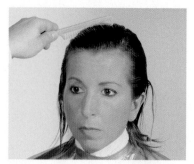
figure 17-21
Comb, divide, and smooth section

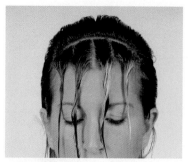
figure 17-22
Divide section into strands

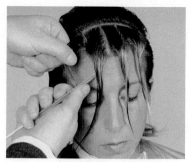
figure 17-23
Ribbon the strand.

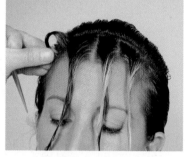
figure 17-24
Direct the strand.

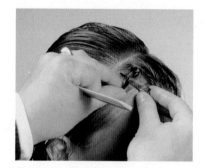
figure 17-25
Anchor curl at base.

- **Barrel curls** have large center openings and are fastened to the head in a standing position on a rectangular base. They have the same effect as stand-up pin curls. A barrel curl's effect is similar to that of a roller, but it does not have the same tension as a roller when it is set.

Creating Volume with Pin Curls

One of the best things about pin curls is they can add volume to the hair. Two types of pin curls that are particularly effective for adding volume are the following:

- **Cascade curls**, also known as *stand-up curls*, are used to create height in the hair design. They are fastened to the head in a standing position to allow the hair to flow upward and then downward. The size of the curl determines the amount of height in the comb out (**figures 17-21** through **17-27**).

 P 17-3 **Wet Set with Rollers** *See page 485*

Create Roller Curls

Rollers are used to create many of the same effects as stand-up pin curls. Rollers have the following advantages over pin curls:

- Because a roller holds the equivalent of two to four stand-up curls, the roller is a much faster way to set the hair.

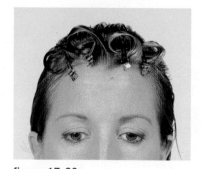
figure 17-26a
Top setting

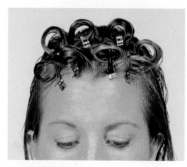
figure 17-26b
Top setting

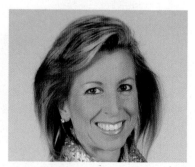
figure 17-27
Comb out as you would a roller set.

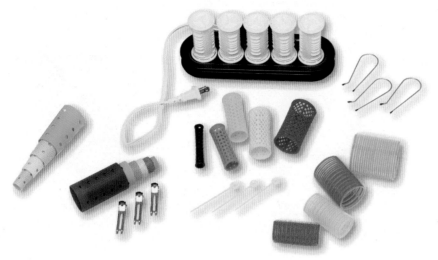

figure 17-28
Rollers (left to right): plastic, mesh, hot, and Velcro

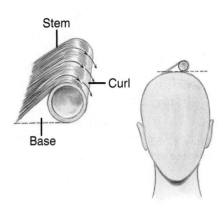

figure 17-29
Parts of a roller curl: base, stem and curl

- The hair is wrapped around the roller with tension, which gives a stronger and longer-lasting set.
- Rollers come in a variety of shapes, widths, and sizes, which broadens the creative possibilities for any style (figure 17-28).

Parts of a Roller Curl

It is important for you to be able to identify the three parts of a roller curl (figure 17-29).

- The **base** is the panel of hair on which the roller is placed. The base should be the same length and width as the roller. The type of base affects the volume.
- The **stem** is the hair between the scalp and the first turn of the roller. The stem gives the hair direction and mobility.
- The **curl**, also known as *circle*, is the hair that is wrapped around the roller. It determines the size of the wave or curl.

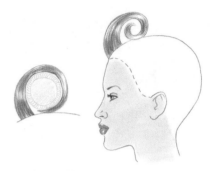

figure 17-30
C-shaped curl

Choosing Your Roller Size

The relationship between the length of the hair and the size of the roller will determine whether the result will be a C shape, wave, or curl. These three shapes are created as follows:

- One complete turn around the roller will create a C-shape curl (figure 17-30).
- One and a half turns will create a wave (figure 17-31).
- Two and a half turns will create curls (figure 17-32).

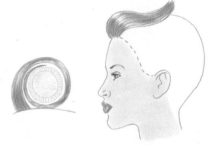

figure 17-31
Wave

Roller Placement

The amount of volume that is achieved depends on the size of the roller and how the roller sits on its base. The general rule of thumb for base control is that the larger the roller, the greater the volume. There are three

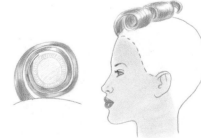

figure 17-32
Curl

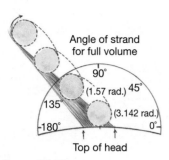

figure 17-33
On-base roller: full volume

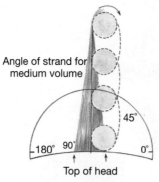

figure 17-34
Half-base roller: medium volume

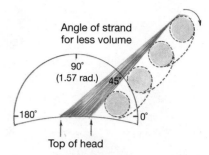

figure 17-35
Off-base roller: less volume

kinds of bases: on base, half base, and off base. **Note:** These bases are also useful when round brushing, using a curling iron/marcel, and backcombing.

- **On base**, also known as *full base*. For full volume, the roller sits directly on its base. Overdirect (higher than 90 degrees) the strand slightly in front of the base and roll the hair down to the base. The roller should fit on the base (**figure 17-33**).

- **Half base**. For medium volume, the roller sits halfway on its base and halfway behind the base. Hold the strand straight up (90 degrees) from the head and roll the hair down (**figure 17-34**).

- **Off base**. For the least volume, the roller sits completely off the base. Hold the strand 45 degrees down from the base and roll the hair down (**figure 17-35**).

Roller Direction

The placement of rollers on the head usually follows the movement of the finished style. For versatility in styling, a downward directional wrap gives options to style in all directions—under, out, forward, or back—while still maintaining volume. To reduce volume, bringing movement closer to the head, use indentation curl placement.

Indentation is the point where curls of opposite directions meet, forming a recessed area. This is often found in flip styles or in bangs (fringes) with a dip or wave movement. Indentation can be achieved using rollers, curling irons, or a round brush.

Hot Rollers

Hot rollers are to be used only on dry hair. They are heated either electrically or by steam and they are a great time saver in the salon. Follow the same setting patterns as with wet setting, but allow the hot roller to stay on the hair for about 10 minutes. A thermal protector can be sprayed on the hair before setting. The result is a curl that is weaker than a wet-set curl, but stronger and longer lasting than can be achieved using a curling iron. Spray-on products are available for application to each section of hair to create a stronger set.

Velcro™ Rollers

Velcro rollers are not allowed by the state board of some states and provinces because they are difficult to clean and disinfect properly. Check with your regulatory agency to determine if you can use them in your state.

Like hot rollers, Velcro rollers are used only on dry hair. Using them on wet hair will snag and pull the hair. If you have a client who needs more body than can be achieved with a round brush, but less volume than a hot roller or wet set will produce, try Velcro rollers. When they are used after blowdrying, Velcro rollers may provide just the amount of volume you need.

Velcro rollers need to stay in the hair for only 5 to 10 minutes, depending on how much set you want in the hair. Follow the same setting patterns as with wet setting, but keep in mind that no clipping is necessary to secure the roller. The Velcro fabric grips the hair well and stays in place on its own.

Mist the entire head with hair spray and then either place the client under a hooded dryer for 5 to 10 minutes or use the diffuser attachment on your blowdryer for the recommended time to give a soft set to the hair. For an even softer look, do not apply heat after the rollers are put in; simply have your client sit for a few minutes. This would be a good time to instruct the client on how she can repeat the process at home in order to maintain the style.

Always remove any hair from Velcro and electric rollers after use. See Chapter 5, Infection Control: Principles and Practices, for instructions on disinfecting multiuse items like rollers.

Master Comb-Out Techniques

A good set leads to a good comb out (figure 17-36). For successful finishes, learn how to shape and mold the hair and then practice fast, simple, and effective methods for comb outs (figure 17-37). If you follow a well-structured system of combing out hairstyles, you will save time and get more consistent results.

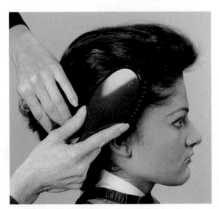

figure 17-36
Brush out the hair.

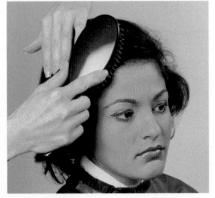

figure 17-37
Direct the hair into desired pattern.

Backcombing and Backbrushing Techniques

Base control is the primary way of establishing the amount of volume in the hair.

Backcombing and backbrushing are also used to lift and increase volume, give direction, as well as to remove indentations caused by roller setting. **Backcombing**, also known as *teasing, ratting, matting,* or *French lacing,* involves combing small sections of hair from the ends toward the scalp, causing shorter hair to mat at the scalp and form a cushion or base. **Backbrushing**, also known as *ruffing* (RUF-ing), is used to build a soft cushion or to mesh two or more curl patterns together for a uniform and smooth comb out.

During the 1950s and 1960s, women typically had their hair wet set and combed out and the set would last an entire week with backcombing and backbrushing. Now these techniques are used for styling updos or for adding a little height to a hairstyle after hot-roller setting or blowdrying.

Backcombing Technique

1. **Section hair.** Starting in the front, pick up a section of hair no more than 1 inch thick and no more than 2- to 3-inches (5 to 7.5 centimeters) wide.

2. **Insert comb.** Insert the fine teeth of your comb into the hair at a depth of about 1½ inches (3.75 centimeters) from the scalp (figure 17-38).

3. **Press comb down.** Press the comb gently down toward the scalp, sliding it down and out of the hair. Repeat this process, working up the section until the desired volume is achieved (figure 17-39).

4. **Create a cushion.** If you wish to create a cushion (base), the third time you insert the comb, use the same sliding motion but firmly push the hair down to the scalp. Slide the comb out of the hair (figure 17-40).

5. **Repeat for volume.** Repeat this process, working up the strand until the desired volume is achieved.

6. **Smooth hair.** To smooth hair that is backcombed, hold the teeth of a comb (or the bristles of a brush) at a 45-degree angle pointing away from you, and lightly move the comb over the surface of the hair (figure 17-41).

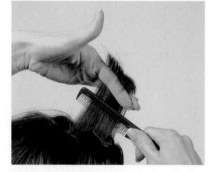

figure 17-38
Insert comb.

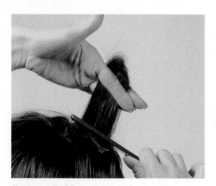

figure 17-39
Press comb down.

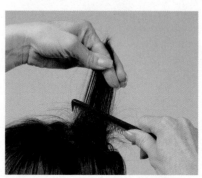

figure 17-40
Create base of backcombed hair.

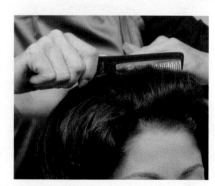

figure 17-41
Smooth hair with comb

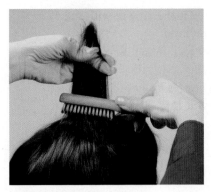

figure 17-42
Roll brush.

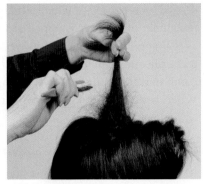

figure 17-43
Remove brush.

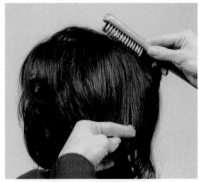

figure 17-44
Blend sections with backcombing.

Backbrushing Technique

1. **Hold strand.** Pick up and hold a strand straight out from the scalp.

2. **Place brush.** Maintaining a slight amount of slack in the strand, place a teasing brush or a grooming brush near the base of the strand. Push and roll the inner edge of the brush with the wrist until it touches the scalp.

3. **Roll brush.** For interlocking to occur, the brush must be rolled (figure 17-42).

4. **Turn brush.** Remove the brush from the hair with a turn of the wrist, peeling back a layer of hair (figure 17-43). The hair will be interlocked to form a soft cushion at the scalp.

5. **Blend hair.** You can create softness and evenness of flow by blending, smoothing, and combing (figure 17-44). Avoid exaggerations and overemphasis. Finished patterns should reflect rhythm, balance, and smoothness of line.

6. **Complete styling.** Final touches make hairstyles look professional, so take your time. After completing the comb out, you can use the tail of a comb to lift areas where the shape and form are not as full as you want them to be. Every touch during the final stage must be very lightly done. When you have completed your finishing touches, check the entire set for structural balance and then lightly spray the hair with a finishing spray.

Understand Hair Wrapping

Hair wrapping is a technique used to keep curly hair smooth and straight while retaining a beautiful shape. Curly hair can be wrapped around the head to give it a smooth, rounded contour, resulting in an effect that is similar to that attained with rollers. When wrapping hair, very little volume is attained because the hair at the scalp is not lifted. If height is desired, you can place large rollers directly at the crown, with the remainder of the hair wrapped around the head.

Wrapping can be done on wet or dry hair. When wrapping dry hair, use a silicone shine product instead of using a gel; this will provide a glossy comb out. On curly hair, wet wrapping creates a smooth, sleek look. When working with very curly hair, press it first, then do a dry hair wrapping.

Ⓟ 17-4 **Hair Wrapping** *See page 487*

After reading the next few sections, you will be able to:

LO❷ **Perform various blowdry styling techniques and learn the proper use of blowdrying tools.**

Finish Hair Using Basic Blowdry Styling

Blowdry styling is the technique of drying and styling damp hair in one operation and it has revolutionized the hairstyling world. Today, women desire hairstyles that require the least possible time and effort to maintain. The selection of styling tools, techniques, and products must relate to the client's lifestyle. Is the client capable of styling her own hair and how much time will she have to do it? As the stylist, you are responsible for guiding and educating the client through this process. To do so, you must first learn all about the tools and products available to you. Remember, the client's first impression of the haircut you have provided will be determined by the quality of the blowdry.

The following are guidelines to follow when blowdry styling:

- Never hold the blowdryer too long in one place.

- Move the blowdryer in a constant back and forth motion unless you are using the cooling button to cool a section.

- Always direct the hot air away from the client's scalp to avoid scalp burns.

- Direct the hot air from the scalp toward the ends of the hair. The hot air should flow in the direction in which the hair is wound; improper technique will rough up the hair cuticle and give the hair a frizzy appearance.

- Because hair stretches easily when it is wet, partially towel dry the hair before blowdrying. This is especially important when you are working with damaged or chemically treated hair. This is not necessary if you are cutting the hair before you blowdry it, as the hair will already be partially dry due to the amount of time it takes to cut it.

✔ **HERE'S A TIP**
Wondering when to use a hood dryer versus a blowdryer to complete your styling? A hood dryer is best used for any kind of wet set—finger waves, pin curls, or rollers. A wet set will last longer than a blown dry style for many people. A blowdry will give a softer result and often takes less time. Choose the best technique in order to achieve the look you want, given the styling techniques you have used.

Tools for Blowdry Styling

The following are the basic tools used for blowdrying techniques.

The Blowdryer

A blowdryer is an electrical appliance designed for drying and styling hair. Its main parts are a handle, slotted nozzle, small fan, heating element, and speed/heat controls. Some blowdryers also come with cooling buttons that are used to help set the hair. The temperature control switch helps to produce a steady stream of air at the desired temperature. The blowdryer's nozzle attachment, or **concentrator**, is a directional feature that creates a concentrated stream of air. The **diffuser** is an attachment that causes the air to flow more softly and helps to accentuate or keep textural definition (figure 17-45).

To keep your blowdryer as safe and effective as possible, always make sure that it is perfectly clean and free of dirt, oil, and hair before use. Dirt or hair in the blowdryer can cause extreme heat and thus burn the hair. The air intake at the back of the dryer must also be kept clear at all times. If the intake is covered and air cannot pass through freely, the dryer element will burn out prematurely.

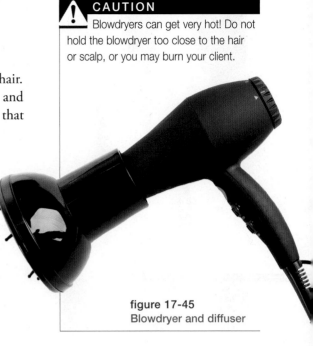
figure 17-45
Blowdryer and diffuser

Combs and Picks

Combs and picks are designed to distribute and part the hair. They come in a wide variety of sizes and shapes to adapt to many styling options (figure 17-46). The length and spacing of the teeth vary from one comb to another. Teeth that are closely spaced remove definition from the curl and create a smooth surface; widely spaced teeth shape larger sections of hair for a more textured surface. Combs with a pick at one end lift the hair away from the head.

Brushes

When choosing a styling brush, take into account the texture, length, and styling needs of the hair that you are working with. Brushes come in many sizes, shapes, and materials (figure 17-47).

- A classic styling brush is a half-round, rubber-based brush. These brushes typically have either seven or nine rows of round-tipped nylon bristles. They are heat resistant, antistatic, and ideal for smoothing and untangling all types of hair. While they are perfect for blowdrying precision haircuts where little volume is desired, they are less suitable for smooth, classic looks.

- Paddle brushes, with their large, flat bases, are well suited for mid-length to longer-length hair. Some have ball-tipped nylon pins and staggered pin patterns that help keep the hair from snagging.

- Grooming brushes are generally oval, with a mixture of boar and nylon bristles. The boar bristles help distribute the scalp oils over the hair shaft, giving it shine. The nylon bristles stimulate the circulation of blood to the scalp. Grooming brushes are particularly useful for adding polish and shine to fine to medium hair, and they are great for combing out updos.

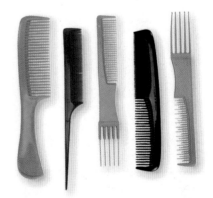
figure 17-46
From left to right: wide-tooth comb, fine-tooth tail comb, styling comb with metal pins, finger-wave comb, teasing comb

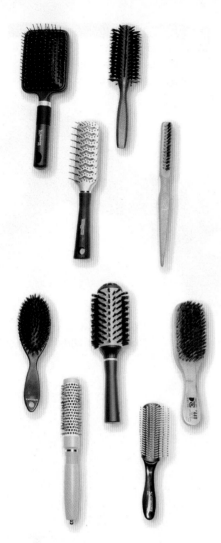

figure 17-47
Brushes: paddle brush, medium round brush, cushion brush, large round brush, vent brush, teasing brush, small round brush, and classic plastic styling brush

- Vent brushes, with their ventilated design, are used to speed up the blowdrying process and they are ideal for blowdrying fine hair and adding lift at the scalp.

- Round brushes come in various diameters. The client's hair should be long enough to wrap twice around the brush. Round brushes often have natural bristles, sometimes with nylon mixed in for better grip. Smaller brushes add more curl; larger brushes straighten the hair and bevel the ends of the hair. Medium round brushes can be used to lift the hair at the scalp. Some round brushes have metal cylinder bases so that the heat from the blowdryer is transferred to the metal base, creating a stronger curl that is similar to those produced with an electric roller. Always use the cooling button on the blowdryer before releasing the section to set the hair into the new shape.

- A teasing brush is a thin, nylon styling brush that has a tail for sectioning, along with a narrow row of bristles. Teasing brushes are perfect for backcombing hair, and the sides of the bristles are ideal for smoothing it into the desired style.

Sectioning Clips

Sectioning clips are usually metal or plastic and have long prongs to hold wet or dry sections of hair in place. It is important to keep the wet hair you are not working on sectioned off in clips so that it does not sit over the dry hair. This is particularly important when drying long hair.

Styling Products

Styling products can be thought of as liquid tools. They give a style more hold, and they can be used to either increase or decrease the amount of curl. They can also be used to add shine. When used correctly, styling products greatly enhance a style.

With so many styling products on the market, stylists need to carefully consider their options before applying one of these products to a client's hair. First, how long does the style need to hold? Under what environmental conditions—dryness, humidity, wind, sun—will the client be wearing the style? You also must consider the type of hair—fine, coarse, straight, curly—when deciding on a product. Heavier products work by causing strands of hair to cling together, adding more pronounced definition, but they can also weigh the hair down, especially fine hair. Styling products range from a light hold to a very firm hold. Determine the amount of support desired and choose accordingly.

Types of Styling Products

- **Foam**, also known as *mousse*, is a light, airy, whipped styling product that resembles shaving foam. It builds moderate body and volume into the hair. Massage it into damp hair to highlight textural movement, or blowdry it straight for styles when body without texture is desired. Foam is good for fine hair because it does not weigh the hair down. It will hold for six to eight hours in dry conditions. Conditioning foams are excellent for drier, more porous hair.

- **Gel** is a thickened styling preparation that comes in a tube or bottle. Gels create the strongest control for slicked or molded styles, and they add distinct texture definition when spread with the fingers. When hair is brushed out, gel creates long-lasting body. Firm hold gel formulations may overwhelm fine hair because of the high resin content. This is not a concern if fine hair is molded into the lines of the style and is not brushed through when dry.

- **Liquid gels**, also known as *texturizers*, are similar to firm hold gels except that they are lighter and less viscous (more liquid) in form. They allow for easy styling, defining, and molding. With brushing, they add volume and body to the style. Good for all hair types, they offer firmer, longer hold for fine hair with the least amount of heaviness and they give a lighter, more moderate hold for normal or coarse hair types. Home-care recommendation regarding styling products is not only professional, but also great customer service. As you style the client's hair, talk about the products you are using to achieve the desired look and why you have chosen them. Have the client hold the product while you demonstrate its uses and benefits. Most clients are eager to learn any and all styling secrets. By discussing and recommending professional products as you use them, you not only educate your client, you also enhance the salon's reputation and help sell its products.

- When **straightening gel** is applied to damp hair (ranging from wavy to extremely curly) and blown dry, it creates a smooth, straight look that provides the most hold in dry outdoor conditions. Straightening gel counters frizz by coating the hair shaft and weighing it down. This is a temporary solution that will last only from shampoo to shampoo. Also, styles that use straightening gel may come undone in extremely humid conditions.

milady pro ™ **LEARN MORE!**

Optional info on **Hair Styling** topics and tutorials can be found at miladypro.com Keyword: *FutureCosPro*

- When sprayed into the roots of fine, wet hair that is then blown dry, **volumizers** add volume, especially at the base. When a vent brush or round brush is used and the hair is not stretched too tightly around the brush, even more volume can be achieved. You may want to add a light gel or mousse to the rest of the hair for more hold, but be careful to avoid the roots and base of hair that has already been treated with volumizer.

- **Pomade** (poh-MAYD), also known as *wax*, adds considerable weight to the hair by causing strands to join together, showing separation in the hair. Used on dry hair, pomade makes the hair very easy to mold, allowing greater manageability. It should be used sparingly on fine hair because of the weight. As a man's grooming product, pomade is excellent on short hair.

- **Silicone** also known as *serum*, adds gloss and sheen to the hair while creating textural definition. Non-oily silicone products are excellent for all hair types, either to provide lubrication and protection to the hair during blowdrying, or to finish a style by adding extra shine. You can mix a couple of drops with most styling products before blowdrying. This application works best on dry, curly, and coarse hair.

DID YOU KNOW?
Graduated Haircuts

Graduated haircuts have either long-layered or short-layered interiors. To blowdry graduated haircuts, use the same basic blowdrying techniques presented in the previous sections, choosing the technique that best suits the length of the hair you are working on.

- **Hair spray**, also known as *finishing spray*, is applied in the form of a mist to hold a style in position. It is the most widely used hairstyling product. Available in both aerosol and pump containers, and in a variety of holding strengths, it is useful for all hair types. Finishing spray is used when the style is complete and will not be disturbed.

- **Thermal protection product**, also known as *heat protection hair care product*, is used on damp hair after you've applied styling product and before blow drying. It protects the hair from heat damage caused by thermal styling tools like blowdryers, flat irons, and curling irons. Thermal protection products can come in a number of forms, including spray, cream, mousse, and serum.

Ⓟ 17-5   **Blowdrying Short, Layered, Curly Hair to Produce Smooth and Full Finish** See page 489

Ⓟ 17-6   **Blowdrying Short, Curly Hair in Its Natural Wave Pattern** See page 493

Ⓟ 17-7   **Diffusing Long, Curly, or Extremely Curly Hair in Its Natural Wave Pattern** See page 495

Ⓟ 17-8   **Blowdrying Straight or Wavy Hair for Maximum Volume** See page 499

Ⓟ 17-9   **Blowdrying Blunt or Long-Layered, Straight to Wavy Hair into a Straight Style** See page 504

Maintain Safety in Thermal Hairstyling

Thermal waving and curling, also known as *Marcel waving*, are methods of waving and curling straight or pressed dry hair using thermal irons and special manipulative techniques (figure 17-48). Thermal irons, which can be either electric or stove heated, have been modernized so successfully that they are more popular today than ever before. These manipulative techniques are basically the same for electric irons or stove-heated irons.

After reading the next few sections, you will be able to:

LO❸   Demonstrate the proper use of thermal irons.

LO❹   Demonstrate the proper use of a flat iron and show an understanding of heat settings.

Thermal Irons

Thermal irons are implements made of quality steel that are used to curl dry hair. They provide an even heat that is completely controlled by the stylist. Electric curling irons have cylindrical barrels ranging from ½ inch

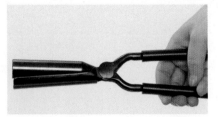

figure 17-48
Conventional thermal (Marcel) iron

to 3 inches in diameter (figure 17-49). Nonelectric thermal irons are favored by many stylists who cater to clients with excessively curly hair because of the larger range of barrel or rod sizes and higher heat capabilities. Nonelectric thermal irons are heated in a specially designed electric or gas stove (figure 17-50).

All thermal irons have four basic parts: (1) rod handle, (2) shell handle, (3) barrel or **rod** (round, solid prong), and (4) **shell** (the clamp that presses the hair against the barrel or rod) (figure 17-51).

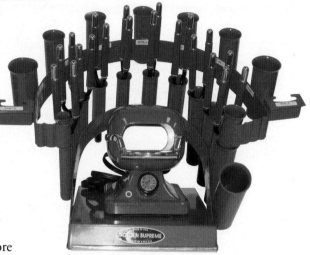

figure 17-49
Electric thermal iron

Flat Irons

Flat irons have two hot plates ranging in size from ½ inch to 3 inches across (figure 17-52). Flat irons with straight edges are used to create smooth, straight styles—even on very curly hair. Flat irons with beveled edges can be manipulated to bend or cup the ends. The edge nearest the stylist is called the inner edge; the one farthest from the stylist is called the outer edge. Modern technology is constantly improving electric curling and flat irons by adding infinite heat settings for better control, constant heat even on high settings, ergonomic grips, and lightweight designs for ease of handling.

It is always important to analyze and understand the condition and texture of hair before you set the heat. Hair that has been bleached is extremely delicate and can break off or melt with excessive heat. Use lower settings for fine hair and higher settings for coarse, curly, and thick hair. Work in ½- to 1-inch (1.25 to 2.5 centimeters) sections and use slow, smooth motions on hair that's a little more resistant. It is always recommended to apply a thermal protection product before the use of any heat appliance. This provides a protective shield and prevents heat damage.

figure 17-50
A modern stove-heated thermal iron and stove

Testing Thermal Irons

After heating the iron to the desired temperature, test it on a piece of tissue paper or a white cloth. Clamp the heated iron over this material and hold for five seconds. If it scorches or turns brown, the iron is too hot

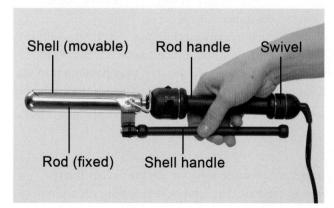

Shell (movable)   Rod handle   Swivel

Rod (fixed)   Shell handle

figure 17-51
The parts of a thermal iron

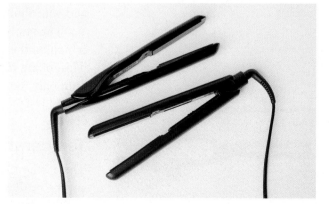

figure 17-52
Flat iron

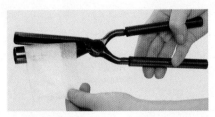

figure 17-53
Testing the heat of a thermal iron

(figure 17-53). Let it cool a bit before using. An overly hot iron can scorch the hair and might even discolor white hair. Remember that fine, lightened, or badly damaged hair withstands less heat than normal hair.

Care of Thermal Irons

Before cleaning a thermal iron, be sure to check the manufacturer's directions for care and cleaning. One way to remove dirt, oils, and product residue is to dampen a towel or rag and wipe down the barrel of the iron with a soapy solution containing a few drops of ammonia. If you are using a nonelectrical thermal iron, immerse the barrel in this solution. Do not clean your iron when it is turned on or when it is still cooling from a previous styling service.

Comb Used with Thermal Irons

The comb should be about 7 inches (17.5 centimeters) long, should be made of hard rubber or another nonflammable substance, and should have fine teeth to firmly hold the hair.

Hold the comb between the thumb and all four fingers of the non-dominant hand, with the index finger resting on the backbone of the comb for better control and one end of the comb resting against the outer edge of the palm. This position ensures a strong hold and a firm movement (figure 17-54).

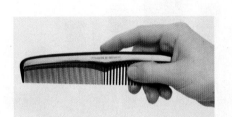

figure 17-54
Holding the comb

After reading the next few sections, you will be able to:

LO⑤ Demonstrate various thermal iron manipulations and explain how they are used.

<table>
<tr><td>⚠ CAUTION</td></tr>
</table>

When using thermal irons on chemically straightened hair, be cautious and test the heat of the iron to avoid causing breakage.

Manipulating Thermal Irons

Hold the iron in a comfortable position that gives you complete control. Grasp the handles of the iron in your dominant hand, far enough away from the joint to avoid the heat. Place your three middle fingers on the back of the lower handle, your little finger in front of the lower handle, and your thumb in front of the upper handle.

The best way to practice manipulative techniques with thermal irons is by rolling the cold iron in your hand, first forward and then backward. This rolling movement should be done without any sway or motion in the arm; only the fingers are used as you roll the handles in each direction (figure 17-55).

Temperature

There is no single correct temperature used for the iron when thermal curling or thermal waving the hair. The temperature setting for an iron depends on the texture of the hair, whether it is fine or coarse, and whether it has been lightened or tinted. Hair that has been lightened

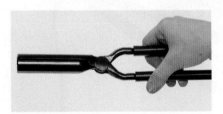

figure 17-55
Rolling the iron

or tinted, as well as white hair, should be curled and waved with a gentle heat. As a rule, coarse and gray hair can withstand more heat than fine hair.

Thermal Curling with Electric Thermal Irons

A modern thermal iron and a hard rubber comb are all you need to give your client curls. Thermal curling, which requires no setting gels or lotions, may be used to great advantage on the following hair types:

- **Straight hair.** Thermal curling permits quick styling because it eliminates the need for rollers (which are placed in wet hair) and a long hair drying process.

- **Pressed hair.** Thermal curling permits styling the hair without the danger of its returning to its former extremely curly condition and it prepares the hair for any desired style.

- **Wigs and hairpieces (human hair).** Thermal curling presents a quick and effective method for styling.

Curling Iron Manipulations

The following is a series of basic manipulative movements for using curling irons. Most other curling iron movements are variations of these basic movements (figures 17-56 through 17-62). Some stylists prefer to use just the little finger, or the little finger plus the ring finger, for this purpose. Either method is correct. The method of holding the iron is a matter of personal preference. Choose the one that gives you the most ease, comfort, and control.

If you want to get really good at using curling irons, the key is to practice manipulating them. Always practice with cold irons. The following four exercises are designed to help you learn the most effective ways to use an iron.

- Because it is important to develop a smooth rotating movement, practice turning the iron while opening and closing it at regular intervals. Practice rotating the iron in both directions—downward (toward you) and upward (away from you) (figure 17-63).

- Practice releasing the hair by opening and closing the iron in a quick, clicking movement.

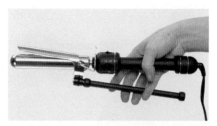

figure 17-56
Use the little finger to open the clamp.

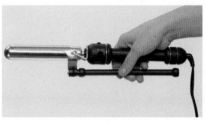

figure 17-57
Use your three middle fingers to close and manipulate the iron.

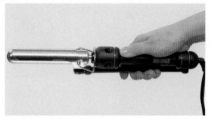

figure 17-58
Shift thumb when manipulating the iron.

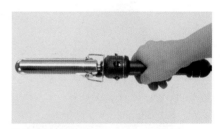

figure 17-59
Close shell and make a one-quarter turn downward

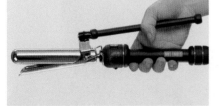

figure 17-60
Iron has made a half turn. Use thumb to open clamp and relax hair tension.

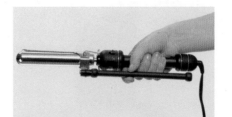

figure 17-61
Rotate iron to three quarters of a complete turn.

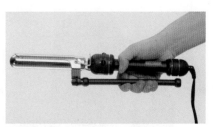

figure 17-62
Full turn

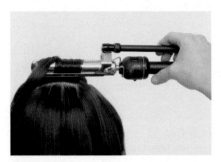

figure 17-63
Rotate while opening and closing
the iron.

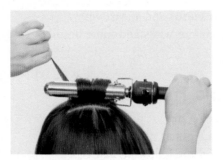

figure 17-64
Guide the hair strand into the center
of curl while rotating the iron.

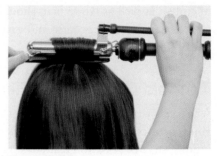

figure 17-65
Remove curl using the comb
as your guide.

- Practice guiding the hair strand into the center of the curl as you rotate the iron. This movement ensures that the end of the strand is firmly in the center of the curl (figure 17-64).

- Practice removing the curl from the iron by drawing the comb to the left and the rod to the right (figure 17-65). Use the comb to protect the client's scalp from burns.

After reading the next few sections, you will be able to:

LO❻ Perform the four basic curl patterns and explain the end result.

The 4 Basic Curl Patterns

There are four basic curl patterns that give a specific end result and are designed for different lengths of hair.

1. The **root curl** creates volume of hair, movement, and a curl formation from roots to ends. It is the most commonly used technique and works best on short or long layered hair (figures 17-66 and 17-67).

2. The **spiral curl** is a method of curling the hair by winding a strand around the rod. It creates a vertical corkscrew effect and works best on one length hair to create volume (figures 17-68 and 17-69).

3. **Waves** create an S pattern and gives texture and volume to the hair. Waves are a popular classic technique that can be applied on any texture and length, usually a surface enhancer.

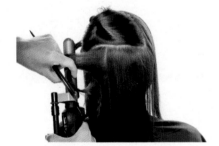

figure 17-66
Insert iron at an angle.

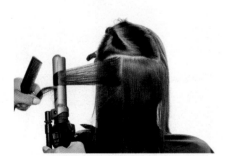

figure 17-67
Rotate iron until hair is wound.

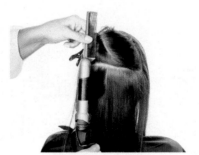

figure 17-68
Hold curl in position.

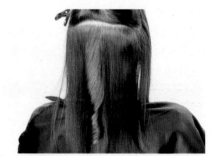

figure 17-69
Finished spiral curl.

4. End curls can be used to give a finished appearance to hair ends. Long, medium-length, or short hair may be styled with end curls. The hair ends can be turned under or over, as desired. The position and direction of the curling iron determine whether the end curls will turn under or over (**figures 17-70** and **17-71**).

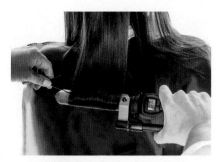

figure 17-70
Turn iron under.

Volume Thermal Iron Curls

Volume thermal iron curls stem from the root curl and are used to create volume or lift in a finished hairstyle. The degree of lift and movement desired determines the type of volume curls to be used.

Volume-Base Thermal Curls

Volume-base curls provide maximum lift or volume, since the curl is placed very high on its base. Section off base as shown. Hold the curl strand at a 135-degree angle. Slide the iron over the strand about ½ inch (1.25 centimeters) from the scalp. Wrap the strand over the rod with medium tension.

Maintain this position for approximately five seconds in order to heat the strand and set the base. Roll the curl in the usual manner and firmly place it forward and high on its base (**figure 17-72**).

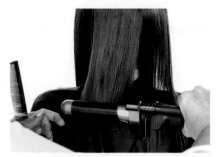

figure 17-71
Turn iron over.

Full-Base Thermal Curls

Full-base curls sit in the center of their base and provide a strong curl with full volume. Section off base as shown. Hold the hair strand at a 125-degree angle. Slide the iron over the hair strand about ½ inch (1.25 centimeters) from the scalp. Wrap the strand over the rod with medium tension. Maintain this position for about five seconds to heat the strand and set the base. Roll the curl in the usual manner, and place it firmly in the center of its base (**figure 17-73**).

Half-Base Thermal Curls

Half-base curls sit half off their base and provide a strong curl with moderate lift or volume. Section off base as shown. Hold the hair at a 90-degree angle. Slide the iron over the hair strand about ½ inch (1.25 centimeters) from the scalp. Wrap the strand over the rod with medium tension. Maintain this position for about five seconds to heat the strand and set the base. Roll the curl in the usual manner, and place it half off its base (**figure 17-74**).

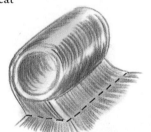
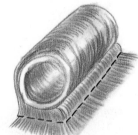

figure 17-72
Volume-base curl

figure 17-73
Full-base curl

Off-Base Thermal Curls

Off-base curls are placed completely off their base and offer a curl option with only slight lift or volume. Section off base as shown previously. Hold the hair at a 70-degree angle then slide the iron over the hair strand about ½ inch (1.25 centimeters) from the scalp. Wrap the strand over the rod with medium tension. Maintain this position for about five seconds to heat the strand and set the base. Roll the curl in the usual manner, and place it completely off its base (**figure 17-75**).

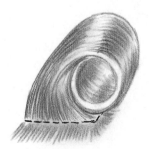
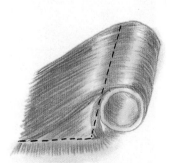

figure 17-74
Half-base curl

figure 17-75
Off base curl

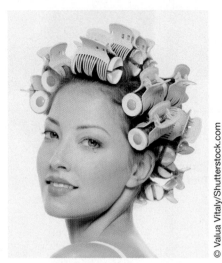

figure 17-76
Model in thermal rollers

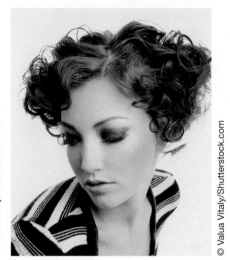

figure 17-77
Finished thermal-curled
short hairstyle

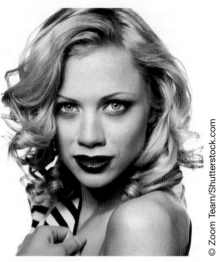

figure 17-78
Finished thermal-curled
medium-length hairstyle

Finished Thermal Curl Settings

For best results when giving a thermal setting, clip each curl in place until the whole head has been curled and is ready for styling (figure 17-76). Brush the hair, working up from the neckline and pushing the waves into place as you progress over the entire head. If the hairstyle is to be finished with curls, do the bottom curls last (figures 17-77 through 17-79).

Using Thermal Irons Safely

Here are some guidelines for the safe use of thermal irons:

* Use thermal irons only after receiving instruction in their use.

* Keep thermal irons clean, especially if hairspray is used before ironing.

* Do not overheat thermal irons because this can damage their ability to hold heat uniformly.

* Test the temperature of the iron on tissue paper or a white cloth before placing it on the hair in order to prevent burning the hair.

* Handle thermal irons carefully to avoid burning yourself or the client.

* Place hot irons in a safe place to cool. Do not leave them where someone might accidentally come into contact with them and be burned.

* When heating a conventional iron, do not place the handles too close to the heater. Your hand might be burned when removing the iron.

* When using a conventional iron, make sure the iron is properly balanced in the heater or it might fall and be damaged or injure someone.

* Use only hard rubber or nonflammable combs. Celluloid combs must not be used in thermal curling, as they are flammable.

* Do not use metal combs; they can become hot and burn the scalp.

* Place a comb between the scalp and the thermal iron when curling or waving hair to prevent burning the scalp.

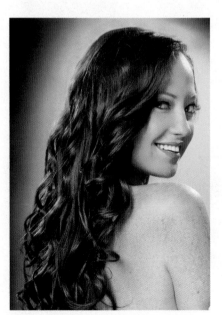

figure 17-79
Finished thermal-curled long hairstyle

- The client's hair must be clean and completely dry to ensure a good thermal curl or wave.

- Do not allow the hair ends to protrude over the iron; this causes fishhooks (hair that is bent or folded).

- When ironing lightened, tinted, or relaxed hair, always use a gentle heat setting.

- Use proper technique when curling the hair to avoid lines of demarcation.

- Always use a thermal protection product to protect the hair from heat damage.

Ⓟ 17-10   **Thermal Waving** *See page 507*

After reading the next few sections, you will be able to:

LO❼   **Describe the three types of hair pressing.**

Thermal Hair Straightening (Hair Pressing)

Thermal hair straightening, or pressing, is a popular service that is very profitable in the salon. When properly done, **hair pressing** temporarily straightens extremely curly or resistant hair by means of a heated iron or comb. A pressing generally lasts until the hair is shampooed. (Permanent or chemical hair straightening is covered in Chapter 20, Chemical Texture Services.) Hair pressing also prepares the hair for additional services such as thermal curling and croquignole (KROH-ken-yohl) thermal curling (the two-loop or Figure 8 technique). A good hair pressing leaves the hair in a natural and lustrous condition and it is not harmful to the hair (**figure 17-80**).

There are three types of hair pressing:

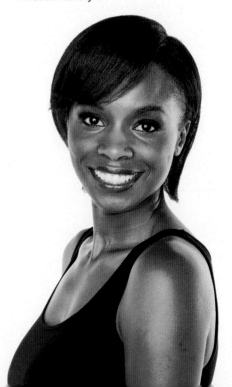

figure 17-80
Pressed hairstyle

- **Soft press**, which removes about 50 to 60 percent of the curl, is accomplished by applying the thermal pressing comb once on each side of the hair. For medium textured hair of average density, use subsections of average size. For coarse hair with greater density, use smaller sections to ensure complete heat penetration and effectiveness. For thin or fine hair with sparse density, use larger sections.

- **Medium press**, which removes about 60 to 75 percent of the curl, is accomplished by applying the thermal pressing comb once on each side of the hair, using slightly more pressure.

- **Hard press**, which removes 100 percent of the curl, is accomplished by applying the thermal pressing comb twice on each side of the hair. A hard press can also be done by first passing a hot thermal iron through the hair. This is called a **double press**.

Prepare for Hair Pressing—Analysis of Hair and Scalp

Before you press a client's hair, you will need to analyze the condition of the hair and scalp. (You may wish to review the steps of "Hair and Scalp Analysis" in Chapter 11, Properties of the Hair and Scalp.) If the client's hair and scalp are not healthy, you should give appropriate advice concerning corrective treatments.

In the case of scalp skin disease, it is not the cosmetologist's job to diagnose the condition, but rather to advise the client to see a dermatologist.

If the hair shows signs of neglect or abuse caused by faulty pressing, lightening, or tinting, recommend a series of conditioning treatments. Failure to correct dry and brittle hair can result in hair breakage during hair pressing. Burned hair strands cannot be conditioned.

Remember to check your client's hair for elasticity and porosity. Under normal conditions, if a client's hair has good elasticity, it can be stretched to about 50 percent of its original length before breaking, when wet. If the porosity is normal, the hair will return to its natural wave pattern when it is wet or moistened.

A careful analysis of the client's hair and scalp should cover the following points:

- Wave pattern
- Length
- Texture (coarse, medium, or fine)
- Feel (wiry, soft, or silky)
- Elasticity
- Color (natural, faded, streaked, gray, tinted, or lightened)
- Condition of hair (normal, brittle, dry, oily, damaged, or chemically treated)
- Condition of scalp (normal, flexible, or tight)

It is important that the cosmetologist be able to recognize individual differences in hair texture, porosity, elasticity, and scalp flexibility. Guided by this information, the cosmetologist can determine how much pressure the hair and scalp can handle without hair breakage, hair loss, or burning from a pressing comb that is too hot.

Hair Texture

Variations in hair texture have to do with the diameter of the hair (coarse, medium, or fine) and the feel of the hair (wiry, soft, or silky). Touching the client's hair and asking about specific hair characteristics will help you determine the best way to treat the hair.

Coarse, extremely curly hair has qualities that make it difficult to press. Coarse hair has the greatest diameter and during the pressing process it requires more heat and pressure than medium or fine hair.

Medium curly hair is the type of hair that cosmetologists deal with most often in the beauty salon. No special problem is presented by this type of hair and this hair type is the least resistant to pressing.

Fine hair requires special care. To avoid hair breakage, use less heat and pressure than you would use on other hair textures.

Wiry, curly hair may be coarse, medium, or fine, and it feels stiff, hard, and glassy. Because of the compact construction of its cuticle cells, hair of this type is very resistant to hair pressing and requires more heat and pressure than other types of hair.

Scalp Condition

The condition of the client's scalp can be classified as normal, tight, or flexible. If the scalp is normal, proceed with an analysis of hair texture and elasticity. If the scalp is tight and the hair coarse, press the hair in the direction in which it grows to avoid injury to the scalp. If the scalp is flexible, remember to use enough tension to press the hair satisfactorily.

Service Notes

Be sure to record the results of your hair and scalp analysis, as well as all pressing treatments, on the client's intake form or service record card.

During your client consultation, question the client about any lightener, tint, gradual colors (metallic), or other chemical treatments that have been used on her hair. As with all services, a release statement should be signed by the client prior to hair pressing in order to protect the school, the salon, and the stylist from liability due to accidents or damage.

Conditioning Treatments

Effective conditioning treatments involve special cosmetic preparations for the hair and scalp thorough brushing and scalp massage. The application of a conditioning treatment usually results in better hair pressing.

A tight scalp can be made more flexible by the systematic use of scalp massage and hair brushing. The client benefits because there is better circulation of blood to the scalp.

Pressing Combs

There are two types of pressing combs: regular and electric. Both should be constructed of good quality stainless steel or brass. The handle is usually made of wood because wood does not readily absorb heat.

The space between the teeth of the comb varies with the size and style of the comb. Closely spaced teeth provide a smooth press. As spacing gets wider, the press gets less smooth.

Pressing combs also vary in size. Shorter combs are used to press short hair; longer combs are used to press long hair.

Tempering The Comb

It may be a good idea to **temper** a new brass pressing comb so that it will hold heat evenly along its entire length and provide consistent results. To temper a new pressing comb, heat the comb until it is extremely hot. Coat the comb in petroleum-base pressing product or pressing oil. Let it cool down naturally and then rinse under hot running water to remove the oil.

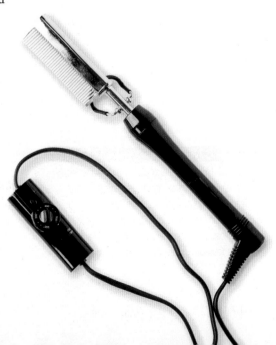

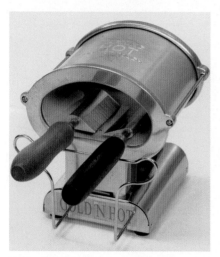

figure 17-81
Electric heater for pressing combs

Tempering the pressing comb also allows you to burn off any polish the manufacturer may have used to coat the comb. If the polish is not burned off, the comb may stick to the hair, causing scorching and breakage.

Heating the Comb

Depending on what they are made of, pressing combs vary in their ability to accept and retain heat. Regular pressing combs may be designed as electrical appliances or to be heated in electric or gas stoves (**figure 17-81**). When heating a pressing comb in a gas stove, point the teeth face up and keep the handle away from the fire.

After heating the comb to the proper temperature, test it on a piece of light paper. If the paper becomes scorched, allow the comb to cool slightly before applying it to the hair.

Electric pressing combs are available in two forms. One comes with an on/off switch; the other is equipped with a thermostat that indicates high or low degrees of heat.

Straightening comb attachments are available for purchase to fit the nozzle of a standard hand-held blowdryer. While these attachments are less damaging than either an electric comb or an oven-heated comb, they may also be less effective at pressing the hair.

Cleaning the Comb

The pressing comb will perform more efficiently if it is kept clean. Wipe the comb clean of loose hair, product, and dust before and after every use. Once all loose hair and clinging dirt are removed, the comb's intense heat keeps it sterile.

With a stove-heated pressing comb (nonelectric), remove the carbon by rubbing the outside surface and between the teeth with a fine steel-wool pad or fine sandpaper. Then place the metal portion of the comb in a hot baking soda solution for about one hour. Rinse and dry the comb thoroughly. The metal will acquire a smooth and shiny appearance.

Pressing Oil or Cream

Prepare the hair for a pressing treatment by first applying pressing oil or cream. Both of these products offer the following benefits:

* Make hair softer

* Prepare and condition the hair for pressing

* Help protect the hair from burning or scorching

* Help prevent hair breakage

* Condition the hair after pressing

* Add sheen to pressed hair

* Help hair stay pressed longer

Hard Press

A hard press is only recommended when the results of a soft or medium press are not satisfactory. The entire comb press procedure is repeated. Pressing oil should be added to hair strands only if necessary. A hard press is also known as a *double comb press*.

> **⚠ CAUTION**
> In case of a scalp burn, immediately apply 1 percent gentian (JEN-chun) violet jelly. Most pharmacies carry gentian violet. It should be noted that gentian violet jelly may cause temporary staining of the skin for a few days due to its violet tint.

Touch-Ups

Touch-ups are sometimes necessary when the hair becomes curly again due to perspiration, dampness, or other conditions. The process is the same as for the original pressing treatment, with the shampoo omitted.

Reminders and Hints for All Pressing Procedures

Good judgment should be used to avoid damage, with consideration always given to the texture of the hair and the condition of the scalp. The client's safety is ensured only when the stylist observes every precaution and takes special care during the actual hair pressing. Listed below are rules of thumb for hair pressing:

- Avoid excessive heat or pressure on the hair and scalp.
- Recommend a conditioning treatment mask, this will help repair and moisturize the hair and scalp, and should typically be done twice a month.
- Avoid too much pressing oil on the hair (it attracts dirt and makes the hair look greasy and artificial).
- Avoid perfumed pressing oil near the scalp if the client has allergies.
- Avoid overly frequent hair pressing.
- Keep the comb clean at all times.
- Avoid overheating the pressing comb if using a stove.
- Test the temperature of the heated comb on a white cloth or paper before applying it to the hair.
- Adjust the temperature of the pressing comb to the texture and condition of the client's hair.
- Use the heated comb carefully to avoid burning the skin, scalp, or hair.
- Prevent the smoking or burning of hair during the pressing treatment by drying the hair completely after it is shampooed and by avoiding excessive application of pressing oil.
- Use a moderately warm comb to press short hair on the temples and back of the neck. You may also use a temple comb, which is about half the size of a regular pressing comb.
- If the hair texture is fine and not too coarse, you may consider using a flat iron on high heat.

Special Considerations

You should take certain precautions and safeguards when dealing with the following special situations:

- **Pressing fine hair.** Follow the same procedure as for normal hair, while avoiding the use of a hot pressing comb or too much pressure. You may want to consider flat ironing on high heat if the curl form is not too wiry. To avoid hair breakage, apply less pressure to the hair near the ends. After completely pressing the hair, style it.

> **⚠ CAUTION**
> Burns and skin rashes are the two general types of injuries that can occur in hair pressing.
>
> Injuries that are the immediate result of hair pressing and that cause physical damage include burned hair that breaks off, burned scalp that causes either temporary or permanent hair loss, and burns on the ears and neck that form scars.
>
> Injuries that are not immediately evident but can cause physical damage later include a skin rash if the client is allergic to pressing oil and the breaking and shortening of the hair due to frequent hair pressings.

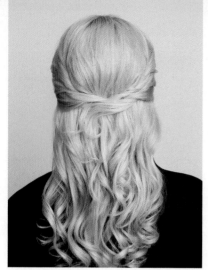

figure 17-82
Tinted, lightened, or gray (unpigmented) hair requires special care when pressing.

- **Pressing short, fine hair.** Extra care must be taken at the hairline. When the hair is extra short, the pressing comb should not be too hot because the hair is fine and will burn easily. A hot comb can also cause painful burns and may result in scars. In the event of an accidental burn, immediately apply 1 percent gentian violet jelly to the burn.

- **Pressing coarse hair.** Apply enough pressure so that the hair remains straightened.

- **Pressing tinted, lightened, or gray (unpigmented) hair.** This hair requires special care. Lightened or tinted hair might require conditioning treatments, depending on the extent to which it has been damaged. Gray hair may be particularly resistant. To obtain good results on gray hair, use a moderately heated pressing comb applied with light pressure. Avoid excessive heat as discoloration or breakage can occur (figure 17-82).

After reading the next few sections, you will be able to:

LO⑧ Understand the importance of preparation, sectioning, pinning, and balance with regard to updos.

LO⑨ Create the two foundational updos for styling long hair.

Creatively Style Long Hair

An **updo**, also known as a *specialty style*, is a hairstyle with the hair arranged up and off the shoulders and secured with implements such as hairpins, bobby pins, and elastics (figure 17-83). Another popular specialty style is a **half updo** also described as *half up*, designed for long or very long hair. This is where half of the hair is pulled back off the face and pinned at or below the crown. Clients usually request updos for special occasions such as weddings, proms, and evening events.

There are a variety of ways to design these looks, but before you begin there are **five key points** you must consider.

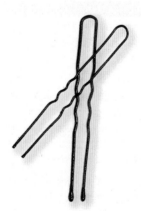

figure 17-83
Hairpins

1. **Preparing** your tools and materials is essential before beginning an updo. A list of tools can be found in the chignon procedure under "implements and materials." Performing an updo on hair that has been washed the previous day is often recommended, as freshly washed hair can be very slippery and difficult to work with. The hair needs to have some grip or the pins and style will not hold. Many stylists also choose to use thermal irons or set the hair in hot rollers prior to doing an updo. The curl allows the hair to be more easily manipulated into rolls or loops and creates a fuller shape. Use a slow-drying aerosol hairspray; it will allow you to work with the hair before it dries.

2. **Sectioning** the hair before you begin allows you to control long hair and a work with cleanliness. Every style has a sectioning pattern; keeping the lines simple will allow you to execute the look in a timely manner and ensure a quality end result.

3. **Pinning** will keep your updo secure, but one thing to remember is that less is more. There are two types of pins: Hairpins are open-ended and can be anchored by bending one end of the pin back so when inserted it automatically locks into place. They work best on hair that has been backcombed or back-brushed, as having a base will prevent them falling out. Bobby pins have a different function as they are used to keep the hair tight to the head and can be interlocked to secure it in place (figure 17-84).

4. **Balance** is often overlooked and can be the difference between a flattering style or one that is not. The head shape, neckline, and facial structure should be analyzed before committing to a look. It is good practice to stand back and away from your work to make sure the balance is right, use the mirror and look at every angle—front, back and profile.

5. **Texture** is what creates the foundation that allows you to build your shape, design your style, and customize it to the individual. With the styling tools and products of today, we can manipulate and create any texture.

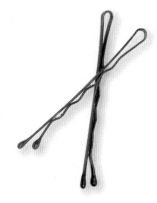

figure 17-84
Bobby pins

The two basic hairstyles described below are the foundation of every updo and long hairstyling. Once mastered, any placement or combination of these techniques will give a unique update to any classic look.

1. The **PonyTail** is the most commonly used hairstyle because of its versatility. It is the foundation for a chignon, bun, and knot, among other designs. It can be placed on various parts of the head and can be worn casual, classic, or trendy.

2. A **French Pleat** (the word *pleat* means "folded" in French) is a classic long hairstyle that is popular in the salon for clients attending formal functions. This basic hairstyle can be applied to straight or curly hair with length below the shoulder. It is one of the more elegant styles and can be adapted for every age group.

figure 17-85
One type of Chignon

Classic Updos

A few classic updo techniques—chignon, bun, and twist— are described below.

• **Chignon** (SHEEN-yahn). A truly classic style, the *chignon knot* has been popular for centuries. It is created out of a simple ponytail and can be dressed up with flowers or ornaments, or kept simple (figure 17-85). If the client's hair is very straight and silky, you may want to first use a large barrel thermal iron or set the hair for 10 minutes in electric rollers, or the style will not last. If the hair is wavy or curly, blowdry the hair straight. If it is extremely curly, you could press the hair first or leave it natural for a textured-looking chignon.

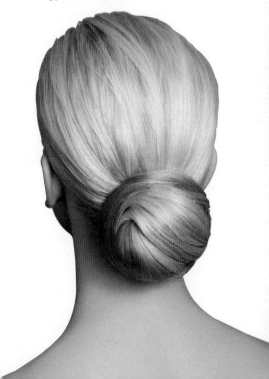

- **Bun.** The classic bun is great for all occasions and can be seen from the red carpet to the runways of fashion week. The foundation technique used for this look is a ponytail and it can sit high or low. It could be twisted around the ponytail or back-brushed and formed into a bun. The bun is secured with an elastic hair band and a few small and large bobby pins, but you can also use accessories to create a personal style.

- **Twist** is also referred to as *French Pleat*. This elegant, sleek look can be worn for any occasion and is very easy to create. The final design creates a look of conical shape. If you are working on straight, fine hair, you may want to first set the hair in electric or Velcro rollers to give it more body.

Ⓟ 17-11 **Chignon** *See page 513*

Ⓟ 17-12 **French Pleat or Twist** *See page 516*

Ⓟ 17-13 **Half Updo** *See page 340*

Perform Formal Styling
Client Consultation

As always, consult with the client first to make sure you understand what she has in mind. Have magazines or look book available that show a lot of updos, such as bridal magazines, or keep a folder of pictures clipped from magazines at your station that show current styles. If you are doing a pre-wedding consultation with a bride, ask the bride to bring her headpiece so that she can try several styles and see how they look. Take photographs to help her decide which style she likes best. Always suggest classic, timeless styles for brides and leave the latest trend for the bridesmaids. This suggestion will be appreciated years later. Keep a photo of the chosen style so that you can duplicate it for the bride's big day.

Express the Artistry of Hairstyling

Hairstyling offers a cosmetologist a wonderful artistic outlet. Once you master the basic styles presented in this chapter, and the foundational techniques these styles require, you will have the technical abilities to experiment and create your own unique and attractive looks.

Styling trends change quickly. In order to offer your clients the latest looks, you may want to consider having a mannequin at home. This will enable you to practice creating the looks you see in magazines and to try out new styling ideas and techniques. Remember, every client's hair presents creative possibilities!

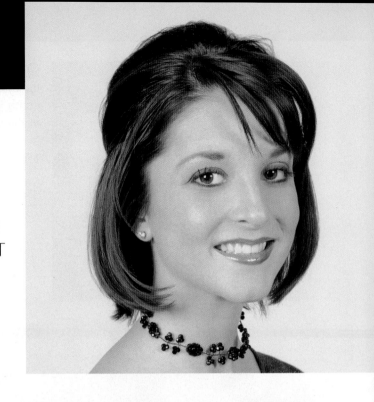

P 17-1

PREPARING HAIR FOR WET STYLING

IMPLEMENTS & MATERIALS

You will need all of the following implements, materials, and supplies:

- ☐ Conditioner
- ☐ Neck strip
- ☐ Plastic cape
- ☐ Shampoo
- ☐ Towels

PREPARATION

Perform:

P 15-1 **Pre-Service Procedure** *See page 340*

PROCEDURE

1. Drape the client for a shampoo service.

2. Shampoo the client's hair and condition if necessary.

3. Towel dry the hair.

4. Remove any tangles with a wide-tooth comb, starting at the ends and working up to the scalp.

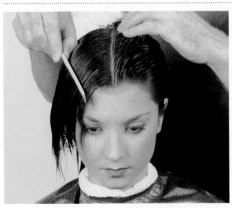

5. Ask the client where they part their hair. Part the hair according to (1) the client's preference, (2) their natural part if that works with your hair design, or (3) create a part anywhere on the head if that better suits the final design.

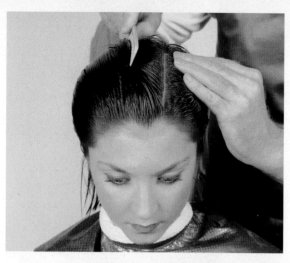

6 Create a clean parting by using the comb and your other hand to separate the hair. Lay the wide-tooth end of a styling comb flat at the hairline and draw the comb back to the end of the desired part.

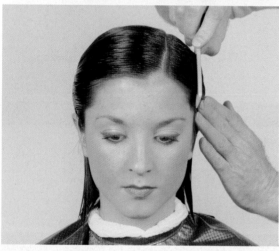

7 Separate the two sides and comb the hair smooth.

8 You are now ready to move on to the next aspect of the service.

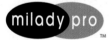 Check out miladypro.com for additional resources and training to enhance your technical skills.   Keyword: *FutureCosPro*

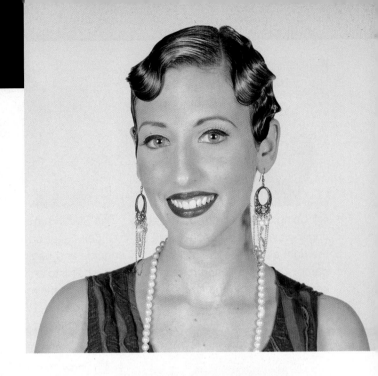

HORIZONTAL FINGER WAVING

IMPLEMENTS & MATERIALS

You will need all of the following implements, materials, and supplies:

- □ Conditioner
- □ Finishing products such as shine or hair spray
- □ Hairnet
- □ Hairpins or clips
- □ Hood dryer
- □ Neck strip
- □ Plastic cape
- □ Shampoo
- □ Styling comb
- □ Towels
- □ Finger-waving lotion or styling gel

PREPARATION

Perform:

P 15-1 **Pre-Service Procedure** *See page 340*

PROCEDURE

1 Drape the client for a shampoo service.

2 Shampoo the client's hair and condition if necessary.

3 Towel dry the hair.

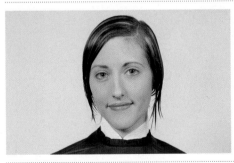

4 Remove any tangles with a wide-tooth comb, starting at the ends and working up to the scalp.

5 Using the wide part of the comb, create a side part from the center of the eye to just in front of the crown. Comb the hair smooth and arrange it according to the planned style.

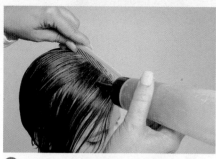

6 Using an applicator bottle, apply finger-waving lotion or liquid gel to the right side while the hair is damp. Comb the lotion through the section and begin the first wave on the top right heavy side.

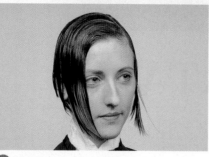

7 Starting at the hairline, use your index finger on your left hand as a guide and begin combing the top of the hair into an S-shape pattern using a circular movement. Work toward the crown in 1½- to 2-inch (3.7 to 5 centimeters) sections at a time.

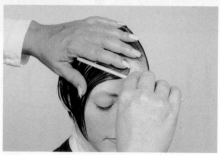

8 To form the first ridge, place the index finger of your left hand directly above the position for the first ridge. With the teeth of the comb pointing slightly upward, insert the comb directly under the index finger.

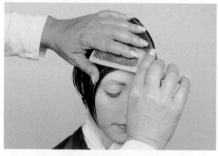

9 Draw the comb forward about 1 inch (2.5 centimeters) along the fingertip. With the teeth still inserted in the ridge, flatten the comb against the head in order to hold the ridge in place.

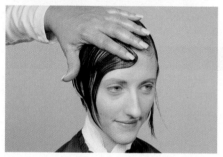

10 Remove your left hand from the client's head and place your middle finger above the ridge with your index finger on the teeth of the comb. Draw out the ridge by closing the two fingers and applying pressure to the head.

11 Do not try to increase the height or depth of a ridge by pinching or pushing with your fingers; such movements will create overdirection of the ridge and uneven hair placement.

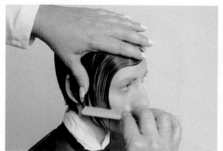

12 Without removing the comb, turn the teeth downward and comb the hair in a semicircular direction to form a dip in the hollow part of the wave. Follow this procedure, section by section, until the crown has been reached, where the ridge phases out.

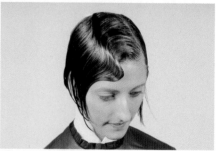

13 The ridge and wave of each section should match evenly, without showing separations in the ridge or in the hollow part of the wave.

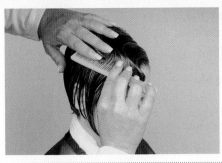

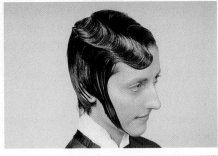

14 To form the second ridge, begin at the crown area and draw the comb from the tip of the index finger toward the base. All movements are followed in a reverse pattern until the hairline is reached, completing the second ridge.

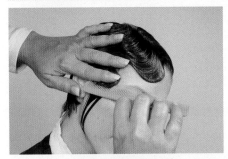

15 Movements for the third ridge closely follow those used to create the first ridge. However, the third ridge is started at the hairline and is extended back toward the back of the head. Continue alternating directions until the right side of the head has been completed.

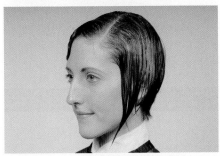

16 Use the same procedure for the left (light) side of the head as you used for finger waving the right (heavy) side of the head. First, shape the hair by combing it in the direction of the first wave.

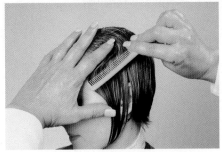

17 Starting at the hairline, form the first ridge, and work section by section, until the second ridge of the opposite side is reached.

18 Both the ridge and the wave must blend, without splits or breaks, with the ridge and wave on the right side of the head.

19 Move to the left side and start with the ridge and wave in the back of the head and proceed, section by section, toward the left side of the face.

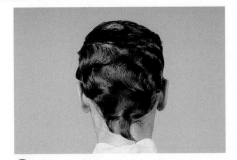

20 Continue working back and forth until the entire head has been completed.

21 Place a net over the hair, secure it with hairpins or clips if necessary, and protect the client's forehead and ears with cotton, gauze, or paper protectors while under the hood dryer. Adjust the dryer to medium heat and allow the hair to dry thoroughly.

22 Remove the client from under the dryer and let the hair cool down. Remove all clips or pins and the hairnet from the hair.

23 Comb out or brush the hair into a soft, waved hairstyle. Add a finishing spray for hold and shine. For a retro look, do not comb or brush the hair.

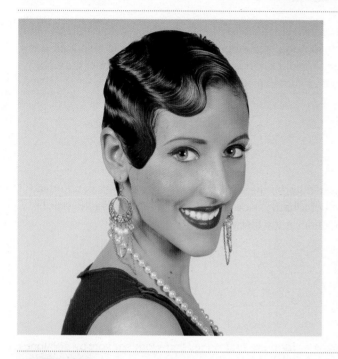

24 Finished look.

POST-SERVICE

Complete:

P 15-2 **Post-Service Procedure** *See page 343*

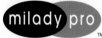 Check out miladypro.com for additional resources and training to enhance your technical skills.   Keyword: *FutureCosPro*

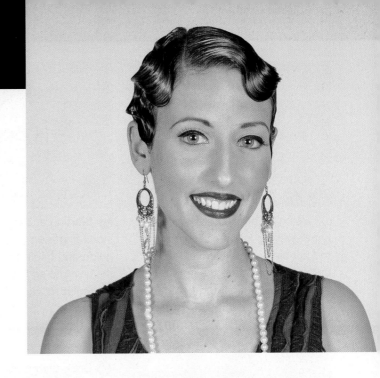

HORIZONTAL FINGER WAVING

IMPLEMENTS & MATERIALS

You will need all of the following implements, materials, and supplies:

- □ Conditioner
- □ Finishing products such as shine or hair spray
- □ Hairnet
- □ Hairpins or clips
- □ Hood dryer
- □ Neck strip
- □ Plastic cape
- □ Shampoo
- □ Styling comb
- □ Towels
- □ Finger-waving lotion or styling gel

PREPARATION

Perform:

P 15-1 **Pre-Service Procedure** *See page 340*

PROCEDURE

1. Drape the client for a shampoo service.

2. Shampoo the client's hair and condition if necessary.

3. Towel dry the hair.

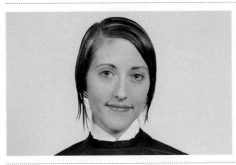

4. Remove any tangles with a wide-tooth comb, starting at the ends and working up to the scalp.

5. Using the wide part of the comb, create a side part from the center of the eye to just in front of the crown. Comb the hair smooth and arrange it according to the planned style.

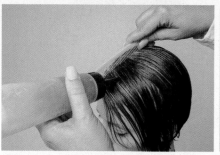

6 Using an applicator bottle, apply finger-waving lotion or liquid gel to the left side of the hair while the hair is damp. Comb the lotion through the section and begin the first wave on the left side of the head.

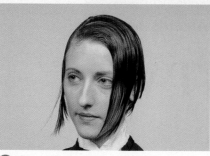

7 Starting at the hairline, use your index finger on your right hand as a guide and begin combing the top of the hair into an S-shape pattern using a circular movement. Work toward the crown in 1½- to 2-inch (3.7 to 5 centimeters) sections at a time.

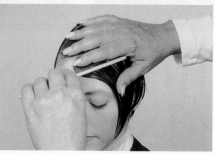

8 To form the first ridge, place the index finger of your right hand directly above the position for the first ridge. With the teeth of the comb pointing slightly upward, insert the comb directly under the index finger.

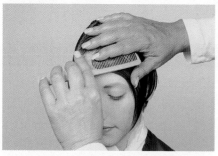

9 Draw the comb forward about 1 inch (2.5 centimeters) along the fingertip. With the teeth still inserted in the ridge, flatten the comb against the head in order to hold the ridge in place.

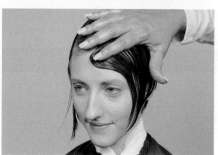

10 Remove your right hand from the client's head and place your middle finger above the ridge with your index finger on the teeth of the comb. Draw out the ridge by closing the two fingers and applying pressure to the head.

11 Do not try to increase the height or depth of a ridge by pinching or pushing with your fingers; such movements will create overdirection of the ridge and uneven hair placement.

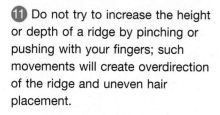

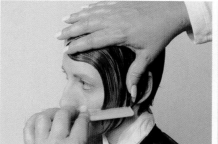

12 Without removing the comb, turn the teeth downward and comb the hair in a semicircular direction to form a dip in the hollow part of the wave. Follow this procedure, section by section, until the crown has been reached, where the ridge phases out.

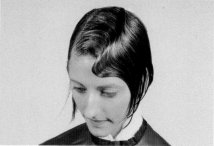

13 The ridge and wave of each section should match evenly without showing separations in the ridge or in the hollow part of the wave. To form the second ridge, begin at the crown area. The movements are the reverse of those followed in forming the first ridge.

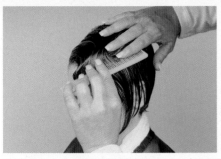

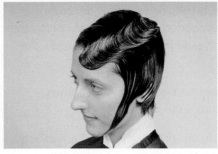

14 To form the second ridge, begin at the crown area and draw the comb from the tip of the index finger toward the base. All movements are followed in a reverse pattern until the hairline is reached, completing the second ridge.

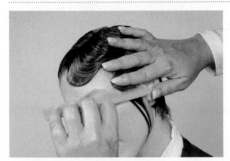

15 Movements for the third ridge closely follow those used to create the first ridge. However, the third ridge is started at the hairline and is extended back toward the back of the head. Continue alternating directions until the right side of the head has been completed.

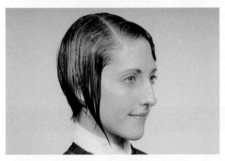

16 Use the same procedure for the left (light) side of the head as you used for finger waving the right (heavy) side of the head. First, shape the hair by combing it in the direction of the first wave.

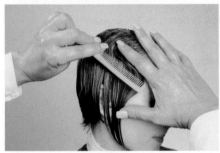

17 Starting at the hairline, form the first ridge and work section by section until the second ridge of the opposite side is reached.

18 Both the ridge and the wave must blend, without splits or breaks, with the ridge and wave on the right side of the head.

19 Move to the left side and start with the ridge and wave in the back of the head and proceed, section by section, toward the left side of the face.

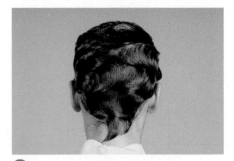

20 Continue working back and forth until the entire head is completed.

21 Place a net over the hair, secure it with hairpins or clips if necessary, and protect the client's forehead and ears with cotton, gauze, or paper protectors while under the hood dryer. Adjust the dryer to medium heat and allow the hair to dry thoroughly.

22 Remove the client from under the dryer and let the hair cool down. Remove all clips or pins and the hairnet from the hair.

23 Comb out or brush the hair into a soft, waved hairstyle. Add a finishing spray for hold and shine. For a retro look, do not comb or brush the hair.

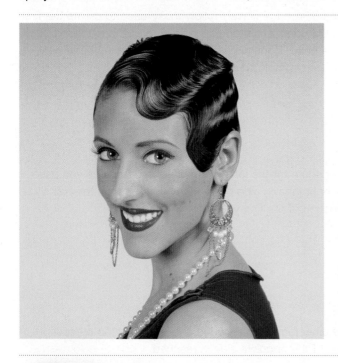

24 Finished look.

POST-SERVICE

Complete:

P 15-2   **Post-Service Procedure** *See page 343*

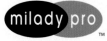 Check out miladypro.com for additional resources and training to enhance your technical skills.   Keyword: *FutureCosPro*

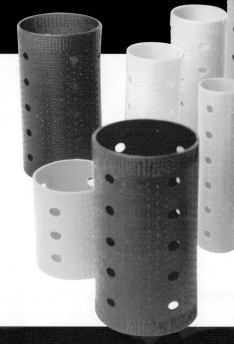
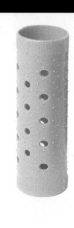

WET SET WITH ROLLERS

IMPLEMENTS & MATERIALS

You will need all of the following implements, materials, and supplies:

- Clips (double or single prong)
- Conditioner
- Finishing products such as shine or hair spray
- Hood dryer
- Neck strip
- Plastic cape
- Plastic rollers of various sizes
- Setting or styling lotion
- Shampoo
- Tail comb
- Towels
- Wide-tooth comb

PREPARATION

Perform:

P 15-1 **Pre-Service Procedure** See page 340

PROCEDURE

1. Drape the client for a shampoo service.

2. Shampoo the client's hair and condition if necessary.

3. Towel dry the hair.

4. Remove any tangles with a wide-tooth comb, starting at the ends and working up to the scalp.

5. Comb the hair in the direction of the setting pattern. Shapings may be used to accent the design.

6. Starting at the front hairline, part off a section the same length and width as the roller.

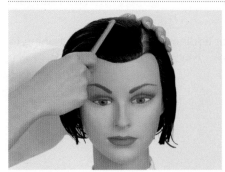

7. Choose the type of base according to the desired volume. Comb the hair out from the scalp to the ends, using the fine teeth of the comb. Repeat several times to make sure that the hair is smooth.

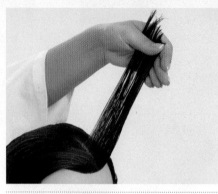

8 Hold the hair with tension between the thumb and middle finger of the left hand. Place the roller below the thumb of the left hand. Do not bring the ends of the hair together. Wrap the ends of the hair smoothly around the roller until the hair catches and does not release.

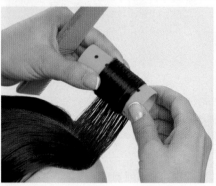

9 Place the thumbs over the ends of the roller and roll the hair firmly to the scalp

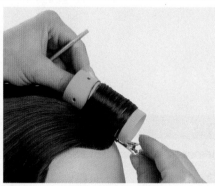

10 Clip the roller securely to the scalp hair.

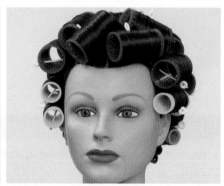

11 Roll the remainder of the hair according to the desired style.

12 Place the client under a hood dryer. Set the dryer at a temperature that is comfortable for the client.

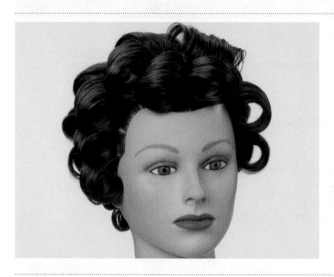

13 When the hair is dry, allow it to cool and then remove the rollers

14 Comb out and style the hair as desired.

POST-SERVICE

Complete:

P 15-2 **Post-Service Procedure** *See page 343*

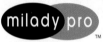
Check out miladypro.com for additional resources and training to enhance your technical skills. Keyword: *FutureCosPro*

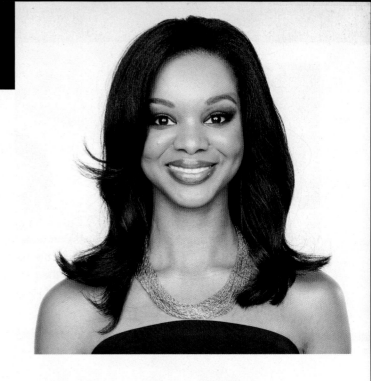

P 17-4

HAIR WRAPPING

IMPLEMENTS & MATERIALS

You will need all of the following implements, materials, and supplies:

- ☐ Boar-bristle paddle brush
- ☐ Bobby pins
- ☐ Conditioner
- ☐ Duckbill clips
- ☐ Hairnet
- ☐ Hood dryer
- ☐ Neck strip
- ☐ Shampoo
- ☐ Styling product (light oil is option)
- ☐ Wide-tooth comb

PREPARATION | PROCEDURE

Perform:

P 15-1 Pre-Service Procedure *See page 340*

1. Drape the client for a shampoo service.

2. Shampoo the client's hair and condition if necessary.

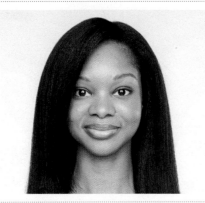

3. Dry and press dry hair.

4. Remove any tangles with a wide-tooth comb, starting at the ends and working up to the scalp.

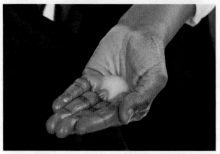

5 Apply a light oil or styling aid to dry hair before wrapping.

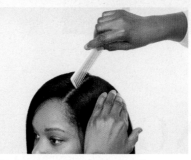

6 Create a parting from the recession area to the crown. Start combing the hair flat and to the right of the parting and hold it down with your hand.

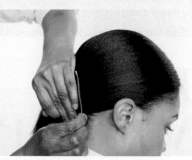

7 Starting on the heavy side of the part, using a natural bristle paddle brush, begin to wrap hair smooth to head shape counterclockwise or in desired style direction. Use duckbill clips or large bobby pins to keep the hair in place while wrapping.

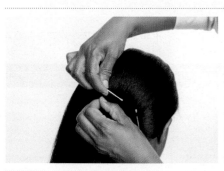

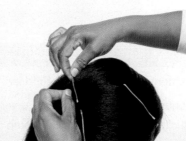

8 Continue wrapping the hair in a clockwise direction around the head. Follow the comb or brush with your hand or use your fingers, smoothing down the hair and keeping it tight to the head as you proceed.

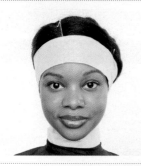

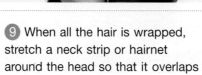

9 When all the hair is wrapped, stretch a neck strip or hairnet around the head so that it overlaps at the ends.

10 Place the client under a hooded dryer until the hair is completely dry, usually 45 minutes to one hour, depending on the hair length. If you have been working on dry hair, leave the hair wrapped for about 17 minutes. The longer the hair is wrapped, the smoother it will be.

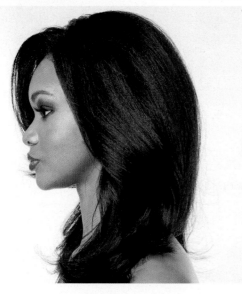

11 Finished look.

POST-SERVICE

Complete:

P 15-2 **Post-Service Procedure** *See page 343*

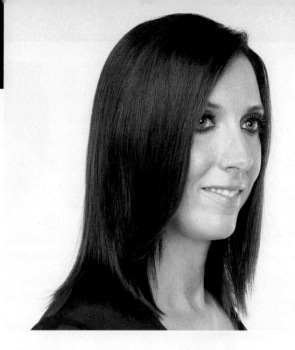

BLOWDRYING SHORT, LAYERED, CURLY HAIR TO PRODUCE SMOOTH AND FULL FINISH

IMPLEMENTS & MATERIALS

You will need all of the following implements, materials, and supplies:

- ☐ Blowdryer with attachments
- ☐ Finishing products such as shine or hair spray
- ☐ Conditioner
- ☐ Neck strip
- ☐ Round brush
- ☐ Sectioning clips
- ☐ Shampoo
- ☐ Styling cape
- ☐ Styling products
- ☐ Towels
- ☐ Wide-tooth comb

PREPARATION

Perform:

P 15-1 **Pre-Service Procedure** *See page 340*

PROCEDURE

1 Drape the client for a shampoo service.

2 Shampoo the client's hair and condition if necessary.

3 Towel dry the hair.

4 Place a clean neck strip on the client and drape with a cutting or styling cape.

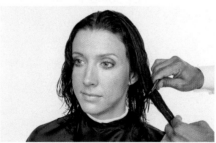

5 Remove any tangles with a wide-tooth comb, starting at the ends and working up to the scalp.

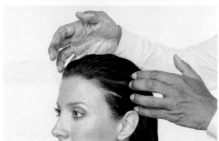

6 Distribute styling product through the hair with your fingers and comb through with a wide-tooth comb.

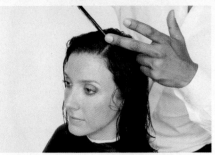

7 Using the comb, mold the hair into the desired shape while still wet.

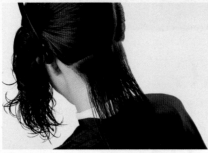

8 Section and part the hair according to the amount of volume desired.

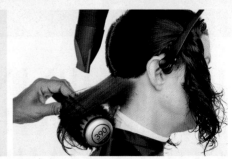

9 Using the techniques that you have learned in roller setting, dry each section at either full base or half base.

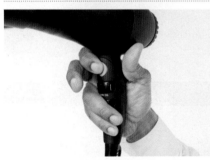

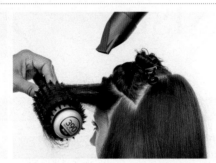

10 For maximum lift, insert the brush on base and direct the hair section up at a 90-degree angle. Roll the hair down to the base with medium tension. Direct the stream of air from the blowdryer over the curl and away from the scalp in a back and forth motion.

11 When the section is completely dry, press the cooling button and cool the section to strengthen the curl formation. Release the curl by unwinding the section from the brush. (Pulling it out could cause the hair to get tangled in the brush.)

12 For less lift at the scalp, begin by holding the section at a 90-degree angle, following the same procedure.

13 Make sure that the scalp and hair are completely dry before combing out the style or the shape will not last. Finish with hair spray.

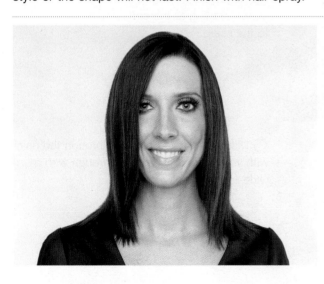

14 Finished look.

POST-SERVICE

Complete:

P 15-2 **Post-Service Procedure** *See page 343*

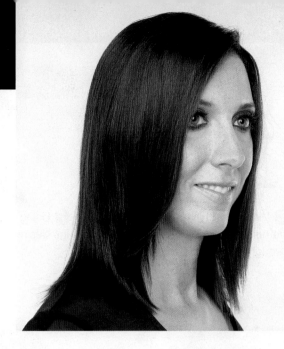

P 17-5 LH

BLOWDRYING SHORT, LAYERED, CURLY HAIR TO PRODUCE SMOOTH AND FULL FINISH

IMPLEMENTS & MATERIALS

You will need all of the following implements, materials, and supplies:

- ☐ Blowdryer with attachments
- ☐ Finishing products such as shine or hair spray
- ☐ Conditioner
- ☐ Neck strip
- ☐ Round brush
- ☐ Sectioning clips
- ☐ Shampoo
- ☐ Styling cape
- ☐ Styling products
- ☐ Towels
- ☐ Wide-tooth comb

PREPARATION

Perform:

P 15-1 **Pre-Service Procedure** *See page 340*

PROCEDURE

1 Drape the client for a shampoo service.

2 Shampoo the client's hair and condition if necessary.

3 Towel dry the hair.

4 Place a clean neck strip on the client and drape with a cutting or styling cape.

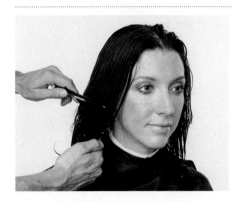

5 Remove any tangles with a wide-tooth comb, starting at the ends and working up to the scalp.

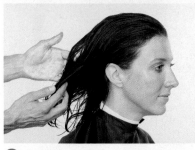

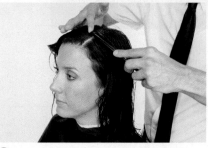

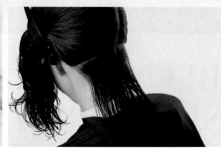

6 Distribute styling product through the hair with your fingers and comb through with a wide-tooth comb.

7 Using the comb, mold the hair into the desired shape while still wet.

8 Section and part the hair according to the amount of volume desired.

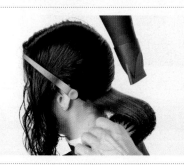

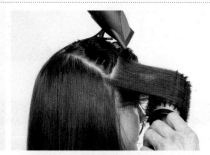

9 Using the techniques that you have learned in roller setting, dry each section either full base or half base.

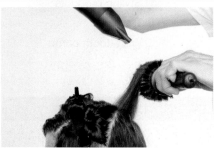

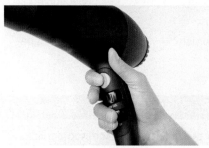

12 For less lift at the scalp, begin by holding the section at a 90-degree angle, following the same procedure.

10 For maximum lift, insert the brush on base and direct the hair section up at a 90-degree angle. Roll the hair down to the base with medium tension. Direct the stream of air from the blowdryer over the curl and away from the scalp in a back and forth motion.

11 When the section is completely dry, press the cooling button and cool the section to strengthen the curl formation. Release the curl by unwinding the section from the brush. (Pulling it out could cause the hair to get tangled in the brush.)

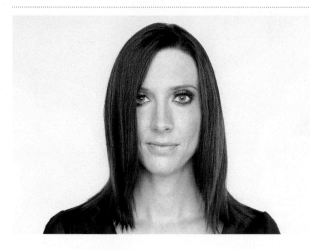

13 Make sure that the scalp and hair are completely dry before combing out the style or the shape will not last. Finish with hair spray.

14 Finished look.

POST-SERVICE

Complete:

P 15-2 **Post-Service Procedure** *See page 343*

BLOWDRYING SHORT, CURLY HAIR IN ITS NATURAL WAVE PATTERN

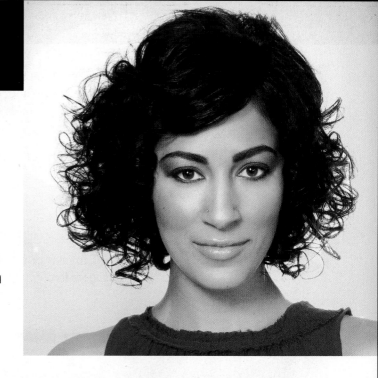

© Tom Carson Photography.

IMPLEMENTS & MATERIALS

You will need all of the following implements, materials, and supplies:

- ☐ Blowdryer with attachments
- ☐ Conditioner
- ☐ Finishing products such as shine or hair spray
- ☐ Neck strip
- ☐ Round brush
- ☐ Sectioning clips
- ☐ Shampoo
- ☐ Styling cape
- ☐ Styling product
- ☐ Towels
- ☐ Wide-tooth comb

PREPARATION

Perform:

P 15-1 **Pre-Service Procedure** *See page 340*

PROCEDURE

1 Drape the client for a shampoo service.

2 Shampoo the client's hair and condition if necessary.

3 Towel dry the hair.

4 Remove any tangles with a wide-tooth comb, starting at the ends and working up to the scalp.

5 Place a clean neck strip on the client and drape with a cutting or styling cape.

6 Apply a liquid gel on the client's hair.

7 Attach the diffuser to the blowdryer.

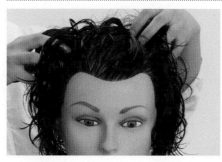

8 With a wide-tooth comb or your fingers, encourage the hair into the desired shape.

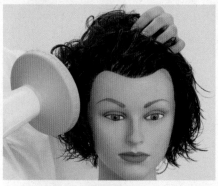

9 Diffuse the hair gently, pressing the diffuser on and off the hair without over-manipulating the hair, until each area of the head is dry.

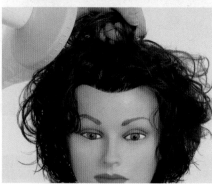

10 To relax or soften the curl, slowly and gently run your fingers through the curl when the hair is almost dry.

11 For a tighter curl, scrunch the hair by placing your hand over a section of hair while it is being diffused, forming a fist with the hair in your hand, using a pulsing motion. Release. Repeat the process until the section is dry.

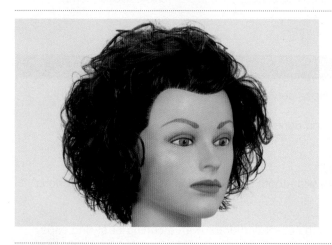

12 For more shine, finish the look with a silicone spray product.

POST-SERVICE

Complete:

P 15-2 **Post-Service Procedure** *See page 343*

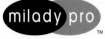 Check out miladypro.com for additional resources and training to enhance your technical skills. Keyword: *FutureCosPro*

DIFFUSING LONG, CURLY, OR EXTREMELY CURLY HAIR IN ITS NATURAL WAVE PATTERN

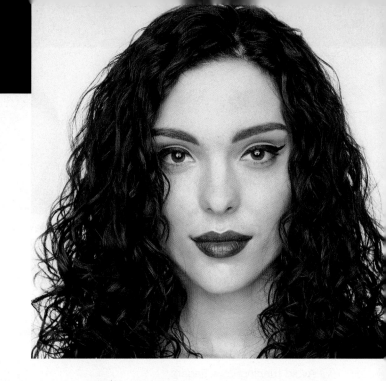

IMPLEMENTS & MATERIALS

You will need all of the following implements, materials, and supplies:

- □ Blowdryer with attachments
- □ Conditioner
- □ Neck strip
- □ Sectioning clips
- □ Shampoo
- □ Styling and finishing products
- □ Styling cape
- □ Towels
- □ Wide-tooth comb

PREPARATION

Perform:

P 15-1 **Pre-Service Procedure** *See page 340*

PROCEDURE

1 Drape the client for a shampoo service.

2 Shampoo the client's hair and condition if necessary.

3 Towel dry the hair.

4 Place a clean neck strip on the client and drape with a cutting or styling cape.

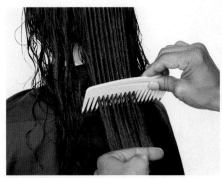

5 Remove any tangles with a wide-tooth comb, starting at the ends and working up to the scalp.

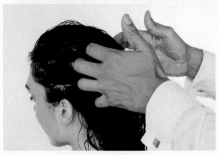

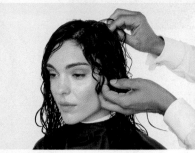

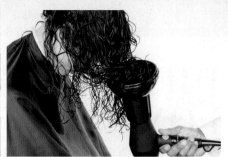

6 Distribute styling product through slightly wet hair with your fingers and comb through with a wide-tooth comb. Always use products designed for this type of hair texture.

7 Position the hair the way the client likes to wear it. Avoid placing a side part before diffusing; it will leave a line of demarcation. If the client wears it to the side, wait until the hair is 100 percent dry before placing a side part.

8 Attach the diffuser to the blowdryer and have the client tilt their head back or bend forward. Diffuse the hair by letting the hair sit on top of the diffuser and pulsing the dryer toward the scalp and then away, repeating until the section is dry.

9 Avoid running your fingers through the hair until its 100 percent dry; doing so will cause the hair to frizz. Once the hair is completely dry, shake the hair, but avoid running your fingers through or using a comb or brush. Use your fingers to separate the curl if necessary.

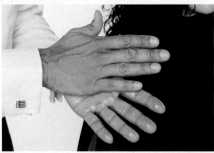

10 Finish by using a serum or shine product and evenly distribute it by gently scrunching the hair, trying not to disturb the curl

11 Finished look.

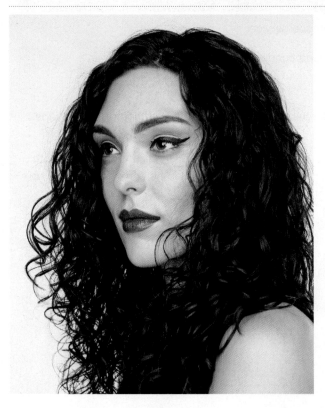

POST-SERVICE

Complete:

P 15-2 **Post-Service Procedure** *See page 343*

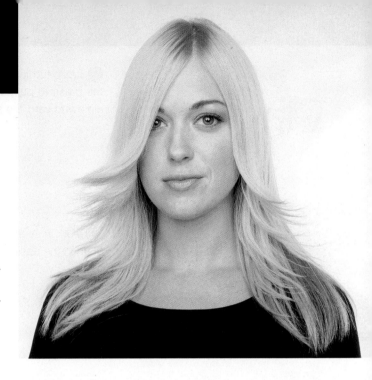

BLOWDRYING STRAIGHT OR WAVY HAIR FOR MAXIMUM VOLUME

IMPLEMENTS & MATERIALS

You will need all of the following implements, materials, and supplies:

- Blowdryer with attachments
- Conditioner
- Neck strip
- Sectioning clips
- Shampoo
- Styling and finishing product
- Styling cape
- Towels
- Vent or classic styling brush
- Wide-tooth comb

PREPARATION

Perform:

P 15-1 **Pre-Service Procedure** *See page 340*

PROCEDURE

1. Drape the client for a shampoo service.

2. Shampoo the client's hair and condition if necessary.

3. Towel dry the hair.

4. Remove any tangles with a wide-tooth comb, starting at the ends and working up to the scalp.

5. Place a clean neck strip on the client and drape with a cutting or styling cape.

6. Apply a mousse, volumizing spray, or lightweight gel.

7. Using a vent brush or classic styling brush, distribute the hair into the desired shape.

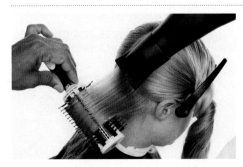

8. Build your shape from the bottom up, working from the nape up toward the crown. When you begin at the nape, hold the hair above the area in a sectioning clip.

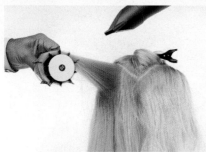

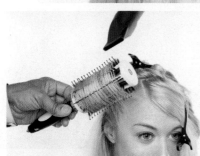

⑨ While turning the brush downward and away from the scalp, allow the brush to pick up a section of hair and begin drying. Direct the airflow toward the top of the brush, moving in the desired direction.

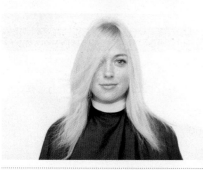

⑩ Work in sections, lifting and drying the sections and then brushing them in the desired direction when they are completely dry.

⑪ Repeat over the entire head, directing the hair at the sides either away or forward. The bang area can be dried either onto the forehead or away from the face.

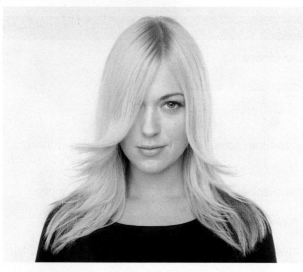

⑫ Finished look.

POST-SERVICE

Complete:

Ⓟ 15-2 **Post-Service Procedure** *See page 343*

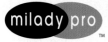

Check out miladypro.com for additional resources and training to enhance your technical skills. Keyword: *FutureCosPro*

BLOWDRYING STRAIGHT OR WAVY HAIR FOR MAXIMUM VOLUME

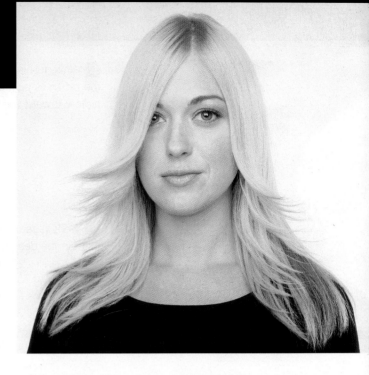

IMPLEMENTS & MATERIALS

You will need all of the following implements, materials, and supplies:

- ☐ Blowdryer with attachments
- ☐ Conditioner
- ☐ Neck strip
- ☐ Sectioning clips
- ☐ Shampoo
- ☐ Styling and finishing product
- ☐ Styling cape
- ☐ Towels
- ☐ Vent or classic styling brush
- ☐ Wide-tooth comb

PREPARATION

Perform:

P 15-1 **Pre-Service Procedure** *See page 340*

PROCEDURE

1. Drape the client for a shampoo service.

2. Shampoo the client's hair and condition if necessary.

3. Towel dry the hair.

4. Remove any tangles with a wide-tooth comb, starting at the ends and working up to the scalp.

5. Place a clean neck strip on the client and drape with a cutting or styling cape.

6. Apply a mousse, volumizing spray, or lightweight gel.

7. Using a vent brush or classic styling brush, distribute the hair into the desired shape.

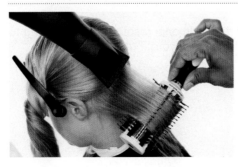

8. Build your shape from the bottom up, working from the nape up toward the crown. When you begin at the nape, hold the hair above the area in a sectioning clip.

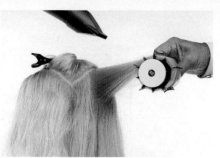

9 While turning the brush downward and away from the scalp, allow the brush to pick up a section of hair and begin drying. Direct the airflow toward the top of the brush, moving in the desired direction.

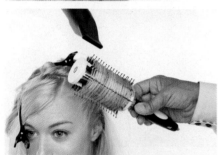

10 Work in sections, lifting and drying the sections and then brushing them in the desired direction when they are completely dry.

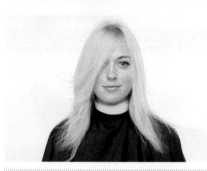

11 Repeat over the entire head, directing the hair at the sides either away or forward. The bang area can be dried either onto the forehead or away from the face.

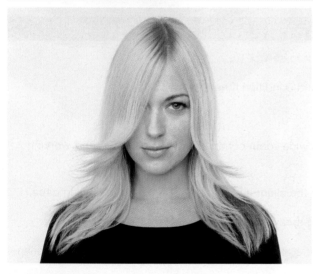

12 Finished look.

POST-SERVICE

Complete:

P 15-2 **Post-Service Procedure** *See page 343*

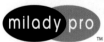 Check out miladypro.com for additional resources and training to enhance your technical skills.   Keyword: *FutureCosPro*

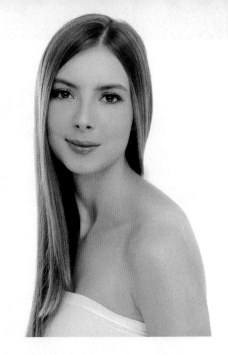

BLOWDRYING BLUNT OR LONG-LAYERED, STRAIGHT TO WAVY HAIR INTO A STRAIGHT STYLE

© Tom Carson Photography.

IMPLEMENTS & MATERIALS

You will need all of the following implements, materials, and supplies:

- ☐ Blowdryer with attachments
- ☐ Conditioner
- ☐ Neck strip

- ☐ Paddle brush
- ☐ Round brush
- ☐ Sectioning clips

- ☐ Shampoo
- ☐ Styling and finishing products
- ☐ Styling cape

- ☐ Towels
- ☐ Wide-tooth comb

PREPARATION

Perform:

Ⓟ 15-1 **Pre-Service Procedure** *See page 340*

PROCEDURE

1 Drape the client for a shampoo service.

2 Shampoo the client's hair and condition if necessary.

3 Towel dry the hair.

4 Remove any tangles with a wide-tooth comb, starting at the ends and working up to the scalp.

5 Place a clean neck strip on the client and drape with a cutting or styling cape.

6 Apply a light gel or a straightening gel.

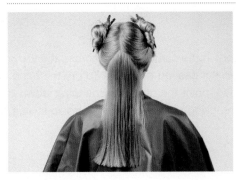

7 Attach the nozzle or concentrator attachment to the blowdryer for more controlled styling. Part and section the hair so that only the section you are drying is not in clips.

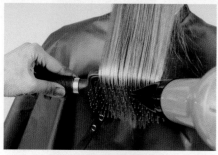

8 Using 1-inch (2.5 centimeters) subsections, start your first section at the nape of the neck and use a classic styling brush to dry the hair straight and smooth. Place the brush under the first section and hold the hair low.

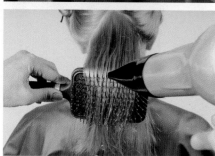

9 Follow the brush with the nozzle of the dryer while bending the ends of the hair in the desired direction, either under or flipped outward. Continue using the same technique, working up to the occipital area in 1-inch (2.5 centimeters) sections.

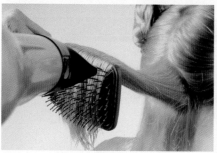

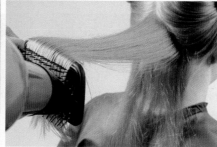

12 After each section is blown dry, follow by using the cooling button on the blowdryer to help set each section and to keep it smooth. For a fuller look, switch to a round brush.

10 To keep the shape flat and straight, use low elevation. For more lift and volume, hold the section straight out from the head or overdirect upward.

11 Work up to the crown, continuing to take 1-inch (2.5 centimeters) sections. On the longer sections toward the top of the crown, you can switch to a paddle brush, using the curve of the brush to add bend to the ends of the hair.

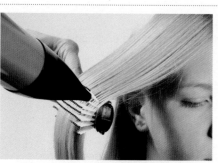

13 Continue by subdividing the hair on the side and start with the section above the ear. Continue working in 1-inch (2.5 centimeters) sections. Hold at a low elevation and follow with the nozzle of the dryer facing toward the ends. Bend the ends under by turning the brush under for a rounded edge, or outward for a flipped edge.

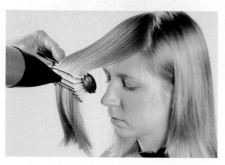

14 Work in the same manner across the top of the head. If there is a bang, dry it in the desired direction. To dry the bang straight and onto the forehead, point the nozzle of the dryer down over the bang and dry it straight, using your fingers or a classic styling brush to direct the hair.

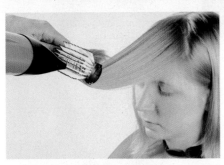

15 To direct the bang away from the face, brush the bang back and push the hair slightly forward with the brush, creating a curved shaping.

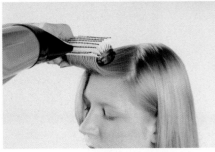

16 Place the dryer on a slow setting and point the nozzle toward the brush. When dry, the bang will fall away from the face and slightly to the side, for a soft look.

17 Finished look.

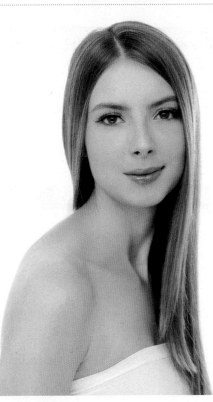

POST-SERVICE

Complete:

P 15-2 **Post-Service Procedure** *See page 343*

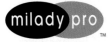

Check out miladypro.com for additional resources and training to enhance your technical skills.   Keyword: *FutureCosPro*

BLOWDRYING BLUNT OR LONG-LAYERED, STRAIGHT TO WAVY HAIR INTO A STRAIGHT STYLE

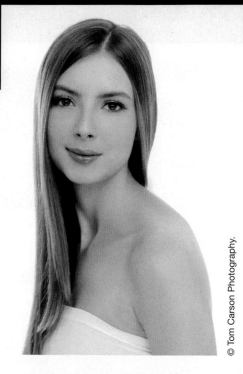

© Tom Carson Photography.

IMPLEMENTS & MATERIALS

You will need all of the following implements, materials, and supplies:

- □ Blowdryer with attachments
- □ Conditioner
- □ Neck strip
- □ Paddle brush
- □ Round brush
- □ Sectioning clips
- □ Shampoo
- □ Styling and finishing products
- □ Styling cape
- □ Towels
- □ Wide-tooth comb

PREPARATION

Perform:

P 15-1 **Pre-Service Procedure** *See page 340*

PROCEDURE

1 Drape the client for a shampoo service.

2 Shampoo the client's hair and condition if necessary.

3 Towel dry the hair.

4 Remove any tangles with a wide-tooth comb, starting at the ends and working up to the scalp.

5 Place a clean neck strip on the client and drape with a cutting or styling cape.

6 Apply a light gel or a straightening gel.

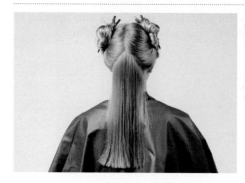

7 Attach the nozzle or concentrator attachment to the blowdryer for more controlled styling. Part and section the hair so that only the section you are drying is not in clips.

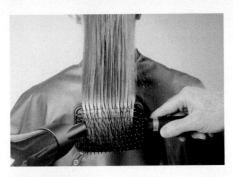

8 Using 1-inch (2.5 centimeters) subsections, start your first section at the nape of the neck and use a classic styling brush to dry the hair straight and smooth. Place the brush under the first section and hold the hair low.

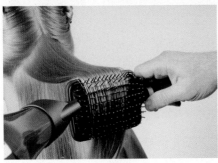

9 Follow the brush with the nozzle of the dryer while bending the ends of the hair in the desired direction, either under or flipped outward.

10 Continue using the same technique, working up to the occipital area in 1-inch (2.5 centimeters) sections. To keep the shape flat and straight, use low elevation. For more lift and volume, hold the section straight out from the head or overdirect upward.

11 Work up to the crown, continuing to take 1-inch (2.5 centimeters) sections. On the longer sections toward the top of the crown, you can switch to a paddle brush, using the curve of the brush to add bend to the ends of the hair.

12 After each section is blown dry, follow by using the cooling button on the blowdryer to help set each section and to keep it smooth. For a fuller look, switch to a round brush.

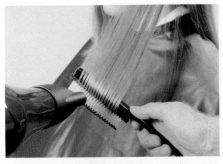

13 Continue by subdividing the hair on the side and start with the section above the ear. Continue working in 1-inch (2.5 centimeters) sections. Hold at a low elevation and follow with the nozzle of the dryer facing toward the ends. Bend the ends under by turning the brush under for a rounded edge, or outward for a flipped edge.

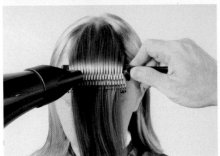

14 Work in the same manner across the top of the head. If there is a bang, dry it in the desired direction. To dry the bang straight and onto the forehead, point the nozzle of the dryer down over the bang and dry it straight, using your fingers or a classic styling brush to direct the hair.

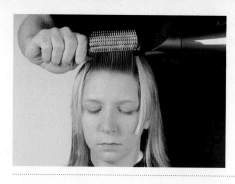

15 To direct the bang away from the face, brush the bang back and push the hair slightly forward with the brush, creating a curved shaping.

16 Place the dryer on a slow setting and point the nozzle toward the brush. When dry, the bang will fall away from the face and slightly to the side, for a soft look.

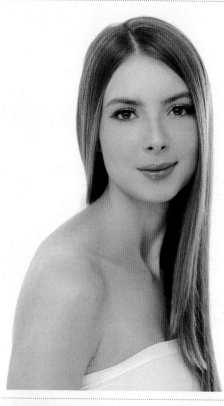

17 Finished look.

POST-SERVICE

Complete:

P 15-2   **Post-Service Procedure** *See page 343*

Check out miladypro.com for additional resources and training to enhance your technical skills.   Keyword: *FutureCosPro*

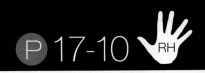
THERMAL WAVING

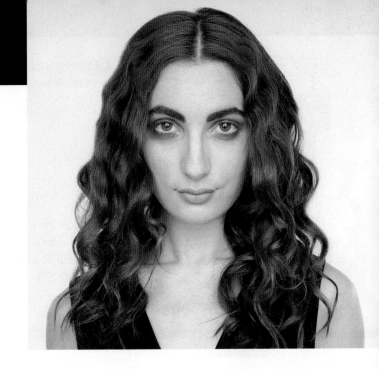

IMPLEMENTS & MATERIALS

You will need all of the following implements, materials, and supplies:

- ☐ Conventional (Marcel) or electric irons
- ☐ Conditioner
- ☐ Hard rubber comb (fine toothed)
- ☐ Shampoo
- ☐ Styling cape and neck strip
- ☐ Towels
- ☐ Wide-tooth comb

PREPARATION

Perform:

P 15-1 **Pre-Service Procedure** *See page 340*

PROCEDURE

1 Drape the client for a shampoo service.

2 Shampoo the client's hair and condition if necessary.

3 Towel dry the hair.

4 Remove any tangles with a wide-tooth comb, starting at the ends and working up to the scalp.

5 Dry the client's hair completely.

6 Drape the client for a dry hair service.

7 Heat the iron.

8 Before beginning the waves, comb the hair in the general shape desired by the client. The natural growth will determine whether or not the first wave will be a left-moving wave or a right-moving wave. The procedure described here is for a left-moving wave.

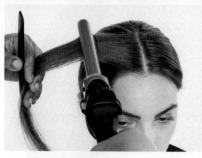

9 With the comb, pick up a strand of hair about 2 inches (5 centimeters) in width. Insert the iron in the hair with the groove facing upward.

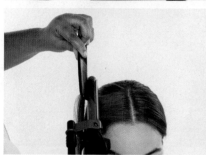

10 Close the iron and give it a ¼-inch (0.625 centimeters) turn forward (away from you). At the same time, draw the hair with the iron about ¼ inch (0.625 centimeters) to the left, and direct the hair ¼ inch (0.625 centimeters) to the right with the comb.

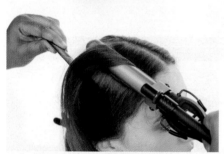

11 Roll the iron one full turn forward and away from you. When doing this, keep the hair uniform with the comb. Keep this position for a few seconds in order to allow the hair to become sufficiently heated throughout.

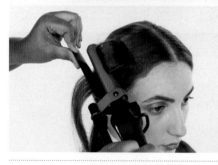

12 Reverse the movement by simply unrolling the hair from the iron and bringing it back into its first resting position. When this movement is completed, you will find the comb resting somewhat away from the iron.

13 Open the iron and place it just below the ridge or crest by swinging the rod of the iron toward you and then closing it. The outer edge of the groove should be directly underneath the ridge just produced.

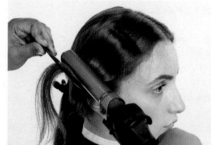

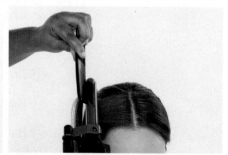

14 Keeping the iron perfectly still, direct the hair with the comb upward about 1 inch (2.5 centimeters), thus forming the hair into a half circle.

15 Without opening the iron, roll it a half turn forward and away from you. In this movement, keep the comb perfectly still and unchanged.

16 Slide the iron down about 1 inch (2.5 centimeters). This movement is accomplished by opening the iron slightly, gripping it loosely, and then sliding it down the strand.

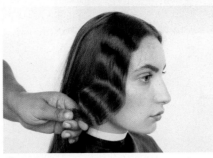

17 After completing step 16, you will find the iron and comb in the correct positions to make the second ridge. This is the beginning of a right-moving wave, in which the hair is directed opposite to that of a left-moving wave.

18 After completely waving one strand of hair, wave the next strand to match. Pick up the strand in the comb and include a small section of the waved strand to guide you as you form a new wave. Be sure to use the same movements to ensure consistency of waves on each section.

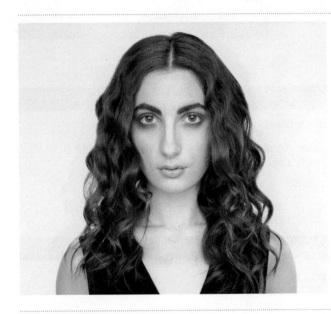

19 Finished look.

POST-SERVICE

Complete:

P 15-2 **Post-Service Procedure** *See page 343*

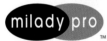 Check out miladypro.com for additional resources and training to enhance your technical skills.   Keyword: *FutureCosPro*

THERMAL WAVING

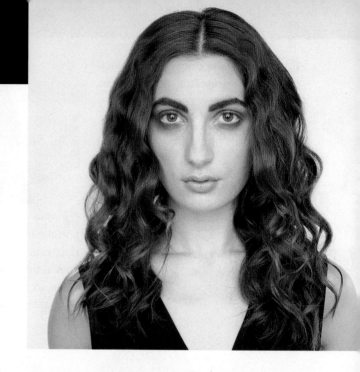

IMPLEMENTS & MATERIALS

You will need all of the following implements, materials, and supplies:

☐ Conventional (Marcel) or electric irons

☐ Conditioner

☐ Hard rubber comb (fine toothed)

☐ Shampoo

☐ Styling cape and neck strip

☐ Towels

☐ Wide-tooth comb

PREPARATION

Perform:

P 15-1 **Pre-Service Procedure** *See page 340*

PROCEDURE

1 Drape the client for a shampoo service.

2 Shampoo the client's hair and condition if necessary.

3 Towel dry the hair.

4 Remove any tangles with a wide-tooth comb, starting at the ends and working up to the scalp.

5 Dry the client's hair completely.

6 Drape the client for a dry hair service.

7 Heat the iron.

8 Before beginning the waves, comb the hair in the general shape desired by the client. The natural growth will determine whether or not the first wave will be a left-moving wave or a right-moving wave. The procedure described here is for a left-moving wave.

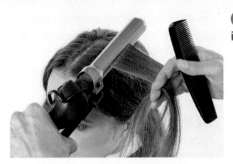

9 With the comb, pick up a strand of hair about 2 inches (5 centimeters) in width. Insert the iron in the hair with the groove facing upward.

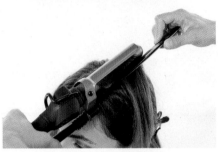

10 Close the iron and give it a ¼-inch (0.625 centimeters) turn forward (away from you). At the same time, draw the hair with the iron about ¼ inch (0.625 centimeters) to the left, and direct the hair ¼ inch (0.625 centimeters) to the right with the comb.

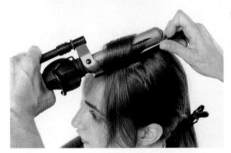

11 Roll the iron one full turn forward and away from you. When doing this, keep the hair uniform with the comb. Keep this position for a few seconds in order to allow the hair to become sufficiently heated throughout.

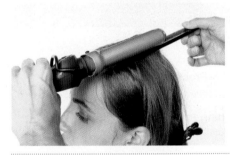

12 Reverse the movement by simply unrolling the hair from the iron and bringing it back into its first resting position. When this movement is completed, you will find the comb resting somewhat away from the iron.

13 Open the iron and place it just below the ridge or crest by swinging the rod of the iron toward you, and then closing it. The outer edge of the groove should be directly underneath the ridge just produced.

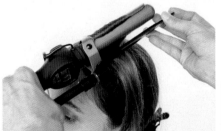

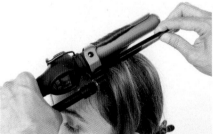

14 Keeping the iron perfectly still, direct the hair with the comb upward about 1 inch (2.5 centimeters), thus forming the hair into a half circle.

15 Without opening the iron, roll it a half turn forward and away from you. In this movement, keep the comb perfectly still and unchanged.

16 Slide the iron down about 1 inch (2.5 centimeters). This movement is accomplished by opening the iron slightly, gripping it loosely, and then sliding it down the strand.

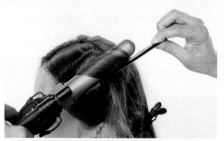

17 After completing step 16, you will find the iron and comb in the correct positions to make the second ridge. This is the beginning of a right-moving wave, in which the hair is directed opposite to that of a left-moving wave.

18 After completely waving one strand of hair, wave the next strand to match. Pick up the strand in the comb and include a small section of the waved strand to guide you as you form a new wave. Be sure to use the same movements to ensure consistency of waves on each section.

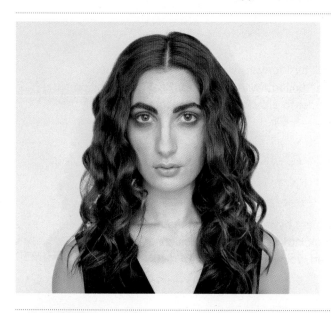

19 Finished look.

POST-SERVICE

Complete:

P 15-2 **Post-Service Procedure** *See page 343*

milady pro ™ Check out miladypro.com for additional resources and training to enhance your technical skills.   Keyword: *FutureCosPro*

CHIGNON

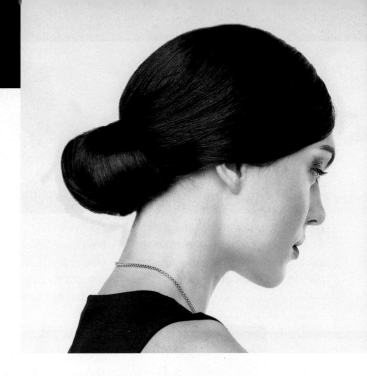

IMPLEMENTS & MATERIALS

You will need all of the following implements, materials, and supplies:

- ☐ Bobby pins
- ☐ Bristle brush
- ☐ Curling iron
- ☐ Elastics

- ☐ Electric or Velcro rollers (optional)
- ☐ Finishing spray
- ☐ Grooming or teasing brush

- ☐ Hairpins
- ☐ Hair spray
- ☐ Neck strip
- ☐ Shampoo

- ☐ Styling cape
- ☐ Tail comb
- ☐ Towels

PREPARATION

Perform:

P 15-1 **Pre-Service Procedure** *See page 340*

PROCEDURE

1 Drape the client; shampoo and towel dry the hair.

2 Re-drape the client with a neck strip and styling cape.

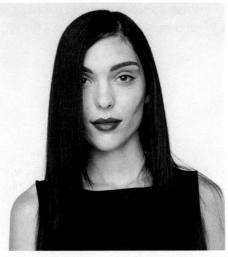

3 Apply the appropriate styling product that will give the hair hold. Blowdry the hair with a brush for a smooth sleek finish.

4 **(Optional)** Set hair in electric or Velcro rollers, depending on the amount of curl or volume you may need.

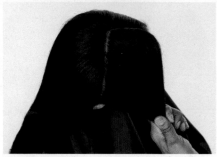

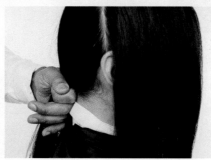

7 Place two bobby pins onto the band and spread them apart, one on each side. Place one bobby pin in the base of the ponytail. Stretch the band around the ponytail base. Place the second bobby pin in the base. Lock the two pins together.

5 Part the hair on desired side. On the heavy side, place a radial section from the back of your side part to the back of the ear.

6 Brush hair into a low ponytail at the nape. Secure the ponytail with an elastic band, keeping the hair as smooth as possible. Use the side of the bristles to smooth the hair.

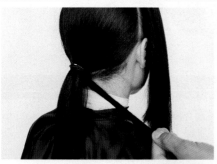

8 Part a small section of hair from the underside of the ponytail, wrap it around the ponytail to cover the elastic, and secure with a bobby pin underneath.

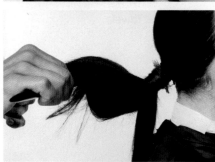

9 Smooth out the ponytail and hold it with one hand, and then begin backbrushing from underneath the ponytail with your other hand. Gently smooth out the ponytail after backbrushing, using the sides of the bristles.

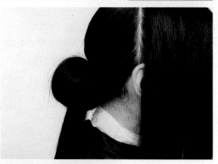

10 Roll the hair under and toward the head to form the chignon. Secure on the left and right undersides of the roll with bobby pins.

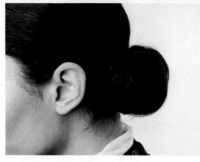

11 Fan out both sides by spreading the chignon with your fingers. Secure with hairpins, pinning close to the head. Use bobby pins if more hold is needed.

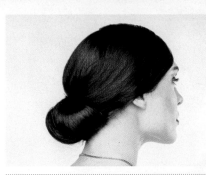

12 Take the remaining section at the front and brush it over in to a side sweep and then wrap around chignon. Finish with a strong hair spray and add flowers or ornaments if desired.

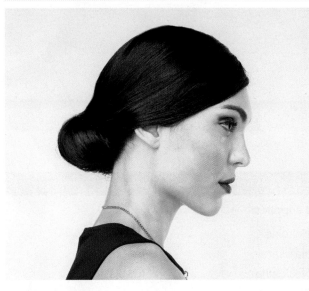

13 Finished look.

POST-SERVICE

Complete:

 15-2 **Post-Service Procedure** *See page 343*

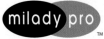 Check out miladypro.com for additional resources and training to enhance your technical skills.   Keyword: *FutureCosPro*

FRENCH PLEAT OR TWIST

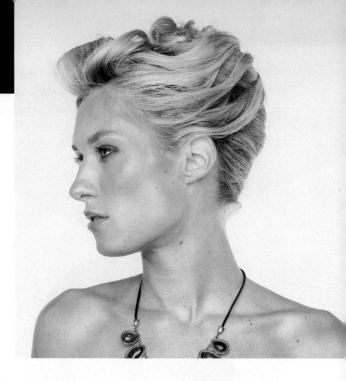

IMPLEMENTS & MATERIALS

You will need all of the following implements, materials, and supplies:

- ☐ Bobby pins
- ☐ Bristle brush
- ☐ Conditioner
- ☐ Convention (Marcel) or electric iron

- ☐ Elastics
- ☐ Electric or Velcro rollers
- ☐ Finishing spray
- ☐ Grooming or teasing brush

- ☐ Hairpins
- ☐ Hair spray
- ☐ Neck strip
- ☐ Shampoo

- ☐ Styling cape
- ☐ Tail comb
- ☐ Towels

PREPARATION

Perform:

P 15-1 **Pre-Service Procedure** *See page 340*

PROCEDURE

1 Drape the client; shampoo and towel dry the hair.

2 Re-drape the client with a neck strip and styling cape.

3 Apply the appropriate styling product that will give the hair a lot of hold. Blowdry the hair, smoothing it with a brush for a sleek finish.

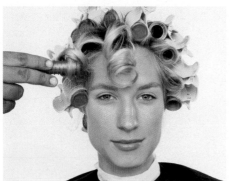

4 Set the hair with a wet set or, if you wish to save time, electric rollers or thermal irons.

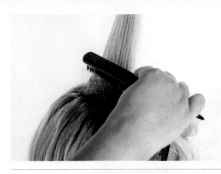

5 Once completely dry, establish a side part from the front hairline to the apex of the head. Divide the front from the back by taking a radial parting from the apex of the head to the top of each ear and clip out of the way. Lightly backcomb the hair in the rear section, building weight throughout till you have accomplished a light packing.

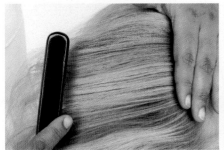

6 Using a grooming or a teasing brush, gently smooth the hair of the back section toward the heavy side. Be sure to not remove all your backcombing.

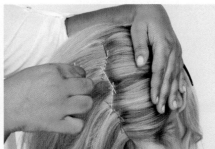

7 Begin pinning the hair at the center of the nape. Move upward with the bobby pins while having the client hold her head completely upright, overlapping the pins by crisscrossing them to lock into place. Continue pinning; stop just below the crown.

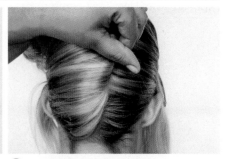

8 With the brush, bring the hair from the left side over the center line (where the bobby pins were placed) and smooth; twist from the center of the nape. Move upward and inward, tucking the ends into the fold as you move up, to create a funnel shape.

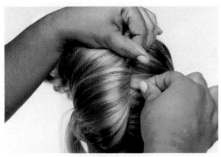

9 Secure with hairpins vertically down into the seam as you work up, hiding the pins in the seam. Move to a side section and lightly backbrush the section. Bring the side section up to last completed section and blend into the fold.

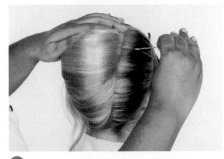

10 Secure with a bobby pin at the top of the side section, leaving the ends out. Repeat on the other side. Fold over while smoothing and pin downward.

11 Backbrush and smooth the remaining side section on the right into the remaining section on the left, just above the top of the twist.

12 Swirl and join this section of hair into the open end of the twist. Use a tail comb or the tail of the backcombing brush to smooth and curl ends into the twist and pin. Take care not to expose the pin.

13 Style the section in the bangs as you wish. This section could also be brought back and added to the crown if your client is more comfortable with all her hair off her face. Or you can sweep the hair loosely to the side and leave the ends hanging softly down.

14 Here is where your creativity and consultation comes into play as you make the best design decision for your client. The hair in the front can be worn off the face, by incorporating it into the top, sides, back, or left out as a side swept bang (fringe). Pieces may be twisted, pinned and placed or backcombed and smoothed, to be worn loose. Spray finished style with a firm hold hair spray and check to make sure there are no exposed pins. Use a tail comb to balance the shape of the pleat.

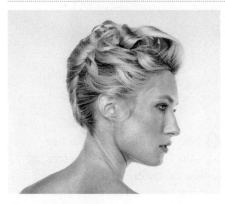 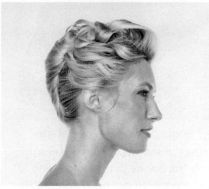 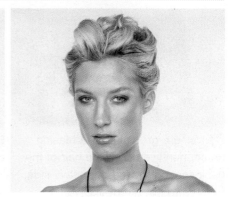

15 Finished look.

POST-SERVICE

Complete:

P 15-2   **Post-Service Procedure** *See page 343*

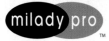 Check out miladypro.com for additional resources and training to enhance your technical skills.   Keyword: *FutureCosPro*

HALF UPDO

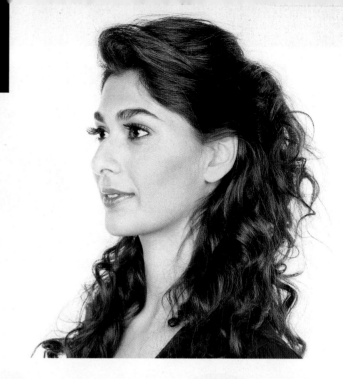

IMPLEMENTS & MATERIALS

You will need all of the following implements, materials, and supplies:

- ☐ Bobby pins, hairpins (same color as client's hair)
- ☐ Bristle brush
- ☐ Conditioner
- ☐ Curling iron
- ☐ Elastics
- ☐ Electric or Velcro rollers
- ☐ Finishing spray
- ☐ Grooming or teasing brush
- ☐ Neck strip
- ☐ Shampoo
- ☐ Styling cape
- ☐ Tail comb
- ☐ Towels
- ☐ Working hair spray

PREPARATION

Perform:

P 15-1 **Pre-Service Procedure** *See page 340*

PROCEDURE

1 Drape the client; shampoo and towel dry the hair.

2 Re-drape the client with a neck strip and styling cape.

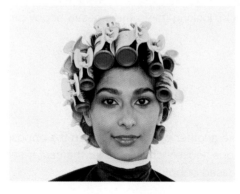

3 Set the hair with a wet set or, if you wish to save time, electric rollers or thermal iron, utilizing any of the three basic curl patters for your desired texture.

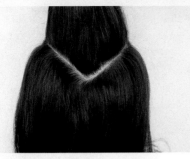

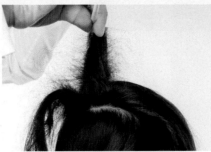

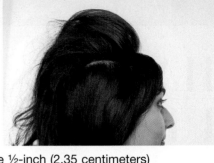

④ Once hair is set, take a large reverse triangle section, starting approximately 2 inches (5 centimeters) from the hairline with the point of the triangle placed just below the crown. Clip the remainder of the hair out of the way.

⑤ Starting at the top of the head, take ½-inch (2.35 centimeters) sections and backcomb or backbrush the entire triangle at the roots—the idea is to create height.

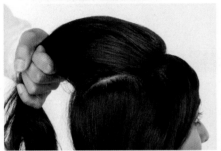

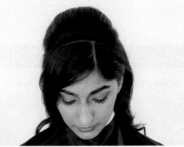

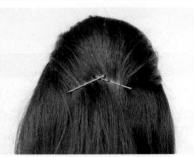

⑥ Smooth out your backcombing by brushing only the surface.

⑦ Gather the hair and place it just below the crown at the point of the triangle. Turn the styling chair and look at the balance and proportion in the mirror. Ask the client if she prefers more or less height, but use your judgment.

⑧ Using bobby pins, secure the hair by crossing your pins so they lock into place. Remove the clips and release the remainder of the hair. Take the section at the top, front hairline at the recession and clip it out of the way.

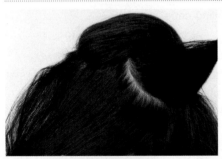

⑨ Starting at the back side, take curved sections from the side of the triangle and loosely cross over the hair that is pinned and secure it with a hairpin, locking it into the crossed bobby pins.

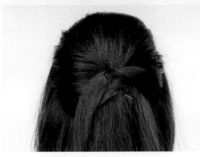

⑩ Take another curved section on the opposite side and repeat the technique, loosely crossing over the center section and pinning into the crossed bobby pins.

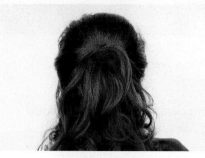

11 Keep repeating this technique until all the sides are off the face, leaving out the hair in front of the triangle. Keep crossing each section at the back until just above the occipital bone.

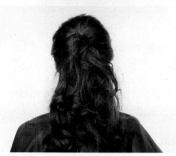

12 At this point, all of the hair at the sides should be pinned at the back with just the front portion remaining. Use your creativity as direction to finish the style. The hair in the front can be worn off the face, by incorporating it into the top, side, or left out as a side swept bang (as shown here). Continue to check your style for balance in the mirror. Step away from your work and look at all the angles.

13 If the client doesn't have bangs, backbrush the front section, smooth it out, and loosely pin it back to one side or you can place a center part. Ask your client what she prefers, but use your best judgment.

14 Arrange the hair at the back with your fingers and check the balance. Avoid using too much hairspray so the hair has movement at the back.

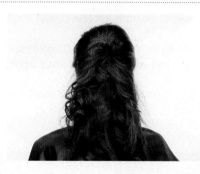

15 Finished look.

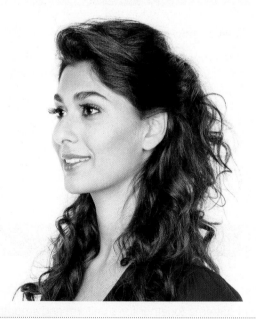

POST-SERVICE

Complete:

P 15-2 **Post-Service Procedure** *See page 343*

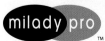

Check out miladypro.com for additional resources and training to enhance your technical skills. Keyword: *FutureCosPro*

REVIEW QUESTIONS

1. What is the purpose of finger waving?

2. What are the three parts of a pin curl?

3. Name the four pin curl bases and their uses.

4. Describe the three kinds of roller curl bases and other useful ways to apply these techniques.

5. What is the purpose of backcombing and backbrushing?

6. How can you avoid burning the client's scalp during blowdrying?

7. List and describe the various styling products used in blowdry styling.

8. How is volume achieved with thermal curls?

9. List at least ten safety measures that must be followed when using thermal irons.

10. Name and describe the three types of hair presses.

11. How do you test the pressing comb before beginning a service?

12. What are the considerations in a hair and scalp analysis prior to hair pressing?

13. Under what circumstances should hair not be pressed?

14. List at least four safety measures that must be followed when pressing the hair.

15. What are the five key points you must consider before beginning an updo?

16. Name the two basic hairstyles considered the foundation of every updo and long hairstyling.

17. Name the four basic curl patterns and their specific end results.

18. Describe a half updo? What length is it designed for?

STUDY TOOLS

- **Reinforce what you just learned:** Complete the activities and exercises in your Theory or Practical Workbook, or your Study Guide.

- **Expand your knowledge:** Search for websites about the topics in this chapter and make a list of additional resources.

- **Study and prepare for your quiz:** Take the chapter test in your Exam Review or your Milady U: Online Licensing Prep.

- **Re-Test your knowledge:** Take the Chapter 17 *Quizzes*!

- **Learn even more:** Look up in a dictionary or search the internet for the definitions of any additional terms you want to learn about.

CHAPTER GLOSSARY

backbrushing	p. 454	Also known as *ruffing* (RUF-ing); technique used to build a soft cushion or to mesh two or more curl patterns together for a uniform and smooth comb out.
backcombing	p. 454	Also known as *teasing, ratting, matting,* or *French lacing*; combing small sections of hair from the ends toward the scalp, causing shorter hair to mat at the scalp and form a cushion or base.

barrel curls	p. 450	Pin curls with large center openings, fastened to the head in a standing position on a rectangular base.
base	p. 451	Stationary, or non-moving, foundation of a pin curl (the area closest to the scalp); the panel of hair on which a roller is placed.
blowdry styling	p. 456	Technique of drying and styling damp hair in a single operation.
bun	p. 474	Also known as a *knot*; the foundation technique used for this look is a ponytail and can sit high or low.
carved curls	p. 449	Also known as *sculptured curls*; pin curls sliced from a shaping and formed without lifting the hair from the head.
cascade curls	p. 450	Also known as *stand-up curls*; pin curls fastened to the head in a standing position to allow the hair to flow upward and then downward.
chignon	p. 473	A classic updo designed around a ponytail; a technique used in formal hairstyling.
circle	p. 446	The part of the pin curl that forms a complete circle; also, the hair that is wrapped around the roller.
closed-center curls	p. 447	Pin curls that produce waves that get smaller toward the ends.
concentrator	p. 457	Nozzle attachment of a blowdryer; directs the air stream to any section of the hair more intensely.
curl	p. 451	Also known as *circle*; the hair that is wrapped around the roller.
diffuser	p. 457	Blowdryer attachment that causes the air to flow more softly and helps to accentuate or keep textural definition.
double press	p. 467	Technique of passing a hot curling iron through the hair before performing a hard press.
end curls	p. 465	Used to give a finished appearance to hair ends either turned under or over.
finger waving	p. 445	Process of shaping and directing the hair into an S pattern through the use of the fingers, combs, and waving lotion.
finger-waving lotion	p. 446	Also known as *liquid gel*; is a type of hair gel that makes the hair pliable enough to keep it in place during the finger-waving procedure.
foam	p. 458	Also known as *mousse*; a light, airy, whipped styling product that resembles shaving foam and builds moderate body and volume into the hair.
French pleat	p. 473	Also known as *classic French twist*; a technique used for formal hairstyling that creates a look of folded hair.
full-base curls	p. 465	Thermal curls that sit in the center of their base; strong curls with full volume.
full-stem curl	p. 447	Curl placed completely off the base; allows for the greatest mobility.
gel	p. 459	Thickened styling preparation that comes in a tube or bottle and creates a strong hold.
hair pressing	p. 467	Method of temporarily straightening extremely curly or unruly hair by means of a heated iron or comb.

hair spray	p. 460	Also known as *finishing spray*; a styling product applied in the form of a mist to hold a style in position; available in a variety of holding strengths.
hair wrapping	p. 455	A technique used to keep curly hair smooth and straight.
half base	p. 452	Position of a curl or a roller that sits halfway on its base and halfway behind the base, giving medium volume and movement.
half-base curls	p. 465	Thermal curls placed half off their base; strong curls with moderate lift or volume.
half-stem curl	p. 447	Curl placed half off the base; permits medium movement and gives good control to the hair.
half updo	p. 472	Hairstyle where half of the hair is pulled back off the face and pinned at or below the crown.
hard press	p. 467	Technique that removes 100 percent of the curl by applying the pressing comb twice on each side of the hair.
indentation	p. 452	The point where curls of opposite directions meet, forming a recessed area.
liquid gels	p. 459	Also known as *texturizers*; styling products that are lighter and less viscous than firm hold gels, used for easy styling, defining, and molding.
medium press	p. 467	Technique that removes 60 to 75 percent of the curl by applying a thermal pressing comb once on each side of the hair, using slightly more pressure than in the soft press.
no-stem curl	p. 447	Curl placed directly on its base; produces a tight, firm, long-lasting curl and allows minimum mobility.
off base	p. 452	The position of a curl or a roller completely off its base for maximum mobility and minimum volume.
off-base curls	p. 465	Thermal curls placed completely off their base, offering only slight lift or volume.
on base	p. 452	Also known as *full base*; position of a curl or roller directly on its base for maximum volume.
open-center curls	p. 447	Pin curls that produce even, smooth waves and uniform curls.
pomade poh-MAYD	p. 459	Also known as *wax*; styling product that adds considerable weight to the hair by causing strands to join together, showing separation in the hair.
ponytail	p. 473	The foundation for a chignon, bun, and knot, and can be worn classic or trendy; can be placed on various parts of the head and is the most commonly used hairstyle because of its versatility.
ribboning RIB-un-ing	p. 449	Technique of forcing the hair between the thumb and the back of the comb to create tension.
ridge curls	p. 449	Pin curls placed immediately behind or below a ridge to form a wave.
rod	p. 461	Round, solid prong of a thermal iron.
root curl	p. 464	A curl pattern that creates volume of hair, movement, and a curl formation from roots to ends.
shaping	p. 447	Section of hair that is molded in a circular movement in preparation for the formation of curls.

shell	p. 461	The clamp that presses the hair against the barrel or rod of a thermal iron.
silicone	p. 459	Also known as *serum*, adds gloss and sheen to the hair while creating textural definition.
skip waves	p. 449	Two rows of ridge curls, usually on the side of the head.
soft press	p. 467	Technique of pressing the hair to remove 50 to 60 percent of the curl by applying the thermal pressing comb once on each side of the hair.
spiral curl	p. 464	Method of curling the hair by winding a strand around the rod.
stem	p. 451	Section of the pin curl between the base and first arc (turn) of the circle that gives the curl its direction and movement; the hair between the scalp and the first turn of the roller.
straightening gel	p. 459	Styling product applied to damp hair that is wavy, curly, or extremely curly and then blown dry; relaxes the hair for a smooth, straight look.
temper	p. 469	A process used to condition a new brass pressing comb so that it heats evenly.
thermal irons	p. 460	Implements made of quality steel that are used to curl dry hair.
thermal protection product	p. 460	Also known as *heat protection hair care product*; is used on damp hair after applying styling product and before blowdrying. It protects the hair from heat damage caused by thermal styling tools like blowdryers, flat irons, and curling irons.
thermal waving and curling	p. 460	Also known as *Marcel waving*; methods of waving and curling straight or pressed dry hair using thermal irons and special manipulative curling techniques.
twist	p. 474	Also known as *French pleat*; a technique used for formal hairstyling that creates a look of conical shape.
updo	p. 472	Hairstyle in which the hair is arranged up and off the shoulders.
volume-base curls	p. 465	Thermal curls placed very high on their base; provide maximum lift or volume.
volumizers	p. 459	Styling products that add volume, especially at the base, when wet hair is blown dry.
waves	p. 464	Create an S pattern and give texture and volume to the hair. Waves are a popular classic technique that can be applied on any texture and length, usually a surface enhancer.

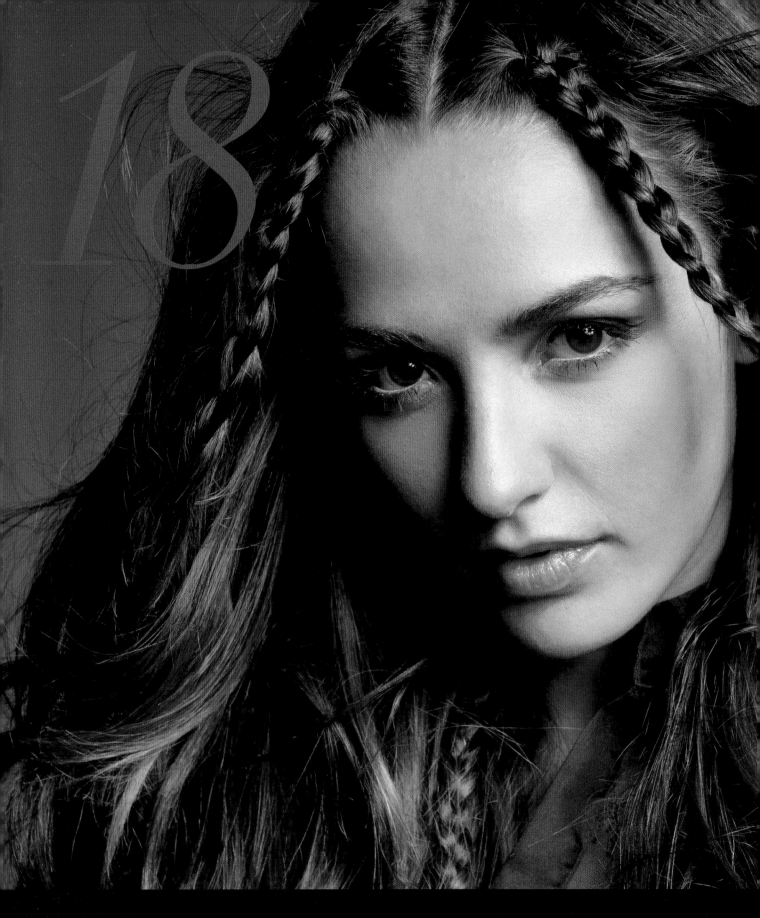

18

BRAIDING AND BRAID EXTENSIONS

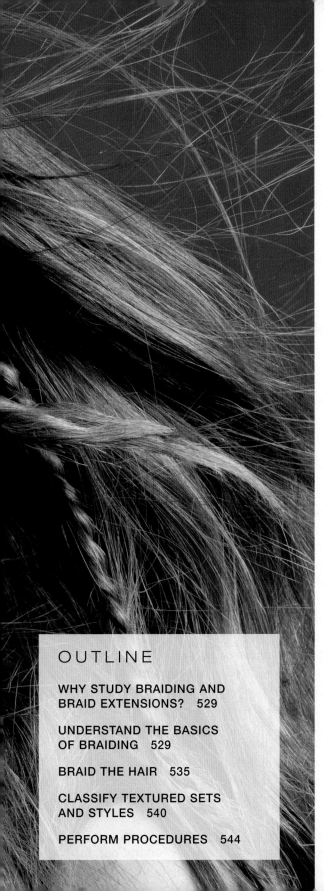

LEARNING OBJECTIVES

After completing this chapter, you will be able to:

LO❶
Know the general history of braiding.

LO❷
Recognize braiding basics and the importance of a consultation.

LO❸
Explain how to prepare the hair for braiding.

LO❹
Describe six types of braiding techniques: rope, fishtail, halo, invisible, single, and single braids with extensions.

LO❺
Demonstrate the procedure for cornrowing.

LO❻
Explain the techniques for textured sets and styles.

LO❼
Demonstrate the procedures for starting locks and lock grooming.

From its origins in Africa to its widespread use today, hair braiding has always played a significant role in grooming and beauty practices. In some African tribes, the statement made by a person's braided style went beyond mere appearance or fashion. Different styles of braiding signified a person's social status within the community. The more important a person's status, the more elaborate his or her braided style appeared. Today, braiding styles continue to communicate important signals about a person's self-esteem and self-image (figure 18-1).

Hair braiding reached its peak of social and esthetic significance in Africa, where it has always been regarded as an art form, handed down from generation to generation. This art form can require an enormous investment of time, with some elaborate styles taking up to an entire day to complete. Because braiding is so time consuming, it is regarded in many African cultures as an opportunity for women to socialize and form relationships. Historically, the first highly decorative braids were seen among African tribes. Many of these tribes, such as the Zulu, were and still are identified by their distinctive hairstyles. As early as 3000 BC, Egyptian women wore braids or plaits decorated with shells, sequins, and glass or gold beads. Ancient paintings from India show women with long, heavy braids. Additional evidence shows that the Anasazi (circa 100 AD), who populated what is now the American Southwest, also favored braids, as did later Native Americans.

The revival of cultural hairstyles in the 1960s and 1970s resulted in the banning of wearing braids in many professions and even high schools, which in turn lead to lawsuits. Suppression was followed by acceptance and mainstream adaptation, and today, braids are as acceptable as any other hairstyle in most modern workplaces.

Braiding salons have sprung up in many areas in the United States. These salons practice what is commonly known as **natural hairstyling**, which uses no chemicals or dyes, and does not alter the natural curl or coil pattern of the hair. While the origins of natural hairstyling are rooted in African heritage, people of all ethnicities appreciate its beauty and versatility. In the twenty-first century, natural hairstyling has brought a diverse approach to hair care. Natural hairstyling can be elaborate, simple, traditional, or trendy. In all cases, offering your clients several different styles of braids can inspire your creativity as a hair artist and create a greater sense of client loyalty.

Some braided styles take many hours to complete. These more complex styles are not disposable hairdos to be casually brushed out. In fact, with proper care, a braided hair design can last up to three months, with six to eight weeks preferable. The investment in time and money is high for both the client and stylist. After you spend hours braiding a client's hair, the last thing you want is to have the client reject it and demand that all the braids be removed. Giving your clients a thorough and detailed consultation is the best way to avoid miscommunications

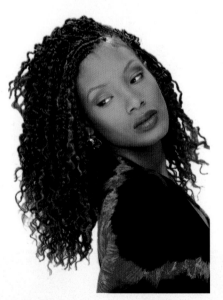

figure 18-1
A contemporary braiding style

Courtesy of Preston Phillips.

and misunderstandings, and will ensure a happy ending to every natural-styling service. Always fill out a client intake form during the initial consultation and update it every time the client returns.

why study

BRAIDING AND BRAID EXTENSIONS?

Cosmetologists should study and have a thorough understanding of the importance of braiding and braid extensions because:

> These services are very popular and consumers are interested in wearing styles specific to their hair texture.

> These techniques provide an opportunity for stylists to express their artistic abilities and to add another high-ticket service to their current service menu!

> All professional cosmetologists should be prepared to work with every type of hair texture and hairstyle trend.

> Working with braid extensions exposes cosmetologists to the fundamental techniques of adding hair extensions, which is another lucrative service for the stylist and the salon.

After reading the next few sections, you will be able to:

LO❷ Recognize braiding basics and the importance of a consultation.

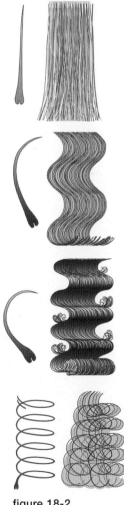

Understand the Basics of Braiding

Before exploring the various braiding techniques, it is important to have a good grasp of braiding basics. During the consultation, you will analyze the condition of your client's hair and scalp, paying particular attention to the hair's type and texture, curl configuration, scalp abrasions, and hair thinning or balding (figure 18-2).

Every client is different. Some clients know exactly what they want in a new style when they come to the salon, others will have no idea of what changes or outcome they are trying to achieve. Performing a thorough client consultation is the best way to understand the needs of the client and provide him or her with the correct braiding services. The consultation is your opportunity to determine what a client wants and needs. As a cosmetologist, it is your duty to personalize every braiding and braiding extension service to enhance each client's individual beauty.

figure 18-2
Wave pattern or coil configuration

Braiding and Textured Hairstyling Consultation

The consultation will consist of the following analysis, test, and recommendations:

- Hair and scalp analysis
- Texture determination
- Elasticity and porosity test
- Style determination
- Product recommendations

Hair And Scalp Analysis

In braiding and other natural hairstyling, texture refers to the following three qualities:

- **Diameter of the hair.** Is the hair coarse, medium, or fine?
- **Feel.** Does the hair feel oily, dry, hard, soft, smooth, coarse, or wiry?
- **Texture determination.** Establish the **wave pattern** or coil configuration. Is the hair straight, wavy, curly, or coiled? A coil is a very tight curl. It is spiral in formation and, when lengthened or stretched, resembles a series of loops. For the purposes of this chapter, the term **textured hair** refers to hair with a tight coil pattern.

In addition to texture, consider the following:

- **Density.** Look for areas where the hair is thin.
- **Condition.** Check for damage and breakage from previous braids or chemical services. Check the hairline for traction alopecia caused by excessive pulling, tight extension braids, or tightly sewn and braided-in weaves.
- **Length.** Make sure that the hair is physically long enough to execute the braiding style.
- **Style determination.** Once the hair and scalp analysis has been completed, it is time to determine which braid style will complement the client's lifestyle and is best for the client's hair texture. Point out braided hairstyles that are of interest to the client, whether it is single box braids, cornrows, or a combination of both braid styles.
- **Product recommendations.** Include instructions on how the client will maintain their hair between salon visits with shampoo, conditioners, and moisturizing regimens. Provide daily and weekly instructions for using sulfate-free and anti-bacterial shampoos, moisturizing leave-in conditioners, essential oil scalp treatments, botanical hair oils, and shine sprays.
- **Scalp health.** Check the condition of the scalp to ensure that it is healthy and properly cared for.
- **Porosity.** Testing the porosity and elasticity of the hair is very important when determining the strength of the hair and the density. Perform a strand test and select several sections of hair strands to test for the porosity and elasticity of the textured hair. To test for the porosity

level, select a small section of hair at the crown section of the head. Holding the hair at the root and at the tip of the hair strand, slide the hair down two to three times slowly and check the porosity of the hair.

- **Elasticity.** Now check for the elasticity of the hair. Select another section of the hair at the crown section of the head and several other sections if the hair texture varies on different sections of the head. Hold the hair with both hands and, using your fingers on the top and bottom of the strand, stretch the hair back and forth to check for the elasticity.

Carefully checking the hair and scalp is essential for a good outcome. If the hair has extremely thin areas, for instance, the braid thickness will be noticeably different in these areas. Check the scalp for any form of alopecia. Areas of the scalp with alopecia are handled differently when choosing the proper braiding technique. In addition, damaged hair should not be braided, since it will further stress the hair. Because everyone has thinner, finer hair around the hairline, you should never choose styles that place excessive tension in this area.

Tools for Braiding

Artists are only as good as their tools, and this adage applies equally to cutting, coloring, and creating natural hairstyles. No matter what length and texture the hair might be, certain tools are essential in order to master various braiding techniques (**figures 18-3** and **18-4**).

- **Boar-bristle brush (natural hairbrush).** Best for stimulating the scalp, as well as removing dirt and lint from locks. Nylon-bristle brushes are not as durable and many snag the hair. However, soft nylon brushes may be an option for fine, soft hair around the hairline.

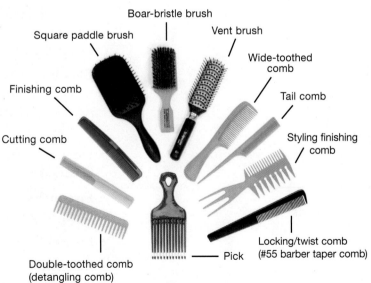

Square paddle brush
Boar-bristle brush
Vent brush
Finishing comb
Wide-toothed comb
Tail comb
Cutting comb
Styling finishing comb
Double-toothed comb (detangling comb)
Pick
Locking/twist comb (#55 barber taper comb)

figure 18-3
Combs and brushes used in braiding

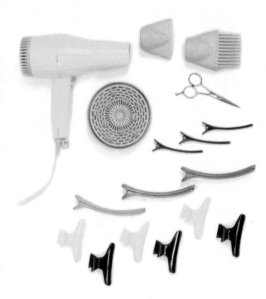

figure 18-4
Clips, blowdryer, diffuser concentrator, nozzle, and scissors

- **Square paddle brush.** This brush is good for releasing tangles, knots, and snarls in short, textured hair and long, straight hair. Square paddle brushes are pneumatic because they have a cushion of air in the head that makes the bristles collapse when they encounter too much resistance. This is key to preventing breakage in fragile textured hair.

- **Vent brush.** This brush has a single or double row of widely spaced pins with protective tips to prevent tearing and breaking the hair. Vent brushes are used to gently remove tangles on wet and wavy or dry and curly hair, as well as on human hair extensions. Always check the protective tips before using a vent brush on the hair. If even only one is missing, discard the brush.

- **Wide-tooth comb.** These are available in a variety of shapes and designs, and they glide through hair with little snarling. The teeth, which range in width from medium to large, have long rounded tips to avoid scratching the scalp. The distance between the teeth is the most important feature of this comb; larger spacing allows textured hair to move between the rows of teeth with ease.

- **Double-tooth comb (detangling comb).** This tool separates the hair as it combs, making it an excellent detangling comb for wet curly hair.

- **Locking/twist comb.** This tool is a #55 barber comb with a smaller angled tooth on one side and a large width on the other end. It allows textured hair to lock and coil easily with various sizes from small, medium, to larger width.

- **Tail comb.** A tail comb is excellent for design parting, sectioning large segments of hair, and opening and removing braids.

- **Finishing comb.** Usually 8 to 10 inches in length, finishing combs are used while cutting. They work well on fine or straight hair.

- **Cutting comb.** This tool is used for cutting small sections. It should be used only after the hair is softened and elongated with a blowdryer.

- **Pick with rounded teeth.** This tool is useful for lifting and separating textured hair. It has long, widely spaced teeth and is commonly made of metal, plastic, or wood.

- **Blowdryer with comb nozzle attachment.** A comb nozzle loosens the curl pattern in textured hair for braiding styles, and it dries, stretches, and softens textured hair. Use a hard plastic comb nozzle because metal attachments become too hot.

- **Diffuser.** Dries hair without disturbing the enhanced curl pattern and finishes the look without dehydrating the hair.

- **Five-inch scissors.** This tool is used for creating shapes and finished looks, and for trimming bangs (fringes) and excess extension material.

- **Long clips.** These clips are used for separating hair into large sections.

- **Butterfly and small clips.** These clips can be used to separate hair into large or small sections.

- **Hood dryer.** Use a hood dryer to remove excess moisture before blowdrying hair completely dry finished braided or locked and textured styles.

- **Steamer.** Use a steamer to deeply hydrate, moisturize, and condition the hair with water vapor. The steam vapor dryer infuses water hydration, opening the cuticle layer of the hair shaft and enabling nourishing, protein conditioners and botanical oils to penetrate deeply into the cortex layer.

- **Small rubber bands, clear elastic bands, or string.** Use these to secure the ends.

  Implements and materials you will need for extensions are listed below:

- **Extension fibers.** These come in a variety of types: Kanekalon®, nylon, rayon, human hair, yarn, lin, and yak.

- **Hackle.** A hackle is a board of fine, upright nails through which human hair extensions are combed; they are used for detangling or blending colors and highlights.

- **Drawing board.** Drawing boards are flat leather pads with very close, fine teeth that sandwich human hair extensions. The pads are weighed down with books, allowing a specific amount of hair to be extracted without loosening and disturbing the rest of the hair during the process of braiding.

Materials for Extensions

A wide variety of fibers are available for the purpose of extending hair. It is important to keep in mind that the fibers you use will largely determine how successful and durable the extension will be. Although it may seem like a good idea to buy the least expensive product, in the long run this may not prove to be the most economical solution—especially if you are buying hair fabric in large quantities. You may get stuck with a lot of material, for instance, that does not give you the results you desire. When buying a new product, buy in small quantities and test the fiber on a mannequin before using it on a client.

The following materials are most commonly used for hair extensions:

- **Human hair.** Human hair is the gold standard for hair extensions. Unfortunately, the human hair market can be a confusing and sometimes deceptive business. Most human hair is imported from Asia, with little information about how it was processed, or even if it is 100 percent human hair. This makes it very important to deal only with suppliers you know and trust (figure 18-5).

- **Kanekalon.** A manufactured, synthetic fiber of excellent quality, Kanekalon is made in a wide variety of types, with different names, colors, and textures. Many companies that offer synthetic hair goods use a line or brand made of Kanekalon. Some Kanekalon fibers are high-heat resistant, some are especially made for

figure 18-5
Human hair is the gold standard for hair extensions.

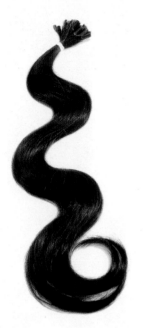

figure 18-6
Kanekalon is a top-of-the-line synthetic fiber used for hair extensions.

braided styles, and others mimic human hair as closely as possible. Durable, soft, and less inclined to tangle than many other synthetics, Kanekalon holds up to shampooing and styling. This durability is one of the reasons it is an extremely popular fiber for use in hair additions and extensions (figure 18-6).

- **Nylon or rayon synthetic.** This product is less expensive than many other synthetics and is available in varying qualities. It reflects light and leaves the hair very shiny. A drawback of nylon and rayon is that both of these fibers have been known to cut or break the surrounding natural hair. In addition, repeated shampooing will make these extensions less durable, and they may melt if high heat, such as that from a hot blowdryer, is applied.

- **Yarn.** Traditional yarn used to make sweaters and hats is now being used to adorn hair. It can be made of cotton or a nylon blend and is very inexpensive and easy to find. Yarn is light, soft, and detangles easily. It is available in many colors, does not reflect light, and gives the braid a matte finish. While yarn may expand when shampooing, it will not slip from the base, making it durable for braids. Be careful when you purchase yarn because some products may appear jet black in the store but actually show a blue or green tint in natural light.

- **Lin.** This beautiful wool fiber imported from Africa has a matte finish and comes only in black and brown. Lin comes on a roll and can be used in any length and size. Keep in mind that this cotton-like fabric is very flammable.

- **Yak.** This strong fiber comes from the domestic ox found in the mountains of Tibet and Central Asia. Yak hair is shaved and processed and used alone or blended with human hair. Mixing human hair with yak hair helps to remove the manufactured shine (figure 18-7).

After reading the next few sections, you will be able to:

LO❸ Explain how to prepare the hair for braiding.

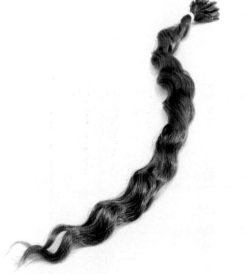

figure 18-7
Yak blends beautifully with human hair.

Prepare the Hair for Braiding: Working with Wet or Dry Hair

In general, it is best to braid curly hair when it is dry. If curly hair is braided wet, it shrinks and recoils as it dries, which may create excess pulling and scalp tension. In turn, the tension can lead to breakage or hair loss from pulling or twisting. If you are using a style that requires your client's hair to be wet while you manipulate it, you must allow for shrinkage in order to avoid damage to the hair and scalp.

Straight, resistant hair is best braided slightly damp or very lightly coated with a wax or pomade to make it more pliable.

- After you shampoo the client's hair, towel blot the hair without rubbing or tension, using several towels if necessary.

- Apply a leave-in conditioner to make combing the hair easier.

- Begin combing at the ends of the hair strand and gently work out the tangles while moving upward toward the scalp. Use a wide-tooth or detangling comb for this purpose.

- Blowdry the hair.

- Wax, pomades, pastes, or lotions can be used to hold the hair in place for a finished look.

- Brush the hair with a large paddle brush, beginning at the ends, just as you did with the comb.

Textured hair presents certain challenges when styling. It is very fragile both wet and dry. Because most braiding styles require the hair to be dry, blowdrying is the most effective way to prepare the hair for the braiding service. Not only does blowdrying quickly dry the hair, it softens it in the process, making it more manageable for combing and sectioning. Blowdrying also loosens and elongates the wave pattern, while stretching the hair-shaft length. This is great for short hair, allowing for easier pick up and manipulation of the hair. Make sure to control the hair while blowdrying to prevent frizzing!

Ⓟ 18-1 | **Preparing Textured Hair for Braiding** *See page 544*

After reading the next few sections, you will be able to:

LO❹ **Describe six types of braiding techniques: rope, fishtail, halo, invisible, single, and single braids with extensions.**

Braid the Hair

Braiding styles are broadly classified as visible and invisible. A **visible braid** is a three-strand braid that is created with an underhand technique. An **underhand technique**, also known as *plaiting*, is one in which the left section goes under the middle strand, then the right section goes under the middle strand. This technique is often used for cornrowing because many braiders believe it creates less tangling. Interestingly, the underhand technique has nothing to do with holding the palms up or down.

An **invisible braid**, also known as an *inverted braid* or *French braid*, is a three-strand braid that is produced with an **overhand technique**. In an overhand technique, the first side section goes over the middle one, then the other side section goes over the middle strand. You can start with either the right or left section; what is key is that the side sections go over the middle section (**figure 18-8**).

The following discussion and procedures will provide you with a basic overview of foundational braiding styles. These techniques are important to master because all of the more advanced and trendy braiding techniques build upon these. Once you have become proficient with these techniques,

milady pro™ **LEARN MORE!**

Optional info on **Styling Textured Hair and Braiding** topics and tutorials can be found at miladypro.com Keyword: *FutureCosPro*

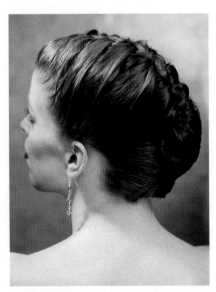

figure 18-8
Braided French twist

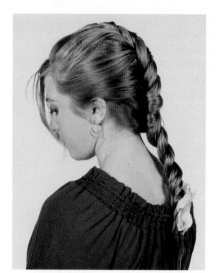

figure 18-9
Rope braid

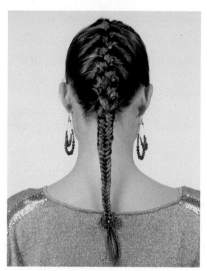

figure 18-10
Fishtail braid

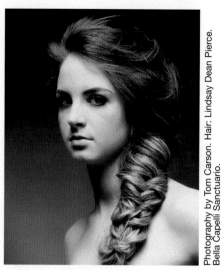

figure 18-11
Stylish fishtail braid

Photography by Tom Carson. Hair: Lindsay Dean Pierce.
Bella Capelli Sanctuario.

your creativity—along with additional training and practice—will allow you to create some of the most complex and beautiful styles you and your clients can imagine.

The procedures begin with the most basic and move on to more complex techniques, including braided extensions.

Rope Braid

The **rope braid** is created with two strands that are twisted around each other. This braid can be done on hair that is all one length or on long, layered hair. Remember to pick up and add hair to both sides before you twist the right side over the left (figure 18-9).

Fishtail Braid

The **fishtail braid** is a simple, two-strand braid in which hair is picked up from the sides and added to the strands as they are crossed over each other (figure 18-10). It is best done on non-layered hair that is at least shoulder length (figure 18-11).

Halo Braids

The **halo braids** are two or three long, simple, inverted, thick cornrows created around the head. The extended long braids are then wrapped around the head and pinned. The top crown is left smooth and neat, while the cornrows are pinned around the head to create a halo effect (figure 18-12).

P 18-2 **Halo Braids** See page 546

Invisible Braid

The invisible braid uses an overhand pick-up technique. It can be done on or off the scalp and with or without extensions. This style is ideal for long

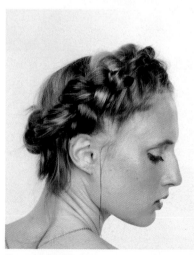

figure 18-12
Halo braid

hair, but it can also be executed successfully on shorter hair with long layers. If you are dealing with straight, layered hair, apply a light coating of wax or pomade to the hair to help hold shorter strands in place (figure 18-13).

Single Braids

Single braids, also known as *box braids* and *individual braids*, are free-hanging braids, with or without extensions, that can be executed using either an underhand or an overhand technique (figure 18-14). The procedure for medium-to-large single braids uses the underhand technique. Single braids can be used with all hair textures and in a variety of ways (figure 18-15). For instance, two or three single braids added to a ponytail or chignon can be a lovely evening look.

The partings or subsections for single braids can be diamond, square, triangular, or rectangular. The parting determines where the braid is placed, and how it moves. Single braids can move in any direction, so make sure to braid in the direction you want the hair to fall. As you braid, you are styling and shaping the finished look.

Single Braids with Extensions

Extensions for single braids come in a wide range of sizes and lengths and are integrated into the natural hair using the three-strand underhand technique. Fibers for extensions can be selected from synthetic hair, yarn, or human hair; the selection is vital in determining the finished style. Braiding must be consistent and close together.

As part of the consultation step, open the package of extension fibers and show them to the client to verify that the color is correct. Remove the fibers from the package and, if necessary, cut them to the desired length. Place half the extension fibers in the bottom portion of the drawing board and sandwich them with the upper portion of board. To secure the hair extensions, place a heavy object on top of the board, such as a large book. This allows you to easily extract the appropriate amount

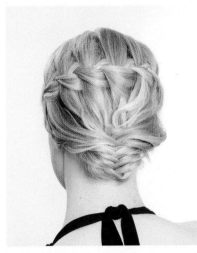

figure 18-13
Invisible braid styled to the side across an invisible/inverted braid tucked under

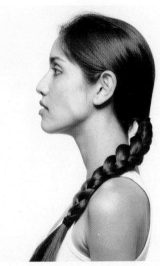

figure 18-14
Single braid

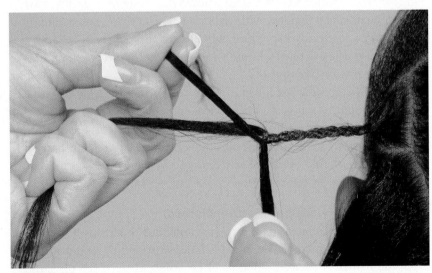

figure 18-15
Single box braids

of fibers for the braids. Hair extensions can also be separated and dispensed by a free-hand method.

When performing single braids with extensions using the hair fibers of human hair, you can create a small invisible knot by looping a small strand of hair around the braid. Pull the hair strand through the loop to create an invisible knot. The alternative method is to just continue braiding down to the desired hair length. To create a bend on the ends of synthetic fibers, wrap the braid ends with a curling rod, then dip all the rodded ends into hot water for 10 to 15 minutes. This method will secure the ends as well as create a spiral curl at the ends of the braid. When braiding children's hair, small elastic bands can be used to hold the ends in place and they can be adorned with beads at the ends. Other optional finishes, such as singeing with a ceramic flat iron or hot gun (i.e. keratin glue hot tool used for fusion weaving), are considered advanced methods and require special training.

Ⓟ 18-3   **Single Braids with Extensions** *See page 549*

After reading the next few sections, you will be able to:

LO⑤   **Demonstrate the procedure for cornrowing.**

Cornrows

Cornrows, also known as *canerows*, are narrow rows of visible braids that lie close to the scalp and are created with a three-strand, on-the-scalp braiding technique (**figure 18-16**). Consistent and even partings are the foundation of beautiful cornrows. Learning to create these partings requires patience and practice. Using a mannequin to practice will help develop your speed, accuracy, and finger and wrist dexterity.

Cornrows are worn by men, women, and children, and can be braided on hair of various lengths and textures. For long, straight hair, large cornrows are a fashionable and elegant hairstyle. Designer cornrows have become increasingly popular, with elaborate designs that demonstrate the stylist's skill and creative expression. The flat, contoured styles can last several weeks when applied without extensions, and up to two months when applied with extensions.

Cornrows typically last for four to six weeks. To ensure healthy hair, cornrows should be removed, shampooed, and conditioned within this time frame. Cornrows with extensions last from six to eight weeks. Layered cornrows should receive touch-ups on individual rows to remain neat and tight, and they should be completely removed by eight weeks to prevent knotting, locking, or thinning hair.

Cornrows with Extensions (Feed-in Method)

Extensions can be applied to cornrows or individual braids with the feed-in method. In this method, the braid is built up strand by strand with extension hair fibers. Excess amounts of extension material can place too much weight on the fragile areas of the hairline and will tighten and pull

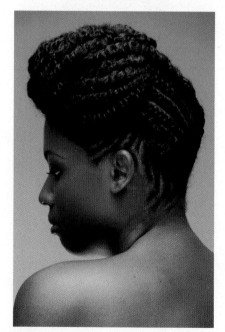

figure 18-16
Sculptured cornrows updo

the hair to leave an unrealistic finished look. By properly applying the correct tension when using the feed-in method, the braid stylist can avoid an artificial look and prevent breakage.

The traditional cornrow is flat, natural, and contoured to the scalp. The parting is important because it defines the finished style. The feed-in method creates a tapered or narrow base at the hairline. Small pieces or strips of extension hair are added to fill in the base, bringing the adjoining braids closer together. This technique takes longer to perform than traditional cornrowing. However, a cornrow achieved by the feed-in method will last longer and look more natural, without placing excessive tension on the hairline. There are several different ways to start a cornrow and feed in extension pieces.

During the cornrow process, when picking up hair at the base, the hair directly underneath the previous revolution must be incorporated into the braid. The hair that you pick up must never come from another panel or from a lower part of the braid. The same is true when executing any braid technique. Overextending or misplacing the beginning of the extension leaves the hair exposed and unsupported, which can lead to breakage and hair loss in that area. This is particularly true when adding extensions at the hairline. If the extension is not made secure by two or three revolutions before picking up, it may shift away from the point of entry. For a professional finish, always trim any ends that may stick up through the braid. Holding your scissors flat, move up the shaft as you trim, making sure that you avoid cutting into the braid.

P 18-4 **Basic Cornrows** *See page 552*

> **⚠ CAUTION**
> Excessive pulling and extremely tight braiding will cause thinning hairlines and alopecia.

↻ ACTIVITY

Braids can be created in different lengths and styled into a variety of updos that suits your client's facial shape. Working with classmates, determine one another's facial shape, based on the following major types. Then experiment with artistic ways to create updos and interwoven braided styles that work with the different types of facial shapes.

- An oval face is egg-shaped and most any braided style suits this facial shape.
- The elongated face is a too-long oval and requires a style with more width at the sides.
- A round face is wide at the cheeks and will benefit from a style with height, such as one in which braids are gathered high on top and secured below the crown in back.
- A square face has a strong, square jawline, which is minimized by allowing longer braids to frame the face.
- Heart-shaped faces are wide at the forehead and narrow at the chin and jaw. Use bangs or sweep braids across the forehead.
- Pear-shaped faces are the opposite of heart-shaped: narrow at the forehead and wide at the chin and jaw. Do the opposite of what is recommended for heart-shaped faces by bringing at least some braids forward to create the illusion of a narrower chin line.

When styling braids for updos, you can coil them around the head, sweep up and intertwine some sections, and then secure them with a braid or band, and even create a side chignon to draw attention away from an elongated face. Use the head shape to guide your style choices, and secure groups of braids by wrapping two or three other braids around them. With some styles, your biggest challenge will be discovering ways to hold up heavy braids (**figure 18-17**).

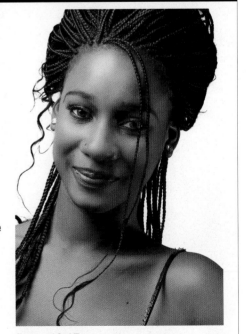

figure 18-17
Upswept braids elongate a slightly wide face shape.

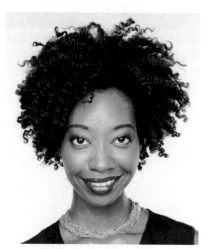

figure 18-18
Example of textured set and style

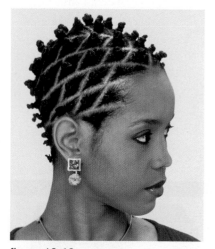

figure 18-19
Bantu knots

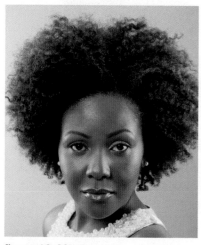

figure 18-20
Braid-out on coily/curly hair

Tree Braids/Interlocking

Tree braiding is a newer way to add hair for a longer look. The client's hair is braided or cornow braided along with hair extensions, but the finished look shows mostly faux hair. Braiders report that tree braids take about four hours, making them faster than some other techniques. Tree braiding techniques are still evolving and there are many ways to do them.

Some braiders add individual strands of hair that are braided along with the natural hair and tied in place about half an inch from the root area. In this technique, a few very short braids can be seen standing up along the front hairline, then the hair extension (long and unbraided) flows freely to create the look of naturally long, straight hair.

Adding long, loose pieces of hair to cornrows can also create tree braids. After a few sections are braided together, a small section of the extension hair is left out of the cornrow to hang free. This technique continues adding hair all along the cornrow. When the look is completed, the free-hanging sections of the extended hair completely conceal the cornrows, creating the look of naturally long, straight or wavy hair, depending on the texture of the extensions.

After reading the next few sections, you will be able to:

LO 6 Explain the techniques for textured sets and styles.

Classify Textured Sets and Styles

There are several **textured set and styles** that are created on natural curly textured hair. Textured sets elongate the natural frizzy hair and produce a smooth, silky curly, wavy and zig-zag pattern when the hair is set wet or dry on natural curly or coily hair textures (figure 18-18).

- **Bantu knot or Nubian knots.** The hair is double-strand twisted or coil twisted and wrapped around itself to make a knot. Knots are secured by bobby pins or elastic bands (figure 18-19).

- **Bantu knot-out style.** Knots can be opened and released to create wavy and fuller loose curls.

- **Braid-out set.** This style involves braiding the hair when either wet or dry and then opening the braid to create a crimped texture-on-texture effect with added volume (figure 18-20).

- **Flat-twist.** The hair is parted in several rows on the entire head. Each section is then divided into two sub-sections and then twisted and interwoven to lie flat on the scalp. Flat-twist can be made in varying patterns with or without extensions.

- **Glamour waves.** Once the hair has a flat-twist set, it must completely dry or the style will appear frizzy. The flat-twist set is untwisted and opened to create a wavy texture.

- **Spiral rod sets.** This set can be achieved with rods, flexi-rods, or curl reformers of all sizes. Hair is wrapped around a vertical rod, moving up the rod in a spiral movement. Hair must completely dry or the style will appear frizzy (figure 18-21).

Coil Styles

- **Coils or comb twists.** Small sections of natural hair that are gelled and spiraled with fingers or a comb to create individual formations of tight, cylindrical coils. The Nubian coils comb technique is styled on naturally curly or textured hair. For this look, hair is curled into a cylindrical shape with a comb or fingers. The comb coil technique is also used to start locks.

- **Coil-out.** Once the hair has been comb coiled into individual coils and then dried completely, the coils are uncoiled or neatly unraveled (figure 18-22). This style is now fuller coils that lift up off the scalp to create a coily textured Afro (figure 18-23). The *Afro* is a style made popular in the 1960s and 1970s of wearing the hair natural, but having it perfectly shaped in mostly a round fashion.

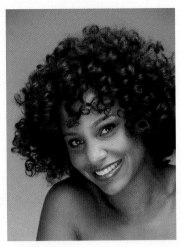
figure 18-21
Spiral rod set

P 18-5 **Nubian Coils:** *Coil Comb Technique* See page 555

Twist Styles

Twist styles also known as *double-strand twist*, start with wet, gelled, or dry hair. The stylist divides the hair into two sections and then overlaps them to create a twisted rope effect (dry) or textured effect (wet). A twist set is a two-part set that can be done on natural hair, transitional hair, twists, extensions, weaves, wigs, and locks. Hair is double-strand twisted and then set on rods. Rods can be placed only at the end of the hair or loc. For a full set, rods can also be placed vertically all the way to the base of the hair. Twist curls on textured hair are achieved by using a double-twist technique. The twisting technique is executed on wet hair to define the textured curls and waves (figure 18-24).

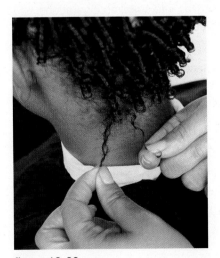
figure 18-22
Coil-out technique

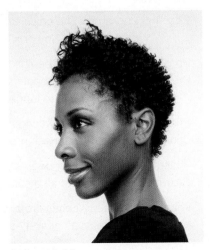
figure 18-23
Coil-out style

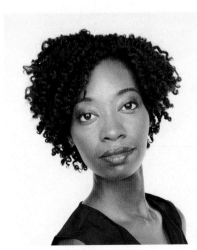
figure 18-24
Two-strand twist

The **twist-out** style involves unraveling the twist to add fullness and a crimped effect. The twist-out's double-strand twists can be made in any size and length. Hair is wet and gel or hair cream is applied to set the textured hair. After hair is dried, twists are opened, finger combed, and styled to create a textured, voluminous Afro.

(P) 18-6   **Twist** *See page 558*

See page 558

After reading the next few sections, you will be able to:

LO **7**   **Demonstrate the procedures for starting locks and lock grooming.**

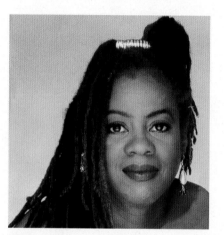

figure 18-25
Locks

Locks

Locks, also known as *dreadlocks* or *locs*, are separate networks of curly, textured hair that have been intertwined and meshed together. Hair locking is achieved without the use of chemicals. The hair locks in several slow phases, which can take from six months to a year depending on the length, density, and coil pattern of the hair (**figure 18-25** and **table 18-1**).

Locks are more than just a hairstyle; they are a cultural expression. There are several ways to cultivate locks, such as double twisting, wrapping with cord, coiling, palm rolling, and braiding. Locks will also form themselves in textured hair that is not combed or brushed out. As demonstrated by the Rastafarians of Jamaica, leaving coily hair to take its own natural course will cause it to intertwine and lock. Cultivated African locks have symmetry and balance.

Courtesy of Preston Phillips.

table 18-1

DEVELOPMENTAL PHASES OF LOCKS

Phase	Characteristics
Phase 1 Beginner Locks	Hair is soft and is coiled into spiral configurations. The coil is smooth and the end is open. The coil has a shiny or a glossy texture.
Phase 2 Pre-Lock Stage	Hair begins to interlace and mesh. The separate units begin to puff up and expand in size. The units are no longer glossy or smooth.
Phase 3 Sprouting Stage	A bulb can be felt at the end of each lock. Interlacing continues.
Phase 4 Growing Stage	Hair begins to regain length. Lock may still be frizzy, but also solid in some areas.
Phase 5 Maturation Stage	Locks are closed at the ends, dense and dull, and do not reflect light. Locks are now much longer.

The four basic methods of locking are:

- **The coil comb technique.** Particularly effective during the early stages of locking while the coil is still open, this method involves placing the comb at the base of the scalp and, with a rotating motion, spiraling the hair into a coil. With each revolution, the comb moves down until it reaches the end of the hair shaft. It offers a tight coil and is excellent on short (1-inch to 3-inch) hair (**figures 18-26** and **18-27**).

- **The palm roll.** This method is the gentlest on the hair, and it works through all the natural stages of locking. Palm rolling takes advantage of the hair's natural ability to coil. This method involves applying gel to dampened subsections, placing the portion of hair between the palms of both hands, and rolling in a clockwise or counterclockwise direction (**figure 18-28**). With each revolution, as you move down the coil shaft, the entire coil is formed (**figure 18-29**). Partings can be directional, horizontal, vertical, or brick-layered. Decorative designs and sculpting patterns are some of the creative options you can choose.

- **Braids or extensions.** Another effective way to start locks involves sectioning the hair for the desired size of lock and single braiding the hair to the end. Synthetic hair fiber, human hair fiber, or yarn can be added to a single braid to form a lock. After several weeks, the braid will grow away from the scalp, at which time the palm roll method can be used to cultivate the new growth to form a lock.

- **Sisterlocks.** An interlocking method that instantly locks any textured hair whether straight, relaxed, wavy, curly, and coily or highly textured using a special tool to achieve the single lock.

Shaping or grooming dreadlocks takes patience and commitment on the part of clients. In the beginning, clients must have frequent professional hair shaping and grooming to ensure a good outcome.

Ⓟ 18-7 **Starting Locks with Nubian Coils** *See page 563*

Ⓟ 18-8 **Cultivating and Grooming Locks** *See page 565*

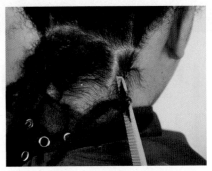
figure 18-26
Spiral the hair with the comb.

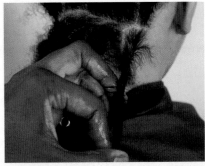
figure 18-27
Finished Lock for lock touch-up using comb coil technique for new growth.

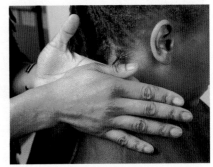
figure 18-28
Roll the hair/lock between the palms.

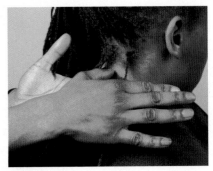
figure 18-29
Roll down the lock shaft.

PREPARING TEXTURED HAIR FOR BRAIDING

You will need all of the following implements, materials, and supplies:

- Blowdry cream or lotion made with botanical, essential oils
- Blowdryer and comb nozzle attachment
- Butterfly clips
- Conditioner (protein or moisturizing)
- Detangling solution (four parts water to one part cream rinse or oil) in spray bottle
- Neck strip
- Shampoo
- Shampoo cape
- Tail comb with large rounded teeth
- Towels

PREPARATION

Perform:

P 15-1 **Pre-Service Procedure** See page 340

PROCEDURE

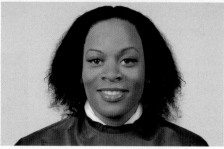

1 Drape the client for a shampoo. If necessary, comb and detangle the hair.

2 Shampoo, rinse, apply conditioner, and rinse thoroughly.

3 Gently towel dry the hair.

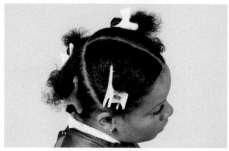

4 Part damp hair from ear to ear across crown and detangle with a tail comb. Use butterfly clips to separate front section from back section.

5 Part the back of head into four to six sections. For thick textured hair, make more sections to allow for increased ease and control. For thinner hair, use fewer sections. The front half of the head, where hair is less dense, can be sectioned in three or more sections. Separate the sections with clips.

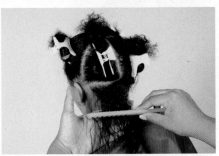

6 Beginning on left section in the back, start combing the ends of the hair first, working your way up to the base of the scalp. As you go along, lightly spray each section with detangling solution if needed. The combing movement should be fast and rhythmic, without creating tension on the scalp. Use a picking motion to comb through the hair.

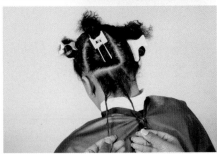

7 After combing thoroughly, divide the section into two equal parts and twist them together to the end to hold the section in place.

8 Continue with the other sections of the hair until the entire head is sectioned.

9 Place the client under a medium-heat hood dryer for 5 to 10 minutes to remove excess moisture.

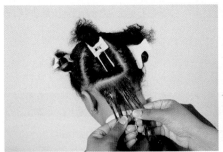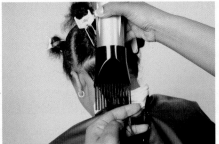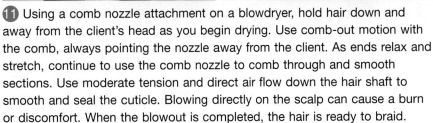

10 Open one of the combed sections. Using fingers, apply blowdry cream to hair from scalp to ends.

11 Using a comb nozzle attachment on a blowdryer, hold hair down and away from the client's head as you begin drying. Use comb-out motion with the comb, always pointing the nozzle away from the client. As ends relax and stretch, continue to use the comb nozzle to comb through and smooth sections. Use moderate tension and direct air flow down the hair shaft to smooth and seal the cuticle. Blowing directly on the scalp can cause a burn or discomfort. When the blowout is completed, the hair is ready to braid.

POST-SERVICE

Complete:

P 15-2 **Post-Service Procedure** *See page 343*

HALO BRAIDS

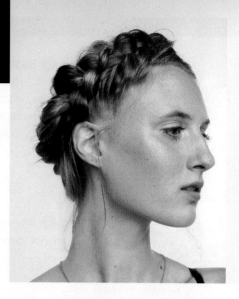

IMPLEMENTS & MATERIALS

You will need all of the following implements, materials, and supplies:

☐ Blowdry cream or lotion made with botanical/ essential oil, shea butter or glycerin base

☐ Boar bristle brush

☐ Butterfly clips

☐ Conditioner (hydration/ protein cocktail or moisturizing)

☐ Detangling solution in spray bottle

☐ Hair accessories or ornamentation (if desired)

☐ Neck strip

☐ Rubber bands, fabric-covered elastics, or other implements for securing the ends

☐ Shampoo

☐ Shampoo cape

☐ Styling and finishing products

☐ Tail comb with large rounded teeth

☐ Clear elastic bands

☐ Towels

PREPARATION

Perform:

P 15-1 **Pre-Service Procedure** *See page 340*

PROCEDURE

① Drape the client for a shampoo. If necessary, comb and detangle the hair.

② Shampoo, rinse, apply conditioner, and rinse thoroughly.

③ Gently towel dry the hair, then blowdry it completely.

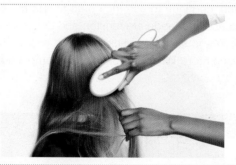

④ Brush the hair with a boar bristle brush or smoothing brush from the center toward the entire hairline.

⑤ On straight hair, mist the hair with a water bottle to dampen the hair. Do not part the hair.

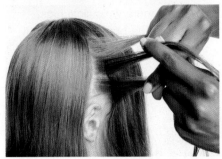

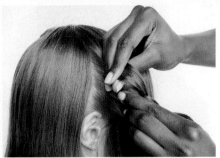

8 Use the overhand technique. In your right hand, gather a section of hair between your thumb and index finger.

6 Start at the ear. Gather three sections of hair into your hands, and begin an inverted braid.

7 In your right hand, gather a section of hair between your thumb and index finger.

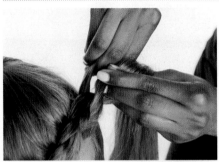

9 The first side section crosses over the middle section. Then the left side section crosses over the middle strand, picking up hair from each side as you create the braid. Note: You can start with either the right or left section. The key is to have the side sections cross over the middle section.

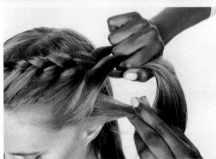

10 Continue the inverted braid around the entire head until you reach the ear.

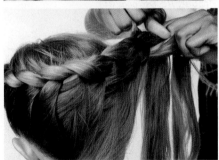

11 Continue braiding the hair until you reach the end of the entire strands.

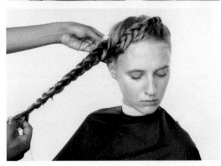

12 Secure with a clear elastic band.

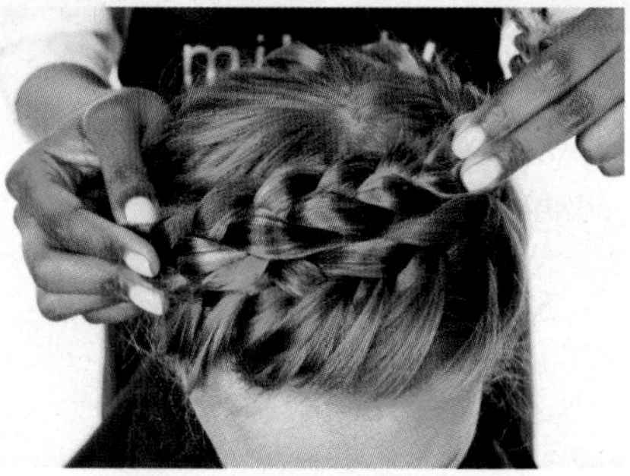

13 Place the long braid around the head on top of the inverted braid.

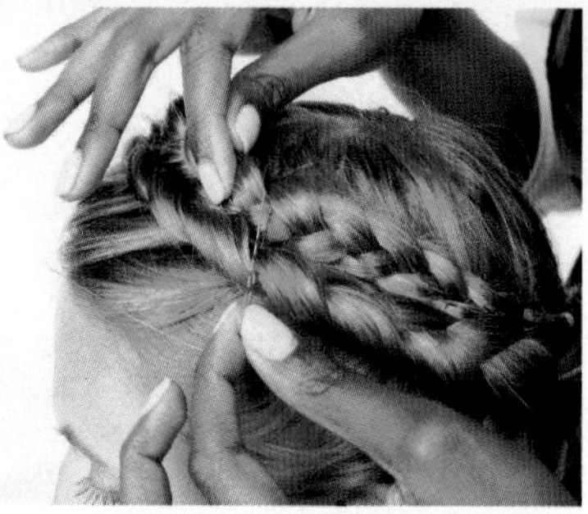

14 Secure the braid with pins.

15 For a more whimsical look, loosen up the braids and pull out some stands of the braid around the head.

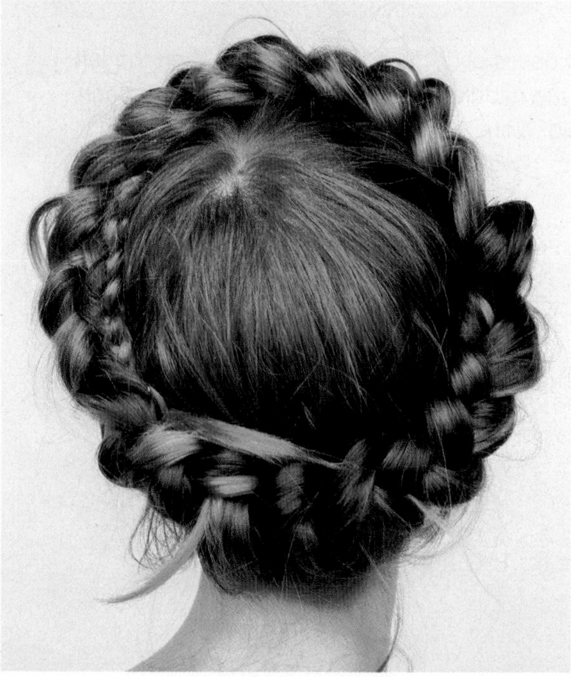

16 Finish off the style with hairspray for hold.

POST-SERVICE

Complete:

P 15-2 **Post-Service Procedure** *See page 343*

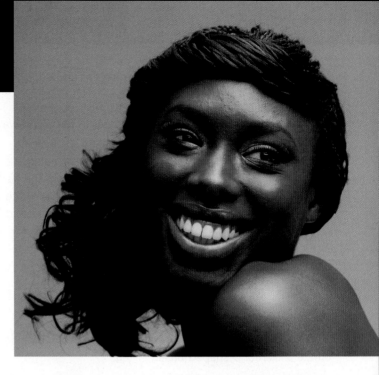

SINGLE BRAIDS WITH EXTENSIONS

IMPLEMENTS & MATERIALS

You will need all of the following implements, materials, and supplies:

- Blowdrying cream or lotion made with botanical/essential oil or glycerin base
- Bobby pins
- Butterfly clips
- Conditioner (hydration/protein cocktail or moisturizing)
- Detangling solution in spray bottle
- Drawing board or tray
- Extension fibers
- Hair accessories or ornamentation (if desired)
- Neck strip
- Oil sheen
- Rubber bands, fabric-covered elastics, or other implements for securing the ends
- Sulfate-free cleansing shampoo
- Shampoo cape
- Styling and finishing products
- Tail comb with large rounded teeth
- Shears
- Barrel curling iron
- Towels

PREPARATION | PROCEDURE

Perform:

P 15-1 **Pre-Service Procedure** *See page 340*

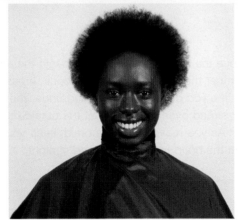

1 Drape the client for a shampoo. If necessary, comb and detangle the hair before shampooing.

2 Shampoo, condition, detangle and separate the hair into four sections, and then blowdry the hair completely.

3 Prepare the extension fibers.

4 Apply a light essential oil to the scalp and massage the oil into the scalp and throughout the hair.

5 Part the hair across the crown from ear to ear. Clip away the front section.

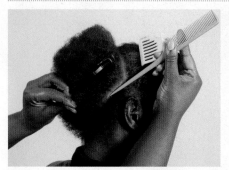

6 Part a diagonal section in the back of the head, at about a 45-degree angle, from the ear to the nape of the neck. You may have to start your partings below the ears to the nape, if the hairline is extended. For a medium-size braid, this section can be from ¼-inch (0.6 centimeters) to 1-inch (2.5 centimeters) wide, depending on the texture and length of the client's hair.

7 Using vertical parts to separate the base into subsections, create a diamond-shaped base.

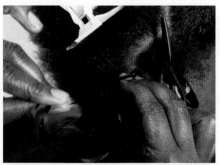

8 Select the appropriate amount of extension fibers from the drawing board or tray. The extension should always be proportional to the section that it is being applied to. For tapered ends, gently pull extension fibers at both sides so that the ends are uneven. Then fold the fibers in half.

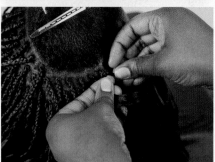

9 Divide the natural hair into three equal sections. Place the folded extension on top of the natural hair, on the outside and center portions of the braid.

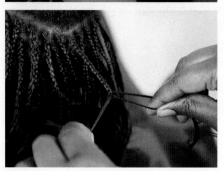

10 Once the extension is in place, begin the underhand braiding technique. Remember that the outer strands should cross under the center strand. Each time you pass an outer strand under the center strand, bring the center strand over tightly so that the outside strand stays securely in the center. As you move down the braid, keep your fingers close to the stitch so that the braid remains tight and straight.

11 Continue to braid to the desired length.

12 The next part is created above the previous section on a diagonal part, moving toward the ear.

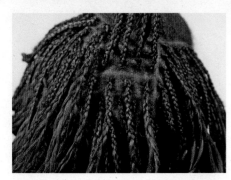

13 After several sections have been completed, alternate the direction of the diagonal to start parting and braiding on the other side of the head. Sections are completed with bricklaying technique.

14 Once the back is finished, create a diagonal or horizontal parting above the ear in the front. As you get closer to the hairline, be aware of the amount of extension hair that is applied to the hairline. Do not add excessive amounts of fiber into a fragile hairline. The fiber should always be proportionate to the hair to which it is being applied.

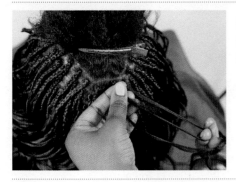

15 Continue braiding on the opposite side of the head. When you reach the crown area, the partings will create a V-shape at the top of the crown. Continue diagonal partings on the crown of the head.

16 After the entire head has been braided, remove all loose hair ends from the braid shaft with shears.

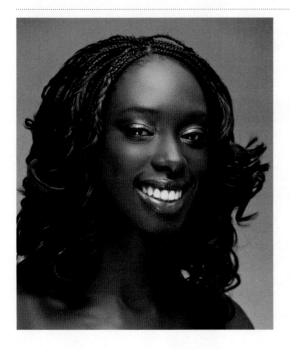

17 If using human hair, spray hair ends with water to activate the wave in the extensions and/or curl with barrel curling iron to create bounce. The finished braids will look quite natural.

POST-SERVICE

Complete:

P 15-2 **Post-Service Procedure** *See page 343*

Clients should visit the salon for post services every two to three weeks to receive a shampoo and steam conditioning treatment and/ or touch-ups on any loose hair extensions.

BASIC CORNROWS

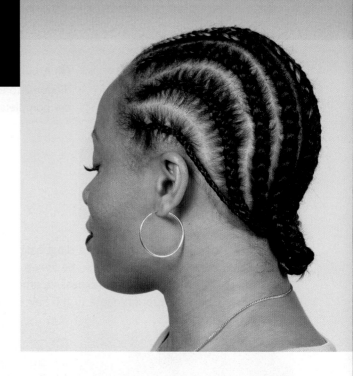

IMPLEMENTS & MATERIALS

You will need all of the following implements, materials, and supplies:

- ☐ Blowdrying cream or lotion made with botanical/essentials oil, shea butter or glycerin base
- ☐ Bobby pins
- ☐ Butterfly clips
- ☐ Conditioner (hydration/ protein cocktail or moisturizing)

- ☐ Detangling solution in spray bottle
- ☐ Drawing board or tray
- ☐ Extension fibers
- ☐ Hair accessories or ornamentation (if desired)
- ☐ Neck strip
- ☐ Oil sheen

- ☐ Rubber bands, fabric-covered elastics, or other implements for securing the ends
- ☐ Sulfate-free cleansing shampoo
- ☐ Shampoo cape
- ☐ Styling and finishing products

- ☐ Tail comb with large rounded teeth
- ☐ Towels

PREPARATION

Perform:

P 15-1 **Pre-Service Procedure** *See page 340*

PROCEDURE

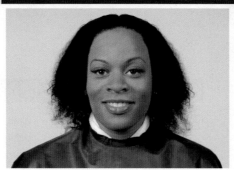

❶ Drape the client for a shampoo. If necessary, comb and detangle the hair before shampooing.

❷ Shampoo, condition, detangle, part, and separate hair into 4 sections, and then blowdry the hair completely.

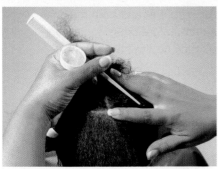 **3** Depending on desired style, determine the correct size and direction of the cornrow base. With tail comb, part hair into 2 inch (5 centimeters) sections (or smaller, depending on the desired style) and apply a light essential oil to the scalp. Massage oil throughout scalp and hair.

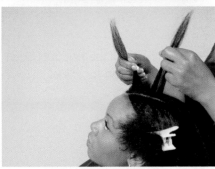 **4** Start by taking two even partings to form a neat row for the cornrow base. With a tail comb, part the hair into a panel; use butterfly clips to keep the other hair pinned to either side.

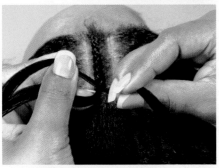 **5** Divide the panel into three even strands. To ensure consistency, make sure that strands are the same size. Place fingers close to the base. Cross the left strand (1) under the center strand (2). The center strand is now on the left and the former left strand (1) is the new center.

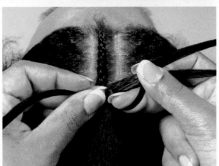 **6** Cross the right strand (3) under the center strand (1). Passing the outer strands under the center strand creates the underhand cornrow braid.

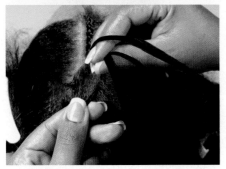 **7** With each crossing under or revolution, pick up a new strand of equal size from the base of the panel and add it to the outer strand before crossing it under the center strand.

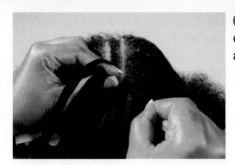

8 As you move along the braid panel, pick up a strand from the scalp with each revolution and add it to the outer strand before crossing it under alternating the side of the braid when you pick up the hair.

9 As new strands are added, the braid will become fuller. Braid to the end.

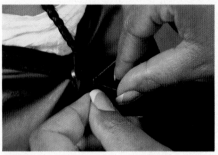

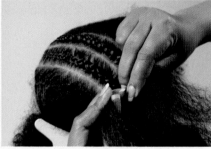

12 Repeat until all the hair is braided and apply oil sheen for shine.

10 Simply braiding to the ends can finish the cornrow; small rubber bands can be used to hold the ends in place when styling for children. Other optional finishes, such as singeing with a flat iron when synthetic hair fibers are attached (heat sealing with a heat gun), are considered advanced methods and require special training.

11 Braid the next panel in the same direction and in the same manner. Keep the partings clean and even.

13 Finished style.

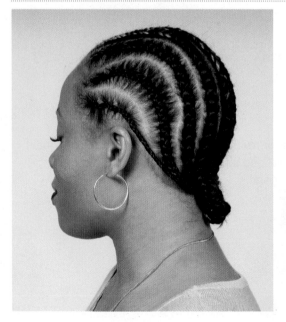

POST-SERVICE

Complete:

P 15-2 **Post-Service Procedure** *See page 343*

Basic cornrows last neatly for three weeks. Clients should visit the salon every three weeks for a complete shampoo, conditioning, and cornrow service.

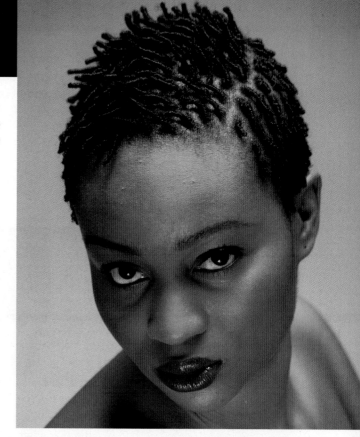

P 18-5

NUBIAN COILS: *COIL COMB TECHNIQUE*

IMPLEMENTS & MATERIALS

You will need all of the following implements, materials, and supplies:

- ☐ Four butterfly clips
- ☐ Barber's comb
- ☐ Holding gel
- ☐ Hood dryer
- ☐ Leave-in conditioner
- ☐ Long duckbill clips
- ☐ Natural botanical oil
- ☐ Shampoo cape
- ☐ Sulfate-free moisturizing shampoo
- ☐ Wide-tooth comb

PREPARATION

Perform:

P 15-1 **Pre-Service Procedure** *See page 340*

PROCEDURE

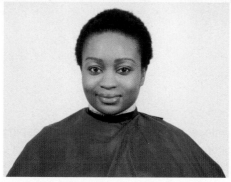

1 Drape the client for a shampoo. If necessary, comb and detangle the hair.

2 Cleanse with sulfate-free shampoo, then condition and rinse.

3 Spray on leave-in conditioner and detangle with a wide-tooth comb.

4 Apply natural botanical oil to the scalp and massage the oil into the scalp.

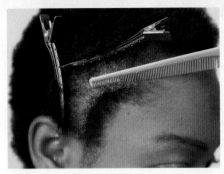

5 Detangle and divide hair into two sections. Clip for control. To create movement, start at the hairline and create a crescent-shape part with smaller end of comb. Apply gel to tip of the comb.

6 Comb through the entire parted section.

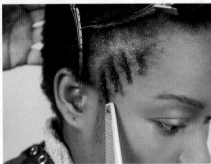

8 Using the comb, twirl hair and place coil end in the direction you would like the hair to lie.

7 At the base, start to rotate or roll-comb with a clockwise rotation, down the hair shaft to the end. The hair is curled toward the end, and the coil lies flat on the scalp.

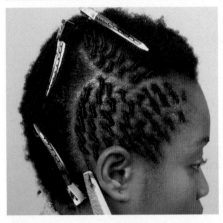

10 The movement can be in multiple directions with dimension. For example, the entire back will move forward from the center back towards the front on both sides, while the top will move upward and forward. Positioning the comb and directing the hair upward will give a different directional movement to the top crown.

11 Once the right back to front section is complete, start on the right side twirling the comb toward the front of the head, in a counterclockwise rotation. The coil style has one continuous movement from front to back.

9 As you move up and around the head, create a sculpting movement which features the head contour.

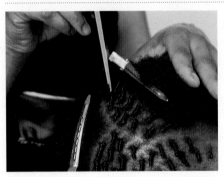

12 Continue coil movement at crown, keeping contours and directions of coil uniform, directing from back to front in a upward and forward direction. The coils will lie flat and point upward.

13 While front coils are still damp, fine tune their direction and make a soft bang.

14 Place the client under the dryer. Add oil for more sheen.

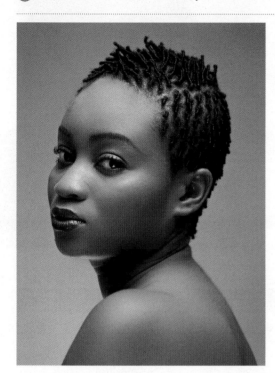

15 Finished style.

POST-SERVICE

Complete:

P 15-2 **Post-Service Procedure** *See page 343*

Coils and coil-out styles last for two to three weeks and can easily start locking the hair if it is not combed out before four weeks.

The hair should be shampooed, conditioned, combed, and detangled every two to three weeks. Comb out coils, shampoo, and use conditioning steam treatments to keep the hair and scalp healthy.

Cleansing the scalp with a tea tree oil solution between salon visits, once weekly, is highly recommended to maintain a healthy scalp.

TWIST

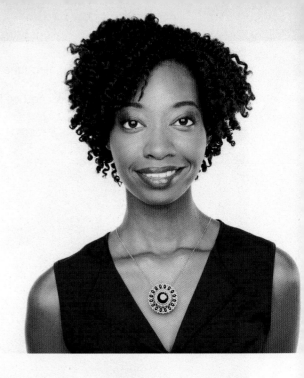

IMPLEMENTS & MATERIALS

You will need all of the following implements, materials, and supplies:

- ☐ Five butterfly clips
- ☐ Blowdryer with nozzle comb attachment
- ☐ Holding gel
- ☐ Hood dryer

- ☐ Leave-in conditioner
- ☐ Long duckbill clips
- ☐ Moisturizing curl-enhancing cream
- ☐ Natural botanical oil

- ☐ Rods
- ☐ Shampoo cape
- ☐ Spray bottle with moisturizing or detangling solution

- ☐ Steamer
- ☐ Sulfate-free moisturizing shampoo
- ☐ Tail comb
- ☐ Wide-tooth comb

PREPARATION

Perform:

P 15-1 **Pre-Service Procedure** *See page 340*

PROCEDURE

1 Drape the client for a shampoo. If necessary, comb and detangle the hair.

2 Cleanse with sulfate-free shampoo, then condition and rinse.

3 Spray on leave-in conditioner and detangle with a wide-tooth comb.

4 Apply natural botanical oil to the scalp and massage the oil into the scalp.

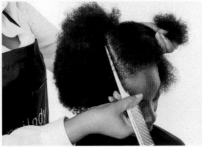

5 Detangle the hair and divide hair into three sections, clipping off the crown.

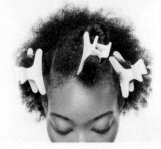

6 Clip all three sections for control.

7 Apply curl-enhancing cream to wet hair on entire head and smooth into hair. If the hair is very tight, blowdry lightly with nozzle comb attachment to stretch the curl pattern. Then, apply product.

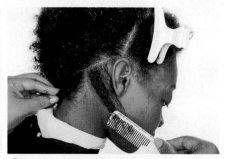

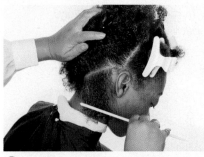

8 Starting on the right side of the head, behind the ear to the nape of the neck, make a 45-degree, ½-inch (1.25 cm.) diagonal parting for small twist or 1-inch (2.5 cm.) sections for medium size twist.

9 Then part a subsection with ½-inch (1.25 cm.) sections for small or larger partings for a medium-size twist.

10

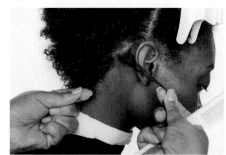

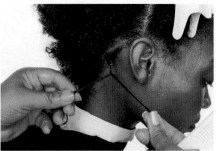

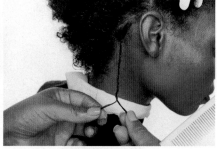

a. Divide the subsection into two equal parts. Overlap both sections to create a twisting movement—a rope-like effect. Apply holding gel to each individual section before you start the twist.

b. Continue twisting hair down the hair shaft.

c. Finish twisting with overlapping twisting movement until you reach the ends of the hair.

11

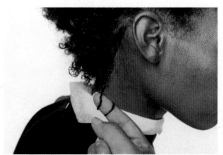

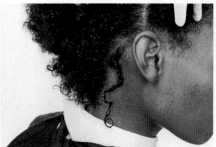

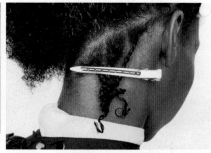

a. Repeat the twisting movement until you reach the end of the hair strands. Then twirl the ends of the hair with your index finger to create a curl. Clip hair off for control.

b. The twist will hang naturally with curls.

c. After you have created a few twists, clip off all twists to secure before moving on the next section.

Remember to make parts in a brick lay formation so the sections will become invisible when the hair lays in between each part.

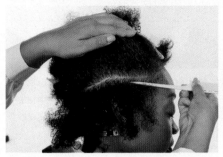 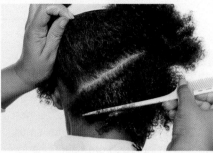 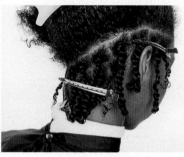

a. Next, make another part of 45 degrees, ½-inch (1.25 centimeters) diagonal above the ear, from the hairline to the back left nape of the neck on the left side of the head.

b. Continue diagonal parts until a V-shape is created with the parts moving up the head. Mist the hair with the water bottle if hair starts drying out. The twist must be created on wet hair for long-lasting hold.

c. Create twists for the entire row and clip each twist off as you move along the row and parted section.

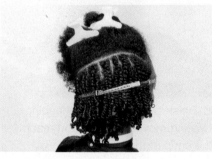

14 Continue these diagonal partings on the right side until you reach the crown area. Clip each row off as you move up the next parted section.

15

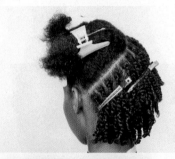

a. Now, move to the left side and continue with a 45-degree, ½-inch (1.25 centimeters) diagonal parting on the left side of the head. Repeat the same parts and sections as the right side.

b. Continue twisting entire left back area of the head.

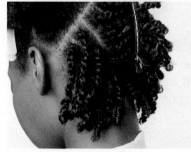

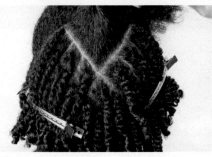

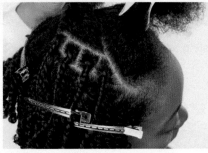

18 Continue with subsections and twisting movement, directing the hair to the left or right side, as desired.

16 Continue moving up the head until you reach the crown area. Notice that the partings will connect exactly with the right side partings to create a V-shape.

17 At the crown, make diagonal parts across the head connecting the parts on the right and left sides of the head.

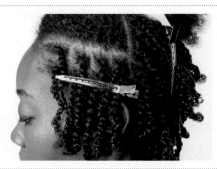

19 If the desired look is laying the hair to the back of the head, start horizontal parts at the back of the crown, and then continue horizontal parts with subsections towards the front hairline.

20 Once entire head is completed and there are straight hair ends, take a few individual twists and rod the ends with two to three rotations. This technique will create consistency and curly ends for the entire head.

21 Place under hood dryer for 30 to 40 minutes, or until entire head is completely dry. Remove the rods.

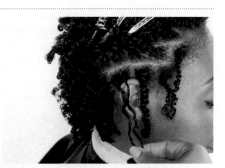

22 Apply light oil and finger style twist.

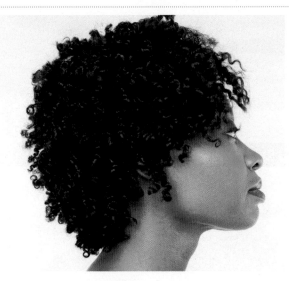

23 Finished style.

24 Create twist-out style using entire twisting method from
Procedure 18-6, steps 1 through 21.

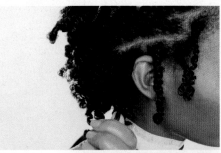

25 Once hair is completely dry, apply light oil and unravel twists
one by one.

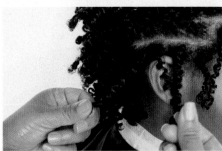

26 Stretch each section of the head by slightly pulling the hair downward
and out with two hands to create free, loose, curly hair with more volume
and movement.

27 To create more fullness and reduce any parts or lines, take a pick or wide-tooth comb.
Place the comb right on the scalp and lift the hair up one inch from the scalp. Do not
disturb the rest of the twist. Gently lift from the scalp for fullness.

28 Finger comb as desired.

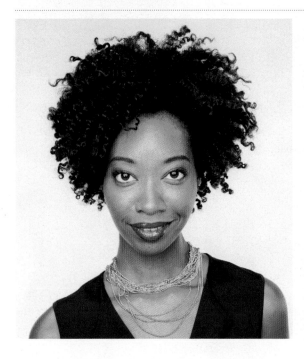

29 Finished style.

POST-SERVICE

Complete:

P 15-2 **Post-Service Procedure** *See page 343*

STARTING LOCKS WITH NUBIAN COILS

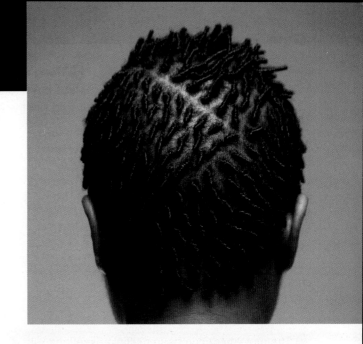

IMPLEMENTS & MATERIALS

You will need all of the following implements, materials, and supplies:

- ☐ Barber's comb
- ☐ Four butterfly clips
- ☐ Holding gel
- ☐ Hood dryer
- ☐ Leave-in conditioner
- ☐ Long duckbill clips
- ☐ Natural botanical oil
- ☐ Shampoo cape
- ☐ Sulfate-free moisturizing shampoo
- ☐ Wide-tooth comb

PREPARATION

Perform:

P 15-1 **Pre-Service Procedure** *See page 340*

PROCEDURE

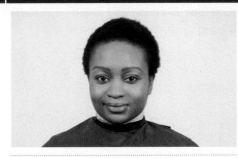

1 Drape the client for a shampoo. If necessary, comb and detangle the hair.

2 Cleanse with sulfate-free shampoo, then condition and rinse.

3 Spray on leave-in conditioner and detangle with a wide-tooth comb.

4 Apply natural botanical oil to the scalp and massage the oil into the scalp.

5 Detangle and divide hair into two sections.

6 Clip for control.

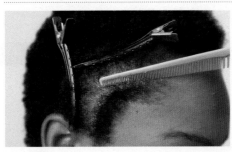

7 To create movement, start at the hairline and create a crescent-shaped part with the smaller end of the comb. Apply gel to the tip of the comb.

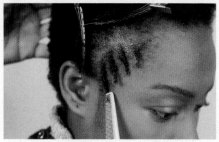

8 Comb the gel through the entire parted section. At the base, start to rotate or roll-comb with a clockwise rotation, down the hair shaft to the end. The hair is curled towards end and coil lies flat on the scalp.

9 Using the comb, twirl hair and place coil end in the direction you would like the hair to lie.

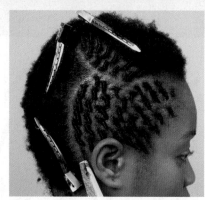

10 As you move up and around the head, create a sculpting movement which features the head contour.

11 The movement can be in multiple directions with dimension. For example, the entire back will move forward from the center back towards the front on both sides, while the top will move upward and forward. Positioning the comb and directing the hair upward will give a different directional movement to the top crown.

12 Once the right back section to front section is complete, start on the right side, twirling the comb toward the front of the head in a counterclockwise rotation.

13 The coil style has one continuous movement from front to back.

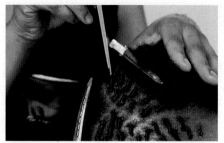

14 Continue coil movement at the crown, keeping contours and directions of coil uniform, directing from back to front in a upward and forward direction. The coils will lie flat and point upward.

15 While front coils are still damp, fine-tune their direction and make a soft bang.

16 Place the client under the dryer. Add oil for more sheen.

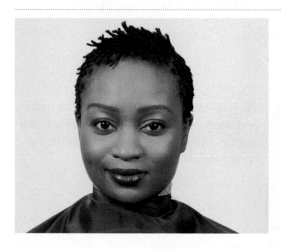

17 Finished style.

POST-SERVICE

Complete:

P 15-2 **Post-Service Procedure** *See page 343*

CULTIVATING AND GROOMING LOCKS

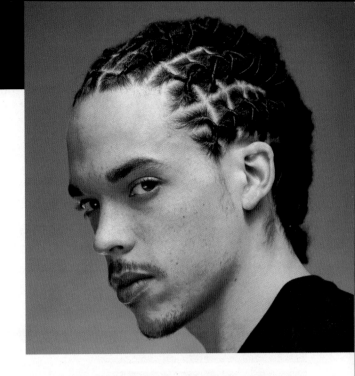

IMPLEMENTS & MATERIALS

You will need all of the following implements, materials, and supplies:

- ☐ Box of small 2 pronged rollerclips
- ☐ Five butterfly clips
- ☐ Herbal rinse
- ☐ Hood dryer
- ☐ Natural botanical oil and light moisturizing conditioner
- ☐ Shampoo cape
- ☐ Steamer
- ☐ Sulfate-free shampoo
- ☐ Tapered barber's comb
- ☐ Water-soluble gel

PREPARATION

Perform:

P 15-1 **Pre-Service Procedure** See page 340

PROCEDURE

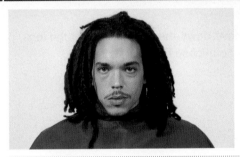

1 Drape the client for a shampoo.

2 Cleanse the hair and scalp with a sulfate-free shampoo.

3 Add light moisturizing conditioner, steam and then rinse locks.

4 Apply oil to the scalp and entire length of lock, and massage the scalp.

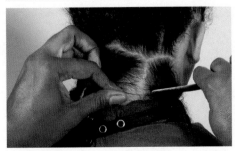

5 Starting at the base of the neck, use the larger end of the barber's comb to square off new growth of locked hair, creating a clean part.

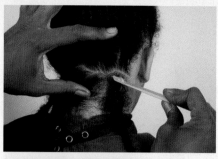

6 Apply gel to the smaller end of the comb. Place a small amount of gel at the new growth base of each lock.

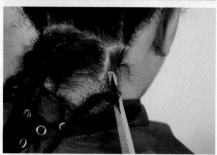

7 Pull down all the loose hair together into the lock with comb and gel. This will compact the loose hair and builds the lock base. Rotate the comb once.

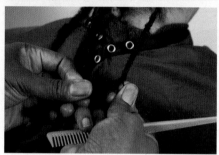

8 Remove the comb and, using two fingers (index finger and thumb), push loose hair together and smooth and then roll hair between fingers.

9 Place the lock between palms of both hands. Pressing gently, rotate the lock in your palm with a back-and-forth motion.

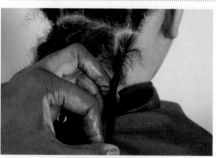

10 Move down the entire length of the lock, palm rolling to smooth loose hair into the lock.

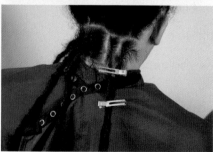

11 Clip off each section at the base if needed and along the length of the lock with a small or large duckbill clip, as you complete palm rolling locks.

12 Once you complete the entire back section, continue to the right and left sides of the head and save the crown section for last.

⓭ Place the client under hood dryer for 30 to 40 minutes until locks are completely dry.

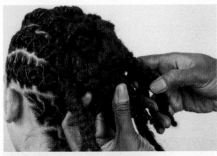

⓮ For dimensional styling, gather several locks and braid hair to create crimped locks or after removal from dryer cornrow entire head of locks with 8 to 10 cornrows. Secure ends with elastic bands.

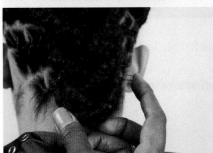

⓯ Then, take the braided locks and create a fishtail braid. Secure with elastic band and tuck fishtail under. Secure with hair pins.

⓰ Spray locks with oil shine.

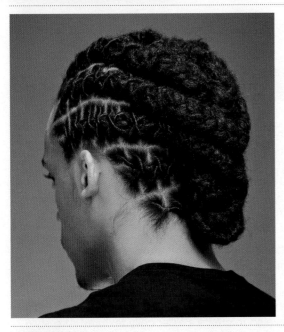

⓱ Finished style.

POST-SERVICE

Complete:

Ⓟ 15-2 **Post-Service Procedure** *See page 343*

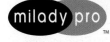 Check out miladypro.com for additional resources and training to enhance your technical skills. Keyword: *FutureCosPro*

REVIEW QUESTIONS

1. What is the most effective way to prepare hair for braiding?

2. What are the steps in creating basic cornrows?

3. List several types of braiding techniques.

4. Name and describe several textured sets and styles.

5. Name and describe the developmental stages of locks.

STUDY TOOLS

- **Reinforce what you just learned:** Complete the activities and exercises in your Theory or Practical Workbook, or your Study Guide.

- **Expand your knowledge:** Search for websites about the topics in this chapter and make a list of additional resources.

- **Study and prepare for your quiz:** Take the chapter test in your Exam Review or your Milady U: Online Licensing Prep.

- **Re-Test your knowledge:** Take the Chapter 18 *Quizzes*!

- **Learn even more:** Look up in a dictionary or search the internet for the definitions for any additional terms you want to learn about.

CHAPTER GLOSSARY

Bantu knot or Nubian knots	p. 540	The hair is double-strand twisted or coil twisted and wrapped around itself to make a knot. Knots are secured by bobby pins or elastic bands.
Bantu knot-out style	p. 540	Knots can be opened and released to create wavy and fuller loose curls.
Braid-out set	p. 540	This style involves braiding the hair when either wet or dry and then opening the braid to create a crimped texture-on-texture effect with added volume.
coils	p. 541	Also known as *comb twist*; small sections of natural hair that are gelled and spiraled with fingers or a comb to create individual formations of tight, cylindrical coils.
coil-out	p. 541	Once hair is comb coiled into individual coils, then dried completely, they are uncoiled or neatly unraveled to create a fuller coily textured Afro style.
coil comb technique	p. 543	A technique with individual formations of cylindrical coils used to create coil styles or locks. This method involves placing the comb at the base of the scalp and, with a rotating motion, spiraling the hair into a coil. With each revolution, the comb moves down until it reaches the end of the hair shaft.
cornrows	p. 543	Also known as *canerows*; narrow rows of visible braids that lie close to the scalp and are created with a three-strand, on-the-scalp braiding technique.
flat-twist	p. 540	Double-strand twists that are interwoven to lie flat on the scalp with various patterns with our without extensions.
fishtail braid	p. 540	Simple two-strand braid in which hair is picked up from the sides and added to the strands as they are crossed over each other.

glamour waves	p. 540	Flat-twist set is unraveled to make a loose, wavy texture on the entire head.
halo braids	p. 536	Two or three long, simple, inverted, thick cornrows created around the head. The extended braids are then wrapped and pinned to make a halo effect.
invisible braid	p. 535	Also known as *inverted braid* or *French braid*; a three-strand braid that is produced with an overhand technique.
locks	p. 542	Also known as *dreadlocks* or *locs*; separate networks of curly, textured hair that have been intertwined and meshed together.
natural hairstyling	p. 528	Hairstyling that uses no chemicals or dyes and does not alter the natural curl or coil pattern of the hair.
nubian knots	p. 540	Also known as *Bantu knots*; hair is double-strand twisted or coil twisted and then wrapped around itself to create a knot and then secured with a pin or elastic band.
overhand technique	p. 535	A technique in which the first side section goes over the middle one, then the other side section goes over the middle strand.
rope braid	p. 536	Braid created with two strands that are twisted around each other.
single braids	p. 537	Also known as *box braids* or *individual braids*; free-hanging braids, with or without extensions, that can be executed using either an underhand or an overhand technique.
spiral rod set	p. 541	This set can be done with rods, flexi-rods, or curl reformers of all sizes. Hair is wrapped around a vertical rod, moving up the rod in a spiral movement.
steamer	p. 533	Used to deeply hydrate, moisturize, and condition the hair with water vapor; infuses water hydration, opening the cuticle layer of the hair shaft and enabling nourishing protein conditioners and botanical oils to penetrate deeply into the cortex layer.
textured set and style	p. 540	Textured sets elongate the natural frizzy hair and make a smooth-silky curl, wavy or zig-zag pattern when the hair is set wet or dry on natural curly or coily hair textures.
textured hair	p. 530	Hair with a tight coil pattern.
twisting	p. 531	A rope effect on individual sections of hair made with a double stranded twist technique done by overlapping two strand sections of hair, to form a candy cane effect.
twist-out	p. 542	A double-stranded twist set is unravel and opened to create a spirally, full-crimped effect.
underhand technique	p. 535	Also known as *plaiting*; a technique in which the left section goes under the middle strand, then the right section goes under the middle strand.
visible braid	p. 535	Three-strand braid that is created using an underhand technique.
wave pattern	p. 530	The coil configuration, of textured hair.
weaving	p. 531	Hair extensions on a weft are sewn or bonded onto a cornrow base to make a longer, fuller head of a natural-looking a hair. There are several methods of weaving from bonding, fusion, braid sew attachment, threading, and tubing.

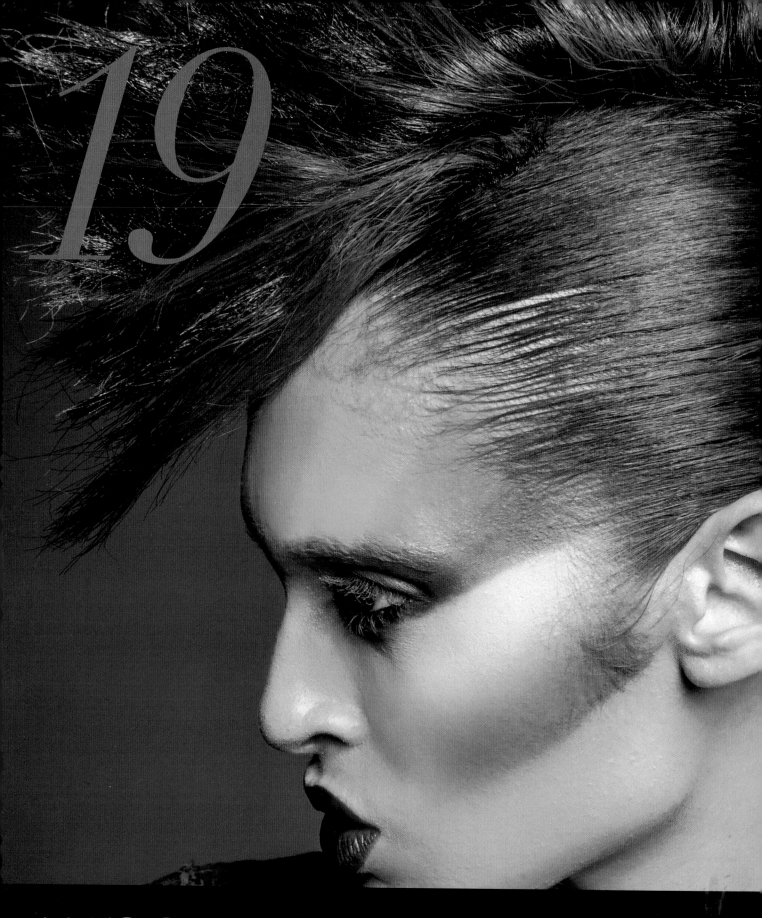

19

WIGS AND HAIR
ADDITIONS

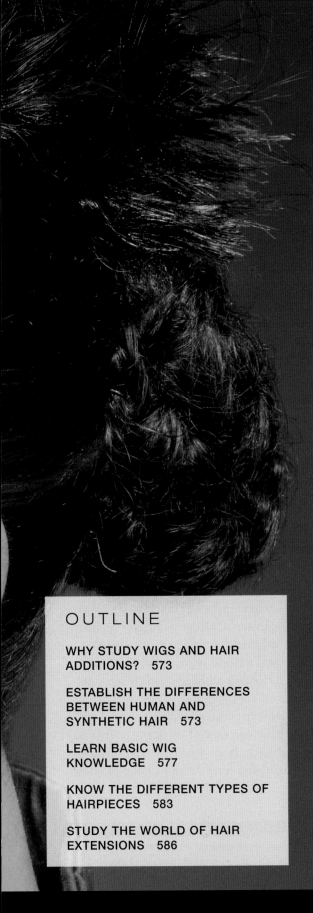

LEARNING OBJECTIVES

After completing this chapter, you will be able to:

LO❶
Understand why cosmetologists should study wigs and hair additions.

LO❷
Explain the differences between human hair and synthetic hair.

LO❸
Examine the two basic categories of wigs.

LO❹
Distinguish several types of hairpieces and their uses.

LO❺
Review several different methods of attaching hair extensions.

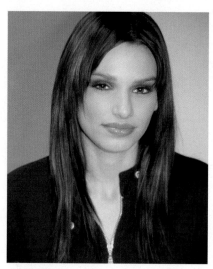

figure 19-1
Client before getting hair extension

Courtesy of www.GarlandDrake.com. Photography by Dixie Dixon, makeup by Kay Castro, Hairstyling by Tony Greenleaf, all for Garland Drake.

From the beginning of recorded history, wigs have played an important role in the world of fashion. The ancient Egyptians shaved their heads with bronze razors and wore heavy black wigs to protect themselves from the sun. In ancient Rome, women wore wigs made from the prized blond hair of barbarians captured from the North. In eighteenth-century England, men wore wigs, called *perukes*, to indicate that they were in the army or navy, or engaged in the practice of law.

In today's fashion-conscious world, wigs and hair additions (a category that includes hairpieces and hair extensions) play an incredibly important role. Working with hair additions can be either a simple retail effort or a highly specialized field. Most clients buy wigs off-the-shelf or on the Internet and rarely have them custom fitted anymore, although there are some opportunities for stylists to cut, color, and care for wigs. Toupees are often custom-made and fitted, using hair-type matches and a perfect mold or exact measurements of the head. Working with toupees takes years of specialized training, which is why much of the toupee business is found in hair replacement centers.

Hair additions range from clip-on hairpieces that salons retail, such as ponytails, chignons, bangs, and even extensions, to elaborately applied extensions in which addition strands are attached individually. In the newest technique, single strands of hair are meticulously hand-tied onto individual strands of the client's hair. In any case, moving beyond clip-in hair additions requires specialized training (figures 19-1 and 19-2).

Each hair extension manufacturer has its own attachment method, and normally you must take the manufacturer's class to be allowed to purchase that manufacturer's extensions. Inventory can be a hefty investment. Even carrying clip-on extensions requires stocking a range of styles and colors, but with every woman in Hollywood wearing them, the demand is high.

The income that hair extension services represent ranges from a small amount for a clip-on ponytail or bang to thousands of dollars for human-hair extensions that are fusion bonded strand-by-strand to the client's hair. Additionally, hair-loss clients and medical clients, such as cancer patients, have very particular needs for hair additions, which you can learn if you choose to specialize.

Because there are many options that require additional training, this chapter gives you a simple, basic overview of the many alternatives available in the world of hair additions. It is a gratifying and lucrative specialty open to any cosmetologist who furthers his or her education.

figure 19-2
The same client, transformed with clip-in extensions.

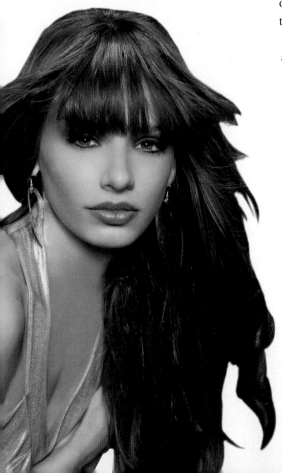

? DID YOU KNOW?

In 1989 the Cosmetic, Toiletry, and Fragrance Association (CTFA) founded the CTFA Foundation, a charitable organization, and established the Look Good...Feel Better program to help cancer patients deal with hair loss. For more information about working with or helping clients with hair loss due to illness, visit the Look Good...Feel Better website at lookgoodfeelbetter.org or call 1-800-395-LOOK.

Courtesy of www.GarlandDrake.com. Photography by Dixie Dixon, makeup by Kay Castro, Hairstyling by Tony Greenleaf, all for Garland Drake.

After reading the next few sections, you will be able to:

LO ❶ Understand why cosmetologists should study wigs and hair additions.

why study
WIGS AND HAIR ADDITIONS?

Cosmetologists should study and have a thorough understanding of wigs and hair additions because:

> The market for products and services related to faux hair has expanded to every consumer group, from baby boomers with fine and thinning hair, to young trendsetters, to celebrities.

> Hair extensions, additions, and customized wigs can be some of the most lucrative services in the salon.

> Each manufacturer has its own systems, but if you understand the fundamentals, you can easily work with any company on the market.

> The skills you develop will open many doors, from working behind the scenes in Broadway shows to working in Hollywood with celebrities who invariably wear faux hair.

After reading the next few sections, you will be able to:

LO ❷ Explain the differences between human hair and synthetic hair.

Establish the Differences Between Human and Synthetic Hair

What is the fastest way to tell if a strand of hair is a synthetic product or real human hair? Pull the strand out of the wig or hairpiece and burn it with a match. Human hair will burn slowly, giving off a distinctive odor. A strand of synthetic fiber, on the other hand, will either ball up and melt, extinguishing itself (a characteristic of a synthetic like Kanekalon®), or it will continue to flame and burn out very quickly (typical of polyester). In either case, it will give off a slight odor.

How can you determine whether real hair or synthetic hair is best for your client? Both have advantages and disadvantages.

Advantages of Human Hair

- More realistic appearance.

- Greater durability.

- Same styling and maintenance requirements as natural hair. Human hair can be custom colored and permed or relaxed to suit the client, and it tolerates heat from a blow dryer, curling iron, flat iron, and hot rollers (figure 19–3).

Disadvantages of Human Hair

- Human hair reacts to the climate in the way that natural hair does. Depending on what type of hair it is, it may frizz or lose its curl in humid weather.

- After shampooing, the hair needs to be reset. This can be a challenge for the client who intends to maintain the hair at home.

- The color will oxidize, meaning that it will fade with exposure to light.

- The hair will break and split if mistreated by harsh brushing, backcombing, or excessive use of heat.

Advantages of Synthetic Hair

- Over the years, the technology used to produce synthetic fibers has greatly improved. Wigs, hairpieces, and extensions made of modacrylic are particularly strong and durable. Top-of-the-line synthetics like Kanekalon®, a modacrylic fiber, simulate protein-rich hair with a natural, lustrous look and feel. These synthetics are so realistic they can even fool stylists (figure 19-4).

- Synthetic hair is a great value. Not only is it very realistic, but it is less expensive than human hair. Both style and texture are set into the hair. Ready-to-wear synthetic hair is very easy for the client to maintain at

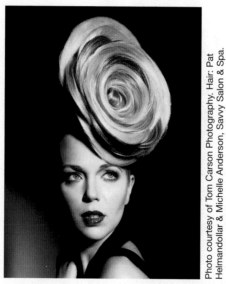

Photo courtesy of Tom Carson Photography. Hair: Pat Helmandollar & Michelle Anderson, Savvy Salon & Spa.

figure 19-3
Human hair additions can add a dramatic touch.

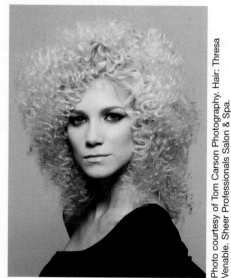

Photo courtesy of Tom Carson Photography. Hair: Thresa Venable. Sheer Professionals Salon & Spa.

figure 19-4
Synthetic additions can be whimsical.

home. Shampooing in cold water will not change the style, nor will exposure to extreme humidity.

- Most synthetic wigs, hairpieces, and extensions are cut according to the latest styles with the cut, color, and texture already set, so all that is required is some detailing, custom trimming, or attachment of the extensions.

- The colors are limitless, ranging from natural to wild fantasy shades. Price is a factor when it comes to color and texture. The cheaper synthetic wigs and hair additions tend to be more solid in color (less tone-on-tone) and the fiber is coarser (polyester based). The higher-end products are a mix of many shades, containing highlights and lowlights for a natural effect.

- Synthetic colors will not fade or oxidize, even when exposed to long periods in the sun.

Disadvantages of Synthetic Hair

- Synthetic hair cannot be exposed to extreme heat (curling irons, flat irons, hot rollers, or the high heat of blow dryers). However, some synthetic hair is coated with a protein base and can tolerate low heat. Always check with the manufacturer and perform a test strand on a small section of the actual synthetic piece.

- Coloring synthetic fibers is not recommended because traditional hair color will not work on them.

- Sometimes synthetic hair is so shiny that it may not look natural. Also, if the hair is thick, it will look unnatural on a fine-haired client.

- Price often has a lot to do with how natural synthetic hair looks. In other words, the most natural-looking synthetic pieces can be expensive.

Quality and Cost

There are pros and cons for both human hair and synthetic hair. The bottom line in both cases is that you get what you pay for.

Ultimately, your success in working with any hair addition will be determined by the quality of the product itself. Do not be fooled by imitations. Inexpensive wigs, hairpieces, and extensions may be great for fun moments or to practice cutting on, but in other situations they can look tacky and unattractive.

The more expensive wigs, hairpieces, and extensions are those made of human hair. Pricing varies as follows:

- European hair is at the top of the line. Virgin hair is the most costly; color-treated virgin hair is very costly as well.

- Virgin human hair from India and Asia, the two regions that provide most of the human hair commercially available, are next in cost. Although, Indian, Asian, and Malaysian Remi/cuticle hair, and Brazilian cuticle hair are still expensive to purchase. Indian hair is usually available in lengths from 12 inches (30 centimeters) to 16 inches (40 centimeters). Asian hair is available in lengths of

12 inches (30 centimeters) to 28 inches (40 centimeters). Indian hair is usually wavy; Asian hair is usually straight.

- Human hair mixed with animal hair is next in expense. The animal hair may be angora, horse, yak, or sheep. Yak hair is taken from the animal's belly and is the purest of whites. Its natural color lends itself to adding fantasy colors, which attract teenagers. Mixed-hair products are often used in theatrical or fashion settings.

- Human hair mixed with synthetic hair finishes the list. The mix is often half human hair and half synthetic hair. These wigs and hairpieces blend the advantages and disadvantages of both and can be a good option if chosen in the best color and texture for the client.

There are several important questions to ask when selecting a hair addition for the client:

- Is the addition made of human hair, animal hair, a mix of both, or is it synthetic or a synthetic blend?

- Is the hair colored, or in its natural state (virgin hair)?

- If the hair is human hair, is it graded in terms of strength, elasticity, and porosity?

- Is the cuticle intact? Cuticle-intact hair is more expensive because the hair has been turned. **Turned hair**, also known as *Remi hair*, is hair in which the root end of every single strand is sewn into the base so that the cuticles of all hair strands move in the same direction: down. The hair is in better condition, and it is much easier to work with because it doesn't tangle easily. Turning is a tedious, time-consuming process that increases the cost of the hair addition.

- Is it **fallen hair** (the opposite of Remi hair), hair that has been shed from the head and gathered from a hairbrush, as opposed to hair that has been cut? Fallen hair is not turned, so the cuticles of the strands will move in different directions. This makes it tangle. With what is called Remi refined hair, the cuticle is partially removed so that it will not lock and mat. This hair tends to be less expensive than Remi hair.

- Is the hair tangle-free? If the cuticle has been removed, this often means you cannot condition the hair because it will tend to mat.

- What is the condition of the hair? Has it been bleached? Can it be colored? Has it been colored with metallic dye?

- Will the hair match the client's hair? Is it similar in type and texture? Is the color-match close enough?

- Can the hair be permed or relaxed?

- If the client is going to maintain her hair at home, will the hair addition last a reasonable amount of time? (Additions should last four to six months in continual use.)

After reading the next few sections, you will be able to:

LO❸ Examine the two basic categories of wigs.

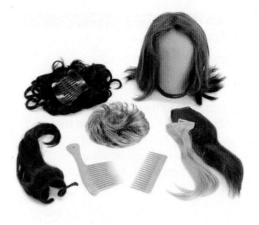
figure 19-5
Wigs and hairpieces come in a wide range of styles and colors.

Learn Basic Wig Knowledge

A **wig** can be defined as an artificial covering for the head consisting of a network of interwoven hair. When a client wears a wig, the client's hair is completely concealed (100 percent coverage). If a hair addition does not fully cover the head, it is either a **hairpiece**, which is a small wig used to cover the top or crown of the head, or a hair attachment of some sort (figure 19-5).

Types of Wigs

There are two basic categories of wigs: cap and capless.

Cap wigs are constructed with an elasticized, mesh-fiber base to which the hair is attached. They are made in several sizes and require special fittings. More often than not, cap wigs are hand-knotted. The front edge of a cap wig is made of a material that resembles the client's scalp, along with a lace extension and a wire support that is used at the temples for a snug, secure fit. Hair is hand-tied under the net (under-knotted) to conceal the cap edge. The sides and back edges contain wire supports, elastic, and hooks for a secure fit. Latex-molded cap wigs are also available; these are prostheses for clients with special needs.

Capless wigs, also known as *caps*, are machine-made from human or artificial hair. The hair is woven into **wefts**, which are long strips of hair with a threaded edge. Rows of wefts are sewn to elastic strips in a circular pattern to fit the head shape. Capless wigs are more popular than cap wigs as they are ready-to-wear and less expensive.

The capless wig is a frame of connected wefts with open areas. To understand the construction of a capless wig, compare a nylon stocking to a fishnet stocking: one has a closed framework (the cap wig), and the other is open (capless). Due to their construction and airiness, capless wigs are extremely light and comfortable to wear (figure 19-6).

In general, capless wigs are healthier, because they allow the scalp to breathe and because they prevent excess perspiration. A cap wig is best

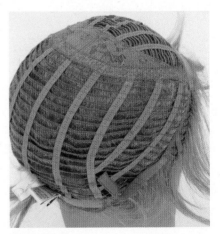
figure 19-6
A capless wig

for clients with extremely thin hair and for clients with no hair because capless wigs will allow a bald scalp to show through. There are many new innovations that make wigs more comfortable and practical than ever, like lace front wigs, which have an incredibly natural-looking hairline. Today's wigs are so well designed and fashionable that many are bought off-the-shelf for immediate wear.

Methods of Construction

- **Hand-tied wigs**, also known as *hand-knotted wigs*, are made by inserting individual strands of hair into mesh foundations and knotting them with a needle. Hand-tying is done particularly around the front hairline and at the top of the head. These wigs have a natural, realistic look and are wonderful for styling. The hand-tied method most closely resembles actual human hair growth, with flexibility at the roots. There is no definite direction to the hair, and it can be combed in almost any direction.

- **Semi-hand-tied wigs** are constructed with a combination of synthetic hair and hand-tied human hair. Reasonably priced, they offer a natural appearance and good durability.

- **Machine-made wigs**, the least expensive option, are made by feeding wefts through a sewing machine, then stitching them together to form the base and shape of the wig. Another favorable characteristic of these wigs is their bounce-back quality; even after shampooing, the style returns. They have the disadvantage of the wefting direction, which restricts styling options.

It is important to be aware of the artificial growth patterns of a wig. Wig construction will determine the direction in which you style the hair. The most flexible and versatile of all patterns is the hand-tied wig. Machine-made wigs are sewn in a specific direction, offering no versatility. If the client likes the style, this is a good thing; if not, the wig is not right for the client.

Taking Wig Measurements

In recent years, working with wigs has become a specialty among salon professionals. As a result, salons have become less and less likely to carry an inventory of wigs, or even to carry a wig catalogue. However, it is advantageous to have a basic understanding of wigs. Here is an overview.

The creation of a custom-made wig begins with taking the client's measurements. Use a soft tape measure, keeping it close to the head without pressure. Always keep a written record of the client's head measurements, and forward a copy to the wig dealer or manufacturer. Each manufacturer has its own form to fill out, which notes the measurements required. Most manufacturers ask for precise specifications of hair shade, quality of hair, length of hair, and type of hair part and pattern. Higher-end companies ask you to include a sample of the client's hair with the order.

If the wig is ready-to-wear, no measuring will be needed because it can be adjusted by tightening or loosening the straps or the elastic in the nape.

Ready-to-wear wigs are more common today. But still, many wigs need to be adjusted to the head and custom styled or trimmed to suit the client.

It is important to choose the proper size for the client's wig to ensure maximum comfort and security. Most adults will wear an average size, although the amount of hair underneath the wig may affect the size requirements.

There are three sizes of wigs: petite, average and large.

1. Petite wigs fit up to 21.5 inches (53.75 centimeters).

2. Average wigs fit heads from 21.5 inches (53.75 centimeters) to 22.5 inches (56.25 centimeters).

3. Large wigs fit heads 22.5 inches (56.25 centimeters) to 24 inches (60 centimeters).

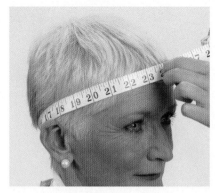
figure 19-7
Measuring the circumference of the head

Measuring the head

Before you measure, make sure to flatten the client's hair down with a brush, so it will not be in the way. Then just lay the tape measure gently around the head. Do not pull or tighten the tape measure to ensure a more accurate measurement.

Wigs should settle into the natural hairline, a few inches above the eyebrows. The back of the wig should come down to the natural hairline (nape) in the back. Most wigs have adjustable tabs or Velcro strips in the back. These tabs allow for adjustments to the circumference of the wig for the best and most comfortable fit.

To determine the size that's right for your client, measure your client's head size by taking the following measurements:

- **Head Circumference:** This measurement is the distance around the head. Circumference = _____ inches. Most wig circumferences can be adjusted up to 1–1½ inches (2.5-3.75 centimeters) (figure 19-7).

- **Front to Nape:** This measurement is the length of the head from the front to the nape of the neck. Front to Nape = _____ inches (figure 19-8).

- **Ear to Ear:** This measurement is the head from the top of one ear, over the crown to the top of the other ear. Ear to Ear = _____ inches (figure 19-9).

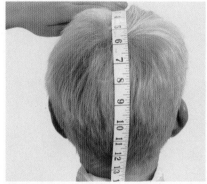
figure 19-8
Measuring from the front to the nape

Blocking the Wig

A **block** is a head-shaped form, usually made of canvas-covered cork or Styrofoam, on which the wig is secured for fitting, coloring, and sometimes styling. Canvas blocks are available in six sizes, from 20 inches (50 centimeters) to 22 inches (56.25 centimeters). The block is best attached to your work area with a swivel clamp, which allows for greater control. However, today most wigs are cut and finished while on the client, and then cleaned and stored on a drying rack. A block is best used for practicing on a wig.

Putting on the Wig

One of the most important steps in the wig service is instructing the client on how to put on the wig. Start by educating the client on the correct

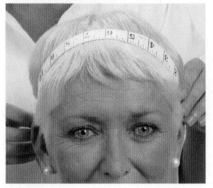
figure 19-9
Measuring from ear to ear over the crown

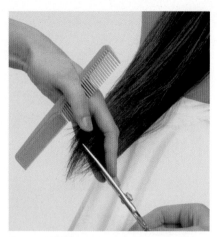

figure 19-10
Free-form cutting with vertical sections

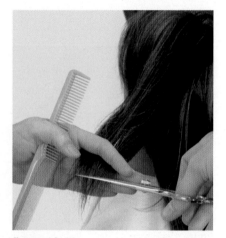

figure 19-11
Free-form cutting with
diagonal sections

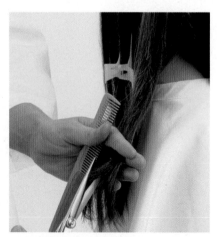

figure 19-12
Free-form cutting with
horizontal sections

method for preparing her hair. The client's skill at securing her hair under the wig cap and making it flat and even will determine how well the wig sits on her head. If the wig does not fit properly—for instance if it is too large and does not have tightening straps or elastic—you can create a small fold or tuck and sew the wig along the inside to create a seam. To shorten the wig from front to nape and remove bulk, create a horizontal tuck or fold across the back. To remove width at the back, create a vertical tuck and sew it in place. Keep in mind that sewing the wig to create a customized fit is a highly specialized art.

Cutting Wigs

When cutting a wig, your general goal is to make the hair look more realistic. As you know, natural hair has many lengths. Even when hair is cut to one length, internally there are various stages of hair growth. Hair that is one-month old and hair that is years-old exist on the same head. The stylist should try to achieve this natural look in the wig. The most effective way to do this is to taper the ends when cutting the wig. The more solid the shape, the more unnatural the hair will look.

When cutting and trimming wigs, you can follow the basic methods of haircutting—blunt, layered, and graduated—using the same sectioning and elevations as on a real head of hair. Or you may do what many top stylists prefer to do, which is to cut free-form on dry hair. The wig should be placed on the block for cutting or, for a realistic cut, the wig should be cut right on the client's head. The comb out and finishing should always be done on the client's head.

If you use free-form cutting, always work toward the weight. Vertical sections create lightness. Diagonal sections create a rounder, beveled edge. Horizontal sections build heavier weight (figures 19-10 through 19-12).

To use this visual approach, begin by cutting a small section and observe how the hair falls. Your next step will be based on how the hair responds.

Draw a diagram of the silhouette or have a photo image handy for reference. These will work as a kind of blueprint for you to follow.

Free-form cutting is usually done on dry hair, which allows you to see how easily the hair will fall. When the hair is wet, it can be hard to judge how the hair will fall.

To practice wig cutting, buy two inexpensive ready-to-wear wigs in the same style. Take a photo for reference purposes. Draw a diagram of the sections, indicating how you are going to cut the wigs. This way, you can rehearse your plan before even picking up the shears.

Begin your practice with the shadow cut. Trim the wigs following the original design that has been pre-cut into the wig, but cut the first wig wet. Then air-dry it and evaluate the style. Trim the second wig, following the same style, but this time cut it dry. Take photos of both results, and evaluate the looks you have achieved with both dry and wet cutting.

You will discover that the wet cutting method was more controlled and technical, while the dry cutting method was freer and more abstract. Often, the more abstract method results in a cut that looks more realistic.

Repeat the above exercise with a razor, thinning shears, and standard haircutting shears using the tapering method only. Compare the results.

Styling the Wig

The important thing to remember when you are styling a wig is that you must never lose sight of the big picture. Some stylists get overly involved in the wig, as if it is a creation that exists apart from the client. This is the wrong approach. A great stylist works with the total person, not just the head. When you have finished styling the wig, step back and ask the client to stand up and walk around so that you can check for balance and proportion and make corrections accordingly.

Most of the hair you will be working with is chemically treated, so it needs to be handled gently. You will achieve the best styling results by following these guidelines:

- When using heat on human hair, always set the styling tool on low.

- Treat the hair gently; do not pull it or otherwise treat it carelessly.

- Traditionally, brushes made with natural boar bristles have been regarded as best for use on human hair. The brush's soft bristles are preferable to sharp-edged synthetic bristles, which can damage hair. Today, however, you will find many synthetic brushes that have smooth, rounded plastic teeth, more like combs, and they are excellent and economical choices. Keep in mind that the key with any brush or comb is to be gentle because hair can be easily damaged.

Use a block when necessary for coloring, perming, relaxing, setting, and basic cut outlining. The comb-out and finishing touches for most modern cuts should be completed on the client's head in order to achieve proper balance and personalization (figure 19-13).

Remember that most clients come into the salon looking for a natural look. Making a wig look believable is very challenging, and to do it well is truly an art form. The areas that must appear the most convincing are the crown, the part, and the hairline. Sometimes, crowns and parts look more natural when they are flat to the head; other times, a more natural look is attained by adding volume to these areas. This will be determined by the style. A general rule is to follow the direction of the knotting and weave, as preset by the wig maker. If you fight the direction, the results may look odd.

Styling Tips for the Hairline

- Choose styling products that have been formulated for color-treated hair. These will work the best, and they are gentlest to human hair. There are also specialized products for wigs. Just remember that whatever you put into the hair will eventually have to be shampooed out.

- If the wig does not have a natural-looking hairline or a lace front, backcomb gently around the hairline. The fluffy effect softens the hairline.

- Release the client's hair around the hairline, and cut and blend it into the wig hair.

The best test to gauge how realistic the wig looks is to use the wind test. This test simulates the wind blowing the client's hair

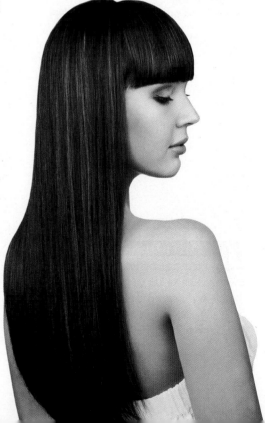

figure 19-13
A natural looking style

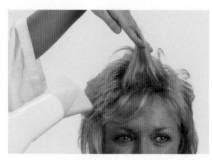

figure 19-14
The wind test

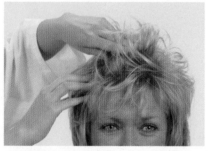

figure 19-15
Style with the fingers for a natural look.

away from her face. Gently blow around the client's face with a blow dryer set at cool and low. Observe how the hairline looks. Does it seem realistic? If so, point out the results to the client, who may be feeling insecure about whether the wig looks natural enough (figure 19-14).

When styling a wig, do not try to make it look perfect. Little imperfections help achieve a realistic look. Use your hands rather than a brush for a more natural look (figure 19-15). Do not plaster the hair down because it will look artificial.

Cleaning the Wig

Clients who bought off-the-shelf wigs may bring them to a salon for cleaning, reshaping, and styling. To clean any wig, always follow the manufacturer's instructions. If shampooing is recommended, use a gentle shampoo, such as one you would use for color-treated hair, or use shampoo specially developed for wigs. Avoid any harsh shampoos with a sulfur base, such as dandruff shampoos. Soak, then gently squeeze the wig and use a drying rack for drying. If you are cleaning a wig made of human hair, you should also condition it.

Coloring Wigs and Hair Additions

All synthetic hair colors used for wigs and hairpieces are standardized according to the 70 colors on the hair color ring used by wig and hairpiece manufacturers. The colors range from black to pale blond. Because most commercially available hair originates in either India or China, the most common natural color level is 1, or black. It is very difficult to lift level 1 to level 10. (See Chapter 21, Haircoloring, for a discussion of hair color levels.) At the other end of the spectrum is white yak hair, which is an excellent base for adding color. Yak hair is especially good to use with fantasy colors that appeal to some younger clients.

If you are going to custom color the hair, use hair that has been decolorized (bleached) through the lifting process, not with metallic dyes. Be sure to check with the manufacturer.

The principles that guide the coloring of natural hair also apply to the art of coloring wigs and hair extensions. As in all disciplines, you must first learn the rules before you break them. Good colorists are not afraid to make mistakes because they have worked hard to learn the basics and know how to correct mistakes.

When coloring a wig, first check to see if the cuticle is intact. Hair in which the cuticle is absent is very porous and will react to color in an extreme manner. Always strand-test the hair prior to a full-color application. Use semipermanent, demipermanent, glaze, rinse, or color mousse products. Use permanent hair color on human hair wigs unless the hair is porous, in which case, semipermanent color is the better choice. (See Chapter 21, Haircoloring, for more detail.)

When coloring a human hair wig or hair addition, conduct regular color checks every five to ten minutes. Remember that the hair you are working on did not come from one head, but from many different heads, so it may be unpredictable. Often, it is easier to color the client's hair to match a hair addition than to color the addition itself.

Perming Wigs and Hair Additions

If you want to perm human hair to match the client's natural wave pattern, you need to know how the hair was colored. Was it decolorized (bleached) or dyed with metallic dye? Do not perm hair that has been colored with a metallic dye.

The permanent wave must be performed with the hair additions off the client's head. For wigs and hairpieces, cover the head form with plastic to protect it from the chemical solutions, pin the wig securely to the head form, and perm as you would a natural head of hair. Perm extensions as they lie flat. (See Chapter 20, Chemical Texture Services, for perming procedures.)

After reading the next few sections, you will be able to:

LO④ **Distinguish several types of hairpieces and their uses.**

Know the Different Types of Hairpieces

In eighteenth-century France, women wore towering hairdos complete with extensions and various apparatuses, such as springs to adjust the height. Some of these coiffures were three-feet high and had elaborate visual elements worked into them such as model ships or gardens. These styles were often untouched for weeks at a time. The bad news is that they sometimes attracted vermin. The moral of this story is that sometimes it is best not to get swept up in current trends or passing fashions. Always be aware of the strength of classic design. Keep it simple, remembering that less is more, and try not to let yourself get carried away.

Hairpieces are an important area of hair additions (**figure 19-16**). They sit on top of the client's head, covering a portion of it, or clip onto another area, such as the nape. They are usually attached by temporary methods. (They are not worn during sleep.) Some, like wiglets that conceal a thinning top, can also be attached with a braid-and-sew technique.

There are many different types of hairpieces, including integration pieces (which are attached with a semipermanent method), toupees (which can be complex and challenging to work with), and fashion hairpieces. Fashion hairpieces include falls, half wigs (falls on a cap that attaches with combs an inch or so behind the hairline and can be used with a headband or with the natural hair combed straight back to conceal the attachment site), wiglets, chignons, bandeaus (falls with a headband attached), cascades (clip-on top curls), ponytails, bangs, and fillers (which add volume to fine hair). Many of the newest fashion hairpieces simply clip on with pressure-sensitive clips, claw clips, or combs. Here, only the major types are covered to give you a general overview. Working with hair additions and hair replacement systems is a specialized art, and many manufacturers have their own attachment systems and training.

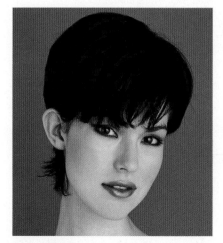

figure 19-16
Hairpieces can look very natural.

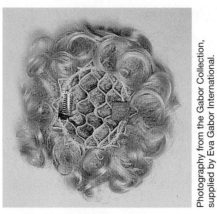

figure 19-17
Integration hairpiece

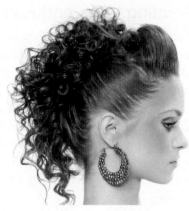

figure 19-18
An integration hairpiece is easy to wear.

The client's hair can be prepared in a number of ways before the hairpiece is attached. It can be tied into a ponytail or bun or twisted into a French twist. It can be blended with the hairpiece or serve as a base for it.

Integration Hairpieces

An **integration hairpiece** is a hairpiece that has openings in the base, through which the client's own hair is pulled to blend with the (natural or synthetic) hair of the hairpiece. These hairpieces are very lightweight, natural-looking products that add length and volume to the client's hair. If your client is wearing hair extensions and would like a change, the integration hairpiece can be a good alternative. It is also recommended for clients with thinning hair, but not for those with total hair loss, as the scalp is likely to show through (**figures 19-17** and **19-18**).

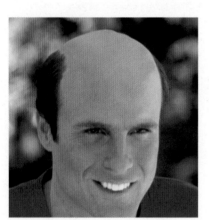

figure 19-19
Male hair-enhancement client

Toupees

While men usually are the clients for toupees, women can also wear these hairpieces. A **toupee** (too-PAY) is a small wig used to cover the top and crown of the head. The fine-net base is usually the most appropriate material for the client with severe hair loss. There are two ways to attach toupees: temporary (tape or clips) or semipermanent (tracks, adhesive, or sewing).

Most wearers of toupees prize the confidence gained from wearing an authentic-looking hairpiece and are prepared to pay a high price for it. The best toupees are custom designed. The top manufacturers offer in-depth instruction for those interested in learning this specialty service (**figures 19-19** and **19-20**).

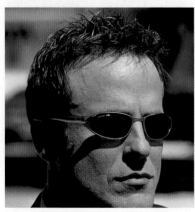

figure 19-20
The same client fitted with a toupee

Fashion Hairpieces

Fashion hairpieces are a great salon product for special occasions or for use as fashion accessories. They include ponytails, chignons, cascades, streaks, bangs, falls/half wigs, and clip-in hair extensions.

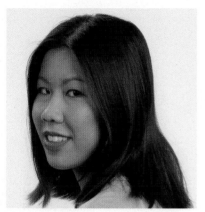

figure 19-21
A client before fitting with
a wraparound ponytail

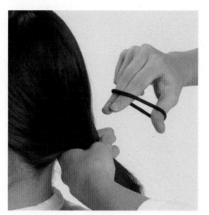

figure 19-22
Client's own ponytail

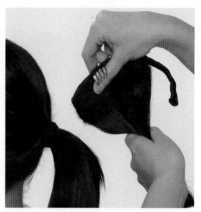

figure 19-23
Attaching the hairpiece

These hairpieces vary in size and usually are constructed on a stiff net base. They are attached, temporarily, with hairpins, clips, combs, bobby pins, or elastic.

Three hair extension methods are:

- **Wraparound Ponytail.** The wraparound ponytail is a long length of wefted hair that covers 10 to 20 percent of the head. It is used as a simple ponytail or in chignons. It is particularly useful for the client who can just get her own hair into a ponytail. (figures 19-21 through 19-25).

- **Cascading Curls.** A cascade of curls is attached with combs. This hair extension fall or attachment allows the client to have longer, fuller cascading curls covering the entire top and back of the head (figures 19-26 through 19-30).

- **Hair Wrap.** A hair wrap is mounted on an elastic loop. It is further secured to the client's own hair with hairpins. This is a simple way to add a little additional hair to a ponytail (figures 19-31 through 19-34).

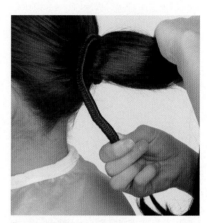

figure 19-24
Wrapping the band around
the ponytail base

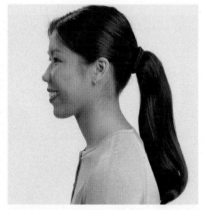

figure 19-25
Same client with a new, much
longer ponytail

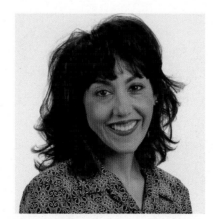

figure 19-26
Client before fitting with
comb-attached curls

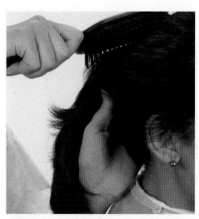

figure 19-27
Brushing the client's hair into
a ponytail

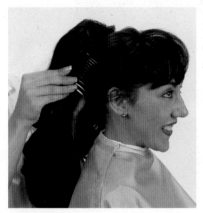

figure 19-28
Attaching the combs

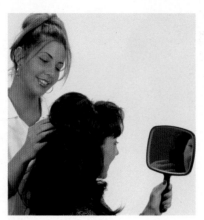

figure 19-29
Adjusting the hairpiece

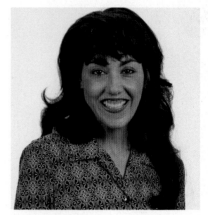

figure 19-30
Cascade of curls

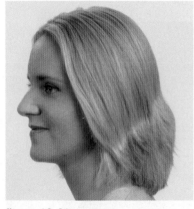

figure 19-31
Client before fitting with a hair wrap

After reading the next few sections, you will be able to:

LO⑤ Review several different methods of attaching hair extensions.

Study the World of Hair Extensions

Hair extensions are hair additions that are secured to the base of the client's natural hair in order to add length, volume, texture, or color. Extensions can be human hair, synthetic hair, or a blend of the two. They are either wefts of hair or strands (small bundles of hair); the latter are attached one-by-one and are usually pre-bonded or keratin-tipped. Unless they are clip-in extensions, they are applied with semipermanent attachment methods.

Hair extensions represent an increasingly popular salon service, not only for clients who are looking for something different but also for those

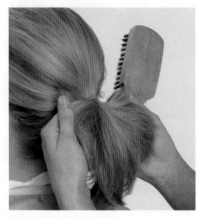

figure 19-32
Brushing client's hair into a ponytail

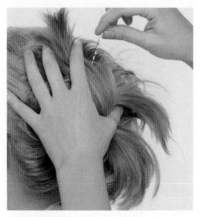

figure 19-33
Securing the hairpiece with hairpins

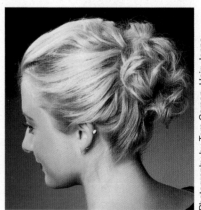

figure 19-34
An easy, dressed-up look

Photography by Tom Carson. Hair: Jenna Kreger & Alyssa Hartrick. The Brown Institute.

who have naturally fine hair or who suffer from hair loss. Hair extensions are extremely popular among celebrities, who never seem to have thin hair and who seem to magically grow their hair long overnight.

Manufacturers generally offer their own method of training in the attachment of hair extensions, but there are certain general guidelines to keep in mind:

- Start by deciding whether you are adding length, thickness, or both.

- Know which final style you are striving to achieve, and map it out. Sketch or visualize a placement pattern.

- As a general rule of thumb, stay 1 inch (2.5 centimeters) away from the hairline at the front, sides, and nape, and 1 inch away from the part.

- With very thin hair, you must be careful that the base does not show through.

- Curly hair tends to expand and can give the illusion of being thicker than it really is. When working with curly hair, you will need to determine whether you are matching the curl or whether you wish to add another curl pattern to the hair.

- Straight, thin hair and curly, thin hair may have similar density, but curly hair will appear thicker. This means you may not need to put as many extensions in curly hair as in straight hair.

- As you now know, there are many different ways to attach hair additions. When it comes to extensions, methods include braid-and-sew, simple bonding (also known as *fusion bonding*), linking, and tube shrinking.

The most important professional approaches to hair addition and extension services should be practiced—always in the following order:

1. Safety for the client's own hair.

2. Comfort—There should be no pulling or pinching; avoid excess tension on the natural hair.

3. Security—Make certain the additions will not fall off. If they are attached with a semipermanent method such as braid-and-sew, bonding, or fusion bonding, be certain that they will last several weeks before they are removed or require readjustment to accommodate the natural hair's growth.

4. Style and fashion.

FOCUS ON

Sharpening Your Skills

In order to achieve a natural look, it is crucial that you blend the client's hair with the hairpiece. You must match both the color and the wave pattern. If the client has naturally wavy hair, it is wise to find a hairpiece with a wave pattern that matches the client's. To match the color, use the color ring. Most hairpieces come in many colors, so it is relatively easy to match to the client's hair. You cannot color a synthetic hairpiece, so any custom coloring to achieve a match must be performed on the client's hair.

Braid-and-Sew Method

In the **braid-and-sew method**, hair extensions are secured to the client's own hair by sewing braids or a weft onto an on-the-scalp braid or cornrow, which is sometimes called the track (figure 19-35). The wefts can also be attached by creating a track, using fiber filler. The filler and hair from the scalp are braided together, using an underhand braiding technique. The filler helps grip the client's own hair and creates a longer-lasting braid, to which you attach the weft. The angle of the track determines how the hair will fall. You may position braids or tracks horizontally, vertically, diagonally, or along curved lines that follow the contours of the head (figure 19-36). The braid-and-sew method can also be used to attach hairpieces.

Partings are determined according to the style you have chosen. The size of the sections is determined by the amount of hair that will be added to the head. Plan the tracks or braids so that the ends will be hidden. It is best to position them 1 inch (2.5 centimeters) behind the hairline to ensure proper coverage.

When sewing on the extension, use only a blunt, custom-designed needle, either straight or curved. These blunt ends will help avoid damage to the hair and will protect you and the client as well. Extensions can be sewn to the track using a variety of stitches.

- **Lock stitch.** A sewing technique used with a curved needle and thread to sew on a weft of hair to a braided cornrow track. This stitch can also be used over the entire length of the track in evenly spaced stitches (figures 19-37 through 19-39).

- **Overcast stitch.** This simple, quick stitch can be used to secure the entire length of the weft to the track. Pass the needle under both the track and the weft, and then bring it back over to make a new stitch. Moving along the track, repeat the stitch until you reach the end of the track. Complete with a lock stitch for security (figures 19-40 and 19-41).

- **Double-lock stitch.** This stitch is much like the lock stitch, but the thread is wound around the needle twice to create the double lock. It is used in the same ways as the lock stitch.

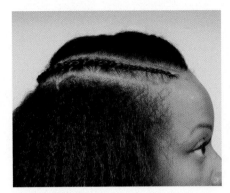
figure 19-35
Cornrow braid track

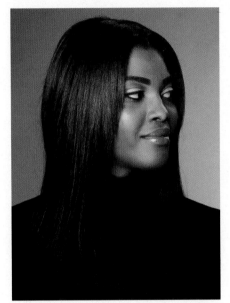
figure 19-36
Hair extensions using the braid-and-sew attachment method

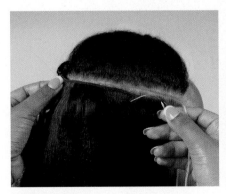
figure 19-37
Sew weft to braid.

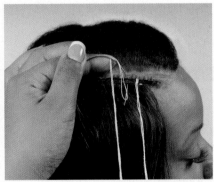
figure 19-38
Wrap the thread around the needle.

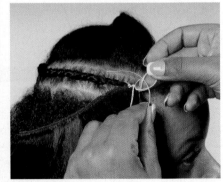
figure 19-39
Form lock stitch.

Photography by Tom Carson. Hair: Kristian Bailey. The Brown Institute.

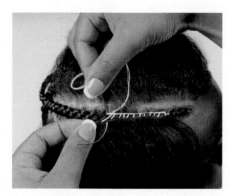

figure 19-40
Finished overcast stitches

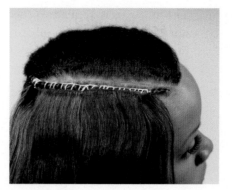

figure 19-41
Complete line of overcast stitching

Advantages

- Advantages of the braid-and-sew method include the fact that, if done correctly, it is a very safe technique (figures 19-42 and 19-43).

- The braid-and-sew attachment method requires no special equipment, and, with practice, you can do it fairly quickly.

Disadvantages

- Drawbacks include, if there is too much tension on the braid, the client's real hair can be damaged.

- Also, the braid-and-sew attachment method is not appropriate for clients who have extremely damaged hair, clients who have baby-fine hair (because breakage can occur), or clients who don't keep their scalps clean.

Bonding Method

In the **bonding** method of attaching hair extensions, hair wefts or single strands are attached with an adhesive or bonding agent.

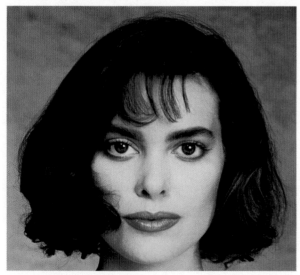

figure 19-42
Before braid and sew extensions

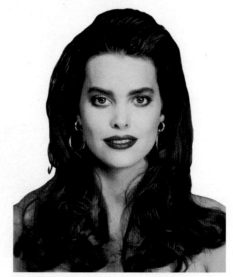

figure 19-43
After braid and sew extensions

The adhesive is applied to the weft with an applicator gun. This gun is not like those available in crafts stores; it is a tool created specifically for bonding.

For bonding, the natural hair should be at least four-inches long. Bonded hair sits snugly on the head, and is fast to apply (figures 19-44 and 19-45). There is, however, a certain degree of slippage. Generally, the bonding product lasts from two to four weeks, depending on factors such as the frequency of shampooing, the oiliness or dryness of the scalp, and the quality of the products used. This means that the client will need to be on a maintenance program that requires salon visits as often as every two weeks. Care must be taken when bonding to avoid working too close to the crown and the parting, or the weft will show through. Working 1 inch (2.5 centimeters) away from the hairline will also keep the wefts from showing. Remember that hair is not a static material; it has a natural swing, and it moves. When the wind blows, it should be the hairline that shows, not the wefts.

Bonded wefts are removed by dissolving the adhesive bond with oil or bond remover. The same technique can be used with loose hair or wefts that are cut into very small sections. This is called **strand bonding**.

Advantages

- Two advantages of bonding are that it can be offered at a very affordable price and the service does not take much longer than the average haircut appointment.

- Also, the client can shampoo with the wefts in, as long as it is done gently.

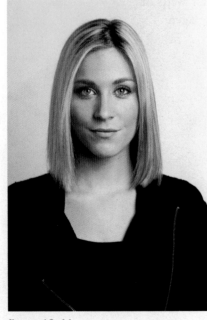

figure 19-44
Client before bonding hair
attachment method

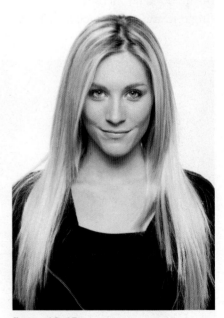

figure 19-45
Client after bonding hair
attachment method

Photography by Tom Carson. Hair: Kathy McCaffrey, Kathy Adams Salon.

Disadvantages

- One drawback of bonding is that some clients may have an allergic reaction to the ingredients in the bonding adhesive. Always perform a patch test prior to the application of bonded extensions, especially when using a latex-based adhesive.

- Also, bonding is not appropriate for clients who have severely damaged hair or those who do not have enough natural hair to hide the wefts. The wefts cannot be exposed to oils or they will slide off.

- In general, bonding should *not* be used to attach wefts that are longer than 12 inches (30 centimeters) to avoid excessive heaviness and the possibility of pulling on the client's natural hair and scalp.

Fusion-Bonding Method

In the **fusion-bonding** method of attaching extensions, individual extension hair is bonded to the client's own hair with a bonding material that is activated by the heat from a special tool. This method, while expensive and extremely time-consuming, harmonizes with the client's natural hair with no uncomfortable or unattractive attachment sites. The bonds are light and comfortable to wear, the hair moves like real hair, and the hair is easy to maintain (**figure 19-46**). The attachment lasts up to four months, almost twice as long as other methods. Removal is quick and painless. The fusion method requires certification training because it is manufacturer specific.

Some fusion-bonding procedures involve wrapping a keratin-based strip around both the client's hair and the extension or applying the bond to the extension first with a special gun-applicator. Today, many of the extensions or addition strands are pre-tipped or keratin-tipped. In fusion bonding, natural strands along a parting are selected and then isolated with a hair shield

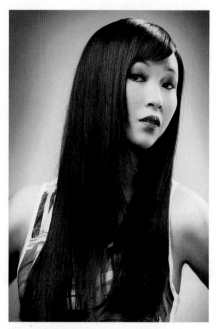

figure 19-46
Hair extensions using the fusion bonding attachment method

Advantages

- One advantage of fusion bonding is that the client's hair will dry more quickly than when bonding full wefts because there is less bulk.

- By using extensions in slightly different colors, you can create the illusion of depth and dimension or a highlighted effect.

- This method also allows for styling versatility.

Disadvantages

- Drawbacks include the fact that the technique is time-consuming.

- The pre-tipped extensions are expensive. Some suppliers will take back the extension hair and re-tip it, which saves costs and reduces waste; others will not. Applying the adhesive or bonding material yourself avoids this issue, but can be messier and even more time-consuming.

Linking

In **linking**, a hook is used to pick up a small amount of hair off a parting. A link is slid on close to the scalp with a special tool. Then an extension or special addition strand is inserted into the link (**figure 19–47**). Once the extension and the natural hair are captured in the link, the link is pinched flat with pliers. Once removed properly with a removal tool (pliers), the extensions can be reused. To use a linking method of attachment, the natural hair should be at least 5 inches (12.5 centimeters)long.

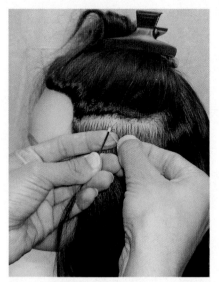

figure 19-47
Linking

Advantages

- Linking offers styling versatility
- The integrity of the natural hair can be maintained if the procedure is done properly.

Disadvantages

- Drawbacks are that this method is expensive and time-consuming.
- Also, the metal links can oxidize (rust).

Tube Shrinking

In tube shrinking, the client's hair and the addition strand are inserted into a tube, which is then heated to shrink it. This method requires special tools and training.

As with all semipermanent attachment methods for hair extensions, various problems can arise. Usually, these problems are caused by the stylist or the client and not the material.

Stylists must follow a logical placement pattern carefully, pay attention to natural growth patterns, and provide complete home-care instructions. Clients must follow home-care instructions carefully to keep the hair neat and clean. They must also return to the salon regularly for maintenance.

Retailing Hair Addition Products

Simple hairpieces are a great retail product for the salon. They can be displayed in fun, creative ways. Because they are fairly easy to attach and remove, they almost sell themselves, particularly to younger, more adventurous clients (**figure 19-48**). Retailing hair additions and related home-care products can mean substantial additional income for you. Offering hair-addition services can be lucrative for the highly trained stylist.

Whether retailing hair goods or offering hair-addition services, keep the following guidelines in mind:

- Identify the client's needs.
- Explain why it would be worthwhile for the client to make the investment.
- Describe the features and benefits of the products you recommend.

Courtesy of www.GarlandDrake.com. Photography by Raymond Drake.

- Discuss product performance and cost.

- Choose high-quality hairpieces and extensions.

- Always believe in your recommendations and stand by your products.

- Price services according to time spent on the service, materials, your expertise, and what the local market will bear.

To be the best, work only with the best. Work with one or two companies that offer a good range of human and synthetic hair, high-quality products, good customer service, and first-rate support, as well as product education through training, seminars, and videos. Always stick with companies that stand by their products.

A Final Thought: Practice, Practice, Practice

Working with hair additions can be one of the most exciting, challenging, and lucrative areas of cosmetology. But to become skilled at this work, you need to take specialized, formal training and practice continually. The more you do, the better you will become. The better you become, the more you will be able to help people look good and feel good about themselves. There is a great satisfaction in being able to do this, particularly when working with people who have suffered the trauma of hair loss and may have given up hope that they could look good again (figure 19-49).

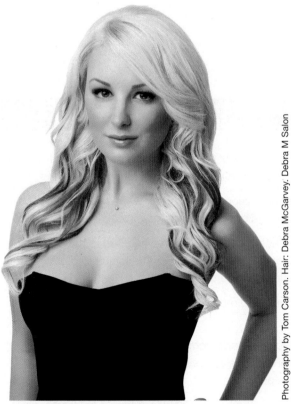

Photography by Tom Carson. Hair: Debra McGarvey. Debra M Salon

figure 19-48
Offering hair addition services can be rewarding and lucrative for the highly trained stylist.

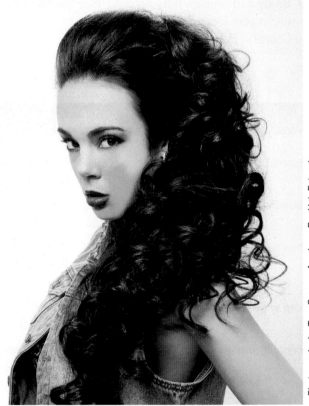

Photography by Tom Carson. Academy Pro Hair Extensions.

figure 19-49
A cascade of curls hair extensions

REVIEW QUESTIONS

1. What are hair extensions?

2. What are the main advantages and disadvantages of human hair and synthetic hair?

3. What are the two basic categories of wigs?

4. What are three types of hairpieces and how are they used?

5. What are fashion hairpieces and list three methods of attachments.

6. What are three primary wig measurements?

7. What are the basic methods of hair cutting and trimming wigs?

8. What are five methods for attaching hair extensions? Describe each.

STUDY TOOLS

- **Reinforce what you just learned:** Complete the activities and exercises in your Theory or Practical Workbook, or your Study Guide.

- **Expand your knowledge:** Search for websites about the topics in this chapter and make a list of additional resources.

- **Study and prepare for your quiz:** Take the chapter test in your Exam Review or your Milady U: Online Licensing Prep.

- **Re-Test your knowledge:** Take the Chapter 19 *Quizzes!*

- **Learn even more:** Look up in a dictionary or search the internet for the definitions for any additional terms you want to learn about.

CHAPTER GLOSSARY

block	p. 579	Head-shaped form, usually made of canvas-covered cork or Styrofoam, on which the wig is secured for fitting, cleaning, coloring, and styling.
bonding	p. 589	Method of attaching hair extensions in which hair wefts or single strands are attached with an adhesive or bonding agent.
braid-and-sew method	p. 588	Attachment method in which hair extensions are secured to the client's own hair by sewing braids or a weft onto an on-the-scalp braid or cornrow, which is sometimes called the track.
cap wigs	p. 577	Wigs constructed of elasticized, mesh-fiber bases to which the hair is attached.
capless wigs	p. 577	Also known as *caps*; machine-made from human or artificial hair which is woven into rows of wefts. Wefts are sewn to elastic strips in a circular pattern to fit the head shape.
fallen hair	p. 576	Hair that has been shed from the head or gathered from a hairbrush, as opposed to hair that has been cut; the cuticles of the strands will move in different directions (opposite of turned or Remi hair).

fusion bonding	p. 591	Method of attaching extensions in which extension hair is bonded to the client's own hair with a bonding material that is activated by heat from a special tool.
hair extensions	p. 586	Hair additions that are secured to the base of the client's natural hair in order to add length, volume, texture, or color.
hairpiece	p. 577	Small wig used to cover the top or crown of the head, or a hair attachment of some sort.
hand-tied wigs	p. 578	Also known as *hand-knotted wigs*; wigs made by inserting individual strands of hair into mesh foundations and knotting them with a needle.
integration hairpiece	p. 584	Hairpiece that has openings in the base through which the client's own hair is pulled to blend with the hair (natural or synthetic) of the hairpiece.
linking	p. 592	Method of attaching hair extensions in which a hook is used to pick up a small amount of hair off a parting. A link is slid on close to the scalp with a special tool. Then an extension or special addition strand is inserted into the link.
machine-made wigs	p. 578	Wigs made by machine by feeding wefts through a sewing machine and then sewing them together to form the base and shape of the wig.
semi-hand-tied wigs	p. 578	Wigs constructed with a combination of synthetic hair and hand-tied human hair.
strand bonding	p. 590	Bonding method with loose hair or wefts that are cut into very small sections
toupee (too-PAY)	p. 584	Small wig used to cover the top or crown of the head.
turned hair	p. 576	Also called *Remi hair*; the root end of every single strand is sewn into the base so that the cuticles of all hair strands move in the same direction: down.
wefts	p. 577	Long strips of human or artificial hair with a threaded edge.
wig	p. 577	Artificial covering for the head consisting of a network of interwoven hair.

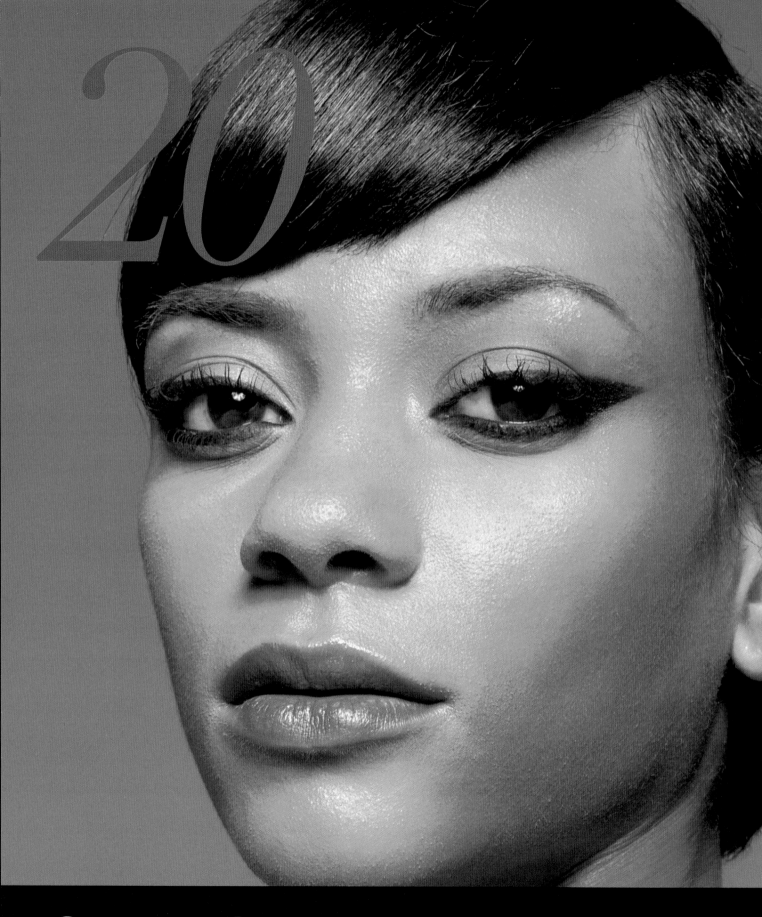

20

CHEMICAL TEXTURE
SERVICES

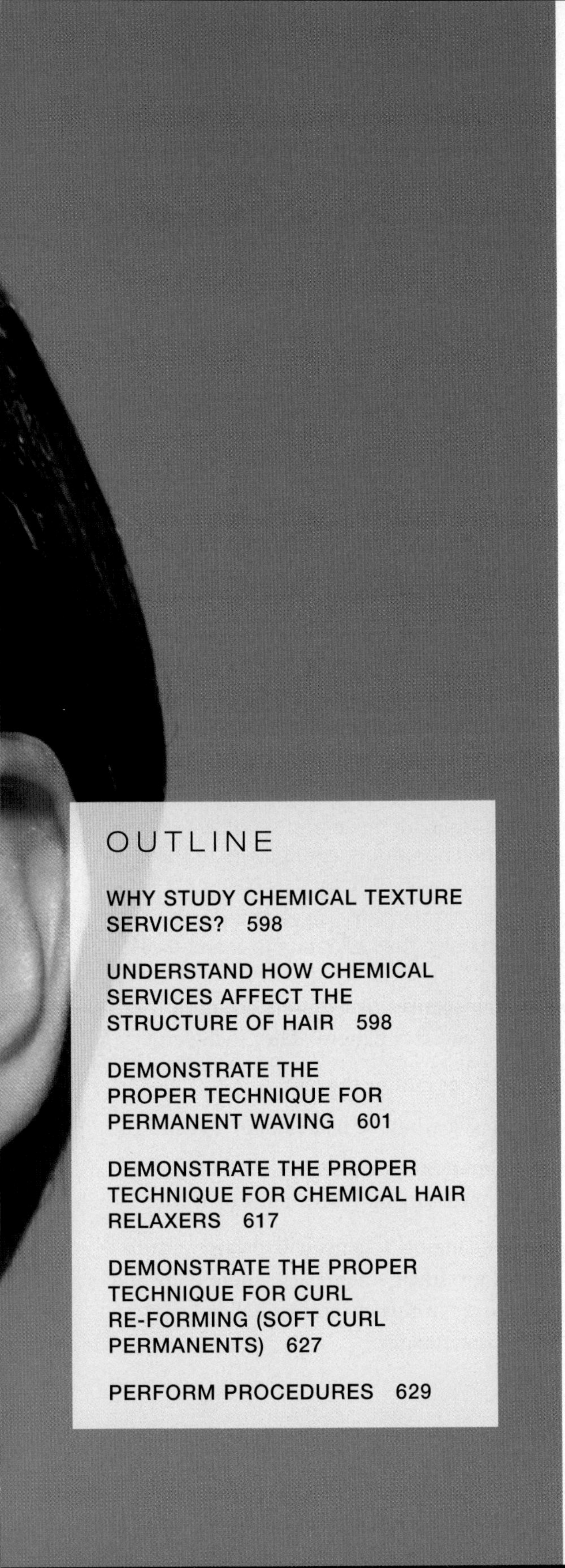

LEARNING OBJECTIVES

After completing this chapter, you will be able to:

LO❶
Explain the four chemical reactions that take place during permanent waving.

LO❷
Explain the difference between an alkaline wave and a true acid wave.

LO❸
Explain the purpose of neutralization in permanent waving.

LO❹
Demonstrate safe and effective perm techniques.

LO❺
Describe how thio relaxers straighten the hair.

LO❻
Describe how hydroxide relaxers straighten the hair.

LO❼
Demonstrate safe and effective hydroxide relaxing techniques.

LO❽
Describe curl re-forming and how it restructures the hair.

OUTLINE

Chemical hair texture services give you the ability to permanently change the hair's natural wave and curl pattern thereby offering clients a variety of styling options that would not otherwise be possible. Texture services can be used to curl straight hair, straighten overly curly hair, or soften tightly coiled hair (figure 20-1).

why study
CHEMICAL TEXTURE SERVICES?

Cosmetologists should study and have a thorough understanding of chemical texture services because:

> Chemical texture services allow stylists the opportunity to offer clients options to change the texture of their hair and explore the fashionable world of hairstyling.

> Knowing how to perform these services accurately, safely, and professionally will help build a trusting and loyal clientele.

> Knowledge builds confidence to offer chemical texture services to all clients.

> Chemical services are among the most lucrative and repetitive services in the salon, and many retail products are specific to hair's texture and condition.

> Without a thorough understanding of chemistry, cosmetologists could damage hair, cause hair loss, and harm their clients and themselves.

Chemical texture services are hair services that cause a chemical change within the hair's natural wave and curl pattern. They include:

- **Permanent waving.** Adding wave or curl to the hair.

- **Relaxing.** Removing curl or waves; leaving the hair smooth and straight.

- **Curl re-forming (soft curl permanents).** Loosening overly curly hair; changing tightly curly or coiled hair into loose curls or waves.

The world of hairstyling is ever changing. Clients will always want to smooth their curly and wavy hair or give their straight hair more body and curl; therefore, mastering the techniques in this chapter will allow you to greatly expand your potential as a cosmetologist.

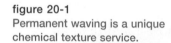

figure 20-1
Permanent waving is a unique chemical texture service.

Understand How Chemical Services Affect the Structure of Hair

Because all chemical texture procedures involve chemically and physically changing the structure of the hair, this chapter begins by reviewing the structure and purpose of each layer of the hair—characteristics of hair that were first discussed in Chapter 11, Properties of the Hair and Scalp.

- **Cuticle.** Tough exterior layer of the hair. It surrounds the inner layers and protects the hair from damage. Although the cuticle is not directly involved in the texture or movement of the hair, texture chemicals must penetrate through the cuticle to their target in the cortex in order to be effective (**figures 20-2** and **20-3**).

- **Cortex.** Middle layer of the hair, located directly beneath the cuticle layer. The cortex is responsible for the incredible strength and elasticity of human hair. Breaking the side bonds of the cortex makes it possible to change the natural wave pattern of the hair.

- **Medulla.** Innermost layer of the hair, often called the *pith* or *core* of the hair. The medulla does not play a role in chemical texture services and may be missing in fine hair.

For more detailed information on the hair's structure, review Chapter 11, Properties of the Hair and Scalp,

Importance of pH in Texture Services

In Chapter 12, Basics of Chemistry, you learned that pH is an abbreviation for potential hydrogen. The symbol *pH* represents the quantity of hydrogen ions. The pH scale measures the acidity and alkalinity of a substance by measuring the quantity of hydrogen ions it contains. The pH scale has a range from 0 to 14. A pH of 7 is neutral, a pH below 7 is acidic, and a pH above 7 is alkaline. The natural pH of hair is between 4.5 and 5.5. Chemical solutions raise the pH of the hair to an alkaline state (**figure 20-4**). This action opens the cuticle layer of the hair and allows the solution to reach the cortex layer, where restructuring occurs. Coarse, resistant hair with a strong, compact cuticle layer requires a highly alkaline chemical solution. Porous, damaged, or chemically treated hair requires a less alkaline solution.

Basic Building Blocks of Hair

To understand how a chemical solution changes the structure of hair, it is important to understand the basic building blocks of hair (**figures 20-5** through **20-8**).

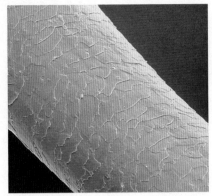

figure 20-2
A healthy cuticle is compact and lies tight against the hair strand. It protects the hair from damage and makes it appear smooth and shiny.

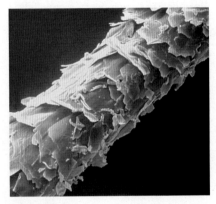

figure 20-3
A damaged cuticle is chipped and does not lie tight again the hair shaft. It cannot adequately protect the hair against damage, so the hair becomes rough, dull, and prone to split ends and breakage.

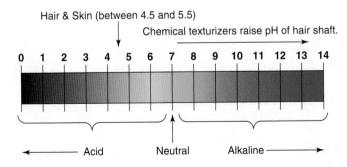

figure 20-4
The importance of pH in texture services

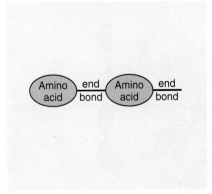

figure 20-5
Peptide bonds (end bonds) link amino acids together in long chains.

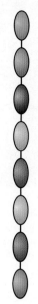

figure 20-6
Polypeptide chains are formed when
amino acids link together.

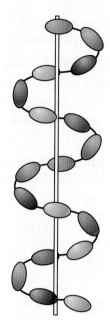

figure 20-7
Keratin proteins are long, coiled
peptide chains.

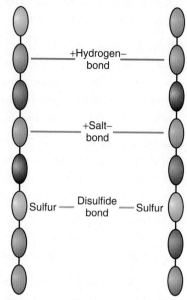

+Hydrogen–
bond

+Salt–
bond

Sulfur — Disulfide
bond — Sulfur

figure 20-8
Side bonds cross-link polypeptide
chains together.

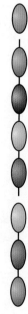

figure 20-9
A correct permanent wave service
only alters the side bonds.

- **Amino acids** are compounds made up of carbon, oxygen, hydrogen, nitrogen, and sulfur.

- **Peptide bonds**, also known as *end bonds*, are chemical bonds that join amino acids together, end-to-end in long chains, to form a polypeptide chain.

- **Polypeptide chains** (pahl-ee-PEP-tyd CHAYNS) are long chains of amino acids joined together by peptide bonds.

- **Keratin proteins** are long, coiled polypeptide chains.

- **Side bonds** are disulfide, salt, and hydrogen bonds that cross-link polypeptide chains together.

Keratin Proteins

Keratin proteins are made of long chains of amino acids linked together end-to-end like beads. The amino acid chains are linked together by peptide bonds (end bonds). These chains of amino acids linked by peptide bonds are called polypeptides. Keratin proteins are made of long, coiled, polypeptide chains, which in turn are comprised of amino acids.

Side Bonds

The cortex is made up of millions of polypeptide chains cross-linked by three types of side bonds: disulfide, salt, and hydrogen. Side bonds are responsible for the elasticity and strength of the hair. Altering these three types of side bonds makes wet setting, thermal styling, permanent waving, curl re-forming, and chemical hair relaxing possible (figure 20-9).

Disulfide Bonds

Disulfide bonds are strong chemical side bonds formed when the sulfur atoms in two adjacent protein chains are joined together. Although there are far fewer disulfide bonds than hydrogen or salt bonds, they are the strongest of the three side bonds, accounting for about one-third of the hair's overall strength. Disulfide bonds are not affected by water; however, boiling water can break and alter their appearance. Although the amount of heat used in conventional thermal styling does not break disulfide bonds, caution must be used when using thermal tools with extreme heat because the high heat can cause irreversible damage to the hair.

Altering the chemical and physical changes in disulfide bonds makes permanent waving, curl re-forming, and chemical hair relaxing possible.

Salt Bonds

Salt bonds are relatively weak physical side bonds that are the result of an attraction between negative and positive electrical charges (ionic bonds); they are easily broken by changes in pH, and they re-form when the pH returns to normal levels. Hydrogen bonds can be broken by water, whereas salt bonds are broken by changes in pH levels. Even though salt bonds are far weaker than disulfide bonds, the hair has so many salt bonds that they account for about one-third of the hair's total strength.

Hydrogen Bonds

Hydrogen bonds are weak physical side bonds that are also the result of an attraction between opposite electrical charges; they are easily broken by water (wet setting) or heat (thermal styling), and they re-form as the hair dries or cools. Although individual hydrogen bonds are very weak, there are so many of them that they, too, account for about one-third of the hair's total strength.

After reading the next few sections, you will be able to:

LO❶ Explain the four chemical reactions that take place during permanent waving.

LO❷ Explain the difference between an alkaline wave and a true acid wave.

LO❸ Explain the purpose of neutralization in permanent waving.

LO❹ Demonstrate safe and effective perm techniques.

Demonstrate the Proper Technique for Permanent Waving

Permanent waving is a two-step process whereby the hair undergoes a physical change caused by wrapping the hair on perm rods; the hair then undergoes a chemical change caused by the application of permanent

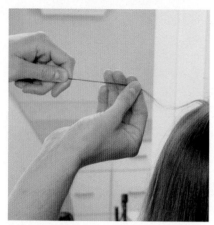

figure 20-10
Elasticity test

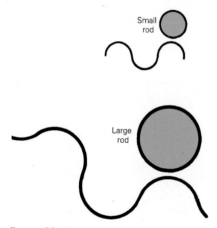

Small rod

Large rod

figure 20-11
The diameter of the rod determines the size of the curl.

waving solution and neutralizer. Because chemical changes are involved, you should always perform an elasticity test before perming the hair (figure 20-10).

When performing a permanent waving service, the size of the rod determines the size of the curl. The shape and type of curl are determined by the shape and type of rod and the wrapping method used (figure 20-11). Selecting the correct perm rod and wrapping method is crucial to creating a successful permanent wave. Perm rods come in a wide variety of sizes and shapes that can be combined with different wrapping methods to provide an exciting range of hairstyling options.

The Chemistry of Permanent Waving

Alkaline permanent waving solutions soften and swell the hair, and they open the cuticle, permitting the solution to penetrate into the cortex. Figure 20-12 illustrates hair saturated with alkaline permanent waving solution (pH 9.4) for 5 minutes. Note the swelling of the cuticle layer. In figure 20-13, hair from the same sample has been saturated with acid-balanced permanent waving solution (pH 7.5) for 5 minutes. Note that there is far less swelling of the cuticle layer.

Reduction Reaction

Once in the cortex, the waving solution breaks the disulfide bonds through a chemical reaction called reduction. A reduction reaction involves either the addition of hydrogen or the removal of oxygen. The reduction reaction in permanent waving is due to the addition of hydrogen.

The chemical process of permanent waving involves the following reactions:

- A disulfide bond joins the sulfur atoms in two adjacent polypeptide chains.

- Permanent wave solution breaks a disulfide bond by adding a hydrogen atom to each of its sulfur atoms.

- The sulfur atoms attach to the hydrogen atom from the permanent waving solution, breaking their attachment to each other.

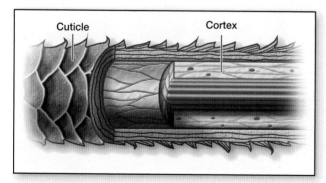

Cuticle   Cortex

figure 20-12
Hair that has been saturated with alkaline waving solution (9.4 pH) for five minutes

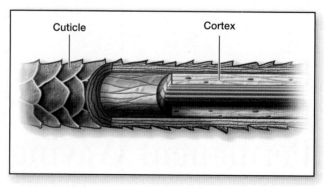

Cuticle   Cortex

figure 20-13
Hair that has been saturated with acid-balanced waving solution (7.5 pH) for five minutes

- Once the disulfide bond is broken, the polypeptide chains can form into their new curled shape. Reduction breaks disulfide bonds (figure 20-14) and oxidation reforms them.

All permanent wave solutions contain a reducing agent. The reducing agent, commonly referred to as *thio*, is used in permanent waving solutions. It contains a *thiol* (THY-ohl), which is a particular group of compounds, along with carboxylic acid.

Thioglycolic acid (thy-oh-GLY-kuh-lik), a colorless liquid with a strong, unpleasant odor, is the most common reducing agent in permanent wave solutions. The strength of the permanent waving solution is determined primarily by the concentration of thio. Stronger perms have a higher concentration of thio, which means that more disulfide bonds are broken compared to weaker perms.

Because acids do not swell the hair nor penetrate into the cortex, it is necessary for manufacturers to add an alkalizing agent. The addition of ammonia to thioglycolic acid produces a new chemical named **ammonium thioglycolate (ATG)** (uh-MOH-nee-um thy-oh-GLY-kuh-layt), which is alkaline and is the active ingredient or reducing agent in alkaline permanents.

The degree of alkalinity (pH) is a second factor in the overall strength of the waving solution. Coarse hair with a strong, resistant cuticle layer needs the additional swelling and penetration that is provided by a stronger and more highly alkaline waving solution.

By contrast, porous hair, or hair with a damaged cuticle layer, is easily penetrated and could be damaged by a highly alkaline permanent waving solution. The alkalinity of the perm solution should correspond to the resistance, strength, and porosity of the cuticle layer.

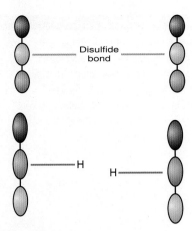

figure 20-14
A reduction reaction breaks disulfide bonds during the permanent waving process.

Types of Permanent Waves

A variety of permanent waves are available in salons today (figure 20-15). Brief descriptions of the most commonly used perms follow.

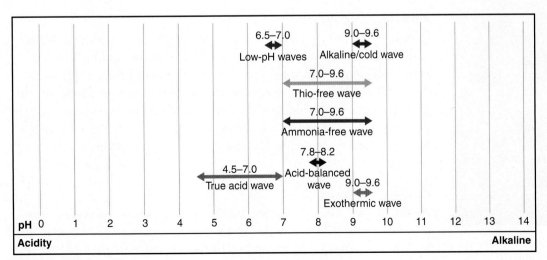

figure 20-15
Depending on the type and formulation, perm solutions can vary from being slightly acidic to highly alkaline.

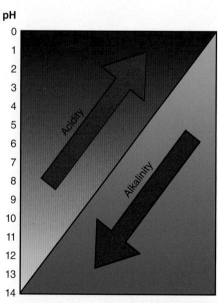

ACTIVITY

Using pH testing strips, test various liquids, including acid waves, acid-balanced waves, lemon juice, and more. Track and evaluate the results for acidity and alkalinity and share with your classmates. Discuss which liquids have a higher or lower pH value?

Alkaline Waves or Cold Waves

Alkaline waves, also known as *cold waves*, were developed in 1941. They have a pH between 9.0 and 9.6. Ammonium thioglycolate (ATG) is the reducing agent, and it processes at room temperature without the addition of heat.

Acid Waves

Glyceryl monothioglycolate (GMTG) (GLIS-ur-il mon-oh-thy-oh-GLY-koh-layt) is the main active ingredient in true acid and acid-balanced waving lotions. It has a low pH and is the primary reducing agent in most acid waves. Most acid waves also contain ATG, just like a cold wave. Although the low pH of acid waves may seem ideal, repeated exposure to GMTG is known to cause allergic sensitivity in both hairstylists and clients.

True Acid Waves

All acid waves have three separate components: permanent waving solution, activator, and neutralizer. The activator tube contains GMTG, which must be added to the permanent waving solution before applying to the hair. The first true acid waves were introduced in the early 1970s. **True acid waves** have a pH between 4.5 and 7.0 and require heat to process; they process more slowly than alkaline waves, and they do not usually produce as firm a curl as alkaline waves. GMTG, which has a low pH, is the active ingredient.

Since acidic solutions contract the hair, you may be wondering how a true acid wave, with a pH below 7.0, can cause the hair to swell. Although a pH of 7.0 is neutral on the pH scale, a pH of 5.0 is neutral for hair. The pH of any substance is always a balance of both acidity and alkalinity. Even the strongest acid also contains some alkalinity. (To review the pH scale, see Chapter 12, Basics of Chemistry.) Acidity increases when alkalinity decreases, and alkalinity increases when acidity decreases (figure 20-16).

Because every step in the pH scale represents a tenfold change in pH, a pH of 7.0 is 100 times more alkaline than the pH of hair (5.0). Even pure water with a pH of 7.0 can damage the hair and cause it to swell.

Acid-Balanced Waves

In order to permit processing at room temperature and produce a firmer curl, the strength and pH of acid waves have increased steadily over the years. Most of the acid waves found in today's salons have a pH between 7.8 and 8.2. Modern acid waves are actually **acid-balanced waves**, which are permanent waves that have a 7.0 or neutral pH; because of their higher pH, they process at room temperature, do not require the added heat of a hair dryer, process more quickly, and produce firmer curls than true acid waves.

Exothermic Waves

An exothermic chemical reaction produces heat. **Exothermic waves** (Eks-oh-THUR-mik WAYVZ) create an exothermic chemical reaction that heats up the waving solution and speeds up the processing.

All exothermic waves have three components: permanent waving solution, activator, and neutralizer. The permanent waving solution

figure 20-16
Acidity increases as alkalinity decreases, and alkalinity increases as acidity decreases.

contains thio, just as in a cold wave. The activator contains an oxidizing agent (usually hydrogen peroxide) that must be added to the permanent waving solution immediately before use. Mixing an oxidizer with the permanent waving solution causes a rapid release of heat and an increase in the temperature of the solution. The increased temperature increases the rate of the chemical reaction, which shortens the processing time.

Endothermic Waves

An endothermic chemical reaction is one that absorbs heat from its surroundings. **Endothermic waves** (en-duh-THUR-mik wayvz) are activated by an outside heat source, usually a conventional hood-type hair dryer.

Endothermic waves will not process properly at room temperature. Most true acid waves are endothermic and require the added heat of a hair dryer.

Ammonia-Free Waves

Ammonia-free waves are perms that use an ingredient that does not evaporate as readily as ammonia, so there is very little odor associated with their use.

Aminomethylpropanol (uh-MEE-noh-meth-yl-pro-pan-all), or AMP, and monoethanolamine (mahn-oh-ETH-an-all-am-een), or MEA, are examples of alkanolamines that are used in permanent waving solutions as a substitute for ammonia. Even though these solutions may not smell as strong as ammonia, they can still be every bit as alkaline and just as damaging. Remember: Ammonia-free does not necessarily mean damage-free.

Thio-Free Waves

Thio-free waves (THY-oh FREE WAYVZ) use an ingredient other than ATG, such as cysteamine (SIS-tee-uh-meen) or mercaptamine (mer-KAPT-uh-meen), as the primary reducing agent. Even though these thio substitutes are not technically ATG, they are still thio compounds.

Although thio-free wave products are often marketed as damage-free, this is not necessarily true. At a high concentration, the reducing agents in thio-free waves can be just as damaging as thio.

Low-pH Waves

The use of sulfates, sulfites, and bisulfites presents an alternative to ATG known as **low-pH waves**. Sulfites work at a low pH. They have been used in perms for years, but they have never been very popular. Permanents based on sulfites are very weak and do not provide a firm curl, especially on strong or resistant hair. Sulfite permanents are usually marketed as body waves or alternative waves.

Selecting the Right Type of Perm

It is extremely important to select the right type of perm for each client. Each client's hair has a distinct texture and condition, so individual needs must always be addressed. After a thorough consultation, you should be able to determine which type of permanent is best suited to your client's

> ⚠ **CAUTION**
> Accidentally mixing the contents of the activator tube with the neutralizer instead of the permanent waving solution will cause a violent chemical reaction that can cause injury, especially to the eyes. So always use caution!

> ⚠ **CAUTION**
> The ingredients, strength, and pH of permanent wave solutions differ among manufacturers and can vary considerably, even within the same category. Always check the manufacturer's instructions and the product's Material Safety Data Sheet (MSDS) for accurate, detailed information.

hair type, condition, and desired results. **Table 20-1** lists the most common types of permanent waves along with recommended hair type for each. These are only general guidelines. Perms for use on color-treated hair are not necessarily safe for damaged or bleached hair. Also, hair that has been treated with a semipermanent color, which coats the hair, is not as porous as hair treated with permanent color and may actually appear more resistant.

Permanent Wave Processing

The strength of any permanent wave is based on the concentration of its reducing agent. In turn, the amount of processing is determined by the strength of the permanent wave solution. If a mild permanent wave solution is used on coarse hair, there may not be enough hydrogen ions to break the necessary number of disulfide bonds, no matter how long the permanent processes. In other words, the perm solution chosen would be incorrect. But the same mild solution may be exactly right for fine hair with fewer disulfide bonds. On the other hand, a strong solution, which releases many hydrogen atoms, may be perfect for coarse hair but too harsh and damaging for fine hair. The amount of processing should be determined by the strength of the solution, not necessarily the perm's processing time.

In permanent waving, most of the processing takes place as soon as the solution penetrates the hair, within the first 5 to 10 minutes. The additional processing time allows the polypeptide chains to shift into their new configuration.

If you find that your client's hair has been overprocessed, it probably happened within the first 5 to 10 minutes of the service, and a weaker

table 20-1

PERMANENT WAVE CATEGORIES

Perm Type	Active Ingredient	Process	Recommended Hair Type
alkaline/cold wave pH: 9.0 to 9.6	ammonium thioglycolate (ATG)	room temperature	coarse, thick, or resistant
exothermic wave pH: 9.0 to 9.6	ammonium thioglycolate (ATG)	exothermic	coarse, thick, or resistant
true acid wave pH: 4.5 to 7.0	glyceryl monothioglycolate (GMTG)	endothermic	extremely porous or very damaged hair
acid-balanced wave pH: 7.8 to 8.2	glyceryl monothioglycolate (GMTG)	room temperature	porous or damaged hair
ammonia-free wave pH: 7.0 to 9.6	monoethanolamine (MEA)/ aminomethylpropanol (AMP)	room temperature	porous to normal
thio-free wave pH: 7.0 to 9.6	mercaptamine/cysteamine	room temperature	porous to normal
low-pH waves pH: 6.5 to 7.0	ammonium sulfite/ammonium bisulfite	endothermic	normal, fine, or damaged

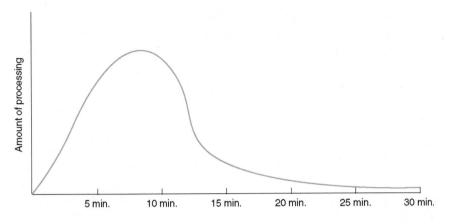

figure 20-17
Average processing times

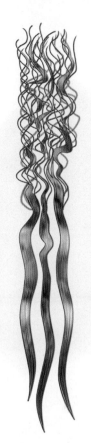

figure 20-18
Overprocessed hair

permanent waving solution should have been used. If the hair is not sufficiently processed after 10 minutes, it may require a reapplication of waving solution. Resistant hair requires a stronger solution, a higher pH, and a more thorough saturation.

It must be noted that saturation of the hair is essential to ensure proper processing for a permanent wave service regardless of the strength of the solution. Resistant hair may not become completely saturated with just one application of waving solution due to the density of the hair's structure. Therefore, reapply the solution slowly and repeatedly until the hair looks wet and stays wet!

Overprocessed Hair

A thorough saturation with a stronger (more alkaline) solution will break more disulfide bonds and process the hair more, but processing the hair more does not necessarily translate into more curl. A properly processed permanent wave should break and rebuild approximately 50 percent of the hair's disulfide bonds (figure 20-17).

If too many disulfide bonds are broken, the hair may not hold the desired curl. Weak hair equals a weak curl. Overprocessed hair usually has a weak curl pattern or may appear to be absolutely straight. Since the hair at the scalp is usually stronger than the hair at the ends, overprocessed hair is usually curlier at the scalp and straighter at the ends (figure 20-18). If the hair is overprocessed, further processing will make it straighter and cause further damage, including breakage.

Underprocessed Hair

Underprocessed hair is the exact opposite of overprocessed hair. If too few disulfide bonds are broken, the hair will not be sufficiently softened and will not hold the desired curl.

Underprocessed hair usually has a very weak curl, but it may also be straight. Since the hair at the scalp is usually stronger than at the ends, underprocessed hair is usually straighter at the scalp and curlier at the ends (figure 20-19). If the hair is underprocessed, further processing will make it curlier.

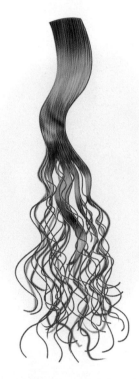

figure 20-19
Underprocessed hair

Permanent Waving (Thio) Neutralization

In permanent waving, **thio neutralization** (THY-oh NEW-truhl-eyez-ay-shun) stops the action of the waving solution and rebuilds the hair into its new curly form. Neutralization performs two important functions:

* Any waving solution that remains in the hair is deactivated (neutralized).

* Disulfide bonds that were broken by the waving solution are rebuilt.

The neutralizers used in permanent waving are oxidizers. In fact, the word *neutralizer* is not accurate because the chemical reaction involved is actually oxidation. The most common neutralizer is hydrogen peroxide. Concentrations vary between 5 volume (1.5 percent) and 10 volume (3 percent).

Thio Neutralization: Stage One The first function of permanent waving (thio) neutralization is the deactivation, or neutralization, of any waving lotion that remains in the hair after processing and rinsing. The chemical reaction involved is called oxidation. Given that water's (H_2O) pH is between 6 and 7, rinsing begins the neutralizing process. Proper rinsing and blotting are important!

Prior to applying the neutralizer, properly rinsing the hair after the permanent has processed removes any remaining perm solution. Oxidative reactions can also lighten hair color, especially at an alkaline pH. To avoid scalp irritation and unwanted lightening of hair color, always rinse perm solution from the hair for at least 5 minutes, and then blot the hair with towels to remove as much moisture as possible. Excess water left in the hair reduces the effectiveness of the neutralizer.

A successful perm requires knowledge, time, and patience:

* Always rinse the hair with warm water, never hot water.

* Always use a gentle stream of water, never a strong blast of water.

* Never apply pressure to the rods while rinsing out the solution.

* Always begin rinsing at the area where you first applied the perm solution; with the most fragile areas typically at the temple and hairline.

* Always check the nape area to ensure that you are thoroughly rinsing the bottom rods.

* Always rinse for the time recommended by the manufacturer.

* Always smell the hair after the recommended time has elapsed; if it still smells like perming solution, continuing rinsing until the odor is gone.

* Always gently blot the hair with a dry towel; never firmly or aggressively blot the hair as it could disrupt the curl-blocking pattern and alter the final wave or curl.

* Always check for excess moisture, especially at the nape of the neck where water tends to accumulate (pull of gravity), prior to neutralizing the hair.

* Always adjust any rods that have become loose or have drifted out of alignment prior to applying the neutralizer.

Some manufacturers recommend the application of a pre-neutralizing conditioner after rinsing and blotting, just before application of the neutralizer. An acidic liquid protein conditioner can be applied to the hair and dried under a warm hair dryer (hair is uncovered, always follow manufacturer's instructions) for 5 minutes or more prior to neutralization. This added step is especially beneficial for very damaged hair because it strengthens the hair prior to neutralization. Always follow the manufacturer's directions and the procedures approved by your instructor.

Thio Neutralization: Stage Two   As discussed previously, permanent waving solution breaks disulfide bonds by adding hydrogen. Thio neutralization rebuilds the disulfide bonds by removing the hydrogen that was added by the permanent waving solution (**figure 20-20a**). The hydrogen atoms are strongly attracted to the oxygen in the neutralizer and release their bond with the sulfur atoms and join with the oxygen (**figure 20-20b**). Each oxygen atom joins with two hydrogen atoms to rebuild one disulfide bond, forming a water molecule. The water is removed in the final rinse. Side bonds are then re-formed into their new shape as different pairs (**figure 20-21**).

Permanent Waving Procedures

Preliminary Test Curls
Preliminary test curls help you determine how your client's hair will react to a perm. It is advisable to do preliminary test curls to assess what the final curl pattern will look like. This is especially important if the hair appears damaged, dehydrated, color treated, or if there is any uncertainty about the results.

Preliminary test curls provide the following information and answer the following questions:

- Correct processing time for the best curl development.

- Results you can expect from the type of perm solution selected.

- Curl results for the rod size and wrapping technique you are planning to use.

- How much color will be removed from the process if the client has color-treated hair.

- Will the integrity of the hair be compromised?

- Did the hair break? Is it dry? frizzy?

- Is the client satisfied with the shape and hold of the curl?

P 20-1   **Preliminary Test Curl for a Permanent Wave**
See page 629

Types of Rods

Concave rods (khan-KAYV RAHDZ) are the most common type of perm rod; they have a smaller diameter

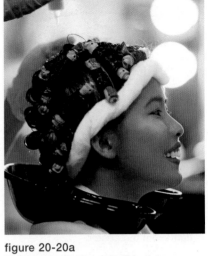
figure 20-20a
Thio neutralization rebuilds the disulfide bonds by removing the hydrogen that was added by the permanent waving solution.

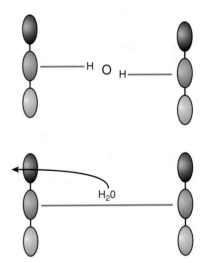
figure 20-20b
Oxidation reaction of thio neutralizers

figure 20-21
New disulfide pairs

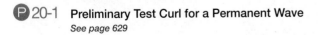

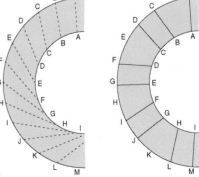

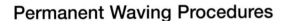

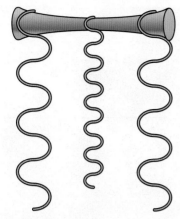

figure 20-22
Concave rods create curl that is tightest in the center.

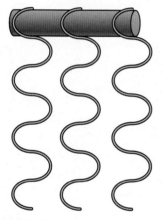

figure 20-23
Straight rods create curl that is tightest on the ends and looser towards the scalp.

in the center that increases to a larger diameter on the ends. Concave rods produce a tighter curl in the center, and a looser curl on either side of the strand (**figure 20-22**).

Straight rods are equal in diameter along their entire length or curling area. This produces a uniform curl along the entire width of the strand (**figure 20-23**).

Both concave and straight rods come in different lengths to accommodate different sections on the head. Short rods, for instance, can be used for wrapping small and awkward sections where long rods would not fit.

Soft bender rods are usually about 12 inches (30.5 centimeters) long with a uniform diameter along the entire length of the rod. These soft foam rods have a flexible wire inside that permits them to be bent into almost any shape (**figure 20-24**).

The **loop rod**, also known as *circle rod*, is usually about 12 inches (30.5 centimeters) long with a uniform diameter along the entire length of the rod. After the hair is wrapped, the rod is secured by fastening the ends together to form a loop (**figure 20-25**).

Today, many perms are performed with large rollers, rag rollers, or other tools in order to achieve large, loose curls and waves. Larger tools are also used for root perms, in which only the base of the hair is permed to create volume and lift without curl.

End Papers

End papers, also known as *end wraps*, are thin, absorbent papers used to control the ends of the hair when wrapping and winding hair on the perm rods. End papers should extend beyond the ends of the hair to keep them smooth and straight and to prevent fishhooks (hair that is bent up at the ends). The most common end-paper techniques are the double flat wrap, single flat wrap, and bookend wrap.

- The **double flat wrap** is a perm wrap in which one end paper is placed under and another is placed over the strand of hair being wrapped.

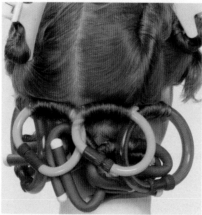

figure 20-24
Loop rods atop soft bender rods

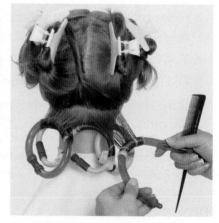

figure 20-25
Loop rods

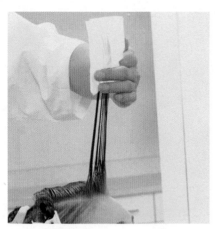

figure 20-26
Double flat wrap

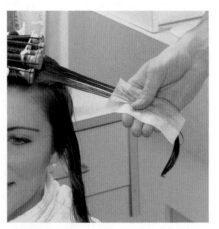

figure 20-27
Single flat wrap

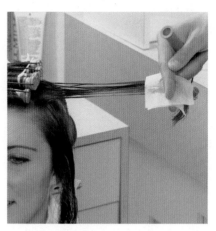

figure 20-28
Bookend wrap

Both papers extend past the hair ends. This wrap provides the most control over the hair ends and also helps keep them evenly distributed over the entire length of the rod (**figure 20-26**).

- The **single flat wrap** is similar to the double flat wrap but uses only one end paper, placed over the top of the strand of hair (**figure 20-27**).

- The **bookend wrap** uses one end paper folded in half over the hair ends like an envelope. The bookend wrap eliminates excess paper and can be used with short rods or with very short lengths of hair. When using this wrap method, be careful to distribute the hair evenly over the entire length of the rod. Avoid bunching the hair in the fold of the paper—hair should be in the center—to produce an even curl (**figure 20-28**).

Sectioning for a Perm

All perm wraps begin by sectioning the hair into panels. The size, shape, and direction of these panels vary based on the wrapping pattern and the type and size of the rod being used. **Base sections** are subsections of panels into which the hair is divided for perm wrapping; one rod is normally placed on each base section (**figure 20-29**). The size of each base section is usually the length and width of the rod being used.

Base Placement

Base placement refers to the position of the rod in relation to its base section; base placement is determined by the angle at which the hair is wrapped. Rods can be wrapped on base, half off base, or off base.

For **on-base placement**, the hair is wrapped 45-degrees beyond perpendicular to its base section, and the rod is positioned on its base (**figure 20-30**). Although on-base placement may result in greater volume at the scalp area, any increase in volume will be lost as soon as the hair begins to grow out. Caution should be used with on-base placement because the additional stress and tension can mark or break the hair.

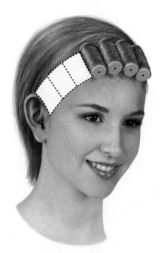

figure 20-29
All perm wraps section the hair into panels. These panels are then divided into base sections.

✓ **HERE'S A TIP**
Keeping the hair evenly damp with water throughout wrapping helps the end papers cling to the hair.

⚠ **CAUTION**
Using a base section that is wider than the perm rod can create an uneven curl pattern and undue tension on the hair.

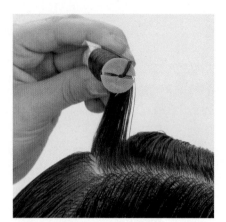

figure 20-30
On-base placement

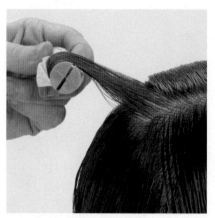

figure 20-31
Half off-base placement

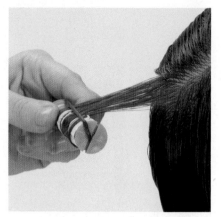

figure 20-32
Off-base placement

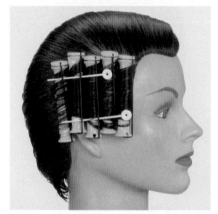

figure 20-33a
Vertical base direction

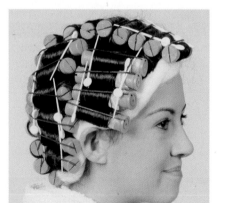

figure 20-33b
Horizontal base direction

In **half off-base placement**, the hair is wrapped at an angle of 90 degrees or perpendicular to its base section, and the rod is positioned half off its base section (figure 20-31). Half off-base placement minimizes stress and tension on the hair.

Off-base placement refers to wrapping the hair at 45 degrees below the center of the base section, so that the rod is positioned completely off its base (figure 20-32). Off-base placement creates the least amount of volume and results in a curl pattern that begins farthest away from the scalp.

Base Direction

Base direction refers to the angle at which the rod is positioned on the head: horizontally, vertically, or diagonally (figures 20-33a and 20-33b); base direction also refers to the directional pattern in which the hair is wrapped. Although directional wraps can be wrapped backward, forward, or to one side, it is important to remember that wrapping with the natural direction of hair growth causes the least amount of stress to the hair. Wrapping against the natural growth pattern can produce a band mark or breakage at the base of the curl.

Wrapping Techniques

There are two basic techniques of wrapping the hair around the perm rod: the croquignole and spiral technique.

A **croquignole perm wrap** (KROH-ken-ohl) is wrapped from the ends to the scalp in overlapping concentric layers (figure 20-34). Because the hair is wrapped perpendicular to the length of the rod, each new layer of hair is wrapped on top of the previous layer, increasing the size (diameter) of the curl with each new overlapping layer. This produces a tighter curl at the ends, and a larger curl at the scalp. Longer, thicker hair increases this effect.

In a **spiral perm wrap** the hair is wrapped at an angle other than perpendicular to the length of the rod (figure 20-35), which causes the hair to spiral along the length of the rod, like the stripes on a candy cane.

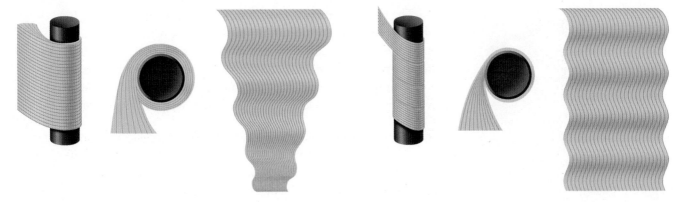

figure 20-34
Croquignole perm wrap

figure 20-35
Spiral perm wrap

A spiral perm wrap may partially overlap the preceding layers. As long as the angle remains constant, any overlap will be uniform along the length of the rod and the strand of hair (figure 20-36). This wrapping technique causes the size (diameter) of the curl to remain constant along the entire length of the strand and produces a uniform curl from the scalp to the ends.

Wrapping Patterns

When doing a permanent waving service, hair is "wrapped" around a hard roller or rod to create curls and waves on straight hair. Wrapping patterns and different types of rods are combined to create a wide variety of specialized perm wraps, thus providing an unlimited array of styling options.For extra-long hair, you may need to use a **double-rod wrap**, also known as *piggyback wrap*, in which the hair is wrapped on one rod from the scalp to midway down the hair shaft (figure 20-37), and another rod is used to wrap the remaining hair strand in the same direction. This allows for better penetration of the processing solution and for a tighter curl near the scalp than that provided by a conventional croquignole wrap.

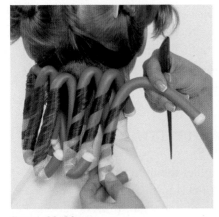

figure 20-36
Spiral wrap on bender rods

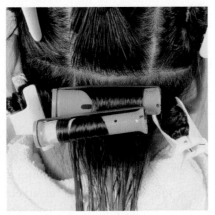

figure 20-37
Piggyback wrap

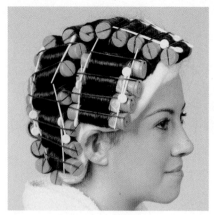

figure 20-38
Basic perm wrapping pattern

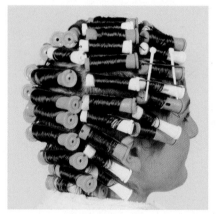

figure 20-39
Curvature perm wrapping pattern

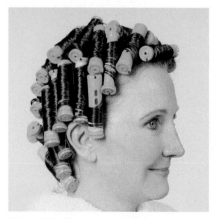

figure 20-40
Bricklay perm wrapping pattern

The **basic permanent wrap**, also known as *straight set wrap*, is a wrapping pattern in which all the rods within a panel move in the same direction and are positioned on equal-sized bases; all the base sections are horizontal and are the same length and width as the perm rod. The **base control** is the position of the tool in relation to its base section, determined by the angle at which the hair is wrapped (figure 20-38).

Ⓟ 20-2   Permanent Wave and Processing Using a Basic Permanent Wrap *See page 631*

In the **curvature permanent wrap**, partings and bases radiate throughout the panels to follow the curvature of the head. This wrapping pattern uses pie-shaped base sections in the curvature areas (figure 20-39).

Ⓟ 20-3   Permanent Wave and Processing Using a Curvature Permanent Wrap *See page 635*

The **bricklay permanent wrap** is similar to the actual technique of bricklaying; base sections are offset from each other row by row, to prevent noticeable splits and to blend the flow of the hair. Different bricklay patterns use different starting points (front hairline, occipital area, and crown), and these starting points affect the directional flow of the hair. The bricklay permanent wrap can be used with various combinations of sectioning, base control, base direction, wrapping techniques, and perm rods (figure 20-40).

Ⓟ 20-4   Permanent Wave and Processing Using a Bricklay Permanent Wrap *See page 638*

The **weave technique** uses zigzag partings to divide base areas. It can be used throughout the entire perm wrap or only in selected areas. This technique is very effective for blending between perm rods with opposite base directions. It can also be used to create a smooth transition from the rolled areas into the unrolled areas of a partial perm. The weave technique can be used with a variety of base directions, wrapping patterns, and perm rods (figure 20-41).

Ⓟ 20-5   Permanent Wave and Processing Using a Weave Technique *See page 640*

The double-rod wrap technique (piggyback wrap), discussed earlier, is a wrap technique whereby extra-long hair is wrapped on one rod from the scalp to midway down the hair shaft. Another rod is then used to wrap the remaining hair strand in the same direction. The upper half of the strand is wrapped around one rod, and then the lower half of the same strand is wrapped around a second rod in an alternate direction and stacked (piggybacked) on top of the first.

Ⓟ 20-6   Permanent Wave and Processing Using a Weave Double-Rod or Piggyback Technique *See page 642*

The double-rod wrap technique doubles the number of rods used. Using more rods increases the amount of curl in the finished perm, making this technique especially effective on long hair. Rods of various diameters may be used to create different effects. The double-rod wrap technique can also be used with a variety of base directions, wrapping patterns, and perm rods.

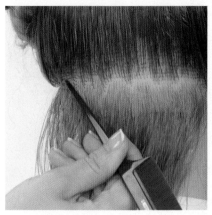

figure 20-41
Weave technique

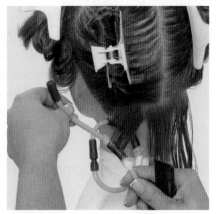

figure 20-42
Spiral perm wrap

In a spiral perm wrap, the hair is wrapped at an angle other than perpendicular to the length of the rod. This wrapping technique produces a uniform curl from the scalp to the ends. Longer, thicker hair will benefit most from this effect (figure 20-42).

Ⓟ 20-7 Permanent Wave and Processing Using a Spiral Wrap Technique *See page 644*

The spiral wrapping technique can be used with a variety of base sections, base directions, and wrapping patterns. Base sections may be either horizontal or vertical length of the hair and do not affect the finished curl. Conventional rods, bendable soft foam rods, and loop rods can all be used for this technique, depending on the length of the rod and the hair.

Partial Perms

If your client wants a perm but does not wish the entire head of hair to be curled, a partial perm may be the answer. Partial perms also allow you to give a perm when some of the hair is too short to roll on rods (figure 20-43).

Partial perms can be used for:

• Male and female clients who have long hair on the top and crown but very short hair with tapered sides and nape.

• Clients who only need volume and lift in certain areas.

• Clients who desire a hairstyle with curls along the perimeter but a smooth, sleek crown.

Partial perms rely on the same techniques and wrapping patterns as those used with other perms, but there are additional considerations:

• In order to make a smooth transition from the rolled section to the unrolled section, use a larger rod for the last rod next to an unrolled section.

• Applying waving solution to unrolled hair may straighten it or make it difficult to style. To protect the unrolled hair, apply a protective barrier cream to the unrolled section before applying the waving lotion.

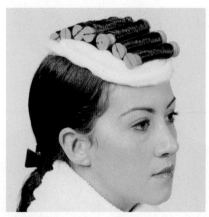

figure 20-43
Partial perm wrap

Perms for Men

Many male clients are looking for the added texture, fullness, style, and low maintenance that only a perm can provide (figure 20-44). Perms help thin hair look fuller, make straight or coarse hair more manageable, and help control stubborn cowlicks. Although men's and women's hairstyles may be different, the techniques for permanent waving are essentially the same.

Safety Precautions for Permanent Waving

- Always protect your client's clothing. Have the client change into a gown, or use a waterproof chemical cape, and double drape with towels to absorb accidental spills.

- Do not give a permanent to any client who has experienced an allergic reaction to a previous permanent.

- Always examine the scalp before the perm service. Do not proceed if there are any skin abrasions or signs of scalp disease.

- Do not perm hair that is excessively damaged or shows signs of breakage.

- Do not attempt to perm hair that has been previously treated with hydroxide relaxers.

- If there is a possibility that metallic haircolor has been previously used on the hair, perform a test for metallic salts.

- Always apply protective barrier cream around the client's hairline and ears prior to applying permanent waving solution.

- Do not dilute or add anything to the waving lotion or neutralizer unless specified in the manufacturer's directions.

- Keep waving lotion out of the client's eyes. In case of accidental exposure, rinse thoroughly with cool water.

- Always follow the manufacturer's directions.

- Wear gloves when applying solutions.

- Immediately replace cotton or towels that have become wet with solution.

- Do not save any opened, unused waving solution or neutralizer. When not used promptly, these chemicals may change in strength and effectiveness.

- Hair that has been permanently waved should be shampooed and conditioned with products formulated for chemically treated hair.

figure 20-44
Many male clients are looking for the added texture, fullness, style, and low maintenance that only a perm can provide.

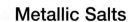

Metallic Salts

Some home haircoloring products contain metallic salts that are not compatible with permanent waving. Metallic salts leave a coating on the hair that may cause uneven curls, severe discoloration, or hair breakage.

Metallic salts are more commonly found in men's haircolors that are sold for home use. Haircolor restorers and progressive haircolors that darken the hair gradually with repeated applications are the most likely to contain metallic salts. If you suspect that metallic salts may be present on the hair, perform the following test.

In a glass or plastic bowl, mix 1 ounce (29.57 milliliters) of 20-volume peroxide with 20 drops of 28-percent ammonia. Immerse at least 20 strands of hair in the solution for 30 minutes. If metallic salts are not present, the hair will lighten slightly and you may proceed with the service. If metallic salts are present, the hair will lighten rapidly. The solution may get hot and give off an unpleasant odor, indicating that you should not proceed with the service.

After reading the next few sections, you will be able to:

LO⑤ Describe how thio relaxers straighten the hair.

LO⑥ Describe how hydroxide relaxers straighten the hair.

LO⑦ Demonstrate safe and effective hydroxide relaxing techniques.

Demonstrate the Proper Technique for Chemical Hair Relaxers

Chemical hair relaxing is a process that rearranges the structure of curly hair into a straighter or smoother form. Whereas permanent waving curls straight hair, chemical hair relaxing straightens curly hair (figure 20-45).

Other than their objectives being quite different, the permanent wave and relaxer services are very similar. In fact, the chemistry of relaxers and permanent wave is exactly the same. Both services change the shape of the hair by breaking disulfide bonds.

The most common types of chemical hair relaxers are ammonium thio, guanidine hydroxide, and sodium hydroxide. It should be noted that thio and guanidine are usually classified as no-lye relaxers and sodium hydroxide is considered to be a lye-based relaxer.

Curly Hair

There are varying degrees and types of curly hair. Some curly hair types are extremely curly, where the hair grows in long twisted spirals, or coils. Cross-sections are highly elliptical and vary in shape and thickness along their lengths. Compared to straight or wavy hair, which tends to possess a

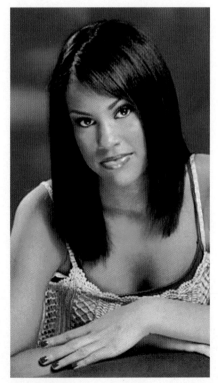

figure 20-45
Relaxed hair

Photography by Tom Carson.

fairly regular and uniform diameter along a single strand, extremely curly hair is irregular, exhibiting varying diameters along a single strand.

The thinnest and weakest sections of the hair strands are located at the twists. These sections are also bent at an extremely sharp angle and will be stretched the most during relaxing. A chain is only as strong as its weakest link, and hair is only as strong as its weakest section. Hair breaks at its weakest point. Extremely curly hair usually breaks at the twists because of the inherent weakness in that section and because of the extra physical force that is required to straighten it.

Thio Relaxers

Thio relaxers (THY-oh ree-LAX-UHRS) use the same ATG that is used in permanent waving but at a higher concentration and a higher pH (above 10). Thio relaxers are also thicker, with a higher **viscosity** (vis-KAHS-ut-ee)—the measurement of the thickness or thinness of a liquid that affects how the fluid flows—making them more suitable for application as a relaxer.

Thio relaxers break disulfide bonds and soften hair, just as in permanents. After enough bonds are broken, the hair is straightened into its new shape, and the relaxer is rinsed from the hair. Blotting comes next, followed by a neutralizer. The chemical reactions of thio relaxers are identical to those in permanent waving.

Thio Neutralization

The neutralizer used with thio relaxers is an oxidizing agent, usually hydrogen peroxide, just as in permanents. The oxidation reaction caused by the neutralizer rebuilds the disulfide bonds that were broken by the thio relaxer.

Thio Relaxer Application

The application steps for thio relaxers are the same as those for hydroxide relaxers, although the neutralization procedure is different. Relaxer may be applied with bowl and brush or the back of a hard rubber comb. Although all thio relaxers follow the same procedures, different application methods are used for virgin relaxers and retouch relaxers.

Follow the same preparation steps as virgin hydroxide relaxers (see page 619) with the possible exception of a light shampoo before a thio relaxer. Do not forget to perform an analysis of the client's hair and scalp. Test the hair for elasticity and porosity on several areas of the head. If the hair has poor elasticity, do not perform a relaxer service.

Ⓟ 20-8 Applying Thio Relaxer to Virgin Hair *See page 647*

Ⓟ 20-9 Thio Relaxer Retouch *See page 650*

Japanese Thermal Straighteners

Japanese thermal straightening, sometimes called thermal reconditioning or TR, combines use of a thio relaxer with flat ironing. When first introduced, they were called thermal ionic reconstructors. Each manufacturer has slightly different procedures. Generally, after the hair is shampooed and conditioned, the straightener is applied to sections, distributed evenly, and processed until the desired degree of curl or frizz reduction is reached. Then the hair is rinsed thoroughly for about 10 minutes, conditioned, and blown dry until it is completely dry. Next, each section is flat ironed; several passes of the flat iron are required for each section. (The added heat and mechanical pressing helps to make these formulas more effective than standard thio relaxers.) The hair is then neutralized and blown dry.

The service can take several hours and is not always appropriate for extremely curly hair or some color-treated hair. Thermal reconditioning is considered a specialty, and many manufacturers require certification in their particular procedure.

Hydroxide Relaxers

The hydroxide ion is the active ingredient in all **hydroxide relaxers**, which are very strong alkalis with a pH over 13. Sodium hydroxide, potassium hydroxide, lithium hydroxide, and guanidine hydroxide are all types of hydroxide relaxers, which can swell the hair up to twice its normal diameter.

Hydroxide relaxers are not compatible with thio relaxers, permanent waving, or soft curl perms due to the difference in chemistry.

Hydroxide relaxers have such a high pH that the alkalinity alone can break the disulfide bonds. The average pH of the hair is about 5, and many hydroxide relaxers have a pH over 13. Since each step in the pH scale represents a tenfold change in concentration, a pH of 13 is 100 million (100,000,000) times more alkaline than a pH of 5 (**figure 20-46**).

Hydroxide relaxers break disulfide bonds differently than in the reduction reaction of thio relaxers. A disulfide bond consists of two bonded sulfur atoms. In **lanthionization** (lan-thee-oh-ny-ZAY-shun), the process by which hydroxide relaxers permanently straighten hair, the relaxers remove a sulfur atom from a disulfide bond and convert it into a lanthionine bond. Lanthionine bonds contain only one sulfur atom. The disulfide bonds that are broken by hydroxide relaxers are broken

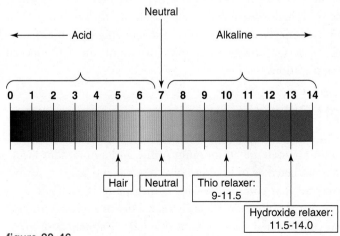

figure 20-46
pH of thio and hydroxide relaxers

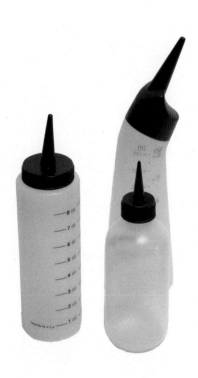

permanently and can never be re-formed. That is why hair that has been treated with a hydroxide relaxer is unfit for permanent waving and will not hold a curl.

Types of Hydroxide Relaxers

Metal hydroxide relaxers are ionic compounds formed by a metal—sodium (Na), potassium (K), or lithium (Li)—which is combined with oxygen (O) and hydrogen (H). Metal hydroxide relaxers include sodium hydroxide (NaOH), potassium hydroxide (KOH), and lithium hydroxide (LiOH).

Although calcium hydroxide (CaOH) is sometimes added to hydroxide relaxers, it is not used by itself to relax hair.

All metal hydroxide relaxers contain only one component and are used exactly as they are packaged in the container; no mixing is necessary. The hydroxide ion is the active ingredient in all hydroxide relaxers. There is no significant difference in the performance of these metal hydroxide relaxers.

Lye-Based Relaxers

Sodium hydroxide (NaOH) relaxers are commonly called lye relaxers. Sodium hydroxide is the oldest, and one of the most common, types of chemical hair relaxer. At one time it was the most popular of hair relaxers, however no-lye relaxers have gained considerable popularity as well. Sodium hydroxide is also known as lye or caustic soda and can cause hair loss and skin burns if used incorrectly.

No-Lye Relaxers

Lithium hydroxide (LiOH) and potassium hydroxide (KOH) relaxers are often advertised and sold as "no mix—no lye" relaxers. Although technically they are not lye, their chemistry is identical, and there is very little difference in their performance.

Guanidine (GWAN-ih-deen) hydroxide relaxers are also advertised and sold as no-lye relaxers. Although technically they too are not lye, the hydroxide ion is still the active ingredient. Guanidine hydroxide relaxers contain two components that must be mixed immediately prior to use. These relaxers straighten hair completely, with less scalp irritation than other hydroxide relaxers. Most guanidine hydroxide relaxers are recommended for sensitive scalps, and they are sold over-the-counter for home use. Although they reduce scalp irritation, they do not reduce hair damage if used incorrectly. They swell the hair slightly more than other hydroxide relaxers, and tend to be more drying on the hair, especially after repeated applications.

Low-pH Relaxers

Sulfites and bisulfites are sometimes used as low-pH hair relaxers. The most commonly used are ammonium sulfite and ammonium bisulfite. Sulfites are marketed as mild alternative relaxers and are compatible with thio relaxers but not compatible with hydroxide relaxers. They do not completely straighten extremely curly hair. Low-pH relaxers are intended for use on color-treated, damaged, or fine hair. See **table 20-2** for a summary of the types and uses of relaxers.

table 20-2

SELECTING THE CORRECT RELAXER

Active Ingredient	pH	Marketed as	Advantages	Disadvantages
sodium hydroxide	12.5–13.5	lye relaxer	very effective for extremely curly hair	may cause scalp irritation and damage the hair
lithium hydroxide and potassium hydroxide	12.5–13.5	no-mix, no-lye relaxer	very effective for extremely curly hair	may cause scalp irritation and damage the hair
guanidine hydroxide	13–13.5	no-lye relaxer	causes less skin irritation than other hydroxide relaxers	with repeated use may dehydrate the hair
ammonium thioglycolate	9.6–10	thio relaxer, no-lye relaxer	compatible with soft curl permanents	strong, unpleasant ammonia smell; with repeated use may dehydrate hair
ammonium sulfite/ ammonium bisulfite	6.5–8.5	low-pH relaxer, no-lye relaxer	less damaging to hair	does not sufficiently relax extremely curly hair

Base and No-Base Relaxers

Hydroxide relaxers are usually sold in base and no-base formulas. **Base cream**, also known as *protective base cream*, is an oily cream used to protect the skin and scalp during hair relaxing. **Base relaxers** require the application of a protective base cream to the entire scalp prior to the application of the relaxer.

No-base relaxers do not require the application of a protective base cream. They contain a protective base cream that is designed to melt at body temperature. As the relaxer is applied, body heat causes the protective base cream to melt and settle out onto the scalp in a thin, oily, protective

---

⚠ CAUTION

Make sure that the client has not had haircoloring containing metallic salts, such as gradual or progressive haircolors, before applying either thio or hydroxide relaxers to the hair. Extreme damage or breakage can occur.

When combining a relaxing service with a permanent or demipermanent hair coloring service, it is always preferable to relax the hair first, and color it two weeks later. Some manufacturers present their demipermanent products as "no lift"—however, all demipermanent haircolor uses low volumes of peroxide or other alkalizing agents, such as MEA, as well as oxidizing agents that gently lighten the hair.

Never use bleaches or high-lift color products on relaxed hair. These combinations have resulted in many lawsuits, immediate and permanent hair loss, scalp burns, and severe damage.

You can use a semipermanent product on the same day as hair relaxing service because these colors contain no ammonia or peroxide. Relax the hair first, check the hair's condition, and then

apply the semipermanent color, following the manufacturer's guidelines and your instructor's directions.

When in doubt, test the hair's strength, and then do a strand test for the color. Accomplished colorists say they use demipermanent and even permanent color products on the same day as relaxing the hair. Permanent color should never be used on the same day as a hair relaxer service! Some manufacturers claim their coloring products allow this; however, same-day chemical services are advanced techniques that depend on the hair's condition, the experience of the stylist, and the specific products used.

Please note that same-day chemical services most always compromise the hair's integrity, whether you are combining hydroxide-based chemicals and haircolor or thio-based chemicals and color. For instance, same-day coloring and Japanese thermal straightening, done incorrectly, can result in extreme and immediate hair breakage.

coating. No-base relaxers are an improvement only on the protection that is provided to the skin by the oils in all hydroxide relaxers. For added protection, protective base cream should always be applied to the entire scalp, hairline, and around the ears, even with no-base relaxers.

Relaxer Strengths

Most chemical hair relaxers are available in three strengths: mild, regular, and super. The difference in strength of hydroxide relaxers parallels the concentration of hydroxide.

- Mild-strength relaxers are formulated for fine, color-treated, or damaged hair. This strength is also used for texturizing hair (leaving some curl and wave in the hair).

- Regular-strength relaxers are intended for normal hair texture with a medium natural curl. This is the most commonly used strength and often produces a smooth, straight hair.

- Super-strength relaxers should be used for maximum straightening on very coarse, extremely curly, and resistant hair. Only select clients should use this strength.

When in doubt, always strand test prior to the actual application. Strand testing will help you choose the proper strength and timing, thereby avoiding damage, breakage, or hair loss.

Periodic Strand Testing (during the actual relaxer application)

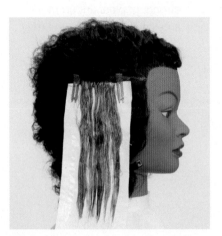

figure 20-47
Sufficiently relaxed strand

Periodic strand testing during processing will help inform you when the hair is sufficiently relaxed. After the relaxer is applied, smooth and gently press the strand to the scalp and remove product using the back of the comb, the applicator brush, or your finger. Be gentle! If the strand remains smooth, with no visible curl pattern, it is sufficiently relaxed. If the curl returns, continue processing. Processing time will vary according to the manufacturer's recommendations, relaxer strength, hair type, condition, and the desired results (**figures 20-47** and **20-48**). Follow the manufacturer's timing guide and your instructor's guidance.

Hydroxide Neutralization

Unlike thio neutralization, **hydroxide neutralization** is an acid–alkali neutralization that neutralizes (deactivates) the alkaline residues left in the hair by a hydroxide relaxer and lowers the pH of the hair and scalp; hydroxide relaxer neutralization does not involve oxidation or rebuilding disulfide bonds. The pH of hydroxide relaxers is so high that the hair remains at an extremely high pH, even after thorough rinsing. Although rinsing is important, rinsing alone does not neutralize (deactivate) the relaxer, nor does it restore the normal acidic pH of the hair and scalp.

As described in Chapter 12, Basics of Chemistry, acids neutralize alkalis. Therefore, the application of an acid-balanced shampoo or a normalizing lotion neutralizes any remaining hydroxide ions to lower the pH of the hair and scalp. Some neutralizing shampoos intended for use after hydroxide relaxers have a built-in pH indicator that changes color to show when the pH of the hair has returned to normal.

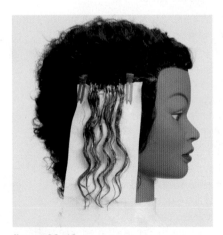

figure 20-48
Insufficiently relaxed strand

Hydroxide Relaxer

Although the same procedure is used for all hydroxide relaxers, application methods vary according to virgin and retouch application:

- A virgin relaxer application should be used for hair that has not had a chemical relaxer service. Since the scalp area and the porous ends will usually process more quickly than the middle of the strand, the application for a virgin relaxer starts ¼ inch (0.6 centimeters) to ½ inch (1.25 centimeters) away from the scalp and includes the entire strand up to the porous ends. To avoid overprocessing and scalp irritation, do not apply relaxer to the hair closest to the scalp or to the ends until the last few minutes of processing.

Ⓟ 20-10   **Applying Hydroxide Relaxer to Virgin Hair** *See page 653*

- A retouch relaxer application should be used for hair that has previously received a chemical relaxer service. The application for a retouch relaxer starts ¼ inch to ½ inch (0.6 to 1.25 centimeters) away from the scalp and includes only the new growth. To avoid overprocessing and scalp irritation, do not apply relaxer to the hair closest to the scalp until the last few minutes of processing. The relaxer should never be applied to hair that is already relaxed.

Ⓟ 20-11   **Hydroxide Relaxer Retouch** *See page 656*

- A texturizing service uses a hydroxide relaxer to reduce the curl pattern by degrees using a mild strength relaxer. The procedure for texturizing is similar to that for relaxing virgin hair and the same precautions apply, only the product is gently combed through using a large-tooth comb. This allows you to observe the curl pattern as it relaxes the curl and creates a natural curly style. Texturizing makes combing and styling tightly-coiled hair easier.

- Most relaxers today recommend the application of a base cream to protect the entire scalp, irrespective of a virgin application or retouch. For a retouch, most manufacturers recommend applying a protective cream or oil to previously relaxed hair to treat the hair while relaxing it and to prevent overlapping. Contemporary hair relaxing often includes the application of a normalizing conditioning lotion after thoroughly rinsing the relaxer out of the hair and prior to using the neutralizing shampoo. **Normalizing lotions** are conditioners with an acidic pH that restore the hair pH before the final neutralizing shampoo.

- All relaxers must include a neutralizing shampoo that must be used after rinsing the relaxer out of the hair. It is an acidic shampoo designed to restore the natural pH of hair and scalp. Some produce a color signal that turns pink if any relaxer residue remains in the hair and turns white when all the relaxer is rinsed out of the hair, so rinse thoroughly!

After a thorough consultation, you should be able to determine which type of relaxer is best suited to your client's hair type, condition, and desired results. **Table 20-2** lists the most common types of relaxers along with selected advantages and disadvantages for each.

Safety Precautions for Chemical Hair Relaxing Service

- Perform a thorough hair analysis and client consultation prior to the service.
- Examine the scalp for abrasions. Do not proceed with the service if redness, swelling, or skin lesions are present.
- Examine the hair for signs of breakage, damage, and extreme dryness. Do not proceed with service if these conditions are present.
- Do not apply a hydroxide relaxer on hair that has been previously treated with a thio relaxer, soft curl perm, or permanent wave.
- Do not apply a thio relaxer or soft curl perm on hair that has been previously treated with a hydroxide relaxer.
- Do not chemically relax hair that has been treated with a metallic dye.
- Do not chemically relax hair that is two shades lighter than natural hair color with permanent color.
- Do not relax hair that has been highlighted or decolorized with bleach.
- Do not relax hair that is color-treated with developer that is 30 to 40 percent.
- Do not shampoo the client prior to the application of a hydroxide relaxer.
- The client's hair and scalp must be completely dry prior to the application of a hydroxide relaxer.
- Apply a protective base cream to avoid scalp irritation.
- Wear gloves during the relaxer application.
- If any solution accidentally gets into the client's eye, flush the eye immediately with cool water and refer the client to a doctor.
- Do not allow chemical relaxers to accidentally come into contact with the client's ears, scalp, or skin.
- Conduct periodic strand tests during the service to monitor the hair's progression.
- Avoid scratching the scalp with your comb or fingernails.
- Do not overlap relaxer onto previously relaxed hair during retouch application.
- Always use proper relaxer strength for hair type as recommended by the manufacturer to avoid hair breakage.
- Do not process hair longer than indicated by the strand test and the manufacturer's recommended timing.
- Thoroughly rinse the relaxer from the hair using warm water. Failure to rinse properly can cause skin irritation and possible hair loss, breakage, and damage.

- Use a neutralizing shampoo to guarantee that the hair and scalp have been restored to their normal pH.

- Always apply a conditioner and comb through using wide-tooth comb after a relaxer service. This will eliminate excessive stretching and remove tangles.

- Use caution when styling relaxed hair with hot tools as relaxed hair may become dehydrated and break.

- Keep accurate and detailed client records of the services performed and the results achieved.

- Have the client sign a release statement indicating that he or she understands the possible risks related to the service.

- You are expected to have a thorough understanding of hair relaxing application, chemical compositions, and precautionary and after-care procedures before performing a relaxer service.

Keratin-Based Straightening Treatments

Keratin-based straightening treatments (also called Brazilian keratin treatments) are available to salon professionals and are widely used. Keratin-based straightening treatments contain silicone polymers and formalin or similar ingredients, which release formaldehyde gas when heated to high temperatures. Some keratin-based straightening treatments marketed as "formaldehyde free" have been found to contain formalin; some other formulas simply use different aldehydes. Do not confuse these treatments with simple "keratin conditioning treatments." Keratin alone will not straighten hair.

Keratin straightening treatments work by fixing the keratin in place in a semipermanent manner; they do not break bonds. Once the treatment is applied, the hair is blown dry, and a flat iron set at 450 degrees Fahrenheit (232.222 Celsius) is used on narrow sections, one by one, to polymerize a coating on the hair. Each section is flat ironed several times, and the procedure takes about two hours or more for longer or very dense hair. Formalin is reactive to proteins and creates a chemical link or bridge with them when heated so as to release formaldehyde.

Depending on the size of the salon, the type of ventilation system in place, and the number of technicians simultaneously performing the service, the formaldehyde released during the process has the potential to exceed the maximum concentration allowed by OSHA (Occupational Safety and Health Administration) of 0.75 parts per million (ppm) over an eight-hour period. Local source capture ventilation is recommended, particularly because the flat ironing takes place so close to both the client's and stylist's face and because the stylist may be exposed to the formaldehyde for long periods of time. Because the coating breaks down over time, the client can be exposed to released vapors even when the treatment itself is complete. This is why it is usually recommended that the client wait at least 72 hours after the treatment before taking a shower. Within this time period, the steam and heat from the shower can accelerate release of the vapors.

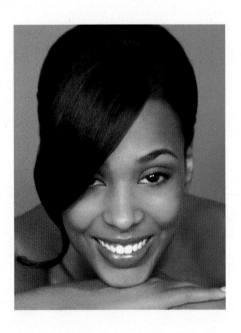

Generally, keratin straightening treatments eliminate up to 95 percent of frizz and curl and last three to five months. They are not usually appropriate for extremely curly, tightly coiled hair. Although this is an advanced treatment, no certification is actually required; nevertheless, most manufacturers do offer specialized training in both the service and the all-important after care. It is vital to follow the manufacturer's directions and inform clients about at-home maintenance care.

It is essential to conduct a detailed consultation before performing a keratin straightening service, so the client will understand what to expect from the service based upon condition of hair, chemical history, and degree of curl.

You will need to discuss the following:

- The client's recent hair history, including all chemical treatments that may still be on the hair and the products used.

- Home-care maintenance during the three-day (72-hour) period after the service is performed, as described below:

  - Usually the hair cannot be shampooed for three days (72 hours) after the service.

  - With most systems, the client should avoid getting any moisture into hair for 72 hours. If the hair gets damp, blowdry immediately and go over lightly with a flat iron on low-heat setting.

  - The client should wear his or her hair down, and should not use pins, clips, ponytail holders, or sunglasses to hold the hair back. The hair must remain in a straight position for 72 hours to maintain its new straightness.

- Determine the length and density of the client's hair before quoting a price.

Pre-Conditioning before a Keratin Straightening Treatment

Pre-conditioning is meant to equalize the porosity of the hair, taking it to a healthier level. For hair that is extremely overprocessed, damaged, or very curly, shampoo and deep condition prior to beginning the service.

Permanent Color/Highlights and Keratin Straightening Treatments

Clients may have a permanent haircolor or highlighting service before the keratin straightening treatments is applied. For those clients, be sure to use a regular/mild shampoo during the haircolor service. Follow the manufacturer's directions regarding the use of a clarifying shampoo before the treatment product is applied.

Do not use a clarifying product on a client that has 70 percent or more highlights.

Toners or Demi-Gloss and Keratin Straightening Treatments

If the client wishes to have a demi-gloss treatment, it should be done at least three to five days after the keratin treatment to prevent color loss and to avoid wetting the newly straightened hair. However, since keratin straightening treatments do coat the hair, a strand test may show that the product you've chosen will not cover the existing cuticle coating to the desired degree.

After reading the next few sections, you will be able to:

LO⑧ Describe curl re-forming and how it restructures the hair.

Demonstrate the Proper Technique for Curl Re-Forming (Soft Curl Permanents)

Curl re-forming does not straighten the hair; it simply makes the existing curl larger and looser. A **soft curl permanent** is a thio-based chemical service that re-formats curly and wavy hair into looser and larger curls and waves. Reformation occurs by wrapping the hair on rods. A soft curl permanent is akin to permanent waving. Often, this type of chemical service is referred to as "a curl" or "curly perm." Soft curl permanents use ATG (ammonium thioglycolate) and oxidation neutralizers just as thio permanent waves do.

Ⓟ 20-12 **Curl Re-Forming (Soft Curl Perm)** *See page 659*

Safety Precautions for Hair Relaxing and Curl Re-Forming

- Perform a thorough hair analysis and client consultation prior to the service. Hair should be in relatively good condition.

- Examine the scalp for abrasions. Do not proceed with the service if redness, swelling, or skin lesions are present.

- Keep accurate and detailed client records of the services performed and the results achieved.

- Have the client sign a release statement indicating that he or she understands the possible risks related to the service.

- Do not apply a hydroxide relaxer on hair that has been previously treated with a thio relaxer.

- Do not apply a thio relaxer or soft curl perm on hair that has been previously treated with a hydroxide relaxer.

- Do not chemically relax hair that has been treated with a metallic dye.

- Do not relax overly damaged hair. Suggest instead a series of reconstruction treatments.

- Do not shampoo the clients hair to the application of a hydroxide relaxer.

- The client's hair and scalp must be completely dry and free from perspiration prior to the application of a hydroxide relaxer.

- Apply a protective base cream to avoid scalp irritation.

- Wear gloves during the relaxer application.

- If any solution accidentally gets into the client's eye, flush the eye immediately with cool water, and refer the client to a doctor.

- Do not allow chemical relaxers to accidentally come into contact with the client's ears, scalp, or skin.

- Perform periodic strand tests during the service to monitor the pace of curl removal.

- Avoid scratching the scalp with your comb or fingernails.

- When performing a hair relaxer service, be sure not to overlap onto previously relaxed hair. Apply to new growth only.

- Thoroughly rinse the chemical relaxer from the hair. Failure to rinse properly can cause excessive skin irritation and possible hair breakage.

- Follow manufacturer's instructions closely when applying a chemical relaxer.

- Use a neutralizing shampoo to guarantee that the hair and scalp have been restored to their normal pH.

Performing texture services involves understanding the chemical process and the precautions. When applied responsibly, your services will be in great demand.

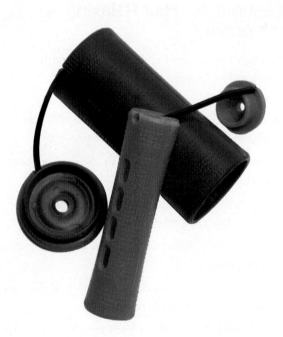

PRELIMINARY TEST CURL FOR A PERMANENT WAVE

IMPLEMENTS & MATERIALS

You will need all of the following implements, materials, and supplies:

- ☐ Applicator bottles
- ☐ Chemical cape
- ☐ Clarifying and acid-balanced shampoo (optional)
- ☐ Conditioner (optional)

- ☐ Cotton coil or rope
- ☐ Disposable gloves
- ☐ End papers
- ☐ Neutralizer
- ☐ Neutralizing bib
- ☐ Perm rods

- ☐ Perm solution
- ☐ Plastic clips for sectioning
- ☐ Plastic tail comb
- ☐ Pre-neutralizing conditioner (optional)

- ☐ Protective barrier cream
- ☐ Roller picks
- ☐ Spray bottle
- ☐ Styling comb
- ☐ Timer
- ☐ Towels

PREPARATION

Perform:

P 15-1 **Pre-Service Procedure** *See page 325*

PROCEDURE

1 Drape the client for shampoo.

2 Gently shampoo and towel dry hair. Avoid irritating the client's scalp. Re-drape the client for a chemical service.

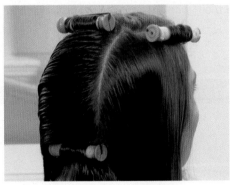

3 Wrap one rod in each different area of the head (top, side, and nape).

4 Wrap a coil of cotton around each rod.

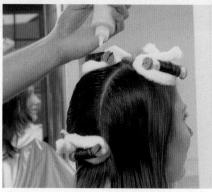

5 Apply perm solution to the wrapped curls. Do not allow perm solution to come into contact with unwrapped hair.

6 Set a timer, and process according to the manufacturer's directions.

7 Check each test curl frequently for proper curl development. Unfasten the rod and unwind the curl about one to two turns of the rod. Do not allow the hair to become loose or completely unwound. Gently move the rod toward the scalp to encourage the hair to fall loosely into the wave pattern.

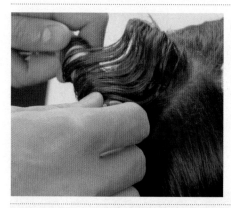

8 Curl development is complete when a firm S is formed that reflects the size of the rod used. Different hair textures will have slightly different S formations. The wave pattern for fine, thin hair may be weak, with little definition. The wave pattern for coarse, thick hair is usually stronger and better defined.

9 When the desired curl has been formed, rinse thoroughly with warm water for at least 5 minutes, blot thoroughly, apply neutralizer, and process according to the manufacturer's directions. Gently dry the hair and evaluate the results. Do not proceed with the permanent if the test curls are extremely damaged or overprocessed. If the test curl results are satisfactory, proceed with the perm, but do not re-perm these preliminary test curls. Rinse and process the test rods, but wait to remove them with the rest of the rods after the perm is completed.

POST-SERVICE

Complete:

P 15-2   **Post-Service Procedure** *See page 343*

PERMANENT WAVE AND PROCESSING USING A BASIC PERMANENT WRAP

IMPLEMENTS & MATERIALS

You will need all of the following implements, materials, and supplies:

- Applicator bottles
- Chemical cape
- Clarifying and acid-balanced shampoo (optional)
- Conditioner (optional)
- Cotton coil or rope
- Disposable gloves
- End papers
- Neutralizer
- Neutralizing bib
- Perm rods
- Perm solution
- Plastic clips for sectioning
- Plastic tail comb
- Pre-neutralizing conditioner (optional)
- Protective barrier cream
- Roller picks
- Spray bottle
- Styling comb
- Timer
- Towels

PREPARATION

Perform:

P 15-1 **Pre-Service Procedure** *See page 340*

PROCEDURE

1. After completing the pre-service procedure, seat the client. If the manufacturer's directions indicate that a shampoo is necessary before the service, then drape the client for a shampoo and gently shampoo and towel dry hair. Avoid irritating the client's scalp.

2. Re-drape the client for a chemical service.

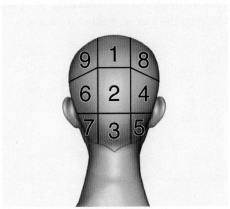

3. Divide the hair into nine panels. Use the length of the rod to measure the width of the panels. Remember to keep the hair evenly damp as you wrap.

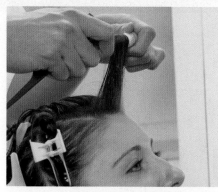

4 **a.** Begin wrapping at the front hairline or crown. Make a horizontal parting the same size as the rod. Using two end papers, roll the hair down to the scalp in the direction of hair growth, and position the rod half off-base.

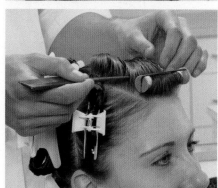

4 **b.** The band should be smooth, not twisted, and should be fastened straight across the top of the rod. Excessive tension may cause band marks or hair breakage.

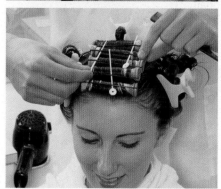

4 **c.** Continue wrapping the remainder of the first panel using the same technique. Option: Insert roller picks to stabilize the rods and eliminate any tension caused by the band.

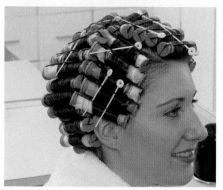

5 Continue wrapping the remaining eight panels in numerical order, holding the hair at a 90-degree angle.

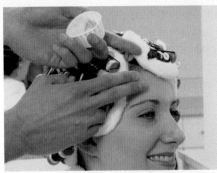

6 Apply protective barrier cream to the hairline and the ears. Apply a coil of cotton around the entire hairline and offer the client a towel to blot any drips. Put on gloves.

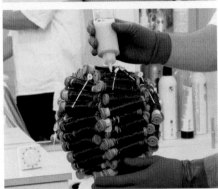

7 Slowly and carefully apply the perm solution to each rod. Ask the client to lean forward while you apply solution to the back area; ask the client to lean back as you apply solution to the front and sides. Avoid splashing and dripping. Continue to apply the solution slowly until each rod is completely saturated. Apply solution to the most resistant area first.

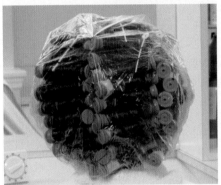

9 Check cotton and towels. If they are saturated with solution, replace them.

10 Process according to the manufacturer's directions. Processing time varies according to the strength of the solution, hair type and condition, and desired results. As a general rule, processing usually takes less than 20 minutes at room temperature.

8 If a plastic cap is used, punch a few holes in the cap and cover all the hair completely. Do not allow the plastic cap to touch the client's skin.

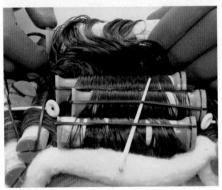

11 Check frequently for curl development. Unwind the rod and check the S pattern formation described in the preliminary test curl procedure. Check a different rod each time!

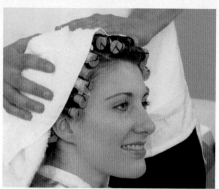

12 When processing is complete, rinse the hair thoroughly for at least 5 minutes. Then towel-blot each rod to remove excess moisture. Option: Some manufacturers recommend the application of a pre-neutralizing conditioner after rinsing and blotting and before applying the neutralizer. Always follow the manufacturer's directions and the procedures approved by your instructor.

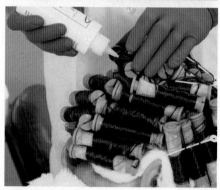

13 Apply the neutralizer slowly and carefully to the hair on each rod. Ask the client to lean forward while you apply solution to the back area, and then to lean back as you apply solution to the front and sides. Avoid splashing and dripping. Continue to apply the neutralizer until each rod is completely saturated.

14 Set a timer for the amount of time specified by the manufacturer.

15 Rinse thoroughly. Remove all of the rods. Option: Shampoo and condition. Always follow the manufacturer's directions and the procedures approved by your instructor.

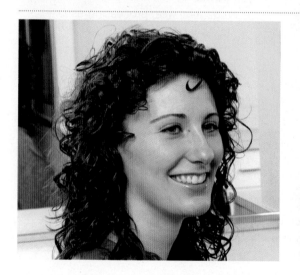

16 Style the hair as desired.

POST-SERVICE

Complete:

P 15-2 **Post-Service Procedure** *See page 343*

PERMANENT WAVE AND PROCESSING USING A CURVATURE PERMANENT WRAP

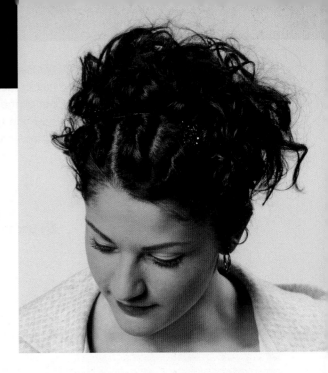

IMPLEMENTS & MATERIALS

You will need all of the following implements, materials, and supplies:

- Applicator bottles
- Chemical cape
- Clarifying and acid-balanced shampoo (optional)
- Conditioner (optional)
- Cotton coil or rope
- Disposable gloves
- End papers
- Neutralizer
- Neutralizing bib
- Perm rods
- Perm solution
- Plastic clips for sectioning
- Plastic tail comb
- Pre-neutralizing conditioner (optional)
- Protective barrier cream
- Roller picks
- Spray bottle
- Styling comb
- Timer
- Towels

PREPARATION | PROCEDURE

Perform:

P 15-1 **Pre-Service Procedure** *See page 340*

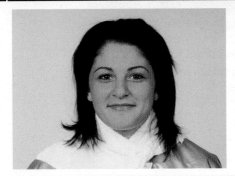

1️⃣ After completing the pre-service procedure, seat the client. If the manufacturer's directions indicate that a shampoo is necessary before the service, then drape the client for a shampoo and gently shampoo and towel dry hair. Avoid irritating the client's scalp.

2️⃣ Re-drape the client for a chemical service.

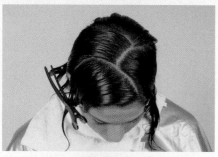

3 Begin sectioning at the front hairline on one side of the part. Comb the hair in the direction of growth. Alternate from side to side as you section out all the curvature panels over the entire head. Sectioning the panels in advance creates a road map that provides direction and gives continuity to the wrapping pattern.

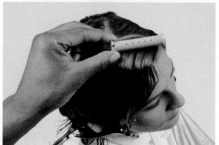

4 Section out individual panels to match the length of the rod.

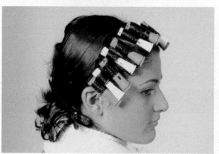

5 Begin wrapping the first panel at the front hairline on one side of the part. Comb out a base section the same width as the diameter of the rod. The base direction should point away from the face. Hold the hair at a 90-degree angle to the head. Using two end papers, roll the hair down to the scalp and position the rod half off-base.

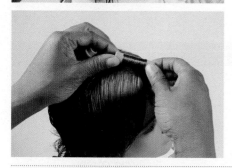

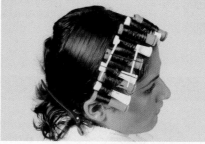

8 When you reach the last rod at the hairline, comb the hair flat at the base and change the base direction. Direct the rod up and toward the base, keeping the base area flat.

6 The remaining base sections in the panel should be wider on the outside of the panel (the side farthest away from the face). Continue wrapping the rest of the rods in the panel, alternating rod diameters.

7 Insert picks to stabilize the rods and eliminate any tension caused by the band.

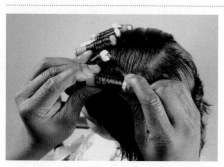

9 Continue by wrapping panel two, which is the front panel on the other side of the part. Repeat the same procedure as on the first panel.

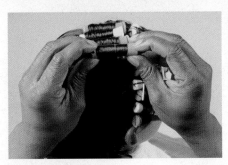

10 Continue with the third panel, which is the panel behind and next to the first panel. Repeat the same procedure until you reach the last two rods at the hairline. Comb the hair flat at the base, and change the base direction. Direct the last two rods up and toward the base, keeping the base area flat.

11 Continue with the fourth panel, on the opposite side of the head, behind and next to the second panel. Repeat the same procedure you used with the third panel. Maintain consistent dampness as you work by re-misting the hair with water if necessary.

12 Follow the same procedure with the fifth panel. The base direction should remain consistent with the pattern already established. The base direction in the back flows around and contours to the perimeter hairline area.

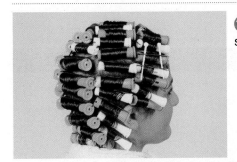

13 All panels should fit the curvature of the head and should blend into the surrounding panels.

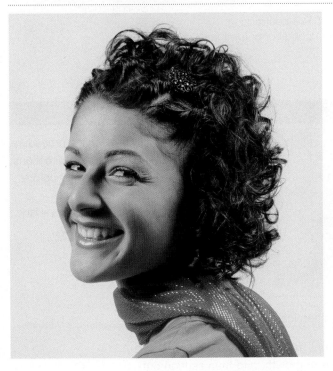

14 Process and style the hair.

POST-SERVICE

Complete:

P 15-2 **Post-Service Procedure** *See page 343*

PERMANENT WAVE AND PROCESSING USING A BRICKLAY PERMANENT WRAP

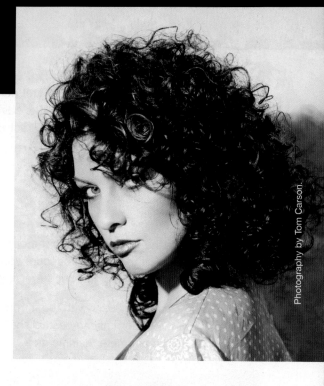

Photography by Tom Carson.

IMPLEMENTS & MATERIALS

You will need all of the following implements, materials, and supplies:

- □ Applicator bottles
- □ Chemical cape
- □ Clarifying and acid-balanced shampoo (optional)
- □ Conditioner (optional)

- □ Cotton coil or rope
- □ Disposable gloves
- □ End papers
- □ Neutralizer
- □ Neutralizing bib
- □ Perm rods

- □ Perm solution
- □ Plastic clips for sectioning
- □ Plastic tail comb
- □ Pre-neutralizing conditioner (optional)

- □ Protective barrier cream
- □ Roller picks
- □ Spray bottle
- □ Styling comb
- □ Timer
- □ Towels

PREPARATION

Perform:

P 15-1 **Pre-Service Procedure** *See page 340*

PROCEDURE

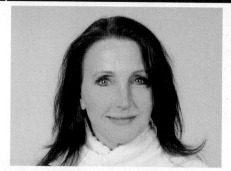

1 After completing the pre-service procedure, seat the client. If the manufacturer's directions indicate that a shampoo is necessary before the service, then drape the client for a shampoo and gently shampoo and towel dry hair. Avoid irritating the client's scalp.

2 Re-drape the client for a chemical service.

3 Begin sectioning at the front hairline on one side of the part. Comb the hair in the direction of growth, and then section out individual panels to match the length of the rod.

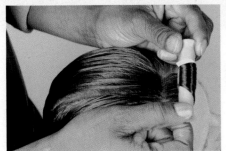

④ Begin by parting out a base section parallel to the front hairline that is the length and width of the rod being used. The base direction is back, away from the face. Hold the hair at a 90-degree angle to the head. Using two end papers, roll the hair down to the scalp and position the rod half off-base.

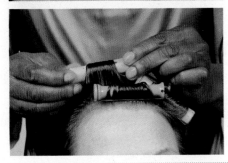

⑤ In the second row directly behind the first rod, part out two base sections for two rods offset from the center of the first rod. Hold the hair at a 90-degree angle to the head. Using two end papers, roll the hair down to the scalp and position the rods half off-base.

⑥ Insert picks to stabilize rods and eliminate any tension caused by the band.

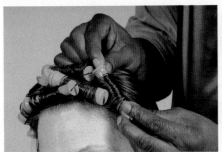

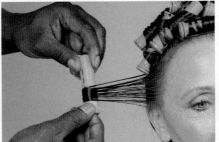

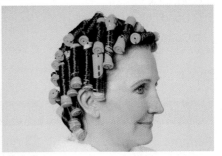

⑦ On the third row, part out a base section at the point where the two rods meet in the previous row. Complete the third row in this manner. This same pattern is used throughout the entire wrap.

⑧ Continue to part out rows that radiate around the curve of the head through the crown area. Maintain even dampness as you work. Extend rows around and down to the side hairline, parting out base sections at the center of the point where the two rods meet in the previous row.

⑨ Stop the curving rows after you have finished wrapping the crown area. Part out horizontal sections throughout the back of the head, and continue with the bricklay pattern. You may need to change the length of the rods from row to row to maintain the pattern.

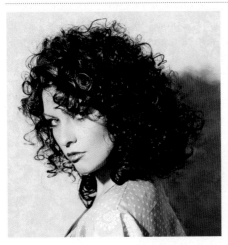

⑩ Process and style the hair.

POST-SERVICE

Complete:

Ⓟ 15-2 **Post-Service Procedure** *See page 343*

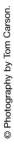
© Photography by Tom Carson.

PERMANENT WAVE AND PROCESSING USING A WEAVE TECHNIQUE

You will need all of the following implements, materials, and supplies:

- ☐ Applicator bottles
- ☐ Clarifying and acid-balanced shampoo (optional)
- ☐ Conditioner (optional)
- ☐ Cotton coil or rope

- ☐ Disposable gloves
- ☐ End papers
- ☐ Neutralizer
- ☐ Neutralizing bib
- ☐ Perm rods
- ☐ Perm solution

- ☐ Plastic clips for sectioning
- ☐ Plastic tail comb
- ☐ Pre-neutralizing conditioner (optional)
- ☐ Protective barrier cream

- ☐ Roller picks
- ☐ Chemical cape
- ☐ Spray bottle
- ☐ Styling comb
- ☐ Timer
- ☐ Towels

PREPARATION

Perform:

P 15-1 **Pre-Service Procedure** See page 340

PROCEDURE

1 After completing the pre-service procedure, seat the client. If the manufacturer's directions indicate that a shampoo is necessary before the service, then drape the client for a shampoo and gently shampoo and towel dry hair. Avoid irritating the client's scalp.

2 Re-drape the client for a chemical service.

3 Begin sectioning at the front hairline on one side of the part. Comb the hair in the direction of growth, and then section out individual panels to match the length of the rod.

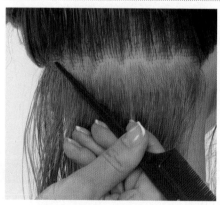

4 Part out one base section the same size as two rods. Comb the entire base section at a 90-degree angle to the head, and use a tail comb to make a zigzag parting along the length of the base section.

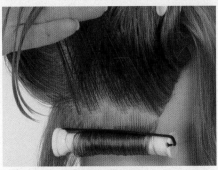

5 a. Using two end papers, roll half of the strand down to the scalp. Maintain even dampness as you work, re-misting the hair with water if necessary.

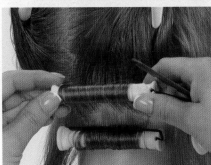

5 b. Comb the remaining half of the base section at a 90-degree angle; use two end papers, and roll the strand down to the scalp.

6 Secure the rods and insert picks to stabilize them and to eliminate any tension caused by the band.

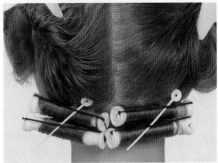

7 Continue with the same procedure in any sections where the effect is desired.

8 Process and style the hair.

POST-SERVICE

Complete:

P 15-2 **Post-Service Procedure** *See page 343*

PERMANENT WAVE AND PROCESSING USING A WEAVE DOUBLE-ROD OR PIGGYBACK TECHNIQUE

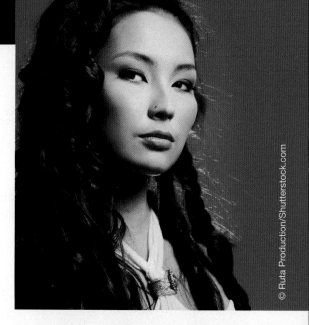

© Ruta Production/Shutterstock.com

IMPLEMENTS & MATERIALS

You will need all of the following implements, materials, and supplies:

- Applicator bottles
- Chemical cape
- Clarifying and acid-balanced shampoo (optional)
- Conditioner (optional)

- Cotton coil or rope
- Disposable gloves
- End papers
- Neutralizer
- Neutralizing bib
- Perm rods

- Perm solution
- Plastic clips for sectioning
- Plastic tail comb
- Pre-neutralizing conditioner (optional)

- Protective barrier cream
- Roller picks
- Spray bottle
- Styling comb
- Timer
- Towels

PREPARATION

Perform:

P 15-1 **Pre-Service Procedure** *See page 340*

PROCEDURE

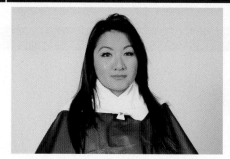

① After completing the pre-service procedure, seat the client. If the manufacturer's directions indicate that a shampoo is necessary before the service, then drape the client for a shampoo and gently shampoo and towel dry hair. Avoid irritating the client's scalp.

② Re-drape the client for a chemical service.

③ Begin sectioning at the front hairline on one side of the part. Comb the hair in the direction of growth, and then section out individual panels to match the length of the rod.

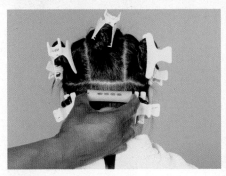

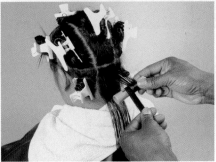

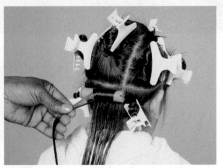

④ **a.** Begin by placing the base rod in the middle of the strand.

④ **b.** Wrap the end of the strand one revolution around the rod while holding it to one side.

⑤ Roll the rod up to the base area, letting the loose ends follow as you roll.

⑥ Insert picks to stabilize the rods and to eliminate any tension caused by the band.

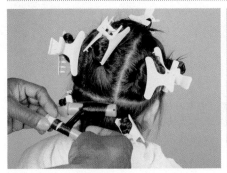

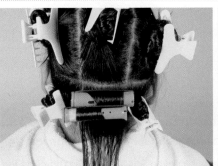

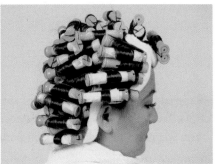

⑦ **a.** Place two end papers on the ends of the strand, position the rod, and roll from the ends toward the base.

⑦ **b.** Secure the end rod on top of the base rod.

⑧ Maintain consistent dampness as you work, re-wetting the hair with water if necessary. Continue with the same procedure in any sections where the effect is desired.

⑨ Process and style the hair.

POST-SERVICE

Complete:

Ⓟ 15-2 **Post-Service Procedure** *See page 343*

PERMANENT WAVE AND PROCESSING USING A SPIRAL WRAP TECHNIQUE

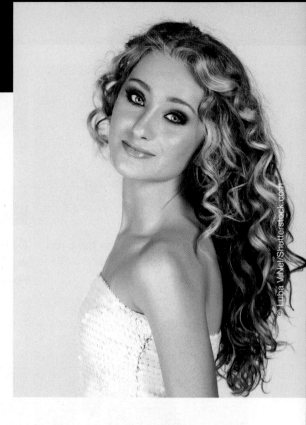

IMPLEMENTS & MATERIALS

You will need all of the following implements, materials, and supplies:

- Applicator bottles
- Chemical cape
- Clarifying and acid-balanced shampoo (optional)
- Conditioner (optional)
- Cotton coil or rope

- Disposable gloves
- End papers
- Neutralizer
- Neutralizing bib
- Perm rods
- Perm solution

- Plastic clips for sectioning
- Plastic tail comb
- Pre-neutralizing conditioner (optional)
- Protective barrier cream
- Roller picks

- Spray bottle
- Styling comb
- Timer
- Towels

PREPARATION | PROCEDURE

Perform:

P 15-1 **Pre-Service Procedure** *See page 340*

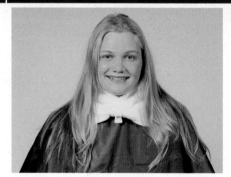

1 After completing the pre-service procedure, seat the client. If the manufacturer's directions indicate that a shampoo is necessary before the service, then drape the client for a shampoo and gently shampoo and towel dry hair. Avoid irritating the client's scalp.

2 Re-drape the client for a chemical service.

3 Begin sectioning at the front hairline on one side of the part. Comb the hair in the direction of growth, and then section out individual panels to match the length of the rod.

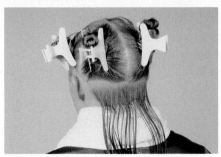

4 Part the hair into four panels, from the center of the front hairline to the center of the nape, and from ear to ear. Section out a fifth panel from ear to ear in the nape area.

5 Section out the first row along the hairline in the nape area. Comb the remainder of the hair up, and secure it out of the way.

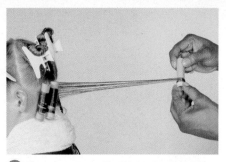

6 Part out the first base section on one side of the first row. Hold the hair at a 90-degree angle to the head. Using one or two end papers, begin wrapping at one end of the rod. Starting the wrap from the right or left side of the rod will orient the curl in that direction.

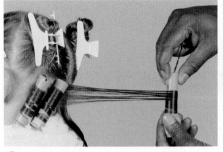

7 Roll the first two full turns at a 90-degree angle to the rod to secure the ends of the hair, and then start spiraling the hair on the rod by changing the angle to an angle other than 90 degrees.

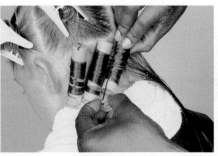

8 Continue to spiral the hair toward the other end of the rod. Roll the hair down to the scalp, position the rod half off-base, and secure it by fastening the ends of the rod together.

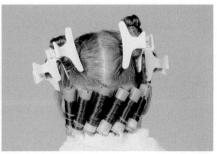

9 Continue wrapping with the same technique, in the same direction, until the first row is completed.

10 Section out the second row above and parallel to the first row. Comb the remainder of the hair up, and secure it to keep it out of the way.

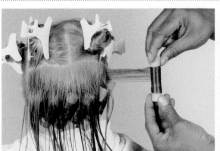

11 Begin wrapping at the opposite side from the side where the first row began, and move in the direction opposite the direction established in the first row.

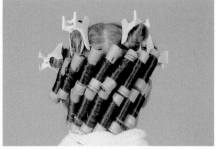

12 Follow the same procedure to wrap the second row, but begin wrapping each rod at the opposite end established in the first row. Maintain consistent dampness as you work, misting the hair with water if necessary. Continue wrapping with the same technique, in the same direction, until the second row is completed.

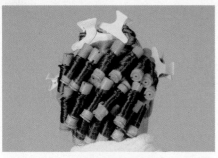

13 a. Section out the third row above and parallel to the second row. Follow the same wrapping procedure, alternating the rows from left to right as you move up the head. This will alternate the orientation of the curl throughout the head.

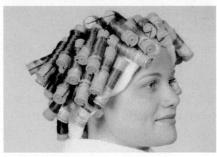

13 b. Complete wrapping.

14 Process and style the hair.

POST-SERVICE

Complete:

P 15-2 Post-Service Procedure *See page 343*

APPLYING THIO RELAXER TO VIRGIN HAIR

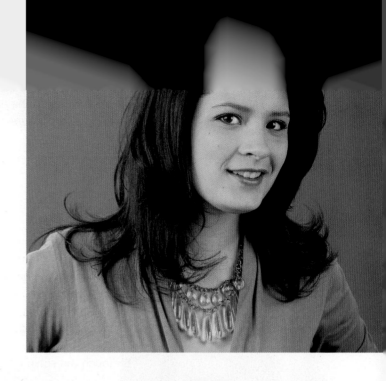

IMPLEMENTS & MATERIALS

You will need all of the following implements, materials, and supplies:

- ☐ Acid-balanced shampoo
- ☐ Applicator brush or tail comb
- ☐ Conditioner
- ☐ Chemical cape
- ☐ Disposable gloves
- ☐ Hard rubber comb
- ☐ Plastic or glass bowl
- ☐ Plastic clips
- ☐ Pre-neutralizing conditioner
- ☐ Protective base cream
- ☐ Spray bottle
- ☐ Styling comb
- ☐ Thio neutralizer
- ☐ Thio relaxer
- ☐ Timer
- ☐ Towels

PREPARATION

Perform:

ⓅⓅ 15-1 Pre-Service Procedure *See page 340*

PROCEDURE

① Perform an analysis of the hair and scalp. Perform tests for porosity and elasticity.

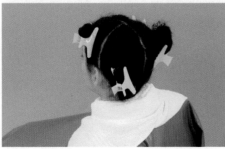

② Drape the client for a chemical service. *The hair and scalp must be completely dry prior to the application of a thio relaxer.*

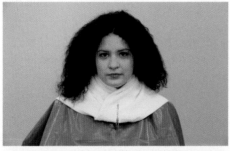

③ Part the hair into four sections, from the center of the front hairline to the center of the nape, and from ear to ear. Clip the sections up to keep them out of the way.

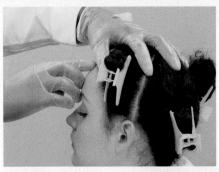

4 Apply protective base cream to the hairline and ears. Option: Take ¼ inch to ½ inch (0.6 to 1.25 centimeters) horizontal partings, and apply a protective base cream to the entire scalp. Always follow the manufacturer's directions and the procedures approved by your instructor.

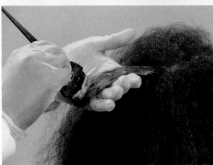

5 Wear gloves on both hands. Begin application in the most resistant area, usually at the back of the head. Make ¼ inch to ½ inch (0.6 to 1.25 centimeters) horizontal subsections, and apply the relaxer to the top of the strand first, and then to the underside. Apply the relaxer with an applicator brush, with the back of the comb, or with your fingers. Apply relaxer ¼ inch to ½ inch (0.6 to 1.25 centimeters) away from the scalp, and up to the porous ends. To avoid scalp irritation, do not allow the relaxer to touch the scalp until the last few minutes of processing.

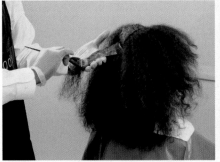

6 Continue applying the relaxer, working your way down the section toward the hairline.

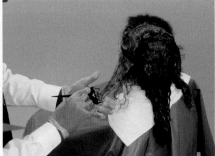

7 Continue the same application procedure with the remaining sections. Finish the most resistant sections first.

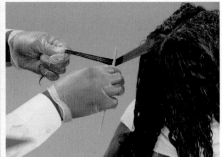

8 After the relaxer has been applied to all sections, use the back of the comb or your hands to smooth each section. Never comb the relaxer through the hair.

9 Process according to the manufacturer's directions. Perform periodic strand tests. Processing usually takes less than 20 minutes at room temperature. Always follow the manufacturer's processing directions.

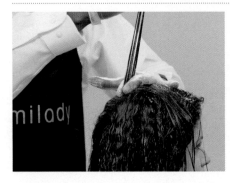

10 During the last few minutes of processing, work the relaxer down to the scalp and through the ends of the hair, using additional relaxer as needed. Carefully smooth all sections using an applicator brush, your fingers, or the back of the comb.

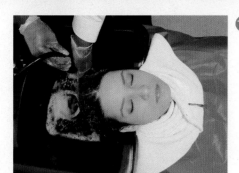

11 Rinse thoroughly with warm water to remove all traces of the relaxer.

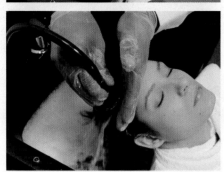

12 Shampoo at least three times with an acid-balanced shampoo. It is essential that all traces of the relaxer be removed from the hair. Optional: Apply the pre-neutralizing conditioner, and comb it through to the ends of the hair. Leave it on for approximately 5 minutes and then rinse. Always follow the manufacturer's directions and the procedures approved by your instructor.

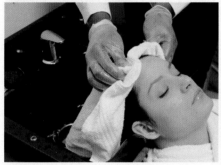

13 Blot excess water from the hair.

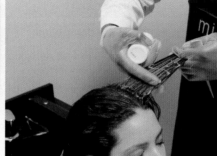

14 Apply thio neutralizer in ¼- to ½ inch (0.6 to 1.25 centimeters) sections throughout the hair and smooth with your hands or the back of the comb.

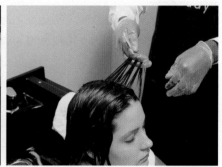

15 Process the neutralizer according to the manufacturer's directions.

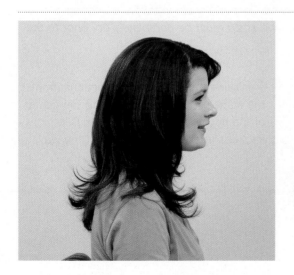

16 Rinse thoroughly. Shampoo, condition, and style.

POST-SERVICE

Complete:

P 15-2 **Post-Service Procedure** *See page 343*

THIO RELAXER RETOUCH

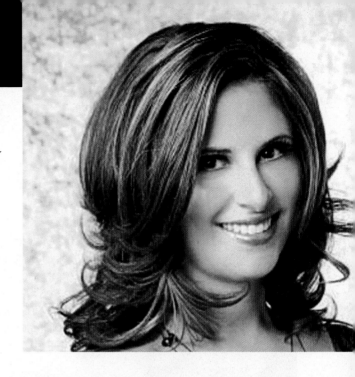

IMPLEMENTS & MATERIALS

You will need all of the following implements, materials, and supplies:

- ☐ Acid-balanced shampoo
- ☐ Applicator brush or tail comb
- ☐ Chemical cape
- ☐ Conditioner
- ☐ Disposable gloves
- ☐ Hard rubber comb
- ☐ Plastic clips
- ☐ Plastic or glass bowl
- ☐ Pre-neutralizing conditioner
- ☐ Protective base cream
- ☐ Spray bottle
- ☐ Styling comb
- ☐ Thio neutralizer
- ☐ Thio relaxer
- ☐ Timer
- ☐ Towels

PREPARATION

Perform:

P 15-1 **Pre-Service Procedure** *See page 340*

PROCEDURE

1️⃣ Perform an analysis of the hair and scalp. Perform tests for porosity and elasticity.

2️⃣ Drape the client for a chemical service. To avoid scalp irritation, do not shampoo the hair prior to a thio relaxer. *The hair and scalp must be completely dry prior to the application of a thio relaxer retouch.*

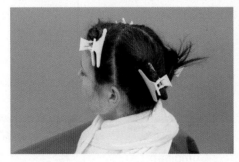

3️⃣ Divide the hair into four sections, from the center of the front hairline to the center of the nape, and from ear to ear. Clip sections up to keep them out of the way.

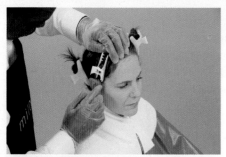

4 Wear gloves on both hands. Apply a protective base cream to the hairline and ears, unless you are using a no-base relaxing product. Option: Take ¼ inch to ½ inch (0.6 to 1.25 centimeters) horizontal partings, and apply protective base cream to the entire scalp.

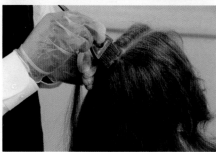

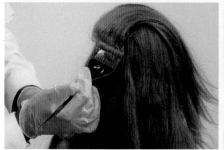

5 Begin application of the relaxer in the most resistant area, usually at the back of the head or under the occipital bone. Make ¼ inch to ½ inch (0.6 to 1.25 centimeters) horizontal subsections, and apply the relaxer to the top of the strand. Apply the relaxer as close to the scalp as possible, but do not touch the scalp with the product. Only allow the relaxer to touch the scalp itself during the last few minutes of processing. To avoid overprocessing or breakage, do not overlap the relaxer onto the previously relaxed hair.

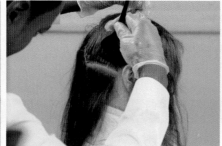

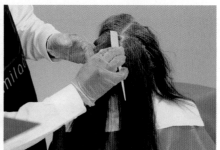

6 Continue applying the relaxer, using the same procedure and working your way down the section toward the hairline.

7 Continue the same application procedure with the remaining sections, finishing the most resistant sections first.

8 After the relaxer has been applied to all sections, use the back of the comb, the applicator brush, or your hands to smooth each section.

9 Process according to the manufacturer's directions. Perform periodic strand tests. Processing usually takes less than 20 minutes at room temperature. Always follow the manufacturer's processing directions.

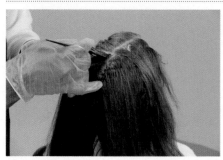

⚠ **CAUTION**
Never intentionally overlap previously relaxed hair as this will result in damage and possible hair breakage!

11 Rinse thoroughly with warm water to remove all traces of the relaxer.

10 During the last few minutes of processing, gently work the relaxer down to the scalp.

⑫ Shampoo at least three times with an acid-balanced shampoo (neutralizer). It is essential that all traces of the relaxer be removed from the hair. If the relaxer product recommends using a pre-neutralizing conditioner, comb it throughout the hair as per the recommendations of the manufacturer. Rinse again and neutralize with acid shampoo. Always follow the manufacturer's directions and the procedures approved by your instructor.

⑬ Blot excess water from hair.

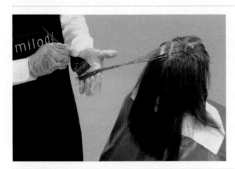

⑭ Apply thio neutralizer in ¼- to ½ inch (0.6 to 1.25 centimeters) sections throughout the hair and smooth with your hands or the back of the comb.

⑮ Process the neutralizer according to the manufacturer's directions.

⑯ Rinse thoroughly. Shampoo, condition, and style.

POST-SERVICE

Complete:

Ⓟ 15-2 **Post-Service Procedure** *See page 343*

APPLYING HYDROXIDE RELAXER TO VIRGIN HAIR

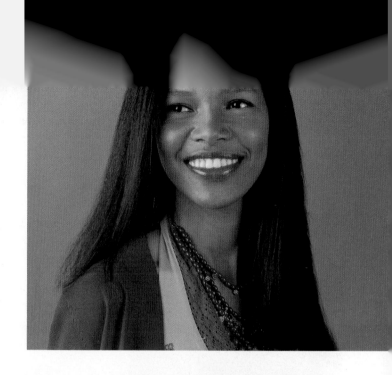

IMPLEMENTS & MATERIALS

You will need all of the following implements, materials, and supplies:

- ☐ Chemical cape
- ☐ Conditioner
- ☐ Disposable gloves
- ☐ Hydroxide relaxer

- ☐ Neutralizing acid-balanced shampoo
- ☐ Plastic clips
- ☐ Plastic or glass bowl

- ☐ Protective base cream
- ☐ Styling comb
- ☐ Tail comb or applicator brush

- ☐ Timer
- ☐ Towels
- ☐ Wide-tooth hard rubber comb

PREPARATION | PROCEDURE

Perform:

ⓟ 15-1 **Pre-Service Procedure** *See page 340*

①	Perform an analysis of the hair and scalp by visually assessing the hair for breakage, sores on the scalp, or any visual signs of irritation. Feel the hair and perform an elasticity test. If hair fails the test for porosity and elasticity, do not perform the relaxer service.

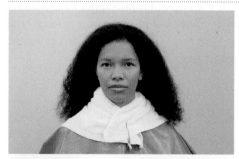

②	Drape the client for a chemical service.

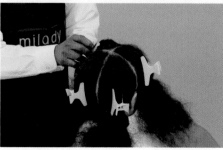

③	To avoid scalp irritation, do not shampoo the hair. *The hair and scalp must be completely dry prior to the application of a hydroxide relaxer.*

④ Part the hair into four sections, from the center of the front hairline to the center of the nape, and from ear to ear. Clip the sections up if necessary to keep hair out of the way.

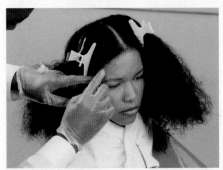

④ **a.** Put on gloves, and apply protective base cream to the hairline and ears.

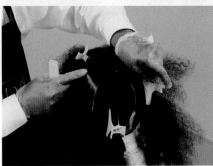

④ **b.** Optional: Take ¼ inch to ½ inch (0.6 to 1.25 centimeters) horizontal partings, and apply a protective base cream to the entire scalp. Always follow the manufacturer's directions and the procedures approved by your instructor. Set timer as indicated by the manufacturer and initial strand test.

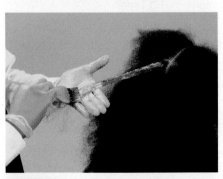

⑤ **a.** Put gloves on both hands. Begin the relaxer application in the most resistant area, usually at the back of the head or nape area. Make ¼ inch to ½ inch (0.6 to 1.25 centimeters) horizontal subsections, and apply the relaxer to the top of the strand first. Do not apply to the scalp.

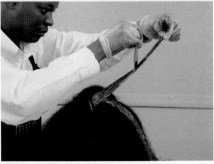

⑤ **b.** Apply relaxer to the underside of the first section using an applicator brush or the back of a tail comb. Apply relaxer ¼ inch to ½ inch (0.6 to 1.25 centimeters) away from the scalp, and up to the porous ends. To avoid scalp irritation, do not allow the relaxer to come near the scalp until the last few minutes of processing.

⑥ Continue applying relaxer to other sections, working your way down the section toward the hairline. Continue the same application procedure with the remaining sections.

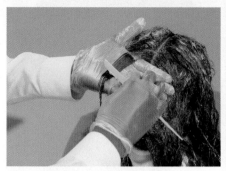

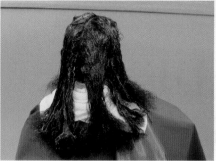

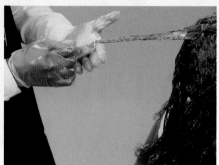

7 After the relaxer has been applied to all sections, use the back of the comb or your hands to smooth each section. Never comb the relaxer through the hair as this may break the hair.

8 Process according to the manufacturer's directions and what your initial strand test indicated regarding timing. Perform periodic strand tests.

9 During the last few minutes of processing, work the relaxer down to the scalp and through the ends of the hair, using additional relaxer as needed. Carefully smooth all sections, using an applicator brush, your fingers, or back of the tail comb.

10 Rinse thoroughly with warm water to remove all traces of the relaxer.

11 If the relaxer comes with a normalizing lotion or conditioner, comb it throughout the hair. Leave it on as indicated by the manufacturer. Rinse thoroughly. Always follow the manufacturer's directions and the procedures approved by your instructor.

12 Shampoo at least three times with an acid-balanced neutralizing shampoo. If you are using a neutralizing shampoo with a color indicator, usually the color will change from pink to white indicating that all traces of the relaxer are removed, and the natural pH of the hair and scalp has been restored.

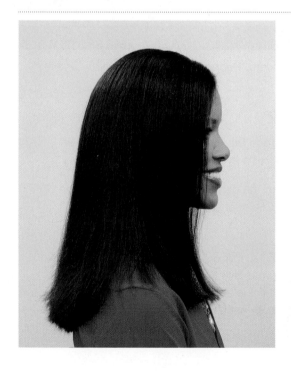

13 Rinse thoroughly, condition, and style as desired.

POST-SERVICE

Complete:

(P) 15-2 **Post-Service Procedure** *See page 343*

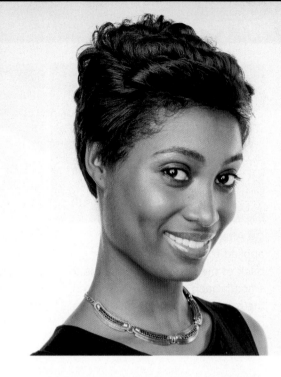

HYDROXIDE RELAXER RETOUCH

IMPLEMENTS & MATERIALS

You will need all of the following implements, materials, and supplies:

- Acid-balanced shampoo
- Chemical cape
- Conditioner
- Disposable gloves
- Hard rubber comb
- Hydroxide neutralizer
- Hydroxide relaxer
- Plastic clips
- Plastic or glass bowl
- Protective base cream
- Spray bottle
- Tail comb or applicator brush
- Timer
- Towels

PREPARATION | PROCEDURE

Perform:

P 15-1 **Pre-Service Procedure** See page 340

1 Perform an analysis of the hair and scalp. Perform tests for porosity and elasticity.

2 Drape the client for a chemical service.

3 To avoid scalp irritation, do not shampoo the hair. *The hair and scalp must be completely dry prior to the application of a hydroxide relaxer retouch.*

4 Divide the hair into four sections, from the center of the front hairline to the center of the nape, and from ear to ear. Clip sections up to keep hair out of the way if necessary.

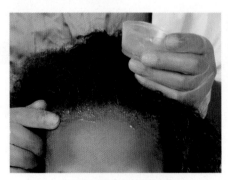

4 **a.** Put on gloves, and apply a protective base cream to the hairline and ears. Put gloves on both hands.

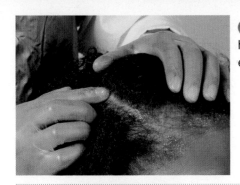

4 b. Optional: Take ¼ inch to ½ inch (0.6 to 1.25 centimeters) horizontal partings and apply protective base cream throughout the entire scalp. Set timer as indicated by the manufacturer for retouch.

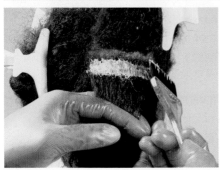

5 Begin application of the relaxer in the most resistant area, usually at the back of the head or nape area. Make ¼ inch to ½ inch (0.6 to 1.25 centimeters) horizontal subsections, and apply the relaxer to the top of the strand. Apply the relaxer as close to the scalp as possible, but do not touch the scalp with the relaxer. Only allow the relaxer to near the scalp during the last few minutes of processing. To avoid overprocessing or breakage, do not overlap the relaxer onto the previously relaxed hair.

6 Continue applying the relaxer, using the same procedure and working your way down the section toward the hairline.

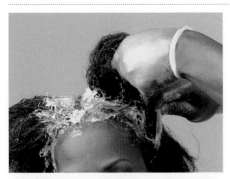

7 Continue the same application procedure with the remaining sections.

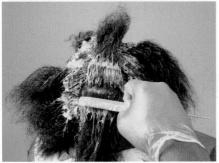

8 After the relaxer has been applied to all sections, use the back of the comb, the applicator brush, or your hands to smooth each section.

9 Process according to the manufacturer's directions. Perform periodic strand tests. Always follow the manufacturer's processing directions.

10 During the last few minutes of processing, gently work the relaxer down to the scalp.

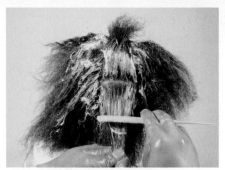

11 Do not relax mid-shaft or ends during the retouch service, as this will cause overprocessing. Option: Oil may be applied to previously relaxed ends to protect from overprocessing caused by overlapping.

12 Rinse thoroughly with warm water to remove all traces of the relaxer. If the relaxer comes with a normalizing lotion or conditioner, comb it through the hair. Leave it on as indicated by the manufacturer and rinse thoroughly. Always follow the manufacturer's directions and the procedures approved by your instructor.

13 Shampoo at least three times with an acid-balanced neutralizing shampoo. If you are using an acid-balanced neutralizing shampoo with a color indicator, usually the color change will go from pink to white indicating all traces of the relaxer have been removed and the natural pH of the hair and scalp has been restored.

13 a. Apply conditioner as per manufacturer's recommendations. Rinse.

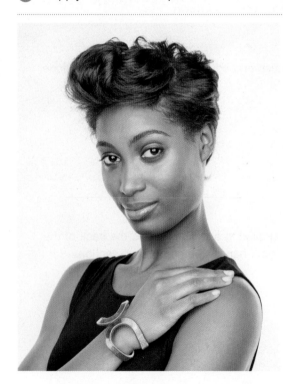

14 Style the hair as desired.

POST-SERVICE

Complete:

P 15-2   **Post-Service Procedure** *See page 343*

CURL RE-FORMING (SOFT CURL PERM)

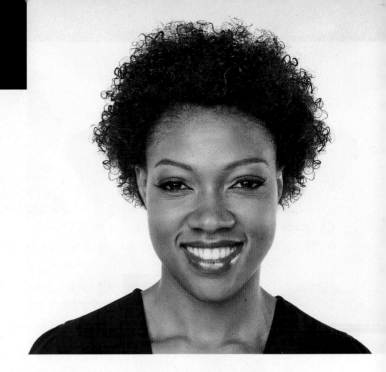

IMPLEMENTS & MATERIALS

You will need all of the following implements, materials, and supplies:

- ☐ Applicator bottle
- ☐ Applicator brush
- ☐ Conditioner
- ☐ Disposable gloves

- ☐ Gentle clarifying shampoo
- ☐ Large-tooth comb
- ☐ Plastic or glass bowl

- ☐ Plastic processing cap
- ☐ Protective base cream
- ☐ Tail comb
- ☐ Thio cream relaxer

- ☐ Thio wrap lotion
- ☐ Thio neutralizer solution

PREPARATION

Perform:

P 15-1 Pre-Service Procedure *See page 340*

> ⚠️ **CAUTION**
> Hair that has been treated with hydroxide relaxers cannot be treated with soft curl permanents. The chemicals are not compatible!

PROCEDURE

1️⃣ Perform an analysis of the hair and scalp. Perform tests for porosity and elasticity. Remember, this procedure requires that the hair and scalp be completely dry. Most manufacturer's directions indicate that a shampoo may be necessary before a soft curl service, if so, drape the client for a shampoo and gently shampoo with a mild shampoo and towel-dry hair. Avoid irritating the client's scalp.

2️⃣ Re-drape the client for a chemical service.

3️⃣ Based on the manufacturer's recommendation for preliminary strand test, conduct strand test to determine proper timing and curl pattern prior to full-head application. Make note of the timing for the Thio cream relaxer, strength used, and rod size.

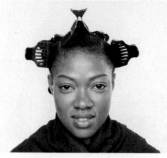
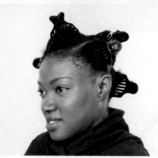
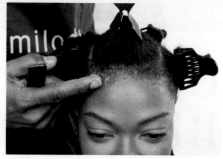

4 Divide the hair into four sections. Clip the sections up to keep them out of the way and for better application of product. Apply a protective base cream to the hairline and ears.

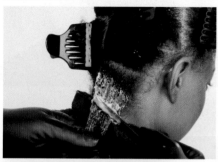

5 Wearing gloves on both hands, begin application of Thio cream relaxer to the most resistant area, usually at the back of the head and nape area. Using an applicator brush or tail comb, apply cream ¼ inch (0.6 to 1.25 centimeters) away from the scalp and topside and underside of the strand. Do not apply to cream to the ends of hair during this step. To avoid possible scalp irritation, do not allow cream to touch the scalp until the last few minutes of processing.

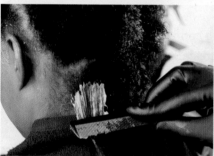
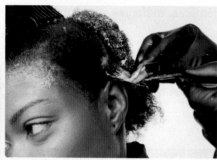

6 Repeat application in remaining sections. Apply Thio cream to the hairline and ends last, since hair is the most fragile in this regoin.

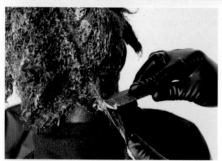

7 Review application of all four quadrants. If necessary, apply more cream until all hair strands are covered. Apply cream to hairline and ends of hair during this step.

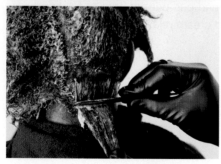

8 After the Thio cream has been applied to all sections, using an applicator brush, the back of the comb, or your hands, begin to smooth each section, starting at the first section where Thio cream was applied. Never comb the cream through the hair.

9 Process according to the manufacturer's directions, and strand test results for timing. Perform periodic strand tests until time has elapsed.

10 During the final remaining minutes of processing, apply the Thio cream to the scalp and through the ends of the hair, using additional cream as needed. Carefully smooth all sections using an applicator brush, your fingers, or the back of the comb.

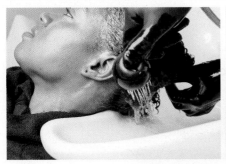 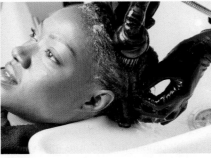

11 Rinse thoroughly with warm water to remove all traces of the Thio cream.

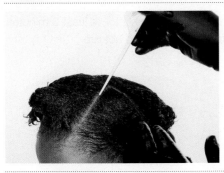

12 After rinsing the hair, towel blot and part it into nine panels. Use the length of the rod to measure the width of the panels. *Review Chapter 20, Understand Permanent Waving, for how to properly wrap hair.*

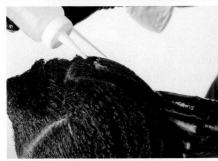 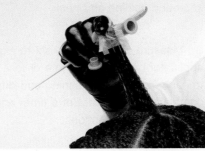 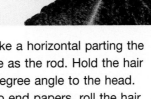

13 a. Wearing gloves, apply thio wrap lotion to each section and roll hair on the appropriate-sized perm rods. Begin wrapping at the most resistant area, usually the nape.

13 b. Make a horizontal parting the same size as the rod. Hold the hair at a 90-degree angle to the head. Using two end papers, roll the hair down to the scalp.

> ⚠ **CAUTION**
> Maintain even dampness as you work.

Position the rod half off-base. Option: Insert roller picks to stabilize the rods and eliminate any tension caused by the band.

13 c. Continue wrapping the remaining eight panels in numerical order using the same technique.

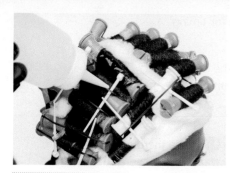

14 Place cotton strip around the hairline and neck to protect client.

15 If the manufacturer or your instructor suggests using a plastic processing cap, cover all the hair completely. Do not allow the plastic cap to touch the client's skin.

16 Process according to manufacturer's directions. Processing time will vary according to the strength of the product, hair type and condition, desired results, and strand test results. Check for proper curl development in 5 minute intervals.

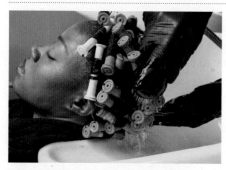

17 When processing is complete, rinse the hair thoroughly for at least 3 minutes. Gently towel blot each rod to remove excess moisture. Do not rub.

18 Re-drape client with fresh cotton strip around hairline and neck.

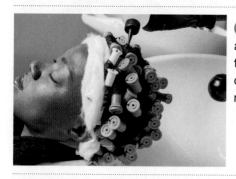

19 Measure approximately six to eight ounces of the Thio neutralizer in an applicator bottle, using more or less as needed. Slowly and carefully apply to each rod. Avoid splashing and dripping. Make sure each rod is completely saturated. Set a timer and neutralize according to the manufacturer's directions.

20 The average time to complete the neutralization process is 10 minutes without the use of a hair dryer.

21 After neutralizing is complete, thoroughly rinse hair with water for about 2 minutes with rods still in the hair. Do not remove rods during rinsing.

22 Gently blot to remove excess water.

23 Remove the rods from the hair, and rinse thoroughly for about 2 minutes.

> ⚠ **CAUTION**
> Hair must not be shampooed for at least 48 hours; otherwise curls will be compromised!

24 Towel dry and apply hydrating conditioner. Using a large-tooth comb, distribute the conditioner throughout the hair.

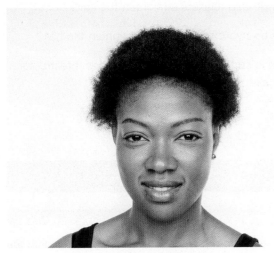

25 Rinse, towel dry, and style as desired.

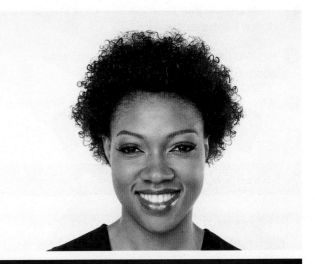

POST-SERVICE

Complete:

Ⓟ **15-2** **Post-Service Procedure** *See page 343*

REVIEW QUESTIONS

1. What are the four chemical reactions that take place during permanent waving?

2. What is the difference between an alkaline wave and a true acid wave?

3. Why do permanent waves need to be neutralized?

4. How do thio relaxers straighten the hair?

5. How do hydroxide relaxers straighten the hair?

6. What is curl re-forming and how does it restructure the hair?

STUDY TOOLS

- **Reinforce what you just learned:** Complete the activities and exercises in your Theory or Practical Workbook, or your Study Guide.

- **Expand your knowledge:** Search for websites about the topics in this chapter and make a list of additional resources.

- **Study and prepare for your quiz:** Take the chapter test in your Exam Review or your Milady U: Online Licensing Prep.

- **Re-Test your knowledge:** Take the Chapter 20 *Quizzes!*

- **Learn even more:** Look up in a dictionary or search the internet for the definitions for any additional terms you want to learn about.

CHAPTER GLOSSARY

acid-balanced waves	p. 604	Permanent waves that have a 7.0 or neutral pH; because of their higher pH, they process at room temperature, do not require the added heat of a hair dryer, process more quickly, and produce firmer curls than true acid waves.
alkaline waves	p. 604	Also known as *cold waves*; they have a pH between 9.0 and 9.6, use ammonium thioglycolate (ATG) as the reducing agent, and process at room temperature without the addition of heat.
amino acids	p. 600	Compounds made up of carbon, oxygen, hydrogen, nitrogen, and sulfur.
ammonia-free waves	p. 605	Perms that use an ingredient that does not evaporate as readily as ammonia, so there is very little odor associated with their use.
ammonium thioglycolate (ATG) uh-MOH-nee-um thy-oh-GLY-kuh-layt	p. 603	Active ingredient or reducing agent in alkaline permanents.
base control	p. 614	Position of the tool in relation to its base section, determined by the angle at which the hair is wrapped.
base cream	p. 621	Also known as *protective base cream*; oily cream used to protect the skin and scalp during hair relaxing.
base direction	p. 612	Angle at which the rod is positioned on the head (horizontally, vertically, or diagonally); also, the directional pattern in which the hair is wrapped.

base placement	p. 611	Refers to the position of the rod in relation to its base section; base placement is determined by the angle at which the hair is wrapped.
base relaxers	p. 621	Relaxers that require the application of protective base cream to the entire scalp prior to the application of the relaxer.
base sections	p. 611	Subsections of panels into which hair is divided for perm wrapping; one rod is normally placed on each base section.
basic permanent wrap	p. 614	Also known as *straight set wrap*; perm wrapping pattern in which all the rods within a panel move in the same direction and are positioned on equal-sized bases; all the base sections are horizontal and are the same length and width as the perm rod.
bookend wrap	p. 611	Perm wrap in which one end paper is folded in half over the hair ends like an envelope.
bricklay permanent wrap	p. 614	Perm wrap similar to actual technique of bricklaying; base sections are offset from each other row by row to prevent noticeable splits and to blend the flow of the hair.
chemical hair relaxing	p. 617	A process or service that rearranges the structure of curly hair into a straighter or smoother form.
chemical texture services	p. 598	Hair services that cause a chemical change that alters the natural wave pattern of the hair.
concave rods khan-KAYV RAHDZ	p. 609	Perm rods that have a smaller diameter in the center that increases to a larger diameter on the ends.
croquignole perm wrap KROH-ken-yohl	p. 612	Perm in which the hair strands are wrapped from the ends to the scalp in overlapping concentric layers.
curvature permanent wrap	p. 614	Perm wrap in which partings and bases radiate throughout the panels to follow the curvature of the head.
disulfide bonds	p. 600	Strong chemical side bonds formed when the sulfur atoms in two adjacent protein chains are joined together.
double flat wrap	p. 610	Perm wrap in which one end paper is placed under and another is placed over the strand of hair being wrapped.
double-rod wrap	p. 613	Also known as *piggyback wrap*; a wrap technique whereby extra-long hair is wrapped on one rod from the scalp to midway down the hair shaft, and another rod is used to wrap the remaining hair strand in the same direction.
end papers	p. 610	Also known as *end wraps*; absorbent papers used to control the ends of the hair when wrapping and winding hair on perm rods.
endothermic waves en-duh-THUR-mik wayvz	p. 605	Perm activated by an outside heat source, usually a conventional hood-type hair dryer.
exothermic waves Eks-oh-THUR-mik WAYVZ	p. 604	Create an exothermic chemical reaction that heats up the waving solution and speeds up processing.
glyceryl monothioglycolate (GMTG) GLIS-ur-il mon-oh-thy-oh-GLY-koh-layt	p. 604	Main active ingredient in true acid and acid-balanced waving lotions.

half off-base placement	p. 612	Base control in which the hair is wrapped at an angle of 90 degrees or perpendicular to its base section, and the rod is positioned half off its base section.
hydrogen bonds	p. 601	Weak physical side bonds that are also the result of an attraction between opposite electrical charges; they are easily broken by water (wet setting) or heat (thermal styling), and they re-form as the hair dries or cools.
hydroxide neutralization	p. 622	An acid-alkali neutralization reaction that neutralizes (deactivates) the alkaline residues left in the hair by a hydroxide relaxer and lowers the pH of the hair and scalp; hydroxide relaxer neutralization does not involve oxidation or rebuild disulfide bonds.
hydroxide relaxers	p. 619	Very strong alkalis with a pH over 13; the hydroxide ion is the active ingredient in all hydroxide relaxers.
keratin proteins	p. 600	Long, coiled polypeptide chains.
lanthionization lan-thee-oh-ny-ZAY-shun	p. 619	Process by which hydroxide relaxers permanently straighten hair; they remove a sulfur atom from a disulfide bond and convert it into a lanthionine bond.
loop rod	p. 610	Also known as *circle rod*; tool that is usually about 12 inches long with a uniform diameter along the entire length of the rod.
low-pH waves	p. 605	Perms that use sulfates, sulfites, and bisulfites as an alternative to ammonium thioglycolate.
metal hydroxide relaxers	p. 620	Ionic compounds formed by a metal (sodium, potassium, or lithium) which is combined with oxygen and hydrogen.
no-base relaxers	p. 621	Relaxers that do not require application of a protective base cream.
normalizing lotions	p. 623	Conditioners with an acidic pH that restore the hair's natural pH before the final neutralizing shampoo.
off-base placement	p. 612	Base control in which the hair is wrapped at 45 degrees below the center of the base section, so the rod is positioned completely off its base.
on-base placement	p. 611	Base control in which the hair is wrapped at a 45-degree angle beyond perpendicular to its base section, and the rod is positioned on its base.
peptide bonds	p. 600	Also known as *end bonds*; chemical bonds that join amino acids together, end-to-end in long chains, to form polypeptide chains.
permanent waving	p. 601	A two-step process whereby the hair undergoes a physical change caused by wrapping the hair on perm rods; the hair then undergoes a chemical change caused by the application of permanent waving solution and neutralizer.
polypeptide chains pahl-ee-PEP-tyd CHAYNS	p. 600	Long chains of amino acids joined together by peptide bonds.
side bonds	p. 600	Disulfide, salt, and hydrogen bonds that cross-link polypeptide chains together.
single flat wrap	p. 611	Perm wrap that is similar to double flat wrap but uses only one end paper, placed over the top of the strand of hair being wrapped.
soft bender rods	p. 610	Tool about 12 inches long with a uniform diameter along the entire length.

soft curl permanent	p. 627	A thio based chemical service that reformats curly and wavy hair into looser and larger curls and waves.
spiral perm wrap	p. 612	Hair is wrapped at an angle other than perpendicular to the length of the rod, which causes the hair to spiral along the length of the rod, similar to the stripes on a candy cane.
straight rods	p. 610	Perm rods that are equal in diameter along their entire length or curling area.
thioglycolic acid	p. 603	The most common reducing agent in permanent wave solutions.
thio neutralization THY-oh NEW-truhl-eyez-ay-shun	p. 608	Stops the action of a permanent wave solution and rebuilds the hair in its new curly form.
thio relaxers THY-oh ree-LAX-UHRS	p. 618	Use the same ammonium thioglycolate (ATG) that is used in permanent waving, but at a higher concentration and a higher pH (above 10).
thio-free waves THY-oh FREE WAYVZ	p. 605	Perm that uses an ingredient other than ATG as the primary reducing agent, such as cysteamine or mercaptamine.
true acid waves	p. 604	Have a pH between 4.5 and 7.0 and require heat to process; they process more slowly than alkaline waves, and they do not usually produce as firm a curl as alkaline waves.
viscosity vis-KAHS-ut-ee	p. 618	The measurement of the thickness or thinness of a liquid that affects how the fluid flows.
weave technique	p. 614	Wrapping technique that uses zigzag partings to divide base areas.

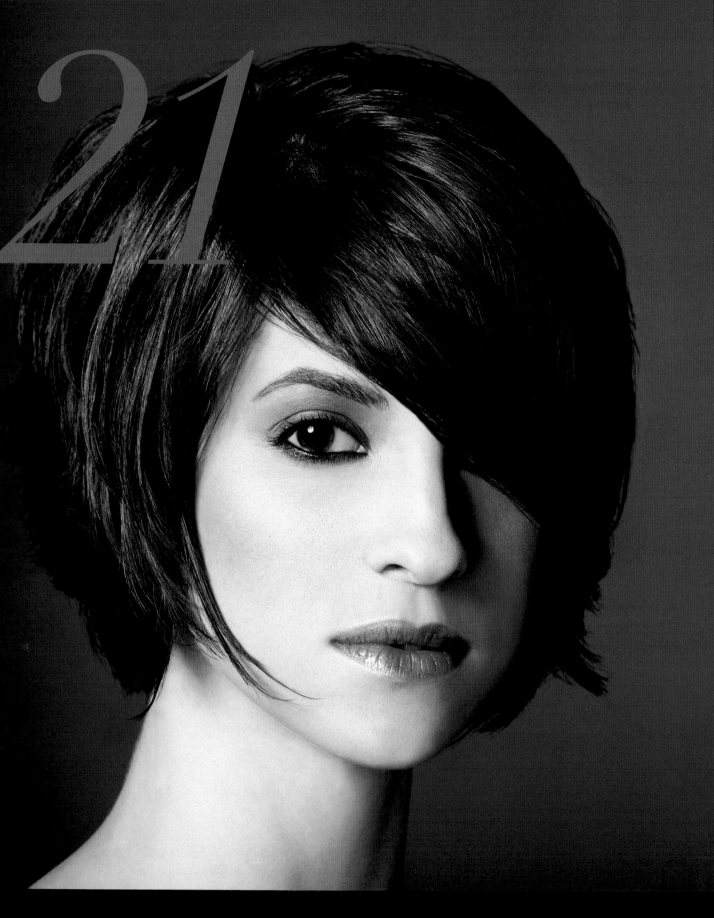

21

HAIRCOLORING

LEARNING OBJECTIVES

After completing this chapter, you will be able to:

LO①

List the reasons why people color their hair.

LO②

Explain how the hair's porosity affects haircolor.

LO③

Understand the types of melanin found in hair.

LO④

Define and identify levels and their role in formulating haircolor.

LO⑤

Identify primary, secondary, and tertiary colors.

LO⑥

Know what roles tone and intensity play in haircolor.

LO⑦

List and describe the categories of haircolor.

LO⑧

Explain the role of hydrogen peroxide in a haircolor formula.

LO⑨

Explain the action of hair lighteners.

LO⑩

List the five key questions to ask when formulating a haircolor.

LO⑪

Understand why a patch test is useful in haircoloring.

LO⑫

Define what a preliminary strand test is and why it is used.

LO⑬

List and describe the procedure for a virgin single-process color service.

LO ⑭
Understand the two processes involved in double-process haircoloring.

LO ⑮
Describe the various forms of hair lightener.

LO ⑯
Understand the purpose and use of toners.

LO ⑰
Name and describe the three most commonly used methods for highlighting.

LO ⑱
Know how to properly cover gray hair.

LO ⑲
Know the rules of color correction.

LO ⑳
Know the safety precautions to follow during the haircolor process.

One of the most creative, challenging, and inspiring salon services is haircoloring. Due to its popularity, it also has the potential for being one of the most lucrative areas in which a stylist can choose to work. You only have to look around while you are dining at a restaurant or standing in line to see a movie to know this is true. Nearly all adults and many teens now color their hair. You will probably find that most of your clients, at some time or another, will want to enhance their hair color, change their hair color, or cover gray. Clients who have their hair colored usually visit the salon every three to twelve weeks. These are the kind of regular guests you want in your client base (figure 21-1).

Why Study
HAIRCOLORING?

Cosmetologists should study and have a thorough understanding of haircoloring because:

> Haircolor services provide stylists and clients with an opportunity for creative expression and artistry.

> Clients increasingly ask for and require excellent haircoloring services to cover gray, to enhance their haircuts, and to camouflage face-shape imperfections.

> Haircolor products employ strong chemical ingredients to accomplish services, so being aware of what these chemicals are and how they work will enable you to safely provide color services for your clients.

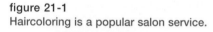
figure 21-1
Haircoloring is a popular salon service.

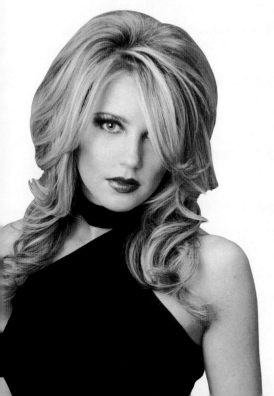

After reading the next few sections, you will be able to:

LO**1** List the reasons why people color their hair.

LO**2** Explain how the hair's porosity affects haircolor.

> **? DID YOU KNOW?**
> **Haircolor** (one word) is a professional, industry-coined term referring to artificial haircolor products and services. **Hair color** (two words) refers to the natural color of hair. For example, you might say of a client, "Mrs. Bailey's natural hair color is brown. The haircolor I am giving her is auburn."

Understand Why People Color Their Hair

It is important to have an understanding of what motivates people to color their hair. This information will help you determine which products and haircolor services are appropriate for your client. A few common reasons clients color their hair include the following:

- Cover up or blend gray (unpigmented) hair.

- Enhance an existing haircolor.

- Create a fashion statement or statement of self-expression.

- Correct unwanted tones in hair caused by environmental exposure such as sun or chlorine.

- Accentuate a particular haircut.

Many people experiment with haircoloring. When a client turns to you for advice and service, you need to have a thorough understanding of the hair structure and how haircoloring products affect it. As a trained professional, you will learn which shades of color are most flattering on your clients and which products and techniques will achieve the desired look.

Review Hair Facts

The structure of the client's hair and the desired results determine which haircolor to use. The hair structure affects the quality and ultimate success of the haircolor service. Some haircolor products may cause a dramatic change in the structure of the hair, while others cause relatively little change. Knowing how products affect the hair will allow you to make the best choices for your client.

Hair Structure

In this section, the structure of hair is quickly reviewed. For an in-depth discussion, see Chapter 11, Properties of the Hair and Scalp.

Hair is composed of the following three major components (**figure 21-2**):

- The cuticle is the outermost layer of the hair. It protects the interior cortex layer and contributes up to 20 percent of the overall strength of the hair.

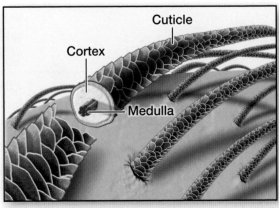

figure 21-2
A cross-section of the hair shaft

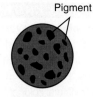

Pigment

Fine textured hair

Medium textured hair

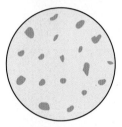

Coarse textured hair

figure 21-3
Melanin distribution according
to hair texture

- The cortex is the middle layer and gives the hair the majority of its strength and elasticity. A healthy cortex contributes about 80 percent to the overall strength of the hair. It contains the natural pigment called melanin that determines hair color. Melanin granules are scattered between the cortex cells like chips in a chocolate chip cookie.

- The medulla is the innermost layer of the hair. It is sometimes absent from the hair and does not play a role in the haircoloring process.

Texture

Hair texture is the diameter of an individual hair strand. Large-, medium-, and small-diameter hair strands translate into coarse, medium, and fine hair textures, respectively. Melanin is distributed differently according to texture. The melanin granules in fine hair are grouped more tightly, so the hair takes color faster and can look darker. Medium-textured hair has an average reaction to haircolor. Coarse-textured hair has a larger diameter and loosely grouped melanin granules, so it can take longer to process (figure 21-3).

Density

Another aspect of hair that plays a role in haircoloring is density. Hair density, the number of hairs per square inch, can range from thin to thick. Density must be taken into account when applying haircolor to ensure proper coverage.

Porosity

Porosity is the hair's ability to absorb moisture. Porous hair accepts haircolor faster, and haircolor application on porous hair can result in a cooler tone than applications on less porous hair. Degrees of porosity are described below:

- **Low porosity.** The cuticle is tight. The hair is **resistant**, which means it is difficult for moisture or chemicals to penetrate. Thus, it requires a longer processing time.

- **Average porosity.** The cuticle is slightly raised. The hair is normal and processes in an average amount of time.

- **High porosity.** The cuticle is lifted. The hair is overly porous and takes color quickly; color also tends to fade quickly. Permed, colored, chemically relaxed, and straightened hair will have a high degree of porosity. Extremely porous hair rejects warmth when color is applied and can process more quickly, which results in deeper color.

Test for porosity:

- Take several strands of hair from four different areas of the head: the front hairline, the temple, the crown, and the nape.

- Hold the strands securely with one hand and slide the thumb and forefinger of the other hand from the ends to the scalp.

- If the hair feels smooth and the cuticle is compact, dense, and hard, it has low porosity. If you can feel a slight roughness, it has average porosity. If the hair feels very rough, dry, or breaks, it has high porosity.

- Observe hair wet and dry to see porosity.

After reading the next few sections, you will be able to:

LO❸ Understand the types of melanin found in hair.

LO❹ Define and identify levels and their role in formulating haircolor.

LO❺ Identify primary, secondary, and tertiary colors.

LO❻ Know what roles tone and intensity play in haircolor.

Identify Natural Hair Color and Tone

Learning to identify a client's natural hair color is the most important step in becoming a good colorist. Natural hair color ranges from black to dark brown to red, and from dark blond to light blond. Hair color is unique to each individual; no two people have exactly the same color. There are three types of melanin in the cortex:

- **Eumelanin** is the melanin that lends black and brown colors to hair.

- **Pheomelanin** is the melanin that gives blond and red colors to hair.

- **Mixed melanin** is a combination of natural hair color that contains both pheomelanin and eumelanin.

Contributing pigment, also known as *undertone*, is the varying degrees of warmth exposed during a permanent color or lightening process. Generally, when you lighten natural hair color, the darker the natural level, the more intense the contributing pigment. This must be taken into consideration before the haircolor selection is made. Haircoloring modifies this pigment to create new pigment.

The Level System

Level is the unit of measurement used to identify the lightness or darkness of a color. Level is the saturation, density, or concentration of color. The level of color answers the following question: How much color?

The **level system** is a system that colorists use to determine the lightness or darkness of a hair color (**figure 21-4**). Haircolor levels are arranged on a scale of 1 to 10, with 1 being the darkest and 10 the lightest. Although the names for the color levels may vary among manufacturers, the important thing is being able to identify the degrees of lightness to darkness (depth) in each level.

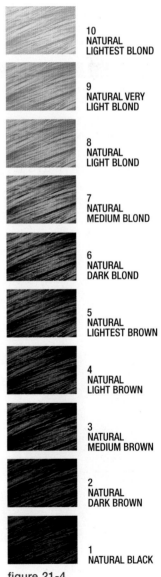

10 NATURAL LIGHTEST BLOND

9 NATURAL VERY LIGHT BLOND

8 NATURAL LIGHT BLOND

7 NATURAL MEDIUM BLOND

6 NATURAL DARK BLOND

5 NATURAL LIGHTEST BROWN

4 NATURAL LIGHT BROWN

3 NATURAL MEDIUM BROWN

2 NATURAL DARK BROWN

1 NATURAL BLACK

figure 21-4
Natural hair color levels

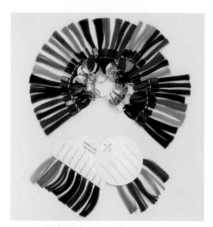

figure 21-5
Manufacturer's swatches are a useful tool.

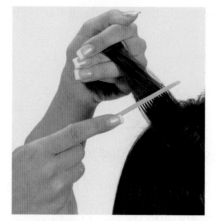

figure 21-6
Take a ½-inch (1.25 centimeters) square section in the crown.

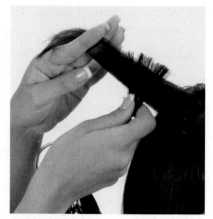

figure 21-7
Hold the color swatch against the hair strand.

Identifying Natural Level

Identifying natural level is the first step in performing a haircolor service. Your most valuable tool is the color wheel. Haircolor swatch books provide a visual representation as well (figure 21-5).

To determine the natural level, perform the following four steps:

1. Take a ½-inch (1.25 centimeters) square section in the crown area and hold it up from the scalp, allowing light to pass through (figure 21-6).

2. Using the natural level-finder swatches provided by the manufacturer, select a swatch that you think matches the section of hair and place it against the hair. Remember, you are trying to determine depth level (darkness or lightness). Do not part or hold the hair flat against the scalp; that will give you an incorrect reading, as the hair will appear darker (figure 21-7).

3. Move the swatch from the scalp area along the hair strand.

4. Determine the natural hair color level.

Identifying Level on Previously Colored Hair

When formulating haircolor, it is as important to be able to identify the level and tone of previously colored hair as it is identifying the natural level. Follow steps one and two above. However, instead of using the natural level finder, use the color swatches provided by the manufacturer.

Gray Hair

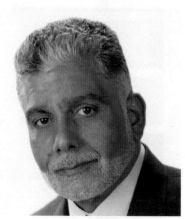

figure 21-8
Many people choose to cover or blend gray hair.

Gray hair is hair that has lost its pigment and is normally associated with aging. Even though the loss of pigment increases as a person ages, few people ever become completely gray-haired (figure 21-8). Most retain a certain percentage of pigmented hair (table 21-1). The gray can be solid or blended throughout the head as in salt-and-pepper hair. Gray hair requires special attention in formulating haircolor. This will be discussed later in the chapter.

table 21-1

DETERMINING THE PERCENTAGE OF GRAY HAIR

Percentage of Gray Hair	Characteristics	Level 5 Natural Hair	
30%	More pigmented than gray hair		Level 5 natural hair with 30% gray
50%	Even mixture of gray and pigmented hair		Level 5 natural hair with 50% gray
70 to 90%	More gray than pigmented; most of remaining pigment is located in the back of the head		Level 5 natural hair with 75% gray
100%	Virtually no pigmented hair; tends to look white		100% gray hair

Color Theory

Color is described as a property of objects that depends on the light they reflect and is perceived (by the human eye) as red, yellow, blue, or other shades. Thus, colors (the light reflected by objects that is perceivable) by definition are in the visible spectrum of light (see Chapter 13, Basics of Electricity). Before you attempt to apply haircoloring products, it is important to have a general understanding of color theory. A **base color** is the predominant tone of a color. Once you have a better understanding of color theory, you will see how each haircolor manufacturer associates base colors with color lines.

The Law of Color

The **law of color** is a system for understanding color relationships. When combining colors, you will always get the same result from the same combination. Equal parts of red and blue mixed together always make violet. Equal parts of blue and yellow always make green. Equal parts of red and yellow always make orange. The color wheels in figures 21-9 through 21-11 will help you understand colors.

COLOR WHEEL

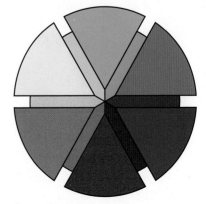

figure 21-9a
A standard color wheel

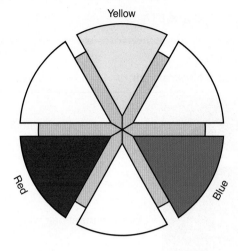

figure 21-9b
Primary colors

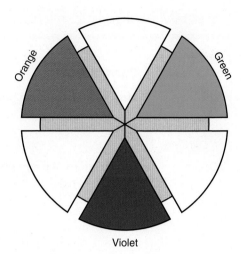

figure 21-10
Secondary colors

Primary Colors

Primary colors are pure or fundamental colors (red, yellow, and blue) that cannot be created by combining other colors. All colors are created from these three primaries. Colors with a predominance of blue are cool colors, whereas colors with a predominance of red and/or yellow are warm colors (figure 21-9a).

Blue is the strongest of the primary colors and is the only cool primary color. In addition to coolness, blue can also bring depth or darkness to any color.

Red is the medium primary color. Adding red to blue-based colors will make them appear lighter; adding red to yellow colors will cause them to appear darker.

Yellow is the weakest of the primary colors. When you add yellow to other colors, the resulting color will look lighter and brighter.

In traditional color theory, when all three primary colors are present in equal proportions, the resulting color is black or dark muddy gray depending on the saturation of the pigment. It is helpful to think of hair color in terms of different combinations of primary colors. Natural brown, for example, has the primary colors in the following proportions: blue-B, red-RR, and yellow-YYY. White can be used to lighten a color. Black can be used to deepen a color.

Secondary Colors

A **secondary color** is a color obtained by mixing equal parts of two primary colors. The secondary colors are green, orange, and violet. Green is an equal combination of blue and yellow. Orange is an equal combination of red and yellow. Violet is an equal combination of blue and red (figure 21-10).

Tertiary Colors

A **tertiary color** (TUR-shee-aye-eer KUL-ur) is an intermediate color achieved by mixing a secondary color and its neighboring primary color on the color wheel in equal amounts. The tertiary colors include blue-green, blue-violet, red-violet, red-orange, yellow-orange, and yellow-green. Natural-

TERTIARY COLORS

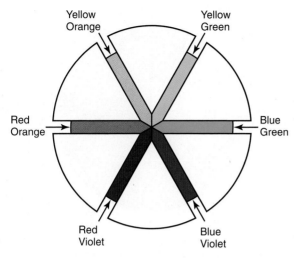

figure 21-11
Tertiary colors

ACTIVITY

Using primary-colored modeling clay—red, blue, and yellow—create secondary and tertiary colors. You will see that if you mix red clay with yellow clay in equal proportions, you will get orange. If you mix red clay with orange clay, what is the result? What happens if you change the proportion of each color? The combinations are endless (figure 21-12).

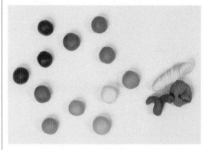

figure 21-12
Creating the color wheel with clay

looking haircolor is made up of a combination of primary colors, secondary colors, and tertiary colors (figure 21-11). When combined, the primary color is always the dominant color. For example, when yellow and orange are combined, the new color is called yellow-orange, not orange-yellow.

Complementary Colors

Complementary colors are primary and secondary colors positioned directly opposite each other on the color wheel. Complementary colors include blue and orange, red and green, and yellow and violet.

Complementary colors neutralize each other (figure 21-13a). When formulating haircolor, you will find that it is often your goal to emphasize or distract from skin tones or eye color. You may also want to neutralize or refine unwanted tones in the hair. Understanding complementary colors will help you choose the correct tone to accomplish these goals.

COLOR WHEEL

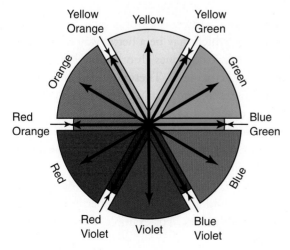

figure 21-13a
Complementary colors neutralize each other.

ACTIVITY

Use a plain sugar cookie to represent the color wheel. Use a dollop of vanilla frosting on a dish, along with red, blue, and yellow food coloring. Mix a small amount of frosting with each primary color. Place it on the (cookie) color wheel. Then mix the two primary colors together to make the secondary color. Continue until the color wheel is completed.

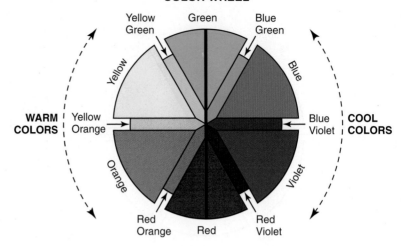

COLOR WHEEL

figure 21-13b
The color wheel divided to represent both warm and cool colors

Here is an easy reference guide for color correction:

- When hair is green...use red to balance.
- When hair is red...use green to balance.
- When hair is blue...use orange to balance.
- When hair is orange...use blue to balance.
- When hair is yellow...use violet to balance.
- When hair is violet...use yellow to balance.

Tone or Hue of Color

The **tone**, also known as *hue*, is the balance of color. The tone or hue answers the question of which color to use based on the client's desired results. These tones can be described as warm, cool, or neutral (figure 21-13b).

Because warm tones reflect more light, they can look lighter than their actual level. These tones are golden, orange, red, and yellow. Some haircolor haircolor manufacturers use words such as *auburn*, *amber*, *copper*, *strawberry*, and *bronze*, which may be a better way to discuss and describe haircolor with the client. Cool tones absorb more light, therefore they can look deeper than their actual level. These tones are blue, green, and violet. Some describe cool tones as smoky or ash to the client. Natural tones are warm tones and are described as sandy or tan.

Intensity refers to the strength of a color. It can be described as soft, medium, or strong. Color intensifiers are tones that can be added to a haircolor formula to intensify the result.

Base color is the predominant tone of a color. Each color is identified by a number and a letter. The number indicates the level and the letter indicates the tone. For example: 6G is level 6–Dark Blond with a G-Gold Base.

When you begin selecting a formula, you must have a good idea of what tones the client likes and dislikes.

Select warm base colors to create brighter colors such as red and gold tones. Select cooler base colors to keep the color result more ash, revealing less gold in the hair. Add a neutral base color to formulate haircolor that will soften and balance colors. Neutral base colors are often used to cover gray hair.

After reading the next few sections, you will be able to:

LO**7** List and describe the categories of haircolor.

Understand the Types of Haircolor

Haircoloring products generally fall into two categories: non-oxidative and oxidative. The classifications of non-oxidative haircolor are temporary and semipermanent (traditional). The classifications of oxidative haircolor are demipermanent (deposit only) and permanent (lift and deposit) (**table 21-2**). All of these products, except temporary color, require a patch test.

table 21-2

REVIEW OF HAIRCOLOR CLASSIFICATIONS AND THEIR USES

Classifications	Uses
Temporary haircolor	Creates fun, bold results and easily shampoos from the hair. Neutralizes yellow hair.
Semipermanent haircolor	Introduces a client to haircolor services. Adds subtle color results. Tones pre-lightened hair.
Demipermanent haircolor	Blends gray hair. Enhances natural color. Tones pre-lightened hair. Refreshes faded color. Filler in color correction.
Permanent haircolor	Changes existing haircolor. Covers gray. Creates bright or natural-looking haircolor changes.

Lighteners, metallic haircolors, and natural colors are also discussed in this chapter. Each of these categories has a unique chemical composition that, in turn, affects the final color result and how long it will last.

All permanent haircolor products and lighteners contain both a developer, or oxidizing agent, and an alkalizing ingredient (See Chapter 12, Basics of Chemistry). The roles of the alkalizing ingredient—ammonia or an ammonia substitute—are as follows:

- Raise the cuticle of the hair so that the haircolor can penetrate into the cortex.

- Increase the penetration of dye within the hair.

- Trigger the lightening action of peroxide.

When the haircolor containing the alkalizing ingredient is combined with the developer (usually hydrogen peroxide), the peroxide becomes alkaline and decomposes, or breaks up. Lightening occurs when the alkaline peroxide breaks up or decolorizes the melanin.

Temporary Haircolors

Temporary haircolors are non-oxidation colors that make only a physical change, not a chemical change, in the hair shaft, and no patch test is required. Because this nonpermanent color has large pigment molecules that do not penetrate the cuticle layer, only a coating of color is deposited which may be removed by shampooing. This form of haircolor may be used in several different situations. For those who wish to neutralize yellow hair or unwanted tones, temporary haircolor is a good choice (figure 21-14). Also, if a person is allergic to aniline colors, this could be an alternative for that client.

Temporary haircolors are available in the following variety of colors and products:

- Color rinses applied weekly to shampooed hair to add color; the hair is styled dry.

- Colored mousses and gels used for slight color and for dramatic effects.

- Hair mascara used for dramatic effects.

- Spray-on haircolor that is easy to apply; used for special effects.

- Color-enhancing shampoos used to brighten, impart slight color, and eliminate unwanted tones.

Semipermanent Haircolor

Traditional **semipermanent haircolor** is a no-lift, deposit-only, non-oxidation haircolor that is not mixed with peroxide and is formulated to last through several shampoos, depending on the hair's porosity. The pigment molecules are small enough to partially penetrate the hair shaft and stain the cuticle layer, but they are small enough to diffuse out of the hair during shampooing, thus fading with each shampoo. Traditional semipermanent haircolor only lasts four to six weeks, depending on how frequently the hair is shampooed. Semipermanent haircolor is a non-oxidation haircolor. It is not

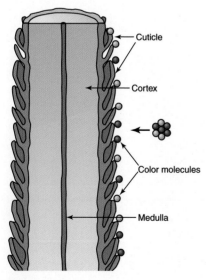

figure 21-14
Action of temporary haircolor

mixed with peroxide, and it only deposits color. It does not lighten the hair, so it does not require maintenance of new growth. Although it is considered gentler than permanent haircolor, it contains some of the same dyes and requires a patch test 24 to 48 hours before application (figure 21-15). Traditional semipermanent colors are used right out of the bottle.

Demipermanent Haircolor

Demipermanent haircolor, also known as *no-lift, deposit-only color*, is formulated to deposit but not lighten color. These products are able to deposit without lifting because they are usually less alkaline (or even acid based) than permanent colors and are mixed with a low-volume developer. Decolorization requires a high pH and a high concentration of peroxide.

Many demipermanent colors use alkalizing agents other than ammonia and oxidizing agents other than hydrogen peroxide. It is important to note that these products are not necessarily any less damaging because of the type of alkalizing agent or oxidizer that is used. If they are milder, it is because the concentration of these active ingredients is lower. A **haircolor glaze** is a common way to describe a haircolor service that adds shine and color to the hair. The word *glaze* is a cosmetic word used to describe the services listed below that can be achieved by using a deposit-only or no-lift color.

Demipermanent haircolors are ideal for the following objectives:

- Introducing a client to a color service (because these products create a change in tone without lightening the natural hair color. They also gently fade so there is typically no line of demarcation as the hair grows.)

- Blending or covering gray.

- Refreshing faded permanent color on the mid-shaft and ends.

- Making color corrections and restoring natural color.

By their very nature, demipermanent haircolors deepen or create a change in tone on the natural hair color (figure 21-16). In recent years, demipermanent haircolors have been used exclusively on the middle of the hair shaft to the ends after permanent color has been applied to the new growth or scalp area. This method of application refreshes the previously colored hair.

Demipermanent haircolor is available as a gel, cream, or liquid. It requires a patch test 24 to 48 hours before application.

Permanent Haircolor

Permanent haircolors lighten and deposit color at the same time and in a single process because they are more alkaline than demipermanent colors and are usually mixed with a higher-volume developer.

Permanent haircolor is used to match, lighten, and cover gray hair. Permanent haircolor products require a patch test 24 to 48 hours before application.

Permanent haircolors contain uncolored dye precursors, which are very small and can easily penetrate into the hair shaft. These dye precursors, called **aniline derivatives** (AN-ul-un DUR-ive-it-ives), contain small,

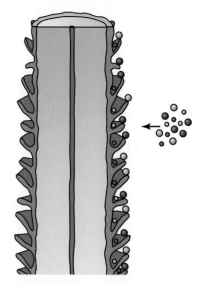

figure 21-15
Action of semipermanent haircolor

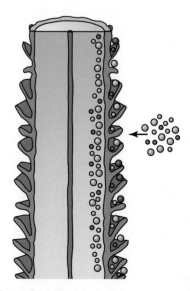

figure 21-16
Action of demipermanent haircolor

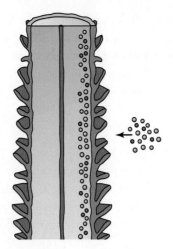

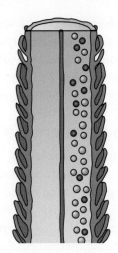

figure 21-17
Action of permanent haircolor

figure 21-18
Permanent haircolor molecules
inside the cortex

uncolored dyes that combine with hydrogen peroxide to form larger, permanent dye molecules within the cortex. These molecules are trapped within the cortex of the hair and cannot be easily shampooed out (**figures 21-17** and **21-18**). Permanent haircolors can also lighten (make a permanent change in) the natural hair color, which is why these products are considered permanent.

A technique called a **soap cap** is a combination of equal parts of a prepared permanent color mixture and shampoo used during the last five minutes of a haircolor service and worked through the hair to refresh the ends.

Permanent haircoloring products are regarded as the best products for covering gray hair. They remove natural pigment from the hair through lightening, while at the same time adding artificial color to the hair. The action of removing and adding color at the same time, which blends gray and non-gray hair uniformly, results in a natural-looking color.

Natural and Metallic Haircolors

Haircolors that are not generally used in the salon, but which you should still be familiar with, are natural or vegetable haircolors and metallic haircolors. Metallic haircolors are also referred to as *gradual colors*. Repeated use of these types of color can create a buildup on the hair causing a grayish or green cast and restrict the application of any chemical service.

Natural Haircolors

Natural haircolors, also known as *vegetable haircolors*, such as henna, are colors obtained from the leaves or bark of plants. They do not lighten natural hair color. The color result tends to be weak, and the process tends to be lengthy and messy. Also, shade ranges are limited. For instance, henna is usually available only in clear, black, chestnut, and auburn tones. Because natural haircolors work by staining the cuticle of the hair shaft, a client who has used natural haircolor may be distressed to find out that many of these chemical products cannot be applied over natural haircolors.

Metallic Haircolor

Metallic haircolors, also known as *progressive haircolors*, are haircolors containing metal salts that change hair color gradually by progressive buildup and exposure to air, creating a dull, metallic appearance. These products require frequent applications and historically have been marketed to men. The main problems are unnatural-looking colors with limited range of colors available and metallic haircolors restrict the application of any chemical service being done on the hair.

> ⚠️ **CAUTION**
> Do not use oxidizing haircolor or haircolor with peroxide on hair that has been treated with metallic hair dye. If you do, the hair will swell and smoke, appearing to be boiling from the inside out.

After reading the next few sections, you will be able to:

LO⑧ Explain the role of hydrogen peroxide in a haircolor formula.

LO⑧ Explain the action of hair lighteners.

Hydrogen Peroxide Developers

A **hydrogen peroxide developer** is an oxidizing agent that, when mixed with an oxidation haircolor, supplies the necessary oxygen gas to develop the color molecules and create a change in natural hair color. **Developers**, also known as *oxidizing agents* or *catalysts*, have a pH between 2.5 and 4.5. Although there are a number of developers on the market, hydrogen peroxide (H_2O_2) is the one most commonly used in haircolor. Keep in mind, there are different forms of peroxide. There are clear liquids that make it easy to apply the product from an applicator bottle. There are cream forms that are used to make a thicker creamy consistency, sometimes for bowl and brush application. Some manufacturers provide dedicated developers that are used with their own specific haircolor products.

Volume measures the concentration and strength of hydrogen peroxide. The lower the volume, the less lift achieved; the higher the volume, the greater the lifting action (**table 21-3**). The majority of permanent haircolor

table 21-3

HYDROGEN PEROXIDE VOLUME AND USES

Volume	When to Use
10-Volume	Used to deposit color or, when less lift is desired, to enhance a client's natural hair color.
20-Volume	Standard volume; will give up to two levels of lift; is used to achieve most results with permanent haircolor and used for complete gray coverage.
30-Volume	Used for additional lift, up to 3 levels, with permanent haircolor.
40-Volume	Up to four levels of lift with standard hair color. Used with most high-lift colors; provides maximum lift in a one-step color service.

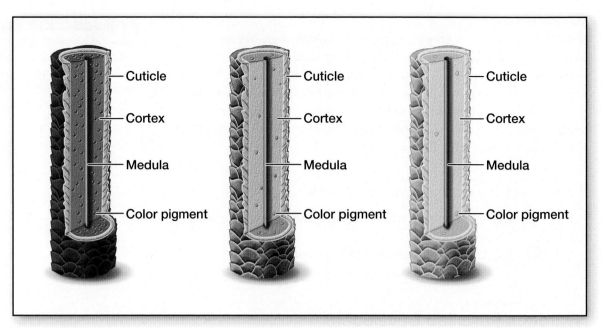

figure 21-19
Haircolor lighteners diffuse pigment.

products use 10-, 20-, 30-, or 40-volume hydrogen peroxide for proper lift and color development (**figure 21-19**). Store peroxide in a cool, dark, dry place.

Volume

Use 10-volume peroxide when less lightening is desired. Use 20-volume peroxide with permanent haircolor, as well as for complete gray coverage. For additional lift, use 30-volume peroxide; and to provide maximum lift in a one-step color service, use 40-volume peroxide.

Lighteners

Lighteners are chemical compounds that lighten hair by dispersing, dissolving, and decolorizing the natural hair pigment. As soon as hydrogen peroxide is mixed into the lightener formula, it begins to release oxygen. This is known as oxidation, a process by which oxygen is released, and it occurs within the cortex of the hair shaft. To achieve a very light, pale blond, it is recommended that you use a **double-process application**, also known as *two-step coloring*, which is a coloring technique requiring two separate procedures in which the hair is pre-lightened before the depositing color is applied. This service includes using a lightener. These products are designed to process up to 90 minutes on the scalp to achieve the desired lift. Once the hair is properly decolorized, the second step is to add soft tone back to the hair, called the toning process. There are products called toners designed in a very light shade palette to add tone to the decolorized hair. Demipermanent colors in a light level, such as a level 8 (Light Blond) to level 10 (Lightest Blond), are also used to tone hair.

Hair lighteners are used to create a light blond shade that is not achievable with permanent haircolor alone, as well as to accomplish the following objectives:

- Lighten the hair prior to application of a final color.

- Lighten hair to a particular shade.

- Brighten and lighten an existing shade.

- Lighten only certain parts of the hair.

- Lighten dark natural or color-treated levels.

- Lighten previously colored hair.

- Lighten hair without simultaneously depositing color.

The Decolorizing Process

The hair goes through different stages of color as it lightens. The amount of change depends on the amount of pigment in the hair, the strength of the lightening product, and the length of time that the product is processed. During the process of decolorizing, natural hair can go through as many as 10 stages (figure 21-20).

Decolorizing the hair's natural melanin pigment allows the colorist to create the exact degree of contributing pigment needed for the final result. Contributing pigment is the varying degree of warmth exposed during the lightening process. First, the hair is decolorized to the appropriate level. Then the new color is applied to deposit the desired color. The natural pigment that remains in the hair contributes to the artificial color that is added. Lightening the hair to the correct stage is essential to a beautiful, controlled, final haircoloring result (figure 21-21).

Toners are traditional semipermanent, demipermanent, and permanent haircolor products that are used primarily on pre-lightened hair to achieve pale and delicate colors. Toners can also be used after dimensional haircolor services. After a highlight service is completed using a lightener, you can tone the hair to create a softer shade of blond. Once the lightener is rinsed, simply towel dry and apply the desired shade of toner over the pre-lightened hair. This will take up to five minutes for the result.

Not all hair will go through all 10 degrees of decolorization. Each natural hair color starts the decolorization process at a different stage. Remember, the goal is to create the correct degree of contributing pigment as the foundation for the final haircolor.

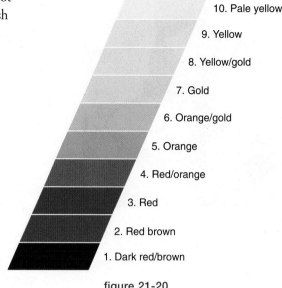

figure 21-20
Ten degrees of decolorization

10. Pale yellow
9. Yellow
8. Yellow/gold
7. Gold
6. Orange/gold
5. Orange
4. Red/orange
3. Red
2. Red brown
1. Dark red/brown

figure 21-21
Level/contributing pigment

      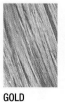 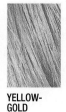 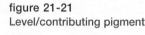

DARK RED-BROWN   RED-BROWN   RED   RED-ORANGE   ORANGE   ORANGE-GOLD   GOLD   YELLOW-GOLD   YELLOW   PALE YELLOW

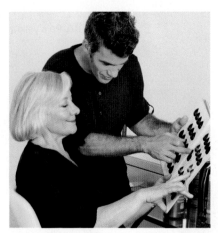

figure 21-22
A client consultation should precede every haircolor service.

Hair cannot be safely lifted past the pale yellow stage with lightener. The extreme diffusion of color necessary to give hair a white appearance causes excessive damage to the hair. The result is that when wet, the hair feels mushy and will stretch without returning to its original length. When dry, the hair is harsh and brittle. Such hair often suffers breakage and will not accept a toner properly. However, this does not mean that only those born with blond hair can be white-blonds. The baby-blond look can be achieved by lightening to pale yellow and neutralizing the unwanted undertone (contributing pigment) with a toner.

Conduct an Effective Haircolor Consultation

A haircolor consultation is the most critical part of the color service (figure 21-22). The consultation is the first important step in establishing a relationship with your client and ensuring you are set up for success. During the consultation, your client will communicate what he or she is looking for in a haircolor service. You will listen carefully, taking in all the information so that you can make an appropriate haircolor recommendation. Allowing sufficient time for the consultation is the single most reliable way to help ensure a client's satisfaction.

See Chapter 4, Communicating for Success, to review and begin the consultation process. As a refresher, incorporate the following steps when conducting a haircolor consultation:

1. Book 15 minutes extra for the consultation with a first time guest. Introduce yourself to the client and welcome him or her to the salon. Give a salon tour. Offer a beverage. During this time with a new client, make sure there are no interruptions.

2. Have the client fill out a client intake form. This allows you to compile a hair history and to note the type of color service the client is looking for. Most salon software programs allow a client profile where you can enter your formulas or special notes about your guest. If the salon does not use a software program, then a haircolor service record card (figure 21-23) is used to document pertinent information on each client. You can also use the service record card to document notes before transcribing them into the online software program after the client leaves. Pay attention to the client's skin and eye color, the condition and length of the client's hair, and the amount of gray in the client's hair.

3. Begin the consultation in an area with proper lighting so that you can accurately determine the client's current hair color. If possible, the walls should be white or neutral.

4. Look at the client directly. Do not look at him or her through the mirror. Ask what the client is thinking about doing with their hair color. Ask questions that require an answer other than yes or no. Encourage the client to talk. Keep the client on track by discussing

> **⚠ CAUTION**
> It is often difficult to lighten dark hair to a very pale blond without causing extreme damage to the hair. The client should be alerted to this danger before you proceed with the service.

> **⚠ CAUTION**
> Medications can affect hair color. In the consultation, determine whether the client is taking any medications. Medical treatments for conditions such as diabetes, high blood pressure, and thyroid problems may all affect the outcome of color services and most other chemical services. Discuss this with your instructor for more information.

HAIRCOLOR SERVICE RECORD CARD

Name _____   Tel. _____

Address _____   City _____

Patch Test: ☐ Negative ☐ Positive   Date _____

Eye Color _____   Skin Tone _____

DESCRIPTION OF HAIR

Form	Length	Texture	Density	Porosity	
☐ straight	☐ short	☐ coarse	☐ low	☐ low	☐ resistant
☐ wavy	☐ medium	☐ medium	☐ medium	☐ average	☐ very resistant
☐ curly	☐ long	☐ fine	☐ high	☐ high	☐ perm. waved

Natural hair color _____

Level	Tone	Intensity
(1-10)	(Warm, Cool, etc.)	(Mild, Medium, Strong)

Scalp Condition

☐ normal   ☐ dry   ☐ oily   ☐ sensitive

Condition

☐ normal   ☐ dry   ☐ oily   ☐ faded   ☐ streaked (uneven)

% unpigmented _____ Distribution of unpigmented _____

Previously lightened with _____ for _____ (time)

Previously tinted with _____ for _____ (time)

☐ original hair sample enclosed   ☐ original hair sample not enclosed

Desired hair color _____

Level	Tone	Intensity
(1-10)	(Warm, Cool, etc.)	(Mild, Medium, Strong)

CORRECTIVE TREATMENTS

Color filler used _____ Conditioning treatments with _____

HAIR TINTING PROCESS

whole head _____ retouch inches (cm) _____ shade desired _____

formula: (color/lightener) _____ application technique _____

Results: ☐ good   ☐ poor   ☐ too light   ☐ too dark   ☐ streaked

Comments: _____

_____

_____

_____

_____

Date	Operator	Price	Date	Operator	Price

figure 21-23
Haircolor service record card

the recent history of his or her hair (over the past six months); remember haircolor history goes back as far as the length of their hair. Hair that is below the shoulder has years of history. Your questions might include the following:

- Are you looking for a temporary or permanent change?
- Do you want color all over or just a few highlights?
- Do you see yourself with a more conservative or dramatic type of color?
- Have you seen so-and-so's (e.g., a TV celebrity) hair? That color would look great on you.
- Do you have any pictures of hair color you like or hair color you don't like?
- Have you ever colored your hair before? When was the last time you colored it?
- How much money do you want to spend on haircolor today?
- Have you had any other chemical services on your hair like a relaxer or keratin treatment? If so, when?
- When you leave the room, do you want your friends to describe you as a blond, a brunette, or a red head?
- How often do you want to be in the salon? Every two weeks or twice a year?

5. Recommend at least two different haircolor options, and always offer the client more than what he or she is asking for. Show pictures of different ranges of colors, from brunette to blond, red, and highlighted colors. Review the procedure and application technique, cost of the service, and follow-up maintenance. Sometimes several steps may be necessary to obtain a haircolor result. A client may love a certain hair color, but may not be able to afford the service. Have a more economical backup solution ready.

6. Be honest and do not promise more than you can deliver. If you are faced with a corrective situation, let the client know what you can accomplish today and how many more visits it will take to achieve the final results that he or she wants.

7. Gain approval from the client.

8. Start the haircolor service.

9. Follow through during the service by educating and informing the client about home care, products, and rebooking. Let the client know what type of shampoo and conditioner is needed to maintain the color. Let the client know how many weeks it will be before they need to come back for another service.

10. Finish completing the client's haircolor service record card (or as part of the client's profile using the salon software program).

Release Statement

A release statement is used by schools and many salons when providing chemical services. Its purpose is to explain to clients that there is a risk

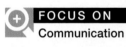

FOCUS ON
Communication

The language you use when discussing haircolor can have a huge impact on how a client perceives haircolor services. Using positive descriptive language to discuss products and services with your clients is an important part of the communication process, and it helps you sell your services. Here are some guidelines:

- Use descriptive language when discussing haircolor (e.g., *soft, buttery blond*; *rich chocolate brown*; *spicy, coppery red*).
- Use positive mood words to convey the benefits of haircoloring to your client (e.g., *sexy, healthy-looking, richer, natural-looking*, and *subtle*).
- Avoid words that can be interpreted negatively such as *bleached, frosted*, and *roots*.

involved in any chemical service and that if the client's hair is in questionable condition, it may not withstand the requested chemical treatment. It also asks that clients provide more information about any prior chemical services that may affect the current color selection and its end result.

To some degree, the release statement is designed to protect the school or salon from responsibility for accidents or damages. A release statement is required for most malpractice insurance. Take note, however, that a release statement is not a legally binding contract and will not clear the cosmetologist of responsibility for what may happen to a client's hair (figure 21-24). If you are unsure about causing excessive damage to the hair, it is wise to decline to perform the service.

figure 21-24
Release form

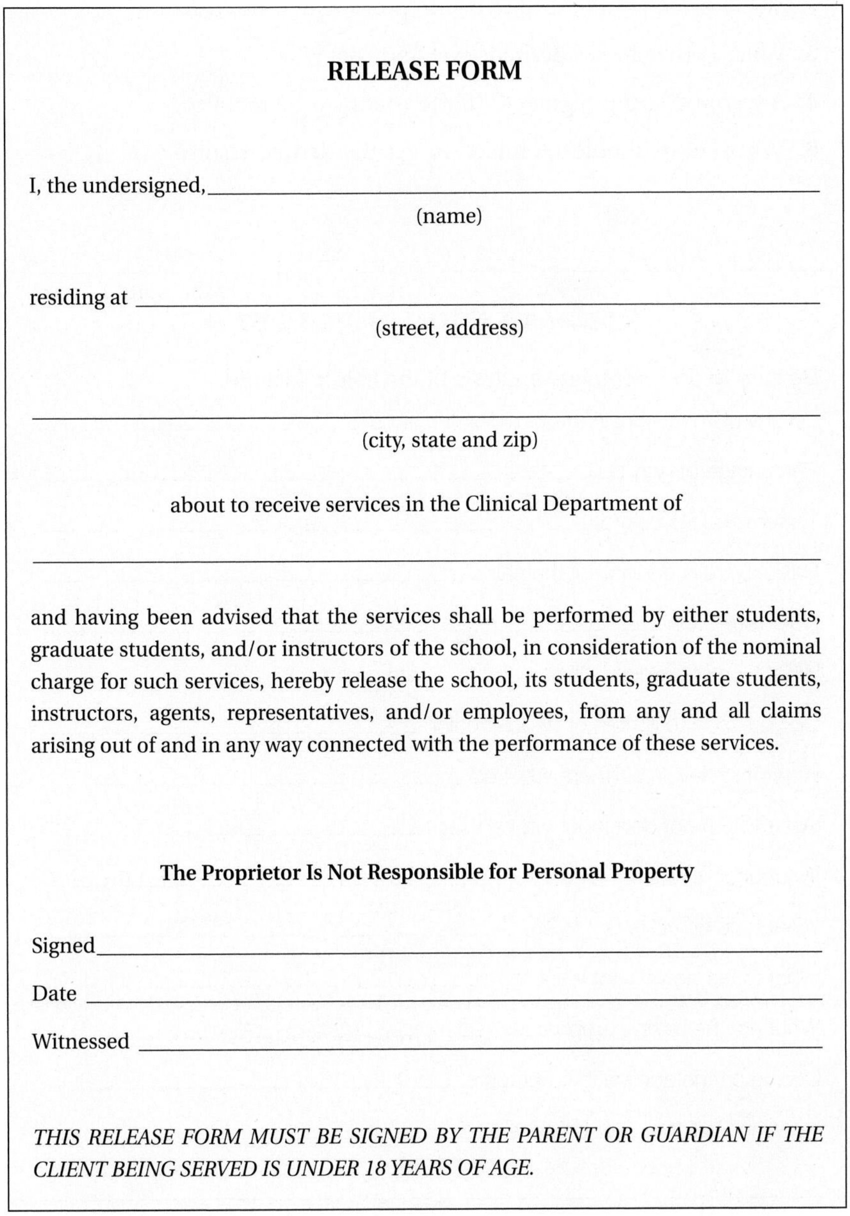

RELEASE FORM

I, the undersigned,_____
(name)

residing at _____
(street, address)

_____
(city, state and zip)

about to receive services in the Clinical Department of

_____

and having been advised that the services shall be performed by either students, graduate students, and/or instructors of the school, in consideration of the nominal charge for such services, hereby release the school, its students, graduate students, instructors, agents, representatives, and/or employees, from any and all claims arising out of and in any way connected with the performance of these services.

The Proprietor Is Not Responsible for Personal Property

Signed_____

Date _____

Witnessed _____

THIS RELEASE FORM MUST BE SIGNED BY THE PARENT OR GUARDIAN IF THE CLIENT BEING SERVED IS UNDER 18 YEARS OF AGE.

After reading the next few sections, you will be able to:

LO ⑩ List the five key questions to ask when formulating a haircolor.

LO ⑪ Understand why a patch test is useful in haircoloring.

Formulate Haircolor

Haircolor formulation is another important aspect of creating a successful haircolor. There are five basic questions that must always be asked when formulating a haircolor. Refer to the additional formulation checklist to cover more details (**figure 21-25**).

1. What is the natural level, and does it include gray hair?
2. What is the level and tone of the previously colored hair?
3. What is the client's desired level and tone?
4. Are contributing pigments (undertones) to be revealed?
5. What colors should be mixed to get the desired result?

FORMULATION CHECKLIST

Be sure to do a complete analysis of the hair to include:

Level and Tone – scalp area, mid-shaft, ends _____

Percentage of gray _____

Texture and Porosity _____

Basic overall condition of the hair _____

Color Selection _____

What type of product will be used to create end result _____

Do you need to lighten or deposit color _____

How many levels of lift are required _____

What volume of developer will be used _____

What undertones are present _____

What tone do you want to see _____

What tones do you not want to see _____

What are the mixing proportions _____

Decide on the application method _____

How long will the color process _____

figure 21-25
Formulation checklist

The combination of the shade selected and the volume of hydrogen peroxide determines the deposit and lifting ability of a haircolor. Always remember to formulate with both lift and deposit in mind in order to achieve the proper balance for the desired end result. A higher-lifting formula, however, may not have enough deposit to cancel the warmth of a client's natural contributing pigment. The volume of hydrogen peroxide mixed with the haircolor product will also influence the lift and deposit.

Mixing Permanent Colors

Your method of mixing permanent colors is determined by the type of application you are using. Permanent color is applied by either the more professional bowl and brush method or the applicator bottle (always follow the manufacturer's directions) (**figures 21-26a** and **21-26b**).

- **Applicator bottle.** Be sure that the applicator bottle is large enough to hold both the color and developer, with enough air space to shake the bottle until the mixture is thoroughly mixed. By lightly squeezing the bottle and covering the top with your finger before shaking, you will prevent color from escaping the bottle after mixing. For a 1:1 ratio, pour 1 ounce of the color into the bottle, add 1 ounce (30 milliliters) of developer, put the top on the bottle, and shake gently. For a 1:2 ratio, pour 1 ounce (30 milliliters) of the color into the bottle, add 2 ounces (60 milliliters) of developer, and mix. The latter ratio is for most permanent high-lift blond colors (**figure 21-27**).

- **Brush and bowl.** Use a nonmetallic mixing bowl. Measure and add the developer into the bowl. Add the color or colors you have selected in the appropriate proportions. Using a plastic whisk or an applicator brush, stir the mixture until it is blended (**figure 21-28**).

Patch Test

When working with haircolor, you must determine whether your clients have any allergies or sensitivities to the mixture. To identify an allergy in a client, the U.S. Food, Drug, and Cosmetic Act requires that a patch test be given 24 to 48 hours prior to each application of an aniline haircolor. A **patch test**, also known as *predisposition test*, is a test for identifying a possible allergy in a client. The color used for the patch test must be the same as the color that will be used for the haircolor service (i.e., if a person is having her or his hair colored with a level 5 with brown and red tones, use that same shade in the patch test). Procedure 21-1 for patch tests should be closely followed.

A negative skin test will show no sign of inflammation and indicates that the color may be safely applied. A positive result will show redness and a slight rash or welt. A client with these symptoms is allergic, and under no circumstances should she receive a haircolor service with the haircolor tested.

Ⓟ 21-1 **Performing a Patch Test** *See page 710*

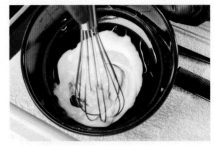

figure 21-26a
Haircolor can be mixed in an applicator bottle or bowl.

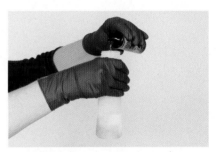

figure 21-26b
Haircolor can be mixed in an applicator bottle or bowl.

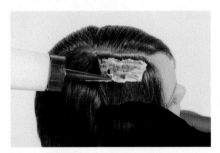

figure 21-27
Applicator bottle

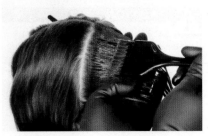

figure 21-28
Application brush and bowl

After reading the next few sections, you will be able to:

LO⓬ Define what a preliminary strand test is and why it is used.

LO⓭ List and describe the procedure for a virgin single-process color service.

LO⓮ Understand the two processes involved in double-process haircoloring.

milady pro ™ **LEARN MORE!**

Optional information on **Haircoloring** can be found at miladypro.com Keyword: *FutureCosPro*

Apply Haircolor

To ensure successful results when performing haircoloring services, the colorist must follow a prescribed procedure and never leave the client unattended while the haircolor is processing. The best color results come from being involved from beginning to end! A clearly defined system makes for the greatest efficiency and the safest and most satisfactory results. Without such a plan, the work will take longer, results will be uneven, and mistakes may be made.

Preliminary Strand Test

Once you have created a color formula for your client, try it out first on a small strand of hair. This preliminary **strand test** determines how the hair will react to the color formula and how long the formula should be left on the hair. The strand test is performed after the client is prepared for the coloring service.

Ⓟ 21-2 **Preliminary Strand Test** *See page 712*

Temporary Colors

There are many methods of applying a temporary color, depending on the product used. Your instructor will help you interpret each manufacturer's directions. One method of applying temporary haircolor is outlined in Procedure 21-3. You may apply colored gels, mousses, foams, or sprays at your workstation after your client has been shampooed. Always use and apply these color products according to the manufacturer's directions.

Ⓟ 21-3 **Temporary Haircolor Application** *See page 714*

Semipermanent Haircolors

Because semipermanent colors do not contain the oxidizers necessary to lift, they only deposit color and do not lighten color. When selecting a semipermanent color, remember that color applied on top of existing color always creates a deeper color and alters the tone.

The porosity of the hair will determine how well these products saturate the hair. Because they are deposit-only, traditional semipermanent colors can build up on the hair ends with repeated applications. A strand test will help determine the formula and processing time before the service.

⚠ **CAUTION**

Colorist dermatitis involves the same types of negative reactions to products as those a client may experience. Since a colorist's hands are in contact with chemical solutions repeatedly during an average day, it is important to take proper precautions. Protect yourself from adverse reactions by wearing gloves until the haircolor product is completely removed from the client's hair.

Demipermanent Haircolor

Demipermanent haircolor is a great way to introduce clients to a color service and to enhance their natural hair color in one easy step.

The application procedure for demipermanent haircolor is similar to that of a traditional semipermanent color, since neither process alters the hair's natural melanin or produces lift. Follow the manufacturer's guidelines for application and processing time for the product you have selected.

Gray hair presents special challenges when formulating demipermanent haircolor. Because there is no lift, the resulting depth of color when covering gray hair may appear too harsh unless you allow for some brightness and warmth in your formulation. Selecting a shade that is one level lighter than the natural color is recommended, so that the gray hair looks somewhat highlighted against the natural color. This will deliver a more natural-looking result.

Hair that has previously received a color service will have a greater degree of porosity, which must also be taken into consideration when formulating and applying a demipermanent haircolor.

P 21-4   **Demipermanent Haircolor Application** *See page 716*

Single-Process Permanent Color

Single-process haircoloring lightens and deposits color in a single application. Examples of single-process coloring are virgin color applications and color retouch applications. A **virgin application** refers to the first time the hair is colored. Pre-lightening or pre-softening is not required with these applications.

P 21-5   Single-Process Color on Virgin Hair *See page 718*

Single-Process Color Retouch

As the hair grows, you will need to apply haircolor to the new growth to keep it looking attractive and to avoid a two-toned effect. This is called a retouch.

The procedure provided for applying color to new growth and to refresh faded ends also includes the application of a **glaze**, a non-ammonia color that adds shine and tone to the hair. For both applications, follow

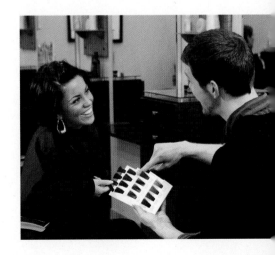

the same preparation steps as for the virgin single-process procedure, including a consultation and patch test.

Ⓟ 21-6 **Permanent Single-Process Retouch with a Glaze** *See page 720*

Steps for applying color to new growth and faded ends:

1. Apply color to the new growth only, being careful not to overlap on previously colored hair. Overlapping can cause breakage and a **line of demarcation**, which is the visible line separating colored hair from new growth.

2. Process color according to your analysis and strand test results.

3. Bringing permanent haircolor through the ends to refresh faded color can cause unnecessary damage to the hair, Instead formulate a demipermanent haircolor for the ends to match the new growth. Work the demipermanent color through to the ends. Then shampoo and condition. Remember that the same color formula used with different volumes of peroxide will produce different results.

Double-Process Haircolor

First, let us discuss the process of **hair lightening**, also known as *bleaching* or *decolorizing*, which is a chemical process involving the diffusion of the natural hair color pigment or artificial haircolor from the hair.

If the client asks for a dramatically lighter color (more than 4 levels), the hair has to be pre-lightened first. Also, to achieve pale or cool colors, it is sometimes more efficient to use a double-process application. By first decolorizing the hair with a lightener and then using a separate product to deposit the desired tone, you will have more control over the coloring process.

Double-process, high-lift coloring, also known as *two-step blonding*, is a technique to create light-blond hair in two steps. The hair is pre-lightened first and then toned. **Pre-lightening** is the first step of double-process haircoloring, used to lift or lighten the natural pigment before the application of toner.

Because the lightening action and the deposit of color are independent of each other, a wider range of haircolor is possible.

You may find that the contributing pigment of the hair can help you in a double-process color application. By pre-lightening the hair to the desired color, you can create a perfect foundation for longer-lasting red colors that avoid muddiness and stay true to tone.

The pre-lightener is applied in the same manner as a regular hair lightening treatment (see the following section). Once the pre-lightening has reached the desired shade, the hair is lightly shampooed, acidified, and towel dried. After a strand test has been taken, the color is then applied in the usual manner.

Using an applicator brush, stir the lightener until it is thoroughly mixed. A creamy consistency provides the best control during application.

Ⓟ 21-7 **Lightening Virgin Hair** *See page 722*

Show How to Use Lighteners

Colorists can choose from three forms of lighteners: oil, cream, and powder. Oil and cream lighteners are considered **on-the-scalp lighteners**, which are lighteners that can be used directly on the scalp by mixing the lightener with activators. New technology has created powder lighteners that can also be used directly on the scalp. Each type has its unique chemical characteristics and formulation procedures. Refer to the manufacturer's directions for best results.

On-the-Scalp Lighteners

Cream, oil, and some powder lighteners are used on-the-scalp because they are easy to apply. Oil lighteners are the mildest type, appropriate when only one or two levels of lift are desired. Because they are so mild, they are also used professionally to lighten dark facial and body hair.

Cream lighteners are strong enough for high-lift blonding, but gentle enough to be used on the scalp. They have the following features and benefits:

- Conditioning agents give some protection to the hair and scalp.

- Thickeners give more control during application.

- Because cream lighteners do not run or drip, overlapping is prevented during retouching services. Cream lighteners may be mixed with activators in the form of dry crystals.

Activators, also known as *boosters*, *protinators*, or *accelerators*, are powdered persulfate salts added to haircolor to increase its lightening ability. Activators are used in powdered off-the-scalp hair lighteners. They are also added to hydrogen peroxide to increase its lifting power. The more activators you use, the lighter the hair will be. Make sure to mix activators according to manufacturer's directions. Each company is different and formulas and strengths will vary from brand to brand. Also keep in mind, activators may increase scalp irritation.

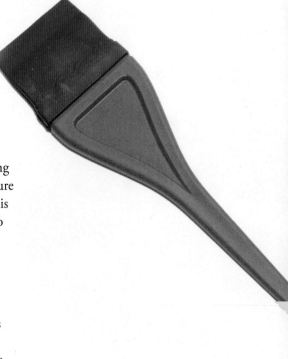

Powdered Off-the-Scalp Lighteners

Off-the-scalp lighteners, also known as *quick lighteners*, are powdered lighteners that cannot be used directly on the scalp. Powdered lighteners are strong, fast-acting lighteners in powdered form. Some powders are designed for on-scalp, double-process blonding. There are other powders that are specifically designed for off-scalp use.

Powdered off-the-scalp lighteners contain persulfate salts for quicker and stronger lightening. They may dry out more quickly than other types of lighteners, but they do not run or drip. Most powder lighteners expand and spread out as processing continues.

Time Factors

Processing time for lightening is affected by the factors listed below:

- The darker the natural hair color, the more melanin it has. The more melanin it has, the longer it takes to lighten the color.

- The amount of time needed to lighten the natural color is also influenced by the hair's porosity. Porous hair of the same color level will lighten faster than hair that is nonporous because the lightening agent can enter the cortex more rapidly.

- Tone influences the length of time necessary to lighten the natural hair color. The greater the percentage of red reflected in the natural color, the more difficult it is to achieve the delicate shades of a pale blond. Ash blonds are especially difficult to achieve because the melanin must be diffused sufficiently to alter both the level and tone of the hair.

- The strength of the lightening product affects the speed and amount of lightening. Stronger lighteners produce pale shades in the fastest time.

- Heat leads to faster lightening. But the stages of lightening must be carefully observed to avoid excessive lift. Excess lift could diffuse so much natural pigment that the toner may not produce the desired color. When this occurs, the toner may absorb too much color or *grab*, giving the hair an unwanted ashy, cool tone.

Preliminary Strand Test

Perform a preliminary strand test prior to lightening in order to determine the processing time, the condition of the hair after lightening, and the end results. Watch the strand carefully for its reaction to the lightening mixture, especially noting any discoloration or breakage. Reconditioning may be required prior to toning. If the color and condition are good, you can proceed with the lightening service. Carefully record all data on the client's service record card, and file it for future use.

If the test shows that the hair is not light enough, increase the strength of the mixture and/or increase the processing time. If the hair strand is too light, decrease the strength of the mixture and/or decrease the processing time.

A patch test must be taken 24 to 48 hours prior to each application of a toner containing aniline derivatives.

Lightener Retouch

New growth is the part of the hair shaft between the scalp and the hair that has been previously colored. New growth will become obvious as the hair grows. When performing a retouch, always lighten the new growth first. The procedure for a lightener retouch is the same as that for lightening a virgin head of hair, except that the mixture is applied only

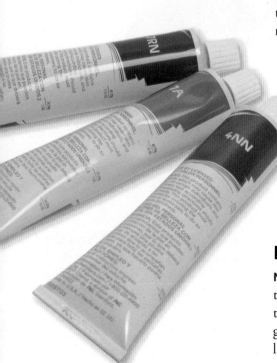

to the new growth as long as that growth is ½ inch (1.25 centimeters) long or less. A cream lightener is generally used for a lightener retouch because it is less irritating to the scalp and its consistency helps prevent overlapping of previously lightened hair. Overlapping can cause severe breakage and lines of demarcation.

Always consult the client's haircolor service record card for information about which lightener formulas have been used in the past, timing, and other matters.

After reading the next few sections, you will be able to:

LO⑯ **Understand the purpose and use of toners.**

Express How to Use Toners

Toners are used primarily on pre-lightened hair to achieve pale, delicate colors. They require a double-process application. The first process is the application of the lightener; the second process is the application of the toner. No-lift, demipermanent haircolors are often used as toners.

The contributing pigment is the color that remains in the hair after lightening. It is essential that you achieve the correct foundation in order to create the right color and degree of porosity required for proper toner development.

Toner manufacturers usually provide literature that indicates the contributing pigment necessary to achieve the color you desire. As a general rule, the paler the color you are seeking, the lighter the contributing pigment needs to be. It is important to follow the literature closely and to understand that overlightened hair will grab the color of the toner. Underlightened hair, on the other hand, will appear to have more red, yellow, or orange than the intended color.

It is not advisable to pre-lighten past the pale-yellow stage. This will create overly porous hair that will not have enough natural pigment left to create the desired effect. Refer to the law of color to select a toner that will neutralize or complement the pre-lightened hair and produce the desired color.

Toner Application

Administer a patch test for allergies or other sensitivities 24 to 48 hours before each toner application. Proceed with the application only if the patch test results are negative and the hair is in good condition.

Your speed and accuracy are both important factors in the application and will determine, to a large extent, whether you get good color results. The procedure for applying low- or non-peroxide toners may vary. Check with your instructor for directions.

> **⚠ CAUTION**
> In all procedures requiring the use of a towel to check for lightening level, make sure that the towel is damp. Blot—do not rub—the strand. Rubbing could cause a roughening of the cuticle, giving a false reading for the entire process.

Ⓟ 21-8 **Toner Application** *See page 724*

After reading the next few sections, you will be able to:

LO ⑰ Name and describe the three most commonly used methods for highlighting.

Create Special Effects Using Haircoloring Techniques

Special effects haircoloring refers to any technique that involves partial lightening or coloring. Coloring for special effects can be thought of as a pure fashion technique. It is a versatile and exciting haircoloring service.

One way you can create special effects is by strategically placing light and dark colors in the hair. **Highlighting** involves coloring some of the hair strands lighter than the natural color to add a variety of lighter shades and the illusion of depth. Subtle highlights do not contrast strongly with the natural color. Light colors cause the light area to advance toward the eye, to appear larger, and to make details more visible.

Reverse highlighting, also known as *lowlighting*, is the technique of coloring strands of hair darker than the natural color. Contrasting dark areas recede, appear smaller, and make detail less visible.

As you begin to expand your knowledge of haircoloring and lightening and to develop your technical ability, you will become more creative. Your instructor will help you master the basic techniques, but the rest is up to you.

The possibilities are limited only by your imagination and your ability to create a finished style that meets the needs of your clients (figure 21-29).

There are several methods for achieving highlights. The three most frequently used techniques follow:

- Cap technique
- Foil technique
- Baliage or free-form technique

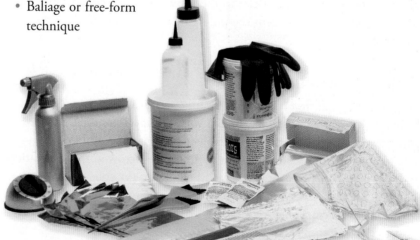

figure 21-29
Lightening tools

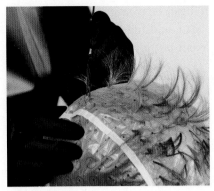
figure 21-30
Pull strands through holes in cap.

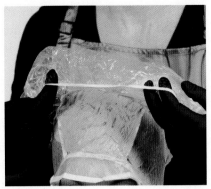
figure 21-31
Cover loosely with plastic cap.

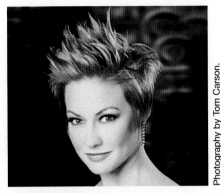
figure 21-32
Cap technique finished look

Cap Technique

The **cap technique** involves pulling clean, dry strands of hair through a perforated cap with a thin plastic or metal hook, and then combing them to remove tangles (figure 21-30). The number of strands pulled through determines the amount of hair that will be highlighted or lowlighted. When only a small number of strands are pulled through, the result will be a subtle look. A more noticeable effect is achieved if many strands are pulled through, and the effect is even more dramatic if larger strands of hair are pulled through.

For highlighting, the hair is usually lightened with a powdered off-the-scalp lightener or a high-lift color, beginning in the area that is most resistant. The lightener is covered for processing (figure 21-31). Once processed, the lightener is removed by a thorough rinse and a shampoo. After towel blotting and conditioning (if necessary), the lightened hair can be toned, if desired (figure 21-32).

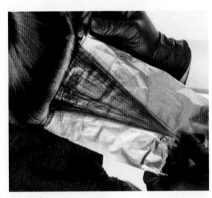
figure 21-33
Slicing

Foil Technique

The **foil technique** involves coloring selected strands of hair by slicing or weaving out sections, placing them on foil or plastic wrap, applying lightener or permanent haircolor, and then sealing them in the foil or plastic wrap for processing. You can also apply permanent haircolor to the strands to create softer, more natural-looking highlights. The same technique can be used for lowlighting. When lowlighting, the use of a demipermanent color is an option.

Placing foil in the hair is an art. It takes practice and discipline. To make it easier, start by working to create clean section blocks on the head. Once you have perfected this, you will fully understand the difference between a slice parting and a weave parting. **Slicing** involves taking a narrow, ⅛-inch (0.3 centimeter) section of hair by making a straight part at the scalp, positioning the hair over the foil, and applying lightener or color (figure 21-33). In **weaving**, selected strands are picked up from a narrow section of hair with a zigzag motion of the comb, and lightener or color is applied only to these strands (figure 21-34).

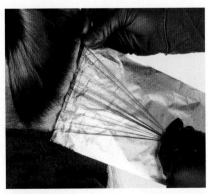
figure 21-34
Weaving

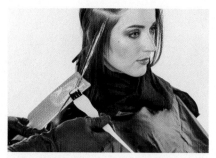

figure 21-35a
Single-, dual-, and three-point baliage technique: single-point application

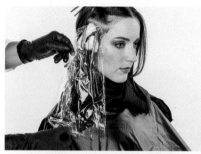

figure 21-35b
Single-, dual-, and three-point baliage technique: Place cotton under painted strand and plastic wrap around section.

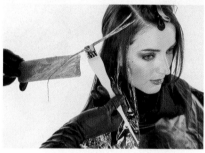

figure 21-35c
Single-, dual-, and three-point baliage technique: dual-point application

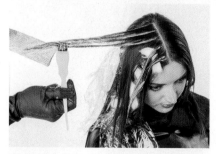

figure 21-35d
Single-, dual-, and three-point baliage technique: three-point application

There are many patterns in which foil can be placed in the hair. There are face-frame, half-head, three-quarter head, and full-head foiling patterns that produce different highlights in different portions of the head.

Ⓟ 21-9   Special Effects Haircoloring with Foil (Full Head) *See page 726*

Baliage Technique

The **baliage** (BAHL-ee-ahj) (sometimes spelled balyage), also known as *free-form technique*, involves the painting of a lightener (usually powdered off-the-scalp lightener) directly onto clean, styled hair. The lightener is applied with an applicator brush or a tail comb from scalp to ends around the head. Some examples of technique for baliage are single-, dual-, and three-point application. After lightener is applied, cotton is placed under the strand and plastic wrap is placed around the section. Hair is then processed according to manufacturer's instructions to desired lightness (figures 21-35 through 21-35d). The finished effects are extremely subtle and are used to draw attention to the surface of the hair (figure 21-36).

Toning Highlighted and Dimensionally Colored Hair

When the hair is decolorized to the desired level during a highlighting service, the use of a toner may not be necessary. However, the use of a pale, soft blond with cool or warm tones does create a finished appearance to the overall color result.

When using a toner on highlighted hair, it is important to consider not only the varying degrees of porosity in the hair, but also the difference in pigmentation from strand to strand that was created by the lightening process. Although an oxidative toner will add color to the highlighted strands, it might also cause a slight amount of lift to the natural or pigmented hair. Perform a strand test to ensure best results.

To avoid affecting the untreated hair, choose from the following options:

- A non-oxidative toner, which contains no ammonia, requires no developer (thus producing no lift of the natural hair color), and is gentle on the scalp and hair.

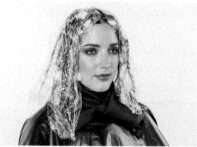

figure 21-35e
Single-, dual-, and three-point baliage technique: Process according to manufacturer's directions to desired lightness.

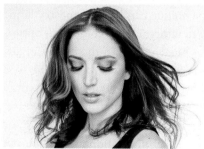

figure 21-36
Baliage technique finished

- Semipermanent color may be used to deposit color without lift. Select a color that is delicate enough to avoid overpowering the pre-lightened hair. Always check the manufacturer's color chart to make sure that the combination of your chosen toner and the contributing pigment will produce the desired color results.

- A demipermanent haircolor may also be used to deposit color. It will not cause additional lightening and lasts longer than temporary or traditional semipermanent colors.

Highlighting Shampoos

- **Highlighting shampoo** colors are prepared by combining permanent haircolor, hydrogen peroxide, and shampoo. They are used when a slight change in hair shade is desired, or when the client's hair processes very rapidly. This process highlights the hair's natural color in a single application. Because highlighting shampoos are made with permanent hair color, aniline is still present in small amounts. Therefore, a patch test is required.

After reading the next few sections, you will be able to:

LO⑱ Know how to properly cover gray hair.

LO⑲ Know the rules of color correction.

Understand the Special Challenges in Haircolor and Corrective Solutions

Each haircoloring service is unique and can present unique challenges. To give each haircoloring service a good start, the colorist must allow enough time for a complete client consultation and analysis of the client's hair. Strand tests must be performed to ensure satisfactory final results. But even the most skilled colorist will occasionally have a problem that can't be predicted. This may be due to the particular structure or condition of the client's hair. The good news is that most haircoloring problems can be resolved or corrected as long as the colorist remains calm.

Gray Hair: Challenges and Solutions

Gray hair is caused by the reduction of pigment in the cortical layer. Gray, white, and salt-and-pepper hair all have characteristics that present unique coloring challenges. For instance, gray hair can turn yellow if the lightener used is not processed long enough. A great many salon coloring

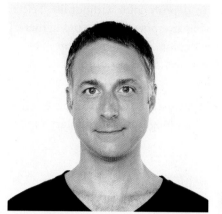

figure 21-37
Gray hair presents certain challenges.

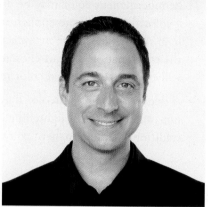

figure 21-38
Many haircolor options cover gray successfully.

services, however, will successfully cover or enhance gray hair if performed correctly (figures 21-37 and 21-38).

Yellowed Hair

A problem that can occur with gray hair is that it can develop a yellow cast, which can be caused by a variety of factors:

- Smoking

- Medication

- Sun exposure

- Hair sprays and styling aids

Lightener and haircolor removers help remove yellow discoloration. Undesired yellow can often be overpowered by the artificial pigments deposited by violet-based colors of an equal or darker level than the yellow.

Formulating for Gray Hair

Gray hair accepts the level of the color applied. However, level 8 or lighter colors may not give complete coverage because of the low concentration of dye found in these lighter colors. Formulations from level 7 and darker will provide better coverage, and can be used to create pastel and blond tones if desired.

For those clients who are 80 to 100 percent gray, a haircolor within the blond range is generally more flattering than a darker shade. This lighter level of artificial color may be selected to give a warm or cool finished color, depending on the client's skin tone, eye color, and personal preference.

One factor to consider when coloring low percentages of gray or salt-and-pepper hair to a darker level is that color on color will always make a darker color. The addition of dark artificial pigment to the natural pigment results in a color that the eye perceives as darker. For this reason, when attempting to cover the unpigmented hair on a salt-and-pepper head, formulate one to two levels lighter than the natural level to ensure a natural result.

table 21-4

SEMIPERMANENT/DEMIPERMANENT COLOR FORMULATION FOR GRAY HAIR

Percentage of Gray Hair	Semipermanent/Demipermanent Color Formulation for Gray Hair
90–100%	Desired level
70–90%	Equal parts desired and one level lighter
50–70%	One level lighter than desired level
30–50%	Equal parts one and two levels lighter
10–30%	Two levels lighter than desired level

For the purposes of a strand test, a manufacturer's product color chart can be used in conjunction with **tables 21-4** and **21-5** to select a color within the proper level.

The gray hair formulation tables provide general guidelines, but there are other considerations to take into account, such as the following:

• Client's personality

• Personal preferences

• Amount of gray hair and its location on the head

You will note that in the tables there are no colors given in the formulations, only the levels of haircoloring and various techniques. Also note that the table does not consider the location of the gray hair. The percentage assumes that the gray hair is equally distributed throughout the entire head. If, for instance, the majority of gray hair is located in the front section of the head, that section would be considered to have more gray hair, with the back portion containing less gray hair. In that instance, you

table 21-5

PERMANENT COLOR FORMULATION FOR GRAY HAIR

Percentage of Gray Hair	Permanent Color Formulation for Gray Hair
90–100%	Desired level
70–90%	Two parts desired level and one part lighter level
50–70%	Equal parts desired and lighter level
30–50%	Two parts lighter level and one part desired level
10–30%	One level lighter

would have to determine what formulation would best suit the client. The gray hair around the face is what the client sees, so it may be wise to formulate based on the percentage of gray hair the client actually sees. The section of hair that surrounds the face is what influences the client's self-image. In some cases, you may want two formulas—one for the area around the face with the most gray and another for the rest of the head.

Tips for Achieving Gray Coverage

- Formulate at a level 7 medium-blond and deeper for best gray coverage.
- Use 20-volume developer.
- Process color for the full processing time, based on manufacturer's instructions.
- Add neutral tones to the formula.
- If 25 percent gray is present, use 25 percent neutral or natural tones in formula.
- If 50 percent gray is present, use 50 percent neutral or natural tones in formula.
- If 75 percent gray is present, use 75 percent neutral or natural tones in formula.

High-lift blond colors are not designed for gray coverage. To create a very light result, formulate at a level 7 for the base color and add some highlights over the color to create a balanced blond on blond result.

Pre-softening

Occasionally, gray hair is so resistant that even when formulation, application, and time are correct, you will find that the coverage is not satisfactory. In such cases, pre-softening becomes necessary. **Pre-softening** is the process of treating gray or very resistant hair to allow for better penetration of color. Pre-softening raises the cuticle layer of the resistant hair to allow for better penetration of color. A pre-softener acts like a stain to the hair. It is applied, processed, and removed. Then the haircolor is applied.

Apply the pre-softening formula to the resistant areas and allow it to stay on the hair for 15 minutes. Refer to manufacturer's directions. While pre-softening the resistant areas, you may mix the final formula and start to apply it to the rest of the head.

Once the resistant hair has been pre-softened, blot the pre-softener color off with a towel and apply the final color formula directly over it. Process per the manufacturer's instructions.

Rules for Effective Color Correction

Sometimes the color may not turn out as expected. Although this can seem disastrous for your client and for you, it does not need to be. Problems can always be corrected. Keep the following guidelines in mind:

- Do not panic. Remain calm.
- Determine the nature of the problem.

- Determine what caused the problem.
- Develop a solution.
- Always take one step at a time.
- Never guarantee an exact result.
- Always strand test for accuracy.

Damaged Hair

Blowdrying, flat irons, wind, harsh shampoos, the sun, salt water, chlorinated water, and chemical services all take their toll on the condition of the hair. Coating compounds such as hair sprays, styling agents, and some conditioners can block/interfere with color penetration. Hair is considered damaged when it has one or more of the following characteristics:

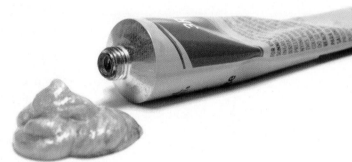

- Rough texture
- Overporous condition
- Brittle and dry to the touch
- Susceptible to breakage
- No elasticity
- Becomes spongy and matted when wet
- Color fades too quickly or grabs too dark

Any of these hair conditions will create problems during a haircoloring, lightening, permanent waving, or hair relaxing treatment. Therefore, damaged hair should receive reconditioning treatments both before and after the application of these chemical services. Tips for dealing with damaged hair are as follows:

- Use a penetrating conditioner that can deposit protein, oils, and moisture-rich ingredients.
- Complete each chemical service by normalizing the pH with an acidic finishing rinse. This will restore the ability of the cuticle to protect the hair.
- Postpone any further chemical service until the hair is reconditioned.
- Schedule the client for between-service conditioning.
- Recommend retail home-care products that will help prepare the hair for the next service.

Fillers

Fillers are used to equalize porosity. Some fillers are ready to use as they come from the manufacturer. Others are a mixture of haircolor and conditioner that your instructor can help you prepare. There are two types of fillers: conditioner fillers and color fillers.

Conditioner fillers are used to recondition damaged, overly porous hair and equalize porosity so that the hair accepts the color evenly from strand to strand and from scalp to ends. They can be applied in a separate procedure or immediately prior to the color application.

Color fillers equalize porosity and deposit color in one application to provide a uniform contributing pigment on pre-lightened hair. Color fillers are used on overly porous, pre-lightened hair to equalize porosity and provide a uniform contributing pigment that compliments the desired finished color. Demipermanent haircolor products are commonly used as color fillers. As a general rule, if you are going three levels or more darker, you will need to use a color filler.

Color fillers accomplish the following goals:

- Deposit color to faded ends and hair shaft.

- Help prepare hair to hold a final color by replacing missing building blocks.

- Prevent streaking and dull appearance.

- Prevent off-color results.

- Produce more uniform, natural-looking color.

- Produce uniform color when coloring pre-lightened hair back to its natural color.

Selecting the Correct Color Filler

All three primary colors must be present to produce a haircolor that looks natural. To correct an unwanted haircolor, always use the primary or secondary color that is missing in the hair. That color is called the complementary color. Remember, complementary colors are directly opposite each other on the color wheel.

Yellow blond hair can be corrected to a natural blond by adding the two missing primary colors, red and blue—in other words, by adding the secondary color violet. Violet cancels yellow. Orange blond hair can be corrected to a natural blond by adding the missing primary color, blue. Blue cancels orange. Adding blue color to yellow hair would make the hair green. Remember that a primary color always cancels a secondary color, and a secondary color always cancels a primary color.

Color fillers may be applied directly from their containers to damaged hair prior to coloring. They may also be added to the haircolor and applied to damaged ends.

Haircolor Tips for Redheads

Red haircolor is exciting and fun, but fading is a common problem with color-treated red hair (**figure 21-39**). A daily shampoo and blowdry, an occasional permanent wave, and/or a few days in the pool or at the beach cause the artificial pigment in red hair to oxidize and fade. It is important to recommend the proper products to maintain the finished haircolor. Tips are summarized below:

- To create warm coppery reds, use a red-orange base color (for example: RO, RG).

- To create hot fiery reds, use red-violet or true red colors (for example: R, RR, RV).

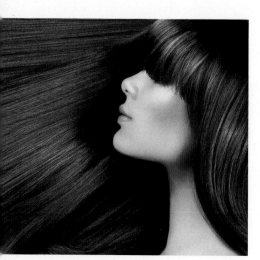

figure 21-39
Vibrant red hair

- After the hair has been colored with a permanent color, always use a demipermanent color to refresh the shaft and ends.

- If gray hair is present, always add the necessary amount of neutral color according to the total amount of color mixed and the desired red level. Always take into account the percent of gray present. As a general rule, follow the guidelines for gray coverage:

  - If 25 percent gray is present, use 25 percent neutral or natural tones in formula.
  - If 50 percent gray is present, use 50 percent neutral or natural tones in formula.
  - If 75 percent gray is present, use 75 percent neutral or natural tones in formula.

- To brighten haircolor, refresh reds with a soap cap of equal parts shampoo and the remaining color formula before rinsing, or mix a demipermanent color and apply it to the ends.

Haircolor Tips for Brunettes

- To avoid orange or brassy tones when lifting brown hair with permanent color, always use a cool blue or green base.

- To avoid unwanted brassy tones, do not lighten more than two levels above the natural color.

- Add one ounce of a natural color to cover gray in brunette hair.

- Natural highlights in brunette hair should be deep or caramel-colored. Blond highlights have too much contrast with brunette hair. Blond highlights do not look natural and require frequent service.

Haircolor Tips for Blonds

Blond haircolor is popular, profitable, and fun. From single-process blond to highlighting, the possibilities are endless. As you work with blond hair, keep the following tips in mind:

- When lightening brown hair to blond, remember that there may be underlying unwanted warm tones.

- When covering gray hair with a blond color, use a level 7 or darker for the best coverage.

- Double-process blonding is the best way to obtain pale blond results.

- If high-lift blonds that lift only 5 levels are used on levels 4 and below, the result may be a color that is too warm or brassy.

- If highlights become too blond or all one color, lowlights or deeper strands can be foiled into the hair to create a more natural color. For lowlights, choose a shade between the highlighted shade and the base color and add gold to your formulation. For example, if the highlighted strands are a level 9 and the base is a level 5, choosing a level 7 gold for the lowlight is a good option. An all-over glaze will add warmth and shine to an overprocessed blond. Choosing shades with gold tones will help to keep the sparkle in pale blonds.

Common Haircolor Solutions

Refresh Faded Color

If the hair appears dull and faded, mix a demipermanent haircolor in the same tonal family as the haircolor formula. Stay within two levels of your formula. Apply all over and check frequently allowing a processing time up to 10 minutes.

Green Cast

If the hair has a buildup of minerals from well water or chlorine, you may want to purify the hair with a product designed to remove the mineral buildup. You can apply a demipermanent color to neutralize any unwanted color that remains in the hair.

Overall Haircolor Is Too Light

This is a result of incorrect formulation. To correct, apply a demipermanent color that is one to two levels darker than the previous formula.

Overall Color Is Too Dark

A simple solution to an overall color that is too dark could be adding a few highlights. This will break up the solid dark color and give an overall appearance of lighter hair. If that idea is not appealing to your guest, you may need to correct the base color. Determine how much of the color needs to be removed. Use a haircolor remover in cases where the hair is too dark because of buildup or formulation. Apply haircolor remover to the areas that need to be lightened. Process for 10 minutes and check development. These removers are designed to remove artificial pigment from the hair. Once you have achieved the desired color, rinse and shampoo.

Restoring Blond to Natural Haircolor

Restoring a client's blond hair back to its natural darker color can be tricky. Even if the client says that she wants to go back to her natural color, she may not like it. She is used to seeing light hair and going too dark could be disastrous. A few tips on how to restore the client's natural color are listed below:

1. If you have a starting regrowth level that is level 6 dark blond and deeper, soften the new growth with a level 6 violet base permanent color with 20 volume. Apply to the scalp area, process for 20 minutes, and rinse. Towel dry. If the starting regrowth level is level 7 medium blond and lighter, soften the regrowth with a level 8 light blond-violet base permanent color with 20 volume. Apply to the scalp area, process for 20 minutes, and rinse. Towel dry.

2. Next, apply a demipermanent glaze with 1 ounce of a level 8 light neutral blond and 1 ounce (30 milliliters) of a level 9 very light blond red-orange. Apply to all the lightened hair. Do not apply to the scalp area. Process for 20 minutes. Rinse and towel dry. This will turn the hair a very light reddish-gold. Do Not Panic!

3. Finally, mix the final deposit-only glaze. If you formulated with level 6 dark blond-violet at the base, use 1½ ounces (44 milliliters) level 6 dark

> **⚠ CAUTION**
> Sometimes hair is so damaged and overly porous that there may be insufficient structure left within the cortex for the artificial pigment to attach to. Hair that looks gun-metal gray is a real danger sign. Hair that is this porous is very fragile and may be close to the breaking point.

neutral blond with ½ ounce (15 milliliters) level 4 light brown gold base. If you formulated with level 8 light violet blond at the base, use 1 ½ ounces (44 milliliters) level 8 light neutral blond with ½ ounce (15 milliliters) level 6 dark golden blond. Apply the chosen formula starting on the pieces that were overlightened from the beginning. Work the color through all over. Process up to 20 minutes, checking it every five minutes.

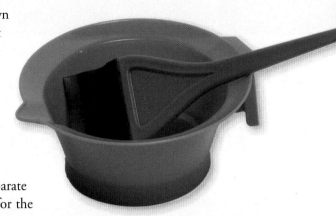

Reevaluate the haircolor at the client's next visit, and determine what is needed to make the color deeper. Apply a separate color to the scalp area and on the remainder of the hair strand for the best results.

After reading the next few sections, you will be able to:

LO⑳ **Know the safety precautions to follow during the haircolor process.**

Know Haircoloring Safety Precautions

- Perform a patch test 24 to 48 hours prior to each application of aniline-derivative haircolor. Apply haircolor only if the patch test is negative.

- Do not apply haircolor if abrasions are present on the scalp.

- Do not apply haircolor if a metallic or compound haircolor is present.

- Do not brush the hair prior to applying color.

- Always read and follow the manufacturer's directions.

- Use cleaned and disinfected applicator bottles, brushes, combs, and towels.

- Protect your client's clothing with proper draping.

- Perform a strand test for color, breakage, and/or discoloration.

- Use an applicator bottle or bowl (glass or plastic) for mixing the haircolor.

- Do not mix haircolor until you are ready to use it; discard leftover haircolor.

- Wear gloves to protect your hands.

- Do not permit the color to come in contact with the client's eyes.

- Do not overlap during a haircolor retouch.

- Use a mild shampoo. An alkaline or harsh shampoo will strip color.

- Always wash hands before and after serving a client.

FOCUS ON
Retailing

Your color client needs to use high-quality salon products at home to help prevent their haircolor from fading. Using the right products increases the longevity of the haircolor, preserves the natural integrity (health) of the hair, and makes your client more likely to return to you for more services. Recommending the right professional products increases your client's satisfaction and your income.

PERFORMING A PATCH TEST

IMPLEMENTS & MATERIALS

You will need all of the following implements, materials, and supplies:

□ Cotton swab   □ Haircolor service record card   □ Mild soap

□ Developer   □ Haircolor product   □ Towel

□ Glass or plastic mixing bowl

PREPARATION

Perform:

P 15-1 **Pre-Service Procedure** *See page 340*

PROCEDURE

1 Select a test area, behind the ear or on the inside of the elbow are good choices.

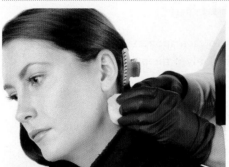

2 Using a mild soap, clean and dry an area about the size of a quarter.

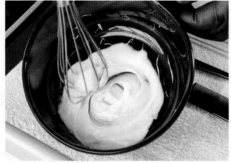

3 Mix a small amount of the same product you plan on using for the service according to the manufacturer's directions.

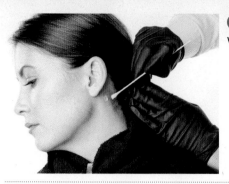

④ Apply a small amount of the haircolor mixture to the test area with a sterile cotton swab.

⑤ Leave the mixture undisturbed for 24 to 48 hours.

⑥ Examine the test area. If there are no signs of redness or irritation, the test result is negative, and you can proceed with the color service.

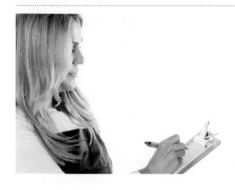

⑦ Record the results on the haircolor service record card.

POST-SERVICE

Complete:

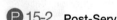 15-2   **Post-Service Procedure** *See page 343*

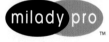   **Check out miladypro.com for additional resources and training to enhance your technical skills. Keyword:** *FutureCosPro*

PRELIMINARY STRAND TEST

IMPLEMENTS & MATERIALS

You will need all of the following implements, materials, and supplies:

- ☐ Bowl and brush
- ☐ Chemical cape
- ☐ Color brushes
- ☐ Developer
- ☐ Glass or plastic mixing bowl

- ☐ Haircolor service record card
- ☐ Plastic sectioning clips
- ☐ Protective gloves
- ☐ Selected haircolor

- ☐ Service record card
- ☐ Shampoo
- ☐ Sheet of foil or plastic wrap
- ☐ Spray bottle containing water

- ☐ Timer
- ☐ Towels

PREPARATION

Perform:

P 15-1 **Pre-Service Procedure** *See page 340*

PROCEDURE

① Perform a scalp and hair analysis.

② Drape client to protect skin and clothing.

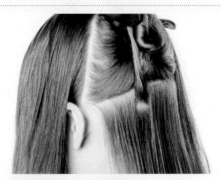

③ Part off a ½-inch (1.25 centimeters) square section of hair in the interior nape area; so it is not visible from the hairline. Using plastic sectioning clips, fasten other hair out of the way.

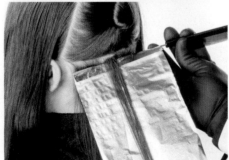

④ Place the hair strand over the foil or plastic wrap and apply the color mixture you plan on using for the service.

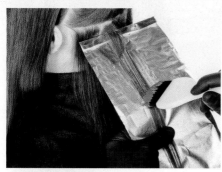

⑤ Follow the application method for the color you will be using to apply the color mixture.

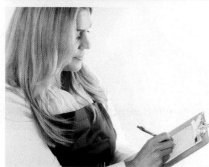

⑥ Check the development at five-minute intervals until the desired color has been achieved. Note the timing on the service record card.

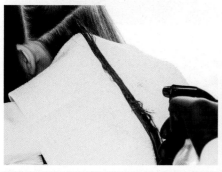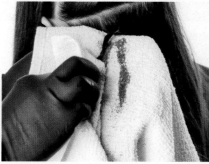

⑦ When satisfactory color has developed, remove the protective foil or plastic wrap. Place a towel under the strand, mist it thoroughly with water, add shampoo, and massage through. Rinse by spraying with water. Dry the hair strand with the towel and observe the results.

⑧ Adjust the formula, timing, or application method as necessary and proceed with the color service.

POST-SERVICE

Complete:

Ⓟ 15-2 **Post-Service Procedure** *See page 343*

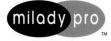 **Check out miladypro.com for additional resources and training to enhance your technical skills. Keyword:** *FutureCosPro*

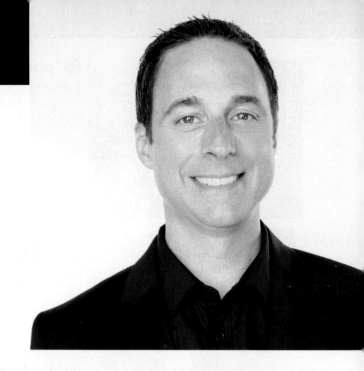

TEMPORARY HAIRCOLOR APPLICATION

IMPLEMENTS & MATERIALS

You will need all of the following implements, materials, and supplies:

- ☐ Bowl and brush
- ☐ Comb
- ☐ Haircolor service record card
- ☐ Protective gloves
- ☐ Shampoo
- ☐ Shampoo cape
- ☐ Temporary haircolor product
- ☐ Timer
- ☐ Towels

PREPARATION

Perform:

P 15-1 **Pre-Service Procedure** *See page 340*

PROCEDURE

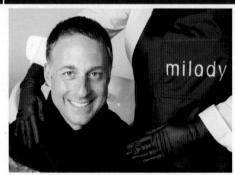

① Drape the client for a haircoloring service. Slide a towel down from the back of the client's head and place lengthwise across the client's shoulders. Cross the ends of the towel beneath the chin and place the cape over the towel. Fasten the cape in the back. Fold the towel over the top of the cape and secure in front.

② Shampoo and towel dry the hair.

③ Make sure the client is comfortably reclined at the shampoo bowl.

④ Put on gloves.

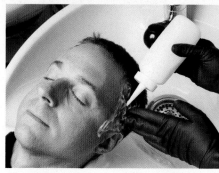

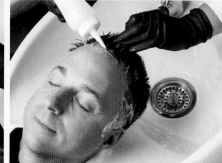

⑤ Put the color into a color bowl and apply with a color brush or as directed by manufacturer's instructions.

⑥ Apply the color and work around the entire head.

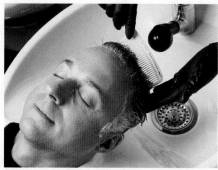

⑧ Do not rinse the hair. Towel-blot excess product.

⑦ Blend the color with your gloved hands or comb it through the hair, applying more color as necessary.

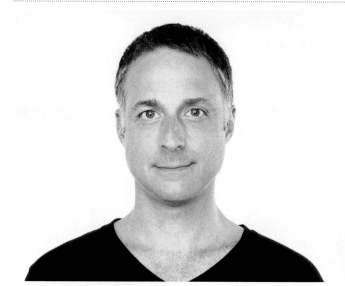

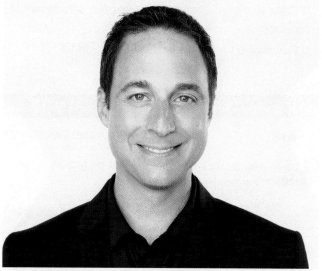

⑨ Proceed with styling and finish.

POST-SERVICE

Complete:

Ⓟ 15-2   **Post-Service Procedure** *See page 343*

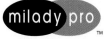 Check out miladypro.com for additional resources and training to enhance your technical skills. Keyword: *FutureCosPro*

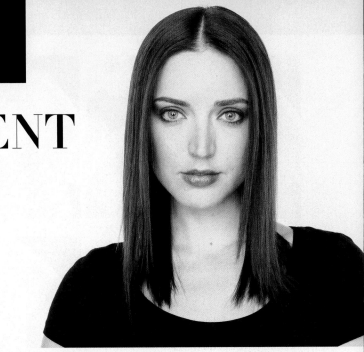

P 21-4

DEMIPERMANENT HAIRCOLOR APPLICATION

IMPLEMENTS & MATERIALS

You will need all of the following implements, materials, and supplies:

- ☐ Chemical cape
- ☐ Color brushes
- ☐ Color chart
- ☐ Comb
- ☐ Conditioner

- ☐ Cotton
- ☐ Glass or plastic bowl
- ☐ Haircolor service record card
- ☐ Plastic cap (optional)

- ☐ Plastic clips
- ☐ Protective cream
- ☐ Protective gloves
- ☐ Selected color
- ☐ Shampoo

- ☐ Timer
- ☐ Towels

PREPARATION

Perform:

P 15-1 **Pre-Service Procedure** *See page 340*

PROCEDURE

1 Shampoo the client's hair with mild shampoo and towel dry.

2 Put on gloves.

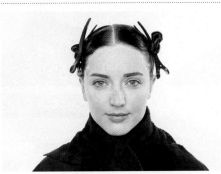

3 Part the hair into four sections—from ear to ear and from front center of forehead to center nape—and apply protective cream around the hairline and over the ears.

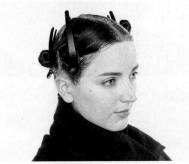

4 Outline the partings with color product.

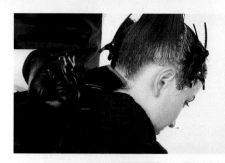
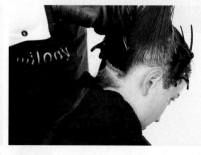
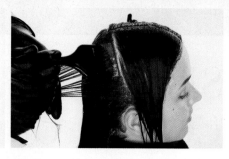

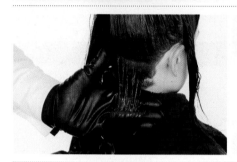

5 Take ½-inch (1.25 centimeter) partings, and apply the color to the new growth or scalp area in all four sections. Take horizontal subsections, starting in the nape of a rear quadrant, repeat on other rear quadrant. When you reach the front, you will take vertical sections applying product so the hair lies away from the face.

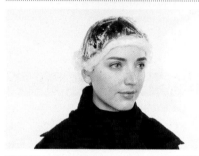
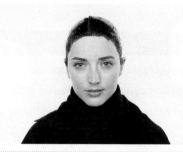

6 After all four sections are completed, work the color through the rest of the hair shaft to the ends until the hair is fully saturated.

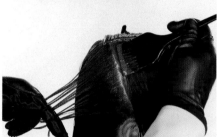

7 Set timer to process. In addition to following the manufacturer's directions, check the haircolor every five minutes as it is processing to ensure you are not overdepositing color on porous hair. Some colors require the use of a plastic cap. To prevent the elastic of the plastic cap from leaving a mark on clients face, place cotton under cap elastic on face and hairline.

8 When processing is complete, massage color into a lather and rinse thoroughly with warm water.

9 Remove any stains from around the hairline with shampoo or stain remover.

10 Shampoo the hair, and condition as needed.

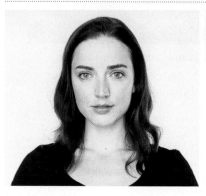
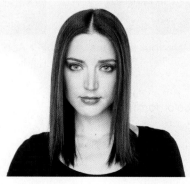

11 Finished look.

POST-SERVICE

Complete:

P 15-2 **Post-Service Procedure** See page 343

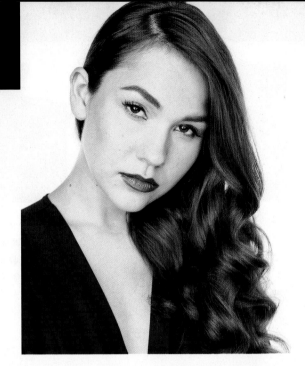

P 21-5

SINGLE-PROCESS COLOR ON VIRGIN HAIR

IMPLEMENTS & MATERIALS

You will need all of the following implements, materials, and supplies:

- ☐ Color brushes
- ☐ Color chart
- ☐ Comb
- ☐ Conditioner
- ☐ Cotton
- ☐ Glass or plastic bowl
- ☐ Haircolor service record card
- ☐ Hydrogen peroxide developer
- ☐ Plastic cap (optional)
- ☐ Plastic clips
- ☐ Protective cream
- ☐ Protective gloves
- ☐ Selected permanent color
- ☐ Shampoo
- ☐ Timer
- ☐ Towels
- ☐ Waterproof cape

PREPARATION

Perform:

P 15-1 **Pre-Service Procedure** *See page 340*

PROCEDURE

1. Drape the client for a haircolor service.

2. Put on gloves.

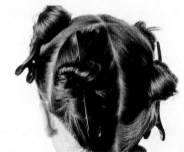

3. Part dry hair into four sections.

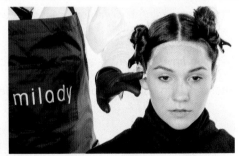

4. Apply protective cream to the hairline and ears.

5. Prepare the color formula.

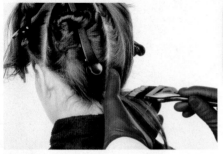

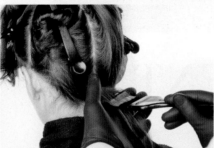

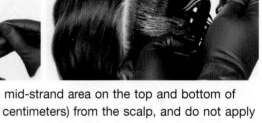

6 Begin application in the section where the color change will be the greatest or where the hair is the most resistant. Here you will take a ¼-inch (0.6 centimeter) horizontal subsection with the tail of the tint brush.

7 Apply color product to the mid-strand area on the top and bottom of subsection. Stay ½ inch (1.25 centimeters) from the scalp, and do not apply if the ends are porous. When you reach the sides, you will switch from horizontal to vertical subsection, starting application at the back of the section.

8 Work your way through all four quadrants. Process according to the strand test results. Check for color development by removing color as described in the strand test procedure.

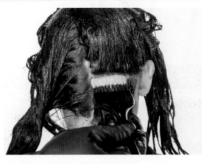

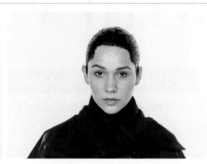

9 Apply color to the hair at the scalp.

10 Work the color through the ends of the hair.

11 Massage color into a lather and rinse thoroughly with warm water.

12 Remove any stains around the hairline with shampoo or stain remover. Use a towel to gently remove stains.

13 Shampoo the hair, and condition as needed.

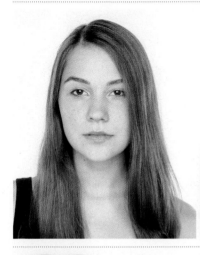

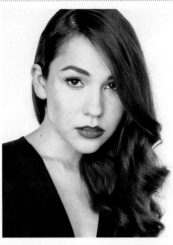

14 Finished look.

POST-SERVICE

Complete:

P 15-2 **Post-Service Procedure** *See page 343*

milady pro™ Check out miladypro.com for additional resources and training to enhance your technical skills. Keyword: *FutureCosPro*

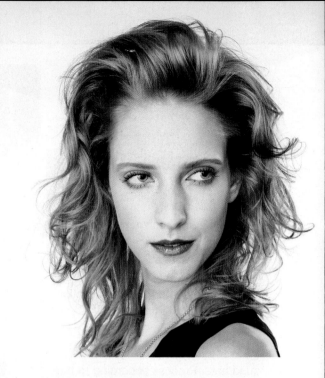

PERMANENT SINGLE-PROCESS RETOUCH WITH A GLAZE

IMPLEMENTS & MATERIALS

You will need all of the following implements, materials, and supplies:

- ☐ Applicator bottle
- ☐ Chemical cape
- ☐ Color brushes
- ☐ Comb
- ☐ Conditioner
- ☐ Cotton
- ☐ Developer
- ☐ Glass or plastic mixing bowl
- ☐ Haircolor ervice record card
- ☐ Plastic cap (optional)
- ☐ Plastic clips
- ☐ Protective cream
- ☐ Protective gloves
- ☐ Selected permanent color
- ☐ Shampoo
- ☐ Timer
- ☐ Towels

PREPARATION

Perform:

P 15-1 **Pre-Service Procedure** See page 340

PROCEDURE

1 Drape the client for a haircolor service.

2 Put on gloves.

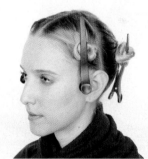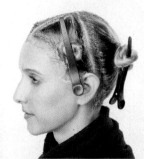

3 Part dry hair into four sections. Apply barrier cream around hairline and ears.

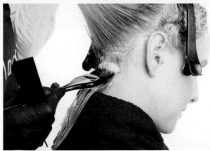

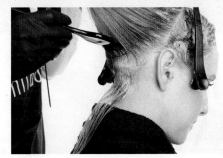

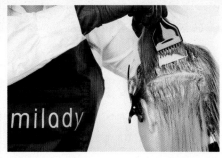

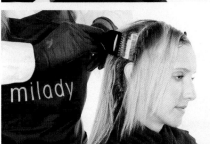

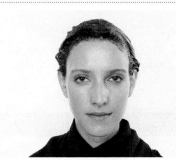

④ Outline all four quadrants with color product. Starting in the nape and working your way up to the crown, apply color product to new growth area using ¼-inch (0.6 centimeter) horizontal subsections. Repeat on the opposite side. When you reach the sides, you will switch from horizontal to vertical subsection, starting application at the back of the section. Be sure to apply product so the hair lies away from the face.

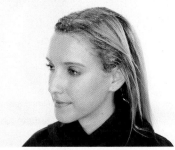

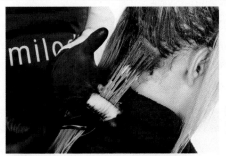

⑤ Complete all four sides and process according to manufacturer's directions. Set a timer for accuracy.

⑥ Prepare a no-lift, deposit-only glaze formula and apply to the mid-strands and ends.

⑦ Work demipermanent glaze through the hair.

⑧ Check haircolor results before rinsing.

⑨ Finished look.

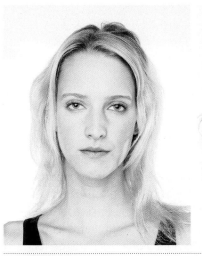

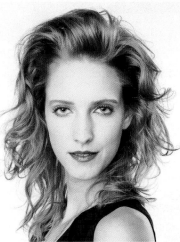

POST-SERVICE

Complete:

Ⓟ 15-2 Post-Service Procedure *See page 343*

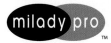

LIGHTENING VIRGIN HAIR

IMPLEMENTS & MATERIALS

You will need all of the following implements, materials, and supplies:

- ☐ Chemical cape
- ☐ Color brushes
- ☐ Comb
- ☐ Conditioner
- ☐ Cotton
- ☐ Glass or plastic mixing bowl
- ☐ Haircolor service record card
- ☐ Hydrogen peroxide developer
- ☐ Lightener
- ☐ Plastic clips
- ☐ Protective cream
- ☐ Protective gloves
- ☐ Shampoo
- ☐ Timer
- ☐ Towels

Note: The colorist in the photographs completed this application using her left hand. The procedure is exactly the same for right-handed or left-handed application.

PREPARATION | PROCEDURE

Perform:

P 15-1 **Pre-Service Procedure** *See page 340*

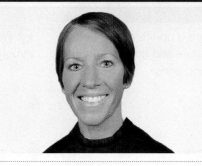

1 Drape the client for a haircolor service.

2 Put on gloves.

3 Part the hair into four sections.

4 Apply a protective cream around the hairline and over the ears.

5 Prepare the lightening formula and use it immediately.

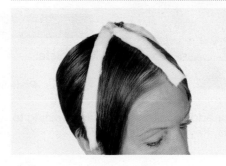

6 An option for a clean and comfortable application is to place cotton around and through all four sections to protect the scalp. Continue by placing strips of cotton at the scalp area along the partings for each subsection. This will prevent the lightener from touching the base of the hair.

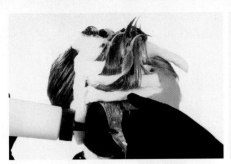

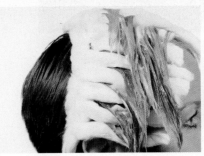

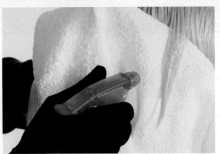

7 Apply the lightener ½ inch (1.25 centimeters) away from the scalp, working the lightener through the mid-strands and up to the porous ends.

8 Continue to apply the lightener. Double-check the application, adding more lightener if necessary. Do not comb the lightener through the hair. The lightener will stop processing if it dries out. Keep the lightener moist during development by reapplying if the mixture dries on the hair.

9 Check for lightening action about 15 minutes before the time indicated by the preliminary strand test. Spray a hair strand with a water bottle and remove the lightener with a damp towel. Examine the strand. If the strand is not light enough, reapply the mixture and continue testing frequently until the desired level is reached.

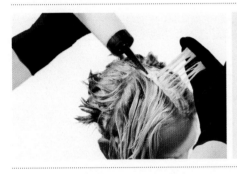

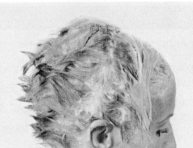

10 Remove the cotton from the scalp area. Apply the lightener to the hair near the scalp with ½-inch (0.3 centimeter) partings.

11 Apply lightener to the porous ends and process until the entire hair strand has reached the desired stage.

12 Rinse the hair thoroughly with warm water. Shampoo gently and condition as needed, keeping your hands under the hair to avoid tangling.

13 Neutralize the alkalinity of the hair with an acidic conditioner. Recondition if necessary.

14 Towel dry the hair, or dry it completely under a cool dryer if required by the manufacturer.

15 Examine the scalp for any abrasions. Analyze the condition of the hair.

16 Proceed with a toner application if desired. (See Procedure 21-8, Toner Application.) If no toner is needed, dry and style the hair.

POST-SERVICE

Complete:

P 15-2 **Post-Service Procedure** *See page 343*

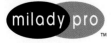

Check out miladypro.com for additional resources and training to enhance your technical skills. Keyword: *FutureCosPro*

TONER APPLICATION

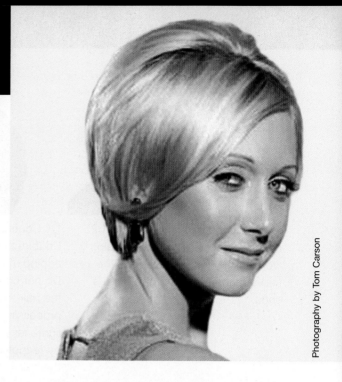

Photography by Tom Carson

IMPLEMENTS & MATERIALS

You will need all of the following implements, materials, and supplies:

- ☐ Applicator bottle
- ☐ Bowl
- ☐ Chemical cape
- ☐ Conditioner
- ☐ Cotton

- ☐ Glass or plastic mixing bowl
- ☐ Haircolor service record card
- ☐ Hydrogen peroxide developer

- ☐ Protective cream
- ☐ Protective gloves
- ☐ Plastic clips
- ☐ Selected toner
- ☐ Shampoo

- ☐ Tail comb
- ☐ Timer
- ☐ Tint brush
- ☐ Towels

Note: This procedure can be performed using an applicator bottle or bowl and tint brush.

PREPARATION PROCEDURE

Perform:

P 15-1 **Pre-Service Procedure** *See page 340*

1. Pre-lighten the hair to the desired stage of decolorization.

2. Shampoo the hair lightly, rinse, and towel dry. Condition as necessary.

3. Put on gloves.

4. Select the desired toner shade.

5. Apply protective cream around the hairline and over the ears.

6. Take a strand test and record the results on the client's service record card.

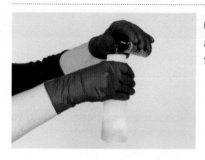

7. If using a toner with developer, mix the toner and the developer in a nonmetallic bowl or bottle, following the manufacturer's directions.

8 Part the hair into four equal sections, using the end of the tail comb or applicator brush. Avoid scratching the scalp.

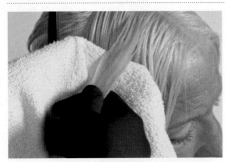

9 Take a strand test. At the crown of one of the back sections, part off ¼-inch (0.6 centimeter) partings and apply the toner from the scalp up to, but not including, the porous ends. If it indicates proper color development, start application in the back at the nape and work application forward.

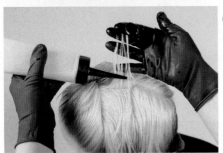

11 If necessary for coverage, apply additional toner to the hair and distribute evenly. Leave the hair loose or cover with a plastic cap if required.

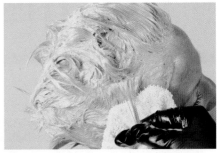

10 Gently work the toner through the ends of the hair, using a tint brush, an applicator bottle, and/or your fingers.

12 Time the procedure according to your strand test. Check frequently until the desired color has been reached evenly throughout the entire hair shaft and ends.

13 Remove the toner by wetting the hair and massaging the toner into a lather.

14 Rinse with warm water, shampoo gently, and thoroughly rinse again.

15 Apply an acidic conditioner to close the cuticle and lower the pH, to help prevent fading.

16 Remove any stains from the skin, hairline, and neck.

17 Style as desired. Use caution to avoid stretching the hair.

18 Finished look.

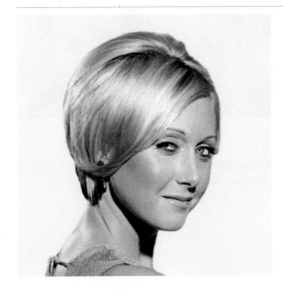

POST-SERVICE

Complete:

P 15-2 **Post-Service Procedure** *See page 343*

SPECIAL EFFECTS HAIRCOLORING WITH FOIL (FULL HEAD)

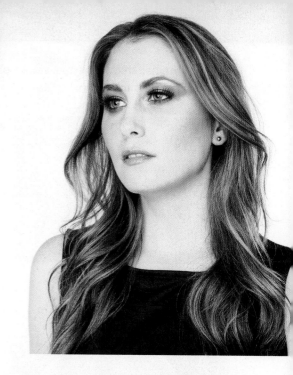

IMPLEMENTS & MATERIALS

You will need all of the following implements, materials, and supplies:

- ☐ Applicator bottle
- ☐ Chemical cape
- ☐ Conditioner
- ☐ Foil
- ☐ Glass or plastic mixing bowl
- ☐ Gloves
- ☐ Haircolor brushes
- ☐ Haircolor service record card
- ☐ Lightener
- ☐ Plastic clips
- ☐ Shampoo
- ☐ Tail comb
- ☐ Timer
- ☐ Towels

PREPARATION

Perform:

P 15-1 Pre-Service Procedure *See page 340*

PROCEDURE

1 Drape the client for a haircolor service.

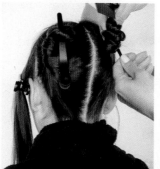 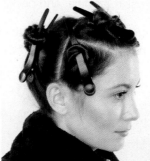 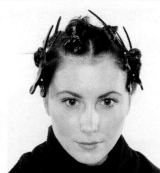

2 Part hair into six sections. Start by dividing the hair into four quadrants, from front hairline to nape and ear to ear. In the front, you will then subdivide your right and left quadrants into a top and side section at the parietal ridge above the ear.

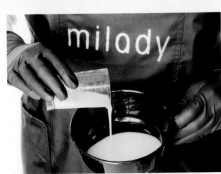

③ Prepare the lightening formula, and use it immediately.

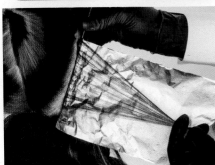

④ With a tail comb, take a thin diagonal slice, following the shape of the hairline, starting in the right back section. From this slice you will then take a fine weave of hair and place a piece of foil under it.

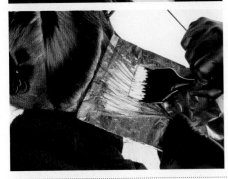

⑤ Holding the hair taut, brush lightener starting from two inches from the top of the foil to the ends, using only enough product to secure foil in place. Work the product up to ¼ inch (0.6 centimeters) from the edge of the foil.

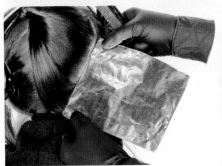

⑥ Fold the foil in half until the ends meet.

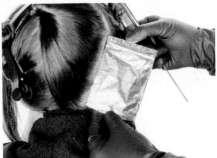

⑦ Fold the foil in half again, using the comb to crease it.

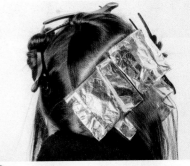

⑧ Take a ¼-inch (0.6 centimeter) subsection in between foils. Clip this hair up and out of the way. Note the contrast in size between the foiled and unfoiled subsections.

⑨ Continue working up the back right side of the head until the section is complete.

⑩ Repeat this procedure on the back left side of the head.

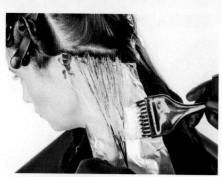

11 Work around the head to the left side area.

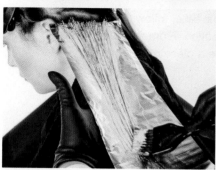

12 Work up the side, bring fine slices of hair into the foil, and apply lightener to the hair.

13 Move to the other side of the head and complete the matching sections.

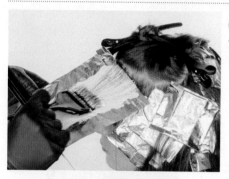

14 Move to the top right side of the head. Take a fine slice of hair from the top of the side section to the center part, following the shape of the hairline. Place it on the foil, and apply lightener.

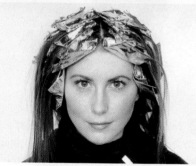

15 Continue toward the top until the last foil is placed. Repeat on the top left side of the head.

16 Allow the lightener to process according to the strand test.

17 Check the foils for the desired lightness.

18 Remove the foils one at a time at the shampoo area. Rinse the hair immediately to prevent the color from affecting the untreated hair.

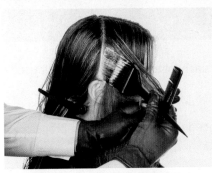

19 Apply a haircolor glaze to the hair, from scalp to ends. A haircolor glaze is an optional service added on to a highlighting to add shine to the finished result.

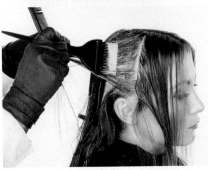

20 Work the glaze into the hair to make sure it is completely saturated, and process per the manufacturer's directions.

21 Rinse the hair, shampoo, condition, and style the hair as desired.

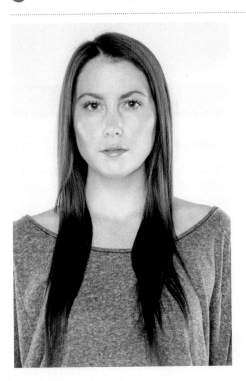

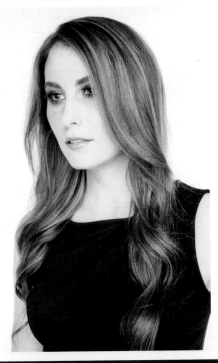

22 Finished look.

POST-SERVICE

Complete:

P 15-2 Post-Service Procedure *See page 343*

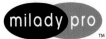

Check out miladypro.com for additional resources and training to enhance your technical skills. Keyword: *FutureCosPro*

REVIEW QUESTIONS

1. Why do people color their hair?

2. How does the hair's porosity affect haircolor?

3. How many types of melanin are found in hair? Describe each.

4. What are levels? What does the level system help you to determine when formulating haircolor?

5. Name the primary, secondary, and tertiary colors.

6. What is the role of tone and intensity in haircolor?

7. What are the categories of haircolor? Briefly describe each one.

8. How does hydrogen peroxide developer work in a haircolor formula?

9. What are the five key questions to ask when formulating a haircolor?

10. Why is a patch test useful in haircoloring?

11. What is a preliminary strand test and why is it used?

12. Explain the action of hair lighteners.

13. What is the procedure for a virgin single-process color service?

14. What are the two processes involved in double-process haircoloring?

15. Name and describe the various forms of hair lightener.

16. What is the purpose of toner? When is it used?

17. What are the three most commonly used methods for highlighting? Describe each.

18. List seven tips for achieving gray coverage.

19. List the rules of color correction.

20. List five safety precautions to follow during the haircolor process.

STUDY TOOLS

- **Reinforce what you just learned:** Complete the activities and exercises in your Theory or Practical Workbook, or your Study Guide.

- **Expand your knowledge:** Search for websites about the topics in this chapter and make a list of additional resources.

- **Study and prepare for your quiz:** Take the chapter test in your Exam Review or your Milady U: Online Licensing Prep.

- **Re-Test your knowledge:** Take the Chapter 21 *Quizzes*!

- **Learn even more:** Look up in a dictionary or search the internet for the definitions for any additional terms you want to learn about.

CHAPTER GLOSSARY

activators	p. 695	Also known as *boosters*, *protinators*, or *accelerators*; powdered persulfate salts added to haircolor to increase its lightening ability.
aniline derivatives AN-ul-un DUR-ive-it-ives	p. 681	Contain small, uncolored dyes that combine with hydrogen peroxide to form larger, permanent dye molecules within the cortex.
Baliage BAHL-ee-ahj	p. 700	Also known as *free-form technique*; painting a lightener (usually a powdered off-the-scalp lightener) directly onto clean, styled hair.
base color	p. 675	Predominant tone of a color.

cap technique	p. 699	Lightening technique that involves pulling clean, dry strands of hair through a perforated cap with a thin plastic or metal hook and then combing them to remove tangles.
color fillers	p. 706	Equalize porosity and deposit color in one application to provide a uniform contributing pigment on pre-lightened hair.
complementary colors	p. 677	A primary and secondary color positioned directly opposite each other on the color wheel.
conditioner fillers	p. 705	Used to recondition damaged, overly porous hair and equalize porosity so that the hair accepts the color evenly from strand to strand and scalp to ends.
contributing pigment	p. 673	Also known as *undertone*; the varying degrees of warmth exposed during a permanent color or lightening process.
demipermanent haircolor	p. 681	Also known as *no-lift deposit-only color*; formulated to deposit but not lift (lighten) natural hair color.
developers	p. 683	Also known as *oxidizing agents* or *catalysts*; when mixed with an oxidation haircolor, supplies the necessary oxygen gas to develop color molecules and create a change in hair color.
double-process application	p. 684	Also known as *two-step coloring*; a coloring technique requiring two separate procedures in which the hair is pre-lightened before the depositing color is applied to the hair.
fillers	p. 705	Used to equalize porosity.
foil technique	p. 699	Highlighting technique that involves coloring selected strands of hair by slicing or weaving out sections, placing them on foil or plastic wrap, applying lightener or permanent haircolor, and then sealing them in the foil or plastic wrap.
glaze	p. 693	A non-ammonia color that adds shine and tone to the hair.
hair color	p. 671	(two words) The natural color of hair.
haircolor	p. 671	(one word) A professional, industry-coined term referring to artificial haircolor products and services.
haircolor glaze	p. 681	Common way to describe a haircolor service that adds shine and color to the hair.
hair lightening	p. 694	Also known as *bleaching* or *decolorizing*; chemical process involving the diffusion of the natural hair color pigment or artificial haircolor from the hair.
highlighting	p. 698	Coloring some of the hair strands lighter than the natural color to add a variety of lighter shades and the illusion of depth.
highlighting shampoo	p. 701	Colors prepared by combining permanent haircolor, hydrogen peroxide, and shampoo.
hydrogen peroxide developer	p. 683	Oxidizing agent that, when mixed with an oxidation haircolor, supplies the necessary oxygen gas to develop the color molecules and create a change in natural hair color.
intensity	p. 678	The strength of a color.
law of color	p. 675	System for understanding color relationships.

level	p. 673	The unit of measurement used to identify the lightness or darkness of a color.
level system	p. 673	System that colorists use to determine the lightness or darkness of a hair color.
lighteners	p. 684	Chemical compounds that lighten hair by dispersing, dissolving, and decolorizing the natural hair pigment.
line of demarcation	p. 694	Visible line separating colored hair from new growth.
metallic haircolors	p. 683	Also known as *progressive haircolors*; haircolors containing metal salts that change hair color gradually by progressive buildup and exposure to air creating a dull, metallic appearance.
mixed melanin	p. 673	Combination of natural hair color that contains both pheomelanin and eumelanin.
natural haircolors	p. 682	Also known as *vegetable haircolors*; colors, such as henna, obtained from the leaves or bark of plants.
new growth	p. 696	Part of the hair shaft between the scalp and the hair that has been previously colored.
off-the-scalp lighteners	p. 695	Also known as *quick lighteners*; powdered lighteners that cannot be used directly on the scalp.
on-the-scalp lighteners	p. 695	Lighteners that can be used directly on the scalp by mixing the lightener with activators.
patch test	p. 691	Also known as a *predisposition test*; test required by the Federal Food, Drug, and Cosmetic Act for identifying a possible allergy in a client.
permanent haircolors	p. 681	Lighten and deposit color at the same time and in a single process because they are more alkaline than no-lift, deposit-only colors and are usually mixed with a higher-volume developer.
pre-lightening	p. 694	First step of double-process haircoloring; used to lift or lighten the natural pigment before the application of toner.
pre-softening	p. 704	Process of treating gray or very resistant hair to allow for better penetration of color.
primary colors	p. 676	Pure or fundamental colors (red, yellow, and blue) that cannot be created by combining other colors.
resistant	p. 672	Hair type that is difficult for moisture or chemicals to penetrate and thus requires a longer processing time.
reverse highlighting	p. 698	Also known as *lowlighting*; technique of coloring strands of hair darker than the natural color.
secondary color	p. 676	Color obtained by mixing equal parts of two primary colors.
semipermanent haircolor	p. 680	No-lift, deposit-only non-oxidation haircolor that is not mixed with peroxide and is formulated to last through several shampoos.
single-process haircoloring	p. 693	Process that lightens and deposits color in the hair in a single application.
slicing	p. 699	Coloring technique that involves taking a narrow, ⅛-inch (0.3 centimeter) section of hair by making a straight part at the scalp, positioning the hair over the foil, and applying lightener or color.

soap cap	p. 682	Combination of equal parts of a prepared permanent color mixture and shampoo used the last five minutes and worked through the hair to refresh the ends.
special effects haircoloring	p. 698	Any technique that involves partial lightening or coloring.
strand test	p. 692	Determines how the hair will react to the color formula and how long the formula should be left on the hair.
temporary haircolor	p. 680	Nonpermanent color whose large pigment molecules prevent penetration of the cuticle layer, allowing only a coating action that may be removed by shampooing.
tertiary color (TUR-shee-aye-ee KUL-ur)	p. 676	Intermediate color achieved by mixing a secondary color and its neighboring primary color on the color wheel in equal amounts.
tone	p. 678	Also known as *hue*; the balance of color.
toners	p. 685	Semipermanent, demipermanent, and permanent haircolor products that are used primarily on pre-lightened hair to achieve pale and delicate colors.
virgin application	p. 693	First time the hair is colored.
volume	p. 683	Measures the concentration and strength of hydrogen peroxide.
weaving	p. 699	Coloring technique in which selected strands are picked up from a narrow section of hair with a zigzag motion of the comb, and lightener or color is applied only to those strands.

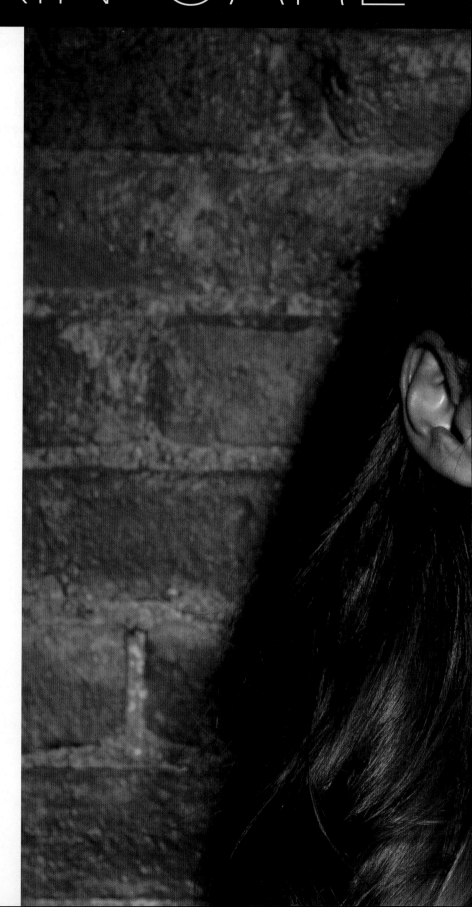

PART 4 SKIN CARE

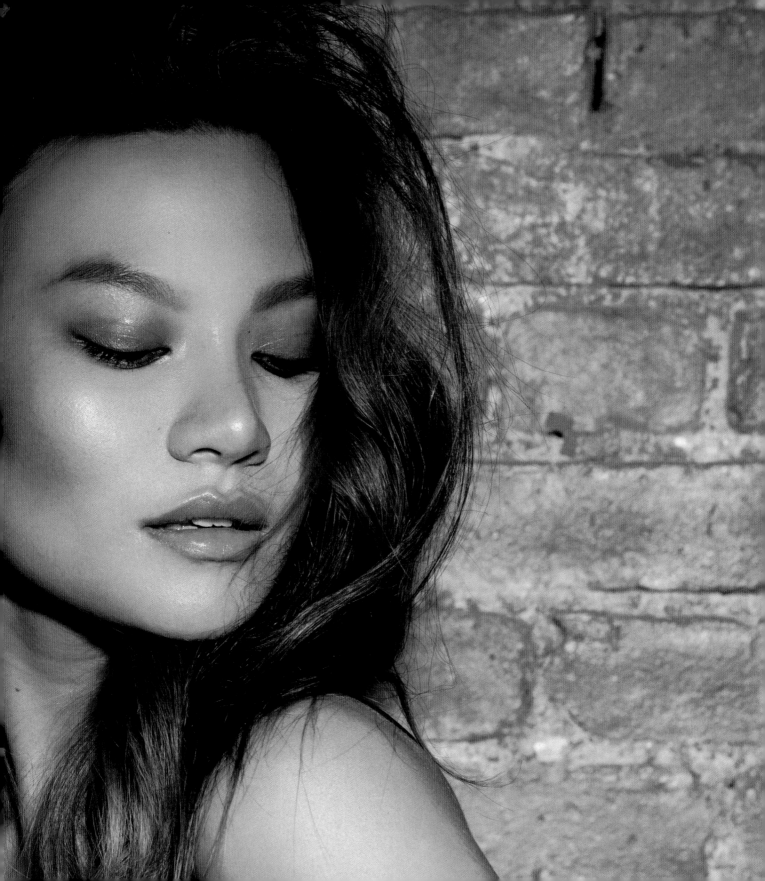

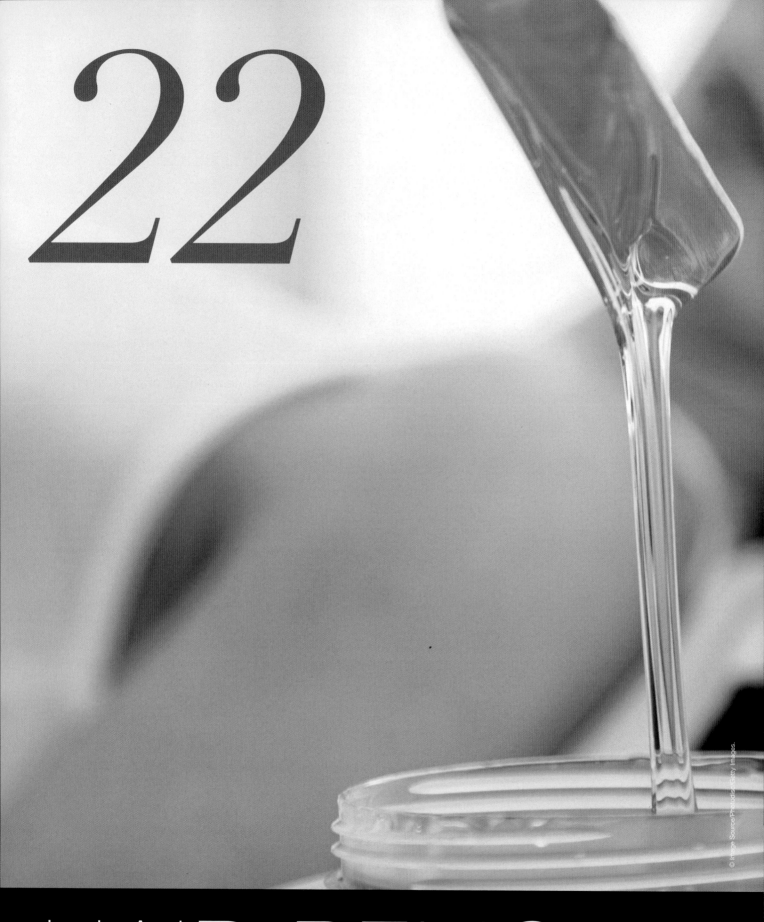

22

HAIR REMOVAL

LEARNING OBJECTIVES

After completing this chapter, you will be able to:

LO❶
Explain the significance of a client intake form used in hair removal services.

LO❷
Name the conditions that contraindicate hair removal in the salon.

LO❸
Identify and describe three methods of permanent hair removal.

LO❹
List the eight methods used for temporary hair removal.

One of the fastest growing services in the salon and spa businesses is hair removal. Once restricted to an occasional lip or brow service, a growing number of clients now want to have their entire face, arms, and legs bare of hair.

Body waxing has gained a tremendous amount of popularity in the last few years. Many clients now have body waxing performed as regularly as getting their hair cut or colored.

The most common form of hair removal in salons and spas is waxing, but with the popularity of these services on the rise, many different methods are now coming into play.

Many men are now frequently requesting hair removal services. It has become a fashion trend for men to have hairless legs, arms, and even chests. Men who participate in sports such as cycling, swimming, body building, and soccer often remove hair from their legs and arms, and occasionally their entire body. The nape of the neck, chest, and back are the most frequent removal requests for men.

Clients with an overabundance of hair are certainly the best candidates for hair removal, although many clients with even just a few unwanted hairs on their arms or legs are now requesting these services. **Hirsuties** (hur-SOO-shee-eez), also known as *hypertrichosis* (hy-pur-trih-KOH-sis), refers to the growth of an unusual amount of hair on parts of the body normally bearing only downy hair, such as the faces of women and the backs of men. **Hirsutism** (HUR-suh-tiz-um) is an excessive growth or cover of hair, especially in women.

Facial and body hair removal has become increasingly popular as evolving technology makes it easier to perform with more effective results. All of the various approaches to hair removal fall into two major categories: permanent and temporary. Salon techniques are generally limited to temporary methods.

why study
Hair Removal?

Cosmetologists should study and have a thorough understanding of hair removal because:

> Removing unwanted hair is a primary concern for many clients, and being able to advise them on the various types of hair removal will enhance your ability to satisfy your clients.

> Offering clients hair removal services that meet their needs and can be scheduled while they are already in the salon can be a valuable extra service you can offer.

> Learning the proper hair removal techniques and performing them safely makes you an even more important part of a client's beauty regimen.

After reading the next few sections, you will be able to:

LO❶ Explain the significance of a client intake form used in hair removal services.

Consult the Client

Before performing any hair removal service, a consultation is always necessary. Ask the client to complete a *client intake form* which is used in skin care services and is a questionnaire that discloses all medications, both topical (applied to the skin) and oral (taken by mouth), along with any known medical issues, skin disorders, or allergies that might affect treatment (**figure 22-1**). Allergies or sensitivities must be noted, highlighted, and documented on the service record card—the client's permanent progress record of services received and products purchased or used. Keep in mind that many changes can occur between client visits. Since a client's last visit, he or she may have been prescribed medications such as antidepressants, hormones, cortisone, medicine for blood pressure or diabetes, or topical prescriptions such as Retin-A®, Renova®, and hydroquinone. A client using any one of these prescriptions may not be a candidate for hair removal. See **figure 22-2** for a sample client intake form.

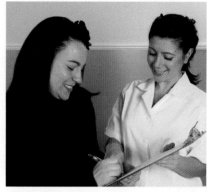

figure 22-1
Filling out a client intake form should be a part of every hair removal service.

Many of these medications cause changes in the skin that can cause epidermal skin to lift during waxing treatment. In other words, the epidermal skin can peel off along with the wax and the hair.

Clients who have autoimmune diseases such as lupus can have reactions to the inflammation caused by waxing, electrolysis, or other hair removal methods.

Clients with conditions such as rosacea or eczema can experience severe inflammation, because these skin conditions are likely to already be inflamed before treatment.

It is imperative that every client sign a release form for the hair removal service you are going to provide. This should be completed prior to every service. It serves as a reminder to the client to really think about any topical or oral medication they might have started since their last visit. See **figure 22-3** for a sample release form. Any changes should be recorded on the service record card.

After reading the next few sections, you will be able to:

LO❷ Name the conditions that contraindicate hair removal in the salon.

Name the Contraindications for Hair Removal

One of the main purposes of a client consultation is to determine the presence of any contraindications for hair removal. Some medical conditions and medications may cause thinning of the skin or make the skin more vulnerable to injury. Waxing clients with these conditions could cause unnecessary inflammation or severe injuries to the skin.

Client history

Name_____

Address_____

City_____ State _____ Zip code_____

Email_____Home phone_____

Cell phone_____Work phone_____

Occupation_____ Referred by_____ Date of birth_____

Is this your first facial treatment?   YES_____   NO_____

Have you been waxed before?   YES_____   NO_____

Do you have acne or frequent blemishes?   YES_____   NO_____

Have you ever used:

RetinA (Tretinoin), Differin (Adapalene), Tazorac (Tazarotene), Azelex?   YES_____   NO_____

Any other topical/dermatological prescription drugs?   YES_____NO_____

Accutane® (isotretinoin)?   YES_____   NO_____

Are you using glycolic or alphahydroxy acids, salicylic acid, or skin bleaching products?   YES_____   NO_____

Have you had microdermabrasion or a chemical peel?   YES_____   NO_____

Have you had laser resurfacing, laser or light treatment, facial injectables, or plastic surgery?   YES_____   NO_____

Do you smoke?   YES_____   NO_____

Do you tan or use tanning beds/booths?   YES_____   NO_____

Are you pregnant?   YES_____   NO_____

Are you nursing?   YES_____   NO_____

Taking birth control pills?   YES_____   NO_____   If so, how long? _____

Have you had skin cancer?   YES_____   NO_____

Do you experience stress?   YES_____   NO_____If so, how often?_____

Do you wear contact lenses?   YES_____   NO_____

Are you under a physician's care?   YES_____   NO_____

Physician's Name_____

Do you have any allergies to cosmetics, foods, or drugs?   YES_____   NO_____

Please list_____

figure 22-2
Client intake form for skin care services

Are you presently using any medications?   YES_____   NO_____

Please list_____

What products do you use presently? _____

Please circle: Soap   Cleansing Milk   Toner   Daily sunscreen   Creams

Other _____

Please circle if you are affected by or have any of the following:

Have had hysterectomy	Herpes	Lupus
Depression or Anxiety	Chronic headaches	Urinary or kidney problems
Seborrhea/Psoriasis/Eczema	Fever blisters/Cold sores	Hepatitis
Asthma	Metal bone pins or plates	Epilepsy
High blood pressure	Sinus problems	Other skin diseases
Pacemaker/Cardiac Problems	Immune disorders	

Please explain above problems or list any significant others:

_____

_____

I understand that the services offered are not a substitute for medical care, and any information

provided by the therapist is for educational purposes only and not diagnostically prescriptive in

nature. I understand that the information herein is to aid the technician in giving better service

and is completely confidential.

SALON POLICIES

1.   Professional consultation is required before initial dispensing of products.

2.   Failure to give 24 hours notice of cancelation of any appointment will result in charges for the service time reserved.

3.   We do not give cash refunds.

I fully understand and agree to the above salon policies.

_____   _____

Client signature   Date

figure 22-2
Client intake form for skin care services (continued)

RELEASE FORM FOR WAXING

I understand that topical creams, medical conditions, and medications which are contraindicated for waxing, and can negatively affect the results of waxing. Certain medications, products, and medical or cosmetic treatments used prior to waxing may result in irritation, skin peeling, blotchiness, pigmentation, and sensitivity.

I understand that I cannot be waxed anywhere on the body if I am taking or have recently taken the prescription drug isotretinoin (Accutane®), prednisolone (prednisone), blood thinners such as Coumadin® (warfarin), and others that have side effects on the condition of the skin.

I understand that I cannot be waxed if I am using topical prescription acne drugs such as Retin-A® (tretinoin), Tazorac® (tazarotene). Differin® (adapalene), or other similar drugs or products that are peeling agents.

I understand that I cannot be waxed if I have recently had any peeling or exfoliation treatment, laser treatments, skin injections, skin or facial surgery.

I understand that I am accepting full responsibility for skin reactions if I do not inform my technician of any and all medical conditions, cosmetic or medical treatments, and medications I am using prior to waxing.

I understand that some redness and/or sensitivity may result. I agree to avoid sun exposure, excessive heat (saunas, hot tubs), and all active products for the next 48 hours or as instructed by the technician.

The hair removal process has been explained and I have had an opportunity to ask questions and receive satisfactory answers.

I consent to be waxed and will not hold the salon or technician responsible for any adverse reactions from treatments or products.

Name (print) _____   Signature _____

Initial below for each visit:

Date: _____ Client initials: _____   Date: _____ Client initials: _____

Date: _____ Client initials: _____   Date: _____ Client initials: _____

Date: _____ Client initials: _____   Date: _____ Client initials: _____

· ·

WAX TREATMENT RECORD

(Cosmetologist to fill out chart notes on back of assessment form for each service)

Client name: _____

Date	Cosmetologist	Wax Service	Notes
9/8/15	Teresa	Brow w/soft wax	New client: shaping for more arch, close-set eyes Tweezed chin No redness

figure 22-3
Sample waxing release form

Clients should not have any waxing or hair removal performed anywhere on the body if they are experiencing any of the following medical conditions or treatments, without first obtaining written permission from their physician:

- Client is using or has used isotretinoin (Accutane) in the last six months.
- Client is taking blood-thinning medications.
- Client undergoing chemotherapy or radiation.
- Client is taking drugs for autoimmune diseases, including lupus.
- Client is taking or has recently taken prednisone or steroids.

- Client has psoriasis, eczema, or other chronic skin diseases.
- Client has a sunburn.
- Client has pustules, papules, or other skin lesions in area to be waxed.
- Client has recently had cosmetic or reconstructive surgery within the previous three months.
- Client has recently had a laser skin treatment on the body.
- Client has severe varicose leg veins.
- Client has hemophilia, bleeding disorders, or circulatory conditions.
- Client has any other questionable medical condition.

Facial waxing should not be performed on clients with any of the following conditions without first obtaining permission from their physician:

- Client has rosacea or very sensitive skin.
- Client has a history of fever blisters or cold sores. (Waxing can cause a flare-up of this condition without medical pretreatment.)
- Client has had a recent chemical peel using glycolic, alpha hydroxy, or salicylic acid, or other acid-based products.
- Client has recently had microdermabrasion.
- Client uses any exfoliating topical medication, including Retin-A®, Renova®, Tazorac®, Differin®, Azelex®, or other medical peeling agent in area to be waxed.
- Client has recently had laser skin treatment or surgical peel.
- Client uses hydroquinone for skin lightening.

If you have any question that your client may have a condition that might be a contraindication for waxing, consult with the client's physician. You may also choose to wax a small area of the skin as a patch test before performing the service.

After reading the next few sections, you will be able to:

LO❸ Identify and describe three methods of permanent hair removal.

Describe Permanent Hair Removal

Although permanent hair removal services are not often offered in salons, it is useful to know the options that exist. Permanent hair removal methods include electrolysis, photoepilation (light-based hair removal), and laser hair removal.

Electrolysis

Electrolysis is the removal of hair by means of an electric current that destroys the growth cells of the hair. The current is applied with a very fine, needle-shaped electrode that is inserted into each hair follicle. This technique must only be performed by a licensed electrologist.

Photoepilation

Photoepilation (FOTO-epp-ihl-aye-shun), also known as *Intense Pulsed Light* (IPL), uses intense light to destroy the growth cells of the hair follicles. This treatment has minimal side effects, requires no needles, and thus minimizes the risk of infection. Clinical studies have shown that photoepilation can provide 50 to 60 percent clearance of hair in 12 weeks. This method can be administered in some salons by cosmetologists and estheticians, depending on state law. Manufacturers of photoepilation equipment generally provide the special training necessary for administering this procedure.

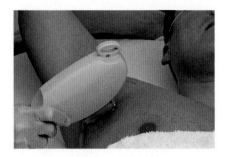

Laser Hair Removal

Lasers are another method for the rapid removal of unwanted hair. In **laser hair removal**, a laser beam is pulsed on the skin, impairing hair growth. It is most effective when used on follicles that are in the growth or anagen phase.

The laser method was discovered by chance when it was noted that birthmarks treated with certain types of lasers became permanently devoid of hair. Lasers are not for everyone; an absolute requirement is that one's hair must be darker than the surrounding skin. Coarse, dark hair responds best to laser treatment. For some clients, this method produces permanent hair removal. For other clients, laser hair removal treatments simply slow down regrowth.

In certain states, cosmetologists or estheticians are allowed to perform laser hair removal under a doctor's supervision. This method requires specialized training, most commonly offered by laser equipment manufacturers.

Laws regarding photoepilation and laser hair removal services vary by state, so be sure to check with your regulatory agency for guidelines.

After reading the next few sections, you will be able to:

LO**4** List the eight methods used for temporary hair removal.

Discuss Temporary Hair Removal

Temporary methods of hair removal, some of which may be offered in the salon or spa, are discussed below.

Shaving

The most common form of temporary hair removal, particularly of men's facial hair, is shaving. The targeted area should be softened by applying a warm, moist towel, and then applying a shaving cream or lotion that has excellent lubrication qualities and calms the skin. An electric clipper may also be used, particularly to remove unwanted hair at the nape of the neck. The application of a pre-shaving lotion helps to reduce any irritation. An electric trimmer can also make short work of unwanted hair at the nape of the neck.

Tweezing

Tweezing is using tweezers to remove hairs, commonly used to shape the eyebrows, and can also be used to remove undesirable hairs from around the mouth and chin. Eyebrow arching is often done as part of a professional makeup service. Correctly shaped eyebrows have a strong, positive impact on the overall attractiveness of the face. The natural arch of the eyebrow follows the orbital bone, or the curved line of the eye socket, but hair can grow both above and below the natural line. These hairs should be removed to give a clean and attractive appearance.

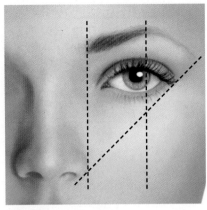
figure 22-4
Guidelines for proper eyebrow shape

Determining the Best Shape for Eyebrows

As with any procedure, always perform a client consultation prior to tweezing or waxing the eyebrows. Determine the client's wishes for final eyebrow shape. If you remove too much hair, it will generally grow back, but regrowth may take several months, and you may end up with an unhappy client who is not likely to return for your services. Conducting a thorough consultation beforehand will help you avoid such mistakes.

To determine the best shape for the brow, hold the base of a comb or spatula against the corner of the nose, with the other end of the comb or spatula extending straight upward toward the eyebrow. This is where the brow should begin. Hold the comb or spatula so it extends from the corner of the nose to the outside corner of the eye and then across the eyebrow. This is where the brow should end.

The high point of the arch of the brow should be near the outside corner of the iris, if the client is looking straight ahead. See **figure 22-4** for an illustration of how these techniques are applied.

Just like a good haircut, the arch and shape of the eyebrows should be well blended and flow in a natural line. Remove the excess brow hair in an even fashion to avoid sharp angles or obvious thinner areas in the brow line. If the client has an uneven brow line, encourage him or her to allow the eyebrows in the thin area to grow back, so that you can help the client achieve a smoother, well-blended, and more natural-looking line.

(P) 22-3   **Eyebrow Tweezing** *See page 753*

Depilatories

A **depilatory** (dih-PIL-uh-Tohr-ee) is a substance, usually a caustic alkali preparation, used for the temporary removal of superfluous hair by dissolving it at the skin's surface. It contains detergents to strip the sebum from the hair and adhesives to hold the chemicals to the hair shaft for the five to ten minutes necessary to remove the hair. During the application time, the hair expands and the disulfide bonds break. Finally, such chemicals as sodium hydroxide, potassium hydroxide, thioglycolic acid, or calcium thioglycolate destroy the disulfide bonds. These chemicals turn the hair into a soft, jelly-like mass that can be scraped from the skin. Although depilatories are not commonly used in salons, you should be familiar with them in the event that your clients have used them.

Depilatories can be inflammatory to skin and should not be used on sensitive skin types or on clients who have contraindications for waxing.

It is a good idea to patch test any depilatory on your client's skin prior to treatment the first time. Select a hairless part of the arm, apply a small amount according to the manufacturer's directions, and leave it on the skin for seven to ten minutes. If there are no signs of redness, swelling, or rash, the depilatory can probably be used safely over a larger area of the skin. Follow the manufacturer's directions for application. For an easy reference guide for which type of hair removal procedure is appropriate for various areas of the body, refer to table 22-1.

Epilators

An **epilator** removes the hair from the bottom of the follicle. Wax is a commonly used epilator and is available in two main forms: hard and soft wax. Both types of wax are made primarily of resins and polymers, but can also be made from sugars, honey, and sometimes beeswax.

Soft wax is applied to the skin and then removed using fabric strips. Hard wax is somewhat thicker and does not require fabric strips for removal. Because waxing removes the hair from the bottom of the follicle, the hair takes longer to grow back. The time between waxings is generally four to six weeks.

Wax is available in various forms including tubs that can be inserted into wax heaters and wax beads that can be melted in a heater. Always check the manufacturer's instructions for heating, using, and removing the particular form of wax, as well as clean-up techniques.

Wax may be applied to various parts of the face and body, such as the eyebrows, cheeks, chin, upper lip, arms, and legs. On male clients, wax may be used to remove hair on the back and nape of the neck. The hair should be at least ¼-inch (0.6 centimeters) long for waxing to be effective. Hair shorter than ¼-inch may not adhere to the wax. If hair is more than ½-inch (1.25 centimeters) long, it should be trimmed before waxing.

Bikini hair removal has also evolved into its own art form, with different designs becoming sought-after services by many clients. **Brazilian bikini waxing**, a waxing technique that requires the removal of all the hair from the front and the back of the bikini area, is a popular style of waxing. The method was named for the completely hairless look required when

table 22-1
APPROPRIATE HAIR REMOVAL PROCEDURES

Body area	Waxing	Tweezing	Depilatories
Face/Upper Lips/Eyebrows	X	X	
Underarms	X		
Arms	X		X
Bikini line	X	X	
Back/shoulders	X	X (after waxing or sugaring)	X
Legs	X		X
Tops of feet/toes	X		X

wearing a Brazilian style bikini. Brazilian bikini waxing requires more specific training than offered in this book. Ask your instructor about advanced courses in Brazilian bikini waxing.

Be aware that removing vellus (lanugo) hair may cause the skin to temporarily feel less soft. When waxing is done properly, the hair will not feel like beard stubble as it grows out.

Before beginning a wax treatment, be sure that the client completes a client intake form (see figure 22-2), and have the client sign a release form (see figure 22-3). Wear disposable gloves to prevent contact with bloodborne pathogens.

Safety Precautions for Waxing

- To prevent burns, always test the temperature of the heated wax before applying to the client's skin. Use a professional wax heater for warming wax. Never heat wax in a microwave or on a stove top. Wax can become overheated and burn the client's skin.

- Use caution so that the wax does not come in contact with the eyes.

- Never double-dip wax. When removing wax from the wax pot, always use a new spatula.

- Do not apply wax over warts, moles, abrasions, or irritated or inflamed skin. Do not remove hair protruding from a mole because the wax could cause trauma to the mole.

- The skin under the arms is sometimes very sensitive. If so, use hard wax.

- Redness and swelling sometimes occur after waxing sensitive skin. Apply an aloe gel and cool compresses to calm and soothe the skin.

Ⓟ 22-4   **Eyebrow Waxing Using Soft Wax** *See page 755*

Ⓟ 22-5   **Lip Waxing Using Hard Wax** *See page 757*

Ⓟ 22-6   **Body Waxing Using Soft Wax** *See page 759*

Threading

Threading, also known as *banding*, is a temporary hair removal method whereby cotton thread is twisted and rolled along the surface of the skin, entwining the hair in the thread and lifting it from the follicle (figure 22-5). The technique is still practiced in many Eastern cultures today. Threading has become increasingly popular in the United States as an alternative to other methods. It requires specialized training.

Sugaring

Sugaring is another temporary hair removal method that involves the use of a thick, sugar-based paste and is especially appropriate for more sensitive skin types (figure 22-6). Sugaring is becoming more popular and produces the same results as soft or hard wax. One advantage with sugaring is the hair can be removed even if it is only ⅛-inch (0.3 centimeters) long.

Removing the residue from the skin is simple, as it dissolves with warm water.

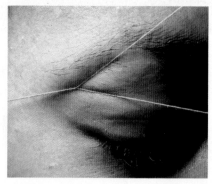
figure 22-5
Threading

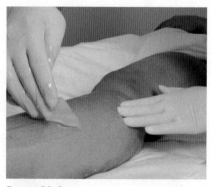
figure 22-6
Sugaring

? DID YOU KNOW?
Threading, sugaring, and specialty waxing, such as Brazilian waxing, are advanced techniques that require additional training and experience. Check with your instructor about advanced training that is often available at trade shows and seminars, as well as through videos.

PRE-SERVICE PROCEDURE

In the morning, the treatment room should be ready to go from the previous night's thorough cleaning and disinfecting. (See "At the End of the Day" in Procedure 22-2, Post-Service Procedure.) The preparations listed below should be performed between every client service.

A. PREPARING THE TREATMENT ROOM

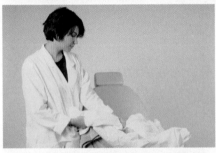

1 Check your room supply of linens (towels and sheets) and replenish as needed. Change the bed or treatment chair linens.

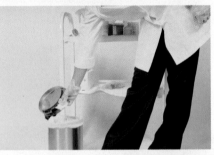

2 Throw away any disposables used during the previous service.

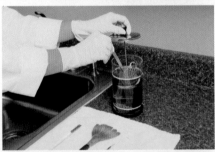

3 Clean and disinfect any used brushes or implements, such as mask brushes, comedo extractors, tweezers, machine attachments, and electrodes.

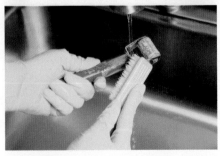

4 Clean and disinfect any machine parts used during the previous service.

⑤ Clean and disinfect counters and the magnifying lamp or lens.

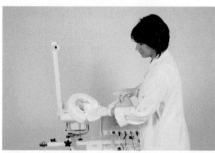

⑥ Check water level on vaporizer as needed.

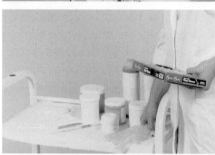

⑦ Replace any disposable implements you may need, such as gloves, sheet cotton, gauze squares, sponges for cleansing and makeup application and removal, disposable makeup applicators (mascara wands, lip brushes, other brushes), spatulas and tongue-depressor wax applicators, cotton swabs, facial tissue, and fabric strips for waxing. Prepare your strips ahead of time by cutting smaller strips for the eye and face areas.

⑧ Prepare to greet your next client.

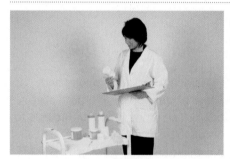

⑨ Review your client schedule for the day. Refresh your mind about each repeat client you will be seeing that day and his or her individual concerns. Make sure you have enough of all the products you will be using that day.

B. PREPARING FOR THE CLIENT

⑩ Retrieve and review the client's intake form and service record card. If the appointment is for a new client, let the receptionist know that the client will need an intake form.

⑪ Organize yourself by taking care of your personal needs before the client arrives—use the restroom, get a drink of water, return a personal call—so that when your client arrives, you can place your full attention on his or her needs. Double-check your room including cleanliness, music, and temperature. Double-check your personal professional appearance including your breath, hair, clothing, and makeup.

⑫ Turn off your cell phone or PDA. Be sure that you eliminate anything that can distract you from your client while he or she is in the salon.

⑬ Take a moment to clear your head of all your personal concerns and issues. Take a couple of deep breaths and remind yourself that you are committed to providing your clients with fantastic service and your full attention.

⑭ Wash your hands following Procedure 5-3, Proper Hand Washing, before going to greet your client.

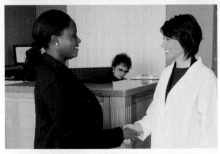

15 Greet your client in the reception area with a warm smile and handshake in a professional manner. Introduce yourself if you've never met. If the client is new, ask them for the intake form he or she filled out in the reception area.

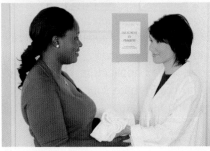

16 Escort the client to the changing area for him or her to change into a smock or robe. Some salons provide disposable slippers that can be worn to and from the dressing room. Make sure you indicate where to securely place personal items. If you do not have a changing room or lockers, he or she will need to change in the treatment room. If the client is only having a lip or brow wax, it is not always necessary to change clothes. Clothing can be protected with proper towel draping.

17 Ask the client to remove all jewelry and put it in a safe place, because you do not want to stop the service for them to remove the jewelry later.

18 Invite the client to take a seat in the treatment chair or to lie down on the treatment table.

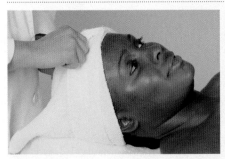
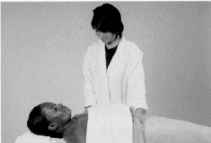

19 Drape the client properly and either place the hair in a protective cap or use a headband and towels to drape the hair properly. Give the client a blanket and make sure she is comfortable before beginning the service.

20 Consult with the new client about his or her concerns, and ask any questions you have concerning their intake form. If the client is returning, ask how their skin has been since the last treatment. Briefly explain your treatment plan to the client.

POST-SERVICE PROCEDURE

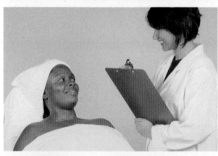

1 After the treatment, ask the client how he or she feels and how their skin feels. Discuss the conditions of the client's skin and what you can do to improve them. Ask if the client has any questions or other concerns. Determine a plan for future visits.

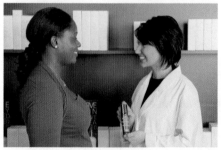

2 Advise client about the importance of proper home care and how the recommended professional products will help to improve the client's skin conditions. Explain each product in the home care step by step.

B. SCHEDULE NEXT APPOINTMENT AND THANK CLIENT

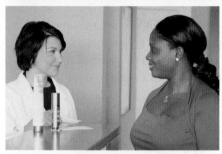

3 Escort the client to the reception desk and write up a service ticket including today's service, recommended products, and when the next service should be. Place all recommended home-care products on the counter.

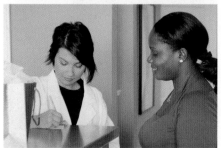

4 After the client has paid for their service and take-home products, ask if you can schedule the next appointment. Write the next appointment time on your business card for the client.

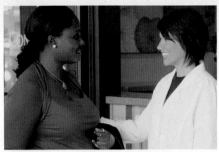

5 Thank the client for the opportunity to work with him or her. Ask the client to feel free to contact you should he or she have any questions or concerns. Thank the client again, shake his or her hand, and wish them a great day.

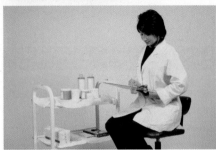

6 Be sure to record service information, observations, and product recommendations on the service record card and be sure you return it to the proper place for filing with the completed client intake form.

AT THE END OF THE DAY

1 Put on a fresh pair of gloves to protect yourself from contact with soiled linens and implements.

2 Turn off and unplug all equipment. Wax heaters must always be turned off nightly for safety as well as not damaging the unused wax.

3 Remove all dirty laundry from the hamper. Spray the hamper with a disinfectant aerosol spray or wipe it down with disinfectant. Mildew grows easily in hampers.

4 Remove all dirty spatulas, used brushes, and other utensils. Most of these should have been removed between clients during the day.

5 Thoroughly clean and disinfect all multiuse tools and implements.

6 Clean and then disinfect all counters, the treatment chair, machines, and other furniture with disinfectant. The magnifying lamp should be cleaned and disinfected on both sides in the same manner.

7 Replenish the room with fresh linens, spatulas, utensils, and other supplies, so it is ready for the next day.

8 Change disinfectant solution.

9 Maintain vaporizer as necessary.

10 Check the room for dirt, smudges, or dust on the walls, on the baseboards, in corners, or on air vents. Vacuum and mop the room with a disinfectant.

11 Spray the air in the room with a disinfectant aerosol spray.

12 Replenish any empty jars. If you are reusing and refilling jars, always use up the entire content of the small jar and thoroughly clean and disinfect the jar before replenishing. Never add cream to a partially used jar.

EYEBROW TWEEZING

You will need all of the following implements, materials, and supplies:

- □ Antiseptic lotion
- □ Cotton balls/pads
- □ Disposable gloves
- □ Emollient cream
- □ Eyebrow brush
- □ Gentle eye makeup remover
- □ Hair cap or headband
- □ Hand-held mirror
- □ Soothing toner
- □ Towels
- □ Tweezers

Perform:

P 22-1 **Pre-Service Procedure** *See page 748*

1️⃣ Put on disposable gloves. Cleanse the eyelid area with cotton balls moistened with gentle eye makeup remover.

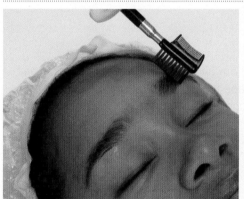

2️⃣ Brush the eyebrows with a small brush to remove any powder or scaliness.

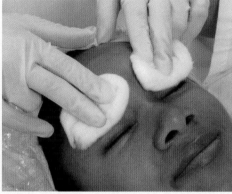

3️⃣ Soften brows. Saturate two pledgets (tufts) of cotton, or a towel with warm water, and place over the brows. Allow them to remain on the brows 1 to 2 minutes to soften and relax the eyebrow tissue. You may soften the brows and surrounding skin by rubbing a small amount of emollient cream into them.

4️⃣ Apply a mild toner on a cotton ball prior to tweezing.

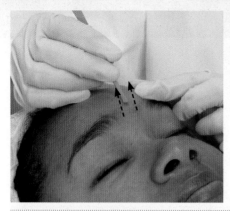

⑤ When tweezing, stretch the skin taut with the index finger and thumb (or index and middle fingers) of your non-dominant hand. Remove the hairs between the brows. Grasp each hair individually with tweezers and pull with a quick motion, always in the direction of growth. Tweeze between the brows and above the brow line first because the area under the brow line is much more sensitive.

⑥ Sponge the tweezed area frequently with cotton moistened with an antiseptic lotion to avoid infection.

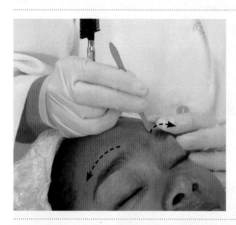

⑦ Brush the hair downward. Remove excessive hairs from above the eyebrow line, being careful to not create a hard line with top of the brow. Shape the upper section of one eyebrow, and then shape the other. Frequently sponge the area with toner.

⑧ Brush the hairs upward. Remove hairs from under the eyebrow line. Shape the lower section of one eyebrow, and then shape the other. Sponge the area with toner. Optional: Apply emollient cream and massage the brows. Remove cream with cool, wet cotton pads.

⑨ After tweezing is completed, sponge the eyebrows and surrounding skin with a toner to soothe the skin.

⑩ Brush the eyebrow hair to its normal position.

POST-SERVICE

Complete:

ⓟ 22-2　**Post-Service Procedure** *See page 751*

EYEBROW WAXING USING SOFT WAX

IMPLEMENTS & MATERIALS

You will need all of the following implements, materials, and supplies:

- ☐ Brow brush
- ☐ Cotton pads and swabs
- ☐ Disposable gloves
- ☐ Fabric strips for hair removal
- ☐ Facial chair
- ☐ Hair cap or headband
- ☐ Mild skin cleanser
- ☐ Roll of disposable paper
- ☐ Single or double wax heater
- ☐ Small disposable spatula or small wooden applicators
- ☐ Soothing emollient or antiseptic lotion
- ☐ Towels for draping
- ☐ Tweezers
- ☐ Wax
- ☐ Wax remover

PREPARATION | PROCEDURE

Perform:

P 22-1 **Pre-Service Procedure** *See page 748*

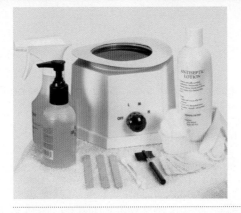

1 Melt the wax in the heater. This should take 10 to 25 minutes, depending on how full the wax pot is and the manufacturer's directions. Wax should have the thickness of caramel sauce. It should not be runny. Runny wax is often too hot and is more likely to drip.

2 Lay a clean towel over the top of the facial chair and then a layer of disposable paper.

3 Place a hair cap or headband on the client's head to keep hair away from the face.

4 Put on disposable gloves.

5 Remove the client's makeup, cleanse the area thoroughly with a mild cleanser, and dry.

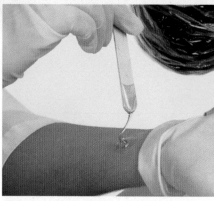

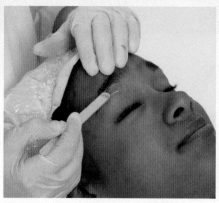

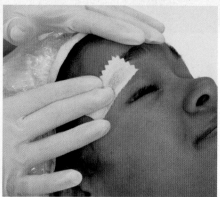

⑥ Test the temperature and consistency of the heated wax by applying a small drop on your inner wrist. It should be warm but not hot, and it should drip smoothly off the spatula.

⑦ With the spatula or wooden applicator, spread a thin coat of the warm wax evenly over the area to be treated, applying in the same direction as the hair growth. Be sure not to put the spatula in the wax more than once. No double dips!

⑧ Apply a fabric strip over the waxed area. Press gently in the direction of hair growth, running your finger over the surface of the fabric three to five times, always in the direction of the hair growth.

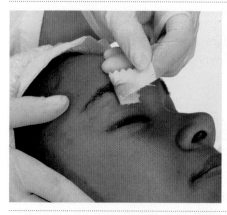

⑨ Gently applying pressure to hold the skin taut with one hand, quickly remove the fabric strip and the wax that sticks to it by pulling it against the direction of hair growth. Do not pull straight up on the strip; doing so could damage or remove the skin.

⑩ Immediately apply pressure to the waxed area with your finger. Hold your finger on the area for approximately 5 seconds to relieve any discomfort.

⑪ Remove any remaining wax residue from the skin with a gentle wax remover.

⑫ Repeat procedure on the area around the other eyebrow.

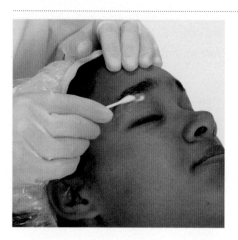

⑬ Cleanse the skin with a mild emollient cleanser and apply an emollient or antiseptic lotion.

POST-SERVICE

Complete:

Ⓟ 22-2   **Post-Service Procedure** *See page 751*

P 22-5

LIP WAXING USING HARD WAX

IMPLEMENTS & MATERIALS

You will need all of the following implements, materials, and supplies:

- ☐ Cotton pads and swabs
- ☐ Disposable gloves
- ☐ Facial chair
- ☐ Hair cap or headband

- ☐ Hard wax
- ☐ Mild skin cleanser
- ☐ Roll of disposable paper

- ☐ Single or double wax heater
- ☐ Small disposable spatula or small wooden applicators

- ☐ Soothing emollient or antiseptic lotion
- ☐ Towels for draping
- ☐ Wax remover

PREPARATION

Perform:

P 22-1 **Pre-Service Procedure** *See page 748*

PROCEDURE

1 Melt the wax in the heater. This should take 10 to 15 minutes, depending on how full the wax pot is and the manufacturer's instructions. Wax should have the thickness of a thick caramel sauce. It should not be runny.

2 Lay a clean towel over the top of the facial chair and then a layer of disposable paper.

3 Place a hair cap or headband on the client's head to keep hair away from the face.

4 Put on disposable gloves.

5 Remove the client's makeup, cleanse the area thoroughly with a mild cleanser, and dry.

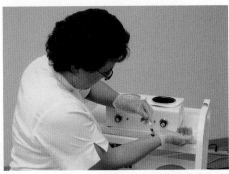

6 Test the temperature and consistency of the heated wax by applying a small drop on your inner wrist. It should be warm but not hot.

7 There are two different techniques for applying hard wax over the lip. Check with your instructor on their preferred method from the choices below:

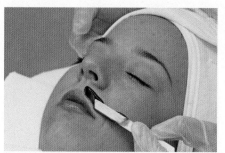

a. With the spatula or applicator, apply the warmed hard wax to the skin over the lip evenly from the center of the lip towards the corner of the mouth, in the same direction as the hair growth, about the thickness of a nickel. Make sure all visible hairs are covered and apply the wax just past where the hair stops growing, creating an edge to lift when removing the wax. It is best to have the pull-tab end where there is no hair underneath.

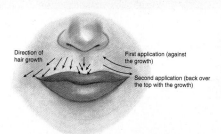

Direction of hair growth

First application (against the growth)

Second application (back over the top with the growth)

b. Alternative method: Another way to perform this step is with the spatula or applicator, first apply the warmed, hard wax about the thickness of a nickel to the skin in the *opposite* direction of hair growth. Go from the corner of the mouth towards the center of the lip. Then, in the same direction as the hair growth, apply the wax in a smooth or figure-eight pattern over the area to be waxed.

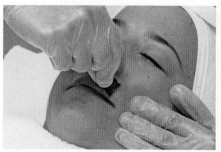

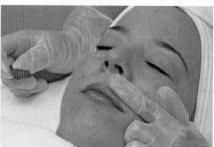

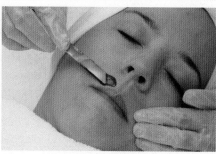

8 Allow the wax to sit for 1 to 2 minutes. If hard wax becomes too dry or cool, it will be brittle and break off when you attempt to remove it. Using your index finger and thumb, gently lift the edge of the wax and pull off the wax in an upwards and inwards movement.

9 Immediately apply pressure to the waxed area with your finger. Hold your finger on the area for approximately 5 seconds to relieve any discomfort.

10 Repeat the application and removal in the same manner to the other side of the lip.

11 Remove any remaining wax residue from the skin with a gentle wax remover.

12 Cleanse the skin with a mild emollient cleanser and apply an emollient or antiseptic lotion.

POST-SERVICE

Complete:

P 22-2 **Post-Service Procedure** *See page 751*

BODY WAXING USING SOFT WAX

IMPLEMENTS & MATERIALS

You will need all of the following implements, materials, and supplies:

- ☐ Disposable gloves
- ☐ Fabric strips for hair removal
- ☐ Facial chair
- ☐ Mild skin cleanser
- ☐ Dusting powder
- ☐ Roll of disposable paper
- ☐ Single or double wax heater
- ☐ Small disposable spatula or small wooden applicators
- ☐ Soothing emollient or antiseptic lotion
- ☐ Towels for draping
- ☐ Soft wax
- ☐ Wax remover

PREPARATION | PROCEDURE

Perform:

P 22-1 **Pre-Service Procedure** *See page 748*

1 Melt the wax in the heater. Be sure the wax is not too hot.

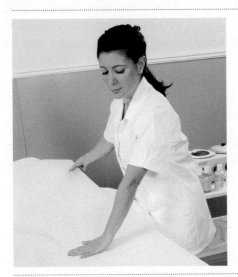

2 Drape the treatment bed with disposable paper or a bed sheet with paper over the top.

3 If bikini waxing, offer the client disposable panties or a small, clean towel.

4 If waxing the underarms, have the client remove her bra and put on a terry wrap. Offer a terry wrap when waxing the legs as well.

5 Assist the client onto the treatment bed and drape with towels.

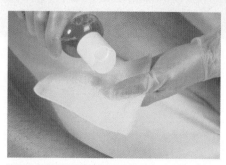

⑥ Apply disposable gloves. Thoroughly cleanse the area to be waxed with a mild cleanser and dry.

⑦ Trim the hair with scissors if it is more than ½-inch (1.25 centimeters) long. Put an extra single–use paper towel under the area to catch the hair and discard it before waxing. This keeps the extra hair from interfering with the wax and easier clean-up.

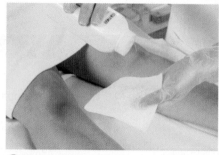

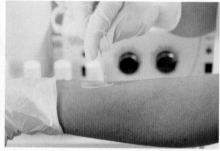

⑧ Apply a light covering of dusting powder.

⑨ Test the temperature and consistency of the heated wax by applying a small drop to your inner wrist.

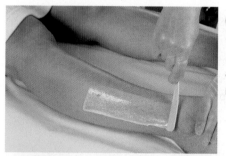

⑩ Using a disposable spatula, spread a thin coat of the warm wax evenly over the skin surface in the same direction as the hair growth. Be sure not to put the spatula in the wax more than once. If the wax strings and lands in an area you do not wish to treat, remove it with lotion designed to dissolve and remove wax.

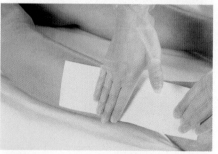

⑪ Apply a fabric strip in the same direction as the hair growth. Press gently but firmly, running your hand back and forth over the surface of the fabric three to five times.

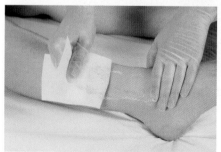

⑫ Gently apply pressure to hold the skin taut with one hand and with the other hand quickly remove the adhering wax in the opposite direction of the hair growth without lifting. Do not pull the fabric strip straight upwards.

13 Apply gentle pressure to the treated area.

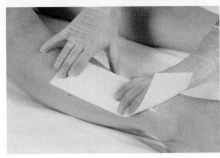

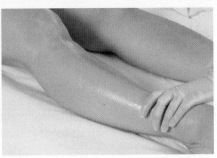

14 Repeat, using a fresh fabric strip every time.

15 Remove any remaining residue of powder from the skin. Cleanse the area with a mild emollient cleanser and apply an emollient or antiseptic lotion.

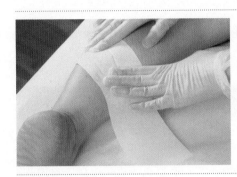

16 For waxing the legs, have the client turn over, and repeat the procedure on the backs of her legs. The entire front leg should be waxed, including the knees, and lotion applied to the front before having the client turn over and continue on the back of the legs. This is to avoid having the client's skin stick to the table.

17 Undrape the client and escort her to the dressing room.

POST-SERVICE

Complete:

P 22-2 **Post-Service Procedure** *See page 751*

• Complete a post-wax consultation and discuss post-wax precautions.

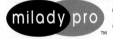
Check out miladypro.com for additional resources and training to enhance your technical skills. Keyword: FutureCosPro

REVIEW QUESTIONS

1. What information should be entered on the client intake form during the consultation?

2. What conditions, treatments, and medications contraindicate hair removal in the salon?

3. What are the two major types of hair removal? Give examples of each.

4. Define electrolysis, photoepilation, and laser removal.

5. Which hair removal techniques should not be performed in the salon without special training?

6. What is the difference between a depilatory and an epilator?

7. Why must a patch test be given before waxing?

8. List safety precautions that must be followed for soft and hard waxing.

9. Define threading and sugaring.

STUDY TOOLS

- **Reinforce what you just learned:** Complete the activities and exercises in your Theory or Practical Workbook, or your Study Guide.

- **Expand your knowledge:** Search for websites about the topics in this chapter and make a list of additional resources.

- **Study and prepare for your quiz:** Take the chapter test in your Exam Review or your Milady U: Online Licensing Prep.

- **Re-Test your knowledge:** Take the Chapter 22 *Quizzes*!

- **Learn even more:** Look up in a dictionary or search the internet for the definitions of any additional terms you want to learn about.

CHAPTER GLOSSARY

Brazilian bikini waxing	p. 746	A waxing technique that requires the removal of all the hair from the front and the back of the bikini area.
depilatory dih-PIL-uh-Tohr-ee	p. 745	Substance, usually a caustic alkali preparation, used for the temporary removal of superfluous hair by dissolving it at the skin surface level.
electrolysis	p. 743	Removal of hair by means of an electric current that destroys the root of the hair.
epilator	p. 746	Substance used to remove hair by pulling it out of the follicle.
hirsuties hur-SOO-shee-eez	p. 738	Also known as *hypertrichosis* (hy-pur-trih-KOH-sis); growth of an unusual amount of hair on parts of the body normally bearing only downy hair, such as the faces of women or the backs of men.
hirsutism HUR-suh-tiz-um	p. 738	Condition pertaining to an excessive growth or cover of hair, especially in women.

laser hair removal	p. 744	Permanent hair removal treatment in which a laser beam is pulsed on the skin, impairing the hair growth.
photoepilation FOTO-epp-ihl-aye-shun	p. 744	Also known as *Intense Pulsed Light*; permanent hair removal treatment that uses intense light to destroy the growth cells of the hair follicles.
sugaring	p. 747	Temporary hair removal method that involves the use of a thick, sugar-based paste.
threading	p. 747	Also known as *banding*; temporary hair removal method that involves twisting and rolling cotton thread along the surface of the skin, entwining the hair in the thread, and lifting it from the follicle.
tweezing	p. 745	Using tweezers to remove hairs.

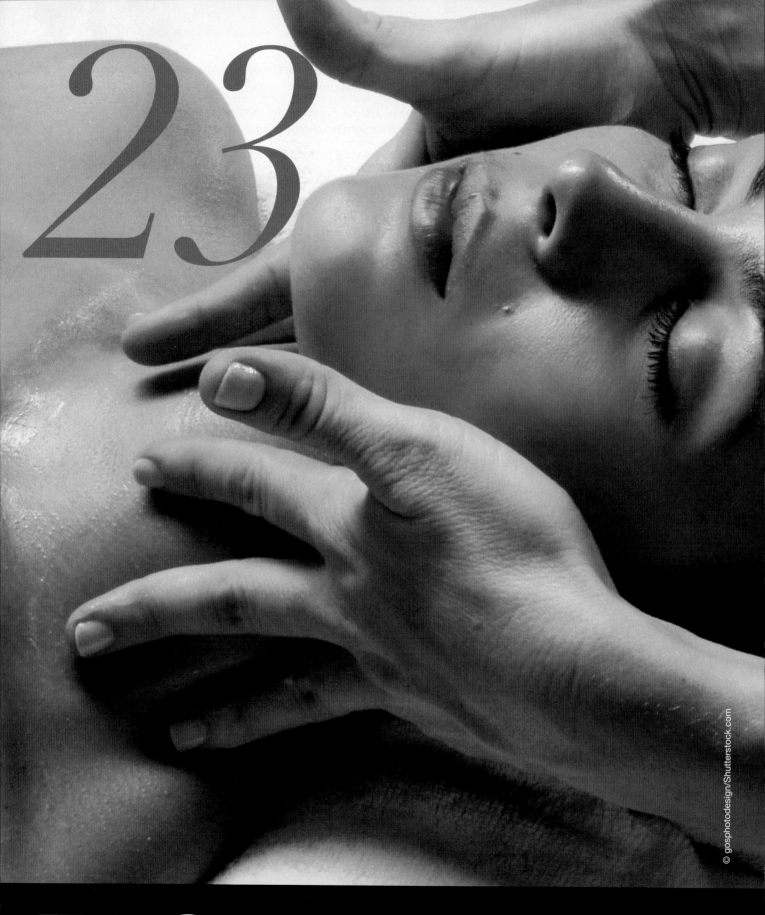

23

FACIALS

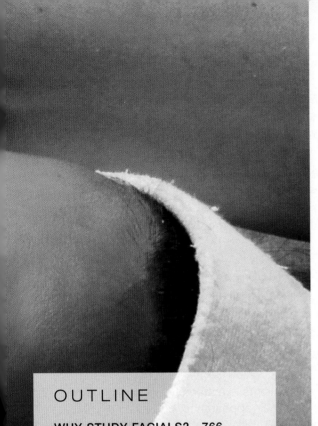

LEARNING OBJECTIVES

After completing this chapter, you will be able to:

LO❶

Explain the pertinent information to gather during a client consultation and skin analysis before performing facial treatments.

LO❷

Identify examples of contraindications that prohibit performing facial treatments.

LO❸

Determine the difference between skin type and skin condition.

LO❹

Name the different categories of skin care products used in facial treatments.

LO❺

Explain the different categories of skin care products used in facial treatments, and provide examples of each.

LO❻

Define why massage is used during a facial.

LO❼

Name and briefly describe the five categories of massage manipulations.

LO❽

Name and describe two types of electrical machines used in facial treatments.

LO❾

Explain how the two types of electrical machines add value to a facial.

LO❿

Know the difference between galvanic and high-frequency treatments used in facial services.

LO⓫

Explain how light therapy is used to treat the skin.

LO⓬

Discuss how aromatherapy is used in the basic facial.

G ood skin care can make a big difference in the way skin looks and in the way a client feels about his or her appearance. A **facial**, also known as a *facial treatment*, is a professional skin treatment that improves the condition and appearance of the skin. Besides being very relaxing, facial treatments can offer many improvements to the appearance of the skin (figure 23-1).

Proper skin care can make oily skin look cleaner and healthier, dry skin look and feel more moist and supple, and aging skin look smoother, firmer, and less wrinkled. A combination of good salon facial treatments and effective, individualized home care will show visible results.

why study
FACIALS?

Cosmetologists should study and have a thorough understanding of facials because:

> Providing skin care services to clients is extremely rewarding, helps busy clients to relax, improves their appearance, and helps clients feel better about themselves.

> Knowing the basics of skin analysis and basic information about skin care products will enable you to offer your clients advice when they ask you for it.

> Although you will not treat a skin disease, you must be able to recognize adverse skin conditions and refer clients to seek medical advice from a physician.

> Learning the basic techniques of facials and facial massage will give you a good overview of, and an ability to perform, these foundational services.

> You may enjoy this category of services and may consider specializing in skin care services. This study will create a perfect basis for making that decision.

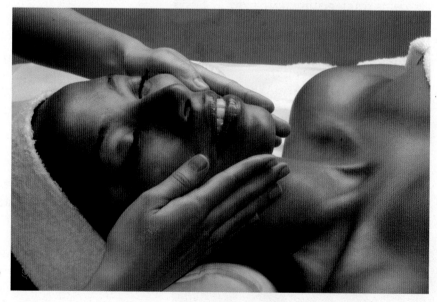

figure 23-1
A facial is a soothing, pleasurable experience for the client.

© gosphotodesign/Shutterstock.com

LO❶ Explain the pertinent information to gather during a client consultation and skin analysis before performing facial treatments.

LO❷ Identify examples of contraindications that prohibit performing facial treatments.

Conduct a Consultation and Skin Analysis

The consultation allows you the opportunity to ask the client questions about his or her health and skin care history, and it allows you to advise the client about appropriate home-care products and treatments. Skin analysis is a very important part of the facial treatment because it determines what type of skin the client has, the condition of the skin, and what type of treatment the client's skin needs.

The salon should designate a quiet area for facial treatments. Not only does the relaxing nature of a facial call for a quiet spot, but also the area needs to be quiet enough that you can conduct a thorough consultation with your client. All facial treatments should begin with a consultation and skin analysis.

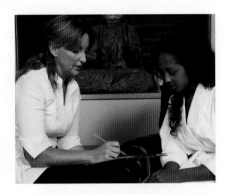

Client Intake Form

Before beginning the consultation and analysis, you must have the client fill out a client intake form (see **figure 22-2** in Chapter 22). The main purpose of the client intake form is to determine whether the client has any contraindications that might prohibit certain skin treatments.

A **contraindication** (kahn-trah-in-dih-KAY-shun) is a condition that requires avoiding certain treatments, procedures, or products to prevent undesirable side effects. For example, if the client is allergic to fragrance, using a scented product would be contraindicated. If a client is using a prescription drug, such as Retin-A® or Tazorac® (both topical drugs that cause skin exfoliation), using other exfoliants in the facial treatment is contraindicated because to do so may injure the skin by causing excessive peeling and inflammation.

Isotretinoin (Accutane), an oral medication for cystic acne, causes thinning of the skin all over the body. Waxing, stimulating treatments, or exfoliation procedures should never be performed on the skin of someone using isotretinoin or someone who has used the drug in the last six months. Because isotretinoin is an oral drug, it stays in the body for several months after the client stops taking it.

The main contraindications to look for are summarized in **table 23-1**.

Clients who have obvious skin abnormalities, such as open sores, fever blisters (herpes simplex), or other abnormal-looking signs should be referred to a physician for treatment. They can be rescheduled after they obtain written approval of facial services.

> ⚠ **CAUTION**
> Cosmetologists do not treat skin diseases. However, as a professional, you must be able to recognize the presence of various skin ailments in order to suggest that the client seek medical advice from a physician.

table 23-1
CONTRAINDICATIONS GRID

Contraindications	What to Avoid	Why?
Isotretinoin (Accutane)	• All waxing anywhere on the body • Any peeling agent or drying agent, including alpha hydroxy acids (AHAs), scrubs, microdermabrasion, and brushing machines	Skin can blister or peel off.
Exfoliating drugs including Retin-A® (Tretinoin), Renova®, Tazorac®, Differin®	• All waxing on the area where the drug is used • Any peeling agent or drying agent, including AHAs, scrubs, microdermabrasion, and brushing machines	Skin can blister or peel off.
Pregnancy	• Electrical treatments • Any questionable treatment without a physician's written permission • Possible sensitivities from waxing	Unknown; general safety precaution
Metal bone pins or plates in the body	• Electrical treatments	Electricity can possibly affect metal.
Heart conditions/pacemaker	• Electrical treatments	Electricity can possibly affect rhythms and pacemakers.
Known allergies	• Avoid known allergens, fragrances.	Allergic reaction can occur.
Seizures or epilepsy	• Electrical or light treatments	Could trigger seizure reaction
Use of oral steroids such as prednisone	• Any stimulating or exfoliating treatment • Waxing	Steroids can cause thinning of the skin which could result in blistering or injury.
Autoimmune diseases such as lupus	• Harsh or stimulating treatments without specific physician permission	Unpredictable reactions in some cases
Diabetes	• General caution advised (many diabetics heal very slowly; obtain physician approval if you are unsure).	None specific
Blood thinners	• Extraction without physician permission • Facial or body waxing without physician permission	May cause bleeding or bruising
Sensitive, redness-prone skin	• Heat • Harsh scrubs • Mechanical treatment • Stimulating massage	Can aggravate redness
Open sores, herpes simplex (cold sores)	• Avoid all treatments until clear with doctor.	Can spread or flare; infectious disease
Recent facial surgery or laser treatment	• Treat with physician's permission only.	Treat with physician's permission only.

Should you ever have any questions regarding a client's treatment and his or her health conditions, always check with the client's doctor first! Remember one simple rule: When in doubt, don't perform the service.

Record-Keeping

During the consultation, keep the client intake form and the service record card at hand so that you can write down all necessary information (figure 23-2). Depending on your place of work, cosmetologists transcribe pertinent information from the intake form onto the service record card. The service record card should contain the following information:

- Client's name, home address, e-mail address, and telephone number
- Client's occupation
- Client's date of birth (useful so that you can determine if any signs of aging are premature)
- Client's medical history and current medications, including whether the client is under the care of a physician or dermatologist
- Contraindications—such as a pacemaker, metal implants, pregnancy, diabetes, epilepsy, allergies, high blood pressure—that call for alternative methods of treatment

SERVICE RECORD CARD				
Name_____			Date of consultation _____	
Address_____			D.O.B. _____	
City_____ State_____ Zip_____			Occupation _____	
Tel. (Home)_____ (Business)_____			Ref. by _____	
Tel. (Cell)_____ (E-mail)_____				
Contraindications				
Medical history				
Current medication				
Previous treatments				
Home care products used				
SKIN TYPE	Oily	Normal	Dry (alipidic)	Combination
SKIN CONDITION	Clogged pores	Sensitive	Dehydrated	Mature
Skin abnormalities				
Remarks				

figure 23-2
Client service record card (front)

SERVICE RECORD					
Date	Type of treatment	By	Products purchased	Observations
2/14	Cleansing, Peel- Relaxing massage	Mary	Moisturizer with sunscreen	
3/16	Cleansing, Peel Modelage mask	Mary	Cleanser, Toner	
4/5	Cleansing, Peel High frequency indirect	Mary	Moisturizer, Foundation #7	
4/26	Cleansing, Peel Massage Alginate mask	John		
5/13	Cleansing, Peel Iontophoresis Paraffin mask	Mary	Night cream for dry skin Lipstick #43	Skin is showing marked improvement.
6/1	Cleansing, Peel Relaxing massage	Mary	Eye contour mask	

figure 23-3
Client service record card (back)

- Information as to whether the client has had facials before and, if so, what kind of treatments were performed

- Information on any skin care products the client is currently using

- Notation of how the client was referred to the salon

- Observations on the client's skin type, skin condition, and any abnormalities of the skin

Figure 23-3 is provided as an example of how to fill out the client service record card to record the date and type of service and/or treatment being performed, the products that are being used, and products purchased by the client for home care. Be sure to note specific products and the date the client purchases so that you can help him or her repurchase if the client forgets product names. The service record card should also have space to allow for recording the results of the analysis and your observations on each visit.

You should record and highlight with a colored pen any important observations or contraindications in the client's service record card. File the completed client intake form and service record card in a secure filing cabinet or system because the client may have revealed information that is private.

Home Care Recommendations

As part of the consultation, do not hesitate to recommend services and products that will be beneficial to the client (**figure 23-4**). Since the client has taken the initiative to come into the salon, they will feel disappointed if you neglect to recommend salon treatments and products, as well as proper home care products for the skin. Also, if you do not recommend professional products, your client may go elsewhere for advice, such as a department store or drugstore. He or she might not get the kind of product you would have advised, and you and the salon will not get the retail income.

Make it clear to your client that if they wish to achieve the best results from a treatment, they must follow a proven routine of skin care at home with products that reinforce the salon treatments. Be careful, however, not to make the client feel that the sole purpose of the consultation is to sell products. Review appropriate and discreet retailing techniques with your instructor to make sure you achieve the right tone with your client.

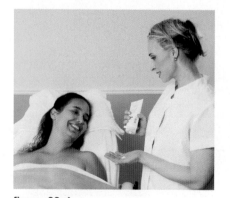

figure 23-4
Recommend skin care products to the client.

After reading the next few sections, you will be able to:

LO ❸ **Determine the difference between skin type and skin condition.**

Determine Skin Type During the Skin Analysis

At this point, you have carefully read the client's intake form and discussed your questions with the client. During the first consultation and before every subsequent facial treatment, it is important to perform a thorough analysis of the client's skin. This initial analysis should take place prior to cleansing. You want to see the skin's natural state before cleansing and then again after cleansing, especially if the client is wearing makeup. If the skin is oily, it will often look shiny or greasy. If the skin is dry, it may look flaky. Table 23-2 lists brief descriptions of basic skin types. Wash your hands thoroughly and perform a dry skin analysis.

Then have the client change into a robe or a wrap and sit in the facial chair. The client's hair should be covered, and any jewelry should be removed by the client and put away in a safe place. Jewelry can get in the way or become soiled or damaged during treatment.

table 23-2

SIGNS AND CONDITIONS ASSOCIATED WITH SKIN TYPES

Skin Type	Signs of Skin Type	Conditions Associated with Skin Type
Oily	Obvious, large pores.	Open and closed comedones, clogged pores. Shiny, thick appearance. Yellowish color. Orange-peel texture.
Dry	Pores very small or not visible.	Tight, poreless-looking skin. May be dehydrated with fine lines and wrinkles; dry and rough to the touch.
Normal	Even pore distribution throughout the skin. Very soft, smooth surface. Lack of wrinkles.	Normal skin is actually very unusual. Most clients have combination skin.
Combination dry	Obvious pores down the center of the face. Pores not visible or becoming smaller toward the outer edges of the face.	May have clogged pores in the nose, chin, and center of the forehead. Dry, poreless toward outside edges of the face.
Combination oily	Wider distribution of obvious or large pores down the center of the face extending to the outer cheeks. Pores become smaller toward edges of the face.	Comedones, clogged pores, or obvious pores in the center of the face.
Acne	Very large pores in all areas. Acne is considered a skin type because it is hereditary.	Presence of numerous open and closed comedones, clogged pores, and red papules and pustules (pimples).

Cosmetologists should avoid wearing jewelry on the hands or arms while administering facial treatments because rings and bracelets may accidentally injure the client or be damaged.

Recline the client in the chair and drape the client using a hair cap, headband, or towels (figure 23-5). Proceed to cleanse the client's skin for a more in-depth inspection. Warm some cleansing milk in your hands and apply the cleanser to the face in upward circular movements. When cleansing the eye area, use a special cleanser made for eye makeup removal. Apply a small amount to the eye areas, being careful not to use so much that it gets in the eyes. Gently remove the cleanser with warm, damp facial sponges or cotton pads. Remember to remove the cleanser using upward and outward movements. When working around the eyes, move outward on the upper lid, and inward on the lower lid.

After thoroughly cleansing the face, apply a cotton eye pad to the client's eyes to avoid exposure to the extreme brightness of the magnifying lamp.

A **magnifying lamp** is a magnifying lens surrounded by a circular light, providing a well-lit, enlarged view of the skin. Magnifying lamps, also sometimes called *loupes* or *"mag" lights*, are used for skin analysis, close inspection of unusual lesions on the skin, extraction of comedones, and hair removal including tweezing, electrolysis, and waxing.

Look through the magnifying lamp at the client's skin. Skin type is determined by how oily or dry the skin is. Skin type is hereditary and cannot be permanently changed with treatments, although the skin may look considerably better after treatment. Skin conditions are characteristics associated with a particular skin type (see table 23-2).

The first thing you should look for is the presence or absence of visible pores (follicles). The amount of sebum produced by the sebaceous glands determines the size of the pores and is hereditary. Obvious pores indicate oily skin areas, and lack of visible pores indicates dry skin.

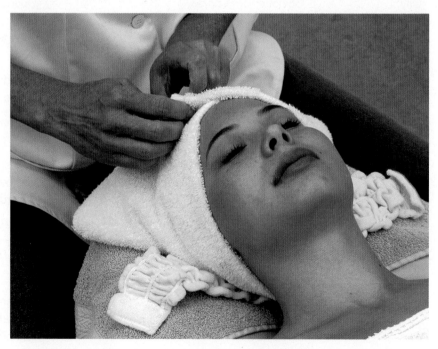

figure 23-5
Draping the hair with a towel

Skin Types

The term **alipidic** (al-ah-PIDD-ic) means lack of lipids, and describes skin that does not produce enough sebum, indicated by absence of visible pores. Alipidic skin, also known as *dry skin*, becomes dehydrated because it does not produce enough sebum to prevent the evaporation of cell moisture. Dehydration indicates a lack of moisture in the skin. Dehydrated skin may be flaky or dry looking, with small, fine lines and wrinkles. It may look like it has a piece of cellophane on top of it. Dehydrated skin also may feel itchy or tight. Dehydration can occur on almost any skin type. The key to truly alipidic skin is the absence of visible pores.

Oily skin that produces too much sebum will have large pores, and the skin may appear shiny or greasy. Pores may be clogged from dead cells building up in the hair follicle, or may contain **open comedones** (KAHM-uh-dohnz), also known as *blackheads*, which are follicles impacted with solidified sebum and dead cell buildup.

Closed comedones are hair follicles impacted with solidified sebum and dead cell buildup that appear as small bumps just underneath the skin's surface.

The difference between open and closed comedones is the size of the follicle opening, called the **ostium** (AH-stee-um). An open comedo has a large ostium, and a closed comedo has a small one.

Extraction (eck-strack-shun) is a procedure in which comedones are removed from the follicles by manual manipulation. The skin is first treated with products and/or equipment that softens the impactions.

Acne

The presence of pimples in oily areas indicates acne (**figure 23-6**). Acne is considered a skin type because the tendency to develop acne is hereditary. Acne is a disorder in which the hair follicles become clogged, resulting in infection of the follicle with redness and inflammation. Acne bacteria are anaerobic, which means they cannot survive in the presence of oxygen. When follicles are blocked with solidified sebum and dead cell buildup, oxygen cannot readily get to the bottom of the follicle where acne bacteria live. Acne bacteria survive from breaking down sebum into fatty acids, which is their only food source. A blocked follicle is an ideal environment for acne bacteria. When acne bacteria flourish from the lack of oxygen and access to a food source such as a blocked follicle filled with sebum, they multiply quickly, eventually causing a break in the follicle wall. This rupture allows blood to come into the follicle, causing redness. Acne papules are red pimples that do not have a pus head. Pimples with a pus head are called pustules. Pus is a fluid inside a pustule, largely made up of dead white blood cells that tried to fight the infection.

Analysis of Skin Conditions

Conditions of the skin are generally treatable. They are generally not hereditary, but they may be associated with a particular skin type.

Dehydration is indicated by flaky areas or skin that wrinkles easily on the surface. Very gently pinching the surface of dehydrated skin will result

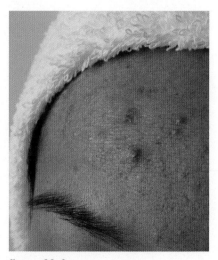

figure 23-6
Acne indicates oily areas.

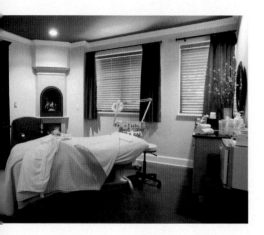

in the visible formation of many fine lines. This is an indication of dehydration. Dehydrated skin can be caused from lack of care, improper or over-drying skin care products, sun exposure, and other causes. Dehydrated skin is treated by using hydrators that help to bind water to the skin surface. These hydrating products should be chosen based on skin type. Hydrators for alipidic skin are generally heavier in texture. Hydrators for oilier skin are lighter weight. Proper hydration of the skin can result in smoother-looking and softer skin.

Most types of hyperpigmentation, or dark blotches of color, are caused by sun exposure or hormone imbalances. Clients who have spent a lot of time in the sun will often have hyperpigmentation. Hyperpigmentation is treated with mild exfoliation and home care products that discourage pigmentation. Daily use of sunscreen and avoidance of sun exposure are very important for this skin type.

Sensitive skin has a thin, red-pink look. Skin will turn red easily, and is easily inflamed by some skin care products. You should avoid strong products or cleansers, fragranced products, and strong exfoliants when treating sensitive skin. Rosacea is a chronic hereditary disorder that can be indicated by constant or frequent facial blushing.

A person with rosacea often has dilated capillaries, telangiectasias (tel-an-jee-EK-tay juhs), which are distended or dilated surface blood vessels, and **couperose** (KOO-per-ohs), which are areas of skin with distended capillaries and diffuse redness.

Rosacea is considered a medical disorder and should be diagnosed by a dermatologist. You should treat a client who has rosacea with very gentle products and treatments, avoiding any treatment that releases heat or stimulates the skin.

Aging and Sun-Damaged Skin

Aging skin has loss of elasticity and the skin tends to sag in areas around the eyes and jawline. Wrinkles may be apparent in areas of normal facial expression. Treatments that hydrate and exfoliate improve the appearance of aging skin.

Sun-damaged skin is skin that has been chronically and frequently exposed to sun over the client's lifetime. Sun-damaged skin will have many areas of hyperpigmentation, lots of wrinkled areas including areas not in the normal facial expression, and sagging skin from damage to the elastic fibers. The skin looks older than it should for the age of the client. It is often confused with aging skin.

A well-planned program combining good home care and advanced and routine facial treatments can help the appearance of aging and sun-damaged skin. Home care programs must be performed diligently and should include products containing ingredients like alpha hydroxy acids, retinol, antioxidants, peptides, as well as the daily use of a broad-spectrum sunscreen. Special treatment programs using alpha hydroxy peels, microdermabrasion, microcurrent treatments, and light therapy can also help greatly improve these skin conditions.

After reading the next few sections, you will be able to:

LO④ Name the different categories of skin care products used in facial treatments.

LO⑤ Explain the different categories of skin care products used in facial treatments, and provide examples of each.

Categorize Skin Care Products

There are many, many types of skin care products available for salon use and for the client's home care. Most skin care products are designed for specific skin types or conditions (**figure 23-7**). Major categories of skin care products are described below.

Cleansers are designed to clean the surface of the skin and to remove makeup. There are basically two types of cleansers: cleansing milks and foaming cleansers.

Cleansing milks are non-foaming, lotion cleansers designed to cleanse dry and sensitive skin types and to remove makeup. They can be applied with the hands or an implement, but they must be removed with a dampened facial sponge, soft cloth, or cotton pad. Ingredients are sometimes added to cleansing milks to make them more specific to a given skin type.

Foaming cleansers are cleansers containing surfactants (detergents) that cause the product to foam and rinse off easily. These products are generally for combination or oilier skin types, although there are some rinse-off cleansers for dry and sensitive skin. Clients love using these products because they can be used quickly and easily in the shower. They have varying amounts of detergent ingredients to treat specific levels of oiliness. Foaming cleansers, like cleansing milks, may have special ingredients to make them more specific for certain skin types. Some have antibacterial ingredients for acne-prone skin.

Toners, also known as *fresheners* or *astringents*, are lotions that help rebalance the pH and remove remnants of cleanser from the skin. They may also contain ingredients that help to hydrate or soothe, and they may sometimes contain an exfoliating ingredient to help remove dead cells. Fresheners and astringents are usually stronger products, often with higher alcohol content, and are used to treat oilier skin types. Toning products are applied with cotton pads after cleansing. Some alcohol-free toners can be sprayed onto the face.

Exfoliants (ex-FO-lee-yahnts) are products that help bring about **exfoliation** (eks-foh-lee-AY-shun), the removal of excess dead cells from the

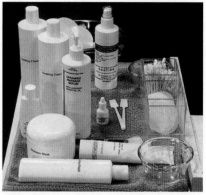

figure 23-7
There are a wide variety of skin care products for every skin type.

> ⚠ **CAUTION**
> It is important to note that the cosmetology professional's domain is the hair and superficial epidermis. Cosmetology professionals must not perform treatments that remove cells beyond the stratum corneum of the epidermis.

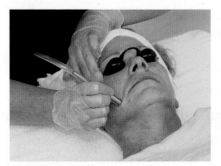

figure 23-8
Microdermabrasion treatment

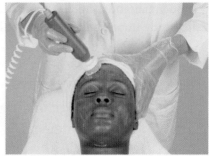

figure 23-9
Using a skin-brushing machine
during a facial treatment

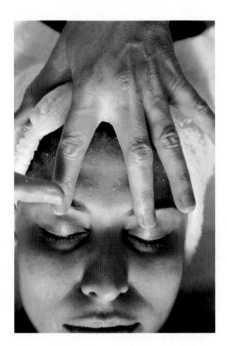

skin surface. Removing dead cells from the surface of the skin allows the skin to look smoother and clearer.

Exfoliants help clear the skin of clogged pores and can improve the appearance of wrinkles, aging, and hyperpigmentation. Cosmetology professionals may use products that remove dead surface cells from the stratum corneum. Deeper, surgical-level peels must only be administered by dermatologists and plastic surgeons.

Exfoliation may be accomplished by using mechanical exfoliants or chemical exfoliants. **Mechanical exfoliants** are products used to physically remove dead cell buildup. **Gommages** (go-mah-jez), also known as *roll-off masks*, are peeling creams that are rubbed off of the skin, and **microdermabrasion scrubs**, scrubs that contain aluminum oxide crystals, along with other granular scrubs, are examples of mechanical exfoliants.

Microdermabrasion can also be used as a machine treatment, which is briefly discussed later in this chapter (figure 23-8). Skin-brushing machines are another example of mechanical exfoliation (figure 23-9).

Chemical exfoliants are products that contain chemicals that either loosen or dissolve dead cell buildup. They are either used for a short time (although some may be worn as a day or night treatment) or combined in a moisturizer. Popular exfoliating chemicals are alpha hydroxy acids (AHAs) (AL-fah hy-DRAHKS-ee AS-uds); these are gentle, naturally occurring acids that remove dead skin cells by dissolving the bonds and intercellular cement between cells. As dead cells are removed from the surface over time, wrinkles appear less deep, skin discolorations may fade,

---

⚠ **CAUTION**

Certain skin conditions can be easily inflamed by mechanical exfoliation. Also, certain medications may thin the skin, making it more susceptible to inflammation, bruising, or blistering. Do not use brushing machines, scrubs, or any harsh mechanical peeling techniques on the following skin types and conditions:

- Skin with many visible capillaries
- Thin skin that reddens easily
- Older skin that is thin and bruises easily or the skin of persons using blood thinning medications
- Skin being medically treated with tretinoin (retinoic acid or Retin-A®), isotretinoin, azelaic acid, adapalene (Differin®), AHA, or salicylic acid (found in many common skin products)
- Acne-prone skin with inflamed papules and pustules

clogged pores are loosened and reduced, new clogged pores are prevented, and skin is smoother and more hydrated. These acids encourage cell renewal, resulting in firmer and healthier-looking skin.

Salon AHA exfoliants, also known as *peels*, contain larger concentrations of AHA, usually around 20 to 30 percent. They should never be used unless the client has been using 10 percent AHA products at home for at least two weeks prior to the higher concentration salon treatment, has no contraindications for exfoliation treatment, and is using a daily facial sunscreen product.

Enzyme peels (EN-zym PEELS), also known as *keratolytic* (kair-uh-tuh-LIT-ik) *enzymes* or *protein-dissolving agents*, are a type of chemical exfoliant that works by dissolving keratin protein in the surface cells of the skin. Usually, enzyme products are made using plant-extracted enzymes from papaya (resulting in an enzyme known as papain [pa-PAIN]) or pineapple (resulting in an enzyme known as bromelain [bro-ma-LAIN]), or they are made from an enzyme derived from beef by-products (resulting in an enzyme known as pancreatin [pan-cree-at-tin]). Enzymes sometimes are blended into scrubs or wearable products, but they are most often designed for use in the salon.

There are two basic types of keratolytic enzyme peels. The first are cream-type enzyme peels (gommage) that usually contain papain. They are applied to the skin and allowed to dry for a few minutes. They form a crust, which is then rolled off the skin (**figure 23-10**).

The second and most popular type of enzyme peel is a powder that is mixed with water in the treatment room and applied to the face. This type of enzyme treatment does not dry the skin and can even be used during a steam treatment.

Proper exfoliation may improve the appearance of the skin in the following ways:

- Reduces clogged pores and skin oiliness
- Promotes skin smoothness
- Increases moisture content and hydration
- Reduces hyperpigmentation
- Decreases uneven skin color
- Eliminates or softens wrinkles and fine lines
- Increases elasticity

In addition, proper exfoliation speeds up cell turnover and allows for better penetration of treatment creams and serums. Makeup applies more evenly on exfoliated skin.

Moisturizers

Moisturizers are products that help increase the moisture content of the skin surface. Moisturizers help diminish the appearance of fine lines and wrinkles. They are basically mixtures of **humectants** (hyoo-MEKK-tents), also known as *hydrators* or *water-binding agents*, which are ingredients that attract water and **emollients** (ee-MAHL-yunts), which are oily or fatty ingredients that prevent moisture from leaving the skin.

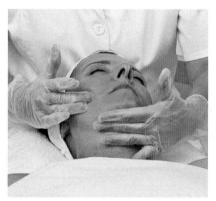

figure 23-10
Rolling a gommage mask off the face

DID YOU KNOW?
A valuable ingredient in moisturizers, particularly in day creams, is sunscreen. Not only does sunscreen guard against premature aging of the skin, but also, when used consistently, it is one of the best ways to help prevent skin cancer.

Moisturizers for oily skin are most often in lotion form and generally contain smaller amounts of emollient. Oilier skin does not need as much emollient because oily skin produces more than adequate amounts of protective sebum.

Moisturizers for dry skin are often in the form of a heavier cream, and they contain more emollients, which are needed by alipidic skin.

All moisturizers may have other ingredients that perform additional functions. These ingredients may include soothing agents for sensitive skin, AHAs or peptides for aging skin, or sunscreens.

Sunscreens and Day Protection Products

Shielding the skin from sun exposure is probably the most important habit to benefit the skin. Cumulative sun exposure causes the majority of skin cancers and prematurely ages the skin.

Most sun exposure over a lifetime is from casual sun exposure. Therefore, every client should be instructed to use a sunscreen every single day! Look for daily moisturizers that contain broad-spectrum sunscreens, which protect against both UVA and UVB light, helping to prevent sunburn, premature aging, and skin cancer. A sun protection factor (SPF) rating of 15 or higher is considered to be adequate strength for daily use. SPF measures how long someone can be exposed to the sun without burning. For example, if someone normally burns in an hour, an SPF-2 sunscreen allows the person to stay in the sun two times as long without burning. Sunscreens with higher SPFs are appropriate for extended outdoor exposure and for sun-sensitive individuals.

Sunscreens are available in lotion, fluid, and cream forms. Lotions are suitable for combination skin, fluids for oily skin, and creams for dry skin.

Night treatments are usually more intensive products designed for use at night to treat specific skin problems. These products are generally heavier than day-use products, and they theoretically contain higher levels of conditioning ingredients.

Serums (SEH-rums) are concentrated products that generally contain higher concentrations of ingredients designed to penetrate the skin and treat various skin conditions (**figure 23-11**). They are typically used at home, and they are applied under a moisturizer or sunscreen. **Ampoules** (am-pyools) are individual doses of serum, sealed in small vials.

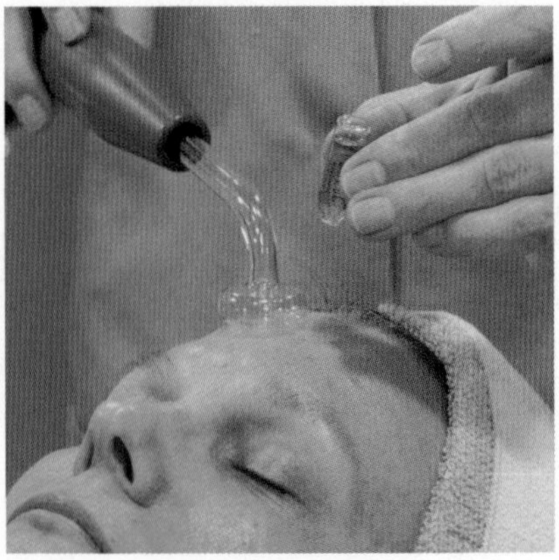

figure 23-11
Skin treatment in an ampoule

Massage creams are lubricants used to make the skin slippery during massage. They often contain oils or petrolatum. If a massage cream is used during a facial treatment, it must be thoroughly removed before any other product can penetrate the skin.

There is a trend toward using treatment products that penetrate the skin during massage. For example, treatment products may be used to increase skin hydration or to soothe redness-prone skin. One of the biggest benefits of massage is that it increases product absorption which, in turn, increases the conditioning effect of treatment products.

Masks

Masks, also known as *masques*, are concentrated treatment products often composed of mineral clays, moisturizing agents, skin softeners, aromatherapy oils, botanical extracts, and other beneficial ingredients to cleanse, exfoliate, tighten, tone, hydrate, and nourish the skin.

- **Clay-based masks** are oil-absorbing cleansing masks that have an exfoliating effect and an astringent effect on oily and combination skin, making large pores temporarily appear smaller. They may have additional beneficial ingredients for soothing, or they may include antibacterial ingredients like sulfur, which are helpful for acne-prone skin.

- **Cream masks** are masks often containing oils and emollients as well as humectants, and they have a strong moisturizing effect. They do not dry on the skin like clay masks do, and they are often used to moisturize dry skin.

- Gel masks can be used for sensitive or dehydrated skin, and they do not dry hard (**figure 23-12**). They often contain hydrators and soothing ingredients, thus helping to plump surface cells with moisture, making the skin look more supple and more hydrated.

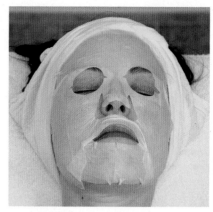

figure 23-12
Gel masks can contain soothing agents for sensitive skin.

- Alginate (al-gin-ate) masks are often seaweed based. They come in a powder form and are mixed with water or, sometimes, serums. After mixing, they are quickly applied to the face. They dry to form a rubberized texture. A **treatment cream**, which is a specialty product designed to facilitate change in the skin's appearance, or a serum is generally applied under alginate masks. The alginate mask forms a seal that encourages the skin's absorption of the serum or treatment cream underneath. Alginate masks are generally used only in the salon.

- **Paraffin wax masks** are specially-prepared facial masks containing paraffin and other beneficial ingredients. They are melted at a little more than body temperature before application. The paraffin quickly cools to a lukewarm temperature and hardens to a candle-like consistency. Paraffin masks are applied over a treatment cream to allow the cream's ingredients to penetrate more deeply into the surface layers of the skin. Eye pads and gauze are used in a paraffin mask application because facial hair could stick to the wax if it is not covered, making the mask difficult and painful to remove.

- **Modelage masks** (MAHD-ul-ahj MAS`KZ) contain special crystals of gypsum, a plaster-like ingredient (**figure 23-13**). As with paraffin masks, modelage masks are used with a treatment cream. Modelage masks are mixed with cold water immediately before application and applied about ¼-inch (0.6 centimeters) thick. After application, the modelage mask hardens. The chemical reaction that occurs when the plaster and the crystals mix with water produces a gradual increase in temperature that reaches approximately 105 degrees Fahrenheit. As the mask is left on the skin, the temperature gradually cools, until it has cooled down completely. The setting time for modelage masks is approximately 20 minutes. Modelage masks sometimes vary in mixing technique or timing. Always follow the manufacturer's instructions for the product you are using.

The heat generated by a modelage mask increases blood circulation and is very beneficial for dry, mature skin or for skin that looks dull and lifeless. This type of mask is not recommended for use on sensitive skin,

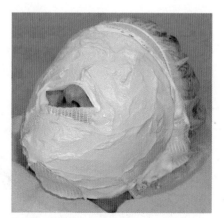

figure 23-13
Modelage mask

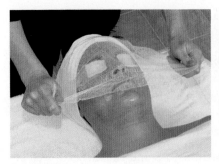
figure 23-14
Placing gauze on the client's face

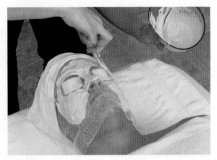
figure 23-15
Applying a mask over the gauze

skin with capillary problems, oily skin, or skin with blemishes. Modelage masks can become quite heavy on the face and should not be applied to the lower neck. These masks should never be used on clients who suffer from claustrophobia, which is a fear of being closed in or confined.

The Use of Gauze for Mask Application

Gauze is a thin, open-meshed fabric of loosely woven cotton (figure 23-14). Masks that have a tendency to run can be applied over a layer of gauze. The gauze holds the mask on the face while allowing the ingredients to seep through to benefit the skin (figure 23-15). Cheesecloth is sometimes used as well. In some cases, it is necessary to apply a second layer of gauze over the mask to keep the ingredients from sliding off. Gauze is also used to keep paraffin and gypsum/plaster masks from sticking to the skin and the tiny hairs on the skin.

To prepare gauze, cut a piece large enough to cover the entire face and neck. Cut out spaces for the eyes, nose, and mouth. Although the client could breathe through the gauze, the cut-out spaces will make breathing more comfortable for the client.

After reading the next few sections, you will be able to:

LO**6**   Define why massage is used during a facial.

LO**7**   Name and briefly describe the five categories of massage manipulations.

Learn the Basic Techniques of a Facial Massage

Massage is the manual or mechanical manipulation of the body by rubbing, gently pinching, kneading, tapping, and other movements to increase metabolism and circulation, to promote absorption, and to relieve pain. Cosmetologists massage their clients to help keep the facial skin healthy and the facial muscles firm.

To master massage techniques, you must have a basic knowledge of anatomy and physiology, as well as considerable practice in performing the various movements. It is important that you use a firm, sure touch when giving a massage. To do this, you must develop flexible hands, a quiet temperament, and self-control.

Keep your hands soft by using creams, oils, and lotions. File and shape your nails to avoid scratching your client's skin. Your wrists and fingers should be flexible, and your palms should be firm and warm. Cream or oil should be applied to your hands to permit smoother and gentler hand movements and to prevent drag or damage to the client's skin.

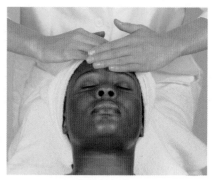
figure 23-16
Digital effleurage on the forehead

Basic Massage Manipulations

All massage treatments combine one or more basic movements or manipulations. Each manipulation is applied to the superficial muscles in a certain way to achieve a certain end. The impact of a massage treatment depends on the amount of pressure, the direction of movement, and the duration of each type of manipulation involved.

The direction of movement is always from the insertion of the muscle toward its origin. The insertion is the portion of the muscle at the more movable attachment (where it is attached to another muscle or to a movable bone or joint). The origin is the portion of the muscle at the fixed attachment (to an immovable section of the skeleton). Massaging a muscle in the wrong direction could result in a loss of resiliency and sagging of the skin and muscles.

Effleurage

Effleurage (EF-loo-rahzh) is a light, continuous stroking movement applied in a slow, rhythmic manner with the fingers (digital effleurage) or the palms (palmar effleurage). No pressure is used. The palms work the large surfaces, and the cushions of the fingertips work the small surfaces, such as those around the eyes (**figure 23-16**). Effleurage is frequently used on the forehead, face, scalp, back, shoulder, neck, chest, arms, and hands for its soothing and relaxing effects. Every massage should begin and end with effleurage.

When performing effleurage, hold your whole hand loosely, and keep your wrist and fingers flexible. Curve your fingers slightly to conform to the shape of the area being massaged, with just the cushions of the fingertips touching the skin. Do not use the ends of the fingertips. They are pointier than the cushions, and will cause the effleurage to be less smooth. Also, the free edges of your fingernails may scratch the client's skin.

Pétrissage

Pétrissage (PEH-treh-sahj) is a kneading movement performed by lifting, squeezing, and pressing the tissue with a light, firm pressure. Pétrissage offers deeper stimulation to the muscles, nerves, and skin glands, and improves circulation. These kneading movements are usually limited to the back, shoulders, and arms.

Although typically used on larger surface areas such as the arms and shoulders, digital kneading can also be used on the cheeks with light pinching movements (**figure 23-17**). The pressure should be light but firm.

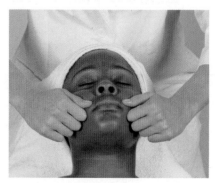
figure 23-17
Pétrissage

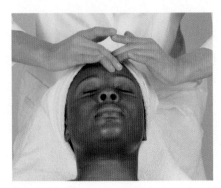

figure 23-18
Friction

When grasping and releasing the fleshy parts, the movements must be rhythmic and never jerky.

Fulling is a form of pétrissage in which the tissue is grasped, gently lifted, and spread out; this technique is used mainly for massaging the arms. With the fingers of both hands grasping the arm, apply a kneading movement across the flesh, with light pressure on the underside of the client's forearm and between the shoulder and elbow.

Friction

Friction (FRIK-shun) is a deep rubbing movement in which you apply pressure on the skin with your fingers or palm while moving it over an underlying structure. Friction has been known to have a significant benefit on the circulation and glandular activity of the skin. Circular friction movements are typically used on the scalp, arms, and hands. Light circular friction is used on the face and neck (**figure 23-18**).

Chucking, rolling, and wringing are variations of friction and are used mainly to massage the arms and legs, as follows:

* **Chucking** is grasping the flesh firmly in one hand and moving the hand up and down along the bone while the other hand keeps the arm or leg in a steady position.

* **Rolling** is pressing and twisting the tissues with a fast back-and-forth movement.

* **Wringing** is a vigorous movement in which the hands, placed a little distance apart on both sides of the client's arm or leg and working downward, apply a twisting motion against the bones in the opposite direction.

Tapotement

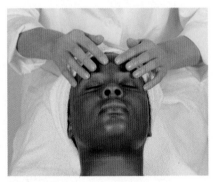

figure 23-19
Tapotement

Tapotement (tah-POH-te-ment), also known as *percussion* (pur-KUSH-un), consists of short, quick tapping, slapping, and hacking movements. This form of massage is the most stimulating and should be applied with care and discretion. Tapotement movements tone the muscles and impart a healthy glow to the area being massaged.

In facial massage, use only light digital tapping. Bring the fingertips down against the skin in rapid succession. Your fingers must be flexible enough to create an even force over the area being massaged (**figure 23-19**).

In **slapping** movements, keeping your wrists flexible allows your palms to come in contact with the skin in light, firm, and rapid slapping movements. One hand follows the other. With each slapping stroke, lift the flesh slightly.

Hacking is a chopping movement performed with the edges of the hands. Both the wrists and hands move alternately in fast, light, firm, and flexible motions against the skin. Hacking and slapping movements are used only to massage the back, shoulders, and arms.

Vibration

Vibration (vy-BRAY-shun) is a rapid shaking of the body part while the balls of the fingertips are pressed firmly on the point of application.

DID YOU KNOW?

Do not talk to your client during the massage except to ask once whether your touch should be more or less firm. Talking eliminates the relaxation therapy of the massage.

Relaxation is achieved through light but firm, slow, rhythmic movements, or very slow, light hand vibrations over the motor points for a short time. Another technique is to pause briefly over the motor points, using light pressure.

The movement is accomplished by rapid muscular contractions in your arms. It is a highly relaxing movement, and should be applied at the end of the massage (figure 23-20). Deep vibration in combination with other classical massage movements can also be produced by the use of a mechanical vibrator to stimulate blood circulation and increase muscle tone.

Physiological Effects of Massage

Before performing a service that includes a facial massage, consult the client's intake form to note and discuss any medical condition that may contraindicate a facial massage. These include cancer, recent facial surgery or laser treatment, facial paralysis, or any skin disease affecting the facial skin. If your client expresses a concern about having a facial massage and has a medical condition, advise him or her to speak with a physician before having the service.

If your client has rosacea, sensitive or redness-prone skin, avoid using vigorous or strong massage techniques.

Clients with acne should not be massaged in any area that has breakouts.

To obtain proper results from a scalp or facial massage, you must have a thorough knowledge of the structures involved, including muscles, nerves, connective tissues, and blood vessels. Every muscle has a **motor point**, which is a point on the skin that covers the muscle where pressure or stimulation will cause contraction of that muscle. Some examples are illustrated in figures 23-21 and 23-22. In order to obtain the maximum benefits from a facial massage, you must consider the motor points that affect the underlying muscles of the face and neck. The location of motor points varies among individuals due to differences in body structure. However, a few manipulations on the proper motor points will relax the client early in the massage treatment.

Skillfully applied massage directly or indirectly influences the structures and functions of the body. The immediate effects of massage are first noticed on the skin. The area being massaged shows increased circulation, secretion, nutrition, and excretion. The following benefits may be obtained by proper facial and scalp massage:

- Skin and all structures are nourished
- Skin becomes softer and more pliable
- Circulation of blood is increased
- Activity of skin glands is stimulated
- Muscle fibers are stimulated and strengthened
- Nerves are soothed and rested
- Pain is sometimes relieved

The recommended frequency of facial or scalp massage depends on the condition of the skin or scalp, the age of the client, and the condition being treated. As a general rule, normal skin or scalp can be kept in

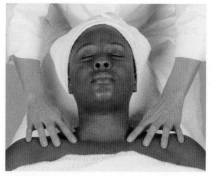
figure 23-20
Vibration on the top of the shoulders

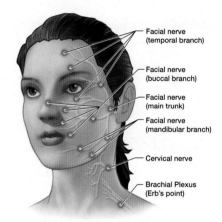
figure 23-21
Motor nerve points of the face

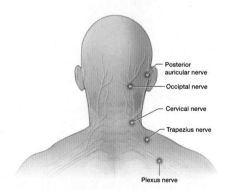
figure 23-22
Motor nerve points of the neck

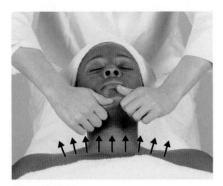

figure 23-23
Chin movement

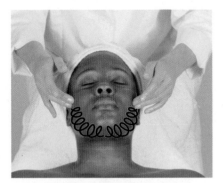

figure 23-24
Circular movement of the lower cheeks

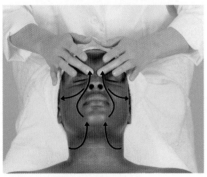

figure 23-25
Mouth, nose, and cheek movements

excellent condition with the help of a weekly massage, accompanied by proper home care.

Facial Manipulations

Because an overview of basic massage/manipulation techniques and guidelines is now complete, the best manipulations to use on the face can be discussed in more depth. When performing facial manipulations, keep in mind that an even tempo, or rhythm, is relaxing. Do not remove your hands from the client's face once you have started the manipulations.

Should it become necessary to remove your hands, feather them off, and then gently replace them with feather-like movements. Remember that massage movements are generally directed from the muscle's insertion toward its origin, in order to avoid damage to muscle tissues.

The following photographs show the different movements that may be used on the various parts of the face, chest, and back. Each instructor may have developed her own routine, however. For example, some instructors and practitioners prefer to start massage manipulations at the chin, while others prefer to start at the forehead. Both are correct. Be guided by your instructor.

Chin movement. Lift the chin, using a slight pressure (figure 23-23).

Lower cheeks. Using a circular movement, rotate from chin to ears (figure 23-24).

Mouth, nose, and cheek movements. Follow the diagram (figure 23-25).

Linear movement over the forehead. Slide fingers to the temples and then stroke up to hairline, gradually moving your hands across the forehead to the right eyebrow (figures 23-26a and 23-26b).

Circular movement over the forehead. Starting at the eyebrow line, work across the middle of the forehead and then toward the hairline (figure 23-27).

Crisscross movement. Start at one side of forehead and work back (figure 23-28).

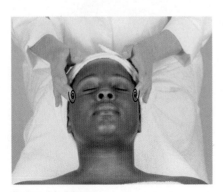

figure 23-26a
Light circular movement over the temples continuing with linear movement over forehead

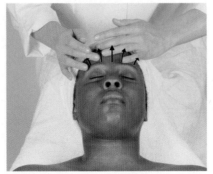

figure 23-26b
Light circular movement over the temples continuing with linear movement over forehead

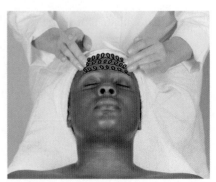

figure 23-27
Circular movement over forehead

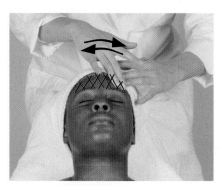

figure 23-28
Crisscross movement

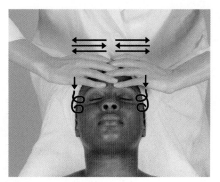

figure 23-29
Stroking (headache) movement

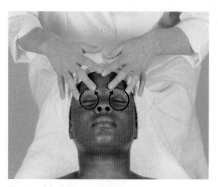

figure 23-30
Brow and eye movement

Stroking (headache) movement. Slide your fingers toward the center of the forehead and then draw your fingers, with slight pressure, toward the temples and rotate (**figure 23-29**).

Brow and eye movement. Place your middle fingers at the inner corners of the eyes and your index fingers over the brows. Slide them toward the outer corners of the eyes, under the eyes, and then back to the inner corners (**figure 23-30**).

Nose and upper cheek movement. Slide your fingers down the nose. Apply a rotary movement across the cheeks to the temples and rotate gently. Slide your fingers under the eyes and then back to the bridge of the nose (**figure 23-31**).

Mouth and nose movement. Apply a circular movement from the corners of the mouth up to the sides of the nose. Slide your fingers over the brows and then down to the corners of the mouth up to the sides of nose. Follow by sliding your fingers over the brows and down to the corners of the mouth again (**figure 23-32**).

Lip and chin movement. From the center of the upper lip, draw your fingers around the mouth, going under the lower lip and chin (**figure 23-33**).

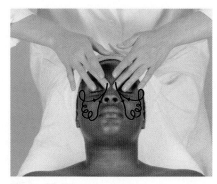

figure 23-31
Nose and upper cheek movement

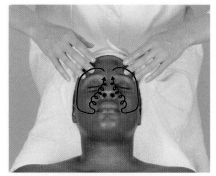

figure 23-32
Mouth and nose movement

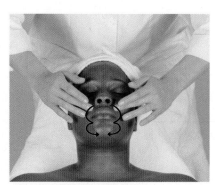

figure 23-33
Lip and chin movement

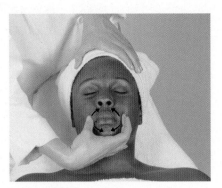

figure 23-34
Optional movement

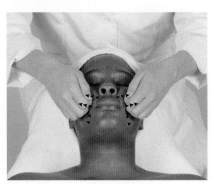

figure 23-35
Lifting movement of cheeks

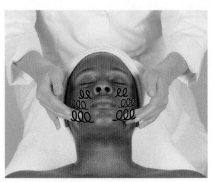

figure 23-36
Rotary movement of cheeks

Optional movement. Hold the head with your left hand, and draw the fingers of your right hand from under the lower lip and around mouth, moving to the center of the upper lip (figure 23-34).

Lifting movement of the cheeks. Proceed from the mouth to the ears, and then from the nose to the top part of the ears (figure 23-35).

Rotary movement of the cheeks. Massage from the chin to the ear lobes, from the mouth to the middles of the ears, and from the nose to the top of the ears (figure 23-36).

Light tapping movement. Work from the chin to the earlobe, from the mouth to the ear, from the nose to the top of the ear, and then across the forehead. Repeat on the other side (figure 23-37).

Stroking movement of the neck. Apply light upward strokes over the front of the neck. Use heavier pressure on the sides of neck in downward strokes (figure 23–38).

Circular movement over the neck and chest. Starting at the back of the ears, apply a circular movement down the side of the neck, over the shoulders, and across the chest (figure 23-39).

Massaging male skin is not all that different from massaging female skin. However, it needs more attention in the areas of the face where there is hair growth. For your male clients, use downward movements in the

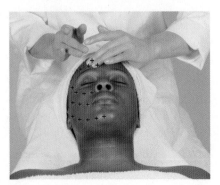

figure 23-37
Light tapping movement

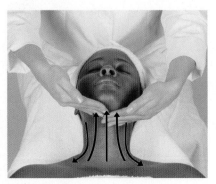

figure 23-38
Stroking movement of neck

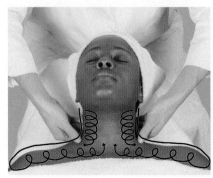

figure 23-39
Circular movement over
neck and chest

beard area. Massaging against hair growth causes great discomfort. Pressure-point massage in the beard area is much appreciated by male clients.

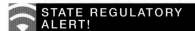
Chest, Back, and Neck Manipulations (Optional)

Some instructors prefer to treat these areas first before starting the regular facial. Apply cleanser, and remove it with a tissue or a warm, moist towel. Then apply massage cream and perform the following manipulations:

Chest and back movement. Use a rotary movement across the upper chest and shoulders. Then slide your fingers to the base of the neck and rotate three times.

Shoulders and back movement. Rotate the shoulders three times. Glide your fingers to the spine and then to the base of the neck. Apply circular movement up to the back of the ear, and then slide your fingers to the front of the earlobe. Rotate three times.

Back massage. To stimulate and relax the client, use your thumbs and bent index fingers to grasp the tissue at the back of the neck. Rotate six times. Repeat over the shoulders. Remove cream with tissues or a warm, moist towel. Dust the back lightly with talcum powder and smooth.

After reading the next few sections, you will be able to:

LO⑧ Name and describe two types of electrical machines used in facial treatments.

LO⑨ Explain how the two types of electrical machines add value to a facial.

Know the Purpose of the Facial Equipment

There are many types of facial equipment that can enhance your ability to perform an outstanding facial treatment. These machines help to increase the efficacy of your products, increase product penetration, and provide for a more complete and relaxing treatment.

We have already mentioned magnifying lamps, which are necessary for both analysis of the skin and procedures such as extraction of comedones and tweezing of excess facial hair.

A facial **steamer** heats and produces a stream of warm steam that can be focused on the client's face or other areas of skin. Steaming the skin helps to soften the tissues, making it more accepting of moisturizers and other treatment products. Steam also helps to relax and soften follicle accumulations such as comedones and clogged follicles, making them easier to extract (**figure 23-40**).

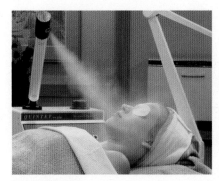

figure 23-40
Facial steamer being used during a facial treatment

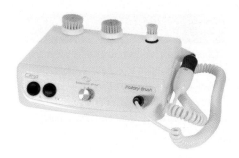

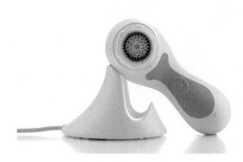

Most steamers work by having a heating coil that boils water. The steam from the boiling water flows through a pipe that can be focused on the area to be treated, normally the face. Only distilled water should be used in most steamers to avoid mineral buildup in the machine. Steam is usually administered at the beginning of the facial treatment. Most clients enjoy steam, but precautions should be taken with clients who have asthma or other breathing disorders.

It is strongly recommended that a professional steamer be used, but if one is not available, a warm steamed towel may be gently wrapped around the face, leaving the nose exposed so the client can breathe comfortably. The towel should be comfortably warm, but not hot. Do not use steamed towels on clients who have sensitive skin, redness-prone skin, rosacea, or claustrophobia.

A **brushing machine** is a rotating electric appliance with interchangeable brushes that can be attached to the rotating head. Brushes of various sizes as well as textures are common. Larger and stiffer brushes are used for back treatment, and smaller and softer brushes are used for the face.

Brushing is a form of mechanical exfoliation, and it is usually administered after or during steam. A fairly thick layer of cleanser or moisturizer should be applied to the face before using the brushing machine.

This applied product provides a buffer for the brushes so that they do not scratch the face, which they might do if the face were completely dry.

Brushing helps remove dead cells from the skin surface, making the skin look smoother and more even in coloration. It also helps to stimulate blood circulation.

Brushing should never be used on clients using keratolytic drugs such as Retin-A®, Differin®, Tazorac®, or other drugs that thin or exfoliate the skin. Clients who have rosacea, sensitive skin, pustular acne, or other forms of skin inflammation or reddening should not have brushing administered. Never use a brushing machine at the same time as another exfoliation technique, such as an AHA treatment or microdermabrasion.

Brushes must be thoroughly cleaned and disinfected between clients.

The skin suction and cold spray machine is used to increase circulation and to jet-spray lotions and toners onto the skin. Skin suction should only be used on non-sensitive and non-inflamed skin.

Spray can be used on almost any skin type. Spray is often used to hydrate the skin and to help clean off mask treatments.

> ⚠ **CAUTION**
> Information regarding facial equipment in this chapter is intended as an overview. You should receive hands-on experience from your instructor before using any facial equipment! Machine models differ; as a result, precautions vary as well. Consult with your instructor and the specific machine manual for safe operation. In some states, use of certain equipment may not be permissible for cosmetologists. Again, check with your instructor to find out what is allowed in your state.

LO **10** Know the difference between galvanic and high frequency treatments used in facial services.

LO **11** Explain how light therapy is used to treat the skin.

How Electrotherapy and Light Therapy Treat the Skin

Galvanic and high-frequency treatment are types of **electrotherapy** (ee-LECK-tro-ther-ah-pee), which is the use of electrical currents to treat the skin.

There are several contraindications for electrotherapy. Electrotherapy should never be administered on heart patients, clients with pacemakers, clients with metal implants, pregnant clients, clients with epilepsy or seizure disorders, clients who are afraid of electric current, or clients with open or broken skin. Furthermore, if you ever have any doubts about whether the client can have electrotherapy safely, request that the client get approval from his or her physician before receiving this therapy.

An electrode is an applicator for directing the electric current from the machine to the client's skin (**figure 23-41**). High-frequency machines require the use of only one electrode. Galvanic machines have two positive electrodes called an anode (AN-ohd), which has a red plug and cord, and a negative electrode called a cathode (KATH-ohd), which has a black plug and cord (**figure 23-42**).

Galvanic current accomplishes two basic tasks. Desincrustation (des-in-cruh-STAY-shun) is the process of softening and emulsifying hardened sebum stuck in the hair follicles. Desincrustation is very helpful when treating oily areas with multiple comedones and most acne-prone skin. Desincrustation products are alkaline fluids or gels that act as solvents for the solidified sebum. These products make extraction of the impactions and comedones much easier. When the negative pole is applied to the face

> ⚠ **CAUTION**
> Do not use the galvanic current on clients who have:
> - Metal implants, a pacemaker, or any heart condition
> - Epilepsy
> - Pregnancy
> - High blood pressure, fever, or any infection
> - Nerve disorders
> - Open or broken skin (wounds, new scars), including pustular acne
> - Fear of electrical current

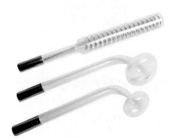

figure 23-41
Various electrodes: mushroom and indirect electrode (spiral)

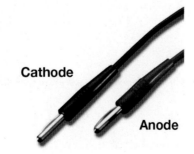

Cathode

Anode

figure 23-42
Cathode and anode

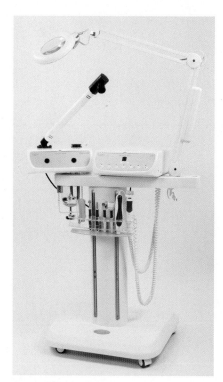

figure 23-43
Five-in-one machine, including galvanic electrodes

over a desincrustation product, the current forces the product deeper into the follicle. The current also produces a chemical reaction that helps to loosen the impacted sebum (**figure 23-43**).

Both electrodes are wrapped in wet cotton. The active electrode is the one that should be applied to the skin. The active electrode—in the case of desincrustation, the negative electrode—is applied to the oily areas of the face for three to five minutes. The positive electrode (in this case, the inactive electrode) is held by the client in her right hand or attached to a pad that is placed in contact with the client's right shoulder (**figure 23-44**). After the desincrustation process has taken place, sebum deposits can easily be extracted with gentle pressure.

Iontophoresis (eye-ahn-toh-foh-REE-sus) is the process of using galvanic current to enable water-soluble products that contain ions to penetrate the skin. Products suitable for iontophoresis will be labeled as such by manufacturers. When the negative current is applied to the face, products with negative ions are able to penetrate the skin, and when the positive current is applied to the face, products with positive ions are able to penetrate the skin. Many ampoules and serums are prepared for iontophoresis.

Again, you must receive thorough hands-on instruction from your teacher before attempting this procedure.

Microcurrent

Microcurrent (MY-kroh-KUR-ent) is a type of galvanic treatment using a very low level of electrical current; it has many applications in skin care and is best known for helping to tone the skin, producing a lifting effect for aging skin that lacks elasticity.

High-Frequency Current

High-frequency current, discovered by Nikola Tesla, can be used to stimulate blood flow and help products penetrate. It works by warming tissues, which allows better absorption of moisturizers and other

> ⚠ **CAUTION**
> Place the passive electrode on the right side of the client's body only (never on the left side) to avoid current flow through the heart.

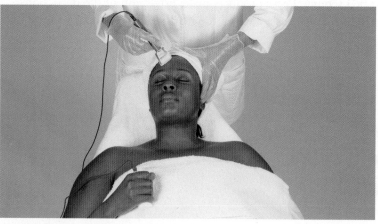

figure 23-44
Client holding a passive electrode

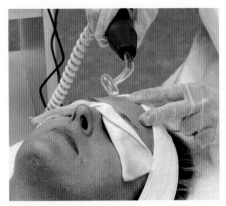

figure 23-45a
Direct application of high frequency

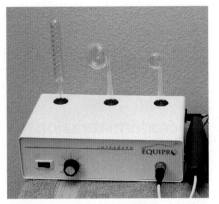

figure 23-45b
The high-frequency machine produces a heat effect that stimulates circulation.

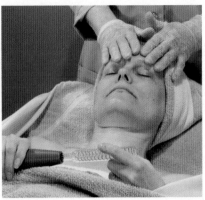

figure 23-46
Indirect application of high frequency

treatment products. High-frequency current can also be applied after extraction or during treatments for acne-prone skin because it has a germicidal effect.

Electrodes for the high-frequency machine are made of glass and contain various types of gas, such as neon, which light up as a color when current is flowing through the electrode. Unlike the galvanic machine, high-frequency treatments require the use of only one electrode. There are several different types of electrodes used with high frequency. The most common is shaped like a mushroom, and it is referred to as a *mushroom electrode* (figures 23-45a and 23-45b).

High frequency can be applied directly to the skin in a technique known as *direct application*. Another application method, known as *indirect massage* or *Viennese massage*, involves the client holding the electrode during treatment, creating an electrical stimulating massage (figure 23-46).

High frequency is applied to the skin as part of the treatment phase of the facial treatment. Again, because machines vary, you should check with your instructor and the manufacturer's manual for instructions for the specific machine you are using.

> ⚠️ **CAUTION**
> The contraindications for galvanic current also apply to both indirect and direct high-frequency current. Furthermore, in order to prevent burns during the treatment, the client should avoid any contact with metal—such as chair arms, stools, jewelry, and metal bobby pins.

Light Therapy

Using light exposure to treat conditions of the skin is known as light therapy. There are several different types of light therapy utilizing various types of light. Traditionally, infrared lamps have been used to heat the skin and increase blood flow. Infrared lights have also been used for hair and scalp treatments.

A popular type of light therapy is called light-emitting diode (LED) treatment (figure 23-47). This treatment uses concentrated light that flashes very rapidly. LEDs were originally developed to help with wound healing. In cosmetology, LED machines are used cosmetically to minimize redness, warm lower-level tissues, stimulate blood flow, and improve skin smoothness. They are applied to improve acne-prone skin. The type and color of the light varies according to treatment objective. Red lights are used to treat aging and redness, and blue light is used for acne-prone skin.

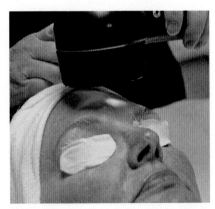

figure 23-47
Light therapy using a LED machine

LEDs are a very safe treatment for most clients, but their use should be avoided on clients who have seizure disorders. Flashing lights have been known to trigger seizures in persons with seizure disorders. Any clients with questionable health conditions should receive written approval from a physician before having an LED treatment.

Microdermabrasion

Microdermabrasion (MY-kroh-dur-muh-BRAY-zhun) is a type of mechanical exfoliation that involves shooting aluminum oxide or other crystals at the skin with a hand-held device that exfoliates dead cells. Microdermabrasion uses a closed vacuum to shoot crystals onto the skin, bumping off cell buildup that is then vacuumed up by suction. Microdermabrasion is a popular treatment because it produces fast, visible results. It is used primarily to treat surface wrinkles and aging skin. Performance of safe and effective microdermabrasion treatments requires extensive training.

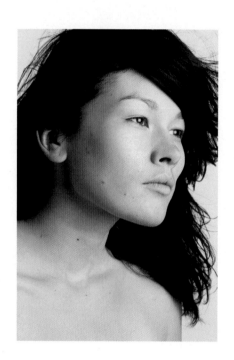

Radharani/Shutterstock.com

Use Facials To Treat Basic and Specialty Skin Types

A professional facial is one of the most enjoyable and relaxing services available to the salon client. Clients who have experienced this very restful, yet stimulating experience do not hesitate to return for more. When clients receive them on a regular basis, the client's skin tone, texture, and appearance are noticeably improved.

Facial treatments fall into one of the following categories:

- **Preservative.** Maintains the health of the facial skin by cleansing correctly, increasing circulation, relaxing the nerves, and activating the skin glands and metabolism through massage.

- **Corrective.** Correct certain facial skin conditions, such as dryness, oiliness, comedones, aging lines, and minor conditions of acne.

As with other forms of massage, facial treatments help to increase circulation, activate glandular activity, relax the nerves, maintain muscle tone, and strengthen weak muscle tissues.

Guidelines for Facial Treatments

Your facial treatments are bound to be successful and to inspire return visits if you follow the simple guidelines summarized below:

- Help the client to relax by speaking in a quiet and professional manner.

- Explain the benefits of the products and service, and answer any questions the client may have.

- Provide a quiet atmosphere, and work quietly and efficiently.

- Maintain neat, clean conditions in the facial work area, with an orderly arrangement of supplies.

- Follow systematic procedures.
- If your hands are cold, warm them before touching the client's face.
- Keep your nails smooth and short to prevent scratching the client's skin.

Another guideline you must always follow is to perform an analysis of your client's skin. After the client is draped and lying on the facial table (also called a facial bed), you should inspect the skin to determine the following:

- Is the skin dry, normal, or oily?
- Are there fine lines or creases?
- Are comedones or acne present?
- Are dilated capillaries visible?
- Is skin texture smooth or rough?
- Is skin color even?

? DID YOU KNOW?

To safely and effectively perform advanced skin care treatments—such as microcurrent, microdermabrasion, and LED light—cosmetologists require advanced, specialized training.

The results of your analysis will determine the products to use for the treatment, what areas of the face need special attention, how mucah pressure to use when massaging, and what equipment should be used.

Basic Facial Application

The steps for performing a basic facial are listed in Procedure 23-1. Some procedures may vary, however, so be guided by your instructor.

The procedure lists the basic implements and materials you will need to perform the basic facial, but you can add other items, such as an alternative head covering, if you wish. There are several types of head coverings on the market. Some are a turban design; others are designed with elastic, like a shower cap. They are generally made of either cloth or paper towels. For the paper towel procedure, be guided by your instructor.

Ⓟ 23-1　**Basic Facial** *See page 796*

Special Problems

There are a number of special problems that must be considered when you are performing a facial. These include dry skin, oily skin and blackheads, and acne.

Dry skin is caused by an insufficient flow of sebum (oil) from the sebaceous glands. The facial for dry skin helps correct this condition. Although it can be given with or without an electrical current, the use of electrical current provides better results.

Ⓟ 23-2　**Facial for Dry Skin** *See page 801*

Oily skin is often characterized by comedones, which are caused by hardened masses of sebum formed in the ducts of the sebaceous glands.

Ⓟ 23-3　**Facial for Oily Skin with Open Comedones (Blackheads)** *See page 803*

Special Notes for Acne-Prone Skin

Minor problem skin and oily skin should respond well to facial treatments. Unresponsive or severe cases of acne need medical treatment, and clients with such conditions should be referred to a dermatologist.

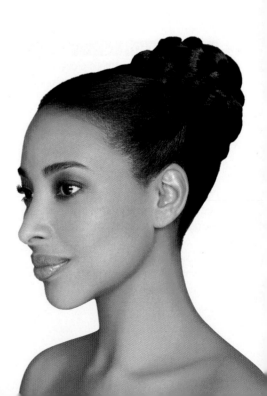

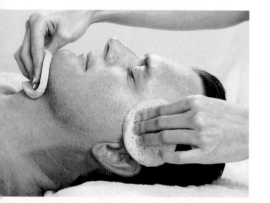

If a client is under medical care, the role of the cosmetologist is to work under the advisement of the client's physician, following the physician's instructions for the type and frequency of facial treatments. Cosmetologists can help these clients with extraction treatments, assist them in choosing proper home-care products and makeup, and help them to understand how to coordinate medications with a home skin care program.

There are numerous topical prescription medications that can make the skin more sensitive and more reactive to skin care products. Always check with the client's dermatologist if you are performing treatments to clients who are under dermatological care.

Because skin with acne contains infectious matter, you must wear protective gloves and use disposable materials such as cotton cleansing pads when working with clients who have acne.

Michaeljung/Shutterstock.com

Facial Treatments for Men

More men are having facial treatments than ever before. Special notes for performing facial treatments on men include always moving with the pattern of the beard; usually these are downwards and outwards movements. Use sponges instead of cotton pads on a man's face, as cotton will get caught in beard hair. Avoid using perfumed products on men. Make sure you have fragrance-free products or neutral-scented products. Advanced courses are available in men's skin treatment.

P 23-4   **Facial for Acne-Prone and Problem Skin** *See page 805*

Consultation and Home Care

Home care is probably the most important factor in a successful skin care program. The key word here is *program*. Clients' participation is essential to achieve results. A program consists of a long-range plan involving home care, salon treatments, and client education.

Every new client should receive a thorough consultation regarding proper home care for his or her skin conditions.

After the first treatment, block out about 30 minutes to explain proper home care for the client.

After the treatment is finished, have the client sit up in the facial chair, or invite the client to move to a well-lighted consultation area. A mirror should be provided for the client, so that he or she can see conditions you will be discussing.

Explain, in simple terms, the client's skin conditions, informing the client of how you propose to treat the conditions. Inform the client about how often treatments should be administered in the salon, and very specifically explain what the client should be doing at home.

You should organize the products you want the client to purchase and use. Explain the use of each one at a time, in the order of use. Make sure to have written instructions for the client to take home.

It is very important to provide clients with products that you believe in and that produce results. Retailing products for clients to use at home is very important for success in the treatment of skin conditions and success in your business.

After reading the next few sections, you will be able to:

LO⑫ Discuss how aromatherapy is used in the basic facial.

Use of Aromatherapy in the Basic Facial

The use of essential oils such as lemon verbena, lavender, and rose is a frequent practice in facial skin care. Many essential oils are also used for **aromatherapy**, the therapeutic use of plant aromas for beauty and health treatment. Aromatherapy is thought to benefit and enhance a person's physical, emotional, mental, and spiritual well-being. Using various oils and oil blends for specific benefits is believed to create positive effects on the body, mind, and spirit (**figure 23-48**).

Essential oils can be used in a variety of ways. Lighting a cinnamon candle in the winter can give the salon a cozy feeling and cheer up both clients and service providers. You can use a spray bottle to diffuse well-diluted essential oils in the treatment room or on the sheets. You can create your own aromatherapy massage oil by adding a few drops of essential oil to a massage oil, cream, or lotion. Always be careful to use essential oils lightly because they can sometimes be overpowering.

> ⚠ **CAUTION**
> Aromatherapy is sometimes used as a healing modality by natural healers who have received extensive training in the properties and uses of essential oils and their aromatherapy benefits. Cosmetologists should never attempt to perform healing treatments with aromatherapy.

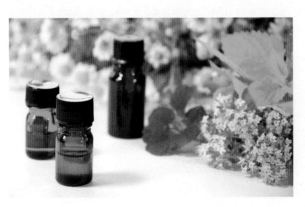

© Botamochy/Shutterstock.com

figure 23-48
Some ingredients for aromatherapy

P 23-1

BASIC FACIAL

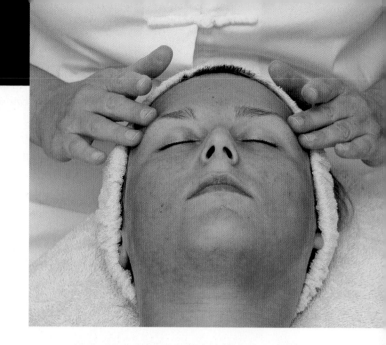

IMPLEMENTS & MATERIALS

You will need all of the following implements, materials, and supplies:

- ☐ Antiseptic lotion
- ☐ Bobby pins/safety pins
- ☐ Bowls
- ☐ Clean sheet or other covering (blanket if necessary)
- ☐ Cleansers and makeup removers
- ☐ Cotton (roll)
- ☐ Cotton pads
- ☐ Cotton swabs and pledgets

- ☐ Disinfectant
- ☐ Disposable gloves
- ☐ Exfoliant
- ☐ Facial gown
- ☐ Facial steamer (optional)
- ☐ Facial table or chair
- ☐ Gauze
- ☐ Headband or head covering
- ☐ Magnifying lamp
- ☐ Mask brush

- ☐ Masks
- ☐ Massage cream or lubricating oil
- ☐ Moisturizers
- ☐ Paper towels
- ☐ Spatulas
- ☐ Sponges
- ☐ Sun-protection products
- ☐ Tissues
- ☐ Toner
- ☐ Towels

- ☐ Trash can
- ☐ Trolley for products and implements

  Optional Items:
- ☐ Infrared lamp
- ☐ Other electrical equipment (towel warmer, etc.)
- ☐ Specialty or intensive-care products (serums, eye creams, extraction supplies)

PREPARATION

Perform:

P 22-1 Pre-Service Procedure *See page 748*

PROCEDURE

① Ask the client to remove any jewelry. Store the client's jewelry in a safe place. Clients may wish to keep their handbags nearby during the facial.

② Show the client to the dressing room and offer assistance if needed. Some salons provide disposable slippers that can be worn to and from the dressing room.

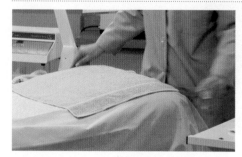

③ Place a clean towel across the back of the facial table to prevent the client's bare shoulders from coming into contact with the bed.

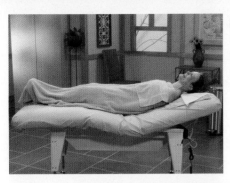

④ If necessary, help the client get onto the facial table. Place a towel across the client's chest, and place a coverlet or sheet over the client's body, folding the top edge of the towel over it. Remove the client's shoes, and tuck the coverlet around the feet.

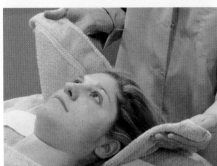

⑤ Fasten a headband lined with tissue, a towel, or other head covering around the client's head to protect their hair. To drape the head with a towel, follow these steps:

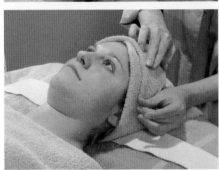

a. Fold the towel diagonally from one of the top corners to the opposite lower corner, and place it over the headrest with the fold facing down. The towel will already be placed on the headrest before the client enters the facial area as described in step 3.

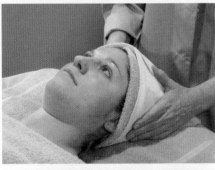

b. When the client is in a reclined position, the back of the head should rest on the towel so that the sides of the towel can be brought up to the center of the forehead to cover the hairline.

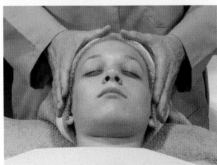

c. Use a headband with a Velcro closure or a pin to hold the towel in place. Make sure that all strands of hair are tucked under the towel, that the earlobes are not bent, and that the towel is not wrapped too tightly.

6 Remove lingerie straps from a female client's shoulders. Alternative method: If client is given a strapless gown to wear, tuck the straps into the top of the gown.

7 If your client wears makeup, use the following steps to remove it. If your client has no makeup, proceed to step 8.

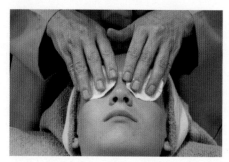

a. Apply a pea-sized amount of eye makeup remover to each of two damp cotton pads and place them on the client's closed eyes. Leave them in place for one minute.

b. Meanwhile, apply another pea-sized amount of eye makeup remover to a damp cotton pad and gently remove the client's lipstick with even strokes from the corners of the lips toward the center. Repeat the procedure until the lips are clean.

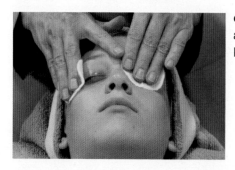

c. Now, remove the eye makeup in the same way, gently stroking down and outward with the cotton pad. Do one eye first, and then the other. Repeat the procedure until the eyelids and lashes are clean.

d. Ask the client to look up, and then remove any makeup underneath the eyes. Always be gentle around the eyes. Never rub or stretch this thin, delicate skin.

8 Remove about one-half teaspoon of cleanser from the container with a clean spatula. Blend it with your fingers to soften it. Starting at the neck with a sweeping movement, use both hands to spread the cleanser. When manipulating the skin, never completely lose touch with the skin.

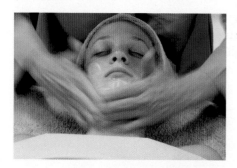

a. Sweep upward on the chin, jaws, cheeks, the base of the nose to the temples, and along the sides and the bridge of the nose. Make small circular movements with your fingertips around the nostrils and sides of the nose.

b. Continue the upward sweeping movements between the brows and across the forehead to the temples. Take additional cleanser from the container with a clean spatula, and blend it with your fingers. Smooth down the neck, chest, and back with long, even strokes.

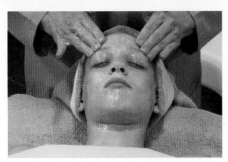

c. Starting at the center of the forehead, move your fingertips lightly in a circle around the eyes to the temples and then back to the center of the forehead.

d. Slide your fingers down the nose to the upper lip, from the temples through the forehead, lightly down to the chin, and then firmly up the jaw line back toward the temples and forehead.

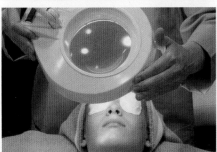

⑨ Remove the cleanser with facial sponges, tissues, moist cotton pads, or warm, moist towels. Start at the forehead and follow the contours of the face. Remove all the cleanser from one area of the face before proceeding to the next. Finish with the neck, chest, and back.

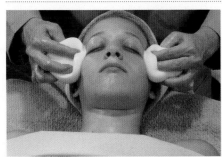

⑩ Analyze the client's skin to determine the products and procedures to be used. Optional: if eyebrow arching is to be done, it should be done at this time. Use warm, moist towels or a facial steamer to moisturize and soften the facial skin, helping to loosen comedones for extraction. If extraction is performed, you must put on disposable gloves for this procedure.

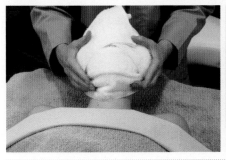 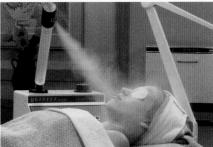

⑪ If you use a steamer, cover the client's eyes with cotton pads moistened with either distilled water or a special eye compress solution. Steam helps to soften superficial lines and increases blood circulation to the surface of the skin.

⑫ Assuming that the client's skin is non-sensitive, exfoliate. Apply a granular scrub to the face and gently massage the scrub in small circular movements for about two minutes. Never use a granular product near the eye area because granules can accidentally get into the eye.

⑬ If you like, this granular scrub can be used during exposure to the facial steamer. Remove the scrub carefully with damp sponges or cotton pads.

⑭ A brushing machine can be used instead of the granular scrub, but remember to apply cleansing milk before using the machine. Check with your instructor to have him or her show you the correct way to use the brushing machine.

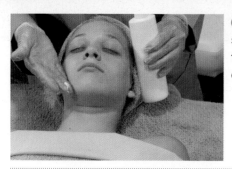

15 Choose a treatment cream, lotion, or massage cream appropriate for the skin type. Using the same procedure as for the cleanser, apply the cream to the face, neck, shoulders, chest, and back. If needed, apply lubrication oil or cream around the eyes and on the neck.

16 Massage the face, using the facial manipulations described in the Facial Massage section of this chapter.

17 Remove the massage cream with warm, moist towels, moist cleansing pads, or sponges. Follow the same procedure as for removing cleanser.

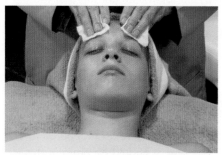

19 Apply a treatment mask formulated for the client's skin condition.

20 Remove some mask from its container with a clean spatula and place it in a little cup or bowl.

18 Sponge the face with cotton pledgets moistened with toner or freshener.

21 Apply the mask with a natural bristle brush, starting at the neck. Use long, slow strokes from the center outward.

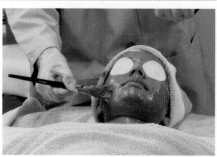

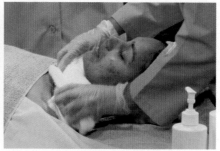

24 Apply toner, astringent, or freshener.

22 Proceed to the jawline and apply the mask on the face from the center outward on half of the face and then on the other half. Allow the mask to remain on the face for 7 to 10 minutes.

23 Remove the mask with wet cotton pledgets, sponges, or towels.

25 Apply a moisturizer or sunscreen.

26 When the service is complete, remove the head covering and show the client to the dressing room, offering assistance if needed.

POST-SERVICE

Complete:

P 22-2 **Post-Service Procedure** *See page 751*

FACIAL FOR DRY SKIN

IMPLEMENTS & MATERIALS

In addition to the items needed for the Basic Facial, you will also need:

- ☐ Eye cream
- ☐ Galvanic or high-frequency machine, depending on treatment
- ☐ Specialized creams, serums, and toners for dry skin

PREPARATION

Perform:

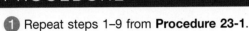 **22-1 Pre-Service Procedure** *See page 748*

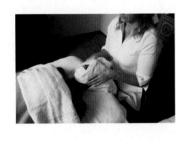

PROCEDURE

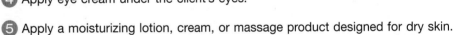

1. Repeat steps 1–9 from **Procedure 23-1**.

2. Focus steam on the face and allow steaming for 5 minutes.

3. During or after steaming, apply a mild granular exfoliating product designed for dry skin. Gently massage with light circular movements. Remove with damp cotton pads, soft sponges, or a warm, moist, soft towel.

4. Apply eye cream under the client's eyes.

5. Apply a moisturizing lotion, cream, or massage product designed for dry skin.

6. Massage the skin with manipulations.

7. If massage cream is used, remove with damp cotton pads, soft sponges, or a warm, moist, soft towel.

8. If you are not using electrotherapy, proceed to step 11.

9. Electrotherapy Option 1, Galvanic Treatment: Apply ionized specialized serum, gel, or lotion. Apply galvanic current as directed by the manufacturer or your instructor.

10. Electrotherapy Option 2, High-Frequency Indirect Current Treatment: Use machine as directed by the manufacturer or your instructor. While the client holds the electrode in his or her hand, perform manipulations for seven to ten minutes. Do not lift your hands from the client's face. Turn off high-frequency machine.

11. Apply additional moisturizing or specialty product for dry skin with slow massage movements.

12 Starting at the neck and using a soft mask brush, apply a soft-setting cream or hydrating gel mask. Make sure you remove the mask from its container with a clean spatula. Mask should be applied from the center outward.

13 Apply cold cotton eye pads. Allow the mask to process for seven to ten minutes. Make sure client is comfortable and warm.

14 Remove the mask with warm, wet cotton pads; sponges; or warm, moist, soft towels.

15 Apply toner for dry skin with cotton pads.

16 Apply moisturizer or sunscreen designed for dry skin.

17 When the service is complete, remove the head covering and show the client to the dressing room, offering assistance if needed.

POST-SERVICE

Complete:

P 22-2 **Post-Service Procedure** *See page 751*

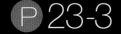

FACIAL FOR OILY SKIN WITH OPEN COMEDONES (BLACKHEADS)

IMPLEMENTS & MATERIALS

In addition to the items needed for the Basic Facial, you will also need:

☐ Desincrustation gel or lotion

☐ Galvanic or high-frequency machine, depending on treatment

☐ Serum, clay-based mask, and toner for oily skin

PREPARATION

Perform:

Ⓟ 22-1 **Pre-Service Procedure** *See page 748*

PROCEDURE

1 Repeat steps 1–7 from **Procedure 23-1**.

2 Apply cleanser designed for oily skin. Gently massage to apply, and then remove with damp cotton pads, soft sponges, or a warm, moist, soft towel.

3 Remove residue with a damp cotton pad or a soft sponge. Do not tone at this time.

4 Focus steam on the face and allow steaming for 5 minutes.

5 During or after steaming, apply a mild granular exfoliating product designed for oily or combination skin. Gently massage with light, circular movements. Remove with damp cotton pads, soft sponges, or a warm, moist, soft towel.

6 Apply a desincrustation lotion or gel to any area with clogged pores. The lotion should generally remain on the skin for five to eight minutes, again, depending on the manufacturer's instructions.

7 Negative galvanic current may be applied over this lotion, depending on the manufacturer's instructions. Remove the preparation with damp cotton pads, soft sponges, or a warm, moist, soft towel.

8 Put on disposable gloves prior to performing extractions. Apply damp cotton pads to the client's eyes to avoid exposure to the glaring light from the magnifying lamp. Cover your fingertips with cotton, and (using the magnifying lamp) gently press out open comedones.

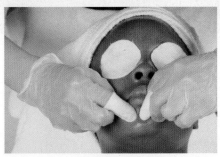

9 Place your middle fingers on either side of the comedone or clogged pore, stretching the skin. Push your fingers down to reach underneath the follicle, and then gently squeeze. Apply the same technique to all sides of the follicle. As an alternative, you may use the same technique using cotton swabs.

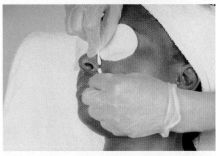

10 Do not extract for more than 5 minutes for the entire face. Never squeeze with bare fingers or fingernails! If galvanic desincrustation was performed prior to extraction, apply positive galvanic current to the face after extractions are complete. This will help to re-establish the proper pH of the skin surface.

11 After extraction is complete, apply an astringent lotion, a toner for oily skin, or a specialized serum designed to be used following extraction. Allow the skin to dry.

12 Unfold gauze across the face and apply direct high-frequency using the mushroom-shaped electrode, according to the machine manufacturer's directions.

13 Extremely oily or clogged skin should not be massaged. If the skin is very clogged, proceed to step 17. If skin is not extremely clogged, apply a hydration fluid or massage fluid designed for oily and combination skin, and perform massage manipulations.

14 Using a mask brush, apply a clay-based mask to all oily areas. To dry areas, such as the eye and neck areas, you may choose to apply a gel mask for dehydrated skin. Allow the mask to process for about 10 minutes. Do not allow the mask to overdry so that it cracks.

15 Remove the mask with damp cotton pads, soft sponges, or a warm, moist, soft towel.

16 Apply toner for oily skin with cotton pads.

17 Apply moisturizer or sunscreen designed for oily or combination skin.

18 When the service is complete, remove the head covering and show the client to the dressing room, offering assistance if needed.

POST-SERVICE

Complete:

P 22-2 **Post-Service Procedure** *See page 751*

FACIAL FOR ACNE-PRONE AND PROBLEM SKIN

IMPLEMENTS & MATERIALS

In addition to the items needed for the Basic Facial, you will also need:

☐ Antibacterial clay or sulfur mask

☐ Desincrustation gel or lotion

☐ Galvanic or high-frequency machine, depending on treatment

☐ Specialized fluids, serums, and toners for acne-prone skin

PREPARATION

Perform:

P 22-1 **Pre-Service Procedure** *See page 748*

PROCEDURE

1. Repeat steps 1–6 from **Procedure 23-1**.

2. Put on disposable gloves. Remove the client's makeup.

3. Apply cleanser designed for oily/acne-prone skin, gently massage to apply, and then remove with damp cotton pads, soft sponges, or a warm, moist, soft towel.

4. Remove residue with damp cotton pad or soft sponge. Do not tone at this time.

5. Focus steam on the face and allow steaming for 5 minutes.

6. Apply a desincrustation lotion or gel to any area with pimples or clogged pores. Negative galvanic current may be applied over this lotion, depending on the manufacturer's instructions. The lotion should generally remain on the skin for 5 to 8 minutes, again, depending on the manufacturer's instructions.

7. Remove the preparation with damp cotton pads, soft sponges, or a warm, moist, soft towel.

8. Extract comedones.

9. After extraction is complete, apply an astringent lotion, a toner for oily skin, or a specialized serum designed for use following extraction. Allow the skin to dry.

10. Unfold gauze across the face and apply direct, high-frequency using the mushroom-shaped electrode, as directed by the machine manufacturer and your instructor.

11. If galvanic desincrustation was performed prior to extraction, apply positive galvanic current to the face after extractions are complete. This will help to re-establish the proper pH of the skin surface.

⑫ Acne-prone skin should not be massaged.

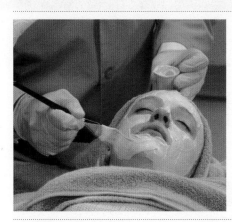

⑬ Using a mask brush, apply an antibacterial or sulfur-based mask to all oily and acne-prone areas. To dry skin, such as the eye and neck areas, you may choose to apply a gel mask for dehydrated skin.

⑭ Allow the mask to process for about 10 minutes. Do not allow the mask to overdry so that it cracks.

⑮ Remove the mask with damp cotton pads, soft sponges, or a warm, moist, soft towel.

⑯ Apply toner for oily skin with cotton pads.

⑰ Apply specialized lotion or sunscreen designed for oily or acne-prone skin.

⑱ When the service is complete, remove the head covering and show the client to the dressing room, offering assistance if needed.

POST-SERVICE

Complete:

Ⓟ 22-2 **Post-Service Procedure** *See page 751*

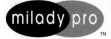 Check out miladypro.com for additional resources and training to enhance your technical skills. Keyword: *FutureCosPro*

REVIEW QUESTIONS

① Explain skin analysis techniques. Why is the skin analysis important?

② What is a contraindication? List five examples.

③ Why is it important to have every client complete a client intake form?

④ Describe the differences between alipidic and oily skin.

⑤ What is the difference between skin type and skin condition?

⑥ Name and explain the different categories of skin care products.

⑦ What are the steps to completing a client consultation?

⑧ Why is massage used during a facial?

⑨ Name and briefly describe the five categories of massage manipulations.

⑩ Name and describe two types of electrical machines used in facial treatments and why these machines add value to a facial.

⑪ Who is not a good candidate for electrical current treatment? Why?

⑫ How can aromatherapy be used in the basic facial?

STUDY TOOLS

• **Reinforce what you just learned:** Complete the activities and exercises in your Theory or Practical Workbook, or your Study Guide.

• **Expand your knowledge:** Search for websites about the topics in this chapter and make a list of additional resources.

• **Study and prepare for your quiz:** Take the chapter test in your Exam Review or your Milady U: Online Licensing Prep.

• **Re-Test your knowledge:** Take the Chapter 23 *Quizzes*!

• **Learn even more:** Look up in a dictionary or search the internet for the definitions of any additional terms you want to learn about.

CHAPTER GLOSSARY

alipidic al-ah-PIDD-ic	p. 773	Literally means "lack of lipids"; describes skin that does not produce enough sebum, indicated by absence of visible pores.
ampoules am-pyools	p. 778	Individual doses of serum, sealed in small vials.
aromatherapy	p. 795	The therapeutic use of plant aromas for beauty and health treatment.
brushing machine	p. 788	A rotating electric appliance with interchangeable brushes that can be attached to the rotating head.
chemical exfoliants	p. 776	Products that contain chemicals that either loosen or dissolve dead cell buildup.
chucking	p. 782	Massage movement accomplished by grasping the flesh firmly in one hand and moving the hand up and down along the bone while the other hand keeps the arm or leg in a steady position.
clay-based masks	p. 779	Oil-absorbing, cleansing masks that have an exfoliating effect and an astringent effect on oily and combination skin, making large pores temporarily appear smaller.

cleansing milks	p. 775	Non-foaming lotion cleansers designed to cleanse dry and sensitive skin types and remove makeup.
contraindication kahn-trah-in-dih-KAY-shun	p. 767	Condition that requires avoiding certain treatments, procedures, or products to prevent undesirable side effects.
couperose KOO-per-ohs	p. 774	Distended capillaries caused by weakening of the capillary walls.
cream masks	p. 779	Masks often containing oils and emollients as well as humectants; have a strong moisturizing effect.
effleurage EF-loo-rahzh	p. 781	Light, continuous stroking movement applied with the fingers (digital) or the palms (palmar) in a slow, rhythmic manner.
electrotherapy ee-LECK-tro-ther-ah-pee	p. 789	The use of electrical currents to treat the skin.
emollients ee-MAHL-yunts	p. 777	Oil or fatty ingredients that prevent moisture from leaving the skin.
enzyme peels EN-zym PEELS	p. 777	Also known as *keratolytic* (kair-uh-tuh-LIT-ik) *enzymes* or *protein-dissolving agents*; a type of chemical exfoliant that works by dissolving keratin protein in the surface cells of the skin.
exfoliants ex-FO-lee-yahnts	p. 775	Products that help bring about exfoliation.
exfoliation eks-foh-lee-AY-shun	p. 775	The removal of excess dead cells from the skin surface.
extraction eck-strack-shun	p. 773	A procedure in which comedones are removed from the follicles by manual manipulation.
facial	p. 766	Also known as a *facial treatment*; a professional skin treatment that improves the condition and appearance of the skin.
foaming cleansers	p. 775	Cleansers containing surfactants (detergents) that cause the product to foam and rinse off easily.
friction FRIK-shun	p. 782	Deep rubbing movement requiring pressure on the skin with the fingers or palm while moving them over an underlying structure.
fulling	p. 782	Form of pétrissage in which the tissue is grasped, gently lifted, and spread out; used mainly for massaging the arms.
gommages go-mah-jez	p. 776	Also known as *roll-off masks*; peeling creams that are rubbed off of the skin.
hacking	p. 782	Chopping movement performed with the edges of the hands in massage.
humectants hyoo-MEKK-tents	p. 777	Also known as *hydrators* or *water-binding agents*; ingredients that attract water.
magnifying lamp	p. 772	A magnifying lens surrounded by a circular light, providing a well-lit, enlarged view of the skin.
masks	p. 778	Also known as *masques*; concentrated treatment products often composed of mineral clays, moisturizing agents, skin softeners, aromatherapy oils, botanical extracts, and other beneficial ingredients to cleanse, exfoliate, tighten, tone, hydrate, and nourish the skin.

massage	p. 780	Manual or mechanical manipulation of the body by rubbing, gently pinching, kneading, tapping, and other movements to increase metabolism and circulation, promote absorption, and relieve pain.
massage creams	p. 778	Lubricants used to make the skin slippery during massage.
mechanical exfoliants	p. 776	Methods used to physically remove dead cell buildup.
microdermabrasion MY-kroh-dur-muh-BRAY-zhun	p. 792	Mechanical exfoliation that involves shooting aluminum oxide or other crystals at the skin with a hand-held device that exfoliates dead cells.
microdermabrasion scrubs	p. 776	Scrubs that contains aluminum oxide crystals.
modelage masks MAHD-ul-ahj MASKZ	p. 779	Facial masks containing special crystals of gypsum, a plaster-like ingredient.
moisturizers	p. 777	Products that help increase the moisture content of the skin surface.
motor point	p. 783	Point on the skin over the muscle where pressure or stimulation will cause contraction of that muscle.
open comedones	p. 773	Also known as *blackheads*; follicles impacted with solidified sebum and dead cell buildup.
ostium AH-stee-um	p. 773	Follicle opening.
paraffin wax masks	p. 779	Specially prepared facial masks containing paraffin and other beneficial ingredients; typically used with treatment cream.
pétrissage PEH-treh-sahj	p. 781	Kneading movement performed by lifting, squeezing, and pressing the tissue with light, firm pressure.
rolling	p. 782	Massage movement in which the tissues are pressed and twisted using a fast back-and-forth movement.
serums SEH-rums	p. 778	Concentrated products that generally contain higher concentrations of ingredients designed to penetrate and treat various skin conditions.
slapping	p. 782	Massage movement in which the wrists are kept flexible so that the palms come in contact with the skin in light, firm, and rapid strokes, one hand after the other, causing a slight lifting of the flesh.
steamer	p. 787	A facial machine that heats and produces a stream of warm steam that can be focused on the client's face or other areas of skin.
tapotement tah-POH-te-ment	p. 782	Also known as *percussion* (pur-KUSH-un); movements consisting of short, quick tapping, slapping, and hacking movements.
toners	p. 775	Also known as *fresheners* or *astringents*; lotions that help rebalance the pH and remove remnants of cleanser from the skin.
treatment cream	p. 779	A specialty product designed to facilitate change in the skin's appearance.
vibration vy-BRAY-shun	p. 782	In massage, the rapid shaking of the body part while the balls of the fingertips are pressed firmly on the point of application.
wringing	p. 782	Vigorous movement in which the hands, placed a little distance apart on both sides of the client's arm or leg, working downward, apply a twisting motion against the bones in the opposite direction.

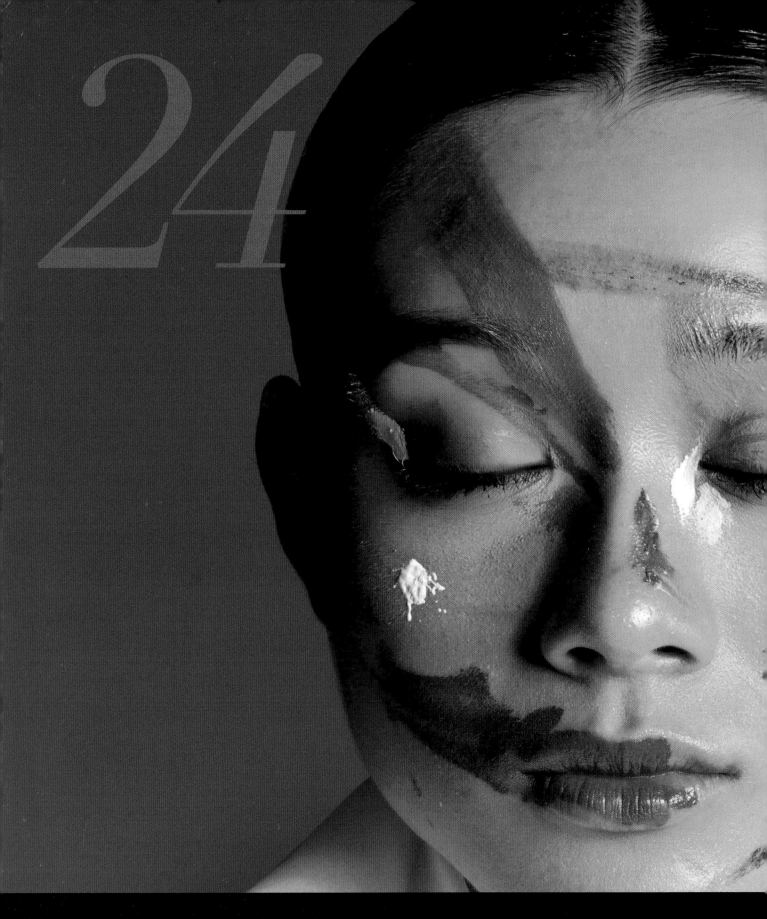

24

FACIAL MAKEUP

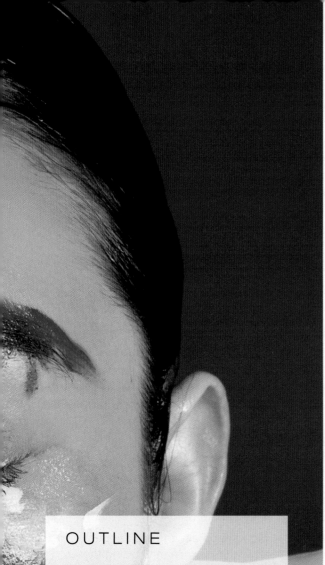

LEARNING OBJECTIVES

After completing this chapter, you will be able to:

LO❶
Describe the various types of cosmetics and their uses for facial makeup.

LO❷
Explain how to use color theory when choosing cosmetics for makeup application.

LO❸
Identify different facial types and summarize basic makeup techniques to alter them.

LO❹
Name and describe the two types of artificial eyelashes.

LO❺
List tips for creating special-occasion makeup for eyes, cheeks, and lips.

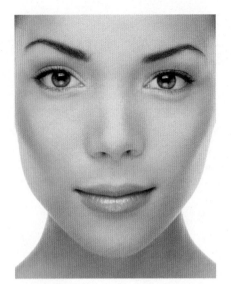

figure 24-1
Makeup enhances your clients' best
features.

The field of makeup artistry is a very rewarding segment of cosmetology. This service produces dramatic results that alter how clients view themselves. Excelling in this field requires the regular application of time-tested techniques, while keeping an eye on current trends. Makeup artists who master a wide range of application methods are able to build a loyal following of diverse clients. The makeup application techniques you employ will vary as greatly as the skin types and personalities of your clients. In the salon setting, many clients request a makeup application that enhances the best features while minimizing those that are less desirable (figure 24-1). Ultimately, the goal of effective makeup application is to enhance the client's individuality, rather than offering a 'make-over' based on some ideal standard.

© Ariwasabi/Shutterstock.com

why study
FACIAL MAKEUP?

Cosmetologists should study and have a thorough understanding of facial makeup because:

> Clients rely on you for advice on how to look their best.

> Basic makeup techniques provide the finishing touch to any hairstyling service.

> A general understanding of facial makeup formulation assists you in understanding when and on whom they should be used.

> Highlighting, contouring, and other face-shape altering techniques will help you accent your clients' best features while minimizing those that are less desirable.

After reading the next few sections, you will be able to:

LO ❶ Describe the various types of cosmetics and their uses for facial makeup.

Describe Facial Makeup and Their Uses

Foundation

Foundation, also known as *base makeup*, is a flesh-toned cosmetic used to minimize the appearance of skin imperfections. It can be used to hide hyperpigmentation (dark spots), acne, and slight birthmarks, among other issues. A makeover session usually begins with foundation application.

Several different formulations are available. The makeup artist may use liquid, stick, cream, or powder foundation; choosing the formula that best suits their client's skin type.

The foundation application process often begins with a **primer** to help disguise less than perfect skin. Some cosmetics companies market a colorless, silicone-based formula meant to simply fill in uneven surfaces of the skin. Color primers were created to actually neutralize skin discolorations (**figure 24-2**). They are available in a variety of shades: green, lavender, and orange-to-peach are the most popular. Green primer helps hide redness in the skin color, lavender is used to reduce a sallow (yellowish) skin appearance, and an orange-to-peach primer cancels out the deep blue in dark spots and discoloration under the eyes.

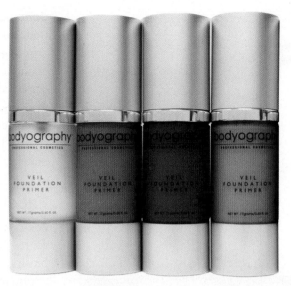

figure 24-2
Color primers neutralize discoloration.

Foundation Chemistry

Liquid and cream forms of makeup are an emulsion of oil and water. These ingredients act as spreading agents and help suspend various *pigments* like titanium dioxide and iron oxides. These pigments are all derived from a natural, mineral source. Liquid foundation is primarily water but often contains an emollient such as an oil or a silicone such as dimethicone. Manufacturers also incorporate emulsifying agents to bind the oil, water, and pigments together. These foundations are either considered to be *water-based*, meaning water in oil, or *oil-based*, meaning oil in water. Often a foundation will contain aluminum or some other drying agent to help the product set quickly when applied to the skin to produce a **matte**, non-shiny finish (**figure 24-3**).

Some liquid foundations are marketed as being oil-free. These are usually intended for oilier skin types. Be sure to check the ingredient deck to ensure the product can be considered **noncomedogenic**, meaning it does not contain ingredients that will clog the follicles, aggravating acne-prone skin.

Cream foundation, also known as *oil-based foundation*, is considerably thicker than a liquid. The thicker the product, the less water it contains. Cream foundations provide heavier coverage and are usually intended for drier, more mature skin types.

All types of foundation offer some form of sun-blocking agent. Even if they do not contain a chemical sunscreen, the pigments alone offer some degree of sun protection.

Mineral makeup is a popular choice in many salons and spas. While there are several liquid mineral lines, this term is most commonly used to describe a highly pigmented powder foundation. The formulations mix binders and flow agents with pigments to provide natural-looking coverage. Powder mineral makeup is usually applied with a large, fluffy brush called a Kabuki brush. When minerals are applied properly, they feel weightless on the skin. Mineral formulations omit questionable ingredients and are popular for clients with acne, rosacea, allergies, or sensitive skin.

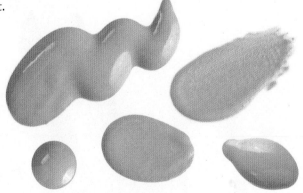

figure 24-3
Foundation

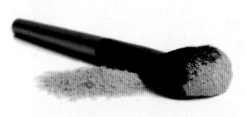

figure 24-4
Loose powder

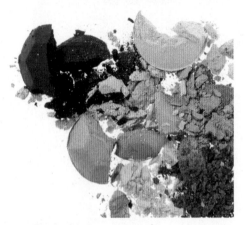

figure 24-5
Eye shadows

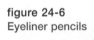

figure 24-6
Eyeliner pencils

© Kubais/Shutterstock.com

© Africa Studio/Shutterstock.com

Concealers

Concealers are used to hide dark eye circles, hyperpigmentation, distended capillaries, and other imperfections. They contain a high concentration of pigment so as to provide greater coverage than foundation. Concealers are packaged in sticks, pencils, tins, jars, or tubes with wands. They are either silicone-based for self-setting light coverage, or oil-based creams for greater coverage. Some of them contain anti-acne ingredients like salicylic acid to control blemishes. Today's concealers are available in a wide range of skin-matching shades.

Face Powders

Face powder is used to create a matte or non-shiny finish. It is used to set the foundation, making it easier to apply other powders, such as blush or bronzer. Face powder is usually a mixture of pigments with talc, cornstarch, or silica and comes in two forms: loose and pressed (**figure 24-4**). Loose powder is easily applied and is best used for setting foundation. Pressed powder is blended with binding agents such as zinc stearate to help it adhere to the skin. This formula is most commonly reserved as the final layer of powder and is perfect for touch-ups. Face powder is often reapplied throughout the day to absorb excess sebum and reduce the shine of oily skin. Powders containing very little pigment are called *translucent*. They are intended to mattify (reduce shine by absorbing oiliness) without adding color. If a colored powder is used, it should match the natural skin tone.

Eye Shadow

Eye shadows are cosmetics used to accentuate the eye shape and compliment eye color. They are available in almost every color of the rainbow, from warm to cool, neutral to bright, and light to dark. Eye shadow is available in cream as well as pressed and loose powder form (**figure 24-5**). They also come in a variety of finishes, including metallic, matte, frost, or shimmer.

Eyeliners

An **eyeliner** is a cosmetic used to define the eyes and make the lash line appear fuller (**figure 24-6**). It is available in pencil, liquid, pressed (cake), gel, or felt-tip pen form and comes in a variety of colors.

Eyeliner pencils consist of a wax (paraffin) or hardened oil base (petrolatum) with a variety of additives to create color. Eyeliner pencils are available in both soft and hard forms for use on the upper and lower eyelids.

Eyebrow Color

Eyebrow pencils, and **eyebrow powders**, are used to add color and shape to the eyebrows. They can be used to darken the eyebrows, correct their shape, or fill in sparse areas. Brow powders are similar to pressed eye shadows and are applied to the brows with a brush. Brow powders cling to eyebrow hairs, making the brows appear darker and fuller.

The chemistry of eyebrow pencils is similar to that of eyeliner pencils. The chemical ingredients in eyebrow powders are similar to those in eye shadows.

Cheek Color

Cheek color, also known as *blush*, is used primarily to add color to the cheeks. Bronzer, another form of cheek color, is often added to give definition and a warm glow. These products come in powder, liquid, gel, and cream forms (**figure 24-7**).

Makeup artists have traditionally used powder blushes; however, cream and gel cheek colors lend a sheer, natural-looking glow. Powder blushes are applied after the foundation and powder have been applied. Creams, liquids, and gels are layered over, and then blended into, the foundation.

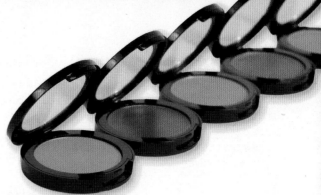

figure 24-7
Powder blush

Lip Color

Lip color, also known as *lipstick* or *lip gloss*, is a waxy cosmetic used to enhance the lips. Lip color is available in a wide variety of colors (**figure 24-8**). Many of them contain skin-friendly ingredients like moisturizers to hydrate the lips or sunscreen to protect against exposure to ultraviolet light.

Lip color is available in many forms, including creams, glosses, pencils, gels, and sticks. These products are a mixture of oils, waxes, and pigments known as lakes or color dyes.

Properly selecting lipstick color takes talent and an understanding of color theory. The lip color must complement the client's hair and eye color as well as current fashion trends. However, classic colors are timeless and therefore never go out of style.

Lip liner is generally applied before the lip color to define the shape of the lips and keep color from bleeding. Lip liners are colored pencils that are available in a variety of sizes. To ensure proper infection control procedures are followed, sharpen the pencil before application, and clean it after each use. Remember to clean and then disinfect your sharpener also!

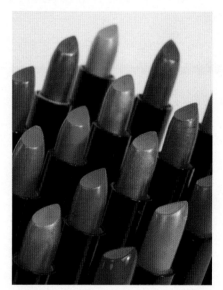

figure 24-8
Lipstick colors

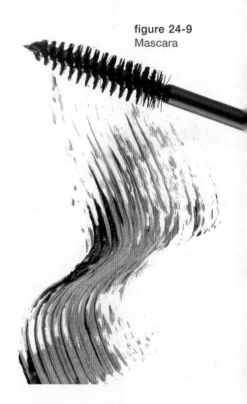

figure 24-9
Mascara

Mascara

Mascara is a cosmetic preparation used to darken, define, and thicken the eyelashes. It is available in liquid, cake, and cream form and in a variety of shades and tints (**figure 24-9**). High-performance mascaras contain rayon

> ### FOCUS ON
> **Retailing**
>
> Lip colors present a huge opportunity for retail. Think of how many lipsticks you own. Most women own several lipsticks, glosses, and pencils. Some carry several at a time in their purses. Suggest a few colors to a client in a variety of finishes. Lip color is a simple way to change a look, and it proves a great way for your client to give herself a treat and brighten her day.

or nylon fibers to lengthen and thicken the hair fibers. Mascara brushes can be straight or curved, with fine or thick bristles. The most popular mascara colors mimic eyelash color in shades of brown and black.

Mascara is a polymer product that is formulated with water, wax, thickeners, film formers, and preservatives. The pigments most commonly used in mascara are carbon black and iron oxides.

Other Cosmetics

Eye makeup removers are special preparations for removing eye makeup. Cleansers are not very effective at removing water-resistant eye makeup. Eye makeup removers are either water-based or oil-based. Water-based removers are comprised of a solution to which other solvents have been added. These types of products are great for correcting little errors during the makeup application process. Oil-based removers are generally used to remove heavy, dramatic makeup and break down the latex glue used to apply false eyelashes.

Greasepaint is a heavy makeup primarily used for theatrical purposes because it does not shift during performances. **Cake makeup**, also known as *pancake makeup*, is a heavy-coverage pressed powder that is applied to the face with a moistened cosmetic sponge. Outside of the theatre setting, these types of products are most commonly used to cover scars and uneven pigmentation.

Makeup Brushes and Other Tools

Makeup brushes come in a variety of shapes and sizes. They are made of synthetic fibers or animal hair.

A makeup brush is divided into three parts: the hair, the ferrule, and the handle (**figure 24-10**). Each part affects the quality, efficacy, and lifespan of the brush.

- *Hair* is the term used for the bristles of makeup brushes.

- **Ferrule** is the metal part that holds the brush intact and supports the strength of the bristles. Look for double crimping, or a ring, around the ferrule to ensure the handle won't loosen.

- The *handle* comes in a wide range of lengths and can be made of wood, acrylic, plastic, or metal.

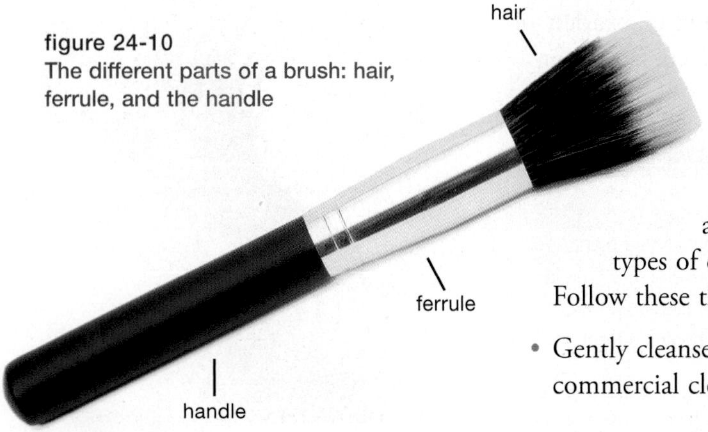

figure 24-10
The different parts of a brush: hair, ferrule, and the handle

hair

ferrule

handle

Caring for Makeup Brushes

Investing in high-quality makeup brushes will ensure they'll be around for years. Take good care of your brushes by cleaning them after each makeup application. While spray-on cleaners can be used to quickly clean brushes, they contain a high level of alcohol and are not recommended for daily use. These types of cleansers dry out brushes over time.

Follow these tips to care for your makeup brushes:

- Gently cleanse brushes with an antibacterial detergent followed by a commercial cleaning solution.

table 24-1

COMMONLY USED MAKEUP BRUSHES AND TOOLS

Standard Brush or Tool	Type of Brush or Tool	Description and Use
	Powder brush	Large, soft brush used to apply powder.
	Blush brush	Smaller, more tapered version of the powder brush; excellent for applying powder cheek color.
	Concealer brush	Usually narrow, firm synthetic brush with a flat edge; used to apply concealer around the eyes and over blemishes
	Lip brush	Similar to the concealer brush, with a more tapered edge.
	Eye shadow brush	Available in a variety of sizes and shapes. The softer and larger the brush, the more diffused the shadow will be. Firm eye shadow brushes are best for depositing a dense layer of color.
	Eyeliner brush	Fine, tapered, firm bristles; used to apply liquid liner or shadow to the lash line.
	Angle brush	Firm, thin bristles; used to apply powder to the eyebrows or eye liner at the lash line.
	Lash comb	Tiny, thin plastic or metal teeth separate eyelashes after mascara application.
	Brow brush (spoolie)	Used to apply mascara to the lashes or brush brows into place.
	Tweezers	Used to groom eyebrows, remove excess facial hair, and apply false eyelashes.
	Eyelash curler	A device used to give lift and curl the upper eyelashes.
	Pencil sharpener	Used before each application of eye or lip liner pencil to ensure ease of application and hygiene.

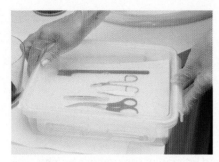

figure 24-11
Store clean, disinfected tools and
implements in a covered container.

- Rinse brushes thoroughly after cleansing.

- Reshape the wet bristles and lay the brushes flat to dry.

- Lay brushes flat on a clean towel until dry and then store them in a clean, closed covered container (figure 24-11).

On a cautionary note: Brushes should always be held under running water with the ferrule (the metal ring that keeps bristles and handle together) pointing downward. If the brush is pointed up, the water may weaken the glue that keeps the bristles in place.

Single-Use Implements

Single-use implements are disposable and should be discarded after <u>one use</u>. These supplies offer clean application every time and prevent the spread of infection. Single use implements include the following items:

Sponges. Available in a variety of sizes and shapes, including wedges and circles, and work well to apply and blend foundation, cream or powder blush, pressed powder, or concealer.

Powder puffs. May be made of velour or cotton and are used to apply and blend powder, powder foundation, or powder blush.

Mascara wands. Used to apply mascara on a client; generally disposable, so as to ensure proper hygiene.

Spatulas. A tool with a wide, flat base; used to remove makeup from containers.

Disposable lip brushes. Used to hygienically apply lip color.

Sponge-tipped shadow applicators. Used to apply shadow and lip color or to blend eyeliner; may be used damp to intensify eye shadow color.

Cotton swabs. May be used to apply shadow, blend eyeliner, apply lip balm, or to correct application mistakes.

Cotton pads or puffs. May be used with toner or makeup removers.

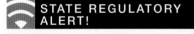
STATE REGULATORY ALERT!

Regulations for cleaning brushes vary from state to state, so check with your regulatory agency.

FOCUS ON
Infection Control for Makeup Application

It is your professional responsibility to prevent the spread of infection. Follow these tips for makeup application to protect your and your client:

- Scrape powders with clean brushes or spatulas onto a clean tissue or tray.
- Do not apply lipstick or gloss directly to the lips from the container or tube. Use a spatula to remove the product, and then apply with a clean brush or disposable applicator.
- Sharpen eye pencils before and after each use on every client.
- While applying eye makeup, sharpen the eye pencil after you finish the client's first eye, before beginning the second eye.

- Properly cleanse hands, multi-use utensils, chairs, and counters between clients with an EPA-approved disinfectant.
- Dispose of any product that you suspect may be contaminated.
- Gracefully refuse to perform a makeup service on any client with a suspected eye infection, or any other possible infection on the face.

After reading the next few sections, you will be able to:

LO ❷ Explain how to use color theory when choosing cosmetics for makeup application.

How to Use Color Theory for Makeup Application

A thorough understanding of color is imperative to becoming an effective makeup artist. Those new to makeup should definitely utilize the color wheel as a guide to makeup application (**figure 24-12**). With practice, you will learn to effortlessly interpret which hues are primary, secondary, and tertiary colors. Professional makeup artists also learn to determine the best selection for their clients by visually grouping products into warm and cool colors. The basics of color theory are discussed in greater detail in Chapter 21, Haircoloring.

Warm and Cool Colors

Warm and cool colors form the basis of all makeup application. Understanding the difference between these two color temperatures enables you to select the proper shade for your client's unique coloring.

As you look at the color wheel, think of it as a tool in determining color choice. There are three main factors to consider when choosing colors for a client:

1. Skin color

2. Eye color

3. Hair color

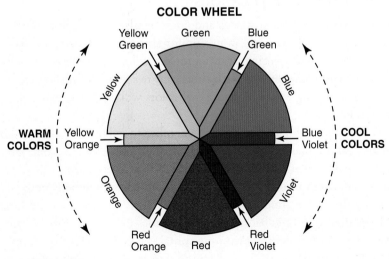

figure 24-12
Color wheel

table 24-2

SKIN COLORS AND TONES

Skin Tones	Skin Colors	
	Warm	Cool
Fair	Yellow, gold, pale peach	Pink or slightly red (ruddy)
Medium	Yellow, yellow-orange, red	Olive (yellow-green)
Deep	Red, orange-brown, red-brown	Dark olive, blue, blue-black

Determining Skin Color

When determining skin color, you must first decide if the skin is fair, medium, or deep. Then determine whether the tone of the skin is warm or cool (use **table 24-2** as a guide). You may not accurately interpret skin tones in the beginning. However with time and practice you will begin to develop this skill.

- **Warm colors** range from yellow and gold to orange, red-orange, most reds, and even some yellow-greens.

- **Cool colors** encompass blues, greens, violets, and blue-reds. You will notice that reds can be both warm and cool. If the red is orange-based, it is warm. If it is blue-based, it is cool. Green is similar: if a green contains more yellow, it is interpreted as being warm; if it contains more blue, it is cool.

You may have heard people refer to a color as having a lot of blue in it. This does not mean that the color is a true blue. Rather, it means that a blue pigment was mixed to create that cosmetic formula. For example deep red lipsticks are manufactured with a blue base.

Selecting Makeup Colors

Now that we have defined warms and cools, it is time to explore the system that will help you feel more comfortable when choosing colors for your clients. To start, pairing warm and cool colors is not recommended. The colors will compete with each other and result in an unbalanced appearance. Staying within one range of colors will ensure a balanced, beautiful look.

When applying makeup, always remember to analyze the client's skin type and choose makeup that will enhance their skin tone, eye and hair color, as well as their features. Keep in mind that, even within this very strategic approach to choosing colors, there are several methods of achieving the desired result.

Regardless of ethnic background, skin varies in color and tone from person to person. A neutral skin tone contains equal elements of warm and cool, no matter how fair or deep the skin is. Remember to always match your foundation color to your client's skin tone, or use the sculpting techniques discussed later in this chapter.

Once you have determined if the skin is fair, medium, or deep, you may choose eye, cheek, and lip products. Select colors to match the skin tone in level, or try to contrast for more impact. Most skin tones are complimented by a wide range of colors. Be cautious when choosing lip, cheek, and eye colors for deep skin tones. Light or flesh-toned shades without enough blue pigment will appear gray or chalky on the skin. Look for products that are rich in pigment when choosing products for use on deep skin tones.

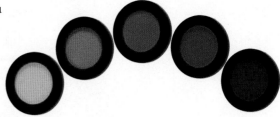
figure 24-13
Complementary colors for blue eyes

Complementary Colors for Eyes

When selecting eye, cheek, and lip colors, neutral tones are always your safest choice. They contain elements of warm and cool, plus they complement any skin tone, eye color, or hair color. Neutral colors range from taupe, to brown, and from gray to white or black. They may have a warm or cool base. For example, plum-brown, charcoal gray, and blue-gray would be considered cool neutrals. An orange-brown would be considered a warm neutral. Matching shadow color with eye color creates a monochromatic field with a less dramatic depth of contrast. Selecting eye shadows in complimentary colors will emphasize the eyes most. You may refer back to the color wheel for additional help in determining complementary eye shadow colors. Remember to coordinate cheek and lip products within the same color family, adding neutrals with warm or cool colors as desired.

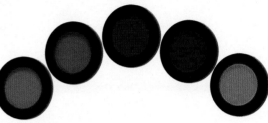
figure 24-14
Complementary colors for green eyes

Complementary color choices for eye colors are summarized below:

Complementary colors for blue eyes. Orange is the complementary color to blue. Because orange contains yellow and red, shadows with any of these colors in them will make eyes look bluer. Common choices include gold, warm orange-browns like peach and copper, red-browns like mauves and plums, and neutrals like taupe or camel (figure 24-13).

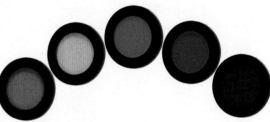
figure 24-15
Complementary colors for brown eyes

Complementary colors for green eyes. Red is the complementary color to green. Because red shadows tend to make the eyes look tired or bloodshot, pure red tones are not recommended. Instead, use brown-based reds or other color options next to red on the color wheel. These include red-orange, red-violet, and violet. Popular choices are coppers, rusts, pinks, plums, mauves, and purples (figure 24-14).

Complementary colors for brown eyes. Brown eyes are neutral and can wear any color. Recommended choices include contrasting colors such as greens, blues, grays, and silvers (figure 24-15).

Adding Cheek and Lip Color

After you have chosen eye makeup, refer to the color wheel (figure 24-12) to coordinate cheek and lip makeup in the same color family. For example, if your client has green eyes, you might recommend an eye shadow in a

table 24-3

DETERMINING HAIR COLOR TONES

Hair Colors	Determining Hair Color Tones	
	Warm	**Cool**
Blond hair	Yellow, orange	White-blond, ash
Red hair	Gold, copper, orange, red	Red-violet, violet
Brown hair	Yellow, gold, orange	Ash
Dark brown/ black hair	Copper, red	Violet, blue

cool plum shade. Select cool colors for the cheeks and lips so that they coordinate with the eye makeup. You could also choose neutrals, as these contain both warm and cool elements and coordinate with any makeup colors.

Hair Color and Eye Color

Hair color needs to be taken into account when determining eye makeup color. For example, if a woman has blue eyes, your instinct might be to select orange-based eye makeup as the complementary color of choice. However, if she has cool blue-black hair, an orange-based color will not be that flattering. In this case, you would choose cool colors that coordinate with the hair color. Looking at the color wheel, start at orange then move along the right side towards the cool end. You will find that red-violets (plums) will be the most flattering choice. As stated earlier, there is a range of colors to choose from for any client. Use **table 24-3** as a general guide.

Mature Skin

Be very careful when selecting color products for older clients who may have uneven, textured skin due to wrinkles or sun damage. Shimmer, glitter, or frosted colors can accent the dry patches or wrinkles typical of mature skin. Stick to muted, softer colors, and avoid creating hard lines (**figure 24-16**).

Expression lines and wrinkles can be minimized with a skin primer and foundation. Apply the skin primer evenly, and then apply the foundation sparingly, in a light, outward, circular motion over the entire face. Care should be taken to remove any foundation that collects in deep recesses and concave areas.

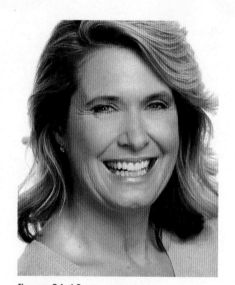

figure 24-16
Makeup for mature skin

© Kurhan/Shutterstock.com

ACTIVITY

Apply makeup to a partner, using color theory to choose and coordinate makeup colors. Have fun and experiment. While a cut and color requires a long-term commitment, makeup does not. Take pictures to track which colors enhance her appearance.

After reading the next few sections, you will be able to:

LO③ Identify different facial types and summarize basic makeup techniques to alter them.

Alter Face Shapes with Makeup

All faces are interesting in their own special ways, but no one is perfect. When you analyze a client's face, you are sure to find that some features are not symmetrical. You might see that the nose, cheeks, lips, or jawline are not the same on both sides, or that one eye is larger than the other, or that the eyebrows might not match. In fact, these tiny imbalances make the face more interesting when properly accented. Face shape altering makeup creates the illusion of nearly perfect proportions wherever desired.

Using proper highlighting and contouring techniques helps define facial features. The basic rule when altering a face shape is that drawing light to an area emphasizes features, while creating a shadow minimizes them (figure 24-17).

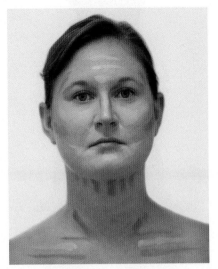
figure 24-17
Highlighting and contouring

- A **highlight** is produced when a product that is lighter than the client's skin tone is placed on the high planes of the face.

- A **contour** is formed when a product that is darker than the client's skin tone is used to create shadows over prominent features so they are less noticeable.

The types of products used to accomplish these highlighting and contouring techniques range from liquid foundation, to cream stick, to loose or pressed powder. It is not recommended that you define every facial feature, as this will tend to look too chiseled and overdone. Before you undertake these types of makeup application techniques, you should have a clear sense of how to analyze face shapes.

Analyzing Face Shape

The primary goal of makeup application is to emphasize the client's most attractive features, while minimizing those that are less appealing. Learning to objectively identify the face shapes and its features takes practice. However, this step is imperative to determining the best makeup for each individual.

Oval-Shaped Face

While all face shapes are attractive in their own way, the oval face with well-proportioned features has long been considered the ideal. The face is divided into three equal horizontal sections.

The first third is measured from the hairline to the tops of the eyebrows. The second third is measured from the tops of the eyebrows to the tip of the nose. The last third is measured from the tip of the nose to the bottom of the chin.

The oval face is approximately three-fourths as wide as it is long (figure 24-18). The ideal distance between the eyes is the width of one eye.

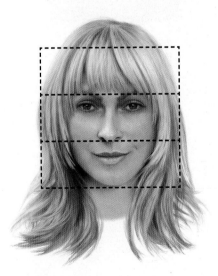
figure 24-18
The oval face can be divided into three equal, horizontal sections.

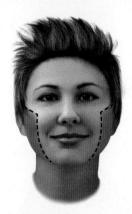

figure 24-19
Round face

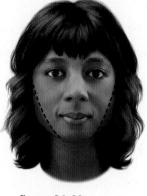

figure 24-20
Square face

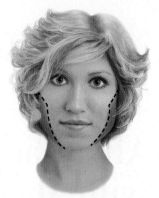

figure 24-21
Triangular face

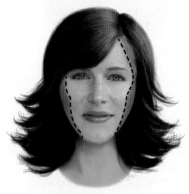

figure 24-22
Heart-shaped face

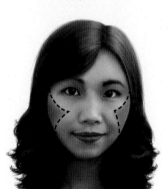

figure 24-23
Diamond-shaped face

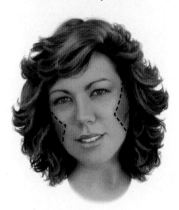

figure 24-24
Oblong face

These are the standard artistic proportions to which you will refer when practicing highlighting and contouring makeup application techniques.

Round Face

The round face is usually broader in proportion to its length than the oval face. It has a rounded chin and hairline. Makeup can be applied to slenderize and lengthen the face (figure 24-19).

Square-Shaped Face

The square face is composed of comparatively straight lines with a wide forehead and square jawline. Makeup can be applied to offset the shape by softening the hard angles of the face (figure 24-20).

Triangular Face

A triangular face is characterized by a jawline that is wider than the forehead. Makeup can be applied to create width at the forehead, slenderize the jawline, and add length to the face (figure 24-21).

Heart-Shaped Face

The heart-shaped face, or inverted triangle has a wide forehead and narrow jawline and pointed chin. Makeup can be applied to minimize the width of the forehead and increase the width of the jawline (figure 24-22).

Diamond-Shaped Face

This face has a narrow forehead. The greatest width is across the cheekbones. A darker foundation or powder can be applied to minimize the width of the outer cheekbone (figure 24-23).

Oblong Face

This face has greater length in proportion to its width than the square or round face. It is long and narrow. Makeup can be applied along the hairline and under the cheekbones to round the forehead and create the illusion of wider cheekbones, making the face appear shorter (figure 24-24).

Altering the Forehead Area

For a low forehead, applying a lighter foundation just above the brows broadens the appearance. For a protruding forehead, applying a darker foundation over the prominent area minimizes the forehead. A suitable hairstyle also goes a long way toward drawing attention away from the forehead (figure 24-25).

Altering the Nose and Chin Areas

For a large or protruding nose, apply a darker foundation along the sides of the nose. This will create a shadow, making the nose appear smaller. Avoid placing cheek color close to the nose.

For a small, flat nose, apply a lighter foundation down the center of the nose, ending at the tip. This will make the nose appear longer. If the nostrils are wide, apply a darker foundation to both sides of the nostrils (figure 24-26).

For a broad nose, use a darker foundation along the sides of the nose and nostrils. Avoid blending this dark tone into the laugh lines. The foundation must be carefully blended (figure 24-27).

To balance a protruding chin and receding nose, shadow the tip of the chin with a darker foundation and highlight the bridge of the nose with a lighter foundation. For a receding chin, highlight the chin by using a lighter foundation than the one used on the face.

For a sagging double chin, use a darker foundation on the sagging portion, and use a natural skin tone foundation on the face (figure 24-28).

Altering the Jawline

The neck and jaw often need additional attention. Clients with a fuller build as well as more mature clients may have what's known as sagging jowls. To contour this area, blend the foundation onto the neck so that the client's skin color is consistent. Then apply a darker shade of foundation over the fullest area of the jaw. This will minimize the lower part of the face (figure 24-29).

To correct a narrow jawline, highlight the thinnest areas with a lighter shade of foundation (figure 24-30). Always set with a translucent powder to avoid transfer onto the client's clothing.

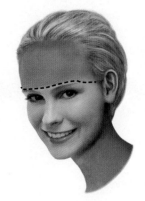

figure 24-25
Placement of corrective makeup for a protruding forehead

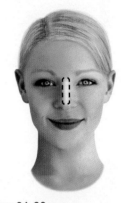

figure 24-26
Placement of corrective makeup for a small, flat nose

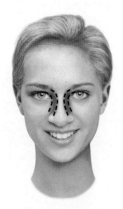

figure 24-27
Placement of corrective makeup for a broad nose

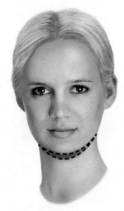

figure 24-28
Placement of corrective makeup for a double chin

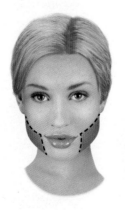

figure 24-29
Placement of corrective makeup for a broad jawline

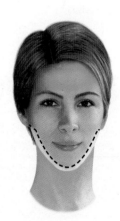

figure 24-30
Placement of corrective makeup for a narrow jawline

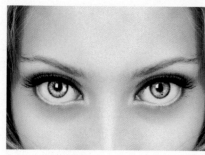

figure 24-31
Round eyes

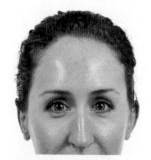

figure 24-32
Close-set eyes

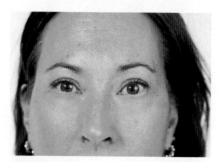

figure 24-33
Hooded eyelids

Altering Eye Shape

The application of eye color can enlarge or minimize certain aspects of the eyes. Learning to implement the proper eye shadow application techniques will enhance the client's overall attractiveness.

Round eyes. This eye shape can be lengthened by extending the shadow beyond the outer corners of the eyes (figure 24-31).

Close-set eyes. If the distance between the eyes is less than the width of one eye, they are too close together. To create space, apply a thin layer of light concealer to the inner corners of the eyes, near the bridge of the nose (figure 24-32).

Protruding or bulging eyes. This can be minimized by blending the deeper color shadow over the prominent part of the upper lid. Blend the color from the outer corners inward towards the center, carrying it just past the creases.

Hooded eyelids (ptosis). Lift the lid at the brow to reveal the natural contours. Holding the lid, apply a slightly deeper shadow through the crease. Blend with a clean brush to minimize any hard lines and create a natural look (figure 24-33).

Small eyes. To make small eyes appear larger, extend the lightest shadow slightly above the upper lash line (figure 24-34).

Wide-set eyes. Apply the shadow from the inner corners of the eyebrows towards the nose, and blend carefully (figure 24-35).

Deep-set eyes. Use bright, light, reflective colors. Create a wash of color across the lid. Use a light-to-medium color along the lash line and outer corners of the eyes (figure 24-36).

Dark circles under eyes. Apply a color correcting concealer over the area to neutralize discoloration. Blend and smooth the product into the surrounding area. Set lightly with translucent powder.

Altering Eyebrows

Reshaping and defining eyebrows is an art unto itself. Well-groomed eyebrows are part of a complete and effective makeup application. If

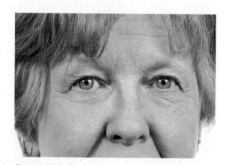

figure 24-34
Small eyes

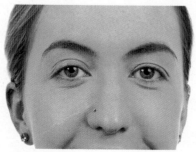

figure 24-35
Wide-set eyes

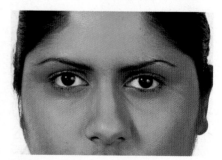

figure 24-36
Deep-set eyes

the eyes are the window to the soul, the eyebrows are the window frame. While brow shape is often dictated by fashion trends, it is ultimately a complete expression of personal style. Thicker brows are seen as being more natural. Thinner brows require more maintenance. Overgrown eyebrows can camouflage the brow bone. Over-tweezed eyebrows can make the face look puffy or protruding, or may give the eyes a surprised look.

When a client wants to learn how to balance their eyebrow shape, begin by removing all unnecessary hairs, then demonstrate how to complete them. When there are spaces between the eyebrow hairs, fill them in with hair-like strokes of an eyebrow pencil or a shadow applied with an angled brush. Brush through the brows with a spoolie or disposable mascara wand to soften the eyebrow color.

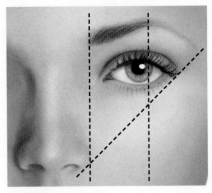

figure 24-37
Ideal brow shape

The ideal eyebrow shape is positioned along three lines (figure 24-37). The client should look straight ahead as you determine each line. The first line runs vertically, from the inner corner of the eye upward. This is where the eyebrow should begin. The second line runs from the outer circle of the iris upward. This is where the highest part of the arch should be. The third line is drawn at an angle from the outer corner of the nose to the outer corner of the eye. This is where the eyebrow should end. Of course, not everyone's eyebrows fit exactly within these measurements. Use them as guidelines to design the ideal brow.

When the arch is too high, remove the superfluous hair from the top of the brow and fill in the lower part with an eyebrow pencil or shadow. Build up the shape by layering color lightly until the desired effect is achieved.

Adjustments to eyebrow shape can also be used to balance the facial features listed below:

Low forehead. A low arch gives more height to a very low forehead.

Wide-set eyes. The eyes can be made to appear closer together by building up the inside corners of the eyebrows. Care must be taken to avoid giving the client a frowning look.

Close-set eyes. To make the eyes appear farther apart, widen the distance between the eyebrows and slightly extend them outward.

Round face. Arch the brows high to make the face appear narrower. Start on a line directly above the inside corner of the eye and extend to the end of the cheekbone.

Long face. Making the eyebrows almost straight can create the illusion of a shorter face. Do not extend the eyebrow lines farther than the outside corners of the eyes.

Square face. The face will appear more oval if there is a high arch on the ends of the eyebrows. Begin the lines directly above the corners of the eyes and extend them outward.

Eyelash Enhancers

There are now treatments available to enhance the eyelashes. Cosmetic lash enhancers are lash lengtheners that contain fibers to make lashes look longer and fuller. Some of these are built into mascaras and some are available as a separate product. Another similar type of product uses a clear polymer to make lashes look thicker.

A prescription drug has now been approved for enhancing lash growth and thickness. Latisse® contains an active drug ingredient called bimatoprost. The drug is applied to the base of the lashes. Most patients using Latisse® see a difference in their lash growth, fullness, and darkness after two to four months of regular use. Latisse® is only available through physicians.

The Lips

Lips can be full, or thin, and are usually uneven. They should be positioned so that the Cupid's bow, the peaks of the upper lip, fall directly in line with the nostrils. In some cases, one side of the lips may be fuller than the other. Table 24-4 illustrates how color can be used on various lip shapes to create the illusion of better proportions.

Skin Tones

For whatever reason, your client may wish to alter their skin tone. This is usually in an attempt to correct ruddy (red) or sallow (yellow) skin.

- For *ruddy skin* (skin that is sensitive, wind-burned, or affected by rosacea), apply a green color corrector or color correcting primer to affected areas, blending carefully. You may then apply a light layer of foundation with a warm, yellow tone to balance the complexion. Set it with translucent powder. Avoid red or pink blush.

- For *sallow skin* (skin that has a yellowish hue), apply a pink-based foundation on the affected areas and blend carefully into the jaw and neck. Set with translucent powder. Avoid yellow-based colors for eyes, cheeks, and lips.

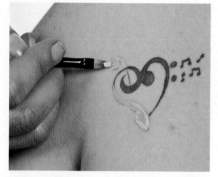

figure 24-38a
Camouflaging covers a tattoo.

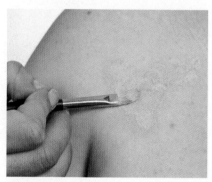

figure 24-38b

Camouflaging Techniques

Camouflaging is a corrective makeup technique used to conceal scars, burns, and pigmentation issues ranging from vitiligo to tattoos (figures 24-38a and 24-38b). These products are available in cream, paste, liquid, and powder. While camouflaging can be achieved with an airbrush, the more common technique involves applying alternating layers of products until the condition is concealed. This form of makeup application is a fairly advanced technique that requires a great deal of practice to master.

Outline the Steps for Basic Makeup Application

Basic makeup application is a step-by-step procedure to enhance your client's features. To accurately interpret their beauty concerns, each session

table 24-4

LIP SHAPES

Lip shape	Corrective Techniques
Thin lower lip	Line just outside the lower lip to make it appear fuller. Fill in with lip color to create balance between the lower and upper lips.
Thin upper lip	Use a liner to outline the upper lip and than fill in with lip color to balance with the lower lip.
Thin upper and lower lips	Outline the upper and lower lips slightly fuller, but do not try to draw for over the natural lip line. Use a lighter color to make lips appear larger.
Cupid bow or pointed upper lip	To soften the peaks of the upper lip, use a natural-color liner to draw a softer curve inside the points. Extend the line to the desired shape. Fill in with lip color.
Large, full lips	Draw a thin line just inside the natural lip line. Use soft, flat lipstick colors that will attract loss attention than frosty or glossy lip colors.
Small mouth and lips	Outline both the upper and lower lips. Fill in lips with soft or frosted colors to make them appear larger.
Drooping corners	Line the lips to build up the corners the mouth. This will minimize the drooping appearance. Fill in lips with the soft color.
Uneven lips	Outline the upper and lower lips with a soft color to create the illusion of matching proportions.
Straight upper lip	Use liner to create a slight dip in the Cupid's bow, directly beneath the nostrils. Fill in with a flattering color.
Fine lines around the lips	Outline the lips with a long-wearing lip pencil, and then fill in with an extended wear lip color to keep lip color from running into fine lines. Lighter colors work better and do not show the lines as much as dark or red colors do.

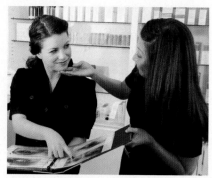

figure 24-39
A client consultation is the first step in gathering pertinent information about the client.

Using a model (or yourself) and two different color applications, divide the face in half. Try different foundations, colors, and intensity on each side. This will give you a visual example of how makeup will work on a face. Actually applying makeup is the best way to learn how to use it.

ACTIVITY

Using a model (or yourself) and two different color applications, divide the face in half. Try different foundations, colors, and intensity on each side. This will give you a visual example of how makeup will work on a face. Actually applying makeup is the best way to learn how to use it.

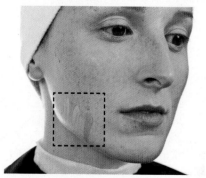

figure 24-40
Apply foundation directly on the jawline to see which color matches.

must start with a consultation. You'll find that lighting affects how well you execute the procedure. Basic makeup is subtle and should look fairly natural in daylight. Select one area as your focal point. Lips, cheeks and eyes should never have to fight for attention.

P 24-1 **Basic Professional Makeup Application** *See page 823*

Client Consultation

As with all other services that take place in the salon, the client consultation is the first step in the makeup application process (figure 24-39). Gather pertinent information about the client, including skin condition, and make note of any skin sensitivities. Listen closely to the client's responses when you ask questions such as: What are your beauty concerns? What is your current makeup regimen? How much time do you spend applying makeup each day? What are your favorite colors? What would you change, if anything, about your current makeup look? This is also the perfect time to assess sensitivity due to contact lenses or allergies. Record this information on a service record card.

After completing the makeup service, fill out and review an instruction sheet for your client to take home. This will remind them of the application techniques, color selection, and product brands to purchase at a later time.

Lighting

Adequate and flattering lighting is essential for both the consultation and the application portions of the makeup process. Be sure your client's face is evenly lit without dark shadows caused by overhead lighting. Daylight is the best choice. If it is necessary to use artificial lighting, a combination of incandescent light (warm bulb light) and fluorescent light (cool industrial tube light) is conducive. If you must choose between the two, incandescent light will be more flattering.

Make sure that the light always shines directly and evenly on the face. And remember, good lighting makes a client look good, and clients who look good are more likely to purchase the products you recommend. When this happens, everyone comes out a winner.

Apply Foundation

Choosing the correct color of foundation is the first step in the application process. The foundation should be as close to the client's natural skin tone as possible. To choose the correct foundation, have the client sit in a well-lit area. Use a cotton swab to apply a small amount of three different skin-matching shades to the jawline (figure 24-40). The color that seems to disappear is the right choice. It is important that the color balances the difference between the skin on the face and neck. If the color of the foundation is too light, it will look dull and chalky. If the color is too dark, it will look muddy and uneven.

After choosing the correct color, use a spatula to remove the makeup from its container. Place the foundation on a palette to avoid contaminating the container. Use a sponge, your finger tips, or a brush to blend the foundation from the center of the face outward, using short downward strokes. There should be no obvious **line of demarcation** (LYN UV dee-mar-KAY-shun) where foundation begins and ends.

- **Cream** foundation is usually applied to the sponge and then blended across the skin.

- **Liquid** foundation is often applied to the skin in small dots across the face and then quickly blended with a sponge or foundation brush.

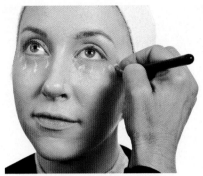

figure 24-41
Apply concealer one shade lighter beneath the eyes using a concealer brush.

Apply Concealer

Select the appropriate type and color of concealer. Be sure that it is no more than two shades lighter than your client's skin. Use a clean spatula to scrape some of the product onto a palette. Using a concealer brush, apply the product over the area that needs concealer. Blend by tapping with the ring finger or sponge. Under the eyes, focus on concealing concave areas and discoloration (**figure 24-41**). When hiding a blemish, avoid applying a color lighter than your client's skin tone as this will draw attention to the area being concealed.

A concealer may be worn alone, without foundation, if chosen and blended correctly. Be sure to use it sparingly and soften the edges so that the complexion looks like clear, even skin rather than a heavy makeup application.

Apply Powder

Apply loose powder with a large powder brush or a disposable powder puff. Remove some loose powder from the container and place it in a disposable cup or tissue. Dip the brush in the powder and fluff it across the face. Make sure all areas of the face are covered, and remove any excess powder (**figure 24-42**). You can also use a disposable cotton ball to apply loose powder.

Powder can also be used to brush out hard edges from blush or eye shadow application. Powder should never look caked, streaked, or blotchy after application.

Pressed powder in compacts is marketed primarily for touch-ups because it can easily be carried in a purse. These products normally come with a powder-puff applicator, which should never be used in the salon because they cannot be easily cleaned and then disinfected.

> **? DID YOU KNOW?**
> Concealer can also be applied with a sponge or cotton swab, but using a synthetic concealer brush produces the most natural result.

Apply Eyebrow Pencil

Sharpen the eyebrow pencil and wipe with clean tissue before each use. Clean the sharpener before each use. Apply the brow color to the brows using short, hair-like strokes. Avoid harsh contrasts between hair and eyebrow color, such as pale blond or silver hair with black eyebrows.

Apply Eyebrow Powder

Scrape powder from the container onto a palette or tissue then, using a clean, angle brush, fill in brows with the same techniques used when

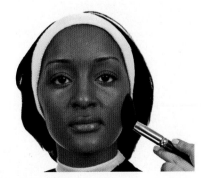

figure 24-42
Apply loose powder with a powder brush to set the foundation.

applying pencil. Many eyebrow kits partner powders with an eyebrow wax to keep hairs in place.

Apply Eye Shadow

When applied to the lids, eye color or shadow makes the eyes appear brighter and more expressive. Selecting colors other than the actual eye color (i.e., a contrasting or complementary color) can enhance the eyes. Accenting natural highlights and contours will also bring more attention to the eyes. Matching eye shadow to eye color creates a flat field of color and should generally be avoided. The only set rules for eye makeup colors are that the chosen colors should enhance the client's eyes. If desired, eye makeup color may be coordinated with the client's clothing. Eye shadow colors are generally referred to as highlight, base, and contour colors.

A *highlight color* is lighter than the client's skin tone and may have a matte or iridescent finish. As the name suggests, highlight colors accent specific areas, such as the brow bone, by making it appear lighter/more prominent.

A *base color* is generally a medium shade that is close to the client's skin tone. It is available in a variety of finishes. The base color is usually applied across the lid, then blended into the crease.

A *contour color* is darker than the client's skin tone. It is applied to minimize unwanted fullness/puffiness, contour the crease, or define the lash line.

Apply Powder Eye Shadow

To apply powder eye shadow, scrape the product onto a palette or tissue with a spatula, and then use an applicator or clean brush. Unless you are altering the shape of the eye, simply apply the color close to the lashes of the upper eyelid, sweeping the color slightly upward and outward. Blend to achieve the desired effect. Many colors can be blended together to achieve a particular effect.

Apply Cream Eye Shadow

To apply cream eye shadow, remove cream shadow with a spatula. Using your ring finger, dab color onto the center of the lid. Smudge a bit with your finger, then use a clean brush to blend upward and outward until you achieve the desired shape. If the cream shadow is not waterproof, you'll need to set the color with powder.

Apply Eyeliners

Most clients prefer eyeliner that is the same color as the lashes or the same color as the mascara for a more natural look. More vibrant colors may be chosen depending on seasonal trends.

Be extremely cautious when applying eyeliner. You must have a steady hand and be sure that your client remains still. Sharpen the eyeliner pencil and wipe it clean before each use to minimize the chance of cross contamination. Remember to also clean the sharpener before each use. Apply to the desired area with short strokes and gentle pressure; the most common placement is close to the lash line (figure 24-43). To use powder shadow as eyeliner, scrape a small amount onto a tissue and apply to the eyes with a clean angle brush. If desired, wet the brush before the application for a more dramatic look.

Apply Blush

After foundation and face powder have been applied, use a clean blush brush to apply color to the cheeks. For a fresh look, color can be applied to the apples of the cheeks, blending outward towards the temples. Never apply blush in a solid circle on the apple of the cheek, beyond the corner of the eye, or blended inward between the cheekbone and the nose. Sweeping blush just below the cheekbones will result in a more chiseled, sophisticated look. Cream and gel blush result in a sheer finish that simulates naturally flushed cheeks. Cream blush is applied before powder so that it blends into the foundation. The application should look soft and natural. It should look as if it fades into the foundation. It is better to apply too little blush than too much. You can always add more if necessary.

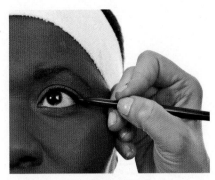

figure 24-43
Apply eyeliner across the eyelid.

Apply Lip Color

Properly applied color should be even and symmetrical on both sides of the mouth. Start by selecting a lip pencil that coordinates well with the chosen lipstick. The liner color should either match the shade of the natural lip or the lipstick. Beginning at the outer corner of the upper lip and working toward the middle, trace the natural lip line. Repeat on the opposite side. Connect the center peaks with rounded strokes, following the natural lip line. Outline the lower lip from the outer corners inwards.

After lining the lips, remove the lip color with a spatula. Resting your ring finger on the client's chin to steady your hand, apply the lip color with a clean brush (figure 24-44). Begin by applying color at the outer corners and work toward the middle of the top lip. Repeat on the opposite side. Then, using the same technique, fill in the bottom lip. Be sure to use rounded strokes when connecting the center peaks known as Cupid's bow. Ask the client to relax her lips and part them slightly. Then ask the client to smile slightly so that you can fill in the corners. Never double dip!

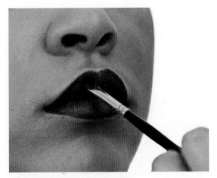

figure 24-44
Using a lip brush to apply lipstick

Apply Mascara

If you are using an eyelash curler, you must curl the lashes before applying mascara. If lashes are curled after mascara, they may break or be pulled out. Use extreme caution whenever using an eyelash curler. Start by crimping at the base of the lash line then continue crimping outward towards the tip. Apply mascara so that it coats even the tiniest hairs at the inner and outer corners of the eyes. Practice mascara application techniques until you feel confident enough to apply it on a client.

Mascara may be used on all lashes, both top and bottom. Using a disposable wand, dip into a clean tube of mascara and apply from the base of the lashes out toward the tips, making sure your client is comfortable throughout the application (figure 24-45). Dispose of the wand, select a new one, and then apply mascara to the other eye. Never double dip!

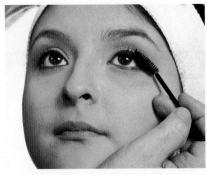

figure 24-45
Apply mascara with a zig-zag motion.

After reading the next few sections, you will be able to:

LO ④   Name and describe the two types of artificial eyelashes.

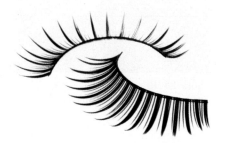

figure 24-46
Strip lashes

Apply Artificial Eyelashes

The use of artificial eyelashes has grown enormously, mainly because the technology has improved dramatically and fashion has become more reliant on these accessories. Clients with sparse lashes and those who wish to enhance their eyes for special occasions are most likely to request this service. The objective is to make the client's own lashes look fuller, longer, and more attractive without appearing unnatural.

Two types of artificial eyelashes are commonly used.

- **Strip lashes** are eyelash hairs on a band that are applied with adhesive to the natural lash line (**figure 24-46**).

- **Individual lashes** are separate artificial eyelashes that are applied to the base of the eyelashes one at a time (**figure 24-47**).

- **Eyelash adhesive** is used to make artificial eyelashes adhere, or stick, to the natural lash line.

Apply Strip Lashes

Strip lashes are available in a variety of sizes, textures, and colors. They are made from human hair, mink, or synthetic fibers attached to a band. Artificial eyelashes are available in natural colors ranging from light to dark brown and black or light to dark auburn, as well as bright, trendy colors. Black and dark brown are the most popular choices. If the length of the eyelash band is too long to fit the curve of the upper eyelid, trim the outside edge. Use your fingers to bend the lash into a horseshoe shape to make it more flexible so that it fits the contour of the eyelid. Never attempt to feather the lashes by nipping them with the points of your scissors. This will result in blunt tips that look unnatural.

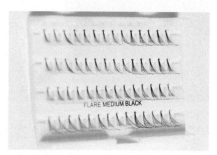

figure 24-47
Individual lashes

Ⓟ 24-2   **False Eyelash Application** *See page 840*

Remove Strip Eyelashes

Strip eyelashes are easily removed with cotton pads saturated with oil-based makeup remover. Hold the pad over the eyes for a few seconds to soften the adhesive. Starting from the outer corner, remove the lashes carefully to avoid pulling out the client's own lashes. Use a cotton swab to remove any makeup and adhesive residue left on the eyelid.

Individual Lashes

Individual eyelash application utilizes tab or cluster (flare) false eyelashes. In this procedure, individual synthetic eyelashes are attached directly to the

⚠ **CAUTION**
Some clients may be allergic to a particular eyelash adhesive. When in doubt, give the client an allergy test or patch test. Put a drop of the adhesive behind one ear. If there is no reaction within 24 hours, you may safely proceed with eyelash application.

© iStock.com/Shariff Che'Lah

base of the client's natural lash line (**figures 24-48** and **24-49**). Follow the manufacturer's instructions for attaching individual lashes.

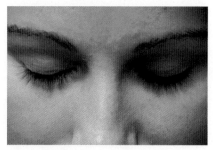

figure 24-48
Client before individual eyelash application

After reading the next few sections, you will be able to:

LO**5** List tips for creating special-occasion makeup for eyes, cheeks, and lips.

How to Use Special-Occasion Makeup

Each time a client requests makeup for a special occasion, you are given an opportunity to showcase your talent. Special occasions require a special arsenal of techniques. You must take into account the environment and mood of the event. For instance, many special occasions are evening events, where lighting is subdued, requiring more dramatic eyes, cheeks, or lips. Using metallic colors can also help accent features for an evening look. If the special occasion will include flash photography—such as a wedding—matte colors are recommended. Products that shimmer may reflect light too much. To create special-occasion makeup, follow the **Basic Makeup Procedure 24-1**, incorporating some of the pointers discussed in the following subsections.

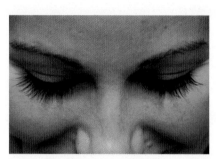

figure 24-49
Client after individual eyelash application

Special-Occasion Makeup for Eyes

Option 1: Striking Contour Eyes

1. Apply the base color from the lashes to the crease with a shadow brush or applicator.

2. Apply medium tone on the lid, blending from lash line to crease with the shadow brush or applicator.

3. Apply medium to deep color in the crease, blending upward and outward, stopping just below the arch.

4. Apply highlight shadow under the brow bone with the shadow brush or applicator.

5. Apply eyeliner on the upper lash line from the outside corner in, tapering as you reach the inner corner. Blend with the small brush or applicator.

6. Apply shadow in the same color as the liner, directly over the liner. This will give longevity and intensity to the liner. Repeat on the bottom lash line, if desired (**figure 24-50**).

7. Apply mascara with a disposable wand

> **HERE'S A TIP**
> Remind the client to take special care with artificial lashes when swimming, bathing, or cleansing the face. Over time, water- and oil-based cleansing products will weaken the adhesive.

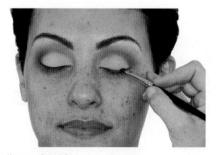

figure 24-50
Contour eyes

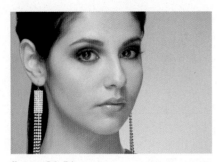

figure 24-51
Smoky eyes

Option 2: Dramatic Smoky Eyes

1. Encircle the eye with dark gray, dark brown, or black eyeliner.

2. Smudge with a small shadow brush or disposable applicator.

3. Using the shadow brush or applicator, apply dark shadow from the upper lash line to the crease, softening and blending as you approach the crease. The shadow should be dark from outer to inner corner. You may choose shimmering- or matte-finish eye shadows.

4. Repeat on the lower lash line, carefully blending any hard edges.

5. If desired, add a highlight color in a shimmering or matte finish to the upper brow area with the shadow brush or applicator.

6. Apply mascara with a disposable wand.

7. Add individual or strip lashes if desired (figure 24-51).

Special-Occasion Makeup for Cheeks

Refer to the "Altering Face Shapes" section for techniques you can use to remedy less attractive aspects of the cheeks. You can also try one of the following steps:

1. Use a darker blush color under the cheekbones to add definition.

2. Apply with a blush brush or applicator, and blend carefully.

3. Add a brighter, lighter cheek color to the apples of the cheeks and blend.

4. Use a cheek color with shimmer or glitter over the cheekbones for highlight.

    Note: You may use cream or powder colors.

Special-Occasion Makeup for Lips

For special occasions, clients may prefer a brighter or darker shade than their everyday lipstick color. You may use shimmer colors or matte colors.

1. Apply liner to the lips. Fill in the lip line with pencil and blot.

2. Apply a similar lipstick color over the entire mouth with a lip brush or disposable applicator.

3. Apply gloss to the center of the lips with a lip brush or disposable applicator (figure 24-52).

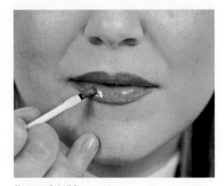

figure 24-52
The perfect pout

DID YOU KNOW?

For those interested in additional instruction and makeup application demonstrations, refer to *Milady Standard Makeup*.

BASIC PROFESSIONAL MAKEUP APPLICATION

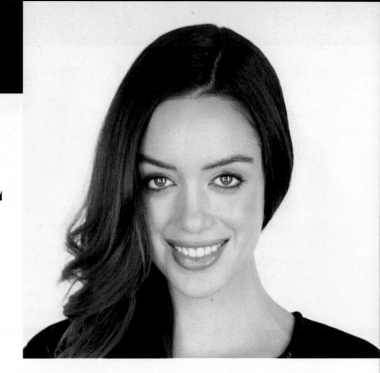

You will need all of the following implements, materials, and supplies:

- Assorted makeup brushes (for concealer, powder, eye shadow, eyeliner, a slanted brush for brows, blush and lip color)
- Cheek colors
- Cleansers
- Concealers
- Cotton pads, puffs, and swabs

- Disposable lip brushes
- Eye shadows
- Eyelash comb
- Eyelash curler
- Eyeliner
- Face powders
- Foundations
- Headband or hair clip
- Lip colors

- Lip liners
- Makeup cape
- Mascara
- Mascara wands
- Moisturizers
- Pencil sharpener
- Serums
- Shadow applicators
- Small makeup palette

- Spatulas
- Sponge wedges
- Sunscreen
- Tissues
- Toner for drier skin
- Towels and draping sheets, if desired

PREPARATION | PROCEDURE

Perform:

P 15-1 **Pre-Service Procedure** See page 340

1 Drape the client and use a headband or hair clip to keep her hair out of her face.

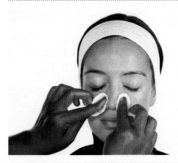

2 Cleanse the face, and then apply toner.

3 Apply a serum, moisturizer, primer, or sunscreen appropriate for client's skin type.

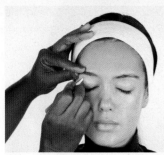 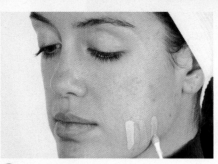 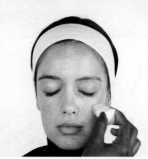

4 Groom eyebrows, if needed. See Chapter 22, Hair Removal for instructions on eyebrow maintenance.

5 Perform a color match test and select the proper type of foundation for the client's skin type. Use a cotton swab to apply a small amount of three different skin-matching shades to the jawline. The color that seems to disappear is the right choice.

6 Place a small amount of the foundation on a palette. Apply foundation from the center of the face blending outward and downward. Blend up to the hairline, removing any excess foundation by blotting with a tissue or sponge.

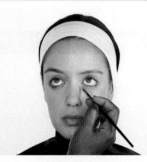 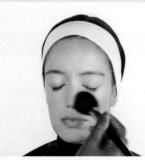 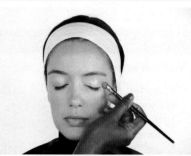

7 Scrape a small amount of concealer with a spatula and place on a palette. Using a synthetic concealer brush or sponge, lightly apply the concealer where needed (under the eyes, over blemishes, over red or dark-colored splotches). Note: Apply all cream and liquid products before powder to ensure even application.

8 Shake the loose powder onto a tissue or palette. Dip a disposable puff or powder brush into the powder and apply to the face. Use a rolling pressing motion with a puff or lightly whisk with a powder brush in a downward and outward motion.

9 Select a complementary eye color in a medium tone. Beginning at the lash line or crease, apply lightly and blend outward with a brush or disposable applicator.

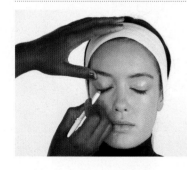

10 Select an eyeliner color that harmonizes with the mascara you will be applying. Lightly pull the outer corner of your client's closed eyelid until taut. Draw a fine line along the entire lash line, tapering in towards the inner corner. Repeat application to the lower lash line if desired. To enhance small eyes, apply liner approximately ¾ of the way from the outer edge of the eye.

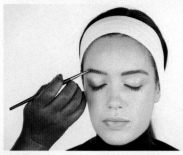

11 Brush the eyebrows into place, and use light, hair-like strokes to apply either a fine-pointed eyebrow pencil or a shadow with a brush. Excess color can be brushed away or removed with a cotton-tipped swab.

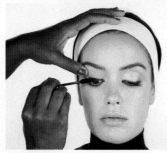

12 Optional step: Apply false lashes before applying the mascara. Refer to **Procedure 24-2, False Eyelash Extensions** for instructions.

13 Use an eyelash curler to curl the lashes. Start by gently crimping at the base of the lash line then continue crimping outward towards the tip to create a natural blend. Apply mascara with a zig-zag motion to coat both sides of the upper lashes. Use an eyelash comb to separate the lashes. Mascara may be applied to the lower lashes as well.

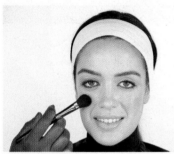

14 Have the client smile and then apply powder cheek color, blending outward and upward toward the temples. Liquid or cream cheek color is applied with a clean applicator before powder and sometimes on bare skin.

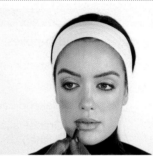

15 Use a freshly sharpened pencil to apply lip liner. Line the lips by beginning at the outer corner of the upper lip and working toward the middle. Repeat on the opposite side. Connect the center peaks using rounded strokes, following the natural line of the lip. Outline the lower lip from the outer corners in.

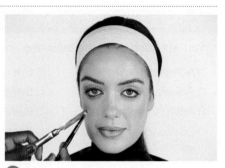

16 Use a spatula to scrape lip color from the container.

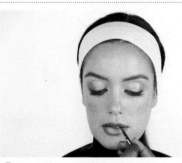

17 Use a lip brush to take the lip color from the spatula and brush it on to the lips, smoothing over any small crevices. Blot the lips with tissue to remove excess product.

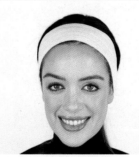

18 Finished makeup application.

POST-SERVICE

Complete:

P 15-2 **Post-Service Procedure**
See page 343

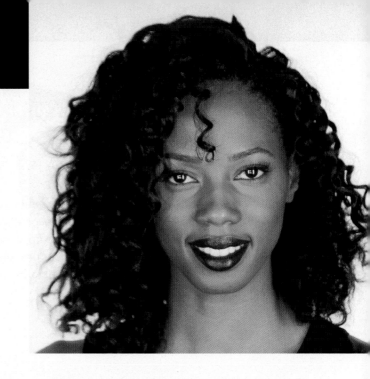

P 24-2

FALSE EYELASH APPLICATION

IMPLEMENTS & MATERIALS

You will need all of the following implements, materials, and supplies:

- ☐ Adhesive tray/holder
- ☐ Adjustable light
- ☐ Artificial eyelashes
- ☐ Disposable mascara wands

- ☐ Eye makeup remover
- ☐ Eyelash brushes
- ☐ Eyelash curler
- ☐ Hand mirror

- ☐ Lash adhesive
- ☐ Mascara
- ☐ Makeup cape
- ☐ Orange stick (wooden pusher)

- ☐ Small scissors
- ☐ Tweezers

A. STRIP EYELASHES

PREPARATION | PROCEDURE

Perform:

P 15-1 **Pre-Service Procedure** *See page 340*

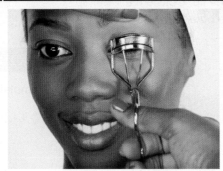

1 Brush the client's eyelashes to make sure they are clean and free of debris. Curl eyelashes with an eyelash curler before applying artificial lashes.

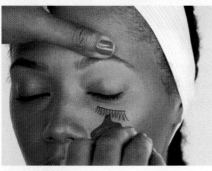

2 Use tweezers to remove lashes from the package. Measure strip lashes by lightly placing them along the client's lash line. Adjust the length by trimming the outer edges of each strip (band).

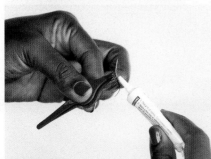

3 Apply a thin layer of lash adhesive to the false eyelash strip and allow a few seconds for it to set.

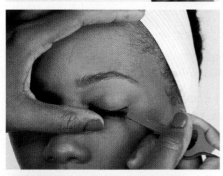

4 Align the strip with the client's lash line, starting at the outer edge of the eye. Use an orange stick (wooden pusher) or the rounded edge of your tweezers to slide the strip right up to the base of the lashes.

Note: Starting with the shorter part of the lash and placing it at the inner corner of the eye toward the nose is also acceptable. The technician starts at the outer lash line in this specific procedure so that the longest areas are aligned. The lash can always taper off to the shortest natural lashes, but not vice-versa.

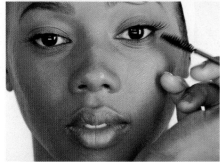

5 Lightly apply mascara to the tips to minimize separation between the false and natural lashes.

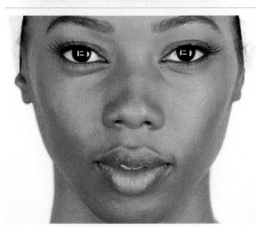

6 Finished strip eyelash application.

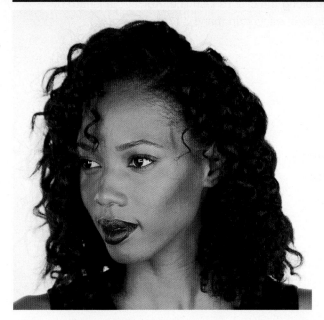

Individual eyelashes create a more natural effect than strip lashes. Altering the placement of various lash lengths can alter the eye shape. Follow these simple steps to apply individual lashes one at a time.

PROCEDURE

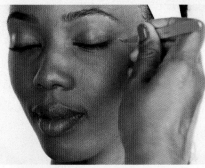

1 Brush the client's eyelashes to make sure they are clean and free of debris. Remove an eyelash cluster or tab from the package with tweezers. Start by applying the longest lashes along the outer edge of the lash line, and one near the center. Fill in the space between them.

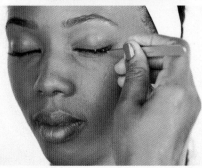

2 Next, proceed to the center of the lash line to apply a row of the medium-length lashes. Use the rounded edge of your tweezers to slide the individual lash right up to the base of the lashes.

3 Once these are in place, proceed to the inner corner of the eye to place the shortest lashes (these are usually called mini lashes).

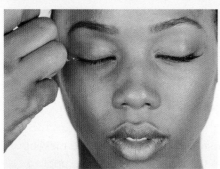

④ Proceed to the other eye and repeat the process.

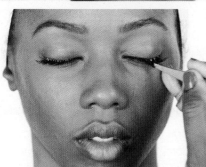

⑤ Take a moment to compare the eyes. Make corrections by filling in spaces until they are balanced.

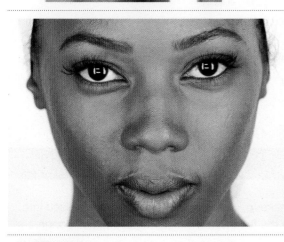

⑥ Finished individual eyelash application

POST-SERVICE

Complete:

Ⓟ 15-2   **Post-Service Procedure** *See page 343*

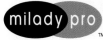

Check out miladypro.com for additional resources and training to enhance your technical skills. Keyword: *FutureCosPro*

1. List eight types of facial cosmetics and how they are used.

2. List the two color temperatures and the range of shades they each encompass.

3. What is the purpose of special-occasion makeup?

4. What is the purpose of face shape altering makeup?

5. Name and describe the two types of artificial eyelashes.

6. List the key cosmetics used in the basic makeup procedure in the order in which they are applied.

STUDY TOOLS

- **Reinforce what you just learned:** Complete the activities and exercises in your Theory or Practical Workbook, or your Study Guide.

- **Expand your knowledge:** Search for websites about the topics in this chapter and make a list of additional resources.

- **Study and prepare for your quiz:** Take the chapter test in your Exam Review or your Milady U: Online Licensing Prep.

- **Re-Test your knowledge:** Take the Chapter 24 *Quizzes*!

- **Learn even more:** Look up in a dictionary or search the internet for the definitions of any additional terms you want to learn about.

CHAPTER GLOSSARY

cake makeup	p. 816	Also known as *pancake makeup*; a heavy-coverage makeup pressed into a compact and applied to the face with a moistened cosmetic sponge.
cheek color	p. 815	Also known as *blush* or *rouge*; used primarily to add a natural-looking glow to the cheeks.
concealers	p. 814	Thick, heavy types of foundation used to hide dark eye circles, dark splotches, and other imperfections.
contour	p. 823	An application technique that creates a shadow over an area, minimizing features.
cool colors	p. 820	Colors that suggest coolness and are dominated by blues, greens, violets, and blue-reds.
eye makeup removers	p. 816	Special preparations for removing eye makeup.
eye shadows	p. 814	Cosmetics applied on the eyelids to accentuate or contour.
eyebrow pencils	p. 814	Pencils used to add color and shape to the eyebrows.
eyebrow powders	p. 814	Powders used to add color and shape to the eyebrows.
eyelash adhesive	p. 834	Product used to make artificial eyelashes adhere, or stick, to the natural lash line.

eyeliner	p. 814	Cosmetic used to outline and emphasize the eyes.
face powder	p. 814	Cosmetic powder, sometimes tinted, that is used to add a matte or non-shiny finish to the face.
ferrule	p. 816	The metal part of the brush that attaches the glued bristles to the handle and adds a certain amount of strength to the bristles.
foundation	p. 812	Also known as *base makeup*; a tinted cosmetic used to cover or even out the coloring of the skin.
greasepaint	p. 816	Heavy makeup used for theatrical purposes.
highlight	p. 823	An application technique that draws light to an area, emphasizing features.
individual lashes	p. 834	Separate artificial eyelashes that are applied to the base of the eyelashes one at a time.
line of demarcation LYN UV dee-mar-KAY-shun	p. 831	An obvious line where foundation begins or ends.
lip color	p. 815	Also known as *lipstick* or *lip gloss*; a paste-like cosmetic used to change or enhance the lip color.
lip liner	p. 815	Colored pencil used to outline the lips and to help keep lip color from bleeding into the small lines around the mouth.
mascara	p. 815	Cosmetic preparation used to darken, define, and thicken the eyelashes.
matte	p. 813	Not shiny.
primer	p. 813	Applied to the skin before foundation to cancel out and help disguise skin discoloration.
strip lashes	p. 834	Eyelash hairs attached to a band that is applied with adhesive to the natural lash line.
warm colors	p. 820	Range of colors from yellow and gold through oranges, red-oranges, most reds, and even some yellow-greens.

Photography by Ted Emmons. Nails by Alisha Rimando Botero, courtesy of Artistic Nail Design.

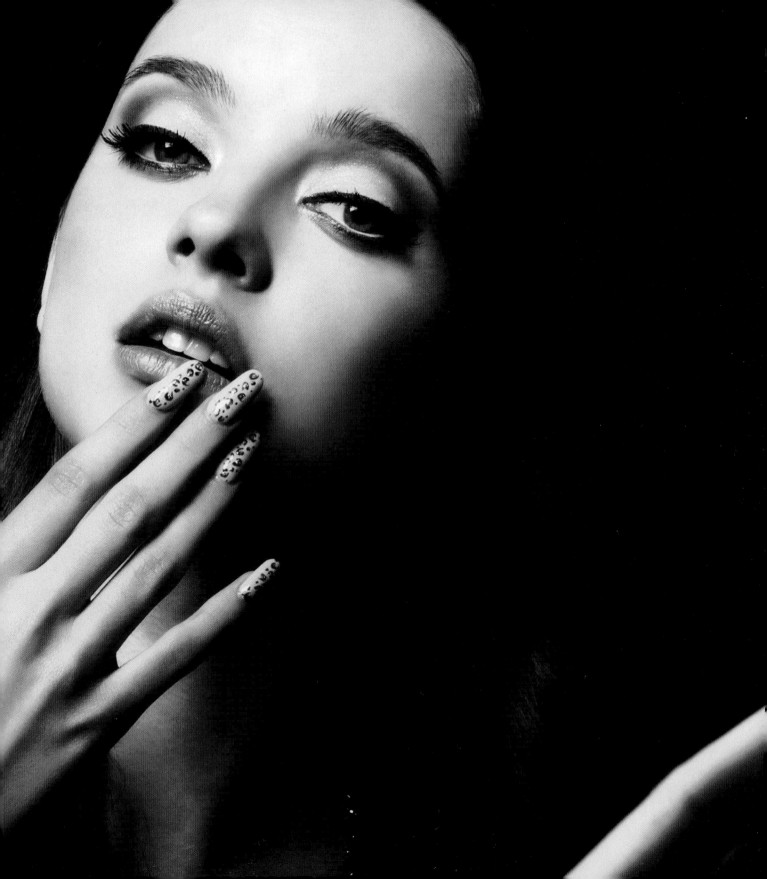

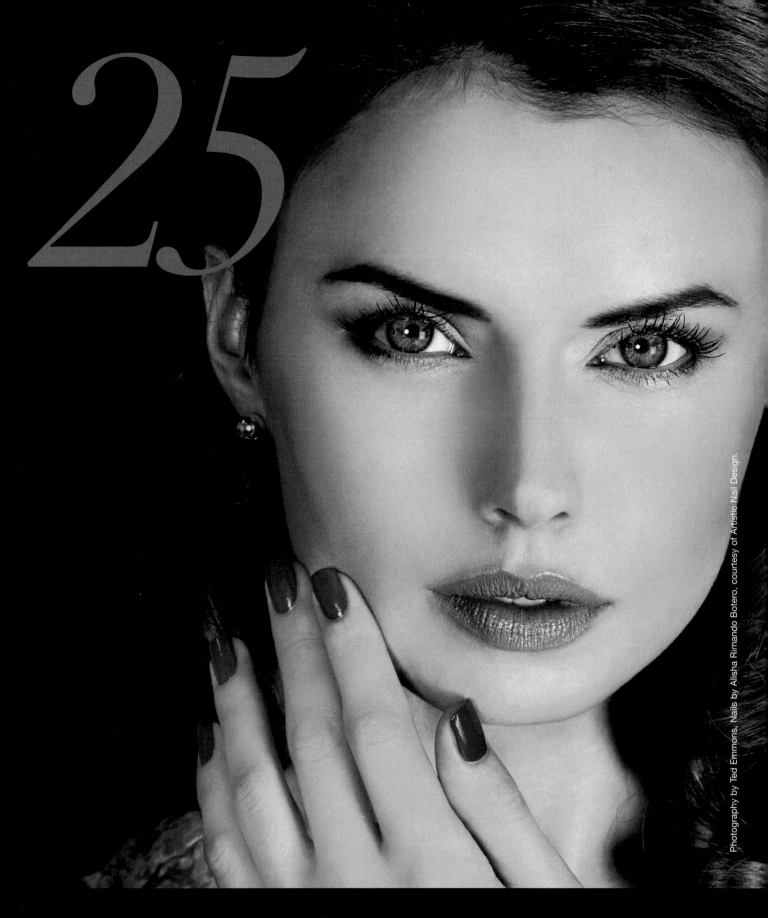

25

MANICURING

Photography by Ted Emmons, Nails by Alisha Rimando Botero, courtesy of Artistic Nail Design.

LEARNING OBJECTIVES

After completing this chapter, you will be able to:

LO①
Define *scope of practice*.

LO②
Describe the potential consequences if a nail technician works outside the state's scope of practice.

LO③
Identify the four types of nail technology tools required to perform a manicure.

LO④
Explain the difference between multiuse (reusable) and single-use (disposable) implements.

LO⑤
Name and describe the three-part procedure used in the performance of the basic manicure.

LO⑥
Explain why a consultation is important before a service in the salon.

LO⑦
List and describe the five basic nail shapes for women.

LO⑧
Describe the most popular nail shape for men.

LO⑨
List the massage movements for performing a relaxing hand and arm massage.

LO⑩
Explain the differences between spa manicures and basic manicures.

LO⑪
Describe how aromatherapy is best used in manicuring services.

LO⑫
Explain the benefits of paraffin wax in manicuring.

849

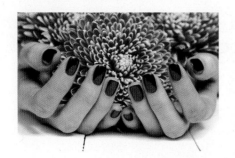

Zoia Kostina/Shutterstock.com

Once you have learned the fundamental techniques in this chapter, you will be officially on your way to providing clients with a professional manicure. A **manicure** is a cosmetic treatment of the hands involving cutting, shaping, and often painting of the nails, removal of the cuticles, and softening of the skin. Manicure and pedicure services are currently the fastest-growing services on salon and spa menus.

why study
MANICURING?

Cosmetologists should study and have a thorough understanding of manicuring because:

> The appearance of nails and hands has become a visual benchmark in our society in the assessment of a person both socially and professionally.

> Fashion continuously changes, and a professional cosmetologist should always stay current to new trends in all facets of the beauty industry.

> Some clients cannot, due to health constraints, maintain their own nails; some just prefer to have a knowledgeable professional perform this task for them.

> Clients love the relaxation and pampering manicures provide.

After reading the next few sections, you will be able to:

LO❶ Define *scope of practice*.

LO❷ Describe the potential consequences if a nail technician works outside the state's scope of practice.

Adhere to State and Government Regulations

During your studies you will be learning about the regulations concerning performing nail services within your state. These regulations are very important to you, as a cosmetologist, and map out what is called your **scope of practice (SOP)**, the list of services that you are legally allowed to perform in your specialty in your state. The SOP may or may not state those services you cannot legally perform. Your instructor will provide important guidelines for your adhering closely to your SOP in your state. Know that if you perform services outside these regulations concerning allowable services, you may lose your license. Also, if damages to a client occur while performing an illegal service, you are fully liable, both professionally and personally.

Occupational Safety and Health Administration (OSHA) also provides guidelines for protecting cosmetologists from chemicals that can affect your health. The main health issue a cosmetologist is prone to is hypersensitivity reactions. To avoid this, the OSHA Hazard Communication Standard requires salon ventilation where chemical services are performed as well as proper personal protective equipment (PPE), which we will continue to discuss throughout this chapter.

After reading the next few sections, you will be able to:

LO③ Identify the four types of nail technology tools required to perform a manicure.

LO④ Explain the difference between multiuse (reusable) and single-use (disposable) implements.

Work with Nail Technology Tools

As a professional cosmetologist, you must learn to work with the tools required for nail services and know all safety, cleaning, and disinfection procedures as defined in your state's regulations.

The four types of nail technology tools that you will incorporate into your services include:

1. Equipment
2. Implements
3. Materials
4. Professional nail products

Equipment

Equipment includes all permanent tools that are not implements that are used to perform nail services.

Manicure Table

A standard manicuring table usually includes a drawer and a shelf (with or without doors) for storing properly cleaned and disinfected implements and professional products (**figure 25-1**). The table can vary in length, but it is usually 36 inches (91.4 centimeters) to 48 inches (121.9 centimeters) long. The width is normally 16 inches (40.6 centimeters) to 21 inches (53.3 centimeters). The surface of the table must be cleaned and disinfected the between clients, so it must be a hard and impenetrable surface, such as Formica or glass, and be kept clear of clutter.

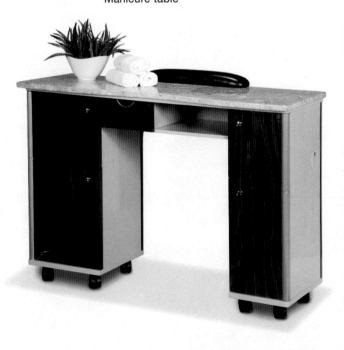

figure 25-1
Manicure table

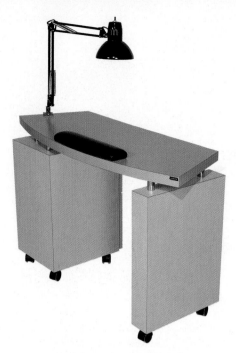

figure 25-2
Manicure table with an adjustable lamp and arm cushion

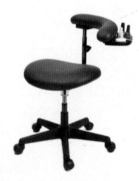

figure 25-3
Technician chair with wheels for maneuverability and hydraulics for height

figure 25-4
Finger bowl for manicures.

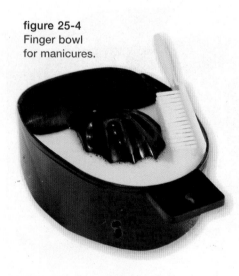

Adjustable Lamp

An adjustable lamp is attached to the table and should use a 40- to 60-watt incandescent bulb or a fluorescent bulb (figure 25-2). Fluorescent bulbs are very popular because they emit a cooler light. Most people prefer true-color fluorescent bulb lamps because they show the skin and polishes in their actual color in natural light. Fluorescent lights also do not heat up objects underneath the lamp as high-watt incandescent bulbs can. Higher temperatures caused by an incandescent bulb can increase the curing speed of some nail enhancement products. Curing too quickly can cause undue cracking and lifting.

Cosmetologist's and Client's Chairs

The cosmetologist's chair should be selected for ergonomics, comfort, durability, resistance to staining, and ease of cleaning. The most appropriate chair has wheels to allow the technician maneuverability and hydraulics to allow adjustment up and down (figure 25-3).

The client's chair must be durable and comfortable. For the comfort of clients, select a chair that has no or low arms on the sides, so that it can be moved closer to the table. This will allow the client's arms to rest on the nail table and prevent the client and cosmetologist from needing to stretch forward. The chair should also have a supportive back so the client can sit comfortably and relax during the service. The client chair should not have wheels, as wheeled chairs are unstable and can cause falling accidents for elderly or weak clients.

Finger Bowls

A finger bowl is used for soaking the client's fingers in warm water to soften the skin and cuticle. Finger bowls can be made of plastic, metal, glass, or even an attractive ceramic. They should be durable and easy to thoroughly clean and disinfect after use on each client (figure 25-4).

Disinfection Container

Although the disinfection container is not required for setting up the manicure table, it is important to have the container readily available for the start and end of the service. A disinfection container must be large enough to hold sufficient liquid disinfectant solution to completely immerse several **service sets**—sets of all the tools that will be used in a service. Containers that do not allow the entire implement (including handles) to be submerged are not acceptable for use in professional salons.

Disinfection containers come in many shapes, sizes, and materials and must have a lid to keep the disinfectant solution from becoming contaminated when not in use. Most containers are equipped with a tray, and lifting the tray by its handle allows the technician to remove the implements from the solution without contaminating the solution or the implements. After the implements are removed from the disinfectant container, they must be rinsed and air- or towel-dried in accordance with the manufacturer's instructions and state regulations.

Disinfectants must never be allowed to come in contact with the skin. If your disinfectant container does not have a lift tray or basket to allow rinsing, always remove the implements with tongs or tweezers and always wear gloves (figure 25-5). It is important to wear gloves when removing and rinsing implements because gloves prevent your fingers from coming into contact with disinfectant solution, which can be irritating to the skin.

Client's Arm Cushion

An 8-inch (20.3 centimeters) to 12-inch (30.5 centimeters) cushion that can be cleaned with soap and water and that is specifically made for the comfort of the client's arm is an option when performing nail services. It must be covered with a fresh, clean towel for each client. A clean towel that is folded or rolled to cushion-size may also be used instead of a commercially purchased cushion.

Service Cushion (Optional)

A foam cushion, higher in the middle and lower on the ends, can be placed between the client and the cosmetologist during a manicure; it is believed to provide more comfort during the service for both parties (**figure 25-7**). It must be fully covered by a fresh, clean towel throughout each service.

Gauze and Cotton Wipe Container

This container holds absorbent cotton, lint-free wipes, or gauze squares for use during the services. This container must have a lid to protect the contents from dust and contaminants.

Trash Containers

A trash container with a self-closing lid should be located next to your workstation (**figure 25-8**). It should be lined with a disposable trash bag and closed when not in use. It must be emptied at the end of each work day, and must be cleaned and disinfected often. A trash container with a self-closing lid is one of the best ways to prevent excessive odors and vapors in the salon.

If a trash receptacle with a self-closing lid is not available, tape or clip a plastic bag to the manicure table for depositing used materials during your manicure. These bags must be emptied after each client departs to prevent product vapors from escaping into the salon air.

Supply Tray (Optional)

A supply tray holds professional nail products, such as polishes, polish removers, and creams. It should be sturdy and easy to clean. Many technicians put every product they need for a service on these trays and then lift it on and off a shelf in their station in one efficient movement for each service. This allows the tabletop to be clear; to maintain a clean, non-cluttered appearance; and makes it easy to clean and disinfect after each service. This tray should also be cleaned and disinfected between clients.

Electric Nail Polish Dryer (Optional)

A nail polish dryer is designed to shorten the time necessary for the client's nail polish to dry. Electric dryers have heaters and fans that blow air onto the nail plates to speed evaporation of solvents from nail polishes, allowing them to harden more quickly. Light bulb-type dryers create warmth to speed drying and work in the same fashion as electric dryers and may or may not have fans.

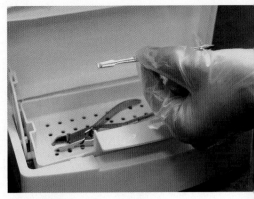
figure 25-5
Disinfection container with removable tray

DID YOU KNOW?

Implements must be properly prepared or prepped with a thorough cleansing before being placed in the disinfectant solution. Implements must be scrubbed with warm water, liquid soap, and a scrub brush, then rinsed and patted dry before placing in the disinfectant liquid (**figure 25-6**). Dirty or improperly prepared implements will not be disinfected in the solution.

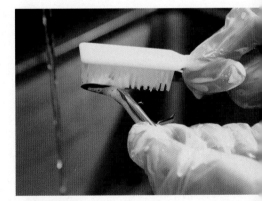
figure 25-6
Scrub implements to prepare for disinfection.

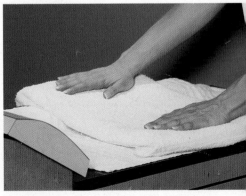
figure 25-7
Service cushion on nail table

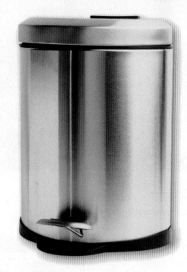

figure 25-8
Metal trash can with self-closing lid

UVA or LED Light (Optional)

UVA (ultraviolet) lamps and LED (light emitting diode) lamps are not designed to dry traditional nail polish. These lamps cure or harden products that contain photoinitiators, which are designed to be sensitive to the UVA wavelength the bulbs emit. These lamps are designed for traditional gels and gel polish curing.

Electric Hand/Foot Mitts (Optional)

These heated mitts, which are available for both hands and feet, are designed to add a special service to a manicure or pedicure. Heated mitts make for a higher-cost service or can be an add-on to a service. After the massage during a pedicure, conditioning lotion or even a mask is applied to the hands or feet, which are then placed in a plastic cover and inserted into the mitts. The warmth aids in penetration of the conditioning ingredients, adds to the comfort of the service, and provides ultimate relaxation for the client.

Terry Cloth Mitts (Optional)

These washable mitts are placed over a client's hands or feet after a penetrating conditioning product and a protective plastic cover has been applied. These mitts are routinely used over paraffin to hold in the heat, or over masks to encourage the natural heat from the skin to enhance the penetration of the product ingredients.

Paraffin Bath (Optional)

A paraffin bath is a special heating unit designed to melt solid paraffin wax into a gel-like liquid and maintain it at a temperature generally between 125 and 130 degrees Fahrenheit (the ideal temperature for application to the hands and feet). Never try to heat the wax in anything other than a paraffin bath designed specifically for this use (**figure 25-9**). This can be very dangerous and may result in painful skin burns or a fire. Read and follow all operating instructions that come with your paraffin bath.

Paraffin, a petroleum by-product that has excellent sealing properties (barrier qualities) to hold moisture in the skin, can be added to manicures and pedicures for an extra charge. Paraffin is used to coat the skin on the hands and feet to hold in the skin's natural moisture in the epidermal layers and thus promoting moisturization of the skin and deeper penetration of other products that have been used on the skin prior to the paraffin.

figure 25-9
Paraffin bath

After basic equipment, the paraffin bath is often the first purchase for many salons and spas. Check the regulations in your state concerning the use of paraffin in salons.

Ventilation System (Optional)

Products used when performing nail services may contain chemicals that can affect a worker's health. Exposure to nail dust and chemical odors and vapors can affect one's breathing and respiratory health. These symptoms do not show immediately, but can sometimes take months or even years to

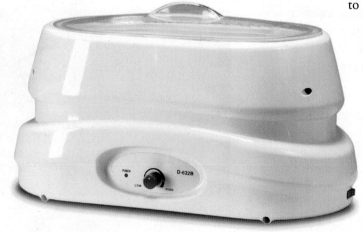

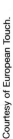

appear. Proper ventilation should be used in the salon to protect nail technicians from becoming overexposed to vapors and dust.

Fans and open windows are actually not substitutes for proper ventilation; they will simply circulate vapors and dust around the room. These do not protect the breathing zone, which is an invisible two-foot sphere around the nail technician's head/face. One of the most effective ways to ensure safe working conditions is local source capture ventilation systems (figure 25-10). These systems are designed to capture vapors and dust at the source and remove them from the air before they have a chance to escape into the salon (figure 25-11a and b). Many types of local exhaust systems are mobile and can be easily transported from one station to another.

Some salons have ventilated tables with filters. In order for these to help air quality, the filters need to be changed regularly. It is best if the tables are vented to the outside.

There are also portable downdraft vent machines that use a powerful fan to pull down and capture chemical vapors and nail dust into a two-stage carbon filter. These carbon filter vent machines sit directly below the nail technician's breathing zone, capturing dust and vapors right at the source. The fan pulls the nail dust and odor down through the filter, leaving odor and chemical-free air at the source.

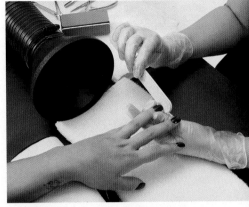

figure 25-10
The best way to control dust in the salon is with a professional source capture ventilation system designed to collect and remove dust particles from the air or to ventilate them to the outdoors.

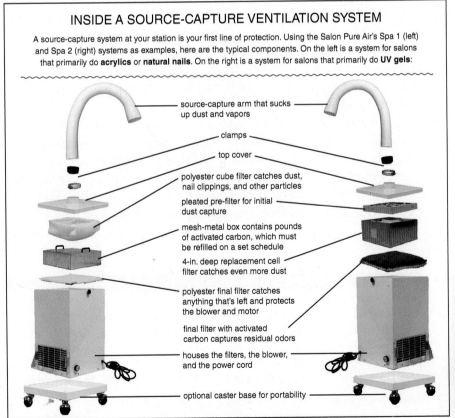

INSIDE A SOURCE-CAPTURE VENTILATION SYSTEM

A source-capture system at your station is your first line of protection. Using the Salon Pure Air's Spa 1 (left) and Spa 2 (right) systems as examples, here are the typical components. On the left is a system for salons that primarily do **acrylics** or **natural nails**. On the right is a system for salons that primarily do **UV gels**:

source-capture arm that sucks up dust and vapors

clamps

top cover

polyester cube filter catches dust, nail clippings, and other particles

pleated pre-filter for initial dust capture

mesh-metal box contains pounds of activated carbon, which must be refilled on a set schedule

4-in. deep replacement cell filter catches even more dust

polyester final filter catches anything that's left and protects the blower and motor

final filter with activated carbon captures residual odors

houses the filters, the blower, and the power cord

optional caster base for portability

Courtesy of Salon Pure Air and NAILS Magazine.

figure 25-11a
The ventilation system should have an activated carbon filter that is a minimum of 3 inches thick for absorption of vapors.

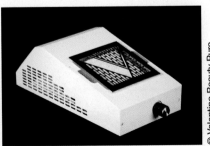

© Valentino Beauty Pure

figure 25-11b
Portable two stage carbon filter ventilation system that captures dust and filters chemical odors.

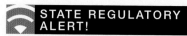
Implements

Implements are tools used to perform your services and are either multiuse or single-use. **Multiuse implements**, also known as *reusable implements*, are generally stainless steel because they must be properly cleaned and disinfected after use on one client and prior to use on another. Less expensive nickel-plated metal implements will corrode during disinfection and sterilization. **Single-use implements**, also known as *disposable implements*, cannot be reused because they cannot be cleaned and disinfected; therefore, they must be thrown away after a single use. It is recommended that cosmetologists have several clean and disinfected service sets of implements available for use at all times.

Multiuse Implements

Multiuse or reusable implements are those that can be reused after infection control procedures have been performed on them. They are metal—stainless steel is recommended if they are to maintain their quality.

Metal Pusher

The **metal pusher**, often incorrectly called a cuticle pusher, is designed to gently scrape cuticle tissue from the natural nail plate. It is not to be used to push back the eponychium (living skin at the base of the natural nail plate that covers the matrix area). Metal pushers must be stainless steel and used carefully to prevent damaging the natural nail and the nail matrix. Improper use on the nail can cause grooving in the nail plate and possible nail growth problems if the nail matrix is accidentally damaged. Improper or careless use of the metal pusher can cause microscopic trauma or injury to the tissues. These injuries are known as **microtrauma**—tiny, often unseen openings in the skin, which can allow microbes to enter the skin, leading to infection.

If you have rough or sharp edges on your metal pusher, use an abrasive to smooth or remove them. This prevents digging into the nail plate or damaging the protective barriers created by the eponychium and cuticle.

When using a metal pusher, hold it the way you would a pencil with the flat end held at a 20- to 30-degree angle from the nail plate. The spoon end is used to carefully loosen and push back the dead cuticle tissue

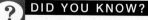

DID YOU KNOW?
A cosmetologist practicing nail procedures full- or part-time will need at least three service sets of quality, stainless-steel implements in order to always have a completely clean and disinfected set ready for use on each client. One set is in the disinfectant, one is being used, and another is ready for use. By always having a set of implements ready, you will ensure that clients will not have to wait for the disinfection process. Remember, it takes approximately 20 minutes to properly clean and then disinfect implements after each use.

These sets can be wrapped in a clean towel and stored in a clean place, or they can be inserted into a sterile pouch before being autoclaved. Open the implements in front of your clients at the start of each service so clients can see that the set has been disinfected prior to their arrival. Refer to your state board guidelines on proper storage of your disinfected or sterilized service sets.

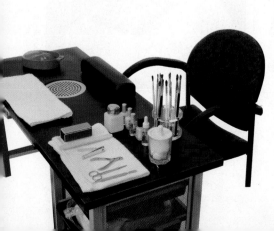

on the nail plate (figure 25-12). To stabilize the hand that is holding the pusher, balance your pinky finger on the hand that is holding the client's finger. This will allow you to have total control while working with the implement.

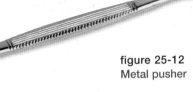

figure 25-12
Metal pusher

Nail Nippers

A **nail nipper** is a stainless-steel implement used to carefully trim away *dead* skin around the nails. It is never used to cut, rip, or tear live tissue because the live nail fold tissue is important to ward off microbes and prevent infection around the nail plate. Nippers must be cleaned and disinfected before use on every client, taking special care to open the hinges for thorough cleaning and disinfecting. Always maintain a sharp edge on your nippers to prevent ripping or tearing of the dead skin, which can cause future hangnails. Cosmetologists must never use their nippers to cut cuticles, as this is a medical procedure.

It is important that you learn the correct use of nail nippers while in school. To use nippers, hold your thumb around one handle and three fingers around the other, with the blades facing the nail plate. Your index finger is placed on the box joint to help control the blade and guide it properly (figure 25-13).

Tweezers

Tweezers are multi-task implements for lifting small bits of debris from the nail plate, retrieving and placing nail art, removing implements from disinfectant solutions, and much more (figure 25-14). They must be properly cleaned and disinfected before use on every client because they may come in contact with a client's skin or nails. They must be stainless steel to allow disinfection after use.

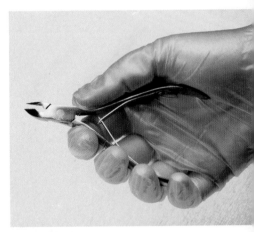

figure 25-13
Nail nipper

Nail Clippers

Nail clippers shorten the free edge quickly and efficiently. If the nails need to be shortened more than the depth of routine filing, they can be cut with nail clippers, clipping from the sides toward the center of the nails to prevent stress to the sides and possible splitting. This clipping will save time during the filing process. File the free edge after using the nail clipper to perfect the shape.

Nail clippers must be properly cleaned and then disinfected before each use on every client. These implements must be stainless steel to be disinfected.

Single-use Implements

Single-use or disposable implements are used once on a client then discarded, preferably while the client can view it being done.

Brushes and Applicators

Any brush, such as those used to apply masks, or applicator, such as those used to scoop product from a container to the skin, that comes into contact with a client's nails or skin during a manicure or pedicure must be properly cleaned and disinfected before use on another client. If it cannot be properly cleaned and disinfected according

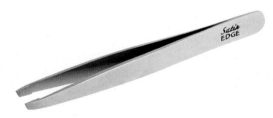

figure 25-14
Tweezers

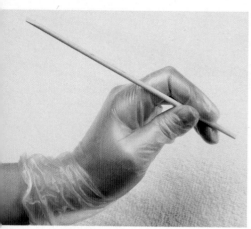

figure 25-15
Wooden pusher

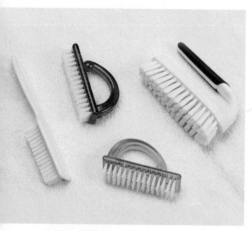

figure 25-16
Nail brushes

to your state's regulations, they must be disposed of after a single use. Check with the manufacturer if you are unsure whether a brush or applicator can be properly cleaned and disinfected.

Nail polish brushes are the exception. They are stored in an oxygen-free, water-free liquid (polish) which does not allow the growth of microbes. With no water or air, they die within a short time. However, microbes just picked up by the brush can be carried to another nail if the brush is immediately used to polish.

Wooden Pusher

The **wooden pusher** is used to remove cuticle tissue from the nail plate, to clean under the free edge of the nail, or to apply products. Hold the stick as you would a pencil with the tip at a 20- to 30-degree angle from the nail plate while pushing the cuticle free (figure 25-15). It is a single-use implement and not intended for reuse or disinfection. Apply nail products by completely wrapping the end of the stick with a small piece of cotton and placing or dipping the cotton tip into the product. If the cotton tip is dipped into product, enough must be retrieved for the entire application. If more product is needed, the cotton on your wooden pusher must be changed to prevent contamination of the product. Using products that have spout lids can shorten time in the application. The spout must not touch the cotton tip, nail plate, or the skin.

Nail Brush

This plastic implement with nylon bristles is used in many ways during nail services (figure 25-16). Clients use a nail brush when they arrive at the salon and perform the hand-washing procedure. Technicians use a nail brush for hand washing between clients. Nail brushes are also used during the manicure to remove debris from the nail plate. Finally—and very importantly—nail brushes are used to scrub the implements clean before disinfection.

Product Application Brushes

Product application brushes can be used to apply nail oils, nail polish, or nail treatments to client's nails. It is recommended that you purchase inexpensive, readily available packages of single-use application brushes to apply products that can support bacterial growth.

Dip enough product from the container for your entire application using the application brush, or pour enough product for the full application into a clean dappen dish, and dip the application brush into this dish throughout the application. Again, these brushes must be disposed of after use on one client.

An exception to this single-use rule is made for brushes used in products that are not capable of harboring or supporting the growth of pathogenic microbes, such as alcohol, nail polish, monomers and polymers, light cured gels, nail primers, dehydrators, bleaches, and so forth. Since these products cannot harbor or support pathogen growth, the brushes do not need to be cleaned and disinfected between each use unless the brush touches a contaminated nail immediately before moving to another nail. Since cosmetologists can only work on healthy nails, contaminated nails should not be an issue. However, a brush is considered contaminated if it is used to apply penetrating nail oil to the nail plate and then placed back into the product, because the products themselves can become contaminated with bacteria and support the growth of pathogens. For this reason, single-use application brushes or droppers should be used to apply oils to the nail plate or surrounding skin.

Materials

Materials and supplies used during a manicure are designed to be single-use and must be replaced for each client. These items are not considered multiuse.

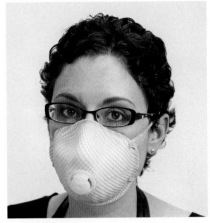

figure 25-17
Inhalation of dusts and vapors can be greatly reduced by wearing a high-quality, properly fitted N-95 dust mask.

Gloves

Gloves are personal protective equipment (PPE), worn to protect the cosmetologist from exposure to microbes during services. Since chemicals can be absorbed through the skin, OSHA recommends nitrile gloves as they protect from chemicals where latex and vinyl do not. If a single client receives both a manicure and a pedicure, a new set of gloves must be worn for each service. In addition, when two services are being performed together, the technician must perform hand washing after removing each set of gloves and before putting on a new set. Many cosmetologists use antimicrobial gel cleanser when cleaning the hands between sets of gloves during the same appointment.

Dust Mask

Use a high quality, properly fitted dust mask when transferring chemicals from one container to another or when buffing or filing nails. It is best to use a round dust mask with a metal strip that you can adjust to fit the bridge of your nose. Properly fitted dust masks rated N-95 are highly effective and a great choice for preventing inhalation overexposure to dusts (figure 25-17). Choose a mask designed specifically for dusts, mists, or molds to ensure the mask will be effective in the salon setting. Paper dust masks protect you from nail filing dust but not chemicals. An air-purifying respirator can be worn to filter chemical vapors or an air-purifying ventilation system can be used at your table. Make sure to purchase a professional air purifier designed for heavy-duty use, not one designed primarily for residential use.

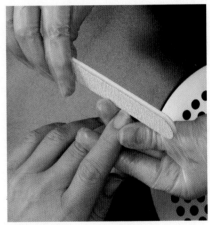

figure 25-18
Typical abrasive nail file

Abrasive Nail Files and Buffers

Abrasive nail files (figure 25-18) and buffers (figure 25-19) are generally single-use only, and they are available in many different types and grits. For example, they come with firm, rigid supporting cores or with padded and very flexible cores. Grits range from less than 180 to over 240 per centimeter. A rule of thumb is the lower the grit, the larger the abrasive particles on the file and the more aggressive its action. Therefore, **lower-grit abrasives** (less than 180 grit) are aggressive and will quickly reduce the thickness of any surface. Lower-grit files also produce deeper and more visible scratches on the surface than do higher-grit. Therefore, lower-grit files must be used with caution and are not used on natural nails since they can cause damage.

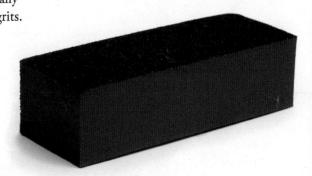

figure 25-19
Abrasive nail block buffer

You must prep the edge of your abrasive files before using them on a client to prevent harm to the client from the sharp edges of the files. These files are stamped from a large sheet of prepared materials, leaving very sharp edges, and these sharp edges are not removed before the files are shipped. You are responsible for removing this damaging edge from every new file.

To prepare a file for use, rub another (clean, unused) file across the edge to remove that sharp edge; this action is referred to as *file prepping*. Many cosmetologists prepare all their new files and then store them in a clean container. If this edge is not removed on new boards, that client is at risk for cuts. Check the corners of buffers as they usually require prepping as well.

Medium-grit abrasives (150 to 180 grit) are used to smooth and refine surfaces, and the 180 grit is used to shorten and shape natural nails. **Fine-grit abrasives** are in the category of 240 and higher grits. They are designed for buffing, polishing, and removing very fine scratches.

miladypro™ **LEARN MORE!**

Optional info on **Manicuring** topics and tutorials can be found at miladypro.com Keyword: *FutureCosPro*

Abrasive boards and buffers typically have one, two, or three different grit surfaces depending on type, use, and style. Some abrasive boards and buffers can be cleaned and disinfected. Check with the manufacturer to see if the abrasive of your choice can be disinfected. All abrasives must be cleaned and disinfected before reuse on another client. Check with your instructor as to whether your state allows abrasive boards and buffers to be disinfected within the SOP. Abrasives that cannot survive the cleaning and disinfection process without being damaged are considered single-use and must be discarded after a single use.

Two-Way or Three-Way Buffer

The two- or three-way buffer abrasive creates a beautiful shine on nails and replaces the chamois that could not be disinfected (**figure 25-20**). These buffers can be shaped like a two-sided nail file, long and narrow, with one or two additional grit abrasives and a final shine surface. They can also be made as a three- or four-sided block buffer. When creating a high shine, begin with the lowest grit abrasive surface, move to the higher grit, and then finish with the shining surface (usually no-grit).

These buffers are generally used on natural nails or in the final steps of the two-color application of monomer liquid and polymer powder nails, such as the French manicure look, for nails that will be worn without polish. Most two- or three-way buffers are single-use only and must be thrown away after each use. The salon or technician must find an inexpensive source for purchasing them if regulations in the state allow the use of these buffers.

figure 25-20
Three-way shine buffers

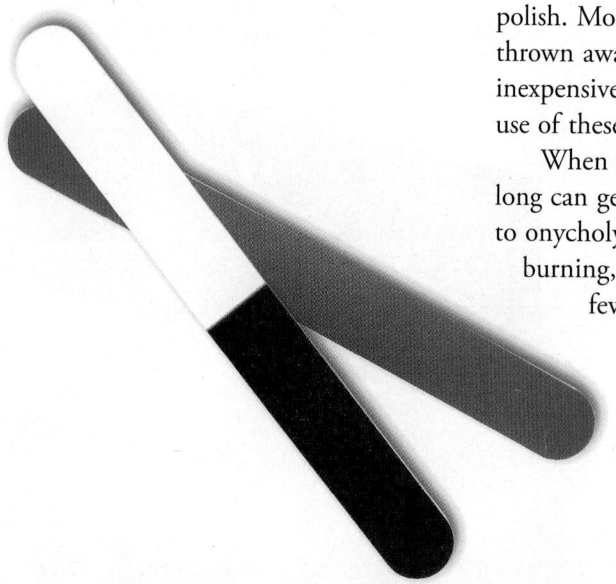

Courtesy of purespadirect.com

When buffing the nail plate, applying excessive pressure or buffing too long can generate excessive and painful heat on the nail bed. This can lead to onycholysis and possible infection. If your client is feeling heat or burning, lighten the pressure, lower the speed of the buffing, and buff fewer times between raising the buffer from the surface.

Single-Use or Terry Cloth Towels

Cloth towels must be laundered between clients, and paper towels must be thrown away after each use. A fresh, clean terry cloth towel or a new disposable paper towel is used by the client after washing his or her hands. Other clean towels are used to cover any surfaces that can become contaminated during each manicure, including the work area. If spills occur on the table, different terry cloth or single-use towels must be used to wipe them from the surface.

Be sure that your towels look clean and are not worn. The best terry cloth towels for use in a personal service are white so they can be bleached during their washing between uses. A towel with stains or holes will affect how your client feels about their service. A dirty towel can cause a client either to not come back or to report your salon to the state board.

Gauze, Cotton Balls, or Plastic-Backed Pads

Lint-free, plastic-backed, fiber or cotton pads are often used to remove nail polish. Plastic backing protects nail professionals' fingertips from overexposure to drying solvents and other chemicals (figure 25-22).

Gauze squares or cotton balls are also popular for removal of nail polish because they are inexpensive and perfectly designed for this and other application tasks. Gauze squares (2" × 2" or 4" × 4"), also called pledgets, have many uses in manicure services, from product removal to application. All these materials must be stored in a manner to prevent dust and debris from contaminating them.

Plastic or Metal Spatulas

A single-use plastic or multiuse metal spatula must be used for removing products from their respective containers to prevent contamination of the products and the spread of disease. If a spatula comes into contact with your or the client's skin, it must be properly cleaned and disinfected before being used again, or it must be replaced. Also, never use the same spatula to remove dissimilar products from different containers because the chemistry of the products may be altered.

Professional Nail Products

As a professional, you need to know how to properly use each nail product, what ingredients it contains, and what it does during use. You must also know how to properly store products and remove them from their containers in a hygienic manner. This section provides basic information regarding several professional nail products that are used during a manicure.

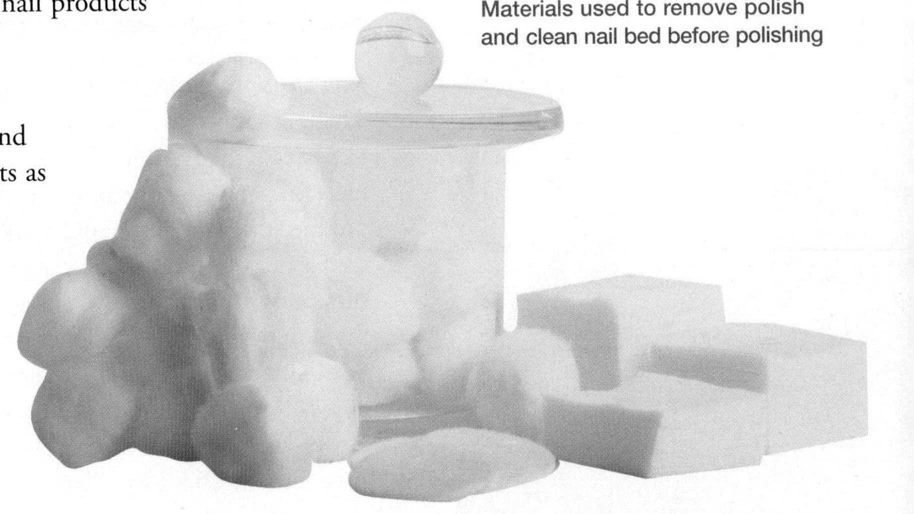

Soap

Soap is used to clean the cosmetologist's and client's hands before a service begins. It acts as an infection control tool during the pre-service hand washing procedure by mechanically removing microbes and debris. Soap is known to remove over 90 percent of pathogenic microbes from the hands, when hand washing is performed properly.

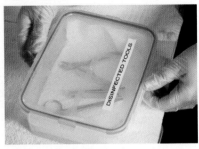

⚠ CAUTION

Abrasives or other implements cannot be stored in a plastic bag or other sealed containers because airtight conditions create the perfect environment for pathogens to grow and multiply before the next use. Always clean, disinfect, and store implements in a clean, unsealed container that allows air to circulate, or roll implements in a towel as a service set (figure 25-21).

figure 25-21
Store disinfected implements in a covered container.

figure 25-22
Materials used to remove polish and clean nail bed before polishing

Liquid soaps (figure 25-23) are recommended and preferred because bar soaps harbor bacteria and can become a breeding ground for pathogenic (disease-producing) bacteria.

Polish Remover

Polish removers are used to dissolve and remove nail polish. There are two types of polish removers available: acetone and non-acetone based products. **Acetone** is a colorless, inflammable liquid, miscible with water, alcohol, and ether, and has a sweetish odor or burning taste; it is used as a solvent. Both acetone-based and non-acetone-based removers may contain additional ingredients such as aloe, vitamin E, or oils to prevent drying of the nail plate and surrounding skin.

Acetone-based polish remover works more quickly and is a better solvent than non-acetone based removers. Non-acetone removers will not dissolve enhancement products as quickly as acetone, so they are preferred when removing nail polish from nail enhancements such as wraps. However, many experienced nail technicians prefer acetone-based removers because, due to their experience, they can work faster removing the polish and feel their speedy work and the rapid evaporation of the acetone prevents the dissolving of the enhancements. Both acetone and non-acetone-based polish removers can be used safely, but both can be drying to the cuticle and surrounding skin. As with all products, read and follow the manufacturer's instructions for use.

When using polish remover, saturate a cotton ball, gauze pad, or plastic-backed cotton pad and hold the saturated cotton on each nail while you silently count to 10. The old polish will now come off easily from the nail plate with a stroking motion, moving toward the free edge. Use a confident, firm touch while removing the polish. Continue until all traces of polish are gone. Complete removal of the polish from the previous manicure is important for client satisfaction. It may be necessary to wrap cotton around the tip of a wooden pusher and wet with polish remover to clean polish away from the nail fold area.

According to OSHA, you must follow instructions for safely disposing of used chemicals. *DO NOT* pour them down the sink or toilet, throw them on the ground or down outside drains, or pour them onto cotton balls. Some chemicals have specific disposal requirements. For example, used liquid acetone must be saved in a fire department-approved metal container and disposed of as hazardous waste.

Nail Creams, Lotions, and Oils

These products are designed to soften dry skin around the nail plate and to increase the flexibility of natural nails. They are especially effective on nails that appear to be brittle or dry, and they are the number one nail product that should be sold to manicure and pedicure clients. **Nail creams** are barrier products because they contain ingredients designed to seal the surface of the skin around the nail and hold in the subdermal moisture in the skin. **Nail oils** are designed to absorb into the nail plate to increase flexibility and into the surrounding skin to soften and moisturize. Typically, oils and lotions can penetrate the nail plate or skin and will have longer-lasting effects than creams, but all three products can be highly effective and useful for clients, especially as daily-use home-care products.

figure 25-23
Use pump bottles of soap at hand washing stations. Do not use bar soaps because they harbor bacteria.

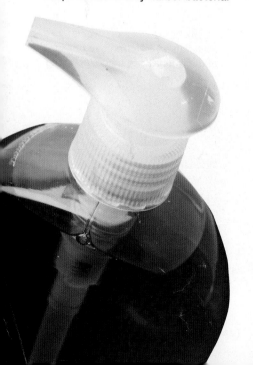

Cuticle Removers

Cuticle removers are designed to loosen and dissolve dead tissue on the nail plate so that this tissue can be more easily and thoroughly removed from the nail plate; therefore, they are inappropriate for contact with the living skin of the eponychium. Typically, these products have a high pH (caustic) and are irritating to the skin. Be careful during application that the cuticle remover is applied to the nail plate and not the surrounding skin.

These products typically contain 2 to 5 percent sodium or potassium hydroxide, with added glycerin or other moisturizing ingredients to counteract the skin-drying effects of the remover. These products must be used in strict accordance with the manufacturer's directions, and skin contact must be avoided where possible to counter the effects of the alkaline ingredients. Excessive exposure of the eponychium to cuticle removers can cause skin and eponychium dryness, leading to hangnails.

To avoid cross contamination, be sure to apply cuticle remover from a clean, sterile palette.

Nail Bleach

These products are designed to apply to the nail plate and under the free edge of natural nails to remove yellow surface discoloration or stains (e.g., tobacco stains). Usually, nail bleaches contain hydrogen peroxide or some other keratin-bleaching agent. Always use these products exactly as directed by the manufacturer to avoid damaging the natural nail plate or surrounding skin.

Apply the bleaching agent to the yellowed nail with a cotton-tipped wooden pusher. Be careful not to apply bleach on your client's skin because it may cause irritation. Wear gloves while bleaching the nails.

Repeat the application if the nails are extremely yellow. You may need to bleach certain clients' nails several times over several services because all of the yellow stain or discoloration may not fade after a single service. If this is true, inform the client so he or she will not be disappointed in your work; suggest a series of treatments to address the problem. Surface stains are removed more easily than those that travel deep into the nail plate. In fact, yellow discoloration that penetrates deep into the nail plate will never be completely removed by nail bleaches. However, the yellowing can be improved.

Colored Polish, Enamel, Lacquer, or Varnish

Colored coatings applied to the natural nail plate are known as *polish*, *enamel*, *lacquer*, or *varnish*. These are all marketing terms used to describe the same types of products containing similar ingredients. There are no real differences in the products.

Polish is a generic term describing any type of solvent-based colored film applied to the nail plate for the purpose of adding color or special visual effects (e.g., sparkles). Polish is usually applied in two coats over a base coat and then followed by a top coat (**figure 25-24**).

When applying nail polish, remove the brush from the bottle and wipe the side of the brush away from you on the inside of the lip of the bottle to remove excess polish. You should have a bead of polish on the

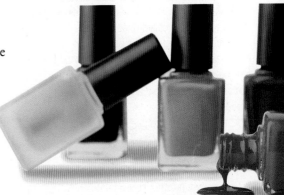

figure 25-24
Polish and top coat for manicure

end of the other side of the brush large enough to apply one layer to the entire nail plate without having to re-dip the brush (unless the nail plate is unusually long or large). Hold the brush at approximately a 30- to 35-degree angle.

Gel Polish Products

A form of nail color that lasts 10 to 21 days is a high-demand salon service that addresses the constant smudging clients experience after a manicure. Developed specifically for natural nails, this light-cured polish will bring your manicure clients back every two weeks for a removal, manicure, and new application. The secret to these gel polish colors is their speedy method of drying or curing under a UV or LED lamp, (see Chapter 29, Light Cured Gels).

The application is basically the same as traditional polishes, although there are nuances that should be learned through education by the manufacturer of the gel. Gel polishes also require a light-cured base coat and top coat that optimally is from the manufacturer that designed the gel polish.

Base Coat

A base coat creates a colorless layer on the natural nail and nail enhancement that promotes adhesion of polish. It also helps to prevent the polish pigments from creating a yellowish stain or other discoloration on the natural nail plate. Some nail plates are especially susceptible to stains from red or dark colors, so the base coat step is important. Base coats are also important to use on nail enhancements under colored polish to prevent surface staining. Base coats usually rely on adhesives, which aid in retaining polish for a longer time. Like nail polishes, base coats contain solvents designed to evaporate. After evaporation, a sticky, adhesion-promoting film is left behind on the surface of the nail plate to increase adhesion of the colored coating.

Nail Hardener

Nail hardeners are used to improve the surface hardness or durability of weak or thin nail plates. If used properly, some nail hardeners can also prevent splitting or peeling of the nail plate. Hardeners can be applied before the base coat or after as a top coat, according to the manufacturer's directions.

There are several basic types of nail hardeners:

Protein hardener is a combination of clear polish and protein, such as collagen. These provide a clear, hard coating on the surface of the nail but do not change or affect the natural nail plate itself. Protein (collagen) has very large molecules that cannot be absorbed into the nail plate.

Other nail hardeners contain reinforcing fibers such as nylon that also cannot be absorbed into the nail plate. Therefore, the protection they provide comes from the coating itself. They are not therapeutic. These products can be used on any natural nail.

The ingredient in hardeners that was once believed to be formaldehyde is actually methylene glycol, an ingredient that creates bridges or cross-links between the keratin strands that make up the natural nail, making the plate stiffer and more resistant to bending and breaking. Methylene glycol is also nonirritating to the skin.

These products are useful for thin and weak nail plates, but should never be applied to nails that are already very hard, rigid, and/or brittle. Methylene glycol hardeners can make brittle nails become so rigid that they may split and shatter. If signs of excessive brittleness or splitting, discoloration of the nail bed, or other signs of adverse nail and skin reactions occur, discontinue use. These products should be used as instructed by the manufacturer until the client's nails reach the desired goal, and then use should be discontinued until the product is needed again. Clients are generally instructed to apply the product daily over nail polish as a top coat, or under nail polish as a base coat when the polish is removed and reapplied. Clients must be instructed to follow the manufacturer's instructions.

Dimethyl urea hardeners (DY-meth-il yoo-REE-uh hard-en-ers) use dimethyl urea (DMU) to add cross-links to the natural nail plate; DMU does not cause adverse skin reactions. These hardeners do not work as quickly as hardeners containing methylene glycol, but they will not over harden nails as those with methylene glycol can with overuse.

Top Coat

Top coats are applied over colored polish to prevent chipping and to add a shine to the finished nail. These products contain ingredients that create hard, shiny films after the solvent has evaporated. Typically, the main ingredients are methacrylic or cellulose-type film formers.

Nail Polish Dryer Products

Nail polish drying accelerators are designed to be used over a top coat to hasten the drying of nail polishes. They are typically applied with a dropper, a brush, or are sprayed onto the surface of the polish. They promote rapid drying by pulling solvents from the nail polish, causing the colored film to form more quickly. These products can dramatically shorten drying time and will reduce the risk of the client smudging the recent polish application.

Hand Creams and Lotions

Hand creams and lotions add a finishing touch to a manicure. Since they soften and smooth the hands, they make the skin and finished manicure look as beautiful as possible. Hand creams are generally designed to be barriers on the skin to help the skin retain its natural moisture. They often contain penetrating ingredients to soften the skin or repair damage. A hand cream's purpose is to make the skin on the hands less prone to becoming dry or cracked. Lotion is generally more penetrating than creams and may treat lower levels of the epidermis. A treatment lotion can be used with warming mitts or paraffin treatments to enhance penetration of the ingredients into the skin.

Nail Conditioners

Nail conditioners contain ingredients to reduce brittleness of the nail. They should be applied as directed by the manufacturer. This treatment is especially useful when applied at night before bedtime. Nail conditioners can be oils, lotions, or creams.

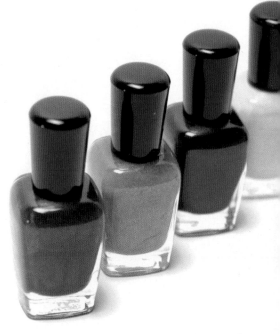

Sunscreens

These lotions radiation contain ingredients that protect the skin from damage by the ultraviolet radiation (UVA) from the sun. UVA is known to cause age spots (hyperpigmentation) on the backs of the hands and damage to the DNA of skin cells. Overexposure to the sun is known as a major cause of aging and skin cancer. Encourage your clients to purchase and use sunscreen on all their exposed skin.

After reading the next few sections, you will be able to:

LO**5** Name and describe the three-part procedure used in the performance of the basic manicure.

LO**6** Explain why a consultation is important before a service in the salon.

LO**7** List and describe the five basic nail shapes for women.

Learn the Necessary Components to Perform the Basic Manicure

The basic manicure is the foundation of all nail technology services, and it is vital that you know and recognize all of the components necessary for making the basic manicure service successful. The information you learn for the basic manicure will serve as your foundation for all of the other nail services you will perform in your career.

Work to get your basic manicure procedure to 30 or 45 minutes at the most, including polishing, before you leave school to make you more hirable and more successful in your career. Practice until you can perform the skills automatically, without considering what is next in the protocol, and you will portray the confidence and professional aura that clients prefer in their cosmetologist (and that salon owners prefer in their employees).

Always start with the left hand, pinky finger when starting a new procedure step. This will help to create a pattern as you practice, which will increase your speed and help you to memorize your steps.

Three-Part Procedure

It is easier to keep track of what you are doing, to remain organized, and to give consistent service if you break your nail care procedures down into three individual parts. These three parts are: pre-service, actual service, and post-service.

A. Pre-Service Procedure

The pre-service procedure is an organized, step-by-step plan for the cleaning and disinfecting of your tools, implements, and materials; for setting up the basic manicuring table; and for meeting, greeting, and escorting your client to your service area.

Ⓟ 25-1   Pre-Service Procedure *See page 880*

B. Service Procedure

The service procedure is an organized, step-by-step plan for accomplishing the actual service the client has requested, such as a manicure, pedicure, or nail tips and wraps.

C. Post-Service Procedure

The post-service procedure is an organized, step-by-step plan for caring for your client after the procedure has been completed. It details helping your client through the scheduling and payment process of the salon and provides information for you on how to prepare for the next client.

Ⓟ 25-2   Post-Service Procedure *See page 884*

Hand Washing

To prevent the spread of communicable disease, it is imperative to wash your hands before and after each client—and to have your clients wash their hands before they sit down at your cleaned and disinfected manicure table. The practice of hand washing before any procedure should be so well taught to your regular clients that they go directly to the washing station before coming to your station.

The Manicure Consultation

The consultation with the client before the manicure, or any other service, is an opportunity for the cosmetologist to know and understand a client's expectations. Do not rush through the consultation—it is an important part of the service! Review the steps of the client consultation in Chapter 4, Communicating for Success.

If the client is new to the salon, he or she should already have filled out the information on the intake form in the waiting room. Use this information to perform the client consultation. In fact, keep the intake form close by throughout the procedure for reference. Look at the forms closely for important responses from the client, and then record your observations after the service on a service record card or using the salon software program.

Always check the client's nails and skin to make sure that they are healthy and that the service you are providing is appropriate. Next, discuss the shape, color, and length of nails that your client prefers. You must be careful not to diagnose a disease or disorder in any way. All information should then be

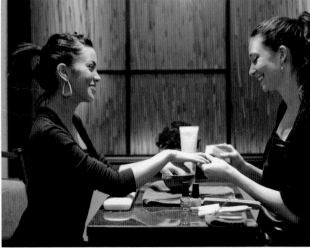

Nail Consultation

Here are a few tips to consider discussing with a client when conducting a consultation with a client for nail services:

1. Evaluate the client's nails for length, strength, and healthiness.
2. Take note of whether they are long, short, or somewhere in between.
3. Notice if the nails are healthy and strong, brittle, or weak.
4. Discuss the client's nail history. Find out what nail services they had in the past, such as manicures, pedicures, or nail enhancements, and ask about the outcome of those services.
5. Examine the shape of the client's nails and nail bed to determine an ideal length and shape for the nails. Also ask the client what nail length and shape they prefer and why they like them.
6. Show the client some photos of finished looks in your nail art books. Also show color wheels and nail art rings. Ask the client to point out the looks and colors they like and the ones they do not like. Ask the client to elaborate as to why they do or do not like them.

7. Make some valid nail service suggestions to the client based on his or her lifestyle and any other relevant characteristics you've learned about them.
8. If the client has expressed any unrealistic expectations or pointed out any unrealistic photos, tactfully explain why certain services may not work for them based on individual characteristics or personal needs.
9. Explain what maintenance services they will need to maintain the service they are receiving and how often they will need to schedule this. Also go over any home maintenance the client will need to perform in order to keep the nails looking their best between salon services.

recorded on the service record card. If there are no health issues observed, continue with the service.

Keep the following considerations in mind: shape of the hands, length of fingers, and shape of the eponychium area. Generally, it is recommended that the shape of the nail's free edge should enhance the overall shape of the fingertips, fingers, and hands of the client. You also need to think about your client's lifestyle; such things as hobbies, recreational activities, and type of work can determine the best nail shape and length.

Basic Nail Shapes for Women

During the consultation, you should discuss the final shape your client wants for her nails, and, of course, you should do your best to please her. Table 25-1 details the five basic shapes that women most often prefer.

Choosing a Nail Color

Polishing is very important for the satisfaction of your clients and for the success of the service, and it may help determine whether clients return to you. Polishing is the last step in a perfect manicure, and it gives your clients a constant visual reminder between visits of the quality of your work. When your clients look at nails that are polished perfectly, they will admire your work and will likely return. If the polish is not applied perfectly, they will have a constant reminder (for a week or more) of a less-than-perfect manicure and may not return.

Many clients will ask for help in choosing a polish color. They may ask, "Do you like this color?" Suggest a shade that complements the client's skin tone by placing the hand on a white towel under your true-color light, then holding the potential polish colors over the skin on the top of the hand. It is best to allow the client to make the choices to ensure their satisfaction. If the manicure is for a special occasion, you might suggest the client pick a color that matches or coordinates with the clothing she will wear; or perhaps the color can represent the holiday, the event, or the season. Some clients will request nail art or other nail fashion enhancements that are popular at the time. Generally, darker shades are appropriate for fall and winter and lighter shades are better for spring and summer; however, this is no longer a hard-and-fast fashion rule. Always have a wide variety of nail polish colors available and the appropriate colors for the French manicure polish techniques.

Applying Polish

The most successful nail polish application is achieved by using four coats. The first, the base coat, is followed by two coats of polish color and one application of top coat to give a protective seal. Applying multiple layers of polish improves the longevity and durability of the overall application (figure 25-25). By building layer upon layer, you will improve adhesion and staying power.

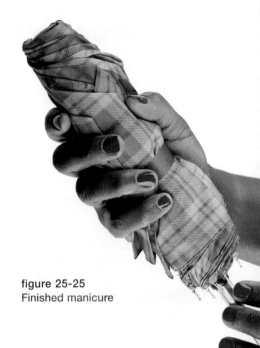

figure 25-25
Finished manicure

table 25-1
BASIC NAIL SHAPES

Shape	Definition
square	The **square nail** is completely straight across the free edge with no rounding at the outside edges.
squoval	The **squoval nail** has a square free edge that is rounded off at the corner edges. If the nail extends only slightly past the fingertip, this shape will be sturdy because there is no square edge to break off, and any pressure on the tip will be reflected directly back to the nail plate, its strongest area. Clients who work with their hands—nurses, computer technicians, landscapers, or office workers—will need shorter, squoval nails.
round	The **round nail** should be slightly tapered and usually should extend just a bit past the fingertip.
oval	The **oval nail** is a conservative nail shape that is thought to be attractive on most women's hands. It is similar to a squoval nail with even more rounded corners. Professional clients who have their hands on display (e.g., businesspeople, teachers, or salespeople) may want longer oval nails.
pointed	The **pointed nail** is suited to thin hands with long fingers and narrow nail beds. The nail is tapered and longer than usual to emphasize and enhance the slender appearance of the hand. Know, however, that this nail shape may be weaker, may break more easily, and is more difficult to maintain than other nail shapes. Rarely are natural nails successful with this nail shape, so they are usually enhancements. They are for fashion-conscious people who do not need the strongest, most durable shape of nail enhancements.

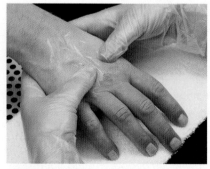
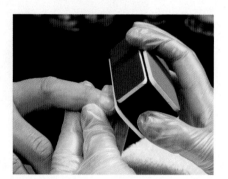
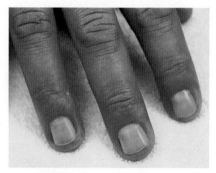

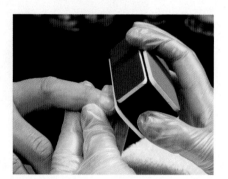

figure 25-26
Buffing a client's nails

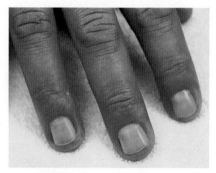

figure 25-27
Round nails are the shape most men choose.

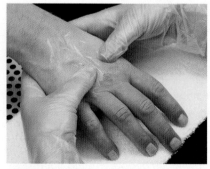

figure 25-28
Beginning a hand massage

The application techniques are the same for all polishes, base coats, and top coats. Apply thin, even coats to create maximum smoothness and minimum drying time. When you have completed the polish application, the nail should look smooth, evenly polished, and shiny.

Ⓟ 25-5   **Polishing the Nails** *See page 893*

After reading the next few sections, you will be able to:

LO❽   Describe the most popular nail shape for men.

How to Cater to a Man's Manicure Service

Since men are becoming more and more interested in their grooming regimens, many now seek services offered for hands and fingernails. A man's manicure is executed using the same procedures as described in the basic manicure, though you omit the colored polish and/or buff the nails with a high-shine buffer (figure 25-26).

Most men tend to go longer between services and will need a little more work than women on their nails and skin. A citrus- or spice-scented hand cream is recommended for the male client rather than a floral scent.

Men's Nail Shapes

Men usually prefer their nails shorter than women do. Round nails are the most common choice for male clients because of their natural appearance. Some men, however, prefer their nails really short, with only a small amount of free edge that is shaped according to the base of the nail plate (figure 25-27).

Men's Massage

Most men enjoy the massage portion of the manicure and want a longer one! Usually men will want a firmer effleurage than women, but that does not mean a deep, sports-type massage—since you are not trained to perform that massage. It just means firmer finger movements on the palm and longer, firmer slides in your effleurage movements (figure 25-28).

Most times, unless the hands are in very poor shape, you can give men a longer massage since polish time is not a factor.

Men's Basic Color: Clear

Men usually prefer buffed nails, clear gloss, or a dull, clear satin coating. This satin-coating nail polish finish is designed especially to help men protect their nails without having nails that appear too polished or feminine (figure 25-29). Although a man may rarely want a shiny top coat or colored nail polish on his nails, you should always discuss his preferences during the client consultation.

You must prepare the nails for polish (remove oils and debris) carefully because peeling or chipping gloss is very annoying to men. Use a base coat under clear to encourage staying power; clear without a base tends to peel. Apply a thin base coat and then one thin coat of clear and a quick-drying top coat or just one coat of base and a satin clear.

Always ask for the next appointment and suggest having a pedicure with the manicure. Most men enjoy pedicures!

Marketing to Men

Since most men are new to professional nail care, include on your service menu and your website a brief written description of what is included in the service and a rundown of the benefits. To target men, you may also want to distribute flyers at local athletic gyms and stores, or other places where men gather. Gift certificates sold to your female clients for their boyfriends and husbands are great marketing tools.

To make men feel more at home in your chair, have men's magazines on hand and be careful that your decor is unisex. Staying open later or opening earlier on chosen days makes it easier for your male clients to schedule appointments. Many salons and spas also have a weekly or biweekly men's night, with no women allowed, so male clients can come in without being among women.

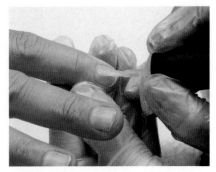

figure 25-29
Most men prefer buffed nails, clear gloss, or a dull clear coating.

After reading the next few sections, you will be able to:

LO**9** **List the massage movements for performing a relaxing hand and arm massage.**

Complete a Hand and Arm Massage

Massage is the manipulation of the soft tissues of the body. It is an ancient therapeutic treatment to promote circulation of the blood and lymph, relaxation of the muscles, and relief from pain. It also has many other benefits. A hand and arm massage, a manicuring specialty, is a service that can be offered with all types of manicures. It is included in all spa manicures, and can be performed on most clients.

A massage is one of the client's highest priorities during the manicure, and often it is the most memorable part of the manicure. Most clients look forward to the soothing and relaxing effects. The massage manipulations should be executed with rhythmic, long, and smooth movements, and you should always have one hand on the client's arm or hand during the movements and the transitions between them. Hand and arm massages are optional during a basic manicure, but it is to the advantage of the cosmetologist to incorporate this special, relaxing segment of a manicure because it is many clients' favorite part of the service.

Before performing a hand and arm massage, make sure that you are sitting in a comfortable position and are not stretching or leaning forward toward your customer. Your posture should be correct and relaxed, and your feet should be parallel and flat on the floor. Sitting or working in an uncomfortable or strained position can cause back, neck, and shoulder injuries.

General Movements

Massage is a series of movements performed on the human body that, in combination, produce relaxation or treatment.

The following movements are usually combined to complete a massage:

- **Effleurage** (EF-loo-rahzh) is a succession of strokes in which the hands glide over an area of the body with varying degrees of pressure or contact.

- Pétrissage (PEH-treh-sahz) or kneading is lifting, squeezing, and pressing the tissue.

- Tapotement (tah-POT-ment) is a rapid tapping or striking motion of the hands against the skin.

- Vibration is a continuous trembling or shaking movement applied by the hand without leaving contact with the skin.

- **Friction** incorporates various strokes that manipulate or press one layer of tissue over another. The hands are placed around the arm with the fingers pointing in opposite directions and then are gently twisted in opposite directions on the arm as one would wring out a washcloth. Perform the movement up and down the forearm, sliding to the new position three to five times (**figure 25-30**).

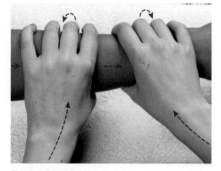

figure 25-30
Friction

The purpose of massage in manicuring is the inducement of relaxation. For that reason, effleurage is the movement that should be perfected, varied, and expertly used. Be sure to hold the client's hand or arm loosely without too much restraint during the massage. A firm but gentle, slow, and rhythmic movement in a predictable routine is the key to a relaxing massage. Moving quickly sends the message to the client that you are hurrying to get the massage over and do not care about providing a good service. Take care not to press or move with pressure over the bones of the arms as this can be quite painful.

Before performing a service that includes a hand and/or arm massage, consult the client's intake form. During the consultation acknowledge and discuss any medical condition your client listed that may be contraindicated for a massage. If they have not discussed massage with their physician, encourage them to do so before performing the service.

Many clients who have high blood pressure (hypertension), diabetes, or circulatory conditions may still have hand and/or arm massage without concern, especially if their condition is being treated by a physician. Hand

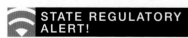

STATE REGULATORY ALERT!

In a few states, your cosmetology license does not permit you to perform a hand or foot massage. Be guided by your instructor concerning your state's mandatory requirements and procedures for massage during nail services.

and/or arm massage is, however, contraindicated for clients with severe, uncontrolled hypertension. Avoid using vigorous or strong massage techniques on clients who have arthritis.

When making decisions about whether to perform a massage on a person who has a medical condition, be conservative. When in doubt, don't include massage as part of your service.

In the traditional manicure, the massage is performed after the basic manicure procedures, right before the polish application. Do not talk to your client during the massage except to ask once whether your touch should be more or less firm. Talking disturbs the relaxation therapy of the massage. If more cream, oil, or lotion is needed during the massage, always leave one hand on the client's hand or arm and retrieve more product with the other. Having your product in a pump container facilitates this important massage technique.

After performing a massage, it is essential that the nail plate be thoroughly cleansed to ensure that it is free from any residue such as oil, cream, wax, or lotion. You can use alcohol, acetone, or nail polish remover to cleanse the nail plate.

(P) 25-4   **Hand and Arm Massage** *See page 890*

After reading the next few sections, you will be able to:

LO⑩   **Explain the differences between spa manicures and basic manicures.**

State the Differences Between Spa Manicures and Basic Manicures

Spa manicures, a step beyond the basic manicure with added specialty techniques and skin treatments, are fast becoming much-requested and desired salon services, but they require more advanced techniques than basic manicures. Cosmetologists who advance their education and knowledge of spa manicures and their specialized techniques will not only make their clients happy, but also find that these manicures are very lucrative as well.

True spa manicures require extensive knowledge not only of nail care, but of skin care as well. Many spa manicures are exceptionally pampering, while others target specific results through the use of advanced skin-care-based methods. Most spa manicures include a relaxing massage, and all spa manicures include some form of exfoliation for not only polishing and smoothing the skin, but also for enhancing penetration of professional products.

? DID YOU KNOW?

Some clients may ask for products that are chemical-free. The truth is that no products are or can be chemical-free—even air and water contain chemicals!

When faced with clients who feel strongly about their beliefs and knowledge—whether their information is correct or not—know your product line and its claims, and offer clients the information so they can make informed decisions.

Spa manicures designed for relaxation may have unique and distinctive names that describe the treatment. For example, "The Rose Garden Rejuvenation Manicure" may incorporate the use of products containing rose oils and may use rose petals for ambiance.

The results-oriented spa manicures, sometimes known as "treatment manicures," may have names that closely represent their purpose such as "The Anti-Aging Manicure" and may incorporate the use of an alpha hydroxy acid–based product for exfoliation and skin rejuvenation, or "The Scrub Manicure" may include longer exfoliation of callused skin. Many spa manicures have more imaginative names, such as "Spot-Be-Gone," for a manicure designed to lighten age spots. Treatment manicures require further training to produce safe and obvious results.

Many clients now base their service decisions on lifestyle choices, such as preferring all-natural products. These clients will seek out spa manicures that meet their needs, and they may ask about the ingredients in the products you are using. In order to know how to answer these questions, you must know whether your product lines make all-natural claims.

The reality is, despite what the product marketing implies, few all-natural products are commercially available due to their short shelf life, and virtually none are chemical-free; even air and water contain chemicals!

One natural alternative is to mix your own products from fresh ingredients. If you choose to create your own fresh products, you may want to make a small batch for each procedure or per day, because they can spoil very quickly and may require refrigeration in the salon.

Additional techniques that may be incorporated into a spa manicure consist of aromatic paraffin treatments, hand masks, and warm, moist-towel applications. When performing any advanced procedures that include oils or cosmetics, always check with your client regarding aroma preferences and allergies.

Theme Manicures

Many salons and spas have developed services around themes. The entire service contains products—from lotions to oils to masks—that support the theme the salon has chosen, and some salons even serve clients themed refreshments during the service.

Examples might include the "Chocolate Wonder Manicure and Pedicure" or the "Pumpkin Fall Festival Manicure and Pedicure." The names and themes of these kinds of services are limited only by your imagination. Let yours go wild and have fun developing these well-received manicures and pedicures. Clients love them!

Waterless Manicures

Waterless manicures eliminate soaking the nails in water and some nail technicians use lotion and heated mitts instead to soften the skin and cuticles. Many clients prefer this manicure and believe it is more relaxing and produces better results than the traditional water manicure. Many technicians prefer it because it eliminates getting water when it is inconveniently available. All manicures (basic, spa, scrub, etc.) can be performed using the dry manicure techniques.

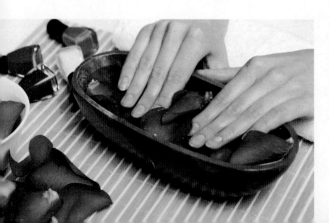

After reading the next few sections, you will be able to:

LO⓫ Describe how aromatherapy is best used in manicuring services.

Indicate Why Aromatherapy is Used During a Nail Service

In the 1870s, Professor René Maurice Gattefossé, a French scientist, discovered the therapeutic use of essential oils, which are inhaled or applied to the skin. These oils are used in manicures, pedicures, and massages to induce such reactions as relaxation or invigoration or to simply create a pleasant fragrance during the service. Many clients enjoy the various aromas, so when it is appropriate, incorporate aromatherapy into your nail services.

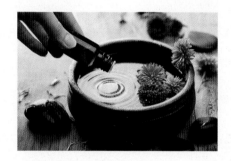

The practice of aromatherapy involves the use of highly concentrated, **essential oils**. These oils are extracted using various forms of distillation from seeds, bark, roots, leaves, wood, and/or resin of plants. Each part of these resources produces a different aroma. For instance, the needles, resin, and wood of a Scotch pine tree all yield a different aroma and, therefore, a different response from the target person. The use of essential oils is limited only by the knowledge of the person controlling their application.

Performing aromatherapy requires study and expert use of the knowledge gained. The oils are very powerful and can produce actual changes in the client. In some countries, the oils are considered medicines and are only prescribed by physicians. Therefore, unless a cosmetologist is prepared to study these oils in-depth, he or she should use blended oils, those that are already mixed and tested, and apply them only as directed.

Summarize the Benefits of Paraffin Wax Treatments

Paraffin wax treatments are designed to trap moisture in the skin while the heat causes skin pores to open to allow deeper penetration of lotions and oils used prior to application. Besides opening the pores, heat from the warm paraffin increases blood circulation and can provide pain relief for those with arthritis or sore muscles. This is considered to be a luxurious add-on service and can be safely performed on most clients.

Be sure to examine the client's intake form during the client consultation to identify any contraindications to wax or the heat involved in the service and to discuss any additional precautions that should be taken for clients with health factors or risks. Generally, you should avoid giving paraffin treatments to anyone who has impaired circulation or skin irritations such as cuts, burns, rashes, warts, or eczema. Senior citizens and chronically ill clients may be more sensitive to heat because of medications or thinning of the skin. In these cases, ask the clients to bring their physician's permission prior to having a paraffin treatment.

When applying paraffin to your clients, there are many different application methods available. Whatever method you choose, be sure that the paraffin bath is not contaminated by direct contact with you or the client's skin. Also remember that once paraffin has been used on a client, it must be discarded. It is against state board regulations to re-melt and reuse paraffin.

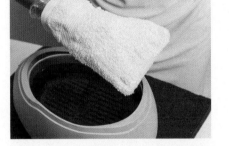

1. Plastic Bag Paraffin Application

An easy way to apply paraffin to hands or feet is by using a metal measuring cup to add equal amounts of warm paraffin to two small, clear plastic bags. Place the bags against the client's hands or feet to check if the temperature is comfortable to them. If the paraffin is too hot, cool it by shaking it in the bag for a few moments. Once the client is comfortable with the temperature, slide the bag onto the client's hand or foot and massage the bag of paraffin against the skin. Once the paraffin has reached the top of the bag, twist and tuck the edge to secure and apply a terry cloth mitt, or wrap with a terry cloth towel. Repeat on the other hand or foot and allow the client to rest for five to ten minutes. To remove, loosen the paraffin from the skin by massaging the bag against the skin and working the paraffin down into the bottom of the bag until all paraffin is removed from the client's skin. Tie a knot in the bag to secure the used paraffin and discard in the trash.

2. Cheesecloth or Paper Towel Paraffin Application

Paraffin dipped cheesecloth or paper towels can also be a luxurious application method. Have the paraffin bath close to the manicure table. It is best if the paraffin is located on a moveable cart for this method. Dip the paper or cheesecloth into the paraffin vertically by holding the corners and then raise up to allow excess paraffin to drip off. Raise and lower the paper towel or cloth three times. As each piece is ready, wrap around the clients hand or arm. Next, cover with a plastic bag or plastic wrap, and wrap in a terry cloth towel or place in a heated mitt.

3. Spray Paraffin

Spray paraffin is also an option for clean application. With this method, a special machine with replaceable paraffin cartridges is used. The warm paraffin is sprayed from the cartridge on the hands and arm and is then placed in plastic mitts or plastic wrap and inserted into terry cloth or electric mitts.

4. Single-Use Commercial Gloves

There are also one-time-use commercial gloves that have paraffin inside. The heating pad inside the glove is activated by massaging it; this heats the paraffin inside. When warm, insert the hands into the heated paraffin mitts, and then discard the mitts when treatment is finished. Be sure to follow manufacturer's directions for all types of paraffin equipment to ensure proper use.

If proper procedures are followed, paraffin will not adversely affect nail enhancements or natural nails. A paraffin wax treatment may be offered before a manicure, during a manicure, or as a stand-alone service. Be guided by your instructor and your state regulations, because some states require the service to be performed before the manicure.

Performing the paraffin wax treatment **before** beginning a manicure has advantages. It allows the client to have their nails polished immediately at the end of the manicure service, and it is a way to pre-soften rough or callused skin.

Many salons and spas have developed manicures that include paraffin treatments during the service. These specialized treatments, such as moisture masks covered in warm paraffin wax, are performed after the massage and before polishing. Performing the paraffin treatment in the middle of the service creates a longer and more relaxed service.

During winter months, paraffin treatments are often requested as a stand-alone service. This service can be on the menu with its own price because clients like the way a paraffin treatment makes their skin feel, as well as the relaxation it provides.

Outline Nail Art Options for Clients

Nail art has never been easier to create. With so many art supplies and mediums available, getting the perfect look is easy and fun. Even basic nail polish can be used to create endless variations of designs.

Polish is one of the most common mediums of nail art used in the salon or spa (**Figure 25-31**). When considering nail art, conservative clients will be more accepting of this medium, as they are used to wearing polish. Polish is most often used to create nail art looks such as French manicures, color fades, color blocking, or marbleizing.

For a traditional **French manicure** look, the nail bed is one color, such as pink, peach, or beige (depending upon the client's skin tone), and the free edge of the nail is another color, such as white. The curved line where the pink and the white meet each other on the nail is called the **smile line**. You can achieve limitless variations to this traditional look just by changing or fading the color.

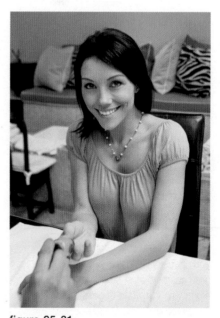

figure 25-31
Relaxed client during a spa manicure

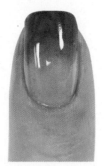

figure 25-32
A color fade can be very
subtle or bold.

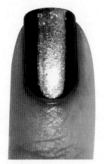

figure 25-33
Color blocking can give
dramatic results.

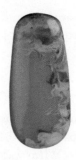

figure 25-34
Marbelizing is a simple nail art technique
that can be done to the entire nail or just
a small portion for a unique design.

Nail art by Alisha Rimando Botero.

With **color fading**, or *color graduation*, one color fades into the other, and the meeting point is a combination of the two. You can achieve this by applying the product more thickly and opaquely and then using the product more thinly and translucently when meeting the other color (**figure 25-32**). For example, if the top third of the nail is dark pink and the bottom third is light pink, then the middle third should be a combination of the two colors. There are multiple ways to achieve this look. Use a sponge or brush to blend colors at the meeting point.

Color blocking is just as it sounds: blocks or sections of color on the nail. Achieve this look by polishing the entire nail with a base color, such as black, and then creating stripes or blocks with another color, such as silver (**figure 25-33**).

Marbleizing is a swirled effect created when you combine two or more colors while wet and then mix them on the nail with a marbleizing tool known as a stylus (**figure 25-34**). A **stylus** is a tool with a solid handle with a rounded ball tip on each end that can range in size (**figure 25-35**). The rounded ball tips are excellent for swirling colors; dotting small circles of color; creating polka dots, eyes, bubbles; and much more. This marbleized effect can be applied over the entire nail or just on a part of the nail for a unique nail art creation.

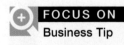
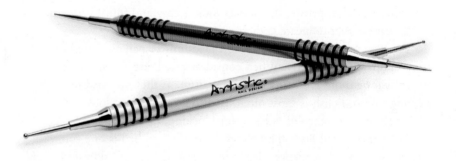

figure 25-35
Stylus tools can be used for marbleizing, creating dot designs, and many other
nail art techniques.

Courtesy of Artistic Nail Design

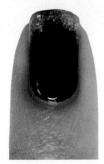

figure 25-36
Variations to the classic French manicure provide endless possibilities.

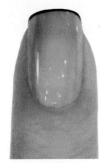

figure 25-37
Clean and classic with a little edge

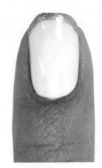

figure 25-38
Bridal white with a hint of glamour

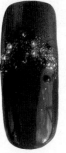

figure 25-39
Create more drama by adding embellishments.

The French Manicure

The French manicure is one of the most popular nail art procedures in the salon and spa today. You must master the technique and variations of it to stay competitive in the marketplace. Try various color combinations, fading techniques, and embellishments to create looks clients will want to try (**figures 25-36** through **25-39**). A French manicure is always an upcharge in any salon or spa and an easy way to create additional income.

Many clients love the application of artistic nail art designs to finish their manicure. The techniques are fun to apply and are only limited by your imagination. Nail art techniques include free-hand designs, airbrush, and even 3-D (**figure 25-40**). They range from simple to complex (**figure 25-41**) and from portrait to modern design. Display your nail art so your clients can see it to open the conversation for adding nail art to your manicures and pedicures.

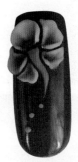
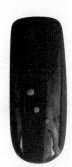

figure 25-40
3-D nail art using liquid monomer and polymer powder

Only the Beginning

During your time in school, it is important that you learn the basic procedures of nail technology, as well as the importance of proper cleaning, disinfection, and other skills necessary for ensuring client safety and enjoyment during nail procedures.

Advanced techniques in manicuring may be learned from your instructor or by attending advanced nail care seminars, reading trade magazines, and attending beauty shows.

figure 25-41
Complex nail art

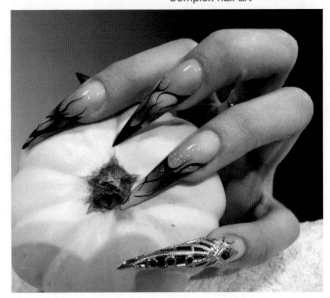

PRE-SERVICE PROCEDURE

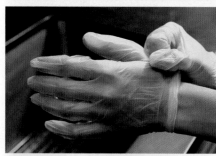

1 It is important to wear gloves while performing this pre-service procedure to prevent possible contamination of the implements by your hands and to protect your skin from the powerful chemicals in the disinfectant solution.

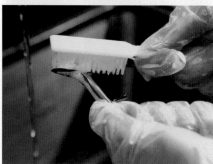

2 Rinse all implements with warm running water, and then thoroughly wash them with soap and a nail brush. Brush grooved areas and open hinged implements to scrub the area.

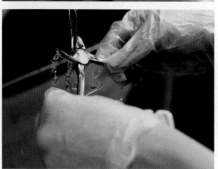

3 Rinse away all traces of soap with warm, running water. The presence of soap in most disinfectants can cause them to become inactive. Dry implements thoroughly with a clean or disposable towel, or allow them to air-dry on a clean towel. Your implements are now properly cleaned and ready to be disinfected.

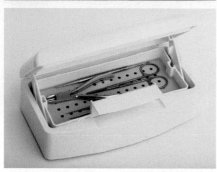

4 Implements must be completely clean and dry before you immerse them in EPA-registered disinfectant solution for the required time (usually 10 minutes). If they are not, your disinfectant may become contaminated or diluted and rendered ineffective. Remember to open hinged implements before immersing them in the disinfectant solution.

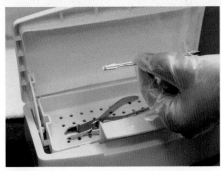 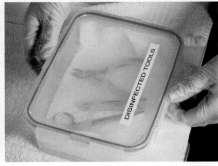 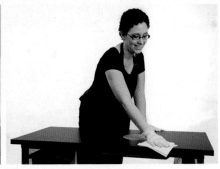

5 Remove implements, avoiding skin contact, and rinse and dry tools thoroughly.

6 Store disinfected implements in a clean, dry container until needed.

7 Clean and then disinfect manicure table and drawer with an appropriate EPA-approved disinfectant.

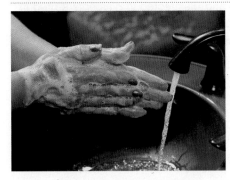

8 Remove gloves and thoroughly wash your hands with liquid soap, rinse, and dry with a clean fabric or single-use towel.

B. BASIC TABLE SETUP

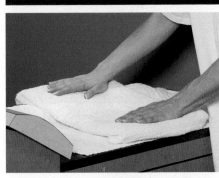

9 Place a clean cloth (preferably a lint-free disposable cloth) down to cover the width of your surface. This cloth can be replaced as needed throughout the service. Take an additional clean cloth and wrap the client's arm cushion. Position the cushion on the edge of the manicure table in front of the client. Be sure to have one end of the towel that is covering the cushion extending toward the client.

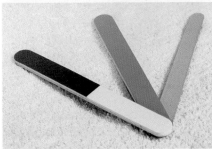

10 Place the abrasives and buffers of your choice on the table to your right if you are right-handed or to the left if left-handed. Note: You will also place the polish your client chooses to the right if you are right-handed, to the left if you are left-handed.

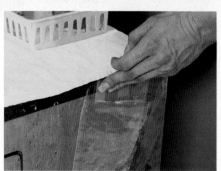

11 If a metal trash receptacle with a self-closing lid is not available, tape or clip a plastic bag that can be closed securely to the right side of the table if right handed, or to the left if left-handed. These bags must be sealed and thrown away after each client to prevent product vapors from escaping into the salon air.

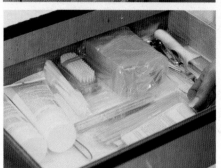

12 The drawer can be used to store the following items for immediate use: cotton balls in their original container or in a fresh plastic bag, abrasives, buffers, nail polish dryer, and other supplies. Never place used materials in your drawer. Only completely cleaned and disinfected implements stored in a sealed container (to protect them from dust and recontamination) and extra materials or professional products should be placed in the drawer. Your drawer should always be organized and clean.

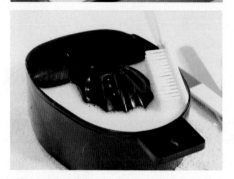

13 Before your client arrives, set out your tools and implements. Then, fill a finger bowl with warm water and place on the left or right of your table. Place your manicure brush next to the finger bowl. You will bring the finger bowl to the middle of the table, when needed.

C. GREET CLIENT

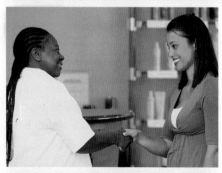

14 Greet your client with a smile, introduce yourself if you've never met, and shake hands. If the client is new, ask him or her for the consultation card she filled out in the reception area.

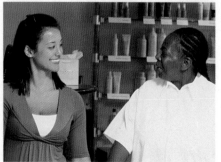

15 Escort your client to the hand washing area and demonstrate the hand washing procedure for them on your own hands. Once you have completed the demonstration, hand your client a fresh nail brush and ask the client to wash his or her hands.

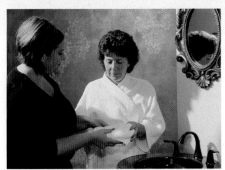

16 Hand your client a fresh paper towel or clean terry cloth towel.

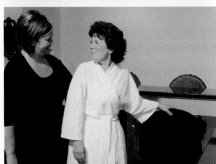

17 Show your client to your work table, and make sure they are comfortable before beginning the service.

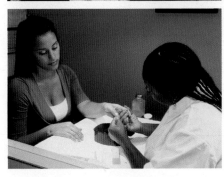

18 Determine what type of service the client is looking for. Look over the client's intake form, perform the needs assessment, and talk to the client about their responses to determine a course of action for the service. Take note of the services to be performed and reiterate everything that you and your client have agreed. Now it is time to perform the service. Remember to put on gloves at the start of each service.

POST-SERVICE PROCEDURE

A. ADVISE CLIENTS AND PROMOTE PRODUCTS

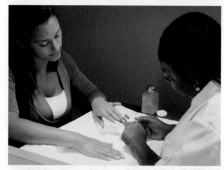

1 Proper home care will ensure that the client's nails look beautiful until he or she returns for another service (in seven to ten days).

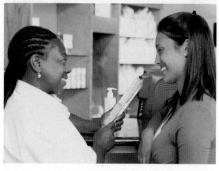

2 Depending on the service provided, there may be a number of retail products that you should recommend for the client to take home. This is the time to do so. Explain why they are important and how to use them.

B. SCHEDULE THE NEXT APPOINTMENT AND THANK THE CLIENT

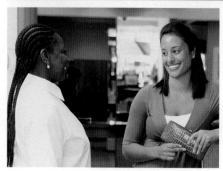

3 Escort the client to the front desk to schedule the next appointment and to collect payment for the service. Set up the date, time, and services. Then write the information on an appointment card and give it to the client.

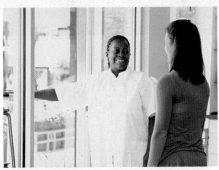

4 Before the client leaves the salon and you return to your station, be sure to thank them for their business.

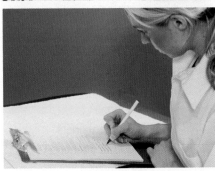

5 Record on the service record card all service information, products used, observations, and retail recommendations. Then file the form in the appropriate place.

C. PREPARE THE WORK AREA AND IMPLEMENTS FOR THE NEXT CLIENT

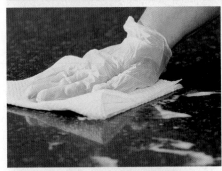

6 Remove your products and tools. Then clean and disinfect your work area, and properly dispose of all used materials.

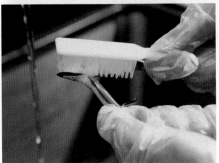

7 Follow steps for cleaning and disinfecting implements in the pre-service procedure. Reset work area with disinfected tools.

PERFORMING A BASIC MANICURE

IMPLEMENTS & MATERIALS

You will need all of the following implements, materials, and supplies on your manicuring table:

- Abrasive nail files and buffers
- Client's arm cushion
- Cuticle removers
- Electric hand/foot mitts (optional)
- Finger bowl

- Gloves
- Gauze and cotton wipe container
- Hand creams and lotions
- Nail creams, lotions, and penetrating nail oils

- Nail hardener
- Polish remover
- Service cushion (optional)
- Single-use towels or terry cloth towels
- Supply tray (optional)

- Terry cloth mitts (optional)
- Trash containers
- Wooden pusher

PREPARATION

Perform:

P 25-1   **Pre-Service Procedure** *See page 880*

PROCEDURE

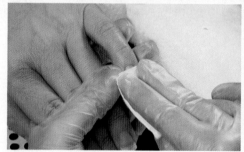

1 Remove the polish and inspect the client's nails. Begin with the little finger of your client's left hand. Saturate a cotton ball, gauze pad, or plastic-backed cotton pad with polish remover and remove existing polish. Continue until all traces of polish are gone. After removal, look closely at the nails to check for abnormalities that could have been hidden by the polish.

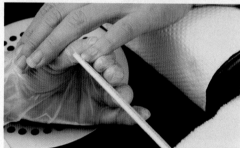

2 Shape the nails. Using a medium grit abrasive board, shape the nails as you and the client have agreed. Start with the left hand, little finger, holding it between your thumb and index finger. File from one side to the center of the free edge, then from the other side to the center of the free edge. Never use a sawing back and forth motion when filing the natural nail, as this can disrupt the nail plate layers and cause splitting and peeling.

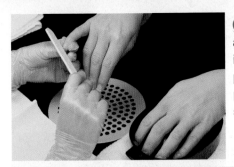

3 Soften the eponychium and cuticle. After filing the nails on the left hand, and before moving on to the right hand, place the fingertips of the left hand in the finger bowl to soak and soften the eponychium (living skin on the posterior and sides of the nail) and cuticle (dead tissue adhered to the nail plate) while you file the nails on the right hand. File the right hand nails the same as you did the left, from the little finger to the thumb.

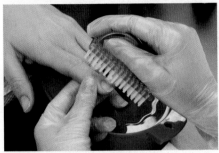

4 Clean the nail surfaces. Brushing the nails with a nail brush removes service debris from the nail surface. After filing the nails on the right hand, remove the left hand from the finger bowl. Holding the left hand above the finger bowl, brush the fingers with your wet nail brush to remove any debris from the fingertips. Use downward strokes, starting at the first knuckle and brushing toward the free edge.

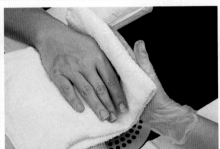

5 Dry the client's hands. Dry the hand with a towel designated as this client's service towel. As you dry, gently push back the eponychium with the towel. Now place the right hand into the finger bowl to soak while you continue with the next step on the left hand.

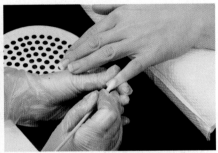

6 Next, you apply cuticle remover. Use a cotton-tipped wooden pusher or cotton swab to carefully apply cuticle remover to the cuticle on each nail plate of the left hand. Do not apply this type of product on living skin as it can cause dryness or irritation. Spread evenly on the nail plate.

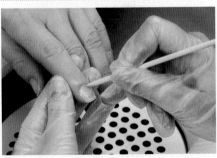

7 Loosen and remove cuticles. After you allow the product to set on the nail for the manufacturer's recommended length of time, the cuticle will be easily removed from the nail plate. Use your wooden pusher or the inside curve of a metal pusher to gently push and lift cuticle tissue off each nail plate of the left hand.

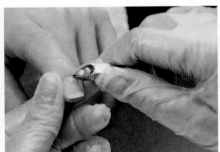

8 Use sharp nippers to remove any loose dead skin (hangnails). Never rip or tear the cuticle tags or the living skin, since this may lead to infection.

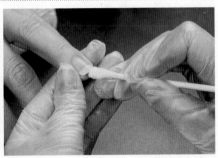

9 Clean under the free edge. Carefully clean under the free edge using a cotton swab or cotton-tipped wooden pusher. Take care to be gentle, as cleaning too aggressively in this area can break the hyponychium seal under the free edge and cause onycholysis. Remove the right hand from the finger bowl, dry the hand, and set it aside.

10 Brush off any debris. Brush the left hand over the finger bowl one last time to remove bits of debris and traces of cuticle remover. It is important that all traces of cuticle remover are washed from the skin because remnants can lead to dryness and/or irritation. Instruct the client to rest the left hand on the table towel.

11 Repeat steps 5 through 10 on the right hand.

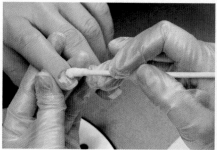

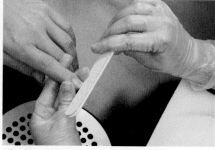

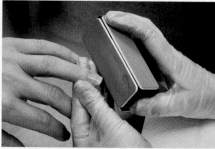

12 Bleach the nails (optional). If the client's nails are yellow, you can bleach them with nail bleach designed specifically for this purpose. Inform the client if his or her nails have deep staining that cannot be completely removed. Note: additional information on nail bleach is found on page 863.

13 Bevel nails. To remove any rough spots on the free edges, bevel (BEH-vel) the underside of the free edge. Hold a medium-grit abrasive board at a 45-degree angle to the underside of the nail and file with an upward stroke. A fine-grit abrasive board or buffer may be preferable for weak nails.

14 Buff (if desired). Use a three-way buffer if planning to end the basic manicure by applying polish. If the client will not be wearing polish, use a four-way buffer to bring the nails to a brilliant shine. Buffing will smooth out any surface scratches and give the natural nail a smooth appearance.

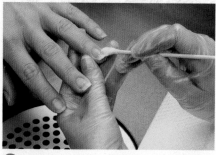

15 Apply nail oil. Use a cotton-tipped wooden pusher, a cotton swab, or an eyedropper to apply nail oil to each nail plate and massage oil into the nail and surrounding skin using a circular motion.

16 Wash and dry client's hands. Thoroughly wash the client's hands and nails with soap and water from your finger bowl, or walk the client to the appropriate hand washing station to have them wash their hands and nails. Either way is acceptable. Dry the client's hands thoroughly with a clean, disposable towel.

17 Apply massage lotion or oil. Follow the hand and arm massage in **Procedure 25-4**.

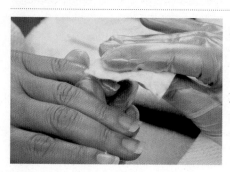

18 Remove traces of oil. After the massage, you must remove all traces of lotion or oil from the nail plate before polishing, or the polish will not adhere well. Use a lint-free wipe saturated with alcohol or polish remover as though you were removing a stubborn, red nail polish. Do not forget to clean under the free edge of the nail plate to remove any remaining massage lotion. The cleaner you get the nail plate, the better the polish will adhere.

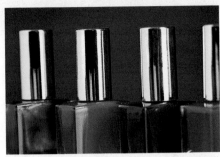

19 Confirm nail color. Most clients will have their polish already chosen before or during the consultation. If not, ask them to choose a color.

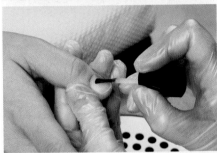

20 Complete **Procedure 25-5, Polishing the Nails.**

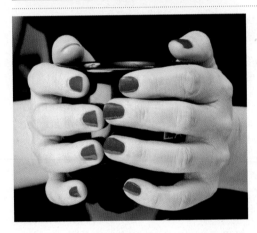

21 You have performed a beautiful, finished manicure.

POST-SERVICE

Complete:

P 25-2 **Post-Service Procedure** *See page 884*

HAND AND ARM MASSAGE

IMPLEMENTS & MATERIALS

In addition to the basic materials on your manicuring table, you will need the following supplies for the hand and arm massage:

☐ Massage lotion, oil, or cream

PREPARATION

Perform:

P 25-3 **Performing a Basic Manicure** *See page 886*

PROCEDURE FOR HAND MASSAGE

1 Start with a hand massage. Depending on which hand you start with, be sure to wrap the other hand in a clean, warm towel.

2 Apply the massage lotion, oil, or cream. Place product in your hand first and rub together to warm, then distribute to the client's hand arm. Enough should be applied to allow movement across the skin without resistance (skin drag). Skin drag is not comfortable for the client.

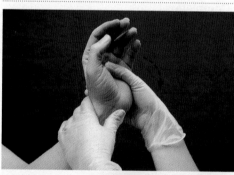

3 **Relaxer movement of wrist.** Place the client's elbow on a cushion covered with a clean towel or a rolled towel. With one hand, brace the client's arm in the wrist area with your non-dominant hand. With your other hand, hold the client's wrist and bend it back and forth slowly and gently but with a firm touch, five to ten times, until you feel that the client has relaxed.

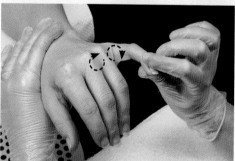

4 **Joint movement of fingers.** Lower the client's arm, brace the arm at the wrist with the left hand, and with your right hand (or dominant hand) start with the little finger, holding it at the base of the nail. Gently rotate fingers to form circles. Work toward the thumb, about three to five times on each finger.

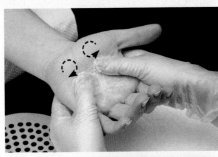

5 **Circular movement on palm.** Place the client's elbow on the cushion or towel near the center of the table and your elbows on the table at the sides of the client's elbow. With your thumbs in the client's palm, rotate them in a circular movement in opposite directions. The circular movements should start from the bottom, center of the hand and move out, up, and across the underside of the fingers, then back down to the bottom, center, in a smooth pattern of altering movements of each thumb over the palm. This pattern becomes rhythmic and relaxing. You can feel the client's hands relax as you perform these movements.

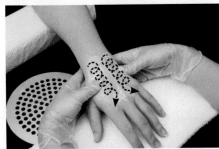

6 **Circular movement on wrist.** This movement is a form of friction massage that is a deep rubbing action and very stimulating. Hold the client's hand with both of your hands, placing your thumbs on top of the client's hand and your fingers below the hand. Move your thumbs in a circular movement in opposite directions from the client's wrist to the knuckle on back of the client's hand. Move up and down, three to five times.

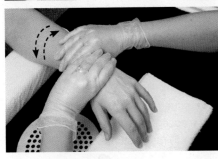

7 **Complete hand massage.** The last time you rotate up, wring the client's wrist by bracing your hands around the wrist and gently twisting in the opposite directions. Now you move onto the opposite hand. Start by wrapping the finished hand in a clean, warm towel, and then unwrap the client's opposite hand to repeat the hand massage steps. Once you've concluded the last movement on this hand, you will have finished the hand massage usually performed in the basic manicure.

PROCEDURE FOR ARM MASSAGE

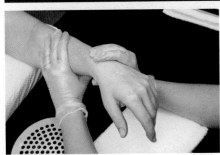

8 **Effleurage of the arm.** Holding the wrist firmly but gently, glide your hand up the arm from wrist to elbow with your palm and fingers on the skin; be certain enough lotion is on the skin to allow a smooth glide of the hand. Cup your movement fingers around the arm, moving up with slight pressure on the skin with your fingers, thumb, and palm to induce relaxation, then move back to the wrist area with a lighter pressure on the skin. Perform this gliding several times. When finishing a movement each time at the top of the arm, rotate the hand to the underside of the arm while pulling the hand back towards you.

Now move to the underarm and perform the same movement. When performing the movement on the underarm, press forward, then at the end release the pressure, gently rotate the hand to the top of the arm, and pull it lightly back toward the hand.

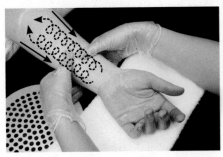

9 **Friction movement on the arms.** A friction massage involves rubbing the muscles against each other. Put the client's arm on the table, palm up with fingers toward you. Your fingers should be underneath the arm, stabilizing it. Rotate your thumbs in opposite directions, starting at the client's wrist and working toward the elbow. When you reach the elbow, slide your hand down the client's arm to the wrist and rotate back up to the elbow three to five times. Turn the client's arm over and repeat three to five times on the top side of the arm.

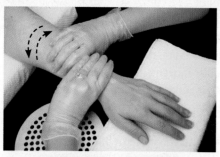

10 **Wringing/friction movement.** Place the arm horizontal on the towel in front of you, with the back of the hand facing up. Place your hands around the arm with your fingers facing the same direction on the arm, and gently twist in opposite directions as you would wring out a washcloth from wrist to elbow. Do this up and down the forearm three to five times.

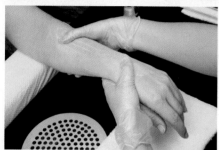

11 **Kneading movement.** Kneading (pétrissage) is a squeezing motion that moves flesh and muscles over the bones beneath in opposite directions, stimulating and increasing blood flow. Place your thumb on the top side of the client's arm so that they are horizontal. Move them in opposite directions, from wrist to elbow and back down to the wrist. Do this three to five times.

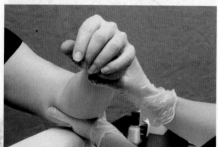

12 **Rotation of elbow.** This is a friction massage movement. Brace the client's arm with your left hand and apply lotion. Cup the elbow with your right hand and rotate your hand over the client's elbow. Do this three to five times. Take care to be very gentle, and do not hit the nerve in the elbow that often is referred to as "the funny bone" as it can be very be painful to the client. To finish the elbow massage, move your left arm to the top of the client's forearm. If the elbow condition reflects that it needs exfoliation, it must be done post massage. Apply a scrub and rotate it around the elbow, remove, and then apply lotion to re-moisturize.

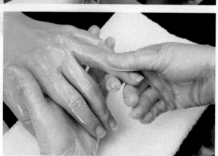

13 **Finger pulls.** Gently slide both hands down the forearm from the elbow to the fingertips as if climbing down a rope. Then, holding the hand with your non-dominant hand, move to the fingertip, and with your thumb on top and pointer finger arched below, gently grab and pull the finger down to the tips. Perform on each finger, little finger to thumb. Perform the movement down the forearm and do finger pulls three to five times on each arm and hand. Understand that this movement should not be performed on clients who have severe arthritis.

If elbow exfoliation is needed, perform it now, then perform the final movement below after re-moisturizing the elbow. Slide the moisturized hands toward the hands and perform the final movement.

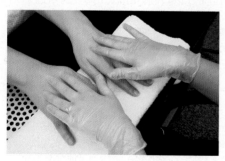

14 **Final movement.** Repeat the arm massage on the opposite arm, remembering to cover and uncover the warm towels as necessary. End the massage with a final feathering off movement. Lay both of the client's hands palm down on the table, cover them with your own hands, palm down on them, and gently press them three times. Then, gently, lift your palms, leaving your fingertips on the base of the hand. Then, with a light-as-a-feather touch, pull your fingers from the back of the hands down the fingers and off the tips of the fingers. Perform two to three times. The client learns quickly this final movement, called "feathering off," is the end of the massage.

POLISHING THE NAILS

IMPLEMENTS & MATERIALS

In addition to the basic materials on your manicuring table, you will need the following supplies:

☐ Base coat

☐ Colored nail polish

☐ Drying product (optional)

☐ Top coat

☐ Ultraviolet or electric nail polish dryer (optional)

PREPARATION   PROCEDURE

Perform:

P 25-3 **Performing a Basic Manicure** *See page 886*

• Before applying polish, have your client put on any jewelry and outerwear he or she may have taken off before the service and get car keys ready. Have the client pay for services now to avoid smudging the polish later.

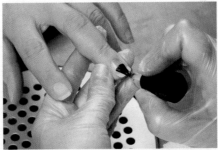

1 Clean nails of oil and other debris. Apply a thin layer of base coat to cover the entire nail plate and the edge.

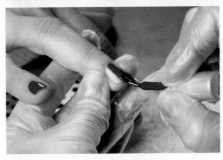

2 Apply polish color by placing the tip of the brush on the nail ⅛" (0.31 cm) away from the cuticle area in the center of the nail. Press the brush onto the nail plate, producing a slight "fanning" of the brush and then push it towards the eponychium. Leave a tiny, rounded margin of unpolished nail at the back of the nail. Pull the brush toward the free edge of the nail, down the center.

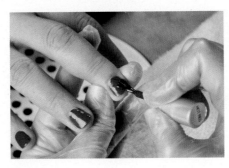

3 Move to each side of the nail and pull in even strokes toward the nail tip.

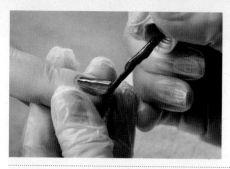

4 After finishing the surface of the nail, move the brush back and forth on the very end of the free edge, barely touching, to apply color to it. This is called "tip sealing" or "tipping" and reduces chipping and layering on the free edges.

5 Apply the second coat of color on all 10 nails.

6 Apply an ample coat of top coat to prevent chipping and to give nails a glossy, finished appearance. Be sure to seal the free edge of each nail with top coat as well.

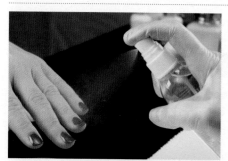

7 If you use a polish-drying product, apply over top coat according to the manufacturer's instructions. After the application, ask the client to be seated at a separate table with his or her hands under a nail dryer or seat the client comfortably away from your table. The drying time should be a minimum of 10 minutes.

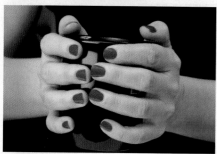

8 Beautifully polished nails.

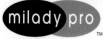 Check out miladypro.com for additional resources and training to enhance your technical skills. Keyword: *FutureCosPro*

REVIEW QUESTIONS

1. Define *scope of practice*.

2. Name the four types of professional nail tools required to perform a manicure.

3. What is the difference between multiuse and single-use implements?

4. What is the three-part procedure, and how is it used in the performance of the basic manicure?

5. Is a consultation necessary each time a client has a service in the salon? Why?

6. Name the basic nail shapes for women.

7. What is the most popular nail shape for men?

8. Which massage movement is most appropriate for a hand and arm massage? Why?

9. What is the difference between a basic manicure and a spa manicure?

10. How is aromatherapy used in manicuring services?

11. Explain the use and benefits of paraffin wax in manicuring.

12. What would be on the manicuring table if it were properly set up?

13. What are the steps in the post-service procedure?

14. What are the steps in a basic manicure procedure?

15. How is nail polish applied properly?

STUDY TOOLS

- **Reinforce what you just learned:** Complete the activities and exercises in your Theory or Practical Workbook, or your Study Guide.

- **Expand your knowledge:** Search for websites about the topics in this chapter and make a list of additional resources.

- **Study and prepare for your quiz:** Take the chapter test in your Exam Review or your Milady U: Online Licensing Prep.

- **Re-Test your knowledge:** Take the Chapter 25 *Quizzes*!

- **Learn even more:** Look up in a dictionary or search the internet for the definitions of any additional terms you want to learn about.

CHAPTER GLOSSARY

acetone	p. 862	A colorless, inflammable liquid; miscible with water, alcohol, and ether; and has a sweetish odor or burning taste. It is used as a solvent.
color blocking	p. 878	Nail art technique that blocks or sections off color on the nail.
color fading	p. 878	Also known as *color graduation*, this nail art technique is when one color fades into the other, and the meeting point is a combination of the two.
dimethyl urea hardeners DY-meth-il yoo-REE-uh hard-dn-ers	p. 865	A hardener that adds cross-links to the natural nail plate. Unlike others containing formaldehyde, DMU does not cause adverse skin reactions.
essential oils	p. 875	Oils extracted using various forms of distillation from the seeds, bark, roots, leaves, wood, and/or resin of plants.

fine-grit abrasives	p. 860	Abrasives 240 grit and higher designed for buffing, polishing, and removing very fine scratches.
French manicure	p. 877	When the nail bed is one color, such as pink, peach, or beige (depending upon the client's skin tone), and the free edge of the nail is another color, such as white.
friction	p. 872	Incorporates various strokes that manipulate or press one layer of tissue over another
implements	p. 856	Tools used to perform nail services. Implements can be multiuse or single-use.
lower-grit abrasives	p. 859	Boards and buffers less than 180 grit that quickly reduce the thickness of any surface.
manicure	p. 850	A cosmetic treatment of the hands involving cutting, shaping, and often painting of the nails, removal of the cuticles, and softening of the skin.
marbleizing	p. 878	A swirled nail art effect when you combine two or more colors while wet and then mix them on the nail with a stylus tool.
massage	p. 871	The manipulation of the soft tissues of the body.
medium-grit abrasives	p. 860	Boards and buffers 150 to 180 grit that are used to smooth and refine surfaces and shorten natural nails.
metal pusher	p. 856	A multiuse implement, made of stainless steel; used to push back the eponychium but can also be used to gently scrape cuticle tissue from the natural nail plate.
microtrauma	p. 856	The act of causing tiny, unseen openings in the skin that can allow entry by pathogenic microbes.
multiuse implements	p. 856	Also known as *reusable implements*; implements that are generally stainless steel because they must be properly cleaned and disinfected between clients.
nail clippers	p. 857	A multiuse implement used to shorten the nail plate quickly and efficiently.
nail creams	p. 862	Barrier products that contain ingredients designed to seal the surface and hold subdermal moisture in the skin.
nail oils	p. 862	Products designed to absorb into the nail plate to increase flexibility and into the surrounding skin to soften.
nail nipper	p. 857	A stainless-steel implement used to carefully trim away dead skin around the nails.
oval nail	p. 869	A conservative nail shape that is thought to be attractive on most women's hands. It is similar to a squoval nail with even more rounded corners.
paraffin	p. 854	A petroleum by-product that has excellent sealing properties (barrier qualities) to hold moisture in the skin.
pointed nail	p. 869	Nail shape suited to thin hands with long fingers and narrow nail beds. The nail is tapered and longer than usual to emphasize and enhance the slender appearance of the hand.
protein hardener	p. 864	A combination of clear polish and protein, such as collagen.

round nail	p. 869	A slightly tapered nail shape; it usually extends just a bit past the fingertip.
scope of practice	p. 850	The list of services that you are legally allowed to perform in your specialty in your state.
service sets	p. 852	Sets of all the tools that will be used in a service.
single-use implements	p. 856	Also known as *disposable implements*; implements that cannot be reused and must be thrown away after a single use.
smile line	p. 877	The curved line where the pink and the white meet each other on a French manicured nail.
square nail	p. 869	A nail shape completely straight across the free edge with no rounding at the outside edges.
squoval nail	p. 869	A nail shape with a square free edge that is rounded off at the corner edges.
stylus	p. 878	A tool with a solid handle with a rounded ball tip on each end that can range in size, used to create nail art.
wooden pusher	p. 858	A wooden stick used to remove cuticle tissue from the nail plate (by gently pushing), to clean under the free edge of the nail, or to apply products.

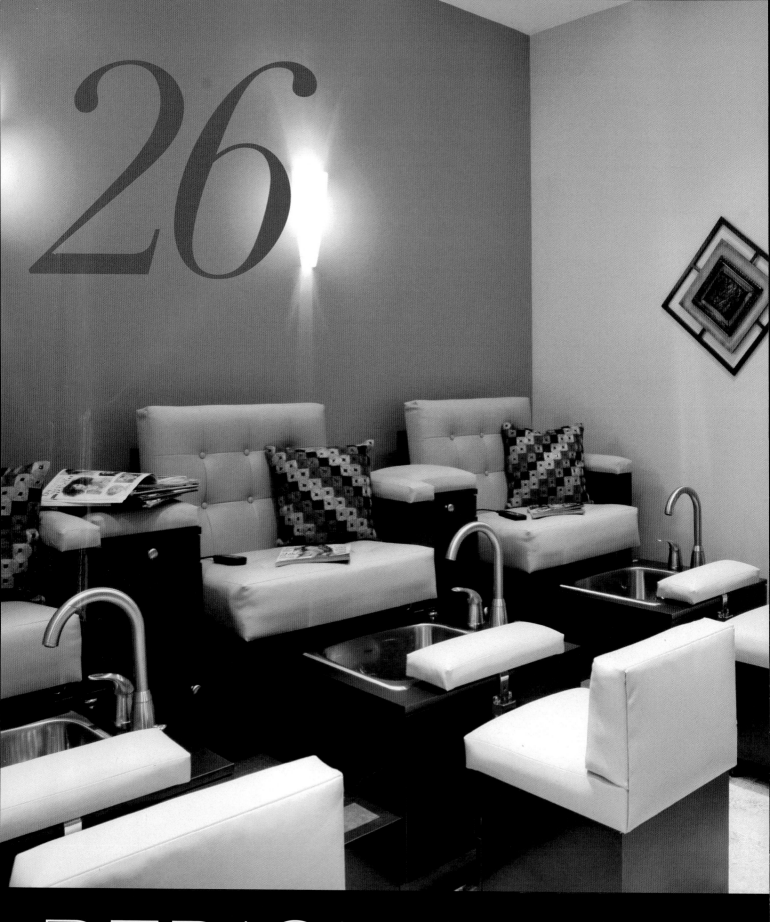

26

PEDICURING

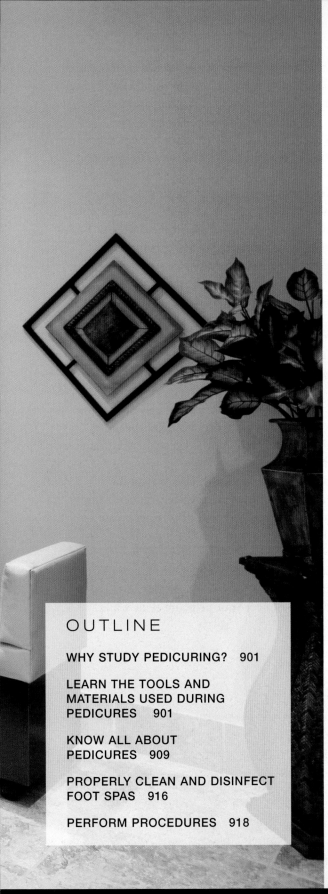

LEARNING OBJECTIVES

After completing this chapter, you will be able to:

LO❶
Describe the equipment used when performing pedicures.

LO❷
Identify materials only used when performing pedicures.

LO❸
Describe the function of callus softener in a pedicure procedure.

LO❹
Explain the differences between a basic pedicure and a spa pedicure.

LO❺
Define *reflexology* and its use during a pedicure procedure.

LO❻
Summarize the importance of cleaning and disinfecting a pedicure bath.

OUTLINE

pedicure is a cosmetic service performed on the feet by a licensed cosmetologist or nail technician. Pedicures can include exfoliating the skin; reducing calluses; and trimming, shaping and polishing the toenails. Often pedicures include a foot and leg massage as well. Though pedicures have been performed as foot care since ancient times and in the beauty industry for decades, they were relatively rare even as recently as the late 1980s.

In the 1990s, with the development of the spa industry and new pampering equipment, techniques, and products, pedicures exploded onto service menus and became the fastest-growing service in the industry. Currently pedicures are a regular ritual in many clients' personal-care regimen. Pedicures are now considered a standard service performed in salons by cosmetologists.

The information in this chapter will provide you with the skills you need to perform beautification and routine care on your clients' feet, toes, and toenails. Pedicures are now a basic part of good foot care and hygiene and are particularly important for clients who are joggers, dancers, and cosmetologists—or for anyone who spends a lot of time standing on his or her feet.

Pedicures are not merely manicures on the feet. Although the basic services are similar, pedicures require specific skills; more knowledge of chronic illnesses, disorders, and diseases; and knowledge of the additional precautions for performing the service.

Pedicures present more potential for damage to clients than do manicures. Experts recommend that you become proficient in performing manicures before learning how to perform pedicures. Pedicures create client loyalty, produce considerable income, and can be important preventive health services for many clients. In short, pedicure services offer something for everyone. Once your clients experience the comfort, relaxation, and value of a great pedicure, they will return for more. For these reasons, you would be wise to perfect your pedicure skills while in school.

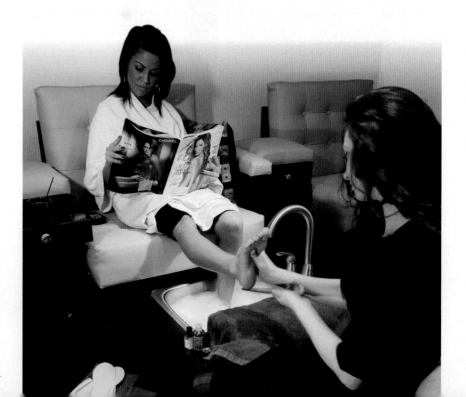

why study
PEDICURING?

Cosmetologists should study and have a thorough understanding of pedicuring because:

> It will enable you to add this very desirable service to your service offerings.

> It is important to differentiate between the various pedicure tools and to know how they are properly used.

> It will allow you to perform a pedicure safely and correctly.

After reading the next few sections, you will be able to:

LO❶ Describe the equipment used when performing pedicures.

LO❷ Identify materials only used when performing pedicures.

LO❸ Describe the function of callus softener in a pedicure procedure.

Learn the Tools and Materials Used During Pedicures

In order to perform pedicures safely, you must learn to work with the tools required for this service and to incorporate all safety, cleaning, and disinfection procedures as written in your state's regulations. The tools include the standard manicure tools plus several that are specific to the pedicure service. Again, the four types of nail technology tools that you will incorporate into your pedicure services include:

* Equipment

* Implements

* Materials

* Professional pedicure products

Equipment

Equipment includes all the permanent tools used to perform nail services that are not implements. Some permanent equipment for performing pedicures is different from that used for manicures.

Pedicure Station

A pedicure station includes a comfortable chair with an armrest and footrest for the client and an ergonomic chair for the cosmetologist.

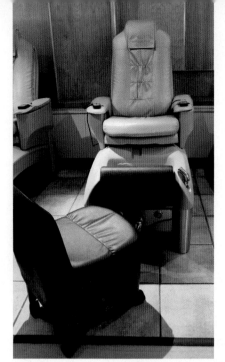

figure 26-1
Comfortable chair and pedicure chair

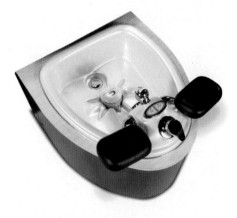

figure 26-2
Sturdy pedicure center with removable and adjustable footrest

Design and location vary according to several factors, such as the size of the area, the size of the pedicure station, the location of the water and low-noise areas in the salon, and the cost of equipment and installation (figures 26-1 through 26-3).

Pedicure Stool and Footrest

Pedicures can present challenges to the service provider in maintaining a healthy posture while performing the service. For that reason, the cosmetologist's pedicuring stool is usually low to make it ergonomically easier for the pedicurist to work on the client's feet. Some stools come with a built-in footrest for the client, making it easier for the stylist to reach the client's feet. Alternately, a separate footrest can be used. Your seat must be comfortable and allow ergonomically-correct positioning (figures 26-4 and 26-5).

Pedicure Foot Bath

The pedicure foot bath varies in design from the basic stainless steel basin to an automatic whirlpool that warms and massages the client's feet (figure 26-6).

The soak bath is filled with comfortably warm water and a product to soak the client's feet. The bath must be large enough to completely immerse both of the client's feet comfortably.

Basin soak baths can be large stainless steel bowls or beautiful ceramic ones. Transportable professional foot baths can be purchased from beauty supply stores or industry manufacturers. They must be manually filled and emptied after each client's service.

A step above the portable water baths is the more customized pedicure unit, which has a removable foot bath and the technician's stool built into one unit. These are more ergonomically designed for the cosmetologist and more professional than sitting on the floor to perform the service. A portable pedicure unit includes a place for the foot bath and a storage area for supplies.

Portable water baths are now available that have inserts that fit inside the bath for containing the water for the feet to soak. A new insert is

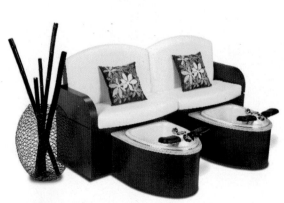

figure 26-3
A fully plumbed station comes with many options.

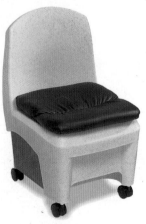

figure 26-4
Low pedicure chair with back support

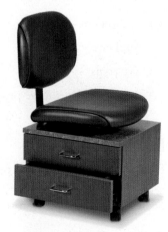

figure 26-5
Pedicure chair with drawers and back support

placed inside the foot bath for each client and then thrown away after the pedicure. The next step up in cost and ease of use is the portable foot basin with built-in whirlpool-action (figure 26-7). These baths add an extra touch to the service with the gentle massaging action the whirlpool. The bath is filled from the sink through attachable hoses. After the service, the bath is drained by pumping the water back into the sink through these hoses. It has a built-in footrest; the surrounding cabinet has areas for storage of pedicure supplies.

The ultimate pedicure foot bath is the fully plumbed whirlpool with the attached pedicure chair, sometimes referred to as a throne-design chair. These units are not portable. They are permanently plumbed to both hot and cold water sources as well as to a drain. Most units have a built-in massage feature in the chair and a warmer, which adds to the relaxation of the client. Recently, many throne-type chairs are available with a self-cleaning and disinfection cycle built into the bath.

Pedicure Carts

Pedicure carts are designed to keep supplies organized. Many different designs are available that include a hard, flat surface for placement of your implements and in-service supplies, as well as drawers and shelves for storage of implements, supplies, and pedicure products. Most are on rollers to allow them to be pushed aside when not in use. Some units include a space for storage of the foot bath. Most take up very little space and greatly aid in organization of the area (figure 26-8).

Electric Foot Mitts (Optional)

These heated mitts, similar to electric manicure mitts but shaped for the feet, are designed to add a special touch to a more-than-basic pedicure. Pedicures in which these are used are a higher-cost service, or they can be included in a lower-cost service for an added fee (an upgrade). After a foot massage, a conditioning lotion or a mask is applied to the feet, and then they are placed in a plastic wrap or cover. Finally, the feet are placed inside the warm, electric foot mitts. A **mask**, also known as a *masque*, is a concentrated treatment product often composed of mineral clays,

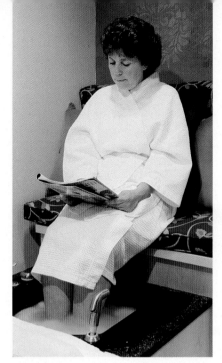
figure 26-6
Self-contained foot bath with hose

STATE REGULATORY ALERT!

Before purchasing any pedicure equipment check with your state board on which pedicure units are permitted. If you are unsure which pedicure unit is which, you can refer to Chapter 5, Infection Control: Principles and Practices, for the section called "Which Foot Spa Do I Have?" on page 91.

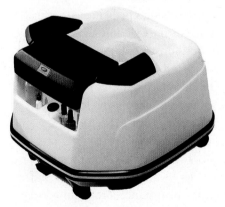
figure 26-7
Typical portable foot bath with a whirlpool fan

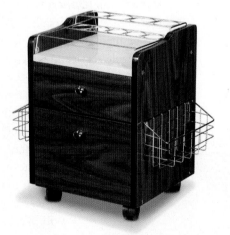
figure 26-8
Pedicure cart with drawers

Courtesy of European Touch.

moisturizing agents, skin softeners, aromatherapy oils, botanical extracts, and other beneficial ingredients to cleanse, exfoliate, tighten, tone, hydrate, and nourish the skin.

The warmth provided by the mitts helps the conditioning agents of the mask penetrate more effectively, adds to the comfort of the service, and provides ultimate client relaxation.

Terry Cloth Mitts (Optional)

These washable and reusable mitts, available for both hands and feet, are placed over a client's feet after a penetrating conditioning product and a plastic cover have been applied. Terry cloth mitts are routinely used over paraffin and a cover, as they hold in the heat provided by the warmed paraffin to encourage the conditioning of the feet or hands by the product. These mitts allow the paraffin to harden to perform its barrier function while electric mitts do not.

Paraffin Bath (Optional)

As discussed in Chapter 25, Manicuring, paraffin is an especially wonderful treatment in a pedicure (figure 26-9).

Although many clients, salon and spa owners, and cosmetologists prefer other paraffin application methods, the traditional method is to dip and re-dip the hands and feet three to four times into the larger paraffin bath. Once paraffin has been used on a client, it must be discarded. It is against state board regulations to re-melt and re-use paraffin. Aside from the other benefits mentioned in Chapter 25, such as relaxation and the warmth to enable penetration of products, the deep, moist heat in the paraffin aids in the reduction of pain and inflammation and promotes circulation to joints affected by arthritis and other chronic problems.

Some unique health precautions for the application of paraffin must be considered for pedicure clients who are chronically ill. Do not provide the paraffin wax treatment to clients with lesions or abrasions, impaired foot or leg circulation, loss of feeling in their feet or legs, or other diabetes-related problems. Further, the skin of elderly clients may be thinner and more sensitive to heat, so a pre-service wax patch test must be performed to ensure the client will be comfortable having the treatment.

Hot Stones (Optional)

Hot stones are generally used in pedicures, not manicures, though they can be incorporated into manicures also. Hot stone pedicures are usually an upscale service included in the massage of the feet and legs. The name, however, is misleading—the stones are not hot, they are merely comfortably warm. The stones are smooth and typically **basalt**, a dark, fine-grained volcanic rock. The movements are up, towards the heart, and are not aggressive. They provide a deep, penetrating, and comforting heat that enhances relaxation and increases circulation.

In many cases, it is recommended that a sheet or towel be placed as barrier in between the stones and skin. Massage therapists, for instance, are required to take a course on stones before they can even receive insurance. Test the warmth of the stones on your arm for

figure 26-9
Paraffin foot bath

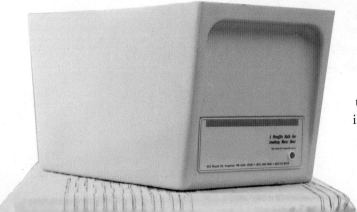

comfort, and then check with the client during your first movement for his or her comfort with the heat.

The stones are scrub-cleaned between clients to prevent transfer of infection, then disinfected. Disinfecting your stones ensures that you do not inadvertently transfer bacteria, fungus, or virus from one client to another. Check with the company you purchased the stones from for their recommendations and policies on disinfection of the stones.

Implements

The implements mentioned in Chapter 25, Manicuring, are used in pedicures also. There are, however, implements that are specific for use in pedicures. Following is a list of these pedicure-specific implements.

Toenail Clippers and Nippers

Toenail clippers are larger than fingernail clippers, with curved or straight jaws specifically designed for shortening toenails. Use only professional toenail clippers made especially for cutting toenails (figure 26-10). They have a wider space between the jaws, allowing them to cut thicker nails. Always clean the clippers well and disinfect them after use. For your client's safety, use only high-quality stainless steel implements made specifically for performing professional pedicures. Professional stainless steel implements will also last longer and make your job easier. Take care not to clip the nails too short and not to break the seal of the hyponychium, an important protection of the toenail unit from infection.

Another professional tool used to shorten toenail length is a toenail nipper. **Toenail nippers** are similar in design to fingernail nippers but are larger, much stronger, and used to trim the toenail as opposed to trimming the excess cuticle (figure 26-11). They have a larger hinge box and longer and thicker jaws. This design allows the toenail nippers to be used in shortening the nail, whereas fingernail nippers are generally for removing dead skin. Toenail nippers must be used carefully to prevent trapping the skin of the toe in the jaws. The tips of the jaws are the cutting area of the jaws. They are held at a 45-degree angle to the nail tip, and small nips of the nail are taken slowly across the free edge to trim the nail.

Curette

A **curette** is an implement with a small, scoop-shaped end that, if carefully used, allows for more efficient removal of debris from the nail folds, eponychium, and hyponychium areas. Curettes are ideal for use around the edges of the big toenail plate (figure 26-12). A double-ended curette, which has a 0.06 inch (1.5 mm) diameter on one end and a 0.1 inch (2.5 mm) diameter on the other, is recommended. Some are made with a small hole, making the curette easier to clean after it has been used.

Curettes require gentle and careful maneuvers to prevent damage to the skin in the nail folds. Never use curettes to cut out tissue or debris that is adhering to living tissues. Cosmetologists must never use curettes with sharp edges because doing so can result in serious injury. Only those with dull or rounded edges are safe and appropriate for use by cosmetologists.

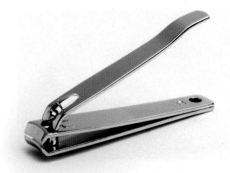

figure 26-10
Toenail clippers are specifically designed for cutting and shortening toenails.

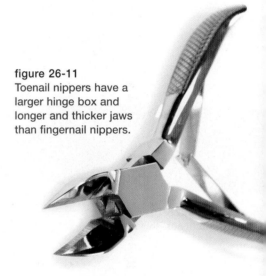

figure 26-11
Toenail nippers have a larger hinge box and longer and thicker jaws than fingernail nippers.

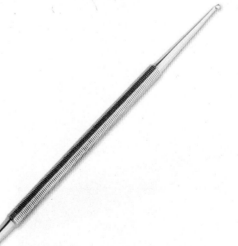

figure 26-12
Double-ended curette

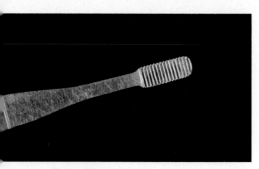

figure 26-13
Nail rasp

To use a curette, place the rounded side of the spoon toward the sidewall of living skin. A gentle scooping motion is then used along the nail plate to remove any loose debris. Take care not to overdo it. Do not use this implement to dig into the soft tissues along the nail fold, as injury may occur. If the tissue is inflamed (i.e., ingrown toenail), the client must be referred to a qualified medical doctor or podiatrist.

Nail Rasp

A **nail rasp** is a metal implement with a grooved edge used for filing and smoothing the edges of the nail plate. Ask your instructor to demonstrate its correct use for you. It is designed to file in one direction and has a filing surface of about ⅛" × ¾" (3.2 mm × 19 mm) attached to a straight or angled metal handle (figure 26-13). The angled rasp is recommended because it is easier to control under the free edge of the nail.

The rasp is placed under the nail, angling the point of the rasp at the center of the nail and the remaining portion toward the side free edge; it is then gently pulled toward the lateral edge of the nail to reduce the sides of the free edge that might grow into the tissues and potentially cause an ingrown nail. This is a prevention tool in the hands of a nail technician. Never use it on nails that are already ingrown; refer clients with ingrown nails to a podiatrist. The rasping process may be repeated to make sure there are no rough edges remaining along the free edge; however, *do not overfile.*

As you become proficient in the use of a nail rasp, you will find it to be an invaluable and time-saving implement as well as an important prevention tool for ingrown toenails. Take special care with this tool: Never use it on the top of the nail or past the hyponichium area of the side of the free edge, as it can roughen the top or damage the skin and initiate infections.

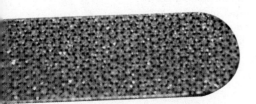

figure 26-14
Metal abrasive file

Pedicure Nail File

For toenails, a medium-grit file will work best for shaping, and a fine-grit file will work best for finishing and sealing the edges. In general, if an abrasive file cannot survive proper cleaning and disinfection procedures without being rendered unusable, it must be considered single-use and be thrown away or given to the client for home use.

Some cosmetologists use a metal file on toenails (figure 26-14). Check with your instructor to find out whether a metal file is legal in your state. Metal files must be either cleaned and then disinfected, or cleaned and then sterilized after each use and before reuse.

Foot Files or Pedicure Paddles

Large **foot files**, also known as *pedicure paddles*, are designed to reduce and smooth thicker foot calluses (figure 26-15). Thicker calluses may be found on the heel, the ball of the foot, and on the side of the great toe. Calluses form from excessive pressure on the foot and provide the extra protection the foot needs. Foot files and paddles are used to reduce and smooth calluses to create softer skin. They are not meant to completely remove the callus, as this can cause the client to have sore or tender feet.

Foot files come in many different grits and shapes. They must be properly cleaned and disinfected between each use or disposed of after a single use if they cannot be disinfected properly.

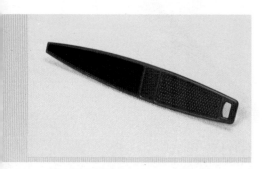

figure 26-15
Foot file for reducing calluses

Many reasonably-priced foot paddles are available for purchase in bulk for single use in pedicures. Foot paddles with disposable and replaceable abrasive surfaces are also available. The handles of these files must be cleaned and disinfected before reuse. Check with your instructor to find out whether these are legal for use in your state.

Materials

All materials mentioned in Chapter 25, Manicuring, are also used in pedicuring. In addition, a few unique materials are used in this service: toe separators and pedicure slippers.

Toe Separators

Toe separators of many designs are available, from foam rubber, one-piece units that fit between the toes to a rope type that is woven between the toes. They are used to keep the toes apart while the technician is polishing the client's nails. The one-piece foam rubber separators are used the most by nail technicians. Toe separators are important for performing a high-quality pedicure (**figure 26-16**). Since toe separators cannot be cleaned and disinfected, a new set must be used on each client and then thrown away or given to the client for at-home use.

Pedicure Slippers

Single-use paper or foam slippers are provided for those clients who have not worn open-toed shoes and want to avoid smudging their newly applied toenail polish or for those that are having other services in the spa. They are specially designed not to touch the nails while being worn (**figure 26-17**).

Professional Pedicure Products

Products for pedicure services include the products discussed in Chapter 25, Manicuring, plus others that are unique to pedicuring. These new product types are:

* Soaks
* Scrubs
* Masks
* Pedicure lotions and creams
* Callus softeners

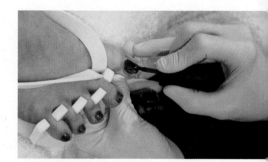

figure 26-16
Toe separators

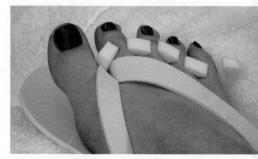

figure 26-17
Pedicure slippers

Foot Soaks

Foot soaks are products that are put into the water in the pedicure bath to soften the skin on the feet during the soak time. A good foot soak product is gentle but effective and thoroughly cleans and deodorizes the feet. Professionally formulated products are designed to properly cleanse without being overly harsh to the skin. Other ingredients may include moisturizers and oils that are designed for use in pedicure baths. The soak sets the stage for the rest of the pedicure, so be sure to use a high-quality product to start your pedicure service on a good note.

Exfoliating Scrubs

These gritty lotions are massaged on the foot and leg to remove dry, flaky skin and reduce calluses. They leave the skin feeling smoother and moisturized. **Exfoliating scrubs** are usually water-based lotions that contain an abrasive as the exfoliating agent. Sea sand, ground apricot kernels, crystals, jojoba beads, and polypropylene beads are all exfoliating agents that may be found in pedicure scrubs. Scrubs also contain moisturizers that help to condition the skin. Cosmetologists must wear gloves when using these products as repeated use will irritate the skin on the hands.

Masks

Masks are concentrated treatment products often composed of mineral clays, moisturizing agents, skin softeners, aromatherapy oils, extracts, and other beneficial ingredients to cleanse, exfoliate, tighten, tone, hydrate, and nourish the skin. They are highly valued by clients. Masks are applied to the skin and remain therefor five to ten minutes to allow penetration of beneficial ingredients (**figure 26-18**). Menthol, mint, cucumber, and other ingredients are very popular in foot-care masks.

Foot Lotions or Creams

Lotions and creams are important to condition and moisturize the skin of the legs and feet, to soften calluses, and to provide slip for massage. They are also formulated as home-care products for maintenance of the service and improvement of the skin. Cosmetologists who work in a podiatry or medical office will be introduced to treatment-level lotions and creams that are associated with the improvement of medical conditions of the feet such as extreme dryness (xerosis). Whether you work in a salon, spa, or medical office, get to know your product line well in order to recommend products to aid the client in maintaining the pedicure benefits.

Callus Softeners

Professional strength **callus softeners** are products designed to soften and smooth thickened tissue (calluses). They are applied directly to the client's calluses and are left on for a short period of time, according to the manufacturer's directions. After the product softens the callus, it is more easily reduced and smoothed with files or paddles.

Callus softeners are potent liquid formulas that are left on the callused area for about five minutes. They are acidic and potentially hazardous, and for that reason safety glasses should be worn whenever using or pouring them. Be sure to wear gloves during their use. Used improperly, these products may cause severe irritation to the nail technician's eyes, hands and

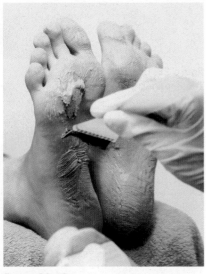

figure 26-18
Foot-care masks are applied to hydrate and nourish the skin.

skin, and they may cause post-service dryness. When used correctly and according to the manufacturer's instructions, they are safe and effective. The three most common active ingredients in callus softeners today are urea, salicylic acid, and potassium hydroxide.

1. **Urea** is an organic compound that has a super-hydrating effect on skin cells. Its function within callus softeners is to over-moisturize and hydrate the tough, thick callus. It is a naturally occurring chemical that is produced within many organisms. Most industrial urea is synthetic and produced from carbon dioxide and ammonia.

2. **Salicylic acid** (sal-uh-SIL-ik AS-ud) is an organic acid that derives originally from the bark of willow trees. It has anti-inflammatory properties and has the ability to break down fats and lipids. As of now, it is the only chemical the FDA has approved to be marketed as a callus "remover," and it acts to lift the dead skin cells off of callus for enhanced filing results. Salicylic acid is also used to treat plantar warts and for exfoliating treatments for acne and psoriasis.

3. **Potassium hydroxide** is an inorganic compound that degrades the protein in the callus cells. This works quickly to soften even the toughest of callus in preparation for filing and reducing. Cuticle removers often contain a small amount of potassium hydroxide to help clean the nail plate of dry, stubborn cuticle.

After reading the next few sections, you will be able to:

LO➍ Explain the differences between a basic pedicure and a spa pedicure.

LO➎ Define *reflexology* and its use during a pedicure procedure.

Know All About Pedicures

Pedicures have become a part of the lifestyle of Americans to the extent that many people get pedicures more often than they have their hair cut. These clients are as choosy about their pedicure as they are about other salon services. As with most beauty procedures, a pedicure is a service that must be practiced and perfected. You must continually search for education and new ideas to keep up with the changes.

Ⓟ 26-1 **Performing the Basic Pedicure** *See page 918*

Choosing Pedicure Products

Many pedicure products are available, but the most synergistic ones (those designed to work well together) are developed systems or lines. These products provide the fastest and easiest ways to develop an optimal

? **DID YOU KNOW?**
The basic pedicure does not include the leg massage, only the foot massage, for two reasons: time and money. Most salons schedule less time for the basic pedicure, allowing less time for massage. Second, higher-cost specialty pedicures must be greatly enhanced to be perceived as worth the higher price. The leg massage is one special addition.

pedicure service. They are available from many manufacturers of professional nail and foot products. Before choosing any one line, check out a variety of product lines, compare them, and then decide for yourself which line is best for your clients.

Always check the quality of the company's educational support and its commitment to the cosmetologists using its products. Find other cosmetologists who use the products and discuss the quality of the company's customer service and its shipping competence, and listen closely to their experiences. Look at your research, and make the decision based on which company best meets your and your clients' needs.

When using a manufacturer's product line, follow its recommendations and suggested procedures because these methods have been tested and found to enhance the effectiveness of the product line.

Service Menu

Tailor your foot-care menu of services to meet the lifestyle and requests of your clientele. For example, if your clientele is mostly younger clients, they will probably love nail art on their toes, while the mature clients are more likely to enjoy paraffin wax treatments.

Shorter services are great menu expanders. Not all clients will want or need a full pedicure. Some clients may only want or need a professional nail trimming. Others may want a pampering massage appointment between their full pedicure services to relieve tension and stress. Some may only want a polish change. List these additional services on your menu with your full pedicures to provide options for your clients.

Interaction During the Service

During the procedure, discuss with your client their foot health, an upgrade they may enjoy, and the products that are needed to maintain the pedicure between salon visits (figure 26-19). However, those that want to

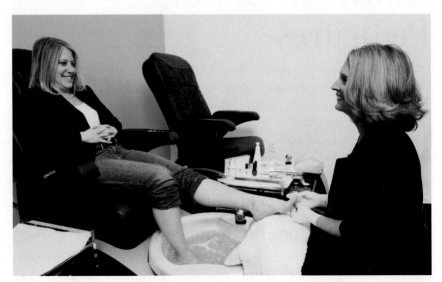

figure 26-19
Discuss foot health and upgrades the client may enjoy throughout the procedure.

drift off should be allowed the peace and tranquility they are seeking. If this is the case, discuss your product recommendations during polishing or when closing the service.

Pedicure clients are often in the salon to relax and be pampered. Offer them refreshment and suggest they sit back and relax, then smile and start the service. Keep your conversation professional; never discuss personal issues, politics, religion, or any other topics that might offend. There should be no distractions for you or the client during the pedicure. Clients purchase this service because of the relaxation it provides. Distractions and too much irrelevant talk can prevent this from happening.

To grow your clientele and to promote the foot health of clients, you must encourage your clients to schedule regular, monthly pedicures. The accepted time between pedicure appointments is generally four weeks because of the slow growth of the toenails. Mention that their feet are in constant use and need routine maintenance. Remind them that proper foot care, through pedicuring, improves both personal appearance and basic foot comfort.

Scheduling

When scheduling a client for a pedicure over the telephone, warn female clients not to shave their legs within 48 hours before the pedicure. Why? Shaving the legs increases the potential presence of tiny microscopic abrasions, and shaving within 48 hours before a pedicure may allow portals of entry for pathogenic microbes, increasing the risk of stinging, irritation, or infection. This policy is an important infection control policy.

To help uphold the policy, post a tasteful sign with the same message in the pedicure area, and place it on your service menu and website where your pedicures are listed. Then, before you place your client's feet in the pedicure soak, ask her when she last shaved her legs—if it was within the last 48 hours, offer her a waterless, basic pedicure that services only her foot and reschedule the pedicure that involves a soak and her legs. It is the responsible thing to do.

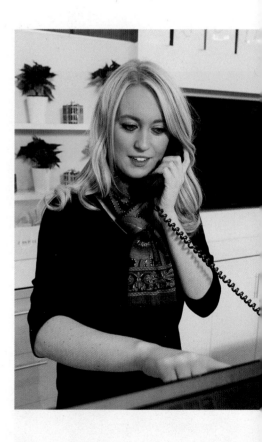

Additionally, as a customer service, when clients are scheduling a pedicure appointment, suggest they wear open-toed shoes or sandals so that polish will not be ruined following the service. Many spas provide single-use pedicure slippers for those who forget to wear open-toed sandals, but a reminder during scheduling is usually appreciated. After all, the appearance of their polish is a priority to most pedicure clients.

Clients dislike waiting for a nail technician who is running late. For that reason, first, it is important to schedule the appointments for the proper length of time for the service. Then, it's your responsibility to know where you should be in a service at a specific time and adjust your service to that timing. That keeps you on time for your next client. An example might be that you should have the consultation and soaking finished within 12 minutes or less after starting the pedicure, then proceed on through the steps at the allotted times until you are polishing 45–50 minutes after beginning a one-hour pedicure in order to be on time for your next client. You may need more time with a client than was scheduled because of the condition of the feet. You will know if this is the

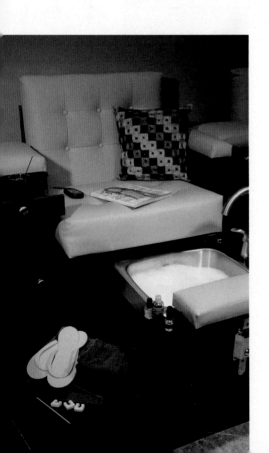

case during the consultation and while evaluating the client's feet. You must tell the client who will take longer that you will do the best you can in the time scheduled, but another pedicure may need to be scheduled to get the feet into good condition. Usually clients with problem feet know that this is the case, and they shouldn't be surprised at the need for another appointment and further work. It is important that you do not work beyond your scheduled time.

By sticking to the appointment time allotted, you will not only be preserving your schedule, you will also be protecting the client. If the client's feet are in bad shape and you work as long as is necessary to get them in optimal condition in only one service, they may become irritated or painful. The best option is to sell the client home-care products to improve the condition of the feet, and schedule another service within one or two weeks.

Series Pedicures

Some improvements in the feet require more than one appointment, this is referred to as a *series*. A situation that may require a series of appointments is callus reduction. When a client comes in with heavy calluses, never use a blade. Not only are blades dangerous and a potential cause of infection, but their use is against the law in most states. Using a blade also stimulates heavier growth of calluses as the skin attempts to grow back quickly to protect the damaged skin.

To reduce calluses during a pedicure and to maintain their reduction, perform a safe amount of exfoliation with a scrub. Apply the new, more effective callus-reduction products on them and use the foot paddle to remove a safe amount of callus. Explain to the client the negatives regarding rushed removal of calluses. Explain that weekly callus reduction appointments for four to six weeks will lower the calluses, and that after that series, the client can receive maintenance pedicures less frequently, about once a month.

During the series appointments, a full pedicure is not performed between the monthly pedicures; the callus-reduction appointment is merely a weekly soak, application of the reduction product for a set time (usually five minutes), reasonable callus reduction, and application of a lotion. It takes about half an hour and should be a less expensive service than an entire pedicure.

At the four-week appointment, a full pedicure is performed with treatments following again. Some clients will require more than the six weeks for a callus reduction series, and this should be explained when the series is suggested. The client can also be sold a glycolic or lactic acid hand and body lotion to use on the feet every other day, and daily use of a lotion containing DMU (dimethyl urea hardeners) should be recommended to soften and prevent the scaly condition from returning. A foot paddle can also be sold to the client for use after showers between treatment appointments. Gloves must be worn during these services.

Another condition that can require weekly treatment is scaly feet. First, however, the client must be sent to a podiatrist to define whether the scaly condition is caused by a fungus. If no fungus is present, the client can return weekly for three to six weeks for a foot exfoliation treatment that includes scrubs and a callus-reduction treatment such as a mask. Remember that masks should be applied all over the feet for one to three minutes, but no longer. These treatments are designed so that the client will have beautiful feet when the series is finished. Home-care products must be recommended to maintain the improved condition.

Spa Pedicure

The pedicure described in **Procedure 26-1, The Basic Pedicure**, is the basis for all other pedicure services. For example, in the basic pedicure, the massage is performed on the foot only, while in the upgrade to a spa pedicure, the massage is performed on the foot and the lower leg (to the knee). An exfoliation is also usually a portion of the spa pedicure, to remove dead cells from the skin on the leg, but may not be in the basic pedicure. This is usually performed prior to the massage or just before a mask.

Another spa pedicure upgrade is the use of a mask on the foot and/or leg. The mask is applied, covered with a wrap or plastic cover, and allowed to set while the client relaxes and the mask's effectiveness increases. A further upgrade would be the incorporation of special products such as aromatherapy, lotions, oils, paraffin, and the addition of other specialty treatments, such as reflexology.

Elderly Clients

Older people need regular, year-round foot care to maintain foot health. Many elderly people cannot reach their feet, cannot see them, or cannot squeeze the nail clippers to trim their own nails. They need continual help in their foot-care maintenance, especially since it can become a health issue. The cosmetologist who offers pedicure services for this segment of the population will be doing these individuals a great service and will find plenty of willing clients in need of their services.

Many of these clients have health issues that require exceptionally gentle care. Never cut their tissues or push back the eponychium as even a microscopic opening, or microtrauma, can be fatal for these clients. Discuss health issues with them; do not perform pedicures on diabetics or on people with circulatory diseases without their physician's permission. Seek training in how to work with these clients so you will know how to work safely on them.

Pedicure Pricing

Most salons and spas will probably have a price list for services. If and when you find yourself in a position to price your own services, a good rule of thumb is to determine the price of your basic pedicure first and then set your prices for more upscale and luxurious pedicures: Do this by increasing the base price of the pedicure according to the value of the added treatments, products, and time it takes you to perform the additional services.

Another great way to upgrade your pedicure service and price is through nail art. Many clients enjoy adding a little something special to their normal pedicure polish, especially if their work prohibits them from

? DID YOU KNOW?
Most salons will have a protocol to follow when finishing services. Follow them closely for two reasons. First, a routine keeps things moving in the salon, and second, clients get used to the closing protocol and know what to expect. If your salon does not have a post-service protocol, or if you work alone, establish one. Clients are more comfortable with a familiar routine.

? DID YOU KNOW?
More expensive pedicures with luxury touches such as masks, paraffin, and mitts should include exfoliation and massage of the legs. The tops of the knees may be included, but the underside of the knees is not included. Exfoliate the leg after the foot is exfoliated, but before the use of the foot file, and then apply a lotion to maintain the softness until the massage.

⚠ CAUTION
When performing a pedicure, do not push back the eponychium with a metal pusher. Compared with the hands, feet are more susceptible to infection, and pushing back the eponychium (or cutting it) can dramatically increase the risk of serious infections on feet. This tool is designed to remove the tissue that may adhere to the surface of the nail plate, not for pushing back the eponychium. This is especially important for clients with diabetes, psoriasis, and other chronic illnesses.

DID YOU KNOW?

You should charge extra for add-on services such as paraffin wax treatments and nail art. Services have dollar value—especially when you consider the time, product expense, skill level, and equipment used. Always be up front about additional service costs, and if a client decides to indulge in one, charge them for it.

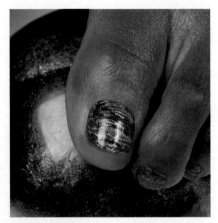

figure 26-20
Gel toenail art

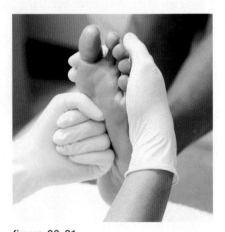

figure 26-21
A foot and leg massage focuses on relaxation.

DID YOU KNOW?

Work on the foot on the client's non-dominant side first. (The dominant side of the body is determined by the side of the client's writing hand.) The foot on the client's dominant side usually needs more soaking and attention. It needs to soak those few extra minutes while you are working on the other foot.

wearing polish or art on their hands. It is easy to get your clients addicted to toenail art by giving the first example at no cost. Once they have it and their friends compliment them, they will want it every time, and you will quickly see an increase in revenue with your existing clientele (figure 26-20). Toenail art is especially popular in sandal season and with formal, open footwear.

Many salons and spas have found that manicure and pedicure packages are well received by their clients and work well for the staff. Manicures and pedicures together are like salt and pepper—although they are different, they go well together.

One great way to sell these packages is to develop theme services for holidays and special events, such as Christmas, Valentine's Day, Mother's Day, prom, weddings, and birthday packages; market them, and you will see your clientele grow.

Pedicure Massage

According to client salon surveys, massage is the most enjoyed aspect of any nail service. Because this is especially true for pedicures, you should spend time developing a technique that you will enjoy giving and that your clients will enjoy receiving.

The definition of *massage i*s the manual or mechanical manipulation of the body by rubbing, gently pinching, kneading, tapping, and other movements. Cosmetologists massage their clients to help keep the facial skin healthy and the facial muscles firm. General body massage sometimes has a therapeutic purpose and sometimes focuses on relaxation. However, massage given during manicures and pedicures definitely focuses on relaxation. The most enjoyable massage is a rhythmic, slow slide with the fingers and palm connecting to the client as much as possible. Maintain a touch connection with the client throughout the massage, sliding the hands from one location to the next in a smooth transition (figure 26-21).

The art of massage has a rich and long history. There are many types of massage, and individuals usually develop their own special styles and techniques. The number of massage routines is as vast as the number of persons performing massages. No matter what techniques you use, perfect them so foot and leg massage becomes second nature to you. During this part of the pedicure, be keenly aware of your client's health, meet any precautionary requirements, and offer a massage that relaxes the client but is not harmful to him or her.

The foot and leg massage is similar to the hand and arm massage that follows a manicure. The massage technique that is used most is effleurage. This technique is even more important for pedicures than manicures because many clients have circulatory issues that may prevent you from using other massage techniques.

Before performing a service that includes a foot and/or leg massage, consult the client's intake form. During the consultation, acknowledge and discuss any medical condition your client listed that may be contraindicated for a foot and/or leg massage. If this is the case, ask the client if they have discussed massage with their physician and if they have not already done so, encourage them to seek their physician's advice as to whether or not a foot and/or leg massage is advisable before performing the service.

Many clients that have high blood pressure (hypertension), diabetes, or circulatory conditions may still have foot and/or leg massage without concern, especially if their condition is being treated and carefully looked after by a physician. Foot and/or leg massage is, however, contraindicated for clients with severe, uncontrolled hypertension. For clients who have circulatory problems such as varicose veins, massaging the foot and/or leg may be harmful because it increases circulation. Ask for written permission from the client's physician before performing this massage.

If your client has sensitive or redness-prone skin, avoid using vigorous or strong massage techniques. This is especially important for clients who have arthritis. When making decisions about whether to perform a foot and/or leg massage on a person who has a medical condition, be conservative. When in doubt, don't include massage as part of your service.

Most of us enjoy being touched, and the art of massage takes a pedicure to a higher level of enjoyment. Many people think foot massage is more special than massage on any other part of the body. Foot massage induces a high degree of relaxation and stimulates blood flow. Be aware of the areas of the feet and legs where the client most enjoys massage, and put a greater emphasis in these areas.

Every massage, whether pedicure or body massage, must end. Feathering is a technique used at the end of a massage to provide a signal for experienced clients that the massage is ending, and to provide a gentle release from the client. At the end of the last movement in the pedicure massage, create a smooth transition by gently placing both of the client's feet onto the footrest, or on another stable surface, and move your palms to the top of the feet with your fingers toward the leg. Press your entire hands three times slowly onto the feet. This should not be a hard press, just a firm push for one to two seconds. After the last press, gently pull your hand toward the tips of the toes with a feather-light touch of your fingertips. Never allow your fingernails to touch the skin. Perform the final feather-off movement only once, and then allow the client to relax a minute or two before moving to the next step of the pedicure.

(P) 26-2   Foot and Leg Massage *See page 918*

Reflexology

Reflexology is a unique method of applying pressure with thumb and index fingers to the hands and feet, and it has demonstrated health benefits. This specialty massage often employs many of the principles of acupressure and acupuncture, and it is considered a science by many technicians.

Reflexology is based on the principle that areas (reflexes) in the feet and hands correspond to all the organs, glands, and parts of the body. It is said that stimulating (pressing) these reflexes or points can reflect positive energy and increase blood flow to the specified areas.

Professional, hands-on training is essential in reflexology for two reasons:

1. The specific touch used in reflexology can be learned only through hands-on training. Clients who have received a reflexology treatment

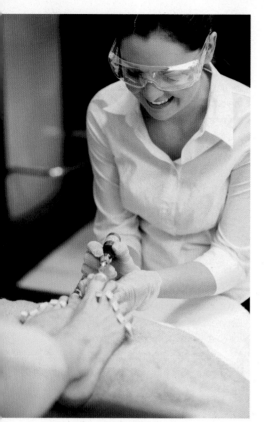

figure 26-22
While working, pay attention to your body's positioning to avoid risk of injury.

from a certified reflexologist recognize the appropriate touch and respond negatively to those who cannot deliver the same treatment because of minimal or no training.

2. An untrained cosmetologist may not be able to produce results for the client, so the client will not be happy about the extra cost and time taken by the service.

If a salon wishes to offer reflexology services to its clients, it is best that the staff or professional receives authentic training and certification in the art of reflexology from a highly recommended reflexologist who is certified by the Reflexology Association of America.

Ergonomics

Pedicures can pose a threat to the health and well-being of cosmetologists who perform them. If technicians are careless about protecting themselves through proper ergonomics, they can develop serious and painful back conditions.

Pay attention to your body's positioning and make sure you are working ergonomically. Always sit in a comfortable position, relaxed and unstrained, to reduce the risk of injury to your back, shoulders, arms, wrists, and hands (figure 26-22). For example, avoid leaning forward or stretching to reach your client's feet. Take a minute to stretch before and after each pedicure to keep your body limber, in-line, and more resistant to injury.

Although it is important to give your client the best possible service, it is also important to keep yourself healthy during the process and to avoid injuries caused by strain or repeated motion.

After reading the next few sections, you will be able to:

LO**6** Summarize the importance of cleaning and disinfecting a pedicure bath.

Properly Clean and Disinfect Foot Spas

Disinfection of the pedicure bath has been discussed and sensationalized in the media—and for good reason. There are specific criteria and steps that must be followed exactly to ensure proper disinfection and infection control. Improper, rushed, or careless cleaning of the pedicure bath may lead to health and safety concerns for salon clients. The salon and the individual technician bear the responsibility for ensuring that proper disinfection occurs and that proper procedures are followed.

Review **Procedure 5-2, Cleaning and Disinfecting Whirlpool, Air-Jet, and Pipeless Foot Spas,** in Chapter 5. The disinfecting procedures have been developed by the Nail Manufacturer's Council (NMC), a group

> **⚠ CAUTION**
> No additive that is added to the water during a pedicure soak kills pathogens and replaces your obligation to clean and disinfect the equipment and implements after the pedicure. Any chemical that is strong enough to adequately kill pathogens is not safe for contact with skin. Disinfectants must never be placed in the foot bath with your client's feet. They can be harmful to the skin.

of nail-care company representatives, and the International Nail Technicians Association (INTA)(a group of professional nail technicians), for cleaning and disinfecting all types of pedicure equipment, including:

- Whirlpool units
- Air-jet basins
- Pipeless foot spas
- Non-whirlpool basins (tubs, footbaths, sinks and bowls)

In addition, salons must always use an EPA-registered hospital disinfectant that the label claims is a broad-spectrum bactericide, virucide, and fungicide (figure 26-23). In addition, many states require salons to record the time and date of each disinfecting procedure in a salon pedicure log or a disinfection log for accountability purposes.

Salon teams are encouraged to incorporate the disinfection procedures discussed in Chapter 5 into their regular cleaning and disinfecting schedules and to display the procedures in the employee areas. Always check your state regulations concerning the required disinfection protocol.

WEB RESOURCES

For more information concerning disinfection and other important topics pertaining to nails, go to probeauty. org /research. This site contains many informational brochures relevant to manicuring and pedicuring. The brochures, which are published in several languages including Vietnamese and Spanish, are written by the leading scientists and technical experts in the industry and are reviewed by other industry leaders before being published.

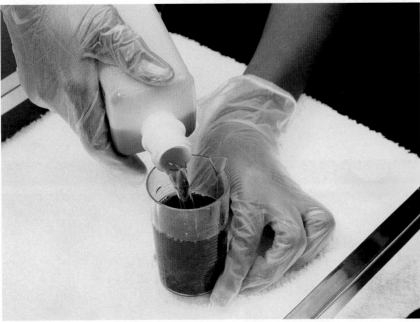

figure 26-23
Use an EPA-registered hospital disinfectant when disinfecting foot baths.

PERFORMING THE BASIC PEDICURE

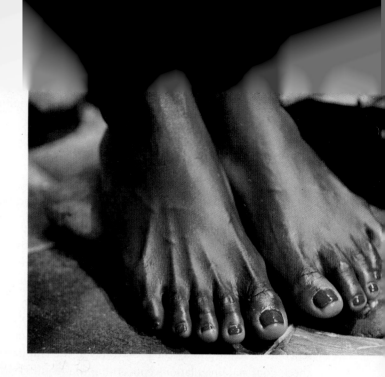

PREPARATION | PROCEDURE

Perform:

Ⓟ 25-1 **Pre-Service Procedure** *See page 880*

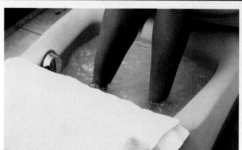

❶ Check the temperature of the pedicure bath for safety. Put on a pair of clean gloves, place the client's feet in the bath, and make sure he or she is comfortable with the water temperature. Allow the feet to soak for 5 to 10 minutes to soften and clean the feet before beginning the pedicure.

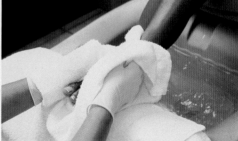

❷ Lift the client's foot you will be working with first from the bath. Using the towels on the footrest, on the pedicure cart, or on your lap, wrap the first towel around the foot and dry it thoroughly. Make sure you dry between the toes. If you are using a basin or portable bath, place the foot on the footrest or on a towel you have placed on your lap.

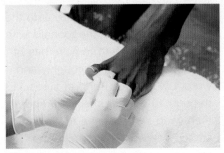

③ First, remove polish from the little toe. Then move across the foot toward the big toe. Complete polish removal is important to a quality pedicure finish.

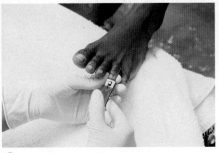

④ Carefully clip the toenails of the first foot straight across and even with the ends of the toes. The big toenail is usually the most challenging to trim. Do not leave any rough edges or "hooks" that might create an opportunity for infections.

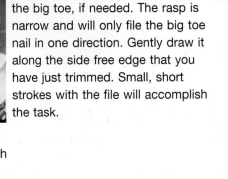

⑤ Carefully use the nail rasp only on the big toe, if needed. The rasp is narrow and will only file the big toe nail in one direction. Gently draw it along the side free edge that you have just trimmed. Small, short strokes with the file will accomplish the task.

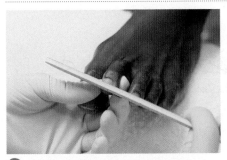

⑥ Carefully file the nails of the first foot with an appropriate single-use and prepped abrasive file. File them straight across, rounding them slightly at the corners. Smooth rough edges with the fine side of an abrasive file.

⑦ After filing, buff the nails to remove any unevenness. Next, apply cuticle remover and callus softener to heavy calluses, and then wrap the foot in a towel, and lay it aside. Remove the other foot from the water and perform steps 2 through 7 on that foot.

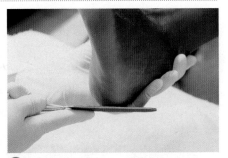

⑧ Remove the first foot from the towel wrap; use a wooden pusher to gently remove any loose, dead tissue. Next, use a foot file to smooth and reduce the thicker areas of calluses. Proceed to exfoliate the foot with a scrub to remove the dry or scaly skin. Use extra pressure on the heels and other areas where more calluses and dry skin build up.

⑨ Place the first foot in the foot bath and rinse off the cuticle remover and callus softener completely. Then lift the foot to above the water and brush the nails with a nail brush. Remove the foot and dry thoroughly.

⑩ Repeat steps 8 and 9 on the other foot.

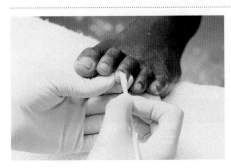

⑪ Unwrap the first foot. Use the single-use, cotton-tipped wooden pusher or product dispenser to reapply cuticle remover to the first foot. Begin with the little toe and work toward the big toe.

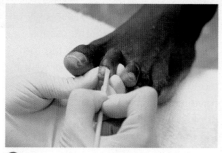

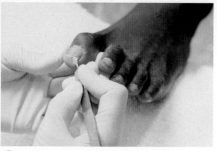

12 Use a clean, lint-free wipe to remove excess cuticle remover. Then carefully remove the cuticle tissue from the nail plate using a wooden or metal pusher, taking care not to break the seal between the nail plate and eponychium. Use a nipper to carefully remove any loose tags of dead skin, but don't cut, rip, or tear living skin; cutting cuticles may lead to serious infection.

13 Next, if necessary, use the curette to gently push the soft tissue folds away from the walls of the lateral nail plate, and gently remove extra build-up of debris between the nail plate and surrounding tissue.

14 Dip your client's first foot into the foot bath and brush the toenails with a nylon nail brush to remove bits of debris. Dry the foot thoroughly and wrap it in a towel. Perform steps 11 through 13 on the other foot, and then wrap that foot in a towel and set it aside while performing the following steps on the first foot.

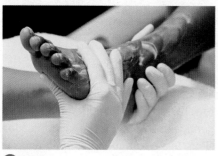

16 Perform a foot massage on the first foot as outlined in **Procedure 26-2, Foot and Leg Massage**. Then rewrap the foot and place it on the towel on the floor or step, wherever appropriate in your salon.

17 Massage the second foot.

15 Apply lotion, cream, or oil to the first foot for skin conditioning and massage. Use a firm touch to avoid tickling your client's feet.

18 Remove traces of lotion, cream, or oil from the nails of both feet with polish remover.

19 Ask the client to put on the sandals she will wear home or provide single-use pedicure slippers. Insert the toe separators, if possible. Apply a nail dehydrator. Then, apply base coat to the nails on both feet, then two coats of color, and finally a topcoat. Apply polish drying product (optional) to prevent smudging of the polish. You may want to escort the client to a drying area and offer him or her refreshment.

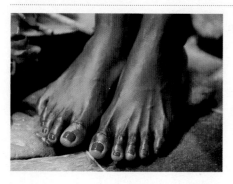

20 Finished look.

POST-SERVICE

Complete:

P 25-2 **Post-Service Procedure** *See page 884*

FOOT AND LEG MASSAGE

These techniques and illustrations provide instruction for massage on the feet and legs. A massage for a basic pedicure will include only the foot, while a spa pedicure will also include the leg massage, up to and including the front of the knee.

IMPLEMENTS & MATERIALS

In addition to the basic materials on your manicuring table, you will need the following for the massage:

□ Gloves   □ Massage oil or lotion

FOOT MASSAGE

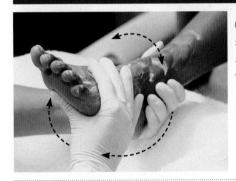

1 Put on a fresh pair of gloves and rest the client's heel on a footrest or stool and suggest that your client relax. Grasp the leg gently just above the ankle and use your other hand to hold the foot just beneath the toes; rotate the entire foot in a circular motion.

2 While holding the ankle, place the palm of your free hand on top of the foot behind the toes. Slide the palm up to the ankle area with gentle pressure and then return to starting position. Repeat three to five times in the middle, then on the sides of the top of the foot.

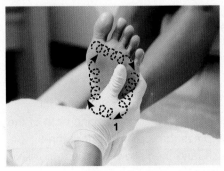

3 Never losing contact with the skin, slide your hands so that the thumbs are on the plantar side of the foot while the fingers are gently holding the dorsal side of the foot, like holding a sandwich. Move one thumb in a firm circular movement, moving from one side of the foot, across, above the heel, up the medial side (center side) of the foot to below the toes, across the ball of the foot and back down the other side of the foot (distal side) to the original position.

④ Repeat the same motions of step 3 with the opposite hand and thumb. The base of the thumbs to the pads of the fingers should be in contact with the skin throughout the movement. Alternate this massage step with each hand and thumb and repeat several times.

⑤ Perform the same thumb movement on the surface of the heels, rotating your thumbs in opposite directions. Repeat three to five times.

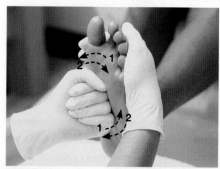

⑥ Place your one hand on top of the foot, cupping it, and make a fist with your other hand. The hand on top of the foot will press the foot toward you while your other hand twists into the instep of the foot. This helps stimulate blood flow and provides relaxation. Repeat three to five times. This is a friction movement. The bottom of the foot is the only place a friction movement is performed in pedicure services.

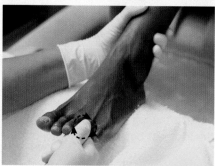

⑦ Start with the little toe, placing the thumb on the top of the toe and curl the index finger underneath the toe. (Your palm is facing up.) Push the fingers and thumb in that position back to the base of the toe, then rotate the thumb and finger in a circular, effleurage movement until the index finger is arched over the top of the toe, and the thumb is underneath. Pull the toe with index finger and thumb outward, away from the foot.

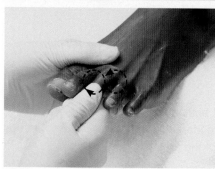

⑧ Hold the tip of the toe, starting with the little toe, and make a figure eight with each toe. Repeat three to five times on each toe and then move to the next. After the last movement on each toe, gently squeeze the tip of each once, and then move on to the next toe.

⑨ Return your hands to the position described in step 4 and repeat steps 3 and 4. Repeat all movements on each foot as many times as you wish, adding other movements that you like to perform, and then move to the other leg/foot.

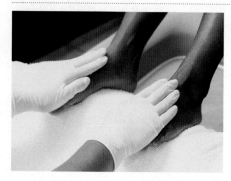

⑩ End the massage with a feathering technique to provide a signal for experienced clients that the massage is ending. Finish by placing both of the client's feet onto the footrest, and firmly press the tops of the feet three times slowly for one to two seconds each, and then allow the client to relax a minute or two before moving to the next step of the pedicure.

11 Once the massage of both feet is completed, you may move on in the pedicure procedure. If you are performing a luxury pedicure, do not perform the feather off movement; slide your hands to the leg and move on to the leg massage after step 9.

LEG MASSAGE

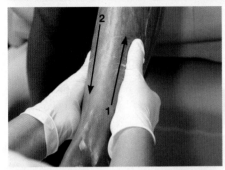

12 Place the foot on the footrest or stabilize it on your lap, then gently grasp the client's leg from behind the ankle with one hand. Perform effleurage movements from the ankle to below the knee on the front of the leg with the other hand. Move up the leg and then lightly return to the original location. Perform five to seven repetitions, then move to the sides of the leg and perform an additional five to seven repetitions.

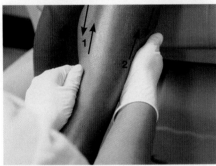

13 Slide to the back of the leg and perform effleurage movements up the back of the leg. Stroke up the leg, then, with less pressure, return to the original location; perform five to seven times.

14 Once the massage of both legs is completed, you may move on in the pedicure procedure.

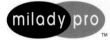

Check out miladypro.com for additional resources and training to enhance your technical skills. Keyword: *FutureCosPro*

REVIEW QUESTIONS

1. List at least five unique pieces of equipment used in pedicures.

2. Describe two specialty materials used when performing pedicures.

3. What is a callus softener and how is it used?

4. Explain the differences between a basic pedicure and a spa pedicure.

5. Define *reflexology* and explain how it is used in pedicuring.

6. Why is cleaning and disinfection of pedicure baths important?

7. List the steps in a basic pedicure.

8. List the steps in a foot and leg massage.

STUDY TOOLS

- **Reinforce what you just learned:** Complete the activities and exercises in your Theory or Practical Workbook, or your Study Guide.

- **Expand your knowledge:** Search for websites about the topics in this chapter and make a list of additional resources.

- **Study and prepare for your quiz:** Take the chapter test in your Exam Review or your Milady U: Online Licensing Prep.

- **Re-Test your knowledge:** Take the Chapter 26 *Quizzes*!

- **Learn even more:** Look up in a dictionary or search the internet for the definitions of any additional terms you want to learn about.

CHAPTER GLOSSARY

basalt	p. 904	A dark, fine-grained volcanic rock used in hot stone massage.
callus softeners	p. 908	Products designed to soften and smooth thickened tissue (calluses).
curette	p. 905	A small, scoop-shaped implement used for more efficient removal of debris from the nail folds, eponychium, and hyponychium areas.
exfoliating scrubs	p. 908	Water-based lotions that contain a mild, gritty-like abrasive and moisturizers to help in removing dry, flaky skin and reduce calluses.
foot files	p. 906	Also known as *pedicure paddles*; large, abrasive files used to reduce and smooth thicker foot calluses.
foot soaks	p. 908	Products containing gentle soaps, moisturizers, and other additives that are used in a pedicure bath to cleanse, deodorize, and soften the skin.
mask	p. 903	Also known as a *masque*; is a concentrated treatment product often composed of mineral clays, moisturizing agents, skin softeners, aromatherapy oils, botanical extracts, and other beneficial ingredients to cleanse, exfoliate, tighten, tone, hydrate, and nourish the skin.
nail rasp	p. 906	A metal implement with a grooved edge that is used for filing and smoothing the edges of the nail plate.

pedicure	p. 900	A cosmetic service performed on the feet by a licensed cosmetologist or nail technician; can include exfoliating the skin and callus reduction, as well as trimming, shaping, and polishing toenails. A pedicure often includes foot massage.
potassium hydroxide	p. 909	An inorganic compound that degrades the protein in the callus cells.
reflexology	p. 915	A unique method of applying pressure with thumb and index fingers to the hands and feet; it has demonstrated health benefits.
salicylic acid sal-uh-SIL-ik AS-ud	p. 909	An organic acid that derives originally from the bark of willow trees.
toe separators	p. 907	Foam rubber or cotton disposable materials used to keep toes apart while polishing the nails. A new set must be used on each client.
toenail clippers	p. 905	Professional implements that are larger than fingernail clippers and have a curved or straight jaw specifically designed for cutting toenails.
toenail nippers	p. 905	Similar in design to fingernail nippers, but are larger, much stronger, and used to trim the toenail as opposed to trimming the excess cuticle.
urea	p. 909	An organic compound that has a super-hydrating effect on skin cells.

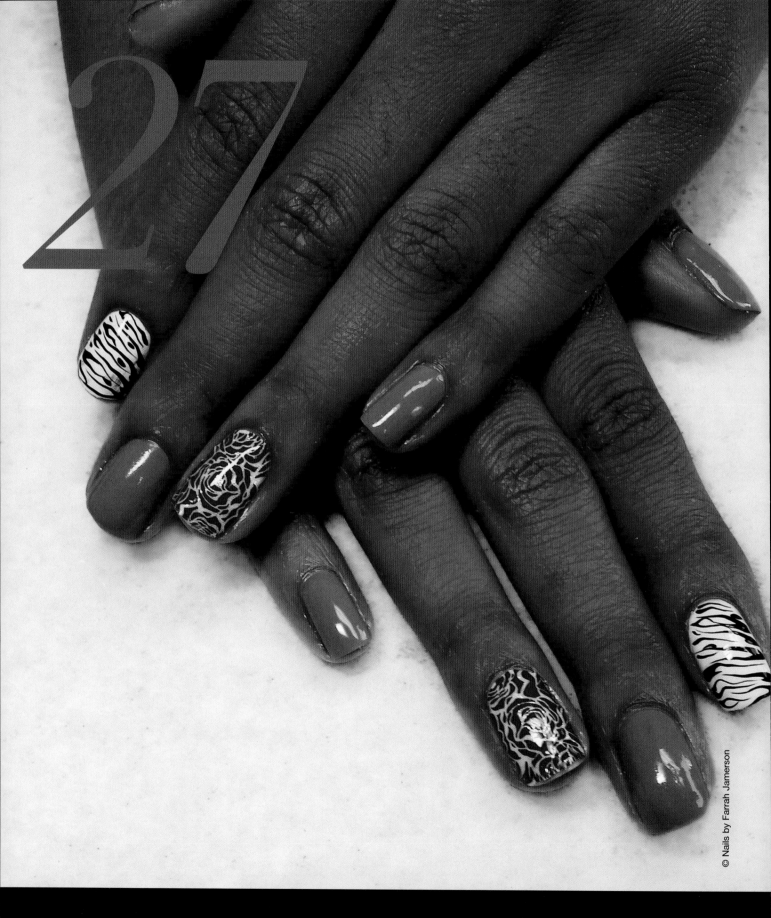

27

NAIL TIPS AND WRAPS

LEARNING
OBJECTIVES

After completing this chapter, you will be able to:

LO❶
In addition to your basic manicure table set up, identify any supplies that are needed for nail tip application and explain their use.

LO❷
Name and describe the three types of nail tips available, and describe the importance of correctly fitting nail tips.

LO❸
Demonstrate the stop, rock, and hold method of applying nail tips.

LO❹
Explain a few methods of applying nail tips.

LO❺
List the types of fabrics used in nail wraps and explain the benefits of using each.

LO❻
Describe the main difference between performing the two-week fabric wrap maintenance and the four-week fabric wrap maintenance.

LO❼
Demonstrate how to remove fabric wraps and what to avoid.

OUTLINE

One of the most popular services that a cosmetologist can offer clients is the opportunity to wear beautiful nails in an almost endless variety of lengths and strengths.

Regardless of whether a client is interested in wearing long, medium, or short nails, she may decide to have nail tips applied over her natural nails for strength and durability. Once a tip is applied, she will have an opportunity to choose from a variety of products that can be layered over the natural nail and the tip to further secure the strength of the nail and its beauty.

why study
NAIL TIPS AND WRAPS?

Cosmetologists should have a thorough understanding of nail tips and wraps because:

> Offering nail extension and wrap services expands your service offerings and enables clients to have a "one stop shop" experience in your salon.

> Learning the proper technique for applying and removing nail tips will help your client keep her natural nails in the best possible health and condition.

> Understanding the types and uses of nail wraps will enable you to determine the appropriate wrap for your clients' specific needs.

> Learning how to safely and correctly apply, maintain, and remove nail tips and wraps will ensure your clients' happiness and loyalty.

After reading the next few sections, you will be able to:

LO❶ In addition to your basic manicure table set up, identify any supplies that are needed for nail tip application and explain their use.

LO❷ Name and describe the three types of nail tips available, and describe the importance of correctly fitting nail tips.

LO❸ Demonstrate the stop, rock, and hold method of applying nail tips.

LO❹ Explain a few methods of applying nail tips.

Learn All You Need to Know About Nail Tips

Nail tips are plastic, pre-molded nails shaped from a tough polymer made from **acrylonitrile butadiene styrene (ABS)** (ak-ruh-loh-NAHY-tril byoo-tuh-DAHY-een STAHY-reen) plastic. They are adhered to the natural nail to add extra length and to serve as a support for nail enhancement products. Tips are combined with an **overlay**, a layer of any kind of nail enhancement product that is applied over the natural nail and tip application for added strength. Nail tips that do not have the reinforcement provided by the overlay are not long-wearing and can break easily.

In addition to the basic materials on your manicuring table, you will need an abrasive board; buffer block; tip adhesive; **tip cutter**, an implement similar to a nail clipper and designed for use on nail tips; **nail dehydrator**, a substance used to remove surface moisture and tiny amounts of oil left on the natural nail plate; and a variety of nail tips for the nail tip application (figure 27-1).

Many nail tips have a shallow depression called a "well" that serves as the point of contact with the nail plate. The **position stop**, the point where the free edge of the natural nail meets the tip, is where the tip is adhered to the nail. If you are using nail tips, you should use your abrasive to shape the free edges of the natural nails to match the shape of the nail tip to the stop point. This will provide a better fit and longer wear of the tip. There are various types of nail tips including partial well, full well, and well-less (no well at all) (figure 27-2).

Nail tips are available in many sizes, colors, and shapes, making it easy to fit each client with precisely the right size and shape tip. Tips can be purchased in large containers of 100 to 500 pieces, as well as in various individual refill sizes. With such a wide assortment, it is easy to fit each client correctly. Make sure when fitting tips to your client that the tips you choose cover the nail plate from sidewall to sidewall exactly. Do not make the mistake of using a tip that is narrower than the nail plate. This can cause the tip to crack at the sides or split down the middle.

Rather than attempting to force a too-small tip onto the nail, it is better to use a slightly larger tip and use an abrasive board to tailor the tip before applying it. You can also trim and bevel the well area before applying the tip to the nail, which can save you blending time. Nail tips

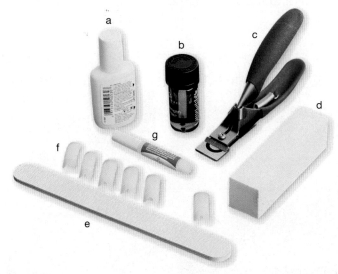

figure 27-1
Supplies needed for nail tip application (clockwise): a) brush-on resin; b) nail dehydrator; c) tip cutters; d) block buffer; e) abrasive file; f) nail tips; g) tip adhesive.

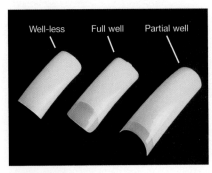

figure 27-2
Nail tips (from left to right): well-less, full well, partial well.

that are pre-beveled require much less filing on the natural nail after application. This also lessens the potential for damage to the natural nail.

The bonding agent used to secure the nail tip to the natural nail is called **nail tip adhesive**. Adhesives can be purchased in either tubes or brush-on containers and are available in several different forms, depending on the thicknesses of the adhesive. For instance, gel adhesives, sometimes referred to as *resin*, are the thickest adhesives and require more time to dry than fast-setting, thinner adhesives, which dry in about five seconds.

Nail adhesives usually come in either a tube with a pointed applicator tip, a one-drop applicator, or as a brush-on. Use care when opening adhesive containers—always point the opening away from your face and away from your client. Cosmetologists and their clients should always wear eye protection when using and handling nail tip adhesives. Even the smallest amount of adhesive in the eyes can be very dangerous and may cause serious injury.

Application of Nail Tips

When using nail adhesive to apply a nail tip to a client, there are a few methods of application.

For a faster, almost immediate set, place enough adhesive on the nail plate to cover the area where the tip will be placed and apply the tip to the nail. You also can use a thin brush-on adhesive and cover the entire nail, then press the tip into it. For a little more time to adjust the tip before it sets, apply the adhesive to the well of the tip, and then apply to the natural nail. This will also ensure there are fewer air bubbles trapped in the adhesive. In either instance, do not apply too much: Less is more when it comes to nail tip adhesives! Do not let adhesive run onto the skin.

When securing the tip to the natural nail, use the stop, rock, and hold method to avoid air bubbles and promote proper adhesion. To perform this method, approach the edge of the nail with the tip at a 45-degree angle. As you slide the tip onto the nail, find the *stop* against the free edge at a 45-degree angle. Rock the tip on slowly by applying steady pressure as you push the tip down to release any air pockets. Hold the tip in place for

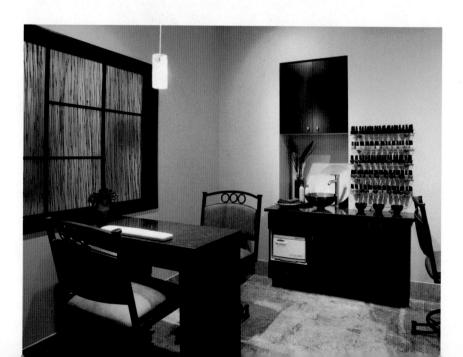

five to ten seconds until the adhesive has dried. This technique also works on well-less tips, followed by positioning on the nail plate and holding it in place for five to ten seconds until the adhesive hardens.

If you applied tips with a well, you will still need additional blending. The contact area will need to be reduced with an abrasive, so that the tip blends in with the natural nail. With a perfect tip application, there should be no visible line where the natural nail stops and the tip begins. To make them match with the surface of the natural nail plate, be sure to take care while filing and blending as this step can cause damage to the natural nail plate if done improperly. Using a medium- to fine-grit file or buffing block file (180 grit or higher), carefully smooth the contact area down until it is flush with the natural nail. Make sure to keep your buffer (or board) flat to the nail as you blend the tip. Never hold the file at an angle because the edge of abrasive may gouge the nail plate and damage it. After you finish blending, remove the shine from the rest of the tip.

Ⓟ 27-1 **Nail Tip Application** *See page 935*

After reading the next few sections, you will be able to:

LO **❺** List the types of fabrics used in nail wraps, and explain the benefits of using each.

Explore the Uses of Nail Wraps

Any method of securing a layer of fabric or paper on and around the nail tip to ensure its strength and durability is called a **nail wrap**. Nail wraps are one type of overlay that can be used over nail tips. Nail wraps are also used to repair or strengthen natural nails or to create nail extensions.

Before applying tips, wraps, or any enhancement service, preparation of the natural nail should include removing the shine with a fine abrasive buffer (240 grit), cleansing the nail, and applying a nail dehydrator. If you accidentally touch or contaminate the freshly prepped natural nail, you must clean it again and reapply nail dehydrator.

Following nail preparation, a **nail wrap resin** is used to coat and secure fabric wraps to the natural nail and nail tip. Wrap resins are made from **cyanoacrylate** (sy-an-oh-AH-cry-late), a specialized acrylic monomer that has excellent adhesion to the natural nail plate and polymerizes in seconds. The wrap resin is meant to penetrate the fabric and adhere it to the nail surface. Wrap resin will not easily penetrate fibers that are contaminated with oil, and those strands become visible in the clear coating. Thus, it is best not to touch the fabric more than you must.

An alternate way to handle the fabric as you adhere and adjust it on the nail is to use a 6" × 4" piece of flexible plastic sheet—a sandwich plastic bag works great—to press fabric onto the nail plate. This will prevent the transfer of oil and debris from your fingers. Changing to an unused portion of the plastic for each finger is necessary. Run this plastic sheet from the cuticle to the free edge after each resin application to ensure that the wrap resin is evenly distributed. This will help prevent air bubbles or areas of bare fabric. Once the fabric is saturated with wrap resin, it will appear almost invisible. (Linen wrap fabric will remain visible because it is quite thick.)

Fabric wrap is a nail wrap made of silk, linen, or fiberglass. Fabric wraps are the most popular type of nail wrap because of their durability. Fabric wraps are cut to cover the surface of the natural nail and the nail tip and are laid onto a layer of wrap resin to build and strengthen the enhancement.

Fabric wraps may be purchased in swatches, rolls, or in packages of pre-cut pieces—some with and some without adhesive backing.

The wrap material is the heart of a nail wrap system and gives this system its unique properties. Nail wraps can be used as an overlay to strengthen natural nails or to strengthen a nail tip application.

- **Silk wraps** are made from a thin natural material with a tight weave that becomes transparent when wrap resin is applied. A silk wrap is lightweight and has a smooth appearance when applied to the nail.

- **Linen wraps** are made from a closely woven, heavy material. It is much thicker and bulkier than other types of wrap fabrics. Nail adhesives do not penetrate linen as easily as silk or fiberglass. Because a linen wrap is opaque, even after wrap resin is applied, a colored polish must be used to cover it completely. Linen is used because it is considered to be the strongest wrap fabric.

- **Fiberglass wraps** are made from a very thin synthetic mesh with a loose weave. The loose weave makes it easy to use and allows the wrap resin to penetrate, which improves adhesion. Even though fiberglass is not as strong as linen or silk, it can create a durable nail enhancement.

- **Paper wraps** are temporary nail wraps made of very thin paper. Paper was one of the very first materials used to create wraps. They are quite simple to use, but they do not have the strength and durability of fabric wraps. For this reason, paper wraps are considered a temporary service and need to be completely replaced each time your client comes in for maintenance. Paper wraps were popular before the 1990s but are rarely used now, having been replaced with silk and fiberglass products.

A **wrap resin accelerator**, also known as *activator*, acts as the dryer that speeds up the hardening process of the wrap resin or adhesive overlay. Wrap resin accelerator is a product specially designed to help any cyanoacrylate glue or wrap resin dry more quickly. Use wrap resin accelerator according to manufacturer's instructions. Keep the wrap resin accelerator off skin to prevent overexposure to the product.

Activators come in several different forms: brush-on bottle, pump spray-on, and aerosol. Activator will dissipate in about two minutes after being applied; during this time, do not apply additional wrap resin or you may find that the activator on the nail causes the wrap resin to harden on the brush, tip of the bottle, or extender. Activator also does not need to be applied after every layer of adhesive. This is an optional step; activator can be used as needed.

In addition to your chosen wrap material, you will need wrap resin and resin accelerator, nail buffer and file, small scissors, plastic, and tweezers to perform a nail wrap overlay (figure 27-3).

Ⓟ 27-2   **Nail Wrap Application** *See page 937*

After reading the next few sections, you will be able to:

LO❻   Describe the main difference between performing the two-week fabric wrap maintenance and the four-week fabric wrap maintenance.

LO❼   Demonstrate how to remove fabric wraps and what to avoid.

Carry Out Nail Wrap Maintenance, Repair, and Removal

Fabric wraps need regular maintenance to keep them looking fresh. In this section, you will learn how to maintain fabric wraps after two weeks and after four weeks. You also will learn how to repair cracks and to remove nail wraps when necessary.

Nail Wrap Maintenance

Nail wraps must have consistent maintenance after the initial application.

Maintenance is the term used for when a nail enhancement needs to be serviced after two or more weeks from the initial application of the nail enhancement product. The maintenance service actually accomplishes two goals: It allows the cosmetologist to 1) apply the enhancement product onto the new growth of nail, commonly referred to as a *fill* or a *backfill*; and 2) structurally correct the nail to ensure its strength, shape, and durability—this is commonly referred to as a *rebalance*.

In a two-week fabric maintenance only resin is applied to the new growth area, where as a four-week fabric maintenance may need the additional stress strip on the new growth area to keep it strong. The maintenance is necessary for the nail's beauty and durability.

Ⓟ 27-3   **Two-week Fabric Wrap Maintenance** *See page 940*

figure 27-3
Supplies needed for nail wrap application (from top to bottom, left to right): a) building resin b) nail dehydrator c) activator d) tweezers e) tip cutters f) tip adhesive g) nail tips h) block buffer i) fiberglass j) abrasive file k) fabric scissors l) plastic sheet m) lint-free wipes.

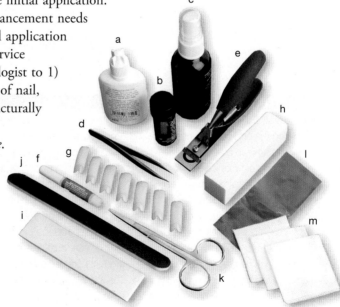

Fabric Wrap Repair

There are circumstances when nail wraps will need to be repaired. In those cases, small pieces of fabric can be used to strengthen a weak point in the nail or to repair a break in the nail.

A **stress strip** is a strip of fabric cut to ⅛-inch (3.12 mm) in length and applied to strengthen a weak point in the nail. A stress strip can be applied across the apex area during the initial wrap application. In this instance, it helps build the arch in the nail and also adds strength. After the stress strip is applied, cover with resin, use activator, and then apply the full fabric strip that overlays the entire nail. Stress strips at the apex are usually only applied when using a thin fabric such as silk or paper. Thin fabrics sometimes need extra strength, and because they are thin, the overlay does not appear too bulky. You would not want to do this technique with linen. A stress strip can also be used to repair or strengthen a weak point in a nail enhancement.

A **repair patch** is a piece of fabric cut to completely cover a crack or break in the nail. Use the four-week fabric wrap maintenance procedure to apply the repair patch.

Ⓟ 27-4   **Four-week Fabric Wrap Maintenance** *See page 943*

Fabric Wrap Removal

There may be times when a client would like to have their nail wraps removed. When this occurs, it is important to remove the wraps as carefully as possible so as not to damage the nail plate. Nail wraps are removed by immersing the entire enhancement into a small glass bowl filled with acetone. Wait for the nail wrap to melt away, and then gently and carefully slide the softened wrap material away from the nail with a wooden pusher. Never nip off the nail tip! This may lead to damage of the nail plate by pulling off layers of the natural nail and can break the seal of the remainder of the enhancement.

Always suggest a manicure after removal of an enhancement to rehydrate the natural nail and cuticle.

Ⓟ 27-5   **Nail Tip & Fabric Wrap Removal** *See page 946*

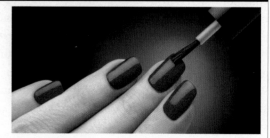

figure 27-4
Host a nail fashion night to introduce customers to the season's most popular colors, latest manicure looks and newest products.

NAIL TIP APPLICATION

In addition to the basic materials on your manicuring table, you will need the following supplies for the Nail Tip Application procedure:

- ☐ Abrasive boards
- ☐ Buffer block
- ☐ Nail dehydrator
- ☐ Nail tip adhesive
- ☐ Nail tips
- ☐ Tip cutter

PREPARATION

Perform:

Ⓟ 25-1 **Pre-Service Procedure** *See page 880*

PROCEDURE

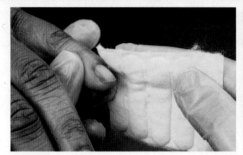

1 Clean the nails and remove existing polish.

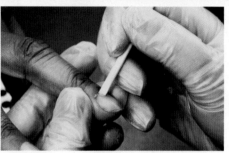

2 Gently push back the eponychium, using a wooden stick, pusher, or other suitable implement, and carefully remove the cuticle tissue from the nail plate.

3 File the free edge of the nails, if needed. Use your 180-grit abrasive or higher to shape the free edges of the natural nails so they match the shape of the nail tip to the stop point.

4 Buff very lightly over the nail plate with a medium-fine abrasive (180- to 240-grit) to remove the shine caused by natural oil and contaminants on the surface of the nail plate. Remove the dust with a clean, dry nail brush.

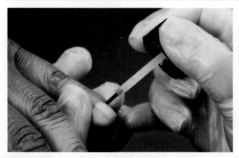

5 Apply nail dehydrator. Be careful not to touch the natural nail with your fingers as any deposit of oils from your fingers could cause lifting of the overlay after it is applied.

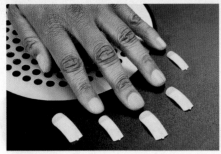

6 Choose properly-sized tips for your client's nail plate and ensure they cover the nail plate from sidewall to sidewall. Put all of the pre-tailored and pre-sized tips in the order of finger position, in front of your client.

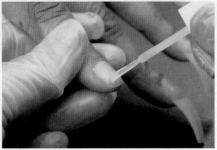

7 Use nail adhesive to apply the properly-sized tips to your client by either applying the adhesive to the natural nail or to the well of the tip.

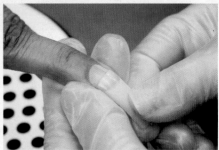

8 Secure the tips onto the client's natural nail using the stop, rock, and hold method.

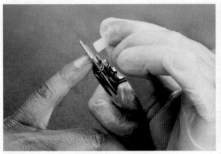

9 Trim the nail tips to the desired length using a tip cutter.

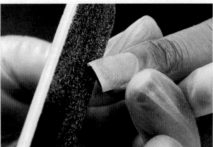

10 If you applied tips with a well, additional blending will be needed. Carefully blend the nail tip with a 180 grit file and buffing block (180- to 240-grit), to carefully smooth the contact area down until it is flush with the natural nail. After you finish blending, remove the shine from the rest of the tip.

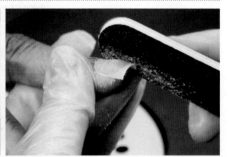

11 Use caution as you shape the nail tip with a 180-grit abrasive. The nail tip contact point is very thin and can break.

12 Your nail tip application process is now complete. Although your client's tips blend with her natural nails, tips should not be worn without an additional nail overlay such as wraps because tips will not be strong enough to wear alone.

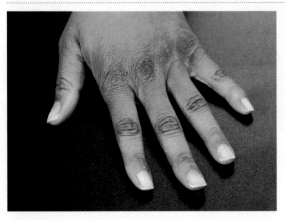

13 Complete set of applied nail tips.

POST-SERVICE

Complete:

P 25-2 **Post-Service Procedure** *See page 884*

NAIL WRAP APPLICATION

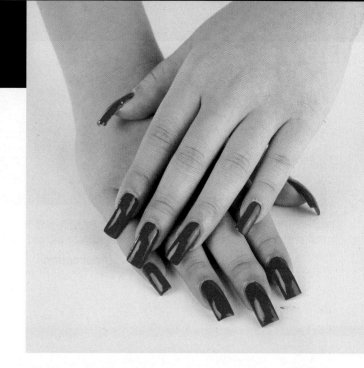

IMPLEMENTS & MATERIALS

In addition to the basic materials on your manicuring table, you will need the following supplies for the Nail Wrap Application procedure:

- ☐ Adhesive-backed fabric
- ☐ Nail buffer
- ☐ Nail dehydrator
- ☐ Small piece of plastic
- ☐ Small scissors
- ☐ Tweezers (optional)
- ☐ Wrap resin
- ☐ Wrap resin accelerator

PREPARATION

Perform:

P 25-1 **Pre-Service Procedure** *See page 880*

PROCEDURE

1 Clean the nails and remove existing polish.

2 Push back the eponychium and remove the cuticle.

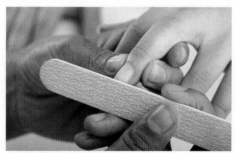

3 File the free edge of the nails, if needed. Use your 180-grit abrasive or higher to shape the free edges of the natural nails so they match the shape of the nail wrap to the stop point.

4 Lightly buff the nail plate with a medium-fine buffer (180-grit to 240-grit) to remove shine caused by the oil found on the natural nail plate. Remove the dust with a clean, dry, disinfected nail brush.

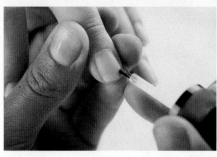

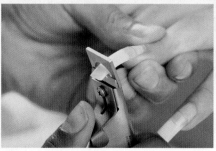

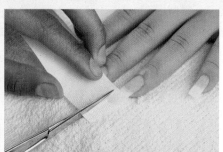

5 Apply a nail dehydrator onto the nail plate.

6 Apply nail tips, if desired. Refer to **Procedure 27-1, Nail Tip Application**.

7 Before removing the backing on the fabric, cut it to the approximate width and shape of the nail entire nail surface. Place custom-cut fabric strips in a row according to the order they will be applied. You may also cut stress strips now if needed to cover the apex area.

Alternatively, if you use pre-cut fabric, pre-size the precut fabric for each nail.

8 Begin with the pinky finger of the left hand and apply the wrap resin to the entire surface of the nail and tip on all 10 fingers. Once completed, return to the first finger to apply the fabric wraps. (If you plan to apply the optional stress strip at the apex area, do this now following the same directions as step 9 to 12.)

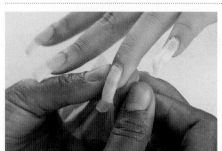

9 Remove the backing from the fabric, and gently fit the fabric over the nail plate, covering the entire nail (use a pair of tweezers to apply the fabric if desired), keeping it ⅟₁₆-inch (1.59 mm) away from the sidewall and eponychium. Use a small piece of thick plastic to press the fabric onto the nail and to smooth it out.

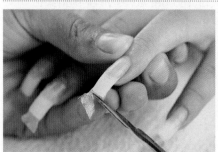

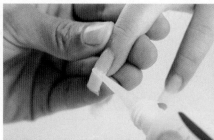

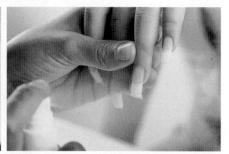

10 Once the fabric is secure on the nail, use small scissors to trim the fabric ⅟₁₆-inch (1.59 mm) away from sidewalls and the free edge. Trimming fabric slightly smaller than the nail plate prevents fabric from lifting and separating from the nail plate.

11 Draw a thin coat of wrap resin down the center of the nail using the extender tip or brush. Press the plastic against the nail at the cuticle and slide down to the free edge to evenly distribute the resin.

12 Use wrap resin accelerator to dry the resin.

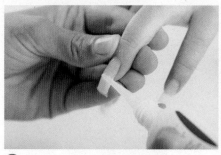

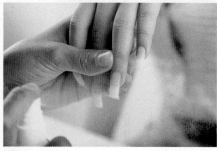

13 Apply and spread a second coat of wrap resin; seal the free edge to prevent lifting and tip separation.

14 Apply wrap resin accelerator.

15 Use a fine (240-grit) abrasive to shape and refine the surface and perimeter. Then, buff the nail wrap with a fine 240 grit buffer to produce a shine. Avoid buffing excessively or for too long, as this can wear through the wrap and weaken it. Remove any dust with a clean, dry, disinfected nail brush.

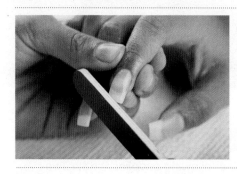

16 If the client prefers, buff to a high shine with a fine (350-grit or higher) shiner buffer.

17 Apply cuticle oil, and then thoroughly wash the nail enhancements. Then apply hand lotion or massage oil and massage the hands and arms.

18 Remove traces of oil using a lint-free wipe with cleanser or non-acetone polish remover.

19 Polish the nails.

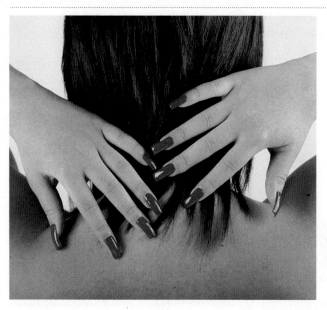

20 Finished look.

POST-SERVICE

Complete:

P 25-2 **Post-Service Procedure** *See page 884*

TWO-WEEK FABRIC WRAP MAINTENANCE

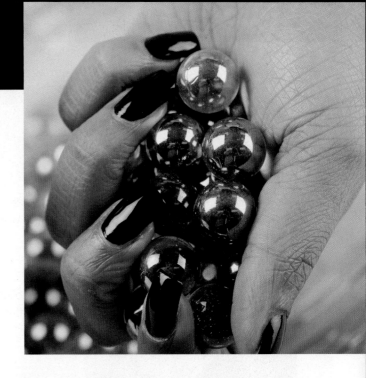

IMPLEMENTS & MATERIALS

In addition to the basic materials on your manicuring table, you will need the following supplies for the Two-Week Fabric Wrap Maintenance procedure:

☐ Abrasive buffer or file   ☐ Nail dehydrator   ☐ Wrap resin   ☐ Wrap resin accelerator

PREPARATION | PROCEDURE

Perform:

P 25-1 **Pre-Service Procedure** *See page 880*

① Use a non-acetone polish remover to remove existing nail polish and to avoid damaging nail wraps. Acetone will break down the wrap resin too quickly.

② Clean the natural nails.

③ Push back the eponychium. If needed, shorten the free edges of the nails with a 180 grit file.

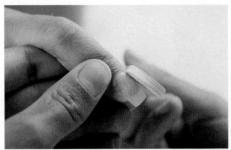

④ Gently file the surface of the wrap nail, including the exposed nail plate, with a 180 to 240 grit file.

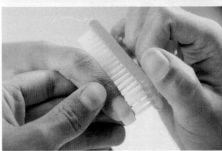

⑤ Remove the dust with a clean, dry nylon nail brush. Proceed to cleanse the nails with a surface cleanser and lint-free wipe. Then apply nail dehydrator to new, natural nail growth area on all 10 nails. Repeat on the right hand.

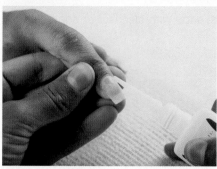

6 Apply a small amount of nail wrap resin to the area of new nail growth, and then continue to spread the wrap resin to the rest of the nail, taking care to avoid touching the skin. Do this for all 10 nails.

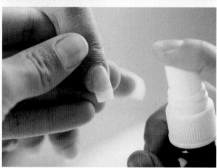

7 Spray, brush, or drop on a wrap resin accelerator that is specifically designed to work with the product you are using. Follow the manufacturer's instructions. Keep the wrap resin accelerator off skin to prevent over-exposure to the product.

8 Apply a second coat of wrap resin to the entire nail plate to strengthen and reseal the nail wrap.

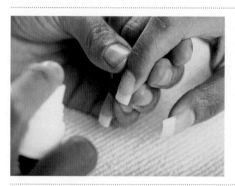

9 Apply a second coat of wrap resin accelerator. Throughout steps 6 through 9 check to make sure the resin is evenly distributed and there are no air bubbles or bare fabric.

10 Use a medium-fine abrasive over the surface of the nail wrap to remove any imperfections, starting with the free edge and then the ridge.

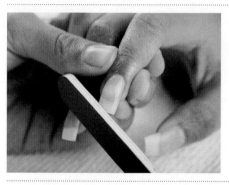

11 If your client prefers, buff to a high shine with a fine-grit buffer (350-grit or higher). Remove any dust with a clean, dry, disinfected nail brush.

12 Apply cuticle oil. Have the client wash and dry their hands. Apply hand lotion or massage oil, and then massage the client's hands and arms.

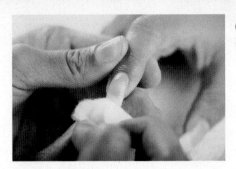

13 Remove traces of oil using a lint-free wipe with cleanser or non-acetone polish remover.

14 Polish the nails.

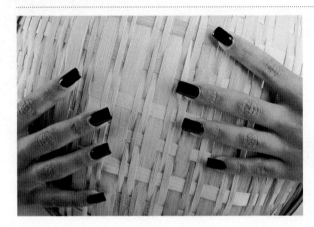

15 Finished Look.

POST-SERVICE

Complete:

P 25-2 **Post-Service Procedure** *See page 884*

FOUR-WEEK FABRIC WRAP MAINTENANCE

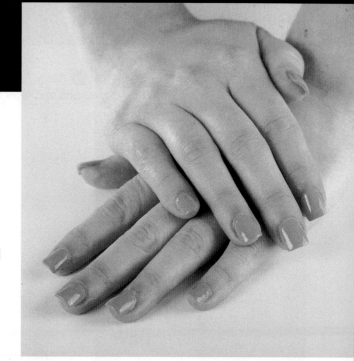

IMPLEMENTS & MATERIALS

In addition to the basic materials on your manicuring table, you will need the following supplies for the Four-Week Fabric Wrap Maintenance procedure:

- ☐ Abrasive buffer or file
- ☐ Adhesive-backed fabric
- ☐ Nail dehydrator
- ☐ Small piece of plastic
- ☐ Small scissors
- ☐ Tweezers (optional)
- ☐ Wrap resin
- ☐ Wrap resin accelerator

PREPARATION

Perform:

P 25-1 **Pre-Service Procedure** See page 880

PROCEDURE

1 Use a non-acetone polish remover to remove existing nail polish and to avoid damaging nail wraps. Acetone will break down the wrap resin too quickly.

2 Push back the eponychium and remove any loosened cuticle.

3 Use a medium- to fine-grit abrasive (180- to 240-grit) to carefully refine the nail surface of the nail until there is no obvious line of demarcation between new growth and fabric wrap. Gently file away any small pieces of fabric that may have lifted since the last service. Avoid damaging the natural nail with the abrasive.

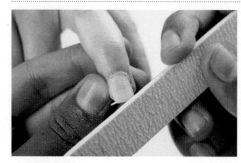

4 Lightly buff the entire nail surface with a medium-fine (180- to 240-grit) buffer to remove the shine. Remove the dust with a clean, dry, nylon nail brush. Cleanse the nails with a surface cleanser and a lint-free wipe.

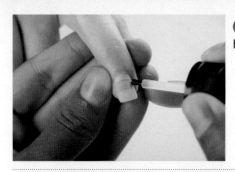

5 Apply nail dehydrator to all 10 nails. Begin with the little finger on the left hand and work toward the thumb. Repeat on the right hand.

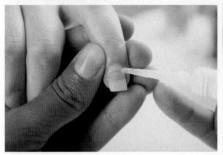

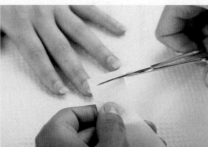

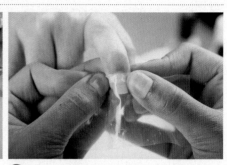

6 Apply a small amount of wrap resin to the fill area and spread throughout the new growth area. Be careful to avoid touching the skin. Apply on all 10 nails.

7 Pre-size the pre-cut silk or fiberglass fabric for each nail, or cut a piece of fabric large enough to cover the new growth area and to slightly overlap the old wrap fabric.

8 Remove the backing from the fabric, and gently fit fabric over the nail plate covering the entire nail (use a pair of tweezers to apply the fabric if desired), keeping it ¹⁄₁₆-inch (1.59 mm) away from the sidewall and eponychium. Use a small piece of thick plastic to press the fabric onto the nail and to smooth it out.

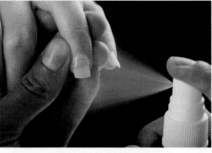

9 Apply another small amount of wrap resin, again avoiding the skin. Use a plastic sheet to help evenly distribute the wrap resin if needed.

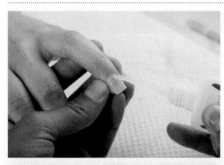

10 Spray, brush, or drip on the wrap resin accelerator on all 10 nails to dry the wrap resin more quickly. Follow the manufacturer's instructions.

11 Apply a second coat of wrap resin to the regrowth area.

12 Apply a second coat of wrap resin accelerator.

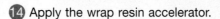

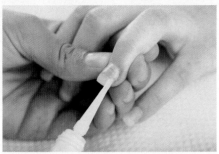

14 Apply the wrap resin accelerator.

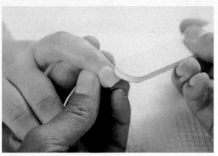

13 Apply a thin coat of nail wrap resin to the entire nail to strengthen and seal wrap.

15 Use a medium-fine abrasive (180- to 240-grit) over the surface of the nail to remove any high spots or other imperfections, starting with the free edge then the ridge. Carefully avoid the skin around the cuticle and sidewalls so that you do not cause cuts or damage.

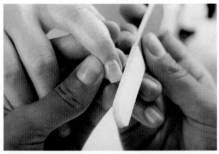

17 Apply cuticle oil. Have the client wash and dry their hands. Apply hand lotion or massage oil, and then massage the client's hands and arms.

18 Use a lint-free wipe and non-acetone polish remover to eliminate traces of oil from the nail so that the polish will adhere.

16 If your client prefers, buff to a high shine with a fine-grit buffer (350-grit or higher). Remove any dust with a clean, dry, disinfected nail brush.

19 Finished look.

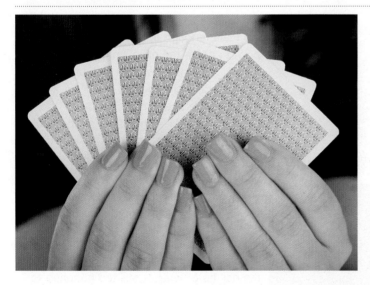

POST-SERVICE

Complete:

P 25-2 **Post-Service Procedure** *See page 884*

NAIL TIP AND FABRIC WRAP REMOVAL

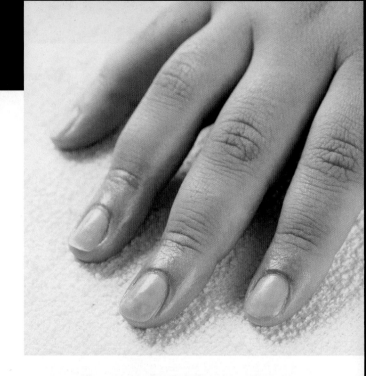

IMPLEMENTS & MATERIALS

In addition to the basic materials on your manicuring table, you will need the following supplies for the Nail Tip and Fabric Wrap Removal procedure:

☐ Buffer block   ☐ Acetone   ☐ Small glass bowl

PREPARATION | PROCEDURE

Perform:

P 25-1 Pre-Service Procedure See page 884

1. Start by applying a thick lotion or barrier cream to the hands and cuticle. This will help protect the surrounding skin prior to soaking in acetone or product remover.

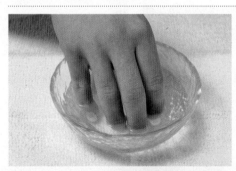

2. Place enough acetone in a small glass bowl to cover the nails. Immerse the client's fingertips in the bowl, making sure that the tips or wraps are covered. Soak for a few minutes. The acetone should be approximately ½-inch (1.28 cm) above the nail tips or wraps.

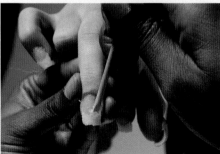

3. Use a wooden pusher to slide softened tips or wraps away from the nail plate.

Be careful not to pry the nail tip or wrap off because you can damage the nail unit. If the nail tip or wrap is still too attached to the nail, have the client soak that nail again for a few more minutes until the entire nail tip or wrap is easily removed.

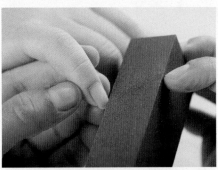

4 Gently buff the natural nails with a fine buffer (240-grit or higher) to remove traces of the wrap resin or any adhesive residue. Then remove any dust with a clean, dry nail brush.

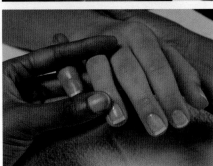

5 Condition the skin surrounding the nail plate with cuticle oil or lotion. Then wash and dry the client's hands and nails.

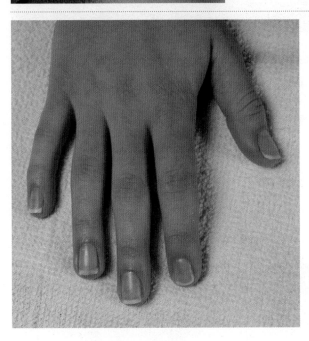

6 Proceed to the desired service. Finished look.

POST-SERVICE

Complete:

P 25-2 **Post-Service Procedure** *See page 884*

REVIEW QUESTIONS

1. What are the supplies, in addition to your basic manicuring table, that you need for nail tip application?

2. What are the types of nail tips available, and why is it important to properly fit them for your client?

3. What types of fabrics are used in nail wraps?

4. What are the benefits of using each of these types of fabric wraps?

5. Describe the stop, rock, and hold method of applying nail tips.

6. Describe the Nail Tip Application Procedure.

7. Describe the Nail Wrap Application Procedure.

8. What is the main difference between performing the two-week fabric wrap maintenance and the four-week fabric wrap maintenance?

9. Describe how to remove nail tips and fabric wraps and what to avoid.

STUDY TOOLS

- **Reinforce what you just learned:** Complete the activities and exercises in your Theory or Practical Workbook, or your Study Guide.

- **Expand your knowledge:** Search for websites about the topics in this chapter and make a list of additional resources.

- **Study and prepare for your quiz:** Take the chapter test in your Exam Review or your Milady U: Online Licensing Prep.

- **Re-Test your knowledge:** Take the Chapter 27 *Quizzes!*

- **Learn even more:** Look up in a dictionary or search the internet for the definitions of any additional terms you want to learn about.

CHAPTER GLOSSARY

acrylonitrile butadiene styrene ak-ruh-loh-NAHY-tril byoo-tuh-DAHY-een STAHY-reen	p. 928	Also known as *ABS*; a common thermoplastic used to make light, rigid, molded nail tips.
cyanoacrylate sy-an-oh-AH-cry-late	p. 931	A specialized acrylic monomer that has excellent adhesion to the natural nail plate and polymerizes in seconds.
fabric wrap	p. 932	Nail wrap made of silk, linen, or fiberglass.
fiberglass wraps	p. 932	Made from a very thin, synthetic mesh with a loose weave.
linen wraps	p. 932	Made from a closely woven, heavy material.
maintenance	p. 933	Term used for when a nail enhancement needs to be serviced after two or more weeks from the initial application of the nail enhancement product.
nail dehydrator	p. 929	A substance used to remove surface moisture and tiny amounts of oil left on the natural nail plate.

nail tip adhesive	p. 930	The bonding agent used to secure the nail tip to the natural nail.
nail tips	p. 928	Plastic, pre-molded nails shaped from a tough polymer made from ABS plastic.
nail wrap	p. 931	A method of securing a layer of fabric or paper on and around the nail tip to ensure its strength and durability.
nail wrap resin	p. 931	Used to coat and secure fabric wraps to the natural nail and nail tip.
overlay	p. 929	A layer of any kind of nail enhancement product that is applied over the natural nail or nail and tip application for added strength.
paper wraps	p. 932	Temporary nail wraps made of very thin paper.
position stop	p. 929	The point where the free edge of the natural nail meets the tip.
repair patch	p. 934	Piece of fabric cut to completely cover a crack or break in the nail.
silk wraps	p. 932	Made from a thin, natural material with a tight weave that becomes transparent when wrap resin is applied.
stress strip	p. 934	Strip of fabric cut to ⅛-inch (3.12mm) in length and applied to the weak point of the nail during the four-week fabric wrap maintenance to repair or strengthen a weak point in a nail enhancement.
tip cutter	p. 929	Implement similar to a nail clipper, designed especially for use on nail tips.
wrap resin accelerator	p. 932	Also known as *activator*; acts as the dryer that speeds up the hardening process of the wrap resin or adhesive overlay.

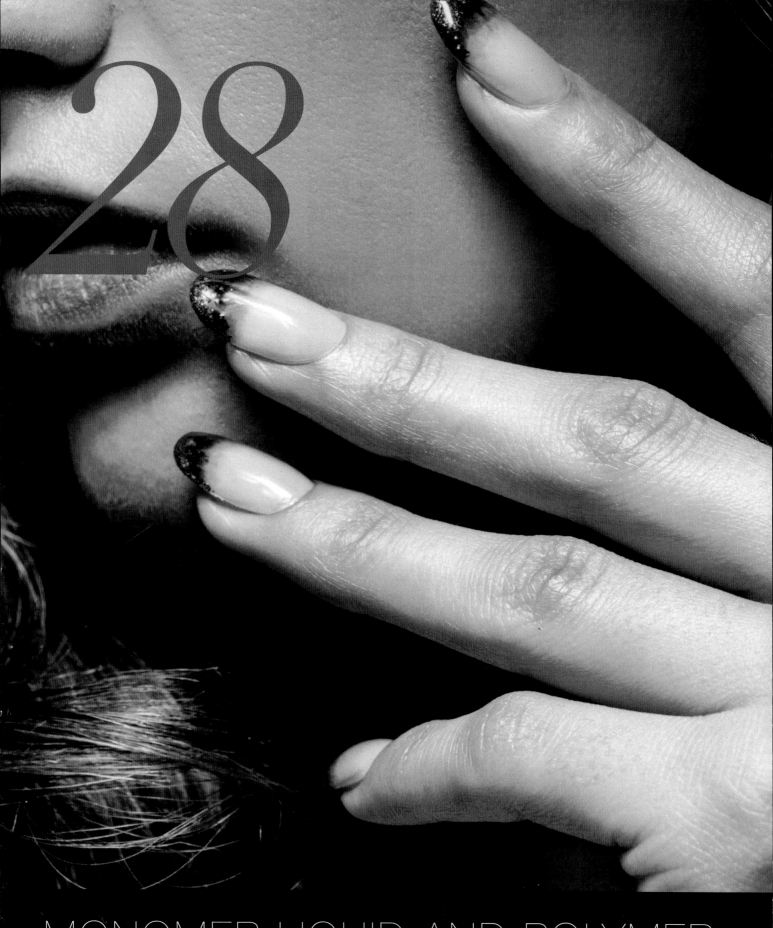

28

MONOMER LIQUID AND POLYMER POWDER NAIL ENHANCEMENTS

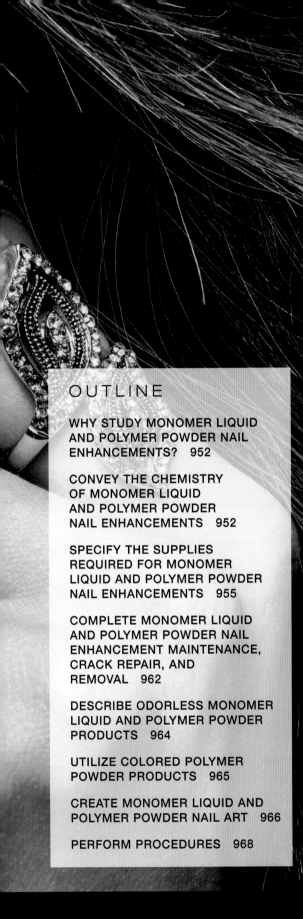

LEARNING OBJECTIVES

After completing this chapter, you will be able to:

LO❶
Explain monomer liquid and polymer powder nail enhancement chemistry and how it works.

LO❷
Name the specific tools, equipment, and supplies required to perform monomer liquid and polymer powder nail enhancements.

LO❸
List the steps to apply nonacid and acid-free nail primers.

LO❹
Explain how to properly store monomer liquid and polymer powder products.

LO❺
Describe the apex, stress area, and sidewall, and tell where each is located on the nail enhancement.

LO❻
Describe how to perform a one-color maintenance service on nail enhancements using monomer liquid and polymer powder.

LO❼
Demonstrate how to perform crack repair procedures.

LO❽
Implement the proper procedure for removing monomer liquid and polymer powder nail enhancements.

LO❾
Describe the general process for using odorless products.

LO❿
List two ways to create nail art from monomer liquid and polymer powder.

why study
MONOMER LIQUID AND POLYMER POWDER NAIL ENHANCEMENTS?

Cosmetologists should study and have a thorough understanding of monomer liquid and polymer powder nail enhancements because:

> Monomer liquid and polymer powder nail enhancements are popular services that will be frequently requested, and clients will expect expert service.

> Monomer liquid and polymer powder nail enhancements are lucrative services. Clients who desire them are committed to their upkeep, so if you earn clients' trust and respect, you will build a loyal clientele.

> Knowing how to properly work with the enhancement material and understanding its chemical makeup will allow you to perform the service safely for you and for your client.

After reading the next few sections, you will be able to:

LO Explain monomer liquid and polymer powder nail enhancement chemistry and how it works.

Convey the Chemistry of Monomer Liquid and Polymer Powder Nail Enhancements

Monomer liquid and polymer powder nail enhancements, also known as *sculptured nails*, are created by combining a chemical known as **monomer liquid** mixed, with **polymer powder**, to form a nail enhancement. The ingredients in two-part monomer liquid and polymer powder enhancement systems belong to a branch of the acrylic family called methacrylates (METH-ah-cry-latz). Keep in mind that other industry literature, product marketing, and the like may use the word *acrylic*.

Mono means one and *mer* stands for units, so a **monomer** (MON-oh-mehr) is one unit called a molecule. *Poly* means many, so **polymer** (POL-i-mehr) means a substance formed by combining many small molecules (monomers) into very long, chain-like structures. This is important to remember, since you will hear these terms many times throughout your career.

Today's monomer liquids and polymer powders come in many colors, including variations of basic pink, white, clear, and natural. These colors can be used alone or blended to create everything from customized shades of pink to match or enhance the color of your client's nail beds, to bold primaries or pastels that can be used to create a wide range of designs and patterns. With these powders, you can create unique colors or designs that can be locked permanently in the nail enhancement. They offer a wonderful way to customize your services or to express your artistry and creativity.

Monomer liquid and polymer powder products can be applied in four basic ways:

1. On the natural nail as a protective overlay

2. Over a nail tip

3. On a form to create a nail extension

4. To create small works of art on top or inside a nail enhancement.

(P) 28-1 **One-Color Monomer Liquid and Polymer Powder Nail Enhancements Over Nail Tips or Natural Nails** *See page 968*

A natural hair and pointed, round, or oval application brush is the best brush to use for applying these products. The brush is immersed in the monomer liquid. The natural hair bristles absorb and hold the monomer liquid like a reservoir. The tip of the brush is then touched to the surface of the dry polymer powder, and, as the monomer liquid absorbs the polymer powder, a small bead of product forms. This small bead is then carefully placed on the nail surface and molded into shape with the brush.

The monomer liquid portion is usually one of three versions of monomer liquid used in the beauty industry: ethyl methacrylate, methyl methacrylate, or odorless monomer liquid. All three often contain other monomers that are used as customizing additives. The industry standards are the ethyl methacrylate monomer liquid (EMA) and the odorless monomer liquid. Methyl methacrylate (MMA) is not recommended for use on nails and is not legal according to the state board rules in some states.

Here are four main reasons why MMA should *not* be used:

1. MMA nail products do not adhere well to the nail plate. To make these products adhere, nail technicians often shred (etch) the surface of the nail. This thins the nail plate and makes it weaker.

2. MMA creates the hardest and most rigid nail enhancements, which makes them very difficult to break. When jammed or caught, the overly-filed and thinned natural nail plate will often break before the MMA enhancement, leading to serious nail damage.

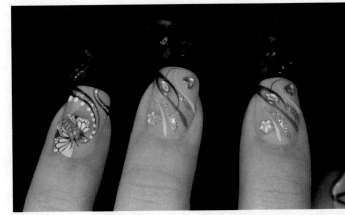

3. MMA is extremely difficult to remove. Since it will not dissolve well in product removers, it is usually pried from the nail plate, creating still more damage.

4. *The FDA says not to use it!* This is clearly the most important reason. The FDA bases' their prohibition on the large number of consumer complaints resulting from the use of MMA nail enhancements in the late 1970's, and they continue to maintain this position today.

For these reasons, the Nail Manufacturers Council and the American Beauty Association have also taken a stance against the use of MMA liquid monomer as an ingredient in artificial nail liquids—not because MMA is toxic, but because it is an unsuitable ingredient. MMA is a widely used monomer with a long history of safe use in medical and dental products. It is fine for making bulletproof windows and shatterproof eyeglasses. However, artificial nails should be beautiful, and they should not damage the natural nail.

It may seem strange that polymer powder is also made mostly from ethyl methacrylate monomer liquid. The polymer powder is made using **polymerization** (POL-i-mehr-eh-za-shun), also known as *curing* or *hardening*, a chemical reaction that creates polymers. In this process, trillions of monomers are linked together to create long chains. These long chains create the tiny round beads of polymer powder of slightly varying sizes. The beads are then poured through a series of special screens that sort the beads by size. The ones that are the right size are separated and then mixed with other special additives and colorants. The final mixture is packaged and sold as polymer powder. It is a surprisingly high-tech process that requires very specific manufacturing equipment, lots of quality control, and scientific know-how to do it right.

Special additives are blended into both the liquid and the powder. These additives ensure complete set or cure, maximum durability, color stability, and shelf life, among other attributes. It is these "custom" additives that make products work and behave differently. The polymer powders are usually blended with pigments and colorants to create a wide range of shades, including pinks, whites, and milky translucent shades, as well as reds, blues, greens, purples, yellows, oranges, browns, and even jet black.

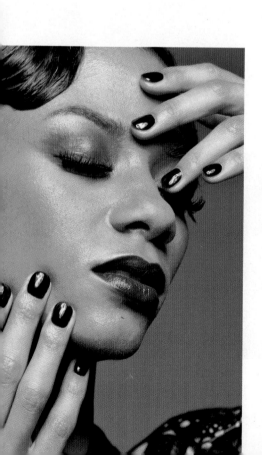

When liquid is picked up by a brush and mixed with the powder, the bead that forms on the end of the brush quickly begins to harden. It is then put into place with other beads and shaped into place as they harden. In order for this process to begin, the monomers and polymers require special additives called *catalysts* (KAT-a-lists), additives designed to speed up chemical reactions. Catalysts are added to the monomer liquid and used to control the set or curing time. In other words, when the monomer liquid and polymer powder are combined, the catalyst (in the liquid) helps control the set-up or hardening time. How? The catalyst energizes and activates the initiators.

The **initiators** found in polymer powder, when activated by a catalyst, will spring into action and cause monomer molecules to permanently link together into long polymer chains. This action is referred to as the polymerization process. Polymerization begins when the liquid in the brush picks up powder from the container and forms a bead. Creating polymers can be thought of as a **chain reaction**, also known as *polymerization reaction*, a process that joins together monomers to create very long polymer chains. Think of it as many dominos, set on their edges and lined up—when you tap the first domino, it hits the next, and so on. This is how polymers form. Once the monomers join together to create a polymer, they do not detach from each other easily.

The initiator that is added to the polymer powder is called benzoyl peroxide (BPO). It is the same ingredient used in over-the-counter acne medicine, except that it has a different purpose in nail enhancement products. BPO is used to start the chain reaction that leads to curing (hardening) of the nail enhancement. There is much less BPO in nail powders than in acne treatments. Diverse nail enhancement products often use different amounts of BPO, since the polymer powders are designed to work specifically with a certain monomer liquid. Some monomer liquids require more BPO to properly cure than others. This is why it is very important to use the polymer powder that was designed for the monomer liquid that you are using. Using the wrong powder can create nail enhancements that are not properly cured and may lead to service breakdown or could increase the risk of your clients developing a skin irritation or sensitivity.

There are many monomer liquid and polymer powder systems available, and you might have to try several in order to find the product that fits best for you and your clients.

After reading the next few sections, you will be able to:

LO❷ Name the specific tools, equipment, and supplies required to perform monomer liquid and polymer powder nail enhancements.

LO❸ List the steps to apply nonacid and acid-free nail primers.

LO❹ Explain how to properly store monomer liquid and polymer powder products.

Specify the Supplies Required for Monomer Liquid and Polymer Powder Nail Enhancements

Just as every type of nail enhancement service requires specific tools, implements, equipment, and supplies, so do monomer liquid and polymer powder nail enhancements. **Figure 28-1** shows examples of those products and supplies. In addition to the supplies in your basic manicuring setup, you will need the following items.

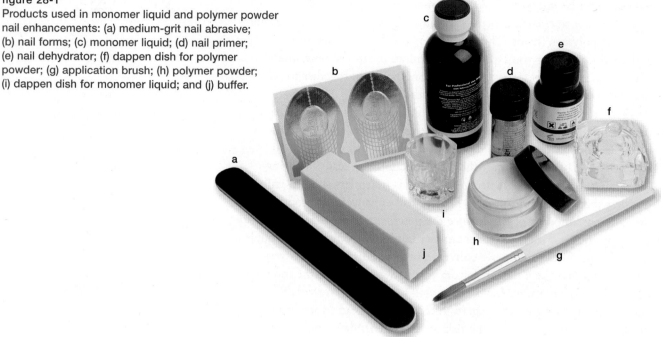

figure 28-1
Products used in monomer liquid and polymer powder nail enhancements: (a) medium-grit nail abrasive; (b) nail forms; (c) monomer liquid; (d) nail primer; (e) nail dehydrator; (f) dappen dish for polymer powder; (g) application brush; (h) polymer powder; (i) dappen dish for monomer liquid; and (j) buffer.

Monomer Liquid

The monomer liquid will be combined with polymer powder to form the nail enhancement. The amount of monomer liquid and polymer powder used to create a bead is called the **mix ratio**. A bead mix ratio can be best described as *dry*, *medium*, or *wet*. If equal amounts of liquid and powder are used to create the bead, it is called a *dry bead*. If twice as much liquid as powder is used to create the bead, it is called a *wet bead*. Halfway between these two is a *medium bead*, which contains one-and-a-half times more liquid than powder. In general, medium beads are the ideal mix ratio for working with monomer liquids and polymer powders. The perfect bead should be smooth, round, and shiny (figure 28-2).

The mix ratio typically ensures proper set and maximum durability of the nail enhancement. For example, if too much flour is added to cookie batter, the cookies will be dry and crumbly; if too little flour is added, the cookies will be soft and gooey. The same holds true for monomer liquids and polymer powders. If too much powder is picked up in the bead, the enhancement will cure incorrectly and may lead to brittleness and/or discoloration. If too little powder is used, the nail enhancement can become weak, and the risk of clients developing skin irritation and sensitivity may increase.

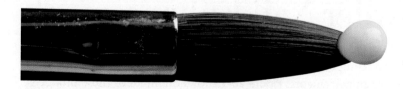

figure 28-2
The perfect bead should be smooth, round, and shiny.

Polymer Powder

Polymer powder is available in white, clear, natural, pink, and many other colors. The color(s) you choose will depend on the nail enhancement method you are using.

Nail Dehydrator

Nail dehydrators remove surface moisture and tiny amounts of oil left on the natural nail plate, both of which can block adhesion. Nail dehydrator should be applied liberally to the natural nail plate only; skin contact should be avoided. This step is a great way to help prevent lifting of the nail enhancement prior to applying primer.

Nail Primer

Nail primer is used on the natural nail prior to product application to assist in adhesion. Primers are used to chemically bond the enhancement product to the natural nail. One end of the primer molecule chemically bonds to the nail protein in the natural nail; the other end of the molecule is a methacrylate, so it bonds to the monomer liquid as it cures.

There are basically two kinds of nail primers for preparing the natural nail for a monomer liquid and polymer powder nail enhancement: *acid-based* and *nonacid* or acid-free primers. Acid-based nail primer (methacrylic acid) was once widely used to help adhere enhancements to the natural nail. Acid-based nail primers are very effective but can cause serious—and sometimes irreversible—damage to the skin and eyes. Never use acid-based nail primer or any other corrosive material without wearing protective gloves and safety eyewear.

Since acid-based nail primer is corrosive to the skin and potentially dangerous to eyes, acid-free and nonacid primers were developed. Acid-free and nonacid primers work as well as or better than acid-based nail primers, and have the added advantage of not being corrosive to skin or eyes. Even so, all nail primer products must be used with caution, and strictly in accordance with the manufacturer's instructions. Skin contact should be avoided during application, and the Safety Data Sheet (SDS) should be referenced for safe handling recommendations and instructions when using these products. Other guidelines to follow when using nail primers are to:

- Never apply nail enhancement product over wet nail primer. This can cause product discoloration and service breakdown.

- Avoid overuse of nail primers.

- Apply primer to the natural nail, but avoid putting it on the nail tips unless instructed by the manufacturer of the nail primer.

- Check your nail primer daily for clarity, to ensure that it does not become contaminated with nail dust and other floating debris, which can dramatically reduce primer effectiveness.

- Never use nail primers that are visibly contaminated with floating debris. To avoid contamination, wipe the primer brush on a clean, dust-free towel before placing the brush back in the bottle.

> **✔ HERE'S A TIP**
>
> Monomer Liquid Bead Mix Ratio Guidelines:
>
> 1 part monomer liquid + 1 part polymer powder = dry bead
>
> 1½ parts monomer liquid + 1 part polymer powder = medium bead
>
> 2 parts monomer liquid + 1 part polymer powder = wet bead

Application of Nail Primer

Manufacturer's instructions for using monomer liquid and polymer powder nail enhancement products may differ slightly from the general guidelines presented in this chapter. You should always use products in accordance with the manufacturer's instructions. If you are in doubt about how to use the products, contact the manufacturer.

- **To apply acid-based nail primers.** Using a tiny applicator brush, insert the brush tip into the nail primer. Touch the brush tip to the edge of the bottle's neck to release the excess primer back into the bottle. Using a light dotting action, carefully dab the brush tip to the center of the properly prepared natural nail. The acid-based primer will spread out and cover the nail plate. Do not use too much product—it will run onto the skin and can cause burns or injury. The brush should hold enough product to treat three or more nails. Let the primer dry to a chalky white before applying enhancement overlay. Be sure to read the label for the manufacturer's suggested application procedures and precautions.

- **To apply nonacid and acid-free nail primers.** Using the applicator brush, insert brush into the nail primer. Wipe excess product from the brush. Using a slightly damp brush, completely cover the nail plate with the primer. Do not use too much product—it will run onto the skin and can cause skin irritation or sensitivity. The brush should hold enough product to treat two or three nails. Be sure the entire nail plate is covered. Before dipping the brush back into the container, gently wipe the brush on a clean table towel so you do not contaminate the bottle with any debris the brush may have picked up. The nail will remain shiny after application; this primer does not dry to a chalky white. Be sure to read the label for the manufacturer's suggested application procedures and precautions.

Abrasives

The term *abrasive* is used to describe nail files and buffers. Although some abrasives have fancy names, they all have a **grit** number. Grit refers to how many grains of sand are on the file per square inch. For example if there were 100 grits of sand per square inch, then the particles would be spread

FOCUS ON

Proper Hand Washing

Always have your clients wash their hands thoroughly with a fingernail brush before any service. Hand sanitizers are an alternative when a hand washing station is not available, but they do not clean the hands. They cannot remove dirt or debris from hands and underneath the nails. They kill some of the bacteria on skin, but not all of it. Hand sanitizers do give clients peace of mind, though. Clients like to see cosmetologists using hand sanitizers, and many clients prefer to use them as well. Keep a high-quality, professional hand sanitizer at your station and offer some to your clients. Let them see you using it, and they will have a greater degree of confidence in the cleanliness of your services. Do not use hand sanitizers in place of hand washing—there is no replacement for proper hand washing.

apart creating a rough surface. If there were 240, the sand particles would be closer together creating a smoother surface. You now understand that the lower the number, the rougher the abrasive will be. The higher the number, the softer it will be. Be aware that the different abrasive core materials will also change how an abrasive works. Plastic and wood cores are used for files and plastic, and sponge cores are used in buffers. The wood will make the abrasive more aggressive, whereas the sponge core will form around the nail and therefore be gentle.

Here is a list of the most common abrasives used for filing, shaping, and buffing nail enhancements (figure 28-3):

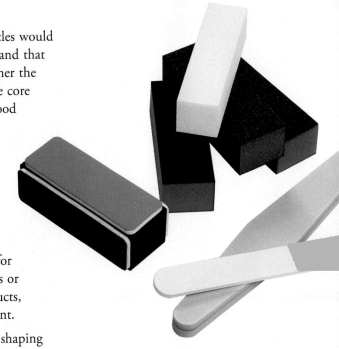

figure 28-3
Assortment of various buffers and shiners

- A course-grit abrasive (100 grit or lower) is strong enough to thin enhancement product to prepare the enhancement for a refill or rebalance. Avoid using coarser, lower-grit abrasives or aggressive techniques on freshly applied enhancement products, as they can damage the soft, freshly created nail enhancement.

- A medium-grit abrasive (150 to 180 grit) is used for initial shaping of the perimeter of the nail, refining the overall surface shape of a nail enhancement, or for smoothing the surface before buffing. If you avoid putting the product on too thick, a 180-grit is usually strong enough to shape the entire nail enhancement.

- A fine-grit abrasive (240 grit or higher) is used for finish filing, refining, and buffing. This grit of file is also used to shape the free edge of a natural nail.

- A **shiner** is a buffer (usually 400/1,000/4,000) used to create a high shine on a natural nail or a nail enhancement when no polish will be worn. This buffer usually has three sides and you must buff the entire nail with the lowest grit side first and then repeat with the other sides to create a glossy shine to the nail. Shiner buffers can also have two sides. In this case, you may want to buff the entire surface of the nail with a 240- or 350-grit buffer prior to buffing with the shiner.

Nail Forms

Nail forms are placed under the free edge of the natural nail and used as a guide to extend the nail enhancements beyond the fingertips for additional length. Single-use (disposable) nail forms often are made of paper or Mylar and coated with adhesive backs. Multiuse (reusable) nail forms are made of pre-shaped plastic or aluminum and can be cleaned and disinfected between clients.

If you are using disposable forms, peel a nail form from its paper backing and, using the thumb and index finger of each of your hands, bend the form into an arch to fit the client's natural nail shape. Slide the form into place and press adhesive backing to the sides of the finger. Check to see that the form is snug under the free edge and level with the natural nail.

If you are using multiuse forms, slide the form into place, making sure the free edge is over the form and that it fits snugly. Be careful not to cut into the hyponychium under the free edge. Tighten the form around the finger by squeezing lightly.

Ⓟ 28-2 Two-Color Monomer Liquid and Polymer Powder Nail Enhancements Using Forms *See page 972*

Nail Tips

Nail tips are preformed nail extensions made from acrylonitrile butadiene styrene (ABS) or tenite acetate plastic and are available in a wide variety of shapes, styles, and colors, including natural, white, and clear. Nail tips are adhered to the tip of the natural nail with a fast-set resin to extend the length. They are not strong enough to wear on their own, so they must be overlaid with an enhancement product.

Ⓟ 27-1 Nail Tip Application *See page 935*

Dappen Dish

The monomer liquid and polymer powder are each poured into a special container called a **dappen dish**. These dishes must have narrow openings to minimize evaporation of the monomer liquid into the air. Do not use open-mouth jars or other containers with large openings. Those types of containers will dramatically increase evaporation of the liquid and can allow the product to be contaminated with dust and other debris. A dappen dish must be covered with a tightly fitting lid when not in use.

Each time the brush is dipped into the dappen dish, the remaining monomer liquid is contaminated with small amounts of polymer powder. So never pour the unused portion of monomer liquid back into the original container. Empty the monomer liquid from your dappen dish after the service, and wipe it clean with a disposable towel. To avoid skin irritation or sensitivity, do not contact skin with the monomer liquid during this process. Wipe the dish clean with acetone, if necessary, before storing in a dust-free location.

figure 28-4
Various sizes of kolinsky, sable, and blended brushes used for applying monomer liquid and polymer powder nail enhancements

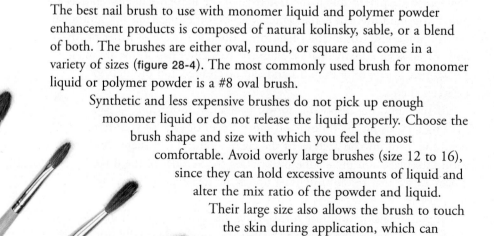

Monomer Liquid and Polymer Powder Application Brush

The best nail brush to use with monomer liquid and polymer powder enhancement products is composed of natural kolinsky, sable, or a blend of both. The brushes are either oval, round, or square and come in a variety of sizes (figure 28-4). The most commonly used brush for monomer liquid or polymer powder is a #8 oval brush.

Synthetic and less expensive brushes do not pick up enough monomer liquid or do not release the liquid properly. Choose the brush shape and size with which you feel the most comfortable. Avoid overly large brushes (size 12 to 16), since they can hold excessive amounts of liquid and alter the mix ratio of the powder and liquid. Their large size also allows the brush to touch the skin during application, which can overexpose your client to the monomer.

Having too much monomer liquid on your brush can increase the risk of accidentally touching the client's skin and may increase the risk of developing skin irritation or sensitivities. Odorless monomer liquid requires less liquid, so using a flat brush that holds less liquid is recommended.

HERE'S A TIP

Avoid wiping your brush too rapidly or too hard against a table towel. This can press hairs against the sharp edge of the metal ferrule that holds the hairs in place and cut them off.

Safety Eyewear

Safety eyewear should be used to protect eyes from flying objects or accidental splashes. There are many types and styles. You can get more information by searching the Internet or contacting a local optometrist, who can also help you with both nonprescription and prescription safety eyewear.

Dust Masks

Dust masks are designed to be worn over the nose and mouth to prevent inhalation of excessive amounts of dust. They provide no protection from vapors.

Protective Gloves

Both disposable and multiuse varieties of protective gloves can be purchased. Several types of materials are used to make these gloves. For many salon-related applications, gloves made of nitrile polymer powder work best.

Storing and Disposing of Monomer Liquid and Polymer Powder Products

Store monomer liquid and polymer powder products in a covered container. Store all polymers and liquids separate from each other in a cool, dark area. Do not store products near heat.

After a service, you must discard used materials. Never save used monomer liquid that has been removed from the original container. Use on one client only. Avoid skin contact with the monomer liquid. If skin contact should occur, wash hands with liquid soap and water.

To dispose of small amounts of monomer liquid, mix them with small amounts of the powder designed to cure them. This is safe for amounts ranging from less than a half-ounce of monomer liquid to quarts or gallons. They should never be disposed of directly into the trash or down the drain. Tiny amounts of monomer liquid left in the dappen dish can be wiped out with a paper towel, placed in a sealed plastic bag, and then disposed of in a metal trash can with a self-closing lid.

After all used materials have been collected from your manicure table, seal them in a plastic bag and discard the bag in a closed waste receptacle. It is important to remove items soiled with enhancement products from your manicuring station after each client. This will help maintain the quality of the air in your salon. Dispose of these items according to local rules and regulations.

LO❺ Describe the apex, stress area, and sidewall, and tell where each is located on the nail enhancement.

LO❻ Describe how to perform a one-color maintenance service on nail enhancements using monomer liquid and polymer powder.

LO❼ Demonstrate how to perform crack repair procedures.

LO❽ Implement the proper procedure for removing monomer liquid and polymer powder nail enhancements.

Complete Monomer Liquid and Polymer Powder Nail Enhancement Maintenance, Crack Repair, and Removal

Regular maintenance helps prevent nail enhancements from lifting or cracking. If the nail enhancements are not regularly maintained, they have a greater tendency to lift, crack, or break, which increases the risk of the client developing an infection or having other problems.

When a cosmetologist has a client with a piece or section of the monomer liquid and polymer powder enhancement that has broken, lifted, or cracked, it is repaired by filing the area and adding monomer liquid and polymer powder to it. This is called a crack repair.

Proper maintenance must be performed every two to three weeks, depending on how fast the client's nails grow.

If you choose to offer nail enhancement services to your clients, proper maintenance is a critical skill for you to learn. Do not let clients go too long without having a proper maintenance service, or you will have many more repairs to perform when they return. Proper maintenance is both safe and gentle to the nail unit and will not result in injury or damage. In the maintenance service, the nail enhancement is thinned down to blend with the new growth area of the natural nail. The apex of the nail is filed away, and the entire nail enhancement is reduced in thickness to prepare for an overlay of new product.

Ⓟ 28-3 **One-Color Monomer Liquid and Polymer Powder Maintenance**
See page 977

Ⓟ 28-4 **Crack Repair for Monomer Liquid and Polymer Powder Nail Enhancements** *See page 980*

Properly Structured Nail Enhancements

Nail enhancements should not only look good, but they should also remain strong and healthy while your client is wearing them. Several areas of the nail must be considered when the nail enhancement is being made to accomplish this. Paying particular attention to the following areas of the nail enhancement will help you to create the look your clients desire and also provide them with the best and longest-lasting nail enhancements.

The **apex**, also known as *arch*, is the area of the nail with the most strength. Having strength in the apex allows the base of the nail, sidewalls, and tip to be thin, yet leaves the nail strong enough to resist frequent chipping or breaking. The apex is usually oval shaped and is located in the center of the nail. The high point is visible no matter where you view the nail (figure 28-5).

The **stress area** is where the natural nail grows beyond the finger and becomes the free edge. This area needs strength to support the extension. This is also the area that you would create your smile line in a two-color method application. A **smile line** is the curved line where the pink and white meet each other on a French manicured nail. It is usually defined by using white polymer on the free edge and pink powder on the nail bed creating a French manicured look.

The **sidewall** runs straight from the cuticle down the side or wall of the nail to the end of the extension. (figure 28-6).

The **nail extension underside** is the actual underside of the nail extension (figure 28-7). The nail extension underside can jut straight out or may dip, depending on the nail style. The nail extension underside should be even, matched on each nail. Undersides should match in length from nail to nail on all fingers. The tip should fit the nail and finger properly, and the underside of the nail extension should be smooth, without any glitches.

The thickness of the nail enhancement should be rather thin if a client is to wear it comfortably while going about her day (figure 28-8). The enhancement should graduate seamlessly from the cuticle to the end of the nail extension, so you do not feel an edge. The sidewalls and the tip's edge should be credit-card thin.

The C-curve of the nail enhancement depends on the C-curve of the natural nail. In the salon, a 35-percent C-curve is the average. The top surface and bottom side should match perfectly. The C-curve will provide structure to the nail so that it appears slender on the hand. More importantly, the C-curve provides strength, like the curve in a bridge or an egg.

To make sure the lengths of the nail extensions and enhancements are appropriate and even, be sure to measure the length of the index, middle, and ring fingers; these should be the same length. The thumb and pinkie fingers should also be in proportion and match.

Monomer Liquid and Polymer Powder Nail Enhancement Removal

There will be circumstances when your client wants to have her monomer liquid and polymer powder nail enhancements removed. Do not worry.

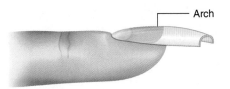

figure 28-5
The arch is the highest point in the center of the nail.

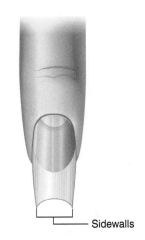

figure 28-6
The sidewall runs straight from the cuticle down the sidewall of the nail to the end of the extension.

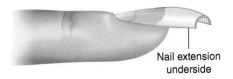

figure 28-7
The nail extension underside will come straight out or drop down a bit depending on the client's natural nail and the look she prefers.

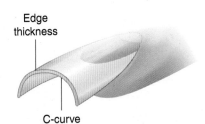

figure 28-8
The thickness of the edge should be credit-card thin, and there should be a consistent C-curve in the nail for strength.

The procedure is simple: Soak the enhancements off of the nail using acetone or the manufacturer's suggested removal solution, remove the enhancement, and complete the service. For client comfort and to avoid product evaporation, you may want to cover the hands with a hand towel during the soaking process.

Nail plates may appear to be thinner after enhancements have been removed. This is generally because there is more moisture in the natural nail plate, which makes them more flexible. It is not an indication that the nail plates have been weakened by the nail enhancement. This excess flexibility will be lost as the natural nails lose moisture over the next 24 hours, and the nail plates will appear to be thicker and more rigid.

P 28-5 **Monomer Liquid and Polymer Powder Nail Enhancement Removal** *See page 982*

After reading the next few sections, you will be able to:

LO 9 Describe the general process for using odorless products.

Describe Odorless Monomer Liquid and Polymer Powder Products

Odorless monomer liquid and polymer powder products are nail enhancement products that have little odor. These products do not necessarily have the same chemistry as all other monomer liquid and polymer powder products. Rather than use ethyl acrylic, these products rely on monomers that have little odor. Even though these products are called "odorless," they do have a slight odor. Generally, if a monomer liquid does not produce a strong enough odor that others in the salon can detect its presence, it is considered to be an odorless product. Those that create a slight odor in the salon are called "low odor."

In general, odorless products must be used with a dry mix ratio (equal parts liquid and powder in bead). If they are too wet when applied, the client risks developing skin irritation or sensitivity. This mix ratio creates a bead that looks frosted on your brush. After it is placed on the nail, it will slowly form into a firm glossy bead that will hold its shape until pressed and smoothed with the nail brush. Wipe your brush frequently to avoid the product sticking to the hairs. Never rewet the brush with monomer liquid. This will change the mix ratio, which can lead to product discoloration, service breakdown, and increased risk of skin irritation and sensitivity. Without re-wetting your brush, use the brush to shape and smooth the surface to perfection.

Odorless products harden more slowly and create a tacky layer called the inhibition layer. This layer can be rolled off or filed away with a 150-grit

To determine whether you have done the best possible job to ensure a smooth, balanced, and symmetrical nail, and that all nails are consistent, try viewing them from the following perspectives.

Top view. Make sure all the perimeter shapes are consistent.

Left side and right side views. Look at the profile of each nail and make sure your apex is consistently located in the correct place and that the apexes match from nail to nail. Also look at the left side and right side of the nail and make sure the extension's underside matches.

Down the center. Look at the degrees of C-curves. Do they match? Is the thinness/thickness of the product consistent and thick enough to withstand wear, or are the nails too thin?

From the client's perspective. Turn the client's hand around and fold the fingers toward the palm of the hand so you can view the top surface from the client's perspective. Sometimes you can see lumps and bumps from this view that you couldn't see when looking at them during application.

Line of light. After the nail is smooth and polished, or after a UV gel sealant has been applied, you can follow the line of light that reflects off the surface of the nail to see whether the nail is really smooth. If the nail surface is not smooth, the line of light will not follow perfectly.

abrasive used from cuticle to free edge. However, avoid skin contact with these freshly filed particles. Some manufacturers also make a resin that brushes on to cure the tacky layer that must be applied immediately after creating the enhancement. This will create a hard surface on the odorless product that makes filing and shaping easier.

Utilize Colored Polymer Powder Products

Polymer powders are now available in a wide range of colors that mimic almost every shade available in nail polish. Nail artistry with colored polymer powder is limited only by your imagination. Some professionals use colors to go beyond the traditional pink and white French manicure combinations and offer custom-blended colors to their clients. They

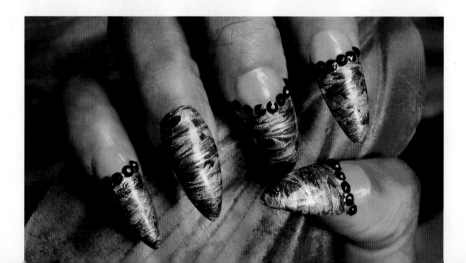

maintain recipe cards so that they can reproduce customized nail enhancements that clients cannot get from anyone else. As with all customized techniques, clients are willing to pay a few dollars more for the special service.

After reading the next few sections, you will be able to:

LO ⑩ List two ways to create nail art from monomer liquid and polymer powder.

Create Monomer Liquid and Polymer Powder Nail Art

Monomer liquid and polymer powder can be used in a variety of ways to create unique nail art. This medium can be challenging to master, but it also has the most versatile results. Designs can be as simple as placing five small beads on a nail to create a three-dimensional flower or fading six or seven colors as thin as paper to create a sunset backdrop for an inlaid design nail.

Three dimensional, or **3-D nail art** describes any art that protrudes from the nail. When applying 3-D art over nail polish, you will want the polish to be dried for at least three minutes before applying the art. You can add a topcoat to the polished nail before you add the art if you would like the art to look matte when complete. Or, you may also add the monomer liquid and polymer powder straight to the polish color, and then seal the nail and art with a shiny topcoat, leaving the entire nail and art with a glossy finish (figure 28-9).

Inlaid designs, designs inside a nail enhancement, are created when nail art is sandwiched between two layers of product while the nail enhancement is being formed. When inlaying flowers in the nail, use the

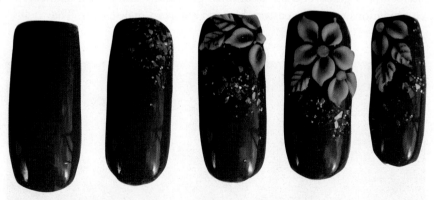

figure 28-9
3-D nail art is a great way to increase income in the salon.

Nail Art by Alisha Rimando Botero.

same technique as in the 3-D flower design except pick up smaller beads and flatten them out so that the size of the flower remains the same, but the flower design will be much thinner. This allows for a layer of clear monomer liquid and polymer powder to cover the design without the nail being too thick (figure 28-10).

Monomer liquid and polymer powder nail art can be used over polish or any other hardened nail enhancement surface. Monomer liquid and polymer powder art does not hold well on a clean, natural nail unless you prep and prime the nail to receive this overlay. If you are working on a surface that can be easily ruined with acetone, be careful not to touch the surface of the nail with the monomer liquid and polymer powder brush too often, or you may damage it. When working on top of a polished nail, you can ruin the polish if you stroke the surface too many times with a brush wet with monomer liquid.

When using monomer liquid and polymer powder for art, there are many brushes and tools available to mold the product into the desired shape. When first beginning to work in this medium, use the same brush you currently use to apply the monomer liquid and polymer powder to nail tips and overlays.

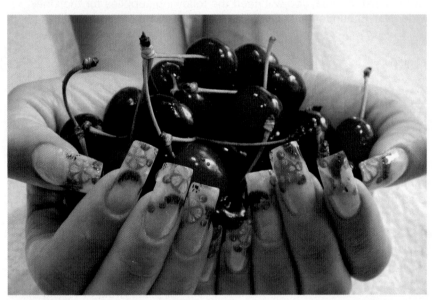

Nails by Massimiliano Braga.

figure 28-10
Inlaid designs are a beautiful addition to your nail menu and promote client loyalty.

ONE-COLOR MONOMER LIQUID AND POLYMER POWDER NAIL ENHANCEMENTS OVER NAIL TIPS OR NATURAL NAILS

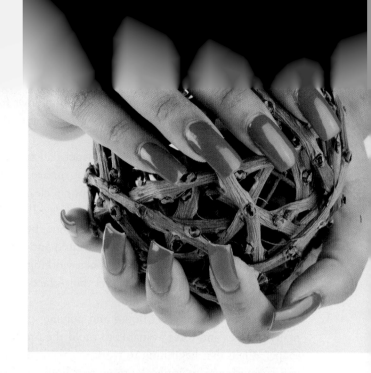

IMPLEMENTS & MATERIALS

In addition to the basic materials on your manicuring table, you will need the following supplies for the One-Color Monomer Liquid and Polymer Powder Nail Enhancements Over Nail Tips or Natural Nails procedure:

- ☐ Abrasives
- ☐ Application brushes
- ☐ Dappen dishes
- ☐ Monomer liquid
- ☐ Nail dehydrator
- ☐ Nail primer
- ☐ Polymer powder
- ☐ Buffer

PREPARATION

Perform:

Ⓟ **25-1** Pre-Service Procedure *See page 880*

PROCEDURE

1 Clean the nails and remove any existing polish, then use a pusher to gently push back the eponychium and carefully remove cuticle tissue from the nail plate. If you are applying nail tips, use a 180-grit abrasive or higher to shape the free edges of the natural nails so they match the shape of the nail tip to the stop point.

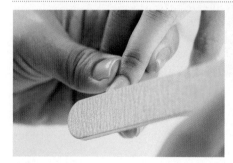

2 Gently file or buff the nail plate with medium/fine abrasive (180- to 240-grit) to remove the shine caused by natural oil on the surface of the nail plate. Avoid over-filing of the nail plate. Remove the nail dust with a clean, dry nail brush and do not touch the surface of the nails with your fingers as you may deposit oils from your fingertips, degrading the cleanliness of the nail. Cleanse the nails with surface cleanser and lint-free wipe.

3 Apply nail dehydrator to nails. Begin with the little finger on the left hand and work toward the thumb.

4 If your client requires nail tips, apply tips as described in **Procedure 27-1, Nail Tip Application** in Chapter 27. Cut tips to desired length.

⑤ Apply nail primer. Release excess primer from the brush and dab the brush to the prepared natural nail only. Always follow the manufacturer's directions. Acid-based nail primer will dry to a chalky white. Acid-free primer will dry to a shiny, sticky surface. Avoid applying primer to the nail tips.

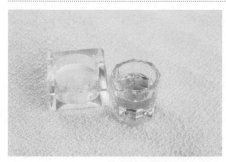

⑥ Pour monomer liquid and polymer powder into separate dappen dishes.

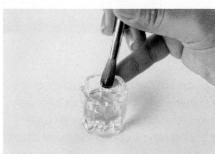

⑦ Dip the brush into the monomer liquid and wipe on the edge of the container to remove the excess.

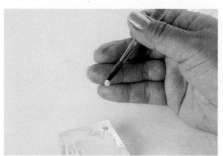

⑧ Dip the tip of the same brush into the polymer powder and rotate slightly. Pick up a bead of product—with a medium-to-dry consistency, not runny or wet—that is large enough for shaping the entire free-edge extension. If you have trouble using a large bead to shape the edge properly, two smaller beads may be easier.

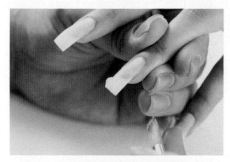

⑨ Place the pink product bead in the center of the free edge of the tip or natural nail. Immediately wipe your brush on the table towel gently to remove any product left in the bristles and bring the brush back to a perfect point.

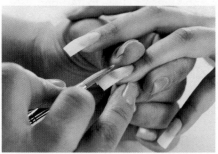

⑩ Use the middle portion or "belly" of your sable brush to press and smooth the product to shape the enhancement's free edge. Do not "paint" the product onto the nail. Pressing and smoothing produces a more natural-looking nail. Keep sidewall lines parallel and avoid widening the tip beyond the natural width of the nail plate.

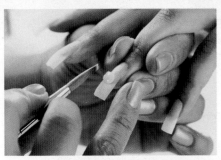

11 Using a medium consistency, place the second bead on the nail plate below the first bead and next to the free edge line in the center of the nail. Immediately wipe your brush gently on the table towel to remove any product left in the bristles and to bring the brush back to a perfect point.

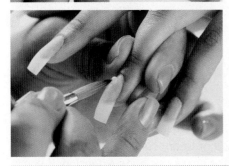

12 Press and smooth the product to the sidewalls, making sure that the product is very thin around all edges. Leave a tiny free margin between the product placement and skin. Avoid placing the product too close to the skin: This may cause the product to lift away from the nail plate or increase the chance of the client developing a skin irritation or sensitivity. Be sure to use a medium consistency mix that is not too wet.

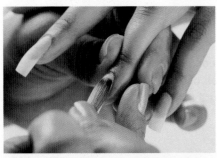

13 Pick up smaller beads of pink polymer powder with your brush and place them at the base of the nail plate, leaving a tiny free margin between the product and the skin. Immediately wipe your brush on the table towel gently to remove any product left in the bristles and to bring the brush back to a perfect point.

14 Use the brush to press and smooth beads over the entire nail plate. Glide the brush over the nail to smooth out imperfections.

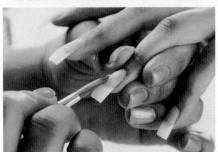

15 Apply more product near the eponychium, sidewalls, and free edge if needed to complete the application. Be sure that the product in these areas remains thin for a natural-looking nail.

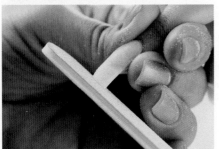

16 Use a 180-grit abrasive to shape the free edge and to remove imperfections. Then refine with medium-fine abrasive (180- to 240-grit).

(17) Buff the nail enhancement with fine-grit buffer (350-grit or higher) until the entire surface is smooth. Use a high-shine buffer if nail polish *will not* be worn. Remove any dust with a clean, dry nail brush before applying oil.

(18) Apply and rub nail oil into the surrounding skin and nail enhancement, massaging briefly to speed up penetration.

(19) Ask the client to wash her hands with soap and water at the hand washing station, or ask her to use the nail brush to clean her nails over a finger bowl. Rinse with clean water to remove soap residue that may cause lifting. Dry thoroughly with a clean, disposable towel.

(20) Apply hand cream and massage the hands and arms. Thoroughly clean each nail of lotion.

(21) Polish nail enhancements depending on your client's preferences.

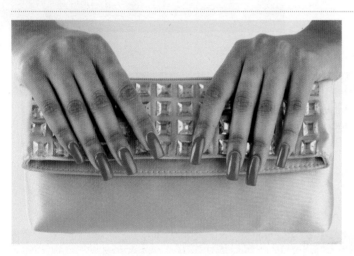

(22) Finished look.

POST-SERVICE

Complete:

(P) 25-2 **Post-Service Procedure** *See page 884*

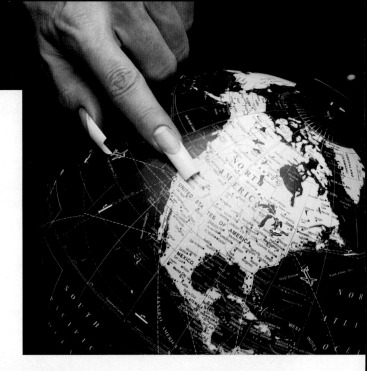

TWO-COLOR MONOMER LIQUID AND POLYMER POWDER NAIL ENHANCEMENTS USING FORMS

IMPLEMENTS & MATERIALS

In addition to the basic materials on your manicuring table, you will need the following supplies for the Two-Color Monomer Liquid and Polymer Powder Nail Enhancements Using Forms procedure:

- ☐ Abrasives
- ☐ Application brushes
- ☐ Dappen dishes
- ☐ Monomer liquid
- ☐ Nail dehydrator
- ☐ Nail forms
- ☐ Nail primer
- ☐ Polymer powder (pink, white and soft white

PREPARATION

Perform:

P 25-1 **Pre-Service Procedure** *See page 880*

PROCEDURE

1 Clean the nails and remove any existing polish.

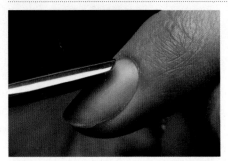

2 Gently push back the eponychium and remove the cuticle tissue from the nail plate.

3 Gently file or buff the nail plate with medium/fine abrasive (180- to 240-grit) to remove the shine caused by natural oil on the surface of the nail plate. Avoid over-filing of the nail plate. Remove the nail dust with a clean, dry nail brush and do not touch the surface of the nails with your fingers, as you may deposit oils from your fingertips, degrading the cleanliness of the nail. Cleanse the nails with surface cleanser and lint-free wipe.

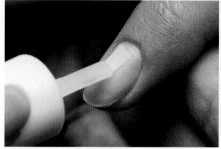

4 Apply nail dehydrator to all nails.

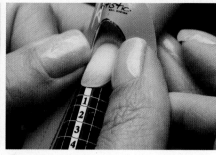

5 Position the nail forms. Further instruction on single-use and multiuse forms are on page p. 959.

6 Apply primer. Release excess primer from the brush and dab the brush to the prepared natural nail only. Always follow the manufacturer's directions. Acid-based nail primer will dry to a chalky white. Acid-free primer will dry to a shiny, sticky surface.

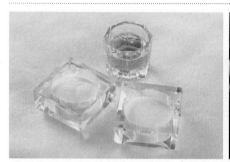

7 Prepare monomer liquid and polymer powder into separate dappen dishes.

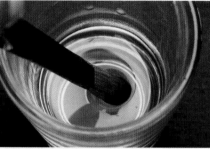

8 Saturate your application brush with monomer liquid and wipe out the excess liquid.

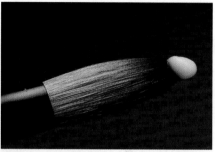

9 Gently wipe your brush to create a flat edge with the hair and dip the tip slightly into the soft white powder to pick up a small bead on one side of the brush.

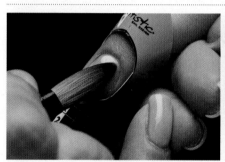

10 Place the bead toward the cuticle area. Press the product at the cuticle line to thin, and angle the brush so that the moon gradually thickens to create an edge.

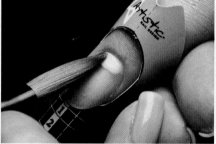

11 Spread the bead from side to side to create the lunula, the whitish, half-moon shape underneath the base of the nail. The edges of the lunula should stop just before the sidewall.

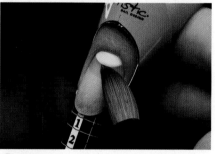

12 Once the product is in place, use the tip of your brush to clean around the edge.

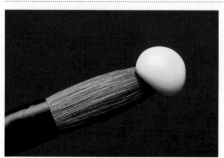

13 Dip the tip of the same brush into the white polymer powder and pick up a bead of product—it should have a dry-to-medium consistency that is large enough to cover the entire free-edge extension up to the edge of the smile line.

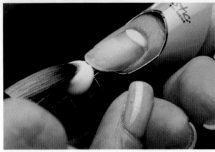

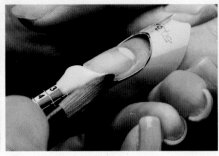

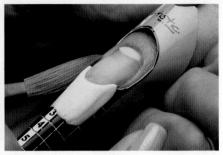

14 Place the white bead in the center of the nail form at the point where the free edge joins the nail form. Wipe your brush gently on a clean or disposable towel while you allow your bead to start to self-level and begin setting up.

15 Use the front of the brush flat to slide the bead to the corners of the natural nail. Then apply pressure to the center of the brush and pull it towards you. This will stretch the thickness of the bead out onto the form to create the extension edge.

16 Use the body of the brush around the perimeter of the nail to shape your extension.

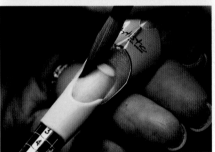

17 Use the tip of the brush to push your smile line into place, and wipe the edge until a crisp, rounded smile line is achieved.

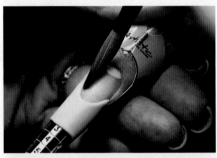

18 Pick up a tiny second bead of white powder, with a drier consistency, and place it on the left corner of the natural nail and brush it toward the smile line and center of the nail. Wipe your brush gently on a clean or disposable towel, and then use the tip of the brush to define the smile line to the corner.

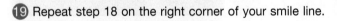

19 Repeat step 18 on the right corner of your smile line.

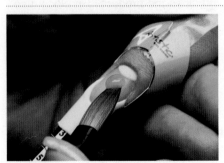

20 Pick up a small bead of pink polymer powder with your brush and place it near the cuticle area of the nail plate. Guide the pink bead towards the cuticle area leaving a tiny free margin between the product and the skin. Smooth out imperfections.

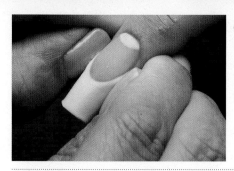

21 When nail enhancement begins to harden, loosen the form and slide it off. The nail enhancements will harden enough to file and shape after several minutes; they should make a clicking sound when lightly tapped with a brush handle. Remove the form and gently press in the sides to narrow the nail as it dries.

22 Repeat Steps 8 through 17 on the remaining nails.

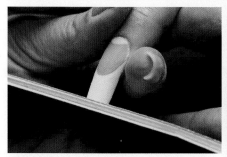

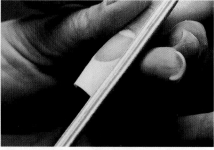

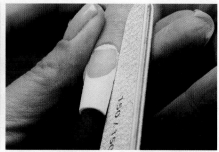

23 Use a medium abrasive (150- to 180-grit) to shape and remove imperfections. Begin by shaping the tip's edge on all nails. Be sure to measure the length so they are consistent.

24 File the left sidewalls and right sidewalls of all nails.

25 File the underside of the nail extensions on both sides of each nail to create a clean, straight lower arch.

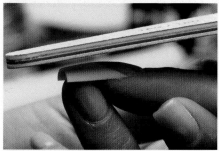

26 Glide the abrasive over the nail with long, sweeping strokes to further shape and perfect the enhancement surface. Remember that the product should be thin near the cuticle, free edge, and sidewalls.

27 Buff the nail enhancements with a 180- to 240-grit buffer. Remove any dust with a clean, dry nail brush before applying oil.

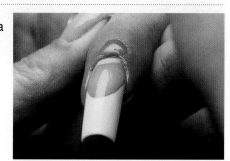

28 Apply and rub nail oil into the surrounding skin and nail enhancement, massaging briefly to speed up penetration.

29 Have your client wash her hands thoroughly with soap, water, and a nail brush to remove dust and chemicals that may be present on the skin. Have the client dry her hands with clean or disposable towel.

30 Apply hand cream and massage the hands and arms.

31 Clean the nail enhancements by removing all traces of lotion from the nail plate with a lint-free wipe saturated with alcohol or polish remover.

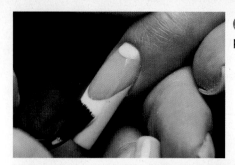

32 Polish the nail with a clear gloss polish depending on your client's preferences.

33 Finished look.

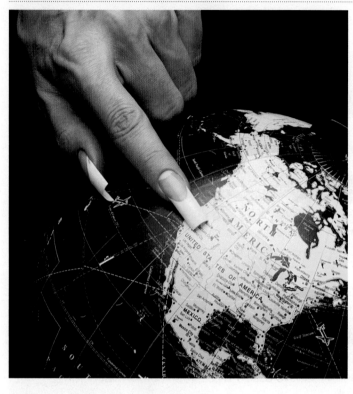

Complete:

P 25-2 **Post-Service Procedure.** *See page 884*

ONE-COLOR MONOMER LIQUID AND POLYMER POWDER MAINTENANCE

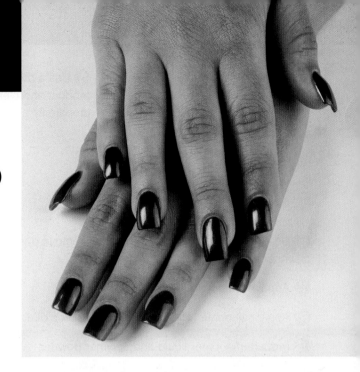

IMPLEMENTS & MATERIALS

In addition to the basic materials on your manicuring table, you will need the following supplies for the One-Color Monomer Liquid and Polymer Powder Maintenance procedure:

☐ Abrasives

☐ Application brushes

☐ Dappen dishes

☐ Monomer liquid

☐ Nail dehydrator

☐ Nail primer

☐ Polymer powder

PREPARATION | PROCEDURE

Perform:

P 25-1 **Pre-Service Procedure** *See page 880*

❶ Remove the existing polish or gel sealant, then use a pusher to gently push back the eponychium and carefully remove cuticle tissue from the nail plate.

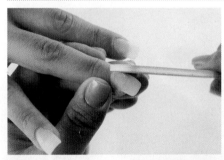

❷ Using a medium-coarse abrasive (150- to 180-grit) flat against the existing product, carefully smooth down the ledge until it is flush with the new growth of nail plate. Smooth out any areas of product that may be lifting or forming pockets. Be careful not to damage the natural nail plate with your abrasive.

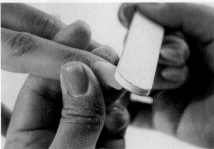

❸ Hold the medium abrasive (150- to 180-grit) flat, and glide it over the entire nail enhancement to reshape, refine, and thin the product at the free edge until the white tip appears translucent.

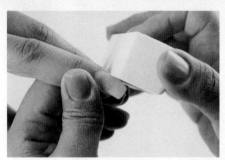

④ Use a medium-fine abrasive (180- to 240-grit) or buffer to smooth the product and blend it into the new growth area. Gently buff the natural nail to prepare it.

⑤ Use a clean nylon manicure brush to remove dust. Cleanse the nails with a surface cleanser and lint-free wipe.

⑥ Apply nail dehydrator to all nails.

⑦ Apply nail primer and follow manufacturer's directions.

⑧ Prepare monomer liquid and polymer powder.

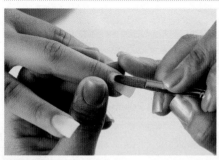

⑨ Pick up one or more small beads of enhancement product and place at the natural nail area, the regrowth.

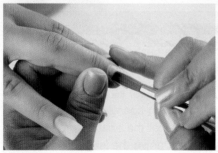

⑩ Use the brush to smooth these beads over the new growth area. Glide the brush over the nail to smooth out imperfections. Enhancement product application near the eponychium, sidewall areas, and free edge must be extremely thin for a natural-looking nail. Be sure to leave a tiny free margin between the nail enhancement product and skin.

⑪ Pick up one or more small beads of enhancement product and place them at the center or apex of the nail.

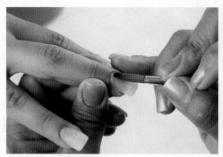

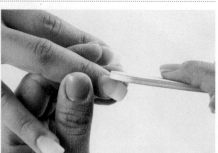

⑫ Use the brush to smooth these beads over the entire nail enhancement. Glide the brush over the nail to smooth out imperfections.

⑬ Allow the nails to harden. Nails are hard when they make a clicking sound when lightly tapped with a brush handle. Once hardened, shape the nail enhancements with an abrasive board.

14 Buff the nail enhancements with a 180- to 240-grit buffer. Remove the dust.

15 Apply and rub nail oil into the surrounding skin and nail enhancement, massaging briefly to speed up penetration.

16 Ask the client to wash her hands with soap and water at the hand washing station, or ask her to use the nail brush to clean her nails over a finger bowl. Rinse with clean water to remove soap residue that may cause lifting. Dry thoroughly with a clean, disposable towel.

17 Apply hand cream and massage the hands and arms. Thoroughly clean each nail of lotion.

18 Polish nail enhancements depending on your client's preferences.

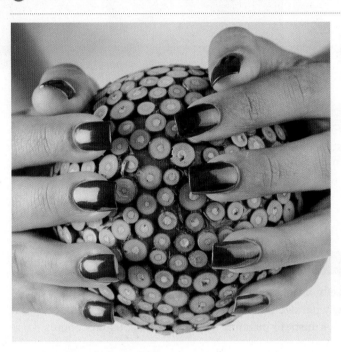

19 Finished look.

POST-SERVICE

Complete:

P 25-2 **Post-Service Procedure.** *See page 884*

CRACK REPAIR FOR MONOMER LIQUID AND POLYMER POWDER NAIL ENHANCEMENTS

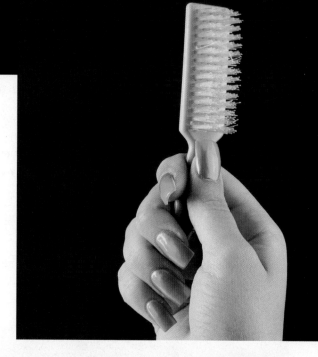

IMPLEMENTS & MATERIALS

In addition to the basic materials on your manicuring table, you will need the following supplies for the Crack Repair for Monomer Liquid and Polymer Powder Nail Enhancements procedure:

☐ Application brushes
☐ Monomer liquid
☐ Nail forms
☐ Polymer powder

☐ Dappen dishes
☐ Nail dehydrator
☐ Nail primer

PREPARATION

Perform:

P 25-1 **Pre-Service Procedure** *See page 880*

PROCEDURE

1 Remove the existing polish or gel sealant, then use a pusher to gently push back the eponychium, and carefully remove cuticle tissue from the nail plate. Depending on nail maintenance needed, refer back to nail maintenance in previous procedures.

2 Gently file the nail surface with a medium/fine abrasive (180- to 240-grit). Avoid over-filing of the nail plate. Remove the nail dust with a clean, dry nail brush.

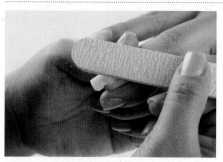

3 File a V-shape into the crack, or file flush to remove the crack. File more than just the crack for extra protection.

4 Buff and remove any dust with a clean, dry nail brush. Apply nail dehydrator to any exposed natural nail in the crack.

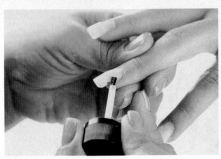

5 Apply nail primer to any exposed natural nail in the crack.

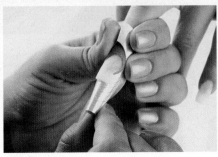

6 If the crack needs support, apply a nail form.

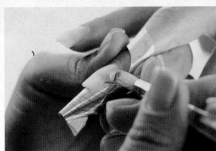

7 Prepare monomer liquid and polymer powder. Pick up one or more small beads of product, and apply them to the cracked area. If you are using the two-color system, be sure to use the correct color of polymer powder.

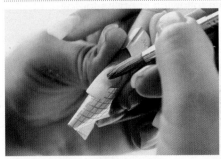

8 Press and smooth the enhancement product to fill the crack. Be careful not to let the product seep under the form.

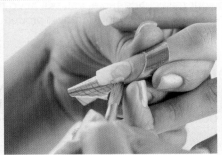

9 Apply additional beads, if needed, to fill in the crack or reinforce the rest of the nail. Shape the enhancement and allow it to harden.

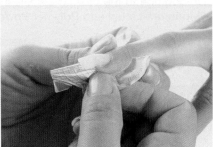

10 Remove the form, if used.

11 Reshape the nail enhancement using a medium abrasive (150- to 180-grit).

12 Buff the nail enhancements with a 180- to 240-grit buffer, then remove dust.

13 Apply and rub nail oil into the surrounding skin and nail enhancement, massaging briefly to speed up penetration.

14 Ask the client to wash her hands with soap and water at the hand washing station, or ask her to use the nail brush to clean her nails over a finger bowl. Rinse with clean water to remove soap residue. Dry thoroughly with a clean, disposable towel.

15 Apply hand cream and massage the hands and arms. Clean the nail enhancements of lotion.

16 Polish nail enhancements depending on your client's preferences.

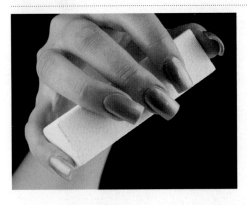

17 Finished repaired nail.

POST-SERVICE

Complete:

P 25-2 **Post-Service Procedure** *See page 884*

MONOMER LIQUID AND POLYMER POWDER NAIL ENHANCEMENT REMOVAL

IMPLEMENTS & MATERIALS

In addition to the basic materials on your manicuring table, you will need the following supplies for the Monomer Liquid and Polymer Powder Nail Enhancement Removal procedure:

☐ Acetone   ☐ Metal or glass bowl   ☐ Hand towel

PREPARATION | PROCEDURE

Perform:

P 25-1 **Pre-Service Procedure** *p. 880*

1 Have the client wash her hands thoroughly, and then remove existing nail polish if applicable. Start by applying a thick lotion or barrier cream to the hands and cuticle. This will help protect the surrounding skin prior to soaking in acetone or product remover.

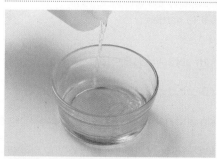

2 Fill the glass bowl with enough acetone or product remover to cover ½-inch (1.27 cm) higher than client's enhancements. One option is to place the bowl inside another bowl of hot water to heat the acetone safely and speed up the removal procedure.

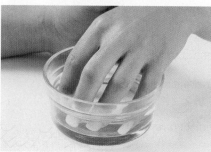

3 Place the client's nails into the bowl and cover the hands with a hand towel if desired. Soak the client's nail enhancements for 20 to 30 minutes or as long as needed to remove the enhancement product. Refer to the manufacturer's directions and precautions for nail enhancement product removal.

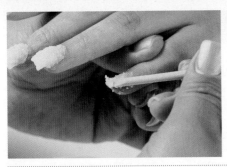

④ Once or twice during the procedure, use a wooden or metal pusher to gently push off the softened enhancement. Repeat until all enhancements have been removed. Do not pry them off with nippers, as this will damage the natural nail plate. Avoid removing enhancements from the acetone or product remover, or they will quickly re-harden, making them more difficult to remove. The key is to leave the nails in the acetone until they fall off and leave the natural nail free of product. Use a plastic-backed cotton pad to remove the remaining product.

⑤ Lightly buff the nails with a 240-grit buffer to smooth any remaining ridges or residue. Remove any dust with a clean, dry nail brush. Cleanse the nails with surface cleanser and lint-free wipes.

⑥ Apply and rub nail oil into the surrounding skin and nail enhancement, massaging briefly to speed up penetration.

⑦ Recommend that the client receive a basic manicure. If client is not receiving a basic manicure, then complete steps 8 and 9.

⑧ Ask the client to wash her hands with soap and water at the hand washing station, or ask her to use the nail brush to clean her nails over a finger bowl. Rinse with clean water to remove soap residue. Dry thoroughly with a clean, disposable towel.

⑨ Apply hand cream and massage the hands and arms. Clean the nails of lotion.

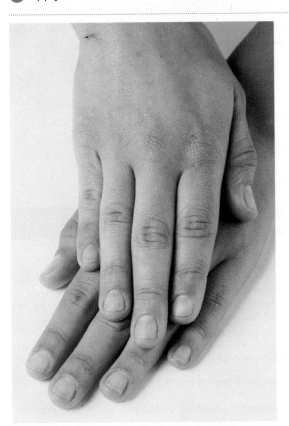

⑩ Finished look.

POST-SERVICE

Complete:

Ⓟ 25-2 **Post-Service Procedure.** *See page 884*

REVIEW QUESTIONS

1. What is the chemistry behind monomer liquid and polymer powder nail enhancements, and how does it work?

2. What are the definitions of *apex*, *stress area*, and *sidewall*, and where is their location on the nail enhancement?

3. What is the proper procedure for applying one-color monomer and polymer nail enhancements over tips and on natural nails?

4. What is the proper procedure for applying two-color monomer and polymer nail enhancements using forms?

5. What is the proper procedure for performing a one-color maintenance service on nail enhancements using monomer liquid and polymer powder?

6. How is a crack repair performed?

7. How are monomer liquid and polymer powder removed from the nail?

8. List a variety of ways to create nail art for monomer liquid and polymer powder.

STUDY TOOLS

- **Reinforce what you just learned:** Complete the activities and exercises in your Theory or Practical Workbook, or your Study Guide.

- **Expand your knowledge:** Search for websites about the topics in this chapter and make a list of additional resources.

- **Study and prepare for your quiz:** Take the chapter test in your Exam Review or your Milady U: Online Licensing Prep.

- **Re-Test your knowledge:** Take the Chapter 28 *Quizzes*!

- **Learn even more:** Look up in a dictionary or search the internet for the definitions of any additional terms you want to learn about.

CHAPTER GLOSSARY

3-D nail art	p. 966	Describes any art that protrudes from the nail.
apex	p. 963	Also known as *arch*; the area of the nail that has all of the strength.
chain reaction	p. 955	Also known as *polymerization reaction*; process that joins together monomers to create very long polymer chains.
dappen dish	p. 960	Special container that holds monomer liquid and polymer powder.
grit	p. 958	Refers to how many grains of sand are on the file per square inch.
initiators	p. 954	Found in polymer powder; when activated by a catalyst, will spring into action and cause monomer molecules to permanently link together into long polymer chains.
inlaid designs	p. 966	Designs inside a nail enhancement.

mix ratio	p. 956	The amount of monomer liquid and polymer powder used to create a bead.
monomer MON-oh-mehr	p. 952	One unit called a molecule.
monomer liquid	p. 952	Chemical liquid mixed with polymer powder to form the sculptured nail enhancement.
monomer liquid and polymer powder nail enhancements	p. 952	Enhancements created by combining monomer liquid and polymer powder.
nail extension underside	p. 963	The actual underside of the nail extension.
nail forms	p. 959	Used as a guide to extend the nail enhancements beyond the fingertip for additional length.
nail primer	p. 957	Used on the natural nail prior to product application to assist in adhesion; used to chemically bond the enhancement product to the natural nail.
odorless monomer liquid and polymer powder products	p. 964	Nail enhancement products that have little odor; must be used with a dry mix ratio (equal parts liquid and powder in bead).
polymer POL-i-mehr	p. 952	Substance formed by combining many small molecules (monomers) into very long, chain-like structures.
polymerization POL-i-mehr-eh-za-shun	p. 954	Also known as *curing* or *hardening*; chemical reaction that creates polymers.
polymer powder	p. 952	Powder in white, clear, pink, and many other colors that is combined with monomer liquid to form the nail enhancement.
shiner	p. 959	A multi sided buffer (usually 400/1,000/4,000 grit) used to create a high shine on a natural nail or a nail enhancement when no polish will be worn.
sidewall	p. 963	The line of the nail enhancement that runs straight from the cuticle down the side or wall of the nail to the end of the extension.
smile line	p. 963	The curved line where the pink and white meet each other on a French manicured nail.
stress area	p. 963	The part of the nail enhancement where the natural nail grows beyond the finger and becomes the free edge. This area needs strength to support the nail extension.

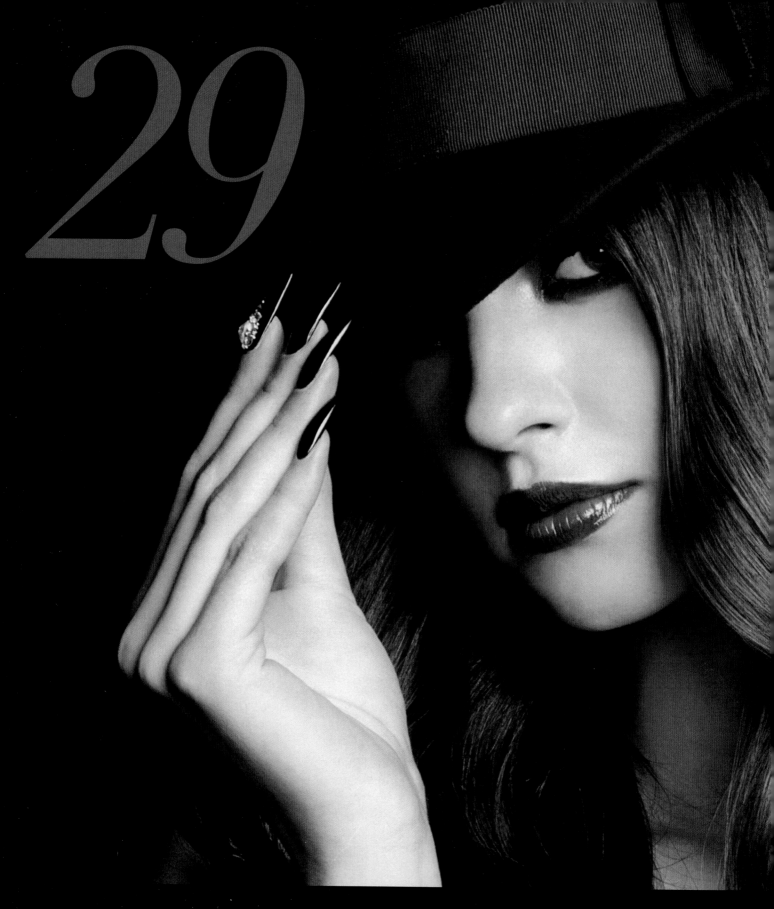

29

LIGHT CURED GELS

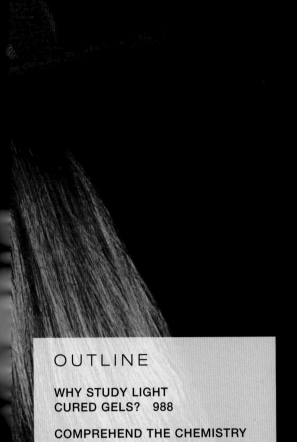

LEARNING OBJECTIVES

After completing this chapter, you will be able to:

LO❶
Describe the chemistry and main ingredients of light cured gels.

LO❷
Explain when you would use a one-color or two-color method for applying UV or LED gels.

LO❸
List the different types of light cured gels used in current systems.

LO❹
Identify the supplies needed for light cured gel application.

LO❺
Determine when to use light cured gels on your client.

LO❻
List the four guidelines that will assist you in choosing the proper light cured gel technology for your client.

LO❼
Discuss the differences between light cured lamps and bulbs.

LO❽
Identify the advantages of using light cured gel polish.

LO❾
Describe how to maintain light cured gel nail enhancements.

LO❿
Explain how to correctly remove hard light cured gels.

LO⓫
Identify the correct way to remove soft light cured gels.

Publisher's note: The term *light cured gels* is used in this chapter to encompass UV and LED gels.

This chapter introduces **light cured gel**, also known as *UV and LED gel*, a type of nail enhancement product that hardens when exposed to a UV and LED light source. Light cured gel is an increasingly popular method for nail enhancement services.

why study
LIGHT CURED GELS?

Cosmetologists should study and have a thorough understanding of light cured gels because:

> Clients may be interested in receiving light cured gel services.

> An understanding of the chemistry of light cured gel products will allow you to choose the best system and products to use in your salon.

> An understanding of how light cured gel nails are made, applied, and cured will allow you to create a safe and efficient salon service.

> Clients often become loyal and steadfast when they receive excellent light cured gel nail services, maintenance, and removal.

After reading the next few sections, you will be able to:

LO❶ Describe the chemistry and main ingredients of light cured gels.

Comprehend the Chemistry of Light Cured Gels

Nail enhancements based on light curing are not traditionally thought of as being methacrylates; however, they are very similar. Like wrap resins, adhesives, monomer liquid, and polymer powder nail enhancements, light cured gel enhancements rely on ingredients from the monomer liquid and polymer powder chemical family. Their ingredients are part of a subcategory of this family called acrylates. Wrap resins are called cyanoacrylates, and monomer liquid and polymer powder nail enhancements are from the same category called methacrylates.

Although most light cured gels are made from acrylates, new light cured gel technologies have been developed that use methacrylates. Like wraps and monomer liquid and polymer powder nail enhancements, light cured gels can also contain monomer liquids, but they rely mostly on a related form called an oligomer. The term *mono* means one, and *poly* means many. *Oligo* means few. An **oligomer** (uh-LIG-uh-mer) is a short chain of monomer liquids that is often thick, sticky, and gel-like and that is not long enough to be considered a polymer. These chains are often referred to as a prepolymer. Nail enhancement monomer liquids are liquids, while polymers are solids. Oligomers are between solid and liquid.

Traditionally, light cured gels rely on a special type of acrylate called a urethane acrylate, while newer light cured gel systems use urethane methacrylates by themselves or in combination with urethane acrylates. **Urethane acrylate** (YUR-ah-thane AK-ri-layt) and **urethane methacrylate** (YUR-ah-thane meth-AK-ri-layt) are the main ingredients used alone or in combination with urethane acrylates to create light cured gel nail enhancements. The term *urethane* refers to the type of starting material that is used to create the most common light cured gel resins. The chemical family of urethanes is known for high abrasion resistance and durability.

Light cured gel resins react when exposed to the UV or LED light source that is recommended for the gel. A chemical called a **photoinitiator** (FOH-toh-in-ish-ee-AY-tohr) initiates the polymerization reaction. The key thing to remember here is that it takes the combination of the resin, photoinitiator, and the proper curing bulb to cause the gel to cure completely. Light cured gel systems employ a single component resin compound that is cured to a solid material when exposed to a UV or LED light source. Light cured gels typically do not use a powder that is incorporated into the gel resin. A few light cured gels on the market incorporate a powder that is sprinkled into the gel, but the rest of the chapter will refer to *gels* as being the more common single-component type.

The difference between light cured gels is the type of photoinitiator used in the formula and the measure of light that photoinitiator responds to. For example, LED gels cure when they are exposed to a certain measure of light found in LED lamps. When the LED gel is directly exposed to this light, it causes the oligomers to start to cure immediately. When exposed for the recommended amount of time, they will cure completely solid.

The photoinitiator found in UV gels cause the gel to cure when directly exposed to UV radiation at that certain measure found in UV lamps (**figure 29-1**). All gels will cure if exposed to natural and florescent or any type of light that is full spectrum, as these contain some measure of the light it takes to cure these gels. The process will just happen slower because they are not getting direct, intense exposure. That is why it is recommended to always keep your containers closed and gel brushes covered, so they do not slowly cure and harden while exposed to light.

Remember that some gels react to UV, some to LED, and some to both. Many still only respond to UV, so be sure to review the manufacturer's recommendations for the type of lamp you will need for the specific product you are using.

Light cured gels can be easy to apply, file, and maintain, and create beautiful, long-lasting nail enhancements (**figure 29-2**). They also have the advantage of having very little or no odor. Although they typically are not as hard as monomer liquid and polymer powder nail enhancements, they are more flexible.

The light cured gel application process differs from other types of nail enhancements. After the nail plate is properly prepared, each layer of

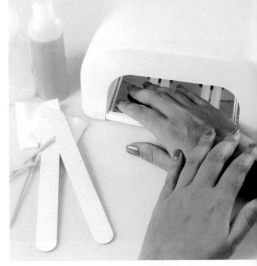

figure 29-1
Position the client's hand in the UV lamp for the required cure time.

DID YOU KNOW?
Ultraviolet light is really not light at all. UV light is really wavelengths of electromagnetic radiation that are just beyond the visible spectrum of light. In this chapter UV light and UV radiation are the same thing.

figure 29-2
Technician applying black gel using a natural hair brush to create a permanent french look to the gel nail enhancements.

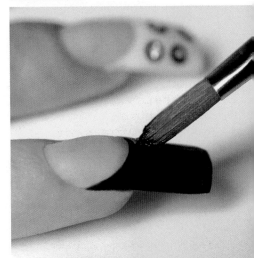

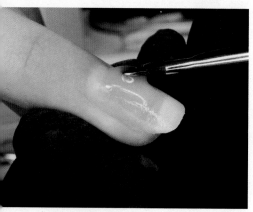

figure 29-3
A cosmetologist in nitrile gloves applies clear gel overlay on natural colored nail tip.

product applied to the natural nail, nail tip, or form requires exposure to a UV or LED light source to **cure**, which means to harden. The UV or LED radiation required for curing comes from a special bulb designed to emit the proper type and intensity of UV or LED radiation.

After reading the next few sections, you will be able to:

LO② Explain when you would use a one-color or two-color method for applying UV or LED gels.

LO③ List the different types of light cured gels used in current systems.

Describe Light Cured Gels

There are many types of light cured gels. Choosing a favorite and relied-upon gel is as important as choosing the monomer liquid and polymer powder system that you prefer. Some cosmetologists favor a gel that is thick and will not level by itself. Other cosmetologists like to use gels that quickly self-level. It is up to you to find the gel that you prefer to use and to learn how to use it well.

The different light cured gels can be described as thin-viscosity gels, medium-viscosity gels, thick-viscosity gels, and building or sculpting gels. Remember that **viscosity** (vis-KAHS-ut-tee) is the measurement of the thickness or thinness of a liquid and that viscosity affects how the fluid flows. Manufacturers have a market name for gels that they make, but most light cured gels fall under these general categories:

- The **one-color method** is the method whereby one color of UV or LED gel is applied over the entire surface of the nail. This method is used for clients who wish to wear colored polish or UV or LED gel polish over the enhancement (figure 29-3).

- The **two-color method** is a method whereby two colors of resin are used to overlay the nail; usually pink and white are used, allowing for a French or American manicure finish in which lacquer is not needed. There are many processes for performing a two-color method over tips or natural nails. The process varies from one gel manufacturer to another and can even vary within one manufacturer's product lines. Consult with the UV or LED gel manufacturer about the product you intend to use before you perform a two-color method.

Ⓟ29-1 **One-Color Method UV or LED Gel on Tips or Natural Nails Finishing With UV or LED Gel Polish** *See page 1002*

Ⓟ29-2 **Two-Color Method UV or LED Gel on Tips or Natural Nails** *See page 1006*

❓ DID YOU KNOW?

It is very common for gel manufacturers to have many colored gels for the two-color method. These pigmented gels can vary in opacity and viscosity. You should follow the manufacturer's recommendations for applying the pigmented gel in a two-color method. Usually, the more opaque gels have thinner viscosities and are applied after the second coat of building gel. The less-opaque pigmented gels are often thicker in viscosity and are applied before the first coat of building gel.

Types of Light Cured Gels

Bonding gels are used to increase adhesion to the natural nail plate, similar to a monomer liquid and polymer powder primer. Bonding gels will vary in consistency and chemical components. The increased adhesion decreases the tendency for enhancements to separate from the natural nail. Some bonding gels contain certain chemicals that smell like a monomer liquid and polymer powder primer, while other bonding gels do not have a strong odor. Light cured gel manufacturers are constantly developing new technology in the formulation of bonding gels. These technologies could make the use of odiferous chemicals obsolete. Some light cured gel manufacturers use air-dry bonding systems. Just because the bonding product may not be cured in a UV or LED lamp does not make it any less effective than a bonding system that is cured in a UV or LED lamp.

When applying primer or bonding gel, insert the brush into the nail primer or bonding gel, wipe off any excess from the brush, and using a slightly damp brush, ensure that the nail plate is completely covered per the manufacturer's recommendations. Avoid using too much product to prevent running into the skin, which can increase the risks of developing skin irritation or sensitivity to the enhancement system.

Building gels include any thick-viscosity resin that allows the cosmetologist to build an arch and curve into the fingernail. When applying this gel, do not pat the gel as you would monomer liquid and polymer powder material; instead, gently brush or float the gel material onto the fingernail. Avoid introducing air into the gel, as this will reduce the strength of the cured gel and may lead to bubbles and cracking.

Always cure each layer of the light cured gel for the time required by the manufacturer's instructions. Curing for too little time can result in service breakdown, skin irritation, and/or skin sensitivity. Improper positioning of the hands inside the bulb also can cause improper curing.

Light cured building gels can be used with self-leveling gels, and if done correctly, this combination can reduce the amount of filing and shaping required to contour the enhancement later in the service. Some light cured building gels have fiberglass strands compounded into the gel during the manufacturing process. These gels typically have hardness and durability properties that closely resemble monomer liquid and polymer powder systems. This type of gel can be very helpful when repairing a break or crack in a client's enhancement.

Self-leveling gels are thinner in consistency than building gels, allowing them to settle and level during application. These gels are used to enhance the thickness of the overlay while providing a smoother surface. Cosmetologists who are experienced in light cured gel application often will choose to apply a building gel first, and then apply a self-leveling gel to create the enhancement, which will help to reduce filing and contouring.

Pigmented gels can be building gels or self-leveling gels that include color pigment. Pigmented building gels can be used earlier in the service to create art or a traditional French manicure look by using a white and pink pigmented gel. To complete this look, you would use the two-color method, which is similar to a two-color monomer liquid and polymer powder process. Self-leveling pigmented gels can also be used near the end

CAUTION

Be careful to not get UV or LED gel products on the skin during application or while you are removing the inhibition layer. Continued over exposure of gel products on the skin can cause a client to become sensitive to the product and could eventually cause an allergic reaction.

DID YOU KNOW?

Light cured gel polishes are also referred to in the industry as *no-chip manicures*, *soak-off gel color*, *soft gels*, and even *power polish*. Despite the assorted names, they are all referring to UV and LED gel polish.

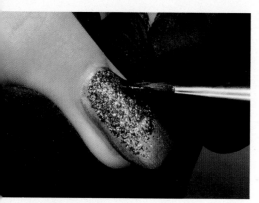

figure 29-4
Gel polish comes in a variety of colors. In this example, the technician wears nitrile gloves while applying gel polish from a pot.

of the application, after filing. Because self-leveling pigmented gels are applied much more thinly, a French manicure look is easily achieved over the filed enhancement, before applying a finishing gel.

Gel polish is a very thin-viscosity gel that is usually pigmented and packaged in a pot or a polish bottle; it is used as an alternative to traditional nail lacquers (**figure 29-4**). Light cured gel polishes do not dry the same way as nail lacquers; they cure in a UV or LED lamp. When gel polish is finished curing, a gloss gel can be applied over it to create a high, lustrous shine. Since the products are cured, the end result appears lacquered but does not have any solvent odor and is immediately dry to the touch. Another advantage of light cured gel polishes is that the color stays without chipping three to four times longer than traditional nail lacquers. Light cured gel polish may be used on natural nails or nail enhancements.

Light cured gels are available in a wide array of colors. They are available in cream and frosted colors, and some even include glitter! These gels can be mixed together to create a few hundred more colors. Light cured gels provide the cosmetologist and client with a wide variety of colors and options for expressing their personality and creativity.

Glossing gel, also known as *sealing gel*, *finishing gel*, or *shine gel*, is used over the finished and filed gel application to create a high shine, in much the same way a top coat would be applied over colored nail polish. Light cured gloss gels do not require buffing and can also be used over a monomer liquid and polymer powder enhancement. There are two types of light cured gloss gels: traditional gloss gels that cure with a sticky inhibition layer that requires cleaning and tack-free gloss gels that cure to a high shine without the inhibition layer.

An **inhibition layer** is a tacky surface left on the nail after a UV or LED gel has cured. Choose the gloss gel that is best for you. Traditional light cured gloss gels do not discolor after prolonged exposure to UV radiation, while tack-free gloss gels often discolor. Many light cured gel manufacturers are developing tack-free gloss gels that do not discolor upon exposure to UV radiation. These advancements may make traditional light cured gloss gels obsolete; but for now, traditional light cured gloss gels still hold the market on non-yellowing performance.

After you have determined how each type of gel behaves on the fingernail, learn how to use the pigmented pink and white gels in the same

ACTIVITY

Acquire samples of gels that are on the market by calling a few popular companies. When you receive the gels, place a small amount of gel on a plastic tip that you have adhered to a wooden stick. Study the gel as it moves over the tip. Try applying the gel in a different way (such as brushing a thin layer, then applying a ball of gel in the stress area). Then observe the gel again. Repeat this procedure with all of the samples. The more you know about how the gels work and behave, the easier it will be for you to apply the gel on your client.

ACTIVITY

We have discussed how gels require a UV or LED light source to cure properly. Gels will not cure if the light cannot penetrate through the gel. If the gel is pigmented, then the pigment can block the transmission of the UV and LED light into the gel and decrease its curing potential.

Place some gel on a disposable form, and spread it using a gel brush. Apply the gel so that you are able to see through it onto the surface of the form. Cure the gel in your UV and LED bulb for the recommended period of time. Clean the surface of the gel to remove the sticky residue—the inhibition layer. Peel the gel from the form and examine the side of the gel that was against the form. If there is a layer of uncured gel, then the gel was applied too thickly. Reapply the gel application thinly and repeat the curing and examination process until you get a full cure.

fashion. Similar to clear gels, pink gels and white gels can be formulated in a variety of viscosities (the measurement of the extent of a liquid to flow), colors, and degrees of opacity. **Opacity** (oh-PAY-sit-ee) is the amount of colored pigment concentration in a gel, making it more or less difficult to see through. If a light cured gel has a high degree of opacity, the gel will be better able to camouflage the nail bed. If a gel has a low degree of opacity, the nail will more clearly show through. There are many different gels on the market, and each of these gels can be combined to give any appearance that you and your client desire.

After reading the next few sections, you will be able to:

LO④ Identify the supplies needed for light cured gel application.

Name the Supplies Required for Light Cured Gels

Just as every type of nail enhancement service requires specific tools, implements, equipment, and supplies, so do light cured gel enhancements. Here is a list of those requirements (**figure 29-5**). In addition to the supplies in your basic manicuring setup, you will need:

- **Light curing gel lamp.** Choose a light curing gel lamp designed to produce the correct amount of UV or LED light needed to properly cure the gel nail enhancement products you use.

- **Application Brush.** Choose brushes with small, flat (or oval) bristles to hold and spread the light cured gels. Ensure gel brushes have caps to protect them from collecting dust and debris as well as shield them

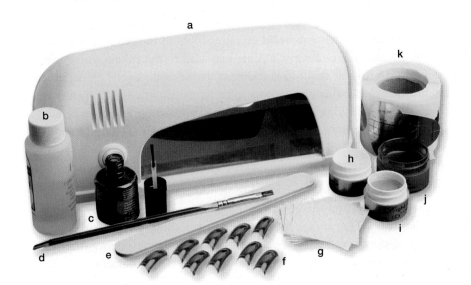

figure 29-5
Supplies needed for a UV gel service (left to right): a) UV lamp; b) cleanser; c) gel primer; d) gel brush; e) abrasive; f) nail tips; g) lint-free nail wipes; h) clear self-leveling gel; i) pink building gel; j) red gel polish; k) nail forms.

from light. Exposure to light can cause the gel to cure in the brush, and then the brush is no longer useable.

- **Gel primer or bonding gel.** Primers and bonding gels are designed specifically to improve adhesion of UV and LED gels to the natural nail plate. Use gel primers as instructed by the manufacturer of the product that you are using.

- **Light cured gel.** This should include pigmented gel(s) for a one-color or two-color service. This will also include a gel that creates a gloss, depending upon the gel system that you choose.

- **Nail forms.** Depending on the manufacturer recommendation, clear plastic forms are sometimes used to allow UV and LED radiation to penetrate from the underside for more complete curing of the free edge. With some brands, a traditional single-use form is acceptable. If using a reusable or multiuse form, remember to clean and disinfect in between uses.

- **Nail tips.** It is important when using nail tips with UV or LED gel to size the tip so that the curve of the tip matches the curve of the nail. If the curves do not match and the tip is spread too flat, then the tip could crack lengthwise down the center. It's also important to ensure the width of the tip measures from one side of the natural nail to the other. If the tip is measured too small it will crack on the side.

- **Nail adhesive.** There are many types of nail adhesives for securing preformed nail tips to natural nails. Select a type and size best suited for your work.

- **Nail dehydrator.** This product removes surface moisture and tiny amounts of oil left on the natural nail plate (both of which can block adhesion) and help prevent lifting of the nail enhancements.

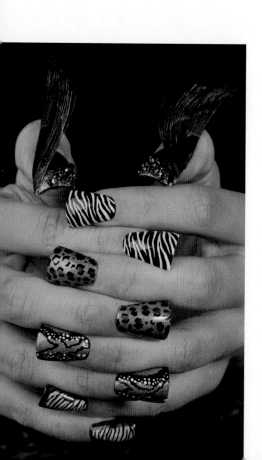

- **Abrasive files and buffers.** Select a medium to fine abrasive buffer (180-240 grit) for natural nail preparation. Choose a medium to fine abrasive file (180- to 240-grit) for smoothing the surface. When contouring the surface, file carefully near the sidewalls and eponychium to avoid injuring the client's skin. Check the free edge thickness and even out imperfections with gentle strokes with the abrasive.

Make certain that you avoid excessive filing of the gel on the sidewalls of the enhancements. Excessive filing may lead to the enhancement being too thin, which can result in cracking at the sidewalls of the enhancement. Remember that nail enhancements must have a slightly rough surface in order for the finishing or glossing gels to adhere, so buffing after surface filing is not necessary. Light cured gel manufacturers may have other recommendations for abrasives; please consult the manufacturer's guidelines for more information on the specific system you are using.

- **A cleansing solution.** Cleansing solutions usually contain isopropanol, and they may contain additional solvents. This solution can be used to cleanse the natural nail as well as to remove the sticky inhibition layer from the gel after curing. The cleansing solution you choose should be the one recommended by the manufacturer.

- **Lint-free cleansing wipes.** Select an appropriate lint-free wipe to cleanse the nail surface. When removing the inhibition layer from light cured gel, avoid cleaning the nail in a manner that would put the gel onto the surface of the skin. Using your cleansing wipe, start at the top of the fingernail nearest the cuticle, and wipe away from the cuticle to the free edge of the fingernail.

Storing Light Cured Gels

When storing light cured gels, ensure the lids are on tight and the containers are upright to avoid leakage. Since light cured gels are light sensitive, meaning light can cure the product, gels should be stored in a dark, cool place to prolong the life of the product.

During a gel procedure, keep the brush and open gel containers away from sunlight, gel lamps, and full-spectrum table lamps to prevent the gel from hardening. When the service is completed, store the application brush away from all sources of UV radiation. Do not leave your open container of gel near a window or a UV or LED lamp. If the gel is exposed to these sources of light, it will cure and become polymerized in the container

---

After reading the next few sections, you will be able to:

LO⑤ Determine when to use light cured gels on your client.

When to Use Light Cured Gels

When to use light cured gels may seem like a question of personal preference, but it really is a question of logic. The general answer could be, "Anytime!" Gel technology has been able to create some very hard, durable, and tough light cured gels. The new light cured resin technology allows light cured gel manufacturers to create tough, durable, and hard products that will perform as well as many of the monomer liquid and polymer powder systems on the market. The answer could easily be, "Never," because there are customers that prefer to wear monomer liquid and polymer powder. It is what they know—they have been wearing these products for years and refuse to change. Most clients will do what you recommend. If you wear and recommend monomer liquid and polymer powder enhancements, that is what most of your clients will wear. If you wear and recommend light cured gels, that will be their preference. You are the professional and, as such, you should recommend a system that you have used and feel will perform best for the client. There may be a situation when you use a system on your client and that is not performing as the two of you would like. It may be best to try something else. Maybe a different gel resin or a change to monomer liquid and polymer powder might be best. The answer to this question remains in your capable hands. It is also possible to use a monomer liquid and polymer powder system for the fill or full-set and to combine that with a light cured gloss gel to create the shine over the enhancement. Pigmented gels, such as light cured gel polishes, may also be used over the monomer liquid and polymer powder system, if that is what you prefer.

There are other factors that will assist you in your choice of gels or acrylics. The salon that you choose to work in or the environment you create in your work area could impact your decision. Gels commonly have fewer odors than acrylics, and if you are trying to create an environment with fewer odors, a gel may be the right choice for you and your clients.

There is one more choice to consider for gels: Consider the new, common gel polishes that are now on the market. Gel polishes are applied in a similar manner to a traditional nail polish but contain less solvent, cure under LED or UV light, and wear longer than traditional nail polish. The choice of when to use a gel polish versus a traditional polish is yours to make with your client. Questions to consider include:

- How easily would your client like the polish to be removed from the fingernail? If the polish is to be removed away from the salon, perhaps a traditional polish should be used.

- How long does the client desire the polish to last? If the polish is meant to remain on the fingernail for two weeks, the best choice is a gel polish.

P 29-3 **Sculpting Light Cured Gel Using Forms** *See page 1009*

P 29-5 **Monomer Liquid and Polymer Powder Nail Enhancements Finished with UV or LED Gel Polish** *See page 1015*

After reading the next few sections, you will be able to:

LO 6 List the four guidelines that will assist you in choosing the proper light cured gel technology for your client.

Choose the Proper Light Cured Gel Technology

There are many gels to choose from to perform your service. Here are a few guidelines that will help you make the best choice:

- If the client has flat fingernails, more building will need to be done to create an arch and curve. This building will be easiest when done with a thicker UV or LED building gel.

- If the client has fingernails that have an arch and curve, then a self-leveling gel may be the best option. Choose the self-leveling gel that you prefer—either a medium- or thick-viscosity gel.

- If your client returns to the salon often with broken enhancements, then a gel that uses fiberglass may be the best product for the next service.

- If a client is in search of manicure with long-lasting polish, a soak-off gel polish will be a great option.

After reading the next few sections, you will be able to:

LO ⑦ Discuss the differences between light cured lamps and bulbs.

Distinguish the Difference Between Light Cured Bulbs and Lamps

What is the difference between a UV bulb and a UV lamp?

A **UV bulb**, also known as *UV light bulb*, is a special bulb that emits UV radiation to cure UV gel nail enhancements. There are a number of bulbs that are used to cure light cured gels: 4-, 6-, 7-, 8-, and 9-watt bulbs.

A **UV lamp** also known as *UV light unit*, is a specialized electronic device that powers and controls UV bulbs to cure UV gel nail enhancements. Lamps that are currently being sold may look similar at first but there are differences, including the number of bulbs in the unit, the distance the bulbs are from the bottom of the unit, and the size of the unit. These factors affect the curing power of the unit.

These bulb and lamp features are similar to **LED**, also known as *light emitting diodes*. These small bulbs emit the correct wave of LED light to cure LED gel products. A **LED lamp** is the electronic device that houses the LED bulbs. Most LED lamps cure gel about four times faster than UV lamps. Remember that the gel must have LED photo-initiators in order to cure in a LED lamp. See manufacturer's directions to see if the product should cure in a UV or LED lamp. Most LED gel products also have UV photo-initiators so they can be cured in either lamp; they just require different cure times. For example, usually a cure time for a gel is 30 seconds in an LED or two minutes in a UV lamp.

Lamps are typically referred to by the number of bulbs inside the lamp multiplied by the wattage. Remember that **lamp wattage** is the measure of how much electricity the bulb consumes, much like miles per gallon tell you how much gasoline a car requires to drive a certain distance. Miles per gallon will not tell you how fast the car can go, just as wattage does not indicate how much UV or LED light a bulb will produce. For example, if a unit has four bulbs in it and each bulb is nine watts, then the lamp is called a 36-watt lamp. Likewise, if the lamp only has three bulbs and each bulb is also nine watts, then it is called a 27-watt lamp. Wattage does not indicate how much UV or LED light a lamp will emit (**figure 29-6**).

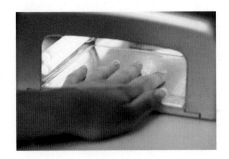

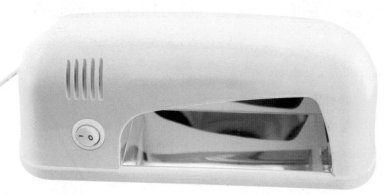

Courtesy of Light Elegance Nail Products

figure 29-6
UV nail lamp

UV and LED gel lamps are designed to produce the correct amount of UV or LED light needed to properly cure the gel nail enhancement products. Light cured gels are usually packaged in small opaque pots or squeeze tubes to protect them from UV and LED light. Even though UV and LED light is invisible to the eye, it is found in sunlight and tanning bulbs. Both true-color and full-spectrum bulbs emit a significant amount of ultraviolet radiation. If the gel product is exposed to these types of ceiling or table bulbs, the product's shelf life may be shortened, causing the product to harden in its container.

Depending on their circuitry, different bulbs produce greatly differing amounts of UV and LED light. This is referred to as the UV and LED bulb intensity or concentration. The intensity will vary from one lamp to the next and is more important than the rating of a UV and LED lamp based on the wattage of the bulb or the number of bulbs in the unit. For these reasons, it is important to use the UV or LED bulb that was designed for the selected UV and LED gel product. This will give you a much greater chance of success and fewer problems. Also, keep in mind that some lamps are designed to cure four fingers at once and recommend that the thumbs be cured separately. There are also lamps that are designed to allow enough light for the thumb to cure with the rest of the hand. These units are usually referred to as five-finger lights. You will need to know this information when using your lamp during the service so that the gels are cured correctly.

UV bulbs will stay violet for years; however, after a few months of use, they may produce too little UV radiation to properly cure the enhancement. Typically, UV bulbs must be changed two or three times per year, depending on frequency of use. If the bulbs are not changed regularly, gels may cure inadequately, meaning the oligomers and additional chemicals are not hardened. This can cause service breakdown, skin irritation, and product sensitivity.

The most common UV bulb that is on the market is a nine-watt bulb. While many of the UV gel systems use the nine-watt bulb, most of the gels can be cured in any manufacturer's 36-watt lamp. A gel that has been specifically designed to cure in a 36-watt lamp may not be able to be cured properly in a 16-watt lamp. The UV gel may become hard when cured in the 16-watt lamp, but it may not become as hard or cure completely. If the gel does not cure completely, it will crack, lift, and separate from the nail. It may not have a high shine, and the client will not be pleased with the service. The result will be similar to a monomer liquid and polymer powder system that has been applied with an incorrect mix-ratio between the liquid and the powder.

LED lights are becoming more common in the salon—most are used to cure the new gel polishes that are applied similarly to a traditional nail polish. These LED lights are not UV and therefore will not cure most of the traditional UV gels to their completed cure strength. There is a wide selection of LED lights on the market, and as such, it is strongly recommended that you use only lights that the manufacturer endorses. Using the wrong LED light source could drastically effect the curing of the LED gel.

While this chapter was being written in 2014, a media release was published that claimed that UV nail curing lights could cause skin cancer[i]. There have been no studies to date that support this claim. Three UV gel manufacturers conducted a series of independent studies that found little to no evidence to support the claim that UV nail lights could cause cancer.

The lamp has as much to do with the proper curing of the UV or LED gel as the bulb! Not all lamps are the same. The differences between the structures of the lamps will alter the curing potential of the unit. For example, if two lamps are similar in every other respect, but lamp A has been constructed with the UV or LED bulbs closer to the fingernails than lamp B, lamp A will have more curing potential than lamp B. Thus, the bulbs are not going to provide the same results. The lamps are both nine-watt and have the same number of bulbs, but lamp A is more powerful than lamp B.

Consult with the gel manufacturer to receive more detailed information on which lamp and bulb will properly cure their light cured gels.

> **✓ HERE'S A TIP**
>
> The heat from the chemical reaction caused when UV or LED gels cure can make some clients uncomfortable. The heat can be controlled by slowly inserting the hand into the UV or LED lamp. This will help to slow the chemical reaction and generate less heat. The heat is a result of the exothermic reaction of the gel as each bond of the polymer is created; the more bonds that are formed when the gel cures, the more heat is generated. In addition, the more bonds that are created when the gel polymerizes, the stronger the gel will be.

After reading the next few sections, you will be able to:

LO **⑧**   **Identify the advantages of using light cured gel polish.**

Specify the Advantages of Light Cured Gel Polish

Light cured gel polish has become a popular service to complement gels and all other enhancement services, including natural nails. Light cured gel polish is a relatively new system that evolved in 2000 with the emergence of new chemistries that became available to the beauty industry. The more popular light cured gel polishes are highly pigmented, which gives these systems the appearance of a traditional solvent-based nail lacquer. Light cured gel polishes are available in hundreds of shades, much the same as traditional nail polish, to suit every client.

Wearing light cured gel polishes instead of traditional nail lacquers does offer great advantages; however, they are removed differently than traditional nail polish. One advantage of light cured gel polishes is that they do not dry—they cure. Cured gel polish systems will not imprint or smudge if the client hits her hands while the nail lacquer is still drying. Another advantage is that the light cured gel polish does not thicken over time because the solvent does not evaporate. Solvent evaporation makes nail lacquers thicken and dry more slowly after the bottle of nail polish has been open for a few months. Since the solvent does not evaporate in light cured gel polish, a container of such polish will last longer.

After reading the next few sections, you will be able to:

LO⑨ Describe how to maintain light cured gel nail enhancements.

LO⑩ Explain how to correctly remove hard light cured gels.

LO⑪ Identify the correct way to remove soft light cured gels.

Relate Nail Art to Light Cured Gels

Light cured gels can be used to create beautiful nail enhancements and can also be a very lucrative nail art medium. There are many colors of pigmented light cured gels on the market today, and by using some simple techniques you can create an array of inlaid art that your clients will love. Inlaid art is art sandwiched between two layers of enhancement products. The finished art is inside the nail. The surface of the nail is smooth, and the nail structure is not compromised by the art inside. It's also fun to add embellishments, such as glitter or confetti to clear UV or LED gel. This technique can be used to create the nail enhancement itself or to apply over a nail enhancement (figure 29-7).

Perform Light Cured Gel Maintenance and Removal

Light cured gel enhancements must be maintained regularly, depending on how fast the client's nails grow. Maintenance service every two weeks is customary for this service.

Gel Maintenance

Begin the maintenance using a medium-grit abrasive file (180-grit) to thin and shape the enhancement. Be careful not to damage the new growth on the natural nail plate with the abrasive when you are preparing the nail for the UV or LED gel maintenance.

Before adding UV or LED gel to the new growth area of the natural nail, be sure to clean the nail with the manufacturer's recommended cleanser or isopropanol (99 percent or better). This removes oils from the fingernail and results in better adhesion of the gel to the nail plate. It is important to remember that you must file with a light touch, because it is usually easier to file light cured gel enhancements than monomer liquid and polymer powder enhancements, as the product is softer and removes easily.

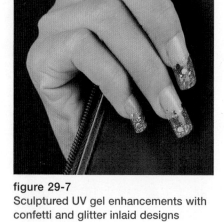

figure 29-7
Sculptured UV gel enhancements with confetti and glitter inlaid designs

Ⓟ 29-4 Light Cured Gel Maintenance *See page 1012*

Light Cured Gel Removal

There are two types of gel, and each employs a different removal method.

- **Hard UV and LED gels**, also known as *traditional gels*, cannot be removed with a solvent, such as acetone. These traditional gels, including colored gels, must be filed off the natural nail to be removed.

- **Soft UV and LED gels**, also known as *soakable gels*, including gel polishes, are removed by soaking in acetone for approximately 5 to 15 minutes or product remover to soften them, allowing the cosmetologist to easily scrape off the loosened gel polish with a wooden stick.

It is important that you read and follow the manufacturer's directions before removing light cured gel nails.

ⓅP 29-6   Light Cured Gel Removal—Hard Gel *See page 1017*

ⓅP 29-7   Light Cured Gel Removal—Soft or Soakable Gel Polishes
See page 1018

✓ HERE'S A TIP

When providing enhancement services, ask whether the client would like enhancements that are removed easily. If the client does, use a soak-off UV or LED gel as the base coat (following the manufacturer's recommendations on that gel product application), and then perform the remainder of the service. Before the client leaves the salon, arrange a date for her to return to have the UV or LED gel removed.

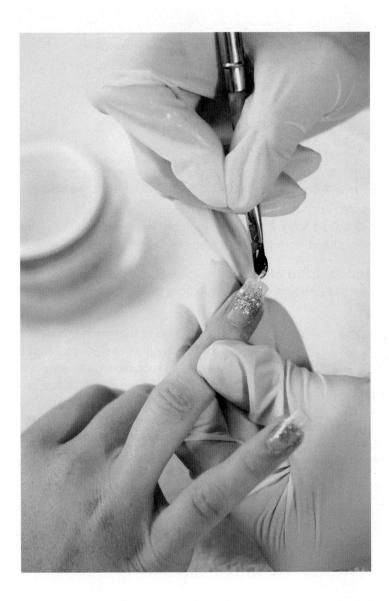

© Andrey_Popov/Shutterstock.com

ONE-COLOR METHOD UV OR LED GEL ON TIPS OR NATURAL NAILS FINISHING WITH UV OR LED GEL POLISH

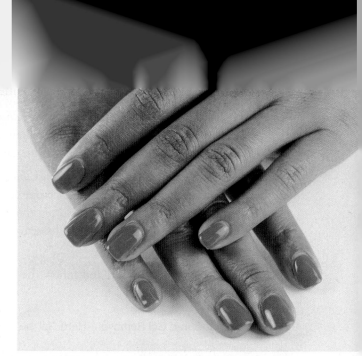

IMPLEMENTS & MATERIALS

In addition to the basic materials on your manicuring table, you will need the following supplies:

- ☐ Cleansing solution
- ☐ Gel brush
- ☑ Lint-free cleansing wipes
- ☐ Nail dehydrator
- ☑ Nail tips and resin
- ☐ Nylon brush (for removing dust)
- ☑ UV or LED gel for the application
- ☐ UV or LED gel lamp
- ☐ UV or LED gel polish
- ☐ UV or LED gel primer or bonding gel

PREPARATION

Perform:

Ⓟ **25-1** Pre-Service Procedure *See page 880*

PROCEDURE

1 Clean the nails with soap and water. Dry the hands thoroughly with a clean disposable towel, and then remove the existing polish. Begin with your client's little finger on the right hand and work toward the thumb. Repeat on the left hand.

2 Apply cuticle remover to the nail plate, if needed. Gently push back the eponychium, and carefully remove cuticle tissue from the nail plate.

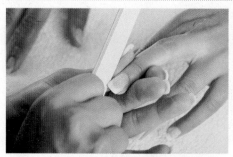

3 Gently file or buff the nail plate with medium/fine abrasive (180- to 240-grit) or the abrasive recommended by the gel manufacturer, to remove the shine on the surface of the nail plate. After filing and/or buffing, remove dust from the nail surface with a clean, dry nylon brush.

4 Use a cleanser and a dehydrator per the manufacturer's recommendation to remove any oils and debris from the fingernail. This increases the adhesive properties of the gel.

5 If your client requires nail tips, apply them according to **Procedure 27-1, Nail Tip Application**, in Chapter 27, Nail Tips and Wraps. Be sure to shorten and shape the tip before the application of the UV or LED gel. During the procedure, the UV gel overlaps the tip's edge to prevent lifting. This seal can be broken during the filing process, allowing the UV gel to peel or lift. Be careful not to break this seal.

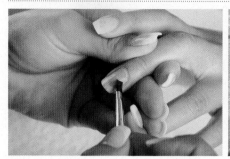
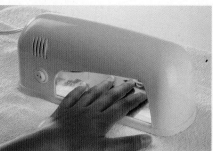
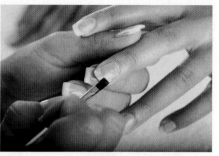

6 If applicable, follow the manufacturer's instructions for applying the bonding gel or primer. Using the applicator brush, insert the brush into the nail primer or bonding gel. Wipe off any excess from the brush, and, using a slightly damp brush, ensure that the nail plate is completely covered per the manufacturer's recommendations. Avoid using too much product to prevent running into the skin.

7 If applicable, cure the bonding gel according to the manufacturer's directions.

8 Gently brush or float the UV or LED gel onto the fingernail surface, including the free edge. Leave a ³⁄₁₆-inch (4.76 mm) gap around the cuticle and sidewall area of the fingernail. Keep the UV or LED gel from touching the cuticle, eponychium, or sidewalls. Apply on four fingers, from pinky to pointer finger.

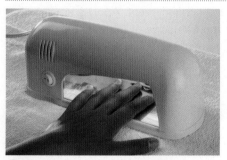

10 Repeat steps 8 and 9 on the left hand, and then repeat the same steps for both thumbs.

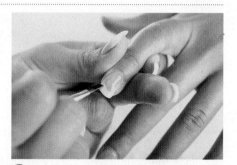

9 Properly position the hand under the UV or LED bulb for the required cure time, as indicated by the manufacturer.

11 Apply a small bead of UV or LED gel to the apex of the nail to create a slight arch. Repeat this application process on the remaining three fingernails.

12 Cure the gel application by properly positioning the hand in the UV or LED lamp for the manufacturer's required cure time.

13 Repeat steps 11 and 12 on the left hand, and then repeat the same steps for both thumbs.

14 Apply a layer of self-leveling gel if needed. This layer is to perfect the shape and add thickness to the enhancement. Cure for the time required by the manufacturer. This step is not necessary when applying to the natural nail.

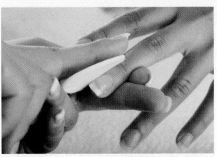

⑮ Remove the inhibition layer by cleaning with the manufacturer's cleanser on a lint-free wipe. Avoid skin contact.

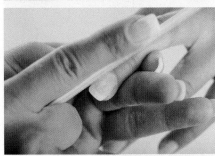

⑯ Using a medium or fine abrasive (180- or 240-grit), refine the surface contour. File carefully near the sidewalls and eponychium to avoid injuring the client's skin. Check the free edge thickness and even out imperfections with gentle strokes.

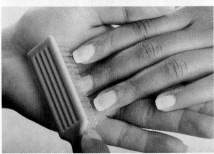

⑰ Remove the dust and filings with a clean and disinfected nylon brush. Cleanse the nails with surface cleanser and a lint-free wipe. Now evaluate the work you just completed and make any necessary adjustments.

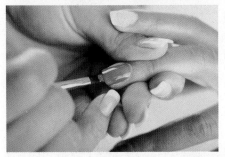

⑱ To add gel polish to the final look, brush the first coat of light cured gel polish thinly over the entire surface of the enhancement. Apply a small amount of the light cured gel polish to the free edge of the fingernail to cap the end and create an even and consistent appearance. Apply to remaining three fingernails.

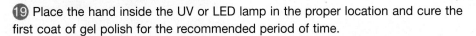

⑲ Place the hand inside the UV or LED lamp in the proper location and cure the first coat of gel polish for the recommended period of time.

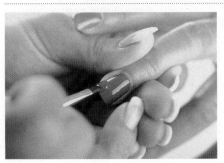

⑳ Repeat steps 18 and 19 on the opposite hand, then repeat the same steps for both thumbs.

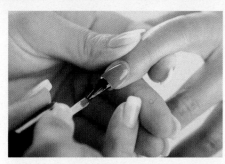

21 Apply UV or LED glossing gel (sealer, gloss, or finisher gel) and cure.

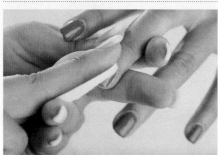

22 Remove the inhibition layer, if required.

23 Apply and rub nail oil into the surrounding skin, massaging briefly to speed up penetration.

24 Ask the client to wash her hands with soap and water at the hand washing station, or ask her to use the nail brush to clean her nails over a finger bowl. Rinse with clean water to remove soap residue. Dry the hands thoroughly with a clean disposable towel.

25 Apply hand cream and massage the hands and arms.

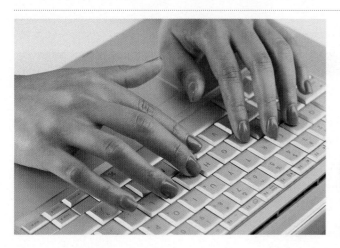

26 Finished look.

POST-SERVICE

Complete:

P 25-2 **Post-Service Procedure** *See page 884*

TWO-COLOR METHOD UV OR LED GEL ON TIPS OR NATURAL NAILS

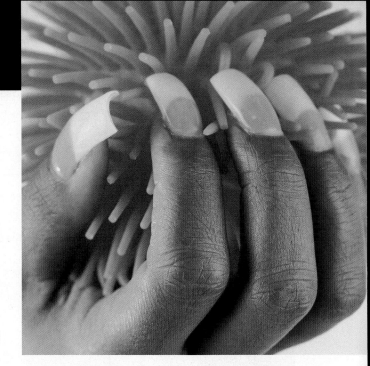

IMPLEMENTS & MATERIALS

In addition to the basic materials on your manicuring table, you will need the following supplies:

□ Cleansing solution

□ Gel brush

□ Lint-free cleansing wipes

□ Nail dehydrator

□ Nail tips

□ Nylon brush

□ Pink UV or LED gel and white UV or LED gel

□ UV or LED gel lamp

□ UV or LED gel primer or bonding gel

PREPARATION

Perform:

P 25-1 **Pre-Service Procedure** *See page 880*

PROCEDURE

1 Clean the nails and remove existing polish.

2 Apply cuticle remover to the nail plate, if needed. Gently push back the eponychium and remove cuticle tissue from the nail plate.

3 Gently file or buff the nails with a medium/fine (180- to 240-grit) buffer or the abrasive recommended by the gel manufacturer, to remove the shine on the surface of the nail plate.

4 Remove the dust from the nail surfaces.

5 Use a cleanser and dehydrator per the manufacturer's recommendation to remove any oils and debris from the fingernail. This increases the adhesive properties of the gel.

6 Apply primer or bonding gel to the natural nail only. Apply nail tips with resin, if desired.

7 Cure bonding gel, if required, following the manufacturer's directions.

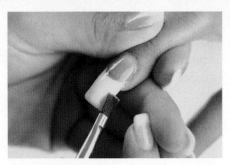

8 Select the desired white gel, and apply it over the tip and along the sidewalls of the fingernail to create the smile line. Be sure to apply this layer of gel thin enough to allow the gel to cure completely through to the surface of the tip. If there is white gel where you do not want it to be, wipe the unwanted gel from the fingernail tip.

9 Using a lint-free nail wipe, pinch the bristles of the brush in the nail wipe to pull off excess gel. Do not use solvents to clean the bristles.

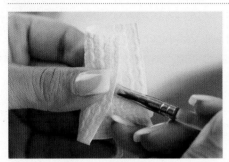

10 Using the tip of your clean gel brush, wipe across the smile line to create a clean, crisp, U-shaped line. Repeat this process until you have the desired smile line. Make certain that all smile lines are uniform from nail to nail before curing the gel.

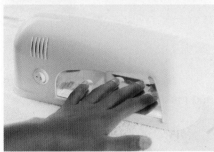

11 Flash cure the white gel one or two fingers at a time in the lamp for the product manufacturer's recommended time. Repeat steps until each finger is cured.

12 If the white gel does not have the same brightness and consistency on all fingers, repeat steps 8-11.

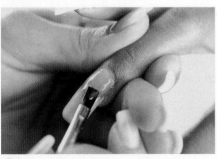

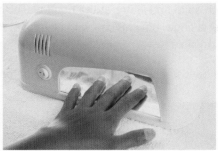

15 Repeat steps 13 and 14 on the left hand, and then repeat the same steps for both thumbs.

13 Gently float a pink-tinted gel onto the fingernail surface, including the free edge. Leave a ³/₁₆-inch (4.76 mm) gap around the cuticle and the sidewall area of the fingernail. Keep the gel from touching the cuticle, eponychium, or sidewalls.

14 After the application of four fingers, cure the pink gel in the UV or LED lamp for the recommended time.

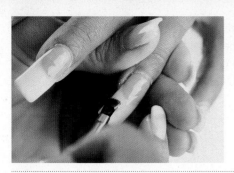

16 Apply a small amount of pink self-leveling gel across the first layer, and float it into place. Float the self-leveling gel over and around the free edge to create a seal. Avoid touching the skin under the free edge to prevent skin irritation and sensitivity. Repeat this application for all four nails.

17 Cure the self-leveling gel.

18 Repeat steps 16 and 17 on the left hand, and then repeat the same steps for both thumbs.

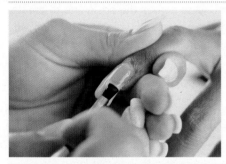

19 Another layer of the UV or LED gel will add thickness to the enhancement if it is desired. Cure the nails.

20 Remove the inhibition layer.

21 Contour the nails with a medium/fine-grit abrasive (180- or 240-grit).

22 Remove the dust with a nylon brush. Evaluate the work you just completed and make any necessary adjustments.

23 Apply the UV or LED gloss gel (sealer, gloss, or finisher gel). Cure the nails.

24 Remove the inhibition layer, if required.

25 Apply and rub nail oil into the surrounding skin, massaging briefly to speed up penetration.

26 Ask the client to wash her hands with soap and water at the hand washing station, or ask her to use the nail brush to clean her nails over a finger bowl. Rinse with clean water to remove soap residue. Dry thoroughly with a clean disposable towel.

27 Apply hand cream and massage the hands and arms. Thoroughly clean each nail of lotion.

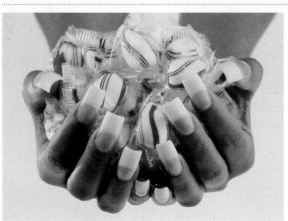

28 Finished look.

POST-SERVICE

Complete:

P 25-2 **Post-Service Procedure** *See page 884*

SCULPTING LIGHT CURED GEL USING FORMS

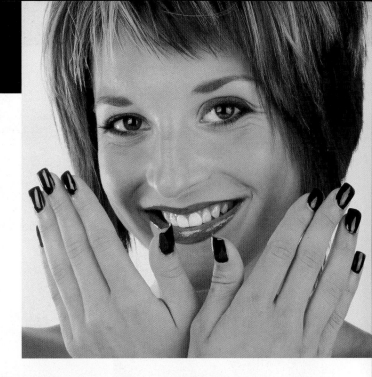

IMPLEMENTS & MATERIALS

In addition to the basic materials on your manicuring table, you will need the following supplies:

- ☐ Cleansing solution
- ☐ Gel brush
- ☐ Lint-free cleansing wipes
- ☐ Nail dehydrator
- ☐ Nail forms
- ☐ UV or LED gel
- ☐ UV or LED gel lamp
- ☐ UV or LED gel primer or bonding gel

PREPARATION

Perform:

P 25-1 **Pre-Service Procedure** *See page 880*

PROCEDURE

1 Clean the nails with soap and water and dry hands thoroughly. Remove the existing polish.

2 Apply cuticle remover to the nail plate if needed. Gently push back the eponychium and remove cuticle from the nail plate. File the free edge of the nails as needed.

3 Gently buff the nails with a medium (180-grit) buffer, or the abrasive recommended by the gel manufacturer, to remove the shine on the surface of the nail plate. Then remove dust using a clean, dry nail brush.

4 Use a cleanser and/or nail dehydrator per the manufacturer's recommendation to remove any oils and debris from the fingernails. This increases the adhesive properties of the gel.

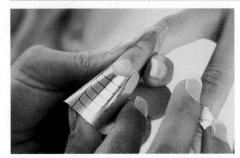

5 Fit forms onto all fingers (as described in Chapter 27, Nail Tips and Wraps).

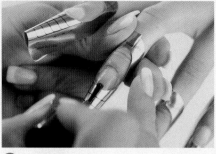

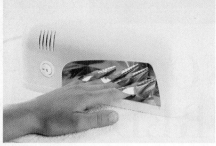

6 Apply the primer or bonding gel.

7 Cure the bonding gel, if required.

8 Repeat steps 6 and 7 on the left hand, and then repeat the same steps for both thumbs.

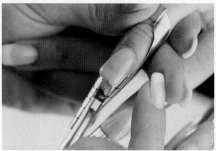

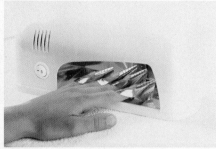

9 Apply the first coat of UV or LED gel (building or self-leveling gel). Consider applying the first coat to one finger at a time to prevent the gel from running.

10 Properly position the hand in the lamp and cure the gel for the required time.

11 Apply a second layer of the UV or LED gel (building or self-leveling gel). Properly position the hand and cure the gel for the required time.

12 If the extension still bends, apply another layer of building or self-leveling UV or LED gel over the entire enhancement and cure. Repeat as needed until the extension doesn't bend.

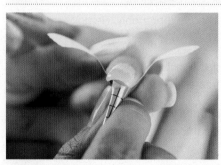

13 Remove the nail forms by pinching the form just before the hyponychium of the finger and then gently pulling the form down and away from the finger.

14 Cure the gel (building or self-leveling gel). Then remove the inhibition layer.

15 Use a medium abrasive (180-grit) to file and shape the free edge of the enhancement.

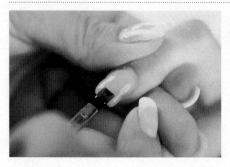

16 Apply another layer of UV or LED gel (building or self-leveling gel), if needed, over the entire enhancement.

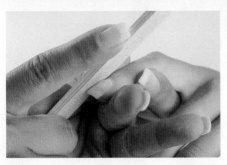

17 File the nails by using a medium/fine abrasive (180- to 240-grit), and refine the surface contour. Be certain to file the enhancement to create an arch and curve in order to optimize the strength of the overlay and create an elegant beauty to the enhancement.

18 Remove the dust. Evaluate your work, and make any necessary adjustments. If finishing with gel polish, do so now, according to Procedure 29-1, steps 18-20, on page 1004. Otherwise, proceed to step 19.

19 Apply the gloss UV or LED gel (sealer, gloss, or finisher).

20 Cure the nail gel.

21 Remove the inhibition layer, if required, with cleanser and a lint-free wipe.

22 Apply and rub nail oil into the surrounding skin and nail enhancement, massaging briefly to speed up penetration.

23 Ask the client to wash her hands with soap and water at the hand washing station, or ask her to use the nail brush to clean her nails over a finger bowl. Rinse with clean water to remove soap residue. Dry thoroughly with a clean, disposable towel.

24 Apply hand cream and massage the hands and arms. Thoroughly clean each nail of lotion.

25 Apply nail polish, if desired.

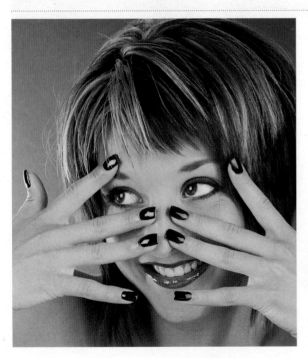

26 Finished look.

POST-SERVICE

Complete:

P 25-2 **Post-Service Procedure** *See page 884*

LIGHT CURED GEL MAINTENANCE

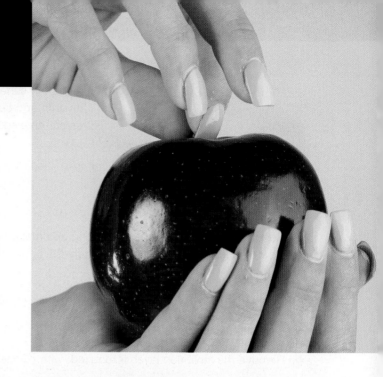

IMPLEMENTS & MATERIALS

In addition to the basic materials on your manicuring table, you will need the following supplies:

- ☐ Cleansing solution
- ☐ Gel brush
- ☐ Lint-free cleansing wipes
- ☐ Nail dehydrator
- ☐ UV or LED gel
- ☐ UV or LED gel lamp
- ☐ UV or LED gel primer or bonding gel

PREPARATION

Perform:

P 25-1 **Pre-Service Procedure** *See page 880*

PROCEDURE

1 Clean the nails with soap and water, and dry the hands thoroughly. Remove the existing polish.

2 Apply cuticle remover to the nail plate if needed. Gently push back the eponychium and remove cuticle from the nail plate.

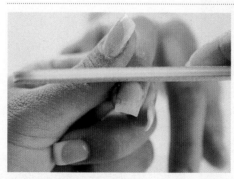

3 File (gently) the nail plate with medium/fine abrasive (180- to 240-grit) to reduce and shape the nail surface.

4 Lightly buff the natural nail regrowth with a medium (180-grit) buffer or the abrasive recommended by the gel manufacturer to remove the shine on the surface of the natural nail plate.

5 Remove dust from the nail surfaces.

6 Use a cleanser and/or dehydrator per the manufacturer's recommendation to remove any oils and debris from the fingernail. This increases the adhesive properties of the gel.

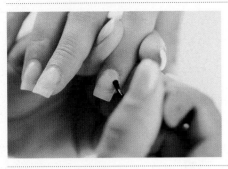

7 Apply primer or bonding gel to the natural nail according to the manufacturer's directions.

8 Cure the bonding gel if required.

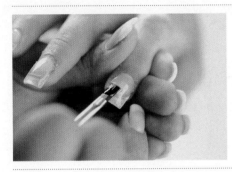

9 Lightly brush the UV or LED gel onto the nail from the natural nail regrowth to the free edge. Keep the gel from touching the cuticle, eponychium, or sidewalls. Apply the gel to the client's right hand, from little finger to pointer finger.

10 Cure the gel on the right hand for the manufacturer's recommended time.

11 Repeat steps 9 and 10 on the left hand. Then repeat the same steps for both thumbs.

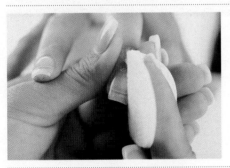

12 Remove the inhibition layer from all nails with cleanser on a lint-free wipe.

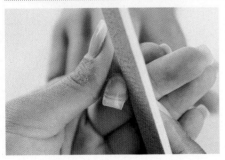

13 File and buff using a medium or fine abrasive (180- to 240-grit). Refine the surface contour. Evaluate the work you just completed, and make any necessary adjustments.

🔢 Remove the dust, and then clean the fingernails. If finishing with gel polish, do so now, according to Procedure 29-1, steps 18-20, on page 1004. Otherwise, proceed to step 15.

⑮ Apply the UV or LED gloss gel (sealer, gloss, or finisher gel).

⑯ Cure the gloss gel.

⑰ Remove the inhibition layer, if required.

⑱ Apply and rub nail oil into the surrounding skin and nail enhancement, massaging briefly to speed up penetration.

⑲ Ask the client to wash her hands with soap and water at the hand washing station or ask her to use the nail brush to clean her nails over a finger bowl. Rinse with clean water to remove soap residue. Dry thoroughly with a clean disposable towel.

⑳ Apply hand cream and massage the hands and arms. Thoroughly clean each nail of lotion.

㉑ Apply nail polish, if desired.

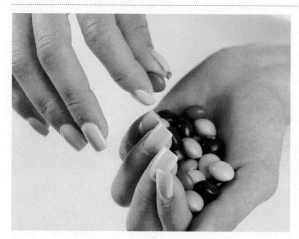

㉒ Finished look.

POST-SERVICE

Complete:

Ⓟ 25-2 **Post-Service Procedure** *See page 884*

MONOMER LIQUID AND POLYMER POWDER NAIL ENHANCEMENTS FINISHED WITH UV OR LED GEL POLISH

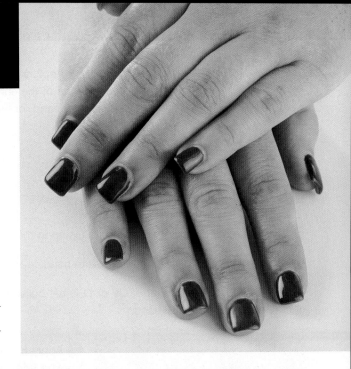

IMPLEMENTS & MATERIALS

In addition to the basic materials on your manicuring table, you will need the following supplies:

- □ Cleansing solution
- □ Gel brush
- □ Lint-free cleansing wipes
- □ Nylon brush
- □ UV or LED gel lamp
- □ UV or LED gel polish
- □ UV or LED gel sealer or top coat

PREPARATION | PROCEDURE

Perform:

P 25-1 **Pre-Service Procedure** *See page 880*

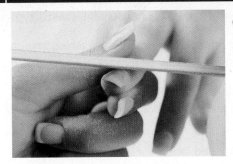

1. Perform monomer liquid and polymer powder application described in Chapter 28, Monomer Liquid and Polymer Powder Nail Enhancements. Once the monomer liquid and polymer powder enhancements have been filed and contoured to the correct shape and length, they will be ready for the gel polish application. Note: Do not buff the nails smooth or use any oils during the filing process as this can prevent adhesion.

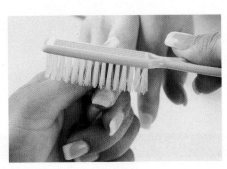

2. Remove the dust and filings with a clean and disinfected nylon brush. Remove any oils that may have been deposited on the fingernails during filing.

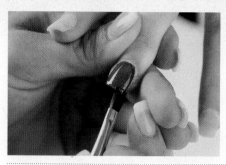

3 Apply a very thin coat of UV or LED gel polish over the entire surface and edge of the enhancement in a brushing technique. Apply to all five nails on one hand, or as recommended by the manufacturer.

4 Place the hand inside the UV or LED lamp in the proper location and cure for the recommended period of time.

5 Repeat steps 3 and 4 on the opposite hand.

6 Apply a second thin coat of UV or LED gel polish over the entire surface of the enhancement on one hand and cure. Repeat on opposite hand.

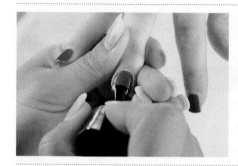

7 Apply the gel polish top gel, sealer, finish, or gloss gel on one hand. Starting from the base of the nail plate, stroke toward the free edge, using polish-style strokes and covering the entire nail surface and edge. Avoid touching the client's skin, as this will cause lifting.

8 Cure the gloss gel.

9 Remove the inhibition layer, if required.

10 Apply and rub nail oil into the surrounding skin and nail enhancement, massaging briefly to speed up penetration.

11 Ask the client to wash her hands with soap and water at the hand washing station, or ask her to use a nail brush to clean her nails over a finger bowl. Rinse with clean water to remove soap residue that may cause lifting. Dry thoroughly with a clean disposable towel.

12 Apply hand cream and massage the hands and arms. Thoroughly clean each nail of lotion.

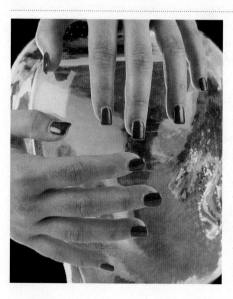

13 Finished look.

POST-SERVICE

Complete:

P 25-2 Post-Service Procedure See page 884

LIGHT CURED GEL REMOVAL—HARD GEL

In addition to the basic materials on your manicuring table, you will need the following supplies:

☐ Abrasives   ☐ Nail buffer   ☐ Nail oil

PREPARATION   PROCEDURE

Perform:

P 25-1 **Pre-Service Procedure** *See page 880*

1. Clean hands and remove polish if applicable.

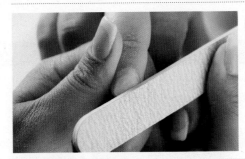

2. Use a medium-grit abrasive (150- to 180-grit) to reduce the thickness of the enhancement on the fingernail. Take care not to file into the natural nail.

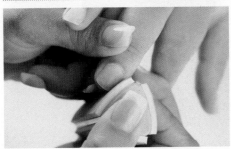

3. Use a fine grit nail buffer (240-grit or higher) to smooth the enhancement. Talk with the client about how to allow the rest of the enhancements to grow out and off of the fingernails. Evaluate the work you just completed, and make any necessary adjustments.

4. While massaging nail oil into the nail and surrounding skin, suggest that your client have natural nail manicures to ensure that the enhancements grow off correctly. Have your client wash her hands and dry thoroughly. Perform an arm and hand massage before completing the service.

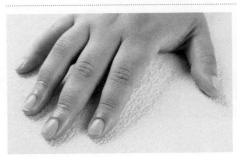

5. Finished look.

POST-SERVICE

Complete:

P 25-2 **Post-Service Procedure** *See page 884*

LIGHT CURED GEL REMOVAL—SOFT OR SOAKABLE GEL POLISHES

IMPLEMENTS & MATERIALS

In addition to the basic materials on your manicuring table, you will need the following supplies:

- ☐ Abrasives
- ☐ Buffer

- ☐ Gel product remover (as recommended by the gel manufacturer)

- ☐ Nail oil
- ☐ Wooden pusher
- ☐ Metal or glass bowl

PREPARATION

Perform:

P 25-1 **Pre-Service Procedure** *See page 880*

PROCEDURE

① Clean hands and remove polish if applicable. Gently file the surface of the gel enhancement or gel polish with a 180-grit file.

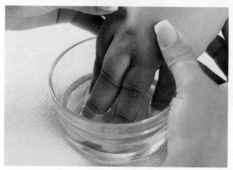

② Pour the soak-off solution into a finger bowl or other glass or metal container so that the level of the remover is sufficient to completely immerse the fingernails in the solution.

③ Soak the client's fingernails in the solution for the manufacturer's recommended period of time.

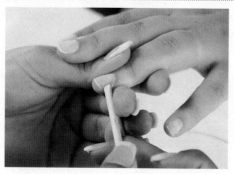

④ Use a wooden stick to ease the gel off the fingernail.

⑤ Lightly buff the fingernail with a fine-grit buffer (240-grit or higher) to remove any remaining gel material from the fingernail area.

⑥ While massaging nail oil into the nail and surrounding skin, evaluate the work you just completed, and make any necessary adjustments. Have your client wash her hands and dry thoroughly. Perform an arm and hand massage before completing the service.

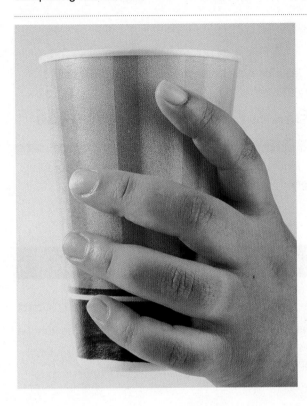

⑦ Finished look.

POST-SERVICE

Complete:

Ⓟ 25-2 **Post-Service Procedure** *See page 884*

REVIEW QUESTIONS

1. Describe the chemistry and main ingredients of light cured gels.

2. When would you use a one-color method of applying light cured gels? When would you use a two-color method for applying light cured gels?

3. What are the different types of light cured gels found in current systems?

4. What supplies are needed for light cured gel application?

5. When should you use light cured gels?

6. When should you use a building gel, a self-leveling gel, or a light cured gel that uses fiberglass?

7. What are the differences between light cured lamps and light cured bulbs?

8. List the steps to use when applying one-color, light cured gel on tips or natural nails.

9. Describe how light cured gels are applied over forms.

10. Describe how to maintain light cured gel nail enhancements.

11. Explain how to correctly remove hard light cured gels.

12. Identify how to correctly remove soft light cured gels.

STUDY TOOLS

- **Reinforce what you just learned:** Complete the activities and exercises in your Theory or Practical Workbook, or your Study Guide.

- **Expand your knowledge:** Search for websites about the topics in this chapter and make a list of additional resources.

- **Study and prepare for your quiz:** Take the chapter test in your Exam Review or your Milady U: Online Licensing Prep.

- **Re-Test your knowledge:** Take the Chapter 29 *Quizzes*!

- **Learn even more:** Look up in a dictionary or search the internet for the definitions of any additional terms you want to learn about.

CHAPTER GLOSSARY

bonding gels	p. 991	Gels used to increase adhesion to the natural nail plate.
building gels	p. 991	Any thick-viscosity adhesive resin that is used to build an arch and curve to the fingernail.
cure	p. 990	To harden.
gel polish	p. 992	A very thin-viscosity, light cured gel that is usually pigmented and packaged in a pot or a polish bottle and used as an alternative to traditional nail lacquers.
glossing gel	p. 992	Also known as *sealing gel*, *finishing gel*, or *shine gel*; these gels are used over the finished light cured gel application to create a high shine.

hard UV and LED gels	p. 1001	Also known as *traditional UV and LED gels*; gels that cannot be removed with a solvent and must be filed off the natural nail.
inhibition layer	p. 992	The tacky surface left on the nail after a light cured gel has cured.
lamp wattage	p. 997	The measure of how much electricity the bulb consumes.
LED	p. 997	Light emitting diode.
LED lamp	p. 997	The electronic device that houses the LED bulbs.
light cured gel	p. 988	Also known as *UV and LED gel*; type of nail enhancement product that hardens when exposed to a UV and LED light.
oligomer uh-LIG-uh-mer	p. 988	Short chain of monomer liquids that is often thick, sticky, and gel-like and that is not long enough to be considered a polymer.
one-color method	p. 990	When one color of gel, usually clear, is applied over the entire surface of the nail.
opacity oh-PAY-sit-ee	p. 993	The amount of colored pigment concentration in a gel, making it more or less difficult to see through.
photoinitiator FOH-toh-in-ish-ee-AY-tohr	p. 989	A chemical that initiates the polymerization reaction.
pigmented gels	p. 991	Any building or self-leveling gel that includes color pigment.
self-leveling gels	p. 991	Gels that are thinner in consistency than building gels, allowing them to settle and level during application.
soft UV and LED gels	p. 1001	Also known as *soakable gels*; these gels are removed by soaking in acetone.
two-color method	p. 990	A method whereby two colors of resin are used to overlay the nail.
urethane acrylate	p. 989	A main ingredient used to create light cured gel nail enhancements.
urethane methacrylate	p. 989	A main ingredient used alone or in combination with urethane acrylates to create light cured gel nail enhancements.
UV bulb	p. 997	Also known as *UV light bulb*; special bulb that emits UV and LED light to cure UV and LED gel nail enhancements.
UV lamp	p. 997	Also known as *UV light unit*; specialized electronic device that powers and controls UV and LED bulbs to cure UV and LED gel nail enhancements.
viscosity vis-KAHS-ut-tee	p. 990	The measurement of the thickness or thinness of a liquid and how the fluid flows.

PART 6 BUSINESS

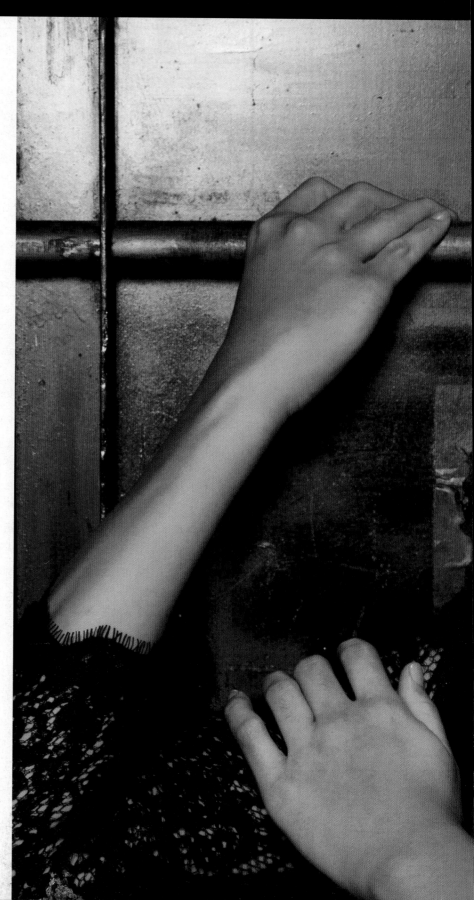

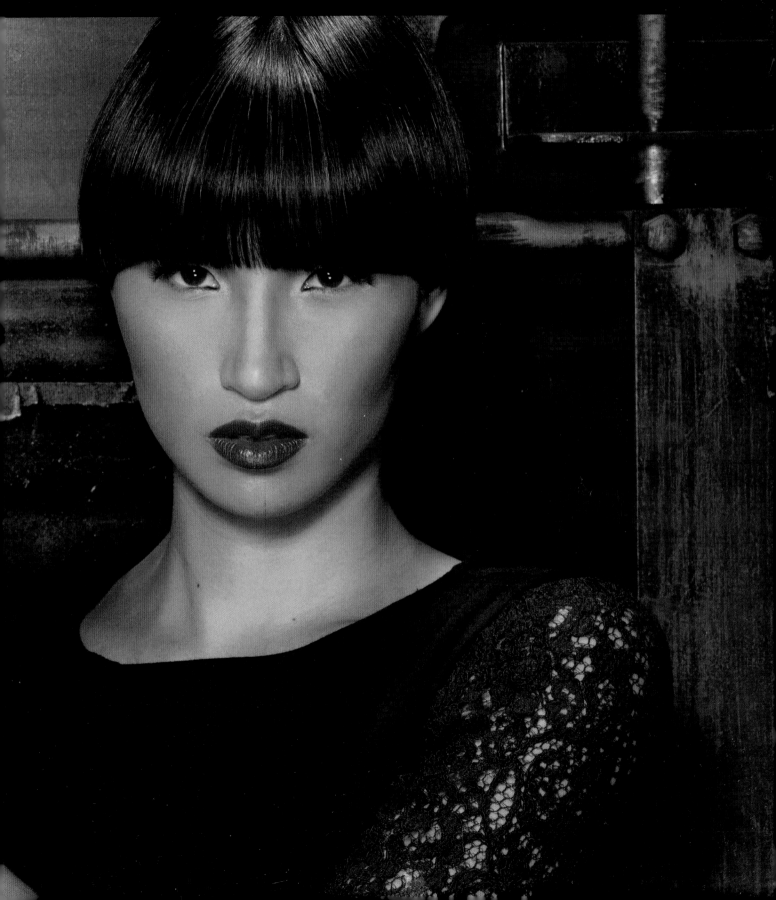

SKILLS

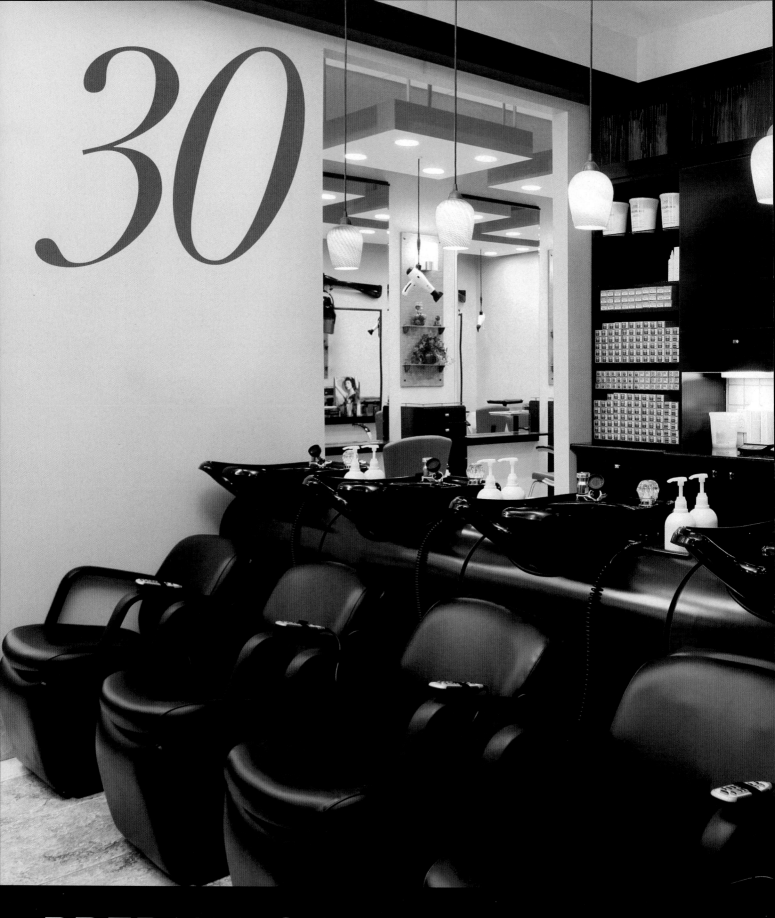

30

PREPARING FOR LICENSURE AND EMPLOYMENT

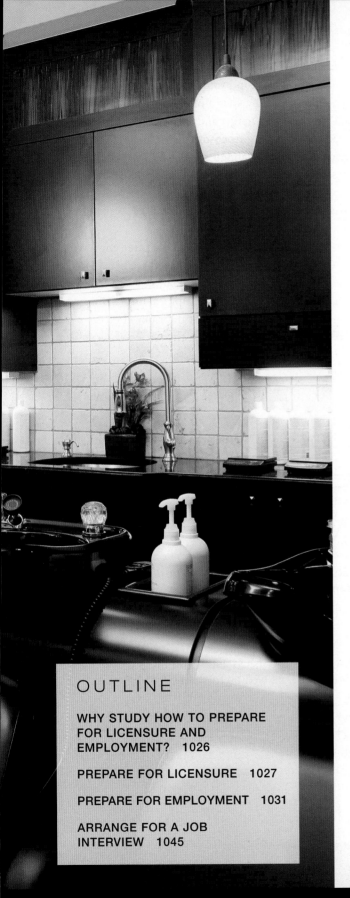

LEARNING OBJECTIVES

After completing this chapter, you will be able to:

LO❶
Describe the process of taking and passing your state licensing examination.

LO❷
Determine your career focus by using the Inventory of Personal Characteristics and Technical Skills.

LO❸
List the different salon business categories.

LO❹
Develop a cover letter, resume, and employment portfolio.

LO❺
Know how to explore the job market, research potential employers, and operate within the legal aspects of employment.

OUTLINE

There are plenty of great jobs out there for energetic, hardworking, talented people. If you look at the top professionals in the cosmetology field, you will find they were not born successful; they achieved success through self-motivation, energy, and persistence. Like you, these stylists began their careers by enrolling in cosmetology school. They were the ones who used their time wisely, planned for the future, went the extra mile, and drew on a reservoir of self-confidence to meet challenges. They owe their success to no one but themselves, because they created it. If you want to enjoy similar success, you must prepare for the opportunities that await you.

No matter what changes occur in the economy, there are often more jobs available for entry-level cosmetology professionals than there are people to fill them. This is a tremendous advantage for you, but you still must thoroughly research the job market in your geographical area before committing to your first job (**figure 30-1**). If you make the right choice, your career will be on the road to success. If you make the wrong choice, it will not be a tragedy, but it may cause unnecessary delay.

why study
HOW TO PREPARE FOR LICENSURE AND EMPLOYMENT?

Cosmetologists should study and have a thorough understanding of how to prepare for licensure and employment because:

> You must pass your State Board Exam to be licensed, and you must be licensed to be hired; therefore, preparing for licensure and passing your exam is your first step to employment success.

> A successful employment search is a job in itself, and there are many tools that can give you the edge—as well as mistakes that can cost you an interview or a job.

> The ability to pinpoint the right salon for you and target it as a potential employer is vital for your career success.

> Proactively preparing the right materials, such as a great resume, and practicing interviewing will give you the confidence that's needed to secure a job in a salon you love.

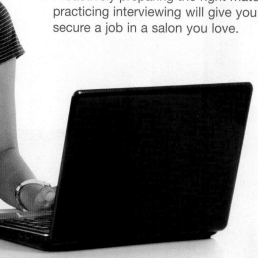

figure 30-1
Job listings are posted online at various job boards.

After reading the next few sections, you will be able to:

LO ❶ Describe the process of taking and passing your state licensing examination.

Prepare for Licensure

Before you can obtain the career position you are hoping for, you must pass your state licensing examinations (usually a written and a practical exam) and secure the required credentials from your state's licensing board by filling out an application and paying a fee. For details on fees, testing dates, requirements, and more, visit the website of your State Board of Cosmetology or your state's department of licensing.

Many factors will affect how well you perform during that licensing examination and on tests in general. They include your physical and psychological state; your memory; your time management skills; and your academic skills, such as reading, writing, note taking, test taking, and general learning.

Of all the factors that will affect your test performance, the most important is your mastery of course content. However, even if you feel that you have truly learned the material, it is still very beneficial to have strong test-taking skills. Being **test-wise** means understanding the strategies for successfully taking tests.

Preparing for the Written Exam

A test-wise student begins to prepare for a test by practicing good study habits and time management. These habits include the following:

- Have a planned, realistic study schedule.
- Read content carefully and become an active studier.
- Keep well-organized notes.
- Develop a detailed vocabulary list.
- Take effective notes during class.
- Organize and review handouts.
- Review past quizzes and tests.
- Listen carefully in class for cues and clues about what could be expected on the test.

More holistic or "whole you" hints to keep in mind include the following:

- Make yourself mentally ready and develop a positive attitude toward taking the test.
- Get plenty of rest the night before the test.
- Dress comfortably and professionally.

DID YOU KNOW?

If you have a physician-documented disability, such as a learning disability, your state may allow you extra time to take the written exam or even provide a special examiner. Ask your instructor and check with your state licensing board. Be certain to make any special arrangements well in advance of the test date.

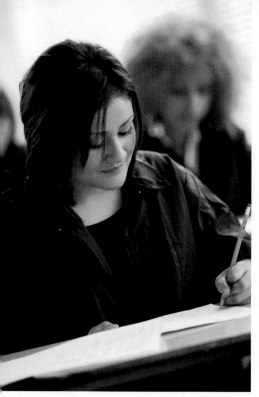

figure 30-2
Candidates taking an in-house school exam

- Anticipate some anxiety (feeling concerned about the test results may actually help you do better).

- Avoid cramming the night before an examination.

- Find out if your state uses computers for the written portion of the test. If so, make certain you are comfortable with computerized test taking.

On Test Day

After you have taken all the necessary steps to prepare for your test, there are a number of strategies you can adopt on the day of the exam that may be helpful (figure 30-2):

- Relax and try to slow down physically.

- Review the material lightly the day of the exam.

- If possible, do a "test drive" to the site before test day if you are unsure of the location. Some exams may be administered at your school and some may be given in alternate locations.

- Arrive early with a self-confident attitude; be alert, calm, and ready for the challenge.

- Read all written directions and listen carefully to all verbal directions before beginning.

- If there are things you do not understand, do not hesitate to ask the examiner questions.

- If possible, skim the entire test before beginning.

- Budget your time to ensure that you have plenty of opportunity to complete the test; do not spend too much time on any one question.

- Wear a watch so that you can monitor the time.

- Begin work as soon as possible, and mark the answers in the test carefully but quickly.

- Answer the easiest questions first in order to save time for the more difficult ones. Quickly scanning all the questions first may clue you in to the more difficult questions.

- Make a note of the questions you skip so that you can find them again later. If the test is administered online you may not be given this option. Some software prevents you from moving forward without answering all questions on the page first. Discuss this with your instructor or the testing facility before taking the exam.

- Read each question carefully to make sure that you know exactly what the question is asking and that you understand all parts of the question.

- Answer as many questions as possible. For questions that cause uncertainty, guess or estimate.

- Look over the test when you are done to ensure that you have read all questions correctly and that you have answered as many as possible.

- Make changes to answers only if there is a good reason to do so.
- Check the test carefully before turning it in. (For instance, you might have forgotten to put your name on it!)

Deductive Reasoning

Deductive reasoning is the process of reaching logical conclusions by employing logical reasoning. Deductive reasoning is a technique that students should learn to use for better test results.

Some strategies associated with deductive reasoning include the following:

- Eliminate options known to be incorrect. The more incorrect answers you can eliminate, the better your chances of identifying the correct answer.

- Watch for key words or terms. Look for any qualifying conditions or statements. Keep an eye out for phrases and words such as *usually, commonly, in most instances, never,* and *always.*

- Study the **stem**, which is the basic question or problem. It will often provide a clue to the correct answer. Look for a match between the stem and one of the choices.

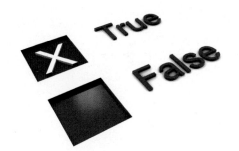

- Watch for grammatical clues. For instance, if the last word in a stem is *an,* the answer must begin with a vowel rather than a consonant.

- Look at similar or related questions. They may provide clues.

- When answering essay questions, watch for words such as *compare, contrast, discuss, evaluate, analyze, define,* or *describe,* and develop your answer accordingly.

- When questions include paragraphs to read and questions to answer, read the questions first. This will help you identify the important information as you read the paragraph.

Understanding Test Formats

There are a few additional tips that all test-wise learners should know, especially with respect to the state licensing examination. Keep in mind, of course, that the most important strategy of test taking is to know your material. Beyond that, consider the following tips on the various types of question formats.

True/False

- Watch for qualifying words (*all, most, some, none, always, usually, sometimes, never, little, no, equal, less, good, bad*). Absolutes (*all, none, always, never*) are generally not true.

- For a statement to be true, the *entire* statement must be true.

- Long statements are more likely to be true than short statements. It takes more detail to provide truthful, factual information.

Multiple Choice

- Read the entire question carefully, including all the choices.

- Look for the best answer; more than one choice may be true.

- Eliminate incorrect answers by crossing them out (if taking the test on the test form).

- When two choices are close or similar, one of them is probably right.

- When two choices are identical, both must be wrong.

- When two choices are opposites, one is probably wrong and one is probably correct, depending on the number of other choices.

- "All of the above" and similar responses are often the correct choice.

- Pay special attention to words such as *not*, *except*, and *but*.

- Guess if you do not know the answer (provided that there is no penalty).

- The answer to one question may be in the stem of another.

Matching

- Read all items in each list before beginning.

- Check off items from the brief response list to eliminate choices.

Essays

- Organize your answer according to the cue words in the question.

- Think carefully and outline your answer before you begin writing.

- Make sure that what you write is complete, accurate, relevant to the question, well organized, and clear.

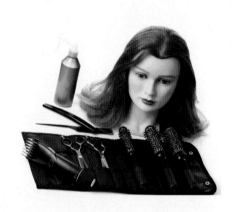

Remember that even though you may understand test formats and effective test-taking strategies, this does not take the place of having a complete understanding of the material on which you are being tested. In order to be successful at taking tests, you must follow the rules of effective studying and be thoroughly knowledgeable of the exam content for both the written and the practical examination.

The Practical Exam

In order to be better prepared for the practical portion of the examination, the new graduate should follow these tips:

- Practice the correct skills required in the test as often as you can.

- Participate in mock licensing examinations, including the timing of applicable examination criteria.

- Familiarize yourself with the content contained in the examination bulletins sent by the licensing agency.

- Make a list of equipment and implements you are expected to bring to the examination.

- Make certain that all equipment and implements are clean and in good working order prior to the exam.

- If allowed by the regulatory or licensing agency, observe other practical examinations prior to taking yours.

- If possible, locate the examination site the day before the exam to ensure that you do not get lost on test day. You can also time your drive the day before, just to make sure you are on time for the actual exam.

- As with any exam, listen carefully to the examiner's instructions, and follow them explicitly.

- Focus on your own knowledge and do not allow yourself to be concerned with what other test candidates are doing.

- Follow all infection control and safety procedures throughout the entire examination.

- Look the part. Every little bit helps; make certain your appearance is neat, clean, and professional.

After reading the next few sections, you will be able to:

LO❷ Determine your career focus by using the Inventory of Personal Characteristics and Technical Skills.

LO❸ List the different salon business categories.

LO❹ Develop a cover letter, resume, and employment portfolio.

Prepare for Employment

When you chose to enter the field of cosmetology, your primary goal was to find a good job after being licensed. Now you need to reaffirm that goal by reviewing a number of important questions.

- What do you really want out of a career in cosmetology?

- What particular areas within the beauty industry are the most interesting to you?

- What are your strongest practical skills? In what ways do you wish to use these skills?

- What personal qualities will help you have a successful career?

One way that you can answer these questions is to copy and complete the Inventory of Personal Characteristics and Technical Skills (**figure 30-3**) on the next page. After you have completed this inventory and identified the areas that need further attention, you can determine where to focus the remainder of your training. In addition, you should have a better idea of what type of establishment would best suit you for your eventual employment.

During your training, you may have the opportunity to network with various industry professionals who are invited to the school as guest speakers. Be prepared to ask them questions about what they like least and

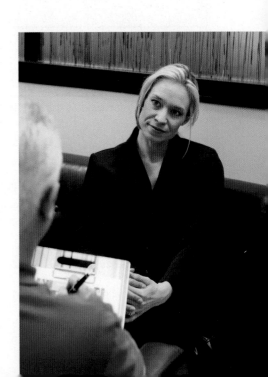

INVENTORY OF PERSONAL CHARACTERISTICS

PERSONAL CHARACTERISTIC	Exc.	Good	Avg.	Poor	Plan for improvement
Posture, Deportment, Poise					
Grooming, Personal hygiene					
Manners, Courtesy					
Communication skills					
Attitude					
Self-motivation					
Personal habits					
Responsibility					
Self-esteem, Self-confidence					
Honesty, Integrity					
Dependability					

INVENTORY OF TECHNICAL SKILLS

TECHNICAL SKILL	Exc.	Good	Avg.	Poor	Plan for improvement
Hair shaping/cutting					
Hairstyling					
Haircoloring					
Texture services, Perming					
Texture services, Relaxing					
Manicuring, Pedicuring					
Artificial nail extensions					
Skin care, Facials					
Facial makeup					
Other					

After analyzing the above responses, would you hire yourself as an employee in your business? Why or why not?

State the short-term goals that you hope to accomplish in 6 to 12 months:

State the long-term goals that you hope to accomplish in 1 to 5 years:

Ask yourself: Do you want to work in a big city or small town? Are you compatible with a sophisticated, exclusive salon or a trendy salon? Which clientele are you able to communicate with more effectively? Do you want to start out slowly and carefully, or do you want to jump in and throw everything into your career from the starting gate? Will you be in this industry throughout your working career, or is this just a stopover? Will you only work a 30- or 40-hour week, or will you go the extra mile when opportunities are available? How ambitious are you, and how many risks are you willing to take?

figure 30-3
Inventory of personal characteristics and technical skills

most in their current positions. Ask them for any tips they might have that will assist you in your search for the right salon. In addition, be sure to take advantage of your institution's in-house placement assistance program if available when you begin your employment search (figure 30-4).

Your willingness to work hard is a key ingredient to your success. The commitment you make now in terms of time and effort will pay off later in the workplace, where your energy will be appreciated and rewarded. Having enthusiasm for getting the job done can be contagious, and when everyone works hard, everyone benefits. You can begin to develop this enthusiasm by establishing good work habits as a student.

How to Get the Job You Want

There are several key personal characteristics that will not only help you get the position you want, but will also help you keep it. These characteristics include the points listed below:

- **Motivation.** This means having the drive to take the necessary action to achieve a goal. Although motivation can come from external sources—parental or peer pressure, for instance—the best kind of motivation is internal.

- **Integrity.** When you have integrity, you are committed to a strong code of moral and artistic values. Integrity is the compass that keeps you on course over the long haul of your career.

- **Good technical and communication skills.** While you may be better in either technical skills or communication skills, you must develop both to reach the level of success you desire.

- **Strong work ethic.** In the beauty business, having a strong **work ethic** means taking pride in your work and committing yourself to consistently doing a good job for your clients, employer, and salon team.

- **Enthusiasm.** Try never to lose your eagerness to learn, grow, and expand your skills and knowledge.

A Salon Survey

According to the U.S. Census Bureau's most recently compiled data as of this printing, there are more than 1.1 million professional salon and spa establishments in the United States alone[i]. These salons employed more than 758,000 active cosmetology professionals[ii]. This year, like every year, thousands of cosmetology school graduates will find their first position in one of the eight basic types of salons described below. As you research salons, focus on the type of salon that you believe will be the best fit for you.

Small Independent Salons

Owned by an individual or two or more partners, this kind of operation makes up the majority of professional salons (figure 30-5). The typical independent salon has five styling stations, but many salons have up to 40. Usually, the owners are hairstylists who maintain their own clientele while

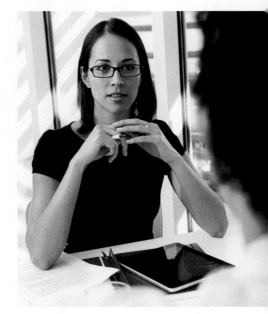

figure 30-4
Your school advisor can help you find employment.

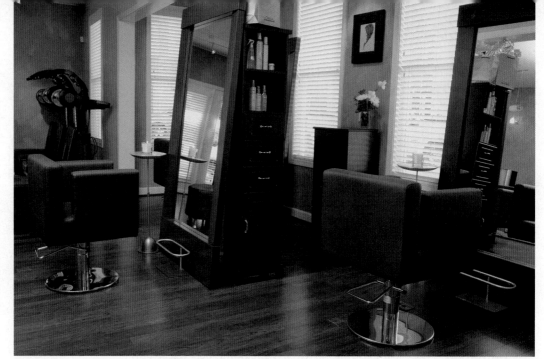

figure 30-5
Perfect 5th in Mooresville, NC is an independent salon.

managing the business. There are nearly as many types of independent salons as there are owners. Their image, decor, services, prices, and clientele all reflect the owner's experience and taste. Depending on the owner's willingness to help a newcomer learn and grow, a beginning stylist can learn a great deal in an independent salon while also earning a good living.

Independent Salon Chains

These are usually chains of five or more salons that are owned by one individual or two or more partners. Independent salon chains range from basic hair salons to full-service salons and day spas. These salons offer everything from low-priced to very high-priced services.

In large high-end salons, stylists can advance to specialized positions in color, nail care, skin care, or other chemical services. Some larger salons also employ education directors and style directors, and stylists are often hired to manage particular locations.

Large National Salon Chains

These companies operate salons throughout the country, and even internationally. They can be budget-priced or value-priced, haircut-only or full service, mid-priced or high-end. Some salon chains operate within department store chains. Management and marketing professionals at the corporate headquarters make all the decisions for each salon, such as size, decor, hours, services, prices, advertising, and profit targets. Many newly licensed cosmetology professionals seek their first jobs in national chain salons because of the secure pay and benefits, additional paid training, management opportunities, and corporate advertising. Also, because the chains are large and widespread, employees have the added advantage of being able to transfer from one location to another.

Franchise Salons

Another chain salon organization, the franchise salon has a national name and a consistent image and business formula that is used at every location. Franchises are owned by individuals who pay a fee to use the name; these individuals then receive a business plan and can take advantage of national marketing campaigns. Decisions such as size, location, decor, and prices are determined in advance by the parent company. Franchises are generally not owned by cosmetologists, but by investors who seek a return on their investment.

Franchise salons commonly offer employees the same benefits as corporate-owned chain salons, including on-the-job training, health-care benefits and advancement opportunities.

Basic Value-Priced Operations

Often located in busy, low-rent shopping center strips that are anchored by a nearby supermarket or other large business, value-priced outlets depend on a high volume of walk-in traffic. They hire recent cosmetology graduates and generally pay them by the hour, sometimes adding commission-style bonuses if an individual stylist's sales pass a certain level. Haircuts are usually reasonably priced and stylists are trained to work fast with no frills.

Mid-Priced Full-Service Salons

These salons offer a complete menu of hair, nail, and skin services along with retail products. Successful mid-priced salons promote their most profitable services and typically offer service and retail packages to entice haircut-only clients. They also run strong marketing programs to encourage client returns and referrals. These salons train their professional styling team to be as productive and profitable as possible. If you are inclined to give more time to each client during the consultation, you may like working in a full-service salon. Here you will have the opportunity to build a relationship with clients that may last over time.

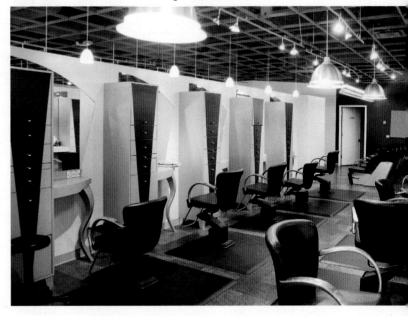

figure 30-6
A high-end salon

High-End Image Salons or Day Spas

This type of business employs well-trained stylists and salon assistants who offer higher-priced services to clients. They also offer luxurious extras such as five-minute head, neck, and shoulder massages as part of the shampoo and luxurious spa manicures and pedicures. Most high-end salons are located in trendy, upscale sections of large cities; others may be located in elegant mansions, high-rent office and retail towers, or luxury hotels and resorts. Clients expect a high level of personal service, and such salons hire professionals whose technical expertise, personal appearance, and communication skills meet their high standards. Medical spas, often owned by physicians, are offshoots of day spas (figure 30-6).

© Paul Matthew Photography/Shutterstock.com

Booth Rental Establishments

Booth renting (also called chair rental) is possibly the least expensive way of owning your own business, but this type of business is regulated by complex laws. For a detailed discussion of booth rental see Chapter 32, The Salon Business.

Resume Development

A **resume** is a written summary of a person's education and work experience. It tells potential employers at a glance what your achievements and accomplishments are. If you are a new graduate, you may have little or no work experience, in which case, your resume should focus on skills and accomplishments. Here are some basic guidelines to follow when preparing your professional resume.

- Keep it simple, limit it to one page.
- Print a hard copy from your electronic version, using good-quality paper.
- Include your name, address, phone number, and e-mail address on both the resume and your cover letter.
- List recent, relevant work experience.
- List relevant education and the name of the institution from which you graduated, as well as relevant courses attended.
- List your professional skills and accomplishments.
- Focus on information that is relevant to the position you are seeking.

The average time that a potential employer will spend scanning your resume before deciding whether to grant you an interview is about 20 seconds. That means you must market yourself in such a manner that the reader will want to meet you. If your work experience has been in an unrelated field, show how the position helped you develop transferable skills. Restaurant work, for example, helps employees develop customer-service skills and learn to deal with a wide variety of customers.

As you list former and current positions on your resume, focus on achievements instead of detailing duties and responsibilities. Accomplishment statements enlarge your basic duties and responsibilities. The best way to show concrete accomplishment is to include numbers or percentages whenever possible. As you describe former and current positions on your resume, ask yourself the following questions:

- How many regular clients did I serve?
- How many clients did I serve weekly?
- What was my service ticket average?
- What was my client retention rate?
- What percentage of my client revenue came from retailing?
- What percentage of my client revenue came from color or texture services?

If you cannot express your accomplishment numerically, can you address which problems you solved or other results you achieved? For instance, did your office job help you develop excellent organizational skills?

This type of questioning can help you develop accomplishment statements that will interest a potential employer. There is no better time for you to achieve significant accomplishments than while you are in school. Even though your experience may be minimal, you must still present evidence of your skills and accomplishments. This may seem a difficult task at this early stage in your working career, but by closely examining your training and school clinic performance, extracurricular activities, and the full- or part-time jobs you have held, you should be able to create a good, attention-getting resume.

For example, consider the following questions:

- Did you receive any honors during your course of training?

- Were you ever selected "student of the month"?

- Did you receive special recognition for your attendance or academic progress?

- Did you win any cosmetology-related competitions while in school?

- What was your attendance average while in school?

- Did you work with the student body to organize any fundraisers? What were the results?

Answers to these types of questions may indicate your people skills, personal work habits, and personal commitment to success (figure 30-7).

Since you have not yet completed your training, you still have the opportunity to make some of the examples listed above become a reality before you graduate. Positive developments of this nature while you are still in school can do much to improve your resume.

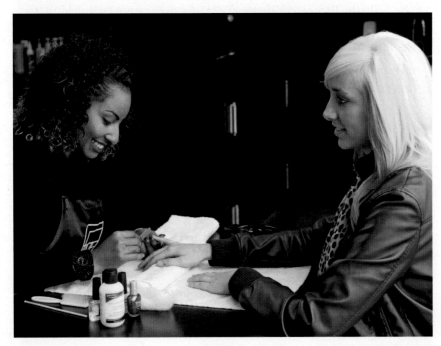

figure 30-7
Excelling in school can help you build a good resume.

The Do's and Don'ts of Resumes

You will save yourself from many problems and a lot of disappointment right from the beginning of your job search if you keep a clear idea in your mind of what to do and what not to do when it comes to creating a resume. Here are some of the do's:

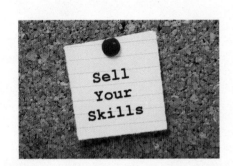

- **Always put your complete contact information on your resume.** If your cell phone is your primary phone, list its number first, and add a land line if you have one.

- **Make it easy to read.** Use concise, clear sentences and avoid overwriting or flowery language.

- **Know your audience.** Use vocabulary and language that will be understood by your potential employer.

- **Keep it short.** One page is preferable.

- **Stress accomplishments.** Emphasize past accomplishments and the skills you used to achieve them.

- **Focus on career goals.** Highlight information that is relevant to your career goals and the position you are seeking.

- **Emphasize transferable skills.** The skills mastered at other jobs that can be put to use in a new position are **transferable skills**.

- **Use action verbs.** Begin accomplishment statements with action verbs such as *achieved, coordinated, developed, increased, maintained,* and *strengthened.*

- **Make it neat.** A poorly structured, badly typed resume does not reflect well on you.

- **Include professional references.** Use only professional references on your resume, and make sure you give potential employers the person's title, place of employment, and telephone number.

- **Be realistic.** Remember that you are just starting out in a field that you hope will be a wonderful and fulfilling experience. Be realistic about what employers may offer to beginners.

- **Always include a cover letter.** See figure 30-16, on page p. 1046, for an example of one, which assumes you have targeted and visited salons in advance, as advised in this chapter.

- **Note any skills with new technologies.** Include software programs, web development tools, and computerized salon management systems.

Here are some of the don'ts for resume writing:

- **Avoid salary references.** Don't state your salary history.

- **Avoid information about why you left former positions.**

- **Don't stretch the truth.** Misinformation or untruthful statements usually catch up with you.

If you don't feel comfortable writing your own resume, consider seeking a professional resume writer or a job coach. There may be employment agencies that can help you as well; many online job-search websites offer easy-to-use resume templates.

Marla Styles

143 Fern Circle • Anytown, USA, 12345 • 123.555.1234 • MarlaStyles@mye-mail.net • StyledToTheNines.blogspot.com

Objective

My objective is to obtain an apprentice position in an upscale salon focusing on haircolor and education so I may become a seasoned hair designer.

Education

ABC Academy of Hair Design Cosmetology, Chicago, IL, May 2015
Awards: Received Award for Best Student Haircut - International Beauty Show 2013

Oak Park River Forest High School, Oak Park, IL, May 2012
Overall GPA: 3.0
Clubs: Paint/Sketch Club, Theater Club, Yearbook Committee

Qualifications

- Creative, energetic and devoted to the cosmetology industry.
- Hold a current Illinois cosmetology license and have a strong knowledge of trends.
- Proven ability to retain clients and was booked solid with requests during my final four months of training.
- Served as mentor to new students of the ABC Academy of Hair Design Cosmetology

Professional Experience

Creative
- Won the student contest for best makeover.
- Developed an outstanding digital portfolio of photos showing cut, color, bridal styles, and makeovers.

Sales
- Increased chemical services to 30 percent of my clinic volume by graduation.
- Named Student of the Month for best attendance, best attitude, highest retail, and most services delivered.

Client Retention
- Developed and retained a school-clinic client base of over 75 individuals, both male and female.

Team Spirit
- Mentored new students and was their peer resource for the first three months of training.
- Volunteered myself as the "go-to person" for other students to consult regarding formal hairstyles.
- Created the official ABC Academy of Hair Design Cosmetology Facebook page, where I regularly shared new industry information.

Administration
- Supervised a student "salon team" that developed a business plan for opening a 12-chair, full-service salon. This project earned an "A" and was recognized for thoroughness, accuracy, and creativity.
- Reorganized a school facial room for greater efficiency and client comfort.
- Led the reorganization of the school dispensary, allowing for increased inventory control and the streamlining of clinic operations.
- Internet savvy with abilities in Microsoft Word, Excel, and PowerPoint.

References
Please see the attached page for references.

figure 30-8
A resume for those with little work experience focuses on achievements.

Review figure 30-8, on page p. 1039, which represents an achievement-oriented resume for a recent graduate of a cosmetology course. Remember that you are a total package, not just a resume. With determination, you will find the right position to begin your cosmetology career. Utilize all available resources during your resume development and job search process. For example, there is an abundance of best practice information available on the Internet, or you can communicate with an individual you may already know who has gone through the hiring process and can provide recommendations. Milady also has fantastic resources that can provide you with additional assistance when you begin your job search. One such Milady online resource to help with resume development and overall job search success is *Beauty & Wellness Career Transitions*.

Employment Portfolio

As you prepare to work in the field of cosmetology, an employment portfolio can be extremely useful. An **employment portfolio** is a collection of photos and documents that reflect your skills, accomplishments, and abilities in your chosen career field. You may choose to have a printed or an online portfolio (figure 30-9).

While the actual contents of the portfolio will vary from graduate to graduate, there are certain items that have a place in any portfolio.

A powerful online or printed portfolio includes the following elements:

- Diplomas, including high school and cosmetology school

- Awards and achievements received while a cosmetology student

- Current resume, focusing on accomplishments

- Letters of reference from former employers

- Summary of continuing education and/or copies of training certificates

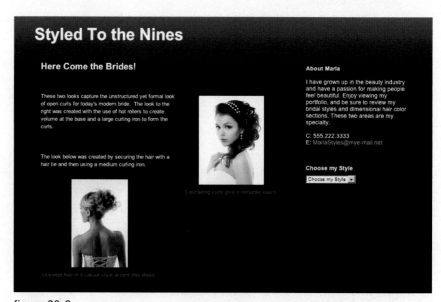

figure 30-9
Bridal showcase in an online employment portfolio (Photo credits: © gromovataya/ Fotolia [Brunette bride]; © furmananna/Fotolia [Blond bride])

- Statement of membership in industry and other professional organizations

- Statement of relevant civic affiliations and/or community activities

- Before-and-after photographs of services that you have performed on clients or models

- Brief statement about why you have chosen a career in cosmetology

- Any other information that you regard as relevant

When you write the statement about why you chose a career in cosmetology, you might include the following elements:

- A statement that explains what you love about your new career

- A description about the importance of teamwork and how you see yourself as a contributing team member

- A description of methods and ideas you would use to increase service and retail revenue (figure 30-10).

Once you have assembled your portfolio, ask yourself whether it accurately portrays you and your career skills. If it does not, identify what needs to be changed. If you are not sure, run it by a neutral party for feedback about how to make it more interesting and accurate. This kind of feedback is also useful when creating a resume. The portfolio, like the resume, should be prepared in a way that projects professionalism.

- For ease of use, you may want to separate sections of a printed portfolio with tabs.

- A bound portfolio should be easy to carry and show to potential employers and clients.

- If you are showing your online portfolio, be sure your electronic device is fully charged and the web page is bookmarked for easy retrieval.

- The photos should all be the same dimensions.

Online Portfolios

If you are technologically savvy or can hire someone to assist you, create a digital portfolio or an online showcase of your work. However, don't expect potential employers to take the extra time to visit a website or view a DVD. Bring along a printed copy of everything you want the employer to see.

Make it a habit to take photos of your work for your portfolio. Bring in models and practice the latest haircut, styling, or coloring techniques. Take compelling before and after photos to show your ability to transform your clients. For ideas, browse the Internet by doing a Google image search for "hairstyling portfolios." Showcase your versatility by providing photos of various hair designs so your potential employer will gain a sense of your abilities.

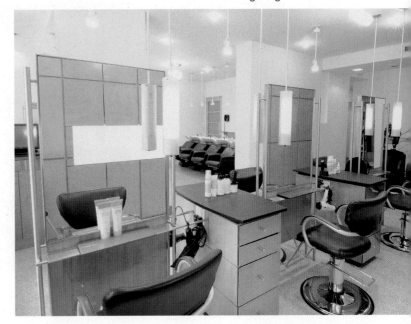

figure 30-10
Prospective colorists should target haircolor specialty salons like Minardi Salon in NYC, which uses Minardi Color Perfect Lighting.

There are many options you can use to create an online or electronic version of your portfolio. You can simply save your photos and scanned documents on a DVD, or you can easily create an online portfolio for free by utilizing a blog. Websites such as blogger.com or wordpress.com offer free blog sites that can easily serve as your online portfolio.

Do your homework, research carefully, and think long-term. You, your portfolio, and web address want to be around for years to come. If creating a website is currently not in your budget, then create a "Fan Page" on Facebook to showcase your work. Remember: Your fan page is your business page and a representation of your professional image.

Targeting the Establishment

One of the most important steps in the process of job hunting is narrowing your search. Listed below are some points to keep in mind when targeting potential employers.

- Accept that your first job will probably not be your dream job. Few people are so fortunate.

- Do not wait until graduation to begin your search. If you do, you may be tempted to take the first offer you receive instead of carefully investigating all possibilities before making a decision.

- Locate a salon that serves the type of clients you wish to serve. Finding a good fit with the clients and staff is critical from the outset of your career (figure 30-11).

- Make a list of area salons or spas. The Internet will be your best source for this. If you are considering relocating to another area, go to anywho.com for a complete listing of businesses in every state, or find top salons in any region or city at citysearch.com. You may also want

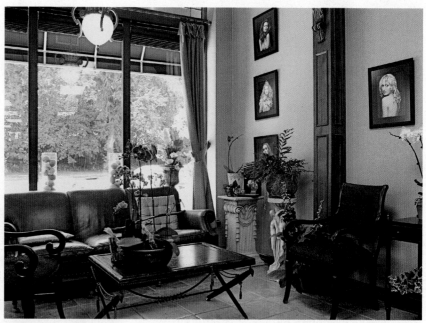

figure 30-11
Independent salons, like Salvatore Minardi in Madison, NJ, reflect the owner's taste, which gives you clues as to whether or not you'll fit in.

Photo by Michael Watson.

to do a Google search for your area of interest and city, using key words such as *haircolor salon Portland*, for example.

- Watch for salons that advertise locally, to get a feel for the market each salon is targeting. Then check the salon's website or see if it is part of a social network, such as Facebook.

- Check out websites and social networking sites for various types of salons. If you contact them, don't waste their time. Get right to the point that you are a student, and ask specific questions about the profession.

- Keep the salon's culture in mind. Do the stylists dress like you? Are the clients in different age groups or just one? Look for the salon that will be best for you and your goals.

Field Research

A great way to find out about potential jobs is to network. Actually get out there, visit salons, and talk to salon owners, managers, educators, and stylists. Whether your first contact is online, in person, or on the phone, sooner or later you'll want to arrange a face-to-face meeting or an exploratory visit to the salon. To set up a salon visit, consider the following:

- If you call, use your best telephone manner; speak with confidence and self-assurance. If you e-mail, be brief, and check spelling and punctuation. Do not text message salon owners or managers, unless they request that you do so.

- Explain that you are preparing to graduate from school in cosmetology, that you are researching the market for potential positions, and that you have a few quick questions.

- If the person is receptive, ask whether the salon is in need of any new stylists, and how many the salon currently employs.

- Ask if you can make an appointment to visit the salon to observe sometime during the next few weeks. If the salon representative is agreeable, be on time! When timing allows, confirm the appointment the day before, via e-mail (figure 30-12).

Remember that a rejection is not a negative reflection on you. Many professionals are too busy to make time for this kind of networking. The good news is that you are bound to discover many genuinely kind people

WEB RESOURCES

To start looking for a cosmetology job, begin at these websites:

Industry specific:
americansalonmag.com
behindthechair.com
modernsalon.com
salonemployment.com
salongigs.com
spaandsalonjobs.com

General:
careerbuilder.com
resumeedge.com
craigslist.org
jobbank.com
jobs.net
monster.com
snagajob.com

Dear Ms. (or Mr.) _____,

This is just a quick reminder that I'll be visiting your salon this Friday, June 12th, at 2:00 PM. I am looking forward to meeting with you, and I am eager to observe your salon and staff at work. If you should need to reach me before that time for any reason, please call or text me at _____, or e-mail me at _____.

Sincerely,
(Your name)

---

figure 30-12
Sample appointment confirmation

who remember what it was like when they started out and who are willing to devote a bit of their time to help others who are beginning their careers.

The Salon Visit

When you visit the salon, take along a checklist to ensure that you observe all the key areas that might ultimately affect your decision making. The checklist will be similar to the one used for field trips that you probably have taken to area salons while in school. Keep the checklist on file for future reference, so that you can make informed comparisons among establishments (figure 30-13).

After your visit, always remember to follow up with a handwritten note or email, thanking the salon representative for his or her time (figure 30-14). Do this even if you did not like the salon and would never consider working there (figure 30-15).

Never burn your bridges. Instead, build a network of contacts who have a favorable opinion of you.

figure 30-13
Salon visit checklist

SALON VISIT CHECKLIST

When you visit a salon, observe the following areas and rate them from 1 to 5, with 5 considered being the best.

_____ **SALON IMAGE:** Is the salon's image consistent and appropriate for your interests? Is the image pleasing and inviting? What is the decor and arrangement? If you are not comfortable or if you find it unattractive, mark the salon off your list of employment possibilities.

_____ **PROFESSIONALISM:** Do the employees present the appropriate professional appearance and behavior? Do they give their clients the appropriate levels of attention and personal service, or do they act as if work is their time to socialize?

_____ **MANAGEMENT:** Does the salon show signs of being well-managed? Is the phone answered promptly with professional telephone skills? Is the mood of the salon positive? Does everyone appear to work as a team?

_____ **CLIENT SERVICE:** Are clients greeted promptly and warmly when they enter the salon? Are they kept informed of the status of their appointment? Are they offered a magazine or beverage while they wait? Is there a comfortable reception area? Are there changing rooms and attractive smocks?

_____ **PRICES:** Compare price for value. Are clients getting their money's worth? Do they pay the same price in one salon but get better service and attention in another? If possible, take home salon brochures and price lists.

_____ **RETAIL:** Is there a well-stocked retail display offering clients a variety of product lines and a range of prices? Do the stylists and receptionist (if applicable) promote retail sales?

_____ **IN-SALON MARKETING:** Are there posters or promotions throughout the salon? If so, are they professionally made, and do they reflect contemporary styles?

_____ **SERVICES:** Make a list of all services offered by each salon and the product lines they carry. This will help you decide what earning potential stylists have in each salon.

SALON NAME: _____

SALON MANAGER: _____

Dear Ms. (or Mr.) _____,

I appreciate having had the opportunity to observe your salon/spa in operation last Friday. Thank you for the time you and your staff gave me. I was impressed by the efficient and courteous manner in which your stylists served their clients. The atmosphere was pleasant, and the mood was positive. Should you ever have an opening for a professional with my skills and training, I would welcome the opportunity to apply. You can contact me at the e-mail address and phone number listed below. I hope we will meet again soon.

Sincerely,

(your name, address, telephone, e-mail address)

figure 30-14
Sample thank-you note

Dear Ms. (or Mr.) _____,

I appreciate having had the opportunity to observe your salon in operation last Friday. I know how busy you and all your staff are, and I want to thank you for the time that you gave me. I hope my presence didn't interfere with the flow of your operations too much. I certainly appreciate the courtesies that were extended to me by you and your staff. I wish you and your salon continued success.

Sincerely,

(your name)

figure 30-15
Thank-you note to a salon at which you do not expect to seek employment

After reading the next few sections, you will be able to:

LO❺ Know how to explore the job market, research potential employers, and operate within the legal aspects of employment.

Arrange for a Job Interview

After you have graduated and completed the first two steps in the process of securing employment—targeting and observing salons—you are ready to pursue employment in earnest. The next step is to contact the establishments that you are most interested in by sending them a resume and requesting an interview. Choosing a salon that is the best match to your skills will increase your chances of success.

Many salons have websites with special employment areas, others post on salon- or job-related websites. Follow instructions exactly for filling out

figure 30-16
Sample resume cover letter

Your Name
Your Address
Your Phone Number

Ms. (or Mr.) _____

Salon Name
Salon Address

Dear Ms. (or Mr.) _____,

We met in August when you allowed me to observe your salon and staff while I was still in cosmetology training. Since that time, I have graduated and have received my license. I have enclosed my resume for your review and consideration.

I would appreciate the opportunity to meet with you and discuss either current or future career opportunities at your salon. I was extremely impressed with your staff and business, and I would like to share with you how my skills and training might add to your salon's success.

I look forward to meeting with you again soon.

Sincerely,
(your name)

forms or sending resumes. (Some salons don't want attachments, such as letters of recommendation or digital portfolios sent with the resumes.) In rare instances, you may need to send a resume and cover letter (figures 30-8 and 30-16) by traditional snail mail. Comply with the salon's guidelines.

Mark your calendar to remind yourself to make a follow-up contact. A week after submitting your resume is generally sufficient. When you call or e-mail, try to schedule an interview appointment. Keep in mind that some salons may not have openings and may not be granting interviews. When this is the case, send a resume, if you have not already, and ask the salon to keep it on file should an opening arise in the future. Be sure to thank your contacts for their time and consideration.

Interview Preparation

When preparing for an interview, make sure that you have all the necessary information and materials in place (figure 30-17), including the following items:

Identification

- Social Security Number
- Driver's license number
- Names, mailing addresses, email addresses and phone numbers of former employers
- Name, phone number and email address of the nearest relative not living with you

PREPARING FOR THE INTERVIEW CHECKLIST

RESUME COMPOSITION
1. Does it present your abilities and what you have accomplished in your jobs and training?
2. Does it make the reader want to ask, "How did you accomplish that?"
3. Does it highlight accomplishments rather than detailing duties and responsibilities?
4. Is it easy to read? Is it short? Does it stress past accomplishments and skills?
5. Does it focus on information that is relevant to your own career goals?
6. Is it complete and professionally prepared?

PORTFOLIO CHECKLIST
_____ Diploma, secondary, and post-secondary
_____ Awards and achievements while in school
_____ Current resume focusing on accomplishments
_____ Letters of reference from former employers
_____ List of, or certificates from, trade shows attended while in training
_____ Statement of professional affiliations (memberships in cosmetology organizations, etc.)
_____ Statement of civic affiliations and/or activities
_____ Before and after photographs of technical skills services you have performed
_____ Any other relevant information
Ask: Does my portfolio portray me and my career skills in the manner that I wish to be perceived? If not, what needs to be changed?

figure 30-17
Preparing for the interview checklist

Interview Wardrobe

Your appearance is crucial, especially since you are applying for a position in the image and beauty industry (figure 30-18). It is recommended that you obtain one or two interview outfits. You may be requested to return for a second interview, hence the need for the second outfit. Consider the following points:

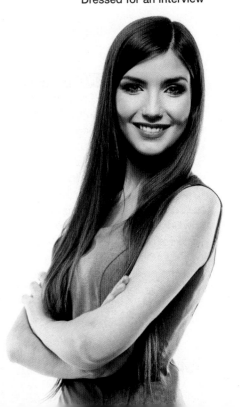

figure 30-18
Dressed for an interview

- Is the outfit appropriate for the position?
- Is it both fashionable and flattering, and similar to what the salon's current stylists wear? (If you haven't visited the salon, walk by or check out its website to gauge its style culture so that you can dress accordingly.)
- Are your accessories both fashionable and functional (for example, not noisy or so large that they would interfere with performing services)?
- Are your nails well groomed?
- Is your hairstyle current? Does it flatter your face and your overall style?
- Is your makeup current? Does it flatter your face and your overall style?
- (For men:) Are you clean shaven? If not, is your beard properly trimmed?
- Is your perfume or cologne subtle (or nonexistent)?
- Are you carrying either a handbag or a briefcase, but not both?

Supporting Materials

- **Resume.** Even if you have already sent a resume, take another copy with you.

- **Facts and figures.** Have ready a list of names and dates of former employment, education, and references.

- **Employment portfolio.** Even if you have just two photos in your portfolio and they are pictures of haircolor and styles you did for friends, bring them along.

Review and Prepare for Anticipated Interview Questions

Certain questions are typically asked during an interview. Being familiar with these questions will allow you to reflect on your answers ahead of time. You might even consider role-playing an interview situation with friends, family, or fellow students. Typical questions include the following:

- Why do you want to work here?

- What did you like best about your training?

- Are you punctual and regular in attendance?

- Will your school director or instructor confirm this?

- What skills do you feel are your strongest?

- In which areas do you consider yourself to be less strong?

- Are you a team player? Please explain.

- Do you consider yourself flexible? Please explain.

- What are your career goals?

- What days and hours are you available for work?

- Are there any obstacles that would prevent you from keeping your commitment to full-time employment? Please explain.

- What assets do you believe that you would bring to this salon and this position?

- What computer skills do you have?

- How would you handle a problem client?

- How do you feel about retailing?

- Would you be willing to attend our company's training program?

- Would you please describe ways that you provide excellent customer service?

- What consultation questions might you ask a client?

- Are you prepared to train for a year before you have your own clients?

Be Prepared to Perform a Service

Some salons require applicants to perform a service in their chosen discipline as part of the interview, and many of these salons require that you bring your own model. Be sure to confirm whether this is a requirement. If it is, make sure that your model is appropriately dressed and properly prepared for the experience and that you bring the necessary supplies, products, and tools to demonstrate your skills.

The Interview

On the day of the interview, try to make sure that nothing occurs that will keep you from completing the interview successfully. You should practice the following behaviors in connection with the interview itself:

- Always be on time or, better yet, early. If you are unsure of the location, find it the day before, so there will be no reason for delays.

- Turn off your cell phone! Do not arrive with ear buds or a hands-free cell phone device in your ear.

- Project a warm, friendly smile. Smiling is the universal language.

- Walk, sit, and stand with good posture.

- Be polite and courteous.

- Do not sit until you are asked to do so or until it is obvious that you are expected to do so.

- Never smoke or chew gum, even if one or the other is offered to you.

- Do not come to an interview with a cup of coffee, a soft drink, snacks, or anything else to eat or drink.

- Never lean on or touch the interviewer's desk. Some people do not like their personal space broached without an invitation.

- Try to project a positive first impression by appearing as confident and relaxed as you can be (**figure 30-19**).

- Speak clearly. The interviewer must be able to hear and understand you.

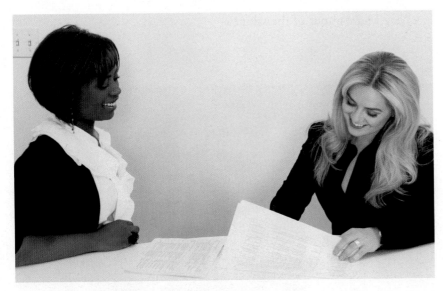

figure 30-19
Interview in progress

- Answer questions honestly. Think about the question and answer carefully. Do not speak before you are ready, and not for more than two minutes at a time.

- Never criticize former employers.

- Always remember to thank the interviewer at the end of the interview.

Another critical part of the interview comes when you are invited to ask the interviewer questions of your own. You should think about those questions ahead of time and bring a list if necessary. Doing so will show that you are organized and prepared. Some questions that you might consider include the following:

- What are you looking for in a stylist?

- Is there a job description? May I review it?

- Is there a salon manual? May I review it?

- How does the salon promote itself?

- How long do stylists typically work here?

- Are employees encouraged to grow in skills and responsibility? How so?

- Does the salon offer continuing education opportunities?

- What does your training program involve?

- Is there room for advancement? If so, what are the requirements for promotion?

- What key benefits does the salon offer, such as advanced training and medical insurance?

- What outside and community activities is the salon involved in?

- What is the form of compensation?

- When will the position be filled?

- May I contact you in a week regarding your decision?

- May I have a tour of the salon?

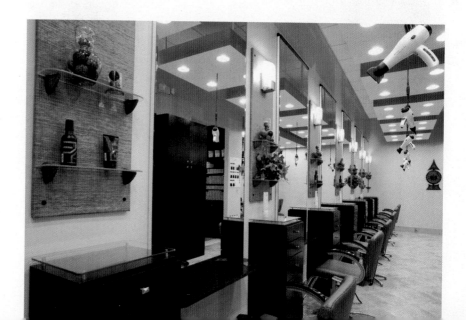

Do not feel that you have to ask all of your questions. The point is to create as much of a dialogue as possible. Be aware of the interviewer's reactions and make note of when you have asked enough questions. By obtaining the answers to at least some of your questions, you can compare the information you have gathered about other salons and choose the one that offers the best package of income and career development.

Remember to follow up the interview with a thank-you note or e-mail. It should simply thank the interviewer for the time he or she spent with you. Close with a positive statement that you want the job (if you do). If the interviewer's decision comes down to two or three possibilities, the one expressing the most desire may be offered the position. Also, if the interviewer suggests that you call to learn about the employment decision, then by all means do so.

Legal Aspects of the Employment Interview

Over the years, a number of legal issues have arisen about questions that may or may not be included in an employment application or interview, including ones that involve race/ethnicity, religion, and national origin, marital status, sexual orientation and if you have children. Generally, there should be no questions in any of these categories. Additional categories of appropriate and inappropriate questions are listed below:

- **Age or date of birth.** It is permissible to ask the age if the applicant is younger than 18. Otherwise, age should not be relevant in most hiring decisions; therefore, date-of-birth questions prior to employment are improper.

- **Disabilities or physical traits.** The Americans with Disabilities Act prohibits general inquiries about health problems, disabilities, and medical conditions.

- **Drug use or smoking.** Questions regarding drug or tobacco use are permitted. In fact, the employer may obtain the applicant's agreement to be bound by the employer's drug and smoking policies and to submit to drug testing.

- **Citizenship.** Employers are not allowed to discriminate because an applicant is not a U.S. citizen. However, employers can request to see a Green Card or work permit.

It is important to recognize that not all potential employers will understand that they may be asking improper or illegal questions. If you are asked such questions, you might politely respond that you believe the question is irrelevant to the position you are seeking, and that you would like to focus on your qualities and skills that are suited to the job and the mission of the establishment.

Employee Contracts

Employers can legally require you to sign contracts as a condition of employment. In the salon business, the most common ones are non-compete and confidentiality agreements. Salon owners often invest a great deal in training, and they don't want you taking all that education to a

? DID YOU KNOW?

These are examples of illegal questions as compared to legal questions:

Illegal Questions
How old are you?
Please describe your medical history.
Are you a U.S. citizen?
What is your native language?

Legal Questions
Are you over the age of 18?
Are you physically able to perform this job?
Are you authorized to work in the United States?
In which languages are you fluent?

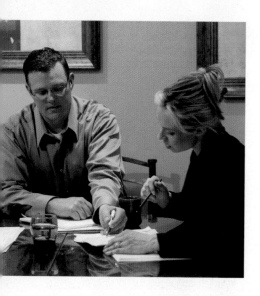

competing salon across the street once your apprenticeship or initial training is complete. Non-compete agreements address this issue, prohibiting you from seeking employment within a given time period and geographic area after you leave employment with them. Often, non-compete agreements also forbid employees from gathering and keeping client records, including client phone numbers. A contract cannot interfere with your right to work, and as a result, these contracts must be very specific and are sometimes controversial. If you are presented with any contract, take it home, read it, and make certain you completely understand it. If you do not completely understand any part of it, consult with a labor-law attorney before signing it.

The Employment Application

Any time that you are applying for any position, you will be required to complete an application, even if your resume already contains much of the requested information. Your resume and the list you have prepared prior to the interview will assist you in completing the application quickly and accurately.

Doing It Right

You are ready to set out on your exciting new career as a professional cosmetologist. The right way to proceed is by learning important study and test-taking skills early and applying them consistently.

Think ahead to your employment opportunities and use your time in school to develop a record of interesting, noteworthy activities that will make your resume more exciting. When you compile a history that shows how you have achieved your goals, your confidence will grow.

Always take one step at a time. Be sure to take the helpful preliminary steps that we have discussed when preparing for employment.

Develop a dynamic portfolio. Keep your materials, information, and questions organized in order to ensure a high-impact interview.

Once you are employed, take the necessary steps to learn all that you can about your new position and the establishment you will be serving. Read all you can about the industry. Attend trade shows and take advantage of as much continuing education as you can manage. Become an active participant in efforts to make the cosmetology industry even better. See Chapter 31, On the Job, to learn some great strategies for ensuring your career success.

As you transition into your new career as a beauty professional, let us Milady continue the journey with you. Be sure to visit the MiladyPro.com website. In addition to helping you prepare for your State Board Exam, MiladyPro.com offers access to materials designed to help you hit the ground running and grow your skill set, assuring long-term success no matter where you may take your career.

REVIEW QUESTIONS

1. What habits and characteristics do test-wise students have?

2. What is deductive reasoning?

3. What are the four most common testing formats?

4. List and describe the different types of salon businesses available to cosmetologists.

5. What is a resume?

6. What is an employment portfolio?

7. List the items that should be included in your employment portfolio.

8. What are some questions that you should never be asked when interviewing for a job?

STUDY TOOLS

- **Reinforce what you just learned:** Complete the activities and exercises in your Theory or Practical Workbook, or your Study Guide.

- **Expand your knowledge:** Search for websites about the topics in this chapter and make a list of additional resources.

- **Study and prepare for your quiz:** Take the chapter test in your Exam Review or your Milady U: Online Licensing Prep.

- **Re-Test your knowledge:** Take the Chapter 30 *Quizzes!*

- **Learn even more:** Look up in a dictionary or search the internet for the definitions of any additional terms you want to learn about.

CHAPTER GLOSSARY

deductive reasoning	p. 1029	The process of reaching logical conclusions by employing logical reasoning.
employment portfolio	p. 1040	A collection, usually bound, of photos and documents that reflect your skills, accomplishments, and abilities in your chosen career field.
resume	p. 1036	Written summary of a person's education and work experience.
stem	p. 1029	The basic question or problem.
test-wise	p. 1027	Understanding the strategies for successful test taking.
transferable skills	p. 1038	Skills mastered at other jobs that can be put to use in a new position.
work ethic	p. 1033	Taking pride in your work and committing yourself to consistently doing a good job for your clients, employer, and salon team.

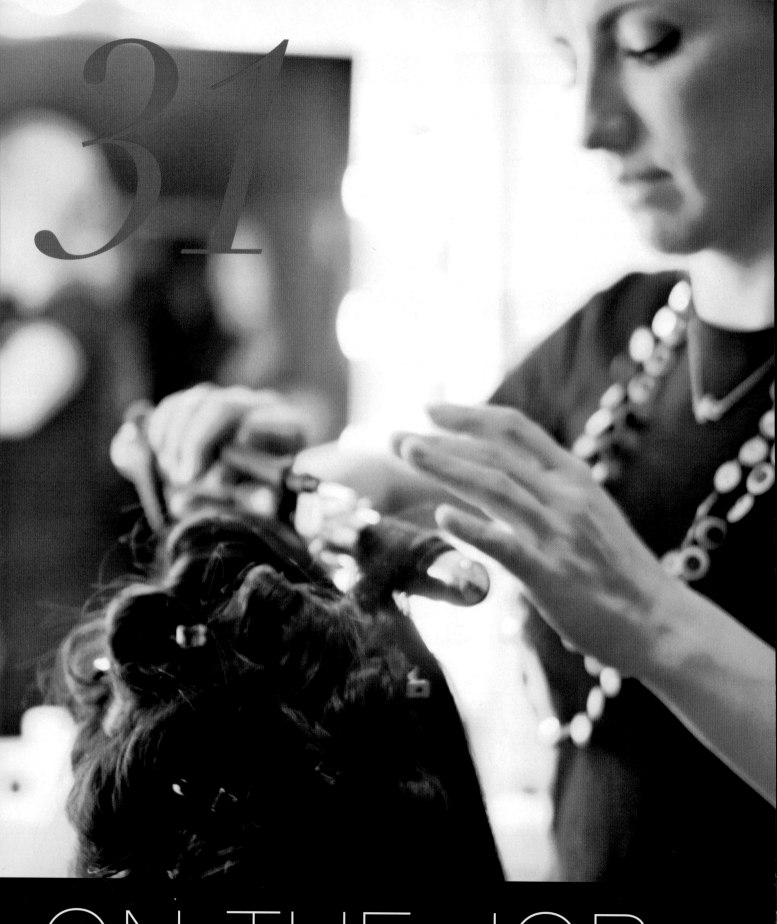

31

ON THE JOB

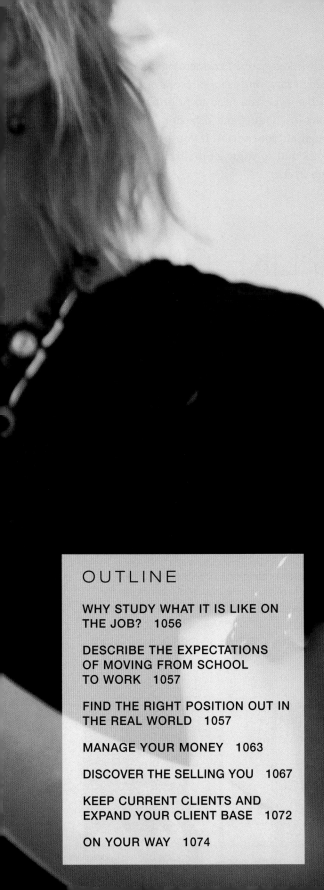

LEARNING OBJECTIVES

After completing this chapter, you will be able to:

LO❶
Describe what is expected of a new employee and what this means in terms of your everyday behavior.

LO❷
List the habits of a good salon team player.

LO❸
Describe three different ways in which salon professionals are compensated.

LO❹
Determine the best way to record your tips and make additional income.

LO❺
Explain the principles of selling products and services in the salon.

LO❻
List the most effective ways to build a client base.

Congratulations! You have worked hard in cosmetology school, passed your state's licensing exam, and been offered your first job in the field. Now, more than ever, you need to prioritize your goals and commit to personal rules of conduct and behavior. These goals and rules should guide you throughout your career. If you let them do so, you can expect to always have work and to enjoy all the freedom that your chosen profession can offer (figure 31-1).

why study
WHAT IT IS LIKE ON THE JOB?

Cosmetologists should study and have a thorough understanding of what it is like on the job because:

> Working in a salon requires each staff member to belong to and work as a team member of the salon. Learning to do so is an important aspect of being successful in the salon environment.

> There are a variety of ways that a salon may compensate employees. Being familiar with each way and knowing how they work will help you to determine if the compensation system at a particular salon can work for you and what to expect from it.

> Once you are working as a salon professional, you will have financial obligations and responsibilities, so learning the basics of financial management while you are building your clientele and business is invaluable.

> As you build your clientele and settle into your professional life, there will be opportunities for you to use a variety of techniques for increasing your income, such as retailing and upselling services. Knowing and using these techniques will help you to promote yourself, build a loyal client base, and create a sound financial future for yourself.

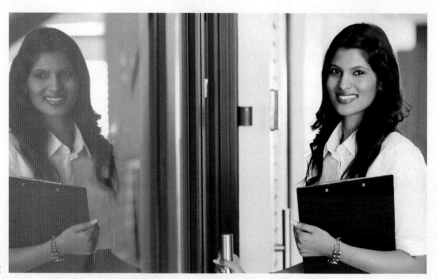

figure 31-1
Getting off to a good start

© michaeljung / Shutterstock.com

After reading the next few sections, you will be able to:

LO**1** Describe what is expected of a new employee and what this means in terms of your everyday behavior.

Describe the Expectations of Moving from School to Work

Making the transition from school to work can be difficult. While you may be thrilled to have a job, working for a paycheck brings with it a number of duties and responsibilities that you may not have considered.

Cosmetology school is a forgiving environment. You are given the chance to do a certain procedure over and over again until you get it right. Making and fixing mistakes is an accepted part of the process, and your instructors and mentors are there to help you. Schedules can be adjusted if necessary, and you are given some leeway in the matter of juggling your personal life with the demands of your schooling.

When you become a salon employee, however, you will be expected to put the needs of the salon and its clients ahead of your own. This means that you must be on time for every scheduled shift, and be prepared to perform whatever services or functions are required of you, regardless of what is happening in your personal life. For example, if someone comes to you with tickets for a concert on a day when you are scheduled to work, you cannot just take the day off. To do so would definitely inconvenience your clients, who might even decide not to return to the salon. It could also burden your coworkers, who might feel resentful if they are asked to take on your appointments.

After reading the next few sections, you will be able to:

LO**2** List the habits of a good salon team player.

LO**3** Describe three different ways in which salon professionals are compensated.

Find the Right Position Out in the Real World

Many cosmetology graduates believe they should be rewarded with a high-paying job, performing only the kinds of services they wish to do, as soon as they graduate from school. It does not work out that way for most people. In a job, you may be asked to do work or perform services that are not your first choice. The good news is that when you are really working in the trenches, you are learning every moment, and there is no substitute for that kind of experience.

What is important is to determine which type of position is right for you by being honest with yourself as you evaluate your skills. If you need help and direction in sorting out the issues around the various workplaces you are considering, ask your instructor for advice. If you chose a salon carefully, based on its culture and the type of salon and benefits you prefer (as discussed in Chapter 30, Preparing for Licensure and Employment), you'll be off to a great start.

Thriving in a Service Profession

The first reality when you are in a service business is that your career revolves around serving your clients. There will always be some people who do not treat others with respect; however, the majority of people you encounter will truly appreciate the work you do for them. They will look forward to seeing you, and they will show their appreciation for your hard work with their loyalty.

Here are some points that will help guide you as you meet your clients' needs:

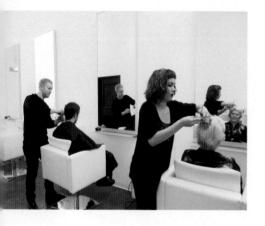

- **Put others first.** You will have to quickly get used to putting your own feelings or desires aside and putting the needs of the salon and the client first. This means doing what is expected of you, unless you are physically unable to do so.

- **Be true to your word.** Choose your words carefully and honestly. Be someone who can be counted on to tell the truth and to do what you say you will do.

- **Be punctual.** Scheduling is central to the salon business. Getting to work on time shows respect not only for your clients, but also for your coworkers who will have to handle your clients if you are late.

- **Be a problem solver.** No job or situation comes without its share of problems. Be someone who recognizes problems promptly and finds ways to resolve them constructively.

- **Be a lifelong learner.** Valued employees continue to learn throughout their careers. Thinking that you are done learning once you are out of school is immature and limiting. Your career might go in all kinds of interesting directions, depending on what new things you learn. This applies to every aspect of your life. Besides learning new technical skills, you should continue gaining more insight into your own behavior and better ways to deal with people, problems, and issues.

Salon Teamwork

Working in a salon requires that you practice and perfect your people skills. A salon is very much a team environment. To become a good team player, you should do your best to practice the following workplace principles:

© bikeriderlondon/Shutterstock.com

- **Strive to help.** Be concerned not only with your own success, but also with the success of others. Be willing to help a teammate by staying a little later or coming in a little earlier.

- **Pitch in.** Be willing to help with whatever needs to be done in the salon—from folding towels to making appointments—when you are not busy servicing clients (figure 31-2).

- **Share your knowledge.** Be willing to share what you know. This will make you a respected member of any team. At the same time, be willing to learn from your coworkers by listening to their perspectives and techniques.

- **Remain positive.** Resist the temptation to give in to maliciousness and gossip.

- **Become a relationship builder.** Just as there are different kinds of people in the world, there are different types of relationships within the salon world. You do not have to be someone's best friend in order to build a good working relationship with that person.

- **Be willing to resolve conflicts.** The most difficult part of being in a relationship is when conflict arises. A real teammate is someone who knows that conflict and tension are bad for the people who are in it, those who are around it, and the salon as a whole. Nevertheless, conflict is a natural part of life. If you can work constructively toward resolving conflict, you will always be a valued member of the team. If you do have a conflict, discuss it with the individual, not with others in the salon.

- **Be willing to be subordinate.** No one starts at the top. Keep in mind that beginners almost always start out lower down in the pecking order.

- **Be sincerely loyal.** Loyalty is vital to the workings of a salon. Salon professionals need to be loyal to the salon and its management. Management needs to be loyal to the staff and clients. Ideally, clients will be loyal to the employee and the salon. As you work on all the team-building characteristics, you will start to feel a strong sense of loyalty to your salon (figure 31-3).

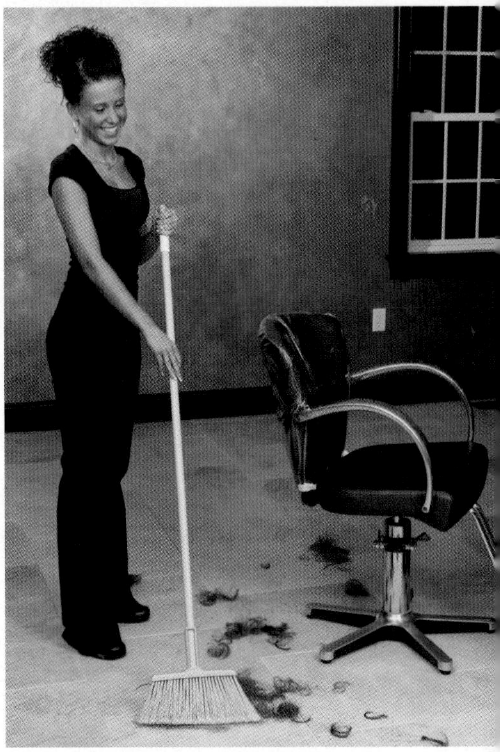

figure 31-2
Pitch in wherever you're needed.

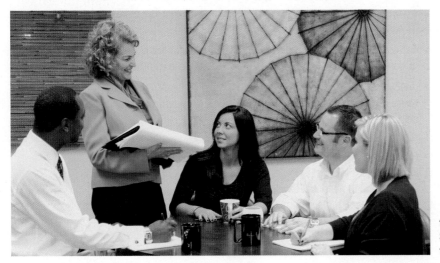

figure 31-3
Staff meetings are essential for building a loyal team.

The Job Description

When you take a job, you will be expected to behave appropriately, perform services asked of you, and conduct your business professionally. In order to do this to the best of your abilities, you should be given a **job description**, a document that outlines all the duties and responsibilities of a particular position in a salon or spa. Many salons have a preprinted job description available. If you find yourself at a salon that does not use job descriptions, you may want to write one for yourself. You can then present this to your salon manager for review, to ensure that you both have a good understanding of what is expected of you.

Once you have your job description, be sure you understand it. While reading it over, make notes and jot down questions you want to ask your manager. When you assume your new position, you are agreeing to do everything as it is written down in the job description. If you are unclear about something or need more information, it is your responsibility to ask.

Remember, you will be expected to fulfill all of the functions listed in the job description. How well you fulfill these duties will influence your future at the salon, as well as your financial rewards.

In crafting a job description, the best salons cover all the bases. They outline not only the employee's duties and responsibilities, but also the attitudes that they expect their employees to have and the opportunities that are available to them. Like the salons that generate them, job descriptions come in all sizes and shapes, and they feature a variety of requirements, benefits, and incentives.

Compensation Plans

When you assess a job offer, your first concern will probably be the compensation, or what you will actually get paid for your work. Compensation varies from one salon to another. There are, however, three common methods of compensation that you are most likely to encounter: salary, commission, and salary plus commission (figure 31-4).

figure 31-4
Compensation for performance

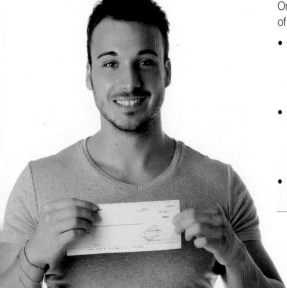

© Stefano Cavoretto/Shutterstock.com

Salary

Being paid an hourly rate is usually the best way for a new salon professional to start out because new professionals rarely have an established clientele. Some salons offer an hourly wage that is slightly higher than the minimum wage to encourage new cosmetologists to take the job and stick with it. In this situation, if you earn $10 per hour and you work 40 hours, you will be paid $400 that week. If you work more hours, you will get more pay. If you work fewer hours, you will get less pay. Regular taxes will be taken out of your earnings.

Remember, if you are offered a set salary in lieu of an hourly rate, that salary must be at least equal to the minimum wage for the number of hours you work. You are entitled to overtime pay if you work more than 40 hours per week. The only exception would be if you were in an official salon management position.

Commission

A **commission** [KAHM-ish-un] is a percentage of the revenue that the salon takes in from services performed by a particular cosmetologist. Commission is usually offered once an employee has built up a loyal clientele. A commission payment structure is very different from an hourly wage, because any money you are paid is a direct result of the total amount of service dollars you generate for the salon. Commissions are paid based on percentages of your total service dollars, and can range anywhere from 25 to 60 percent, depending on your length of time at the salon, your performance level, and the benefits that are part of your employment package.

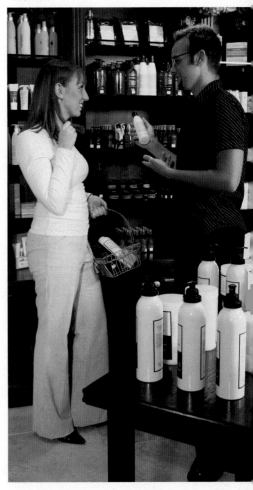

figure 31-5
Commissions on retail sales boost income.

Suppose, for example, that at the end of the week when you add up all the services you have performed, your total is $1,000. If you are at the 50 percent commission level, then you would be paid $500 (before taxes). Keep in mind that until you have at least two years of servicing clients under your belt, you may not be able to make a living on straight commission compensation. Additionally, many states do not allow straight commission payments unless they average out to at least minimum wage.

Salary Plus Commission

A salary-plus-commission structure is another common way to be compensated in the salon business. It basically means that you receive both a salary and a commission. This kind of structure is often used to motivate employees to perform more services, thereby increasing their productivity. For example, imagine that you earn an hourly wage that is equal to $300 per week, and you perform about $600 worth of services every week. Your salon manager may offer you an additional 25 percent commission on any services you perform over your usual $600 per week. Or perhaps you receive a straight hourly wage, but you can receive as much as a 15 percent commission on all the retail products you sell. Sometimes, salons call this structure salary plus bonus. With this structure, your salary is actually based on an average of what you would have made if you were paid commission, but you also get a bonus on anything over and above. You can see how this kind of structure quickly leads to significantly increased compensation (figure 31-5).

Accepting a commission-paying position in a salon can have its positives and negatives for new cosmetologists. If you think you have enough clients to work on commission and can make enough of a paycheck to pay your expenses, then go ahead and give it a try—it could be a great way to work into better commission scales or even booth renting. (As of this printing, Pennsylvania and New Jersey forbid booth renting by law, but other states may regulate licensing differently; always check.)

If you don't think you can make enough money being paid solely on a commission basis, then take a job in a salon that is willing to pay you an hourly wage until you build your client base. After you have honed your technical skills and built a solid client base, you can consider working on commission.

Beauty pros can increase their chances of building a solid and loyal clientele more quickly if they:

- Live in a large city or choose areas within their cities that have a large number of potential clients.
- Select a location where the competition for clients is less saturated.
- Have advanced training, skills, and certifications.
- Have and use their artistic abilities.
- Employ marketing and publicity strategies.
- Concentrate on an unusual niche within the beauty business (teens, for example).

Tips

When you receive satisfactory service at a hotel or restaurant, you are likely to leave your server a tip. It has become customary for salon clients to acknowledge beauty professionals in this way, too. Some salons have a tipping policy; others have a no-tipping policy. This is determined by what the salon feels is appropriate for its clientele.

Tips are income in addition to your regular compensation and must be tracked and reported on your income tax return. Reporting tips will be beneficial to you if you wish to take out a mortgage or another type of loan and want your income to appear as strong as it really is.

As you can see, there are a number of ways to structure compensation for a salon professional. You will probably have the opportunity to try each of these methods at different points in your career. When deciding whether a certain compensation method is right for you, it is important to be aware of what your monthly expenses are and to have a personal financial budget in place. Budget issues are addressed later in this chapter.

Employee Evaluation

The best way to keep tabs on your progress is to ask for feedback from your salon manager and key coworkers. Most likely, your salon will have a structure in place for evaluation purposes. Commonly, evaluations are scheduled 90 days after hiring, and then once a year after that. But you should feel free to ask for help and feedback any time you need it. This feedback can help you improve your technical abilities, as well as your customer-service skills.

Ask a senior stylist to sit in on one of your client consultations and to make note of areas where you can improve. Ask your manager to observe your technical skills and to point out ways you can perform your work more quickly and more efficiently. Have a trusted coworker watch and evaluate your skills when it comes to selling retail products. All of these evaluations will benefit your learning process enormously.

Find a Role Model

One of the best ways to improve your performance is to model your behavior after someone who is having the kind of success that you wish to have (figure 31-6). Watch other stylists in your salon. You will easily be able to identify who is really good and who is just coasting along. Focus on the skills of the ones who are really good. What do they do? How do they treat their clients? How do they treat the salon staff and manager? How do they book their appointments? How do they handle their continuing education? What process do they use when formulating color or selecting a product? What is their attitude toward their work? How do they handle a crisis or conflict?

Go to these professionals for advice. Ask for a few minutes of their time, but be willing to wait for it, because it may not be easy to find time to talk during a busy salon workday. If you are having a problem, explain your situation, and ask if the mentor can help you see things differently. Be prepared to listen and not argue your points. Remember that you asked for help, even when what your coworker is saying is not what you want to

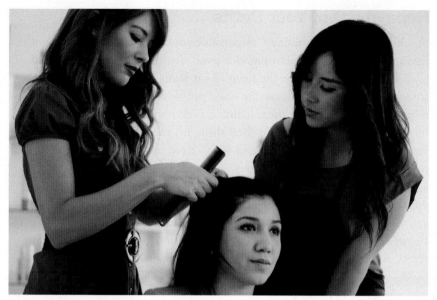

figure 31-6
Identify a role model from whom you can learn best practices.

hear. Thank your coworker for his or her help, and reflect on the advice you have been given.

A little help and direction from skilled, experienced coworkers will go a long way toward helping you achieve your goals.

After reading the next few sections, you will be able to:

LO④ Determine the best way to record your tips and make additional income.

Manage Your Money

Although a career in the beauty industry is very artistic and creative, it is also a career that requires financial understanding and planning. Too many cosmetology professionals live for the moment and do not plan for the future. They may end up feeling cheated out of the benefits that their friends and family in other careers are enjoying.

In a corporate structure, the human resources department of the corporation handles a great deal of the employees' financial planning for them. For example, health and dental insurance, retirement accounts, savings accounts, and many other items may be automatically deducted and paid out of the employees' salary. Most beauty professionals, however, must research and plan for all of those expenses on their own. This may seem difficult, but in fact it is a small price to pay for the kind of freedom, financial reward, and job satisfaction that a career in cosmetology can offer. And the good news is that managing money is something everyone can learn to do.

milady pro LEARN MORE!

Optional info on **Budget** topics and tutorials can be found at miladypro.com
Keyword: *FutureCosPro*

Repayment of Your Debts

In addition to making money, responsible adults are also concerned with paying back their debts. Throughout your life and your career, you will undoubtedly incur debt in the form of car loans, home mortgages, or student loans. While it is easy for some people to merely ignore their responsibility in repaying these loans, it is extremely irresponsible and immature to accept a loan and then shrug off the debt. Not paying back your loans is called defaulting, and it can have serious consequences regarding your personal and professional credit. Legal action can be taken against you if you fail to repay your loans. The best way to meet all of your financial responsibilities is to know precisely what you owe and what you earn so that you can make informed decisions regarding your finances. Before committing to a loan, make sure you understand the payment terms, interest rate, and what you realistically can afford.

Reporting Your Income

As you enter your new career and work to become established, you most likely will be in a commissioned or salaried structure. When you receive your paycheck, taxes and other deductions will already be taken according to your state. When you complete your yearly state taxes, it is critical that you report cash tips and other income that is not shown on your paycheck. Other income may be from performing work outside of the salon, such as doing services on location for weddings, parties, or in a private residence. There are serious legal consequences for not reporting such income including:

• Fines and even potentially jail time.

• Decreasing your borrowing power as it is based on your reported income.

• Reducing the amount of Social Security benefits for retirement.

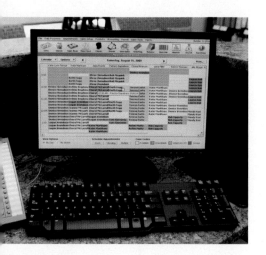

FOCUS ON
Salon Technology

Today, it is common for most salons to utilize computer technology to support their salon. The increasing number of computerized salons could be advantageous for technology-savvy students. You may be able to master salon software programs more easily than other stylists. These programs now handle cash flow management, inventory tracking, payroll automation, client appointment books, performance evaluation tracking, and more. Just remember, these client records are usually considered the salon's property. Additionally, cost-effective, online continuing education is increasingly popular.

If you are accustomed to working with technology, you may be able to help a salon set up e-mail access, a website, social networking pages, and more. With many clients enjoying the freedom of online booking and text-message appointment reminders, and with salons benefiting from e-mail or even electronic marketing programs, the more you understand technology, the better. Today, hair care manufacturers even have special educational programs you can access on your mobile phone and social networking pages where you can swap haircolor formulas or ask for instant help.

- Lowering the Bureau of Labor's endorsement as a sustainable industry leading to lower federal loans and grants available.

The best way to record your tips and additional income is to keep a daily log. At the end of each week, add the total amount of your additional income. Next, add the total for the month and keep this on a single page in the front of your log book. At the end of the year, you will be able to easily report your total cash income for your taxes. Ethical stylists make a commitment to report their income accurately at the end of each year so they avoid the potential audits from state authorities.

Personal Budget

It is amazing how many people work hard and earn very good salaries but never take the time to create a personal budget. Many people are afraid of the word *budget*, because they think that it will be too restrictive on their spending or that they will have to be mathematical geniuses in order to work with a budget. Thankfully, neither of these fears is rooted in reality.

Personal budgets range from being extremely simple to extremely complex. The right one for you depends on your needs. At the beginning of your career, a simple budget should be sufficient. To get started, take a look at the worksheet in **figure 31-7** on page 1066. It lists the standard monthly expenses that most people have to budget. It also includes school loan repayment, savings, and payments into an individual retirement account (IRA).

Keeping track of where your money goes is one step toward making sure that you always have enough. It also helps you to plan ahead and save for bigger expenses such as a vacation, your own home, or even your own business. All in all, sticking to a budget is a good practice to follow faithfully for the rest of your life.

Giving Yourself a Raise

Once you have taken some time to create, use, and work with your personal budget, you may want to look at ways in which you can have more money left over after paying bills. You might automatically jump to the most obvious sources, such as asking your employer for a raise or asking for a higher percentage of commission. While these tactics are certainly valid, you will also want to think about other ways to increase your income. Here are a few tips:

- **Spend less money.** Although it may be difficult to reduce your spending, it is certainly one way to increase the amount of money that is left over at the end of the month. These dollars can be used to invest, save, or pay down debt.

- **Work more hours.** If possible, choose times when the salon is busiest, which are the most convenient for clients. Come early and stay late to accommodate clients' booking needs. Saturday is a peak workday in most salons.

- **Increase service prices.** It will probably take some time before you are in a position to increase your service prices. For one thing, to do so, you need a loyal **client base**, customers who are loyal to

ACTIVITY

Go through the budget worksheet and fill in the amounts that apply to your current living and financial situation. If you are unsure of the amount of an expense, put in the amount you have averaged over the past three months, or give it your best guess. You may need to have three or four months of employment history in order to complete the income item, but fill in what you can. If the balance is a minus number, start listing ways you can decrease expenses or increase income.

Personal Monthly Budget Worksheet

A. Expenses

1. Monthly rent (or share of the rent) $_____
2. Car payment   _____
3. Car insurance   _____
4. Auto fuel/upkeep and maintenance   _____
5. Electricity   _____
6. Gas   _____
7. Health insurance   _____
8. Entertainment (movies, dining, etc.)   _____
9. Groceries   _____
10. Dry cleaning   _____
11. Personal grooming   _____
12. Prescriptions/medical   _____
13. Cell phone   _____
14. Internet/television/home phone   _____
15. Student loan   _____
16. IRA   _____
17. Savings deposit   _____
18. Other expenses   _____

TOTAL EXPENSES $_____

B. Income

1. Monthly take-home pay   _____
2. Tips   _____
3. Other income   _____

TOTAL INCOME $_____

C. Balance

Total Income (B)   _____

Minus Total Expenses (A)   _____

BALANCE $_____

figure 31-7
A budget worksheet

a particular cosmetologist, which in this instance is you. Also, you must have fully mastered all the services that you are performing. But if you have a loyal client base and service mastery, there is nothing wrong with increasing your prices every year or two, as long as you do so by a reasonable amount. Do a little research to determine what your competitors are charging for similar services, and increase your fees accordingly.

- **Retail more.** Most salons pay a commission on every product you recommend and sell to your clients. If you sell more products, you make more money!

Seek Professional Advice

Just as you will want your clients to seek out your advice and services for their hair care needs, sometimes it is important for you to seek out the advice of experts, especially when it comes to your finances. You can research and interview financial planners who will be able to give you advice on reducing your credit card debt, on how to invest your money, and on retirement options. You can speak to the officers at your local bank, who may be able to suggest bank accounts that offer you greater returns or flexibility with your money, depending on what you need.

When seeking out advice from other professionals, be sure not to take anyone's advice without carefully considering whether the advice makes sense for your particular situation and needs. Before you buy into anything, be an informed consumer about other people's goods and services.

- How do your expenses compare to your income?
- What is your balance after all your expenses are paid?
- Were there any surprises for you in this exercise?
- Do you think that keeping a budget is a good way to manage money?
- Do you know of any other methods people use to manage money?

After reading the next few sections, you will be able to:

LO⑤ Explain the principles of selling products and services in the salon.

Discover the Selling You

Another area that touches on the issue of you and money is selling. As a salon professional, you will have enormous opportunities to sell retail products and upgrade service tickets. **Ticket upgrading**, also known as *upselling services*, is the practice of recommending and selling additional services to your clients. These services may be performed by you or other professionals licensed in a different field (**figure 31-8**). **Retailing** is the act of recommending and selling products to your clients for at-home use. These two activities can make all the difference in your economic picture.

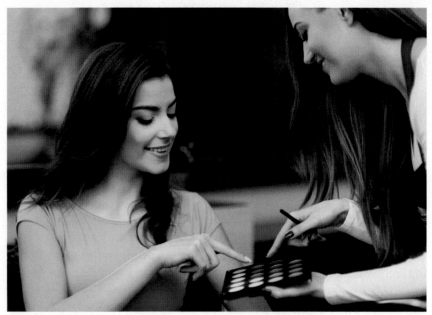

figure 31-8
Your client may wish for a makeup service as well as hairstyling.

The following dialogue is an example of ticket upgrading. In this scene, Judy, the stylist, suggests an additional service to Ms. King, her client, who has just had her hair styled for a wedding she will be attending that evening.

Read the script yourself and change the words to make them fit your personality. Then try it the next time you feel that an additional service could help one of your clients.

Judy: I'm really glad you like your new hairstyle. It will be perfect with the formal dress you described.

Ms. King: I don't know. To tell you the truth, I don't get dressed up all that often, and putting the look together was harder than I thought it would be.

Judy: Yes, I know what you mean. Have you given some thoughts about your makeup for tonight, Ms. King?

Ms. King: Well, actually, I was sort of wondering about that. My dress is cobalt blue and I'm not really sure about my lipstick and eye shadow. Got any ideas?

Judy: Let me get our makeup artist and see if she is available for a consultation. She is excellent. If she has an opening, maybe you might have your makeup done for the event. This way you don't need to worry. Not only does she do an excellent job, she even sends you home with a touch-up kit. Shall I get her for you?

Ms. King: Definitely. That sounds terrific!

Judy: Have you already made arrangements for your mani-pedi? Marie, one of our nail techs, does amazing treatments and can do an express polish change if that's all you need. That will ensure that your total look is the best it can be.

Ms. King: I think that's a great idea. Thanks for the suggestion!

Principles of Selling

Some salon professionals shy away from sales. They think that it is being pushy. A close look at how selling works can set your mind at ease. Not only can you become very good at selling once you understand the principles behind it, but you can also feel good about providing your clients with a valuable service.

To be successful in sales, you need ambition, determination, and a pleasing personality. The first step in selling is to sell yourself. Clients must like and trust you before they will purchase beauty services, cosmetics, skin or nail care items, shampoos and conditioners, or other merchandise.

Remember, every client who enters the salon is a potential purchaser of additional services or merchandise. Recognizing the client's needs and preferences lays the foundation for successful selling (figure 31-9).

To become a proficient salesperson, you must be able to apply the following principles of selling salon products and services:

• Be familiar with the features and benefits of the various services and products that you are trying to sell, and recommend only those that the client really needs. You should try and test all the products in the salon yourself.

• Adapt your approach and technique to meet the needs and personality of each client. Some clients may prefer a soft sell that involves informing them about the product, without stressing that they purchase it. Others are comfortable with a hard-sell approach that focuses emphatically on why a client should buy the product.

• Be self-confident when recommending products for sale. You become confident by knowing about the products you are selling and by believing that they are as good as you say.

• Generate interest and desire in the customer by asking questions that determine a need.

figure 31-9
When you have multiple retail displays, everyone who comes into the salon has the potential to be a retail client.

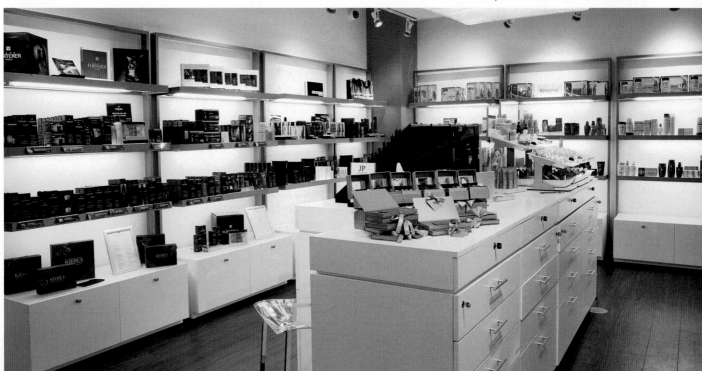

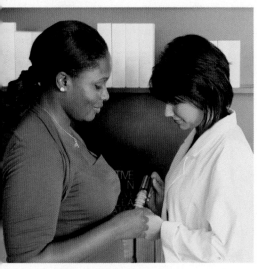

figure 31-10
Demonstrate a product's benefits.

- Never misrepresent your services or products. Making unrealistic claims will only lead to your client's disappointment, making it unlikely that you will ever again make a sale to that client.

- Do not underestimate the client's intelligence or her knowledge of her own beauty regimen or particular needs.

- To sell a product or service, deliver your sales talk in a relaxed, friendly manner. If possible, demonstrate use of the product (**figure 31-10**).

- Recognize the right psychological moment to close any sale. Once the client has offered to buy, quit selling. Do not oversell; simply praise the client for making the purchase and assure the client that he or she will be happy with it.

The Psychology of Selling

Most people have reasons for doing what they do, and when you are selling something, it is your job to figure out the reasons that will motivate a person to buy. When dealing with salon clients, you will find that their motives for buying salon products vary widely. Some may be concerned with issues of vanity. (They want to look better.) Some are seeking personal satisfaction. (They want to feel better about themselves.) Others need to solve a problem that is bothersome. (They want to spend less time maintaining their hair.)

Sometimes a client may inquire about a product or service but still be undecided or doubtful. In this type of situation, you can help the client by offering honest and sincere advice. When you explain a salon service to a client, address the results and benefits of that service. Always keep in mind that the best interests of the client should be your first consideration. You will need to know exactly what your client's needs are, and you need to have a clear idea as to how those needs can be fulfilled. Refer to the sample dialogues in this section—one involves ticket upgrading, and the other involves retailing, both of which demonstrate effective selling techniques.

FOCUS ON
Overcoming Objections

Making sales won't always be easy. Sometimes a client is stuck on a haircolor that isn't flattering. Other times, he or she may not feel convinced a product is any better than a drugstore brand or the client may have a genuine price objection.

To overcome an objection, reword the objection in a way that addresses the client's need. For instance, let's say you recommend a shampoo based on the fact that your client has dry hair and she just had it colored. In response, she says she already has a shampoo for color-treated hair.

First, acknowledge what she said. Then reword her objection that she already has the right shampoo in a different way, which gets her thinking. For example:

"Yes, it's good to use a shampoo for color-treated hair. I did notice that your hair is still dry, even before I colored it. This shampoo not

only protects your color from fading, it will definitely moisturize it more, which is what adds the shine you told me you wanted. I can leave it at the front desk, so you can think about it."

If the objection is a price objection, base your reaction on the client's. For strong objections, acknowledge the price and offer a free sample, if you can. If the objection is moderate, acknowledge it and reiterate the product's benefits.

"It is a little more expensive, but if you really want your color to last and your hair to be silky and shiny, this is the best product I've ever found. We used it on you at the back bar today. See what you think, and let me know."

Always state things in terms of the client's benefit, based on the information you gathered during the consultation.

Here are a few tips on how to get the conversation started on retailing products:

- Ask all your clients what products they are using for home maintenance of their hair, skin, and nails.

- Discuss the products you are using as you use them. For instance, tell the client why you are using the particular mousse or spray gel and what it will do for him or her. Also explain how the client should use the product at home.

- Place the product in the client's hands whenever possible or have the product in view (figure 31-11).

- Advise the client about how the recommended service will provide personal benefit (more manageable hairstyling or longer-lasting haircolor, for instance).

- Keep retail areas clean, well lit, and appealing.

- Inform clients of any promotions and sales that are going on in the salon.

- Be informed about the merits of using a professional product, as opposed to generic store brands.

- If you have time, offer a quick styling lesson. If your client has difficulty home styling, he or she will appreciate your guidance. After demonstrating, watch as the client mimics the recommended styling technique, so you can guide them.

While you realize that retailing products is a service to your clients, you may not be sure how to go about it. Imagine the following scenes and see how Lisa highlights the benefits and features of a product to her client, Ms. Steiner. Notice that price is not necessarily the most important factor.

Scenario: Meet a Need

Ms. Steiner: I really love my new haircolor. When should I have it redone? I hope it stays this red.

Lisa: You should come back in four weeks for a retouch. By then, you'll have had time to think about those highlights I suggested. I'm also going to suggest you use color-safe shampoo and conditioner to keep your color vibrant between now and your next visit. Red is the quickest color to fade, and these products will keep the color intact.

Ms. Steiner: Is that what you used on me today? It smelled great.

Lisa: I love that scent, too. Also, in addition to protecting the color, the shampoo is also very hydrating. The conditioner adds shine and seals the cuticle. The next time I see you, your hair should be almost as vibrant as it is now.

Ms. Steiner: Great!

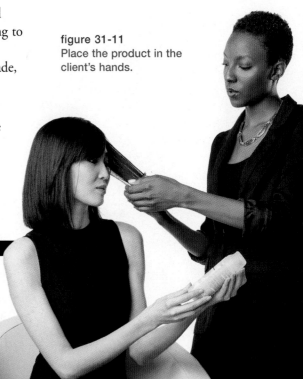

figure 31-11
Place the product in the client's hands.

ACTIVITY

Pick a partner from class and role-play the dynamics of a sales situation. Take turns being the customer and the stylist. Evaluate each other on how you did, with suggestions about where you can improve. Then try this exercise with someone else because no two customers are the same.

Keep Current Clients and Expand Your Client Base

Once you have mastered the basics of good service, take a look at some marketing techniques that will expand your client base, the customers that keep coming back to you for services.

The following are only a few suggestions; there are many others that may work for you. The best way to decide which techniques are most effective is to try several!

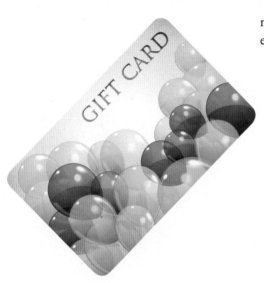

- **Birthday cards.** Ask clients for their birthday information (just the month and day, not the year) on the client consultation card, and then use it as a tool to get them into the salon again. About one month prior to the client's birthday, send a card with a special offer. Make it valid only for the month of their birthday. This form of advertisement is not expensive, and it is always greatly appreciated.

- **Provide consistently good service.** It seems basic enough, but it is amazing how many professionals work hard to get clients, and lose them because they rush through a service, leaving clients feeling dissatisfied. Providing good-quality service must always be your first concern.

- **Be reliable.** Always be courteous, thoughtful, and professional. Be at the salon when you say you will be there, and do not keep clients waiting. (See Chapter 4, Communicating for Success, for tips on how to handle the unavoidable times when you are running late.) Give your clients the hair length and style they ask for, not something else. Recommend a retail product only when you have tried it yourself and know what it can and cannot do.

- **Be respectful.** When you treat others with respect, you become worthy of respect yourself. Being respectful means that you do not gossip or make fun of anyone or anything related to the salon. Negative energy brings everyone down, especially you.

- **Be positive.** Become one of those people who always sees the glass as half full. Look for the positive in every situation. No one enjoys being around a person who is always unhappy.

- **Be professional.** Sometimes a client may try to make your relationship more personal than it ought to be. It is in your best interest, and your client's best interest, not to cross that line. Remember that your job is to be the client's beauty advisor, not a psychiatrist, a marriage counselor, or a buddy.

- **Ask for your clients' e-mail addresses.** E-mail is now the preferred mode of communication for many people. In fact, many clients now prefer to book appointments using e-mail.

© maximmmmum/Shutterstock.com

- **Utilize social media.** The Internet is a powerful medium to build your reputation and attract new clients. Utilize social media tools such as Facebook and Yelp to establish your credibility, showcase your work, and provide a space for satisfied clients to recommend you. Create a Facebook page dedicated to your business, and make it a place to share beauty tips, trends, and information and promotions. Post before and after photos to illustrate your skills. Always gain approval from your clients before sharing their photos. Yelp is a powerful tool to build your credibility. If the salon has a Yelp listing, be sure to utilize it as a way to build your business. Satisfied clients are able to post a review of your services and provide a rating of their overall experience. It is always in good practice to casually invite your clients to provide a review, however, it is not ethical to pressure anyone to do so.

- **Business card referrals.** Make up a special business card with your information on it, but leave room for a client to put her name on it as well. If your client is clearly pleased with your work, give her several cards. Ask her to put her name on them and to refer her friends and associates to you. For every card you receive from a new customer with her name on it, give her 10 percent off her next salon service, or a complimentary added service to her next appointment. This gives the client lots of motivation to recommend you to others, which in turn helps build up your clientele (**figure 31-12**).

- **Local business referrals.** Another terrific way to build business is to work with local businesses to get referrals. Look for clothing stores, florists, gift shops, and other small businesses near your salon. Offer to have a card swap and commit to referring your clients to them when they are in the market for goods or services that your neighbors can provide, if they will do the same for you. This is a great way to build a feeling of community among local vendors and to reach new clients you may not be able to otherwise.

- **Public speaking.** Make yourself available for public speaking at local women's groups, the PTA, organizations for young men and women, and anywhere else that will put you in front of people in your community who are all potential clients. Put together a short program (20 to 30 minutes) in which, for example, you might discuss professional appearance with emphasis in your chosen field and other grooming tips for people looking for jobs or who are already employed.

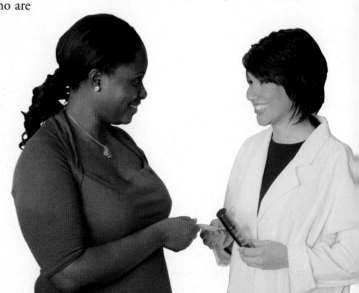

figure 31-12
Referral cards help build your client base.

Rebooking Clients

The best time to think about getting your client back into the salon is while they are still in your salon. It may seem a little difficult to assure your client that you are concerned with their satisfaction on this visit while you are talking about their next visit, but the two go together. The best way to encourage your client to book another appointment before he or she leaves is to simply talk with the client, ask questions, and listen carefully to their answers.

During the time that you are working on a client's hair, for instance, talk about the condition of their hair, their hairstyling habits at home, and the benefits of regular or special salon maintenance. You might raise these issues in a number of ways.

Scenario: Color Client

"Mrs. Rivera, your color will need to be retouched in four weeks, and I know you have a trip planned next month. I want to assure we get you in. Shall I book a retouch for your next visit?"

Scenario: Haircutting Client

"Mr. Ross, since your son is getting married next month, I can set up an appointment for the week before the wedding so you can be sure to get in. Will that work for you?"

Again, you will want to listen carefully to what your clients tell you during their visit, because they will often give the careful listener many good clues as to what is happening in their lives. That will open the door to a discussion about their next appointment.

On Your Way

Your first job in the beauty industry will most likely be the most difficult. Getting started in this business means spending some time on a steep learning curve. Be patient with yourself as you transition from the "school you" to the "professional you." Always remember that in your work life, as in everything else you do, practice makes perfect. You will not know everything you need to know right at the start, but be confident in the fact that you are graduating from cosmetology school with a solid knowledge base. Make use of the many generous and experienced professionals you will encounter, and let them teach you the tricks of the trade. Make the commitment to perfecting your technical and customer service skills.

Above all, always be willing to learn. If you let the concepts that you have learned in this book be your guide, you will enjoy your life and reap the amazing benefits of a career in cosmetology (figure 31-13).

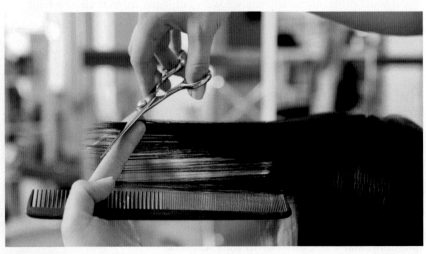

figure 31-13
Make career satisfaction your goal.

© Tyler Olson/Shutterstock.com

REVIEW QUESTIONS

1 What is expected of a new salon employee, and what are two things you must do every day?

2 What are six habits of a good salon team player?

3 What are the three most common methods of salon compensation you're likely to encounter?

4 What are five principles of selling salon products and services? Explain them.

5 What are six ways to expand your client base?

STUDY TOOLS

- **Reinforce what you just learned:** Complete the activities and exercises in your Theory or Practical Workbook, or your Study Guide.

- **Expand your knowledge:** Search for websites about the topics in this chapter and make a list of additional resources.

- **Study and prepare for your quiz:** Take the chapter test in your Exam Review or your Milady U: Online Licensing Prep.

- **Re-Test your knowledge:** Take the Chapter 31 *Quizzes*!

- **Learn even more:** Look up in a dictionary or search the internet for the definitions of any additional terms you want to learn about.

CHAPTER GLOSSARY

client base	p. 1065	Customers who are loyal to a particular cosmetologist.
commission KAHM-ish-un	p. 1061	A percentage of the revenue that the salon takes in from services performed by a particular cosmetologist, usually offered to that cosmetologist once the individual has built up a loyal clientele.
job description	p. 1060	Document that outlines all the duties and responsibilities of a particular position in a salon or spa.
retailing	p. 1067	The act of recommending and selling products to your clients for at-home use.
ticket upgrading	p. 1067	Also known as *upselling services*; the practice of recommending and selling additional services to your clients.

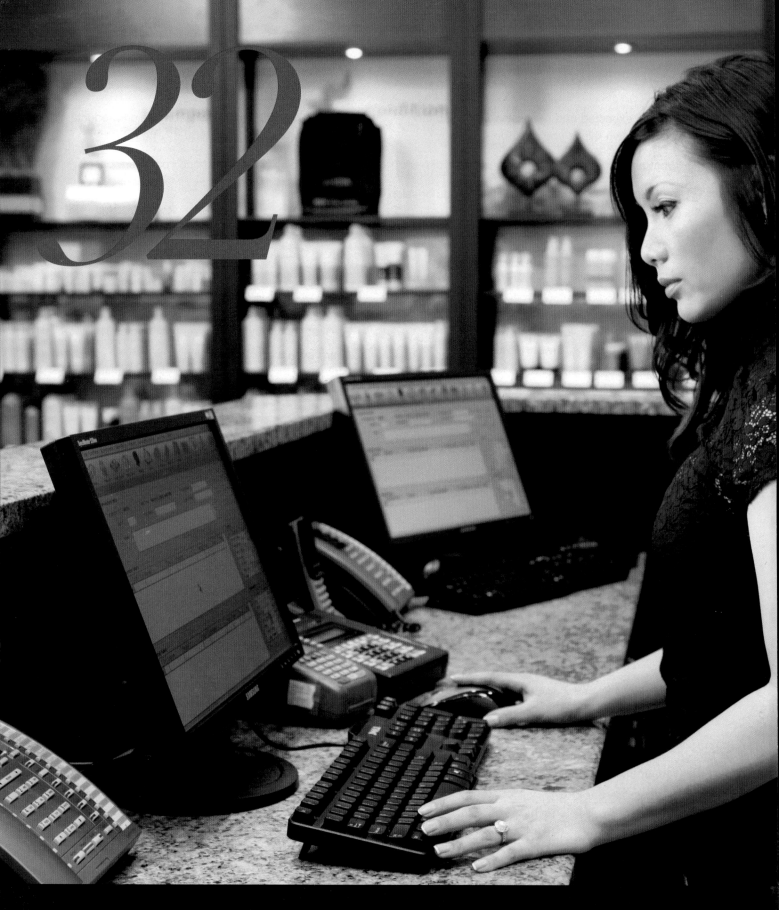

32

THE SALON BUSINESS

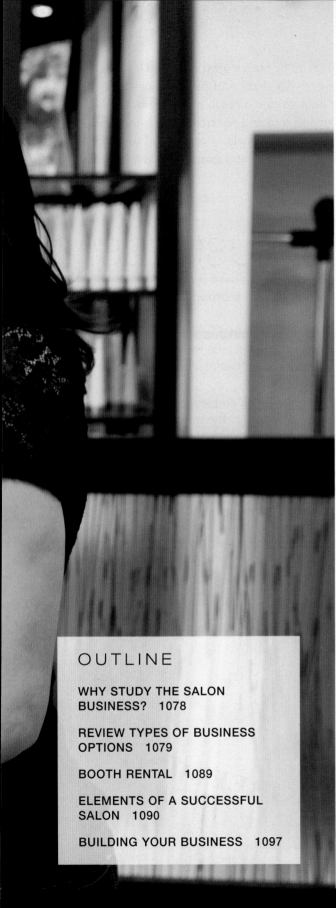

LEARNING OBJECTIVES

After completing this chapter, you will be able to:

LO❶
Identify two options for going into business for yourself.

LO❷
List the basic factors to be considered when opening a salon.

LO❸
Compare the types of salon ownership.

LO❹
Recognize the information that should be included in a business plan.

LO❺
Explain the importance of record keeping.

LO❻
Examine the responsibilities of a booth renter.

LO❼
Distinguish the elements of successful salon operations.

LO❽
Validate why selling services and products is a vital aspect of a salon's success.

The better prepared you are to be both a great artist and a successful businessperson, the greater your chances of success (figure 32-1).

Entire books have been written on each of the topics touched on in this chapter, so be prepared to read and research your business idea extensively before making any final decisions about opening a business. The following information is only meant to be a general overview.

why study
THE SALON BUSINESS?

Cosmetologists should study and have a thorough understanding of the salon business because:

> As you become more proficient in your craft and your ability to manage yourself and others, you may decide to become an independent booth renter or even a salon owner. In fact, most owners are former stylists.

> Even if you spend your entire career as an employee of someone else's salon, you should have a familiarity of the rules of business that affect the salon. It is also important to look at your career behind the chair as your own business.

> To become a successful entrepreneur, you will need to attract employees and clients to your business and maintain their loyalty over long periods of time.

> Even if you think you will be involved in the artistic aspect of salons forever, business knowledge will serve you well in managing your career and professional finances, as well as your business practices.

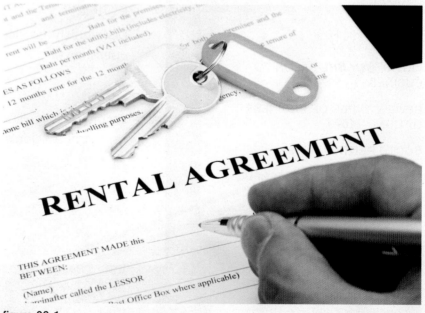

figure 32-1
Opening your own salon or spa is a big step.

Review Types of Business Options

If you reach a point in your life when you feel that you are ready to become your own boss, you will have two main options to consider: (1) owning your own salon, or (2) renting a booth in an existing salon.

Both options are extremely serious undertakings that require significant financial investment and a strong line of credit. Salon owners have a very different job than hairdressers. Typically, owners continue to work behind the chair while they manage the business. This is extremely time consuming, and there is no guarantee of profits, which is why salon ownership is definitely not for everyone. Owning your own salon and renting a booth have different pros and cons.

Opening Your Own Salon

Opening your own salon is a huge undertaking—financially, physically, creatively, and mentally—because you will face challenges that are complex and unfamiliar to you. Before you can open your doors, you'll need to decide what products to use and carry, what types of marketing and promotions you will employ, the best method and philosophy for running the business and creating a culture, and whom to hire if you need additional staff.

Regardless of the type of salon you hope to open, you should carefully consider basic issues and perform basic tasks, as outlined in the following section.

Create Your Brand identity

Creating your brand identity from at the start is essential in building a unique, successful business. To create your brand, start by identifying a few simple concepts to use as building blocks for your brand identity.

- What is your point of difference? What is going to make a client want to visit your business vs. the one across the street?

- What are you selling? Every salon sells haircuts and haircolor; think beyond the obvious. Are you selling a luxury experience, a family-friendly environment, or a cost-conscious express service?

- What is your aesthetic? Will there be a consistent color, theme, or uniform for your staff?

Identifying the answers to the three main questions above will solidify your concepts and serve as reference. Refer to them frequently for inspiration, guidance, and a reminder of what your business is built upon.

Create a Vision and Mission Statement for the Business with Goals

A **vision statement** is a long-term picture of the long-term goals for the business, what it is to become, and what it will look like when it gets there. A mission statement is a guide to the actions of the organization: It spells out the overall goals, provides a path, and contains the core values to help guide decision making. The mission statement lays the foundation for how your company's strategies are created. **Goals** are an essential set of benchmarks that, once achieved, help you to realize your mission and your vision. It is important to set realistic goals for both the short term and long term.

Create a Business Timeline

While initially you will be concerned with the first two aspects of the timeline, once your business is successful you will need to think about the others as well.

- **Year One:** It could take a year or more to determine and complete all of the aspects of starting the business.

- **Years Two to Five:** This time period is for tending to the business, its clientele, and its employees and for growing and expanding the business so that it is profitable.

- **Years Five to Ten:** This time period, if successfully achieved, can be for adding more locations, expanding the scope of the business (for example, adding spa services), construction of a larger space, or anything else you or your clients need and want.

- **Years 11 to 20:** In this time period, you may want to move from being a working cosmetologist into a full-time manager of the overall business and to begin planning for your eventual retirement.

- **Year 20 Onward:** This may be the perfect time to consider selling your successful business or changing it in some way, such as taking on a junior partner and training him or her to take over the day-to-day operations of the business so you can have time away from the business to explore interests or hobbies.

Determine Business Feasibility

Determining whether or not the business you envision is feasible means addressing certain practical issues. For example, do you have a special skill or talent that can help you set your business apart from other salons in your area? Does the town or area in which you are planning to locate the business offer you the appropriate type of clientele for the products and services you want to offer? Based on what you envision for the business, how much money will you need to open the business? Is this funding available to you?

Choose a Business Name

The name you select for your business explains what it is and can also identify characteristics that set your business apart from competitors in the marketplace. The name you select for your business will also influence how clients and potential clients perceive the business. The name will create a picture of your business in clients' minds, and once that picture exists it can be very difficult to change it if you are not satisfied. In addition, once your business is named, it is complicated to make all of the legal, banking, and tax changes if you change your mind.

Choose a Location

You will want to base your business location on your primary clientele and their needs. Select a location that has good visibility, high traffic, easy access, sufficient parking, and handicap access (figure 32-2).

Written Agreements

Many **written agreements** and documents govern the opening of a salon, including leases, vendor contracts, employee contracts, and more. All of these written agreements detail, usually for legal purposes, who does what and what is given in return. You must be able to read and understand them. Additionally, before you open a salon, you must develop a **business plan** (BIZ-nez plahn), a written description of your business as you see it today and as you foresee it in the next five years (detailed by year). A business plan is more of an agreement with yourself, and it is not legally binding. However, if you wish to obtain financing, it is essential that you have a business plan in place first. The plan should include a general description of the business and the services that it will provide; area **demographics** (dem-oh-graf-iks), which consist of information about a specific population, including data on race, age, income, and educational attainment; expected salaries and cost of related benefits; an operations plan that includes pricing structure and expenses, such as equipment, supplies, repairs, advertising, taxes, and insurance; and projected income and overhead expenses for up to five years. A certified public accountant (CPA) can be invaluable in helping you gather accurate financial information. The Chamber of Commerce in your proposed area typically has information on area demographics.

Business Regulations and Laws

Business regulations and laws (BIZ-nez reg-U-lay-shuns AND LAWZ), are any and all local, state, and federal regulations and laws that you must comply with when you decide to open your salon or rent a booth. Since the laws change from year to year and vary from state to state and from city to city, it is important that you contact your local authorities regarding business licenses, permits, and other regulations, such as zoning and business inspections. Additionally, you must know and comply with all federal Occupational Safety and Health Administration (OSHA) guidelines, including those requiring that information about the ingredients of cosmetic preparations be available to employees. OSHA requires Safety Data Sheets (SDSs) for this purpose. There are also many federal laws that apply to hiring and firing, payment of benefits, contributions to employee entitlements (for example, social security and unemployment), and workplace behavior.

Understanding the laws and rules of owning a salon is imperative to running a successful business. The laws and rules not only lay the foundation of acceptable guidelines regarding hiring and firing, they also build a framework for day to day policies and procedures and safety. Not following the laws and rules can result in costly fines and heavy penalties. It is important to become very familiar with the local, state, and federal laws and rules before you open your business.

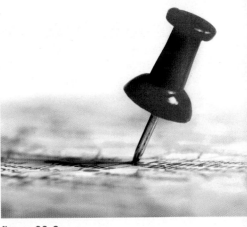

figure 32-2
Location. Location. Location. Your salon should have good visibility and high pedestrian traffic.

When you open your business, you will need to purchase **insurance** that guarantees protection against financial loss from malpractice, property liability, fire, burglary and theft, and business interruption. You will need to have disability policies as well. Make sure that your policies cover you for all the monetary demands you will have to meet on your lease.

Salon Operation

Business or **salon operation** refers to the ongoing, recurring processes or activities involved in the running of a business for the purpose of producing income and value.

Record Keeping

Record keeping is the act of maintaining accurate and complete records of all financial activities in your business.

Salon Policies

Salon policies are the rules and regulations adopted by a salon to ensure that all clients and associates are being treated fairly and consistently. Even small salons and booth renters should have salon policies in place.

After reading the next few sections, you will be able to:

LO❸ Compare the types of salon ownership.

Types of Salon Ownership

A salon can be owned and operated by an individual, a partnership, or a corporation or franchise. Before deciding which type of ownership is most desirable for your situation, research each option thoroughly. There are excellent reference tools available, and you can also consult a small business attorney for advice.

Individual Ownership

If you like to make your own rules and are responsible enough to meet all the duties and obligations of running a business, individual ownership may be the best arrangement for you.

The **sole proprietor** (SOHL PRHO-pry-eh-tohr) is the individual owner and, most often, the manager of the business who:

• Determines policies and has the last say in decision making.

• Assumes expenses, receives profits, and bears all losses.

Partnership

Partnerships may mean more opportunity for increased investment and growth. They can be magical if the right chemistry exists, or they can be disastrous if you find yourself linked with someone you wish you had known better in the first place. Your partner can incur losses or debts that you may not even be aware of unless you use a third-party accountant. Trust is just one of the requirements for this arrangement.

In a **partnership** business structure, two or more people share ownership—although not necessarily equally.

- One reason for going into a partnership arrangement is to have more **capital**, or money to invest in a business; another is to have help running your operation.

- Partners also pool their skills and talents, making it easier to share work, responsibilities, and decision making (**figure 32-3**).

- Keep in mind that partners must assume one another's liability for debts.

Corporation

A **corporation** (KOR-pour-aye-shun) is an ownership structure controlled by one or more stockholders. Incorporating is one of the best ways that a business owner can protect her or his personal assets. Most people choose to incorporate solely for this reason, but there are other advantages as well. For example, the corporate business structure saves you money in taxes, provides greater business flexibility, and makes raising capital easier. It also limits your personal financial liability if your business accrues unmanageable debts or otherwise runs into financial trouble.

Characteristics of corporations are generally as follows:

- Corporations raise capital by issuing stock certificates or shares.

- Stockholders (people or companies that purchase shares) have an ownership interest in the company. The more stock they own, the bigger that interest becomes.

- You can be the sole stockholder (or shareholder), or you can have many stockholders.

- Corporate formalities, such as director and stockholder meetings, are required to maintain a corporate status.

- Income tax is limited to the salary that you draw and not the total profits of the business.

- Corporations cost more to set up and run than a sole proprietorship or partnership. For example, there are the initial formation fees, filing fees, and annual state fees.

- A stockholder of a corporation is required to pay unemployment insurance taxes on his or her salary, whereas a sole proprietor or partner is not.

Franchise Ownership

A franchise is a form of business organization in which a firm that is already successful (the franchisor) enters into a continuing contractual relationship with other businesses (franchisees) operating under the franchisor's trade name in exchange for a fee. When you operate a franchise salon, you usually operate under the franchisor's guidance and must adhere to a contract with many stipulations. These stipulations ensure that all locations in the franchise are run in a similar manner, look the same way, use the same logos, and, sometimes, even train the same way or carry the same retail products.

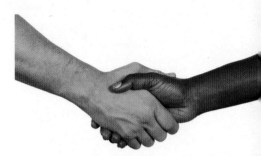

figure 32-3
Partners share the rewards and the responsibilities.

? DID YOU KNOW?

When you open your own business, you should consult with an attorney and an accountant before filing any documents to legalize your business. It is helpful to find these kinds of professionals who have previous experience in the salon business. Your attorney will advise you of the legal documents and obligations that you will take on as a business owner, and your accountant can inform you of the ways in which your business may be registered for tax purposes.

Franchises offer the advantage of a known name and brand recognition, and the franchisor does most of the marketing for you. Also, many have protected territories, meaning another franchise salon with the same name cannot open up within your fixed geographic area. However, franchise agreements vary widely in what you can and cannot do on your own. Owning a franchise is no guarantee of making a profit, and you should always research the franchise, talk to other owners of the franchise's salons, and have an attorney read the contract and explain anything you do not understand, including your precise obligations and arrangements for paying the franchise fee. In most cases, whether or not you are profitable, you must pay the fee.

After reading the next few sections, you will be able to:

LO ④ Recognize the information that should be included in a business plan.

Business Plan

Regardless of the type of salon you plan to own, it is imperative to have a thorough and well-researched business plan. Remember, the business plan is a written plan of a business as it is seen in the present and envisioned in the future, and it follows your business throughout the entire process from start-up through many years in the future. Many, many books, classes, DVDs, and websites offer much more detailed information than can be provided here, but below is a sampling of the kinds of information and materials that a business plan should include.

- **Executive Summary.** Summarizes your plan and states your objectives.
- **Vision Statement.** A long-term picture of what the business is to become and what it will look like when it gets there.
- **Mission Statement.** A description of the key strategic influences of the business, such as the market it will serve, the kinds of services it will offer, and the quality of those services.
- **Organizational Plan.** Outlines employees and management levels and also describes how the business will run administratively.
- **Marketing Plan.** Outlines all of the research obtained regarding the clients your business will target and their needs, wants, and habits.
- **Financial Documents.** Includes the projected financial statements, actual (historical) statements, and financial statement analysis.
- **Supporting Documents.** Includes owner's resume, personal financial information, legal contracts, and any other agreements.
- **Salon Policies.** Even small salons and booth renters should have policies that they adhere to. These ensure that all clients and employees are treated fairly and consistently.

Purchasing an Established Salon

Purchasing an existing salon could be an excellent opportunity, but, as with anything else, you have to look at all sides of the picture. If you

? DID YOU KNOW?
Your accountant may suggest that your business become an S Corporation (Small Business Corporation), which is a business elected for S Corporation status through the IRS. This status allows the taxation of the company to be similar to a partnership or sole proprietor as opposed to paying taxes based on a corporate tax structure. Or your accountant may suggest that your business become registered as an LLC (Limited Liability Company), which is a type of business ownership combining several features of corporation and partnership structures. Owners of an LLC also have the liability protection of a corporation. An LLC exists as a separate entity, much like a corporation. Members cannot be held personally liable for debts unless they have signed a personal guarantee.

choose to buy an established salon, seek professional assistance from an accountant and a business lawyer (figure 32-4). You can purchase all the assets of a salon, or some or all of its stock. It is important to know, if you purchase an established salon, you are not purchasing the staff or clientele. There is no guarantee that with new ownership the staff will be retained or that the clients will continue to return. In general, any agreement to buy an established salon should include the following items:

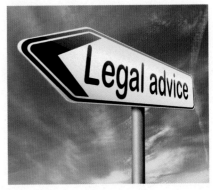

figure 32-4
A lawyer specializing in leases and business sales is a good source of professional advice.

- A financial audit to determine the actual value of the business once the current owner's bookings are taken out of the equation. Often, the salon owner brings in the bulk of the business income, and it is unlikely you will retain all the former owner's clients without a lot of support and encouragement from that former owner. Any existing financial statements should also be audited.

- Written purchase and sale agreement to avoid any misunderstandings between the contracting parties.

- Complete and signed statement of inventory (goods, fixtures, and the like) indicating the value of each article.

- If there is a transfer of a note, mortgage, lease, or bill of sale, the buyer should initiate an investigation to determine whether there are defaults in the payment of debts.

- Confirmed identity of owner.

- Use of the salon's name and reputation for a definite period of time.

- Disclosure of any and all information regarding the salon's clientele and its purchasing and service habits.

- Disclosure of the conditions of the facility. If you are buying the actual building, a full inspection is in order, and many other legalities apply. Be guided by your realtor and attorney.

- Non-compete agreement stating that the seller will not work in or establish a new salon within a specified distance from the present location.

 ACTIVITY

Form student groups to plan the practical side of your own salons. Divide into teams. Designate certain tasks to specific team members, or decide if everyone will work on every task as a group.

- Each group should perform the following tasks:
- Decide on a name for their salon.
- Determine what services will be offered.
- Create fun signage for the salon's exterior.
- Write a vision statement for their salon.
- Write a mission statement for their salon.
- Create an organizational plan and a marketing plan for their salon.

Most students will not be able to develop complex budgets, but if you feel up to it, decide on a specific budget and allocate it to key areas, such as decorating, equipment, supplies, and personnel. Ask your instructors to provide feedback about whether your budget is realistic.

- An employee agreement, either formal or informal, that lets you know if the employees will stay with the business under its new ownership. Existing employee contracts should be transferable.

Drawing Up a Lease

In most cases, owning your own business does not mean that you own the building that houses your business. When renting or leasing space, you must have an agreement between yourself and the building's owner that has been well thought out and well written. The lease should specify clearly who owns what and who is responsible for which repairs and expenses. You should also secure the following:

- Exemption of fixtures or appliances that might be attached to the salon so that they can be removed without violating the lease.

- Agreement about necessary renovations and repairs, such as painting, plumbing, fixtures, and electrical installation.

- Option from the landlord that allows you to assign the lease to another person. In this way, obligations for the payment of rent are kept separate from the responsibilities of operating the business, should you decide to bring in another person or owner.

Protection Against Fire, Theft, and Lawsuits

- Ensure that your business has adequate locks, fire alarm system, burglar alarm system, and surveillance system.

- Purchase liability, fire, malpractice, and burglary insurance, and do not allow these policies to lapse while you are in business.

- Become thoroughly familiar with all laws governing cosmetology and with the safety and infection control codes of your city and state.

- Keep accurate records of the number of employees, their salaries, lengths of employment, and Social Security numbers as required by various state and federal laws that monitor the social welfare of workers.

- Ignorance of the law is no excuse for violating it. Always check with your regulatory agency if you have any questions about a law or regulation.

Business Operations

Whether you are an owner or a manager, there are certain skills that you must develop in order to successfully run a salon. To run a people-oriented business, you need:

- An excellent business sense, aptitude, good judgment, and diplomacy.
- Knowledge of sound business principles.

Because it takes time to develop these skills, you would be wise to establish a circle of contacts—business owners, including some salon owners—who can give you advice along the way. Consider joining a local entrepreneurs' group or your city's Chamber of Commerce in order to extend the reach of your networking. The Chamber of Commerce is a local organization of businesses and business owners whose goal is to promote, protect, and further the interests of businesses in a community.

Smooth business management depends on the following factors:

- Sufficient investment capital
- Efficiency of management
- Good business procedures
- Strong computer skills
- Cooperation between management and employees
- Trained and experienced salon personnel (**figure 32-5**)
- Excellent customer service delivery
- Proper pricing of services (**figure 32-6**)

Allocation of Money

As a business operator, you must always know where your money is being spent. A good accountant and an accounting system are indispensable. The figures in **table 32-1** serve as a guideline, but may vary depending on locality.

After reading the next few sections, you will be able to:

LO ⑤ Explain the importance of record keeping.

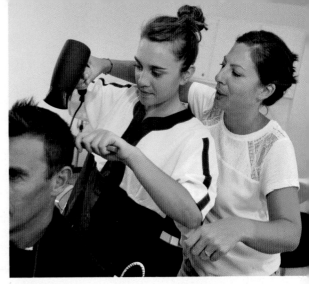

figure 32-5
Coaching a new stylist

The Importance of Record Keeping

Good business operations require a simple and efficient record system. Proper business records are necessary to meet the requirements of local, state, and federal laws regarding taxes and employees. Records are of value only if they are correct, concise, and complete. Proper bookkeeping methods include keeping an accurate record of all income and expenses. Income is usually classified as receipts from services and retail sales. Expenses include rent, utilities, insurance, salaries, advertising, equipment, and repairs. Retain all check stubs, cancelled checks, receipts, and invoices. A professional accountant or a full-charge bookkeeper is recommended to help keep records accurate (**table 32-1**). Please note table 32-1 is a generalization, and percentages can vary from city to city. For example, rent in New York City may be a different percentage of sales than in Duluth, Minnesota.

The term *full-charge bookkeeper* refers to someone who is trained to do everything from recording sales and payroll to generating a profit-and-loss statement. The most important part of record keeping is having the ability to defend your business in the case of an audit by the federal or state government and to have accurate proof of all sales made and taxes paid.

Purchase and Inventory Records

The purchase of inventory and supplies should be closely monitored. Purchase records help you maintain a perpetual

figure 32-6
Example of service menu of a high end image salon (See Chapter 30, Preparing for Licensure and Employment, for description).

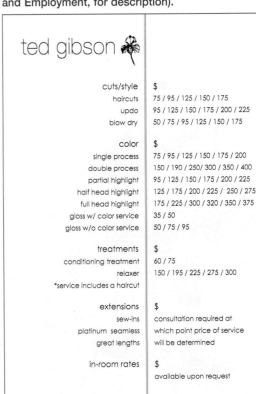

ted gibson	
cuts/style	$
haircuts	75 / 95 / 125 / 150 / 175
updo	95 / 125 / 150 / 175 / 200 / 225
blow dry	50 / 75 / 95 / 125 / 150 / 175
color	$
single process	75 / 95 / 125 / 150 / 175 / 200
double process	150 / 190 / 250/ 300 / 350 / 400
partial highlight	95 / 125 / 150 / 175 / 200 / 225
half head highlight	125 / 175 / 200 / 225 / 250 / 275
full head highlight	175 / 225 / 300 / 320 / 350 / 375
gloss w/ color service	35 / 50
gloss w/o color service	50 / 75 / 95
treatments	$
conditioning treatment	60 / 75
relaxer	150 / 195 / 225 / 275 / 300
*service includes a haircut	
extensions	$
sew-ins	consultation required at
platinum seamless	which point price of service
great lengths	will be determined
in-room rates	$
	available upon request
	pricing does not include gratuities

table 32-1

FINANCIAL BENCHMARKS FOR SALONS IN THE UNITED STATES

Expenses	Percent of Total Gross Income
Salaries and Commissions (Including Payroll Taxes)	53.5
Rent	13.0
Supplies	5.0
Advertising	3.0
Depreciation	3.0
Laundry	1.0
Cleaning	1.0
Light and Power	1.0
Repairs	1.5
Insurance	0.75
Telephone	0.75
Miscellaneous	1.5
Total Expenses	85.0
Net Profit	15.0
Total	100.0

Courtesy Kopsa Otte CPAs & Advisors in York, NE, nationally known as the only accounting firm that specializes in salons and spas.

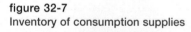

figure 32-7
Inventory of consumption supplies

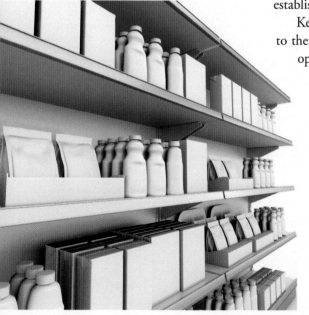

inventory, which prevents overstocking or a shortage of needed supplies, and they alert you to any incidents of theft. Purchase records also help establish the net worth of the business at the end of the year.

Keep a running inventory of all supplies, and classify them according to their use and retail value. Those to be used in the daily business operation are **consumption supplies** (KON-sump-shun sup-LYZ) (figure 32-7). Those to be sold to clients are **retail supplies**. Both categories have different tax responsibilities, so be sure to check with your accountant that you are charging the proper taxes.

Service Records

Always keep service records or client cards that describe treatments given and merchandise sold to each client. Using a salon-specific software program for this purpose is highly recommended. All service records should include the name and address of the client, the date of each purchase or service, the amount charged, the products used, and the results obtained. Clients' preferences and tastes should also be noted. For more information on filling out these cards, and for examples of a client record card, see Chapter 4, Communicating for Success.

© Gepardu/Shutterstock.com

Booth Rental

Booth rental (BOO-th ren-tal), also known as *chair rental* is renting a booth or a station in a salon. This practice is popular in salons all over the United States. Many people see booth rental or renting a station in a salon as a more desirable alternative to owning a salon.

In a booth rental arrangement, a professional generally rents a station or work space in a salon for a weekly fee paid to the salon owner. A booth renter is solely responsible for his or her own clientele, supplies, record keeping, and accounting and has the ability to be his or her own boss with very little capital investment.

Booth rental is a desirable situation for many cosmetologists who have large, steady clientele and who do not have to rely on the salon's general clientele to keep busy. Unless you are at least 70 percent booked all the time, however, it may not be advantageous to rent a booth.

Although it may sound like a good option, booth renting has its share of obligations, such as:

- Keeping records for income tax purposes and other legal reasons.
- Paying all taxes, including higher Social Security (double that of an employee).
- Carrying adequate malpractice insurance and health insurance.
- Complying with all IRS obligations for independent contractors. Go to irs.gov and search for independent contractors.
- Using your own telephone and booking systems.
- Collecting all service fees, whether they are paid in cash or via a credit card.
- Creating all professional materials, including business cards and a service menu.
- Purchasing of all supplies, including back-bar and retail supplies and products.
- Tracking and maintaining inventory.
- Managing the purchase of products and supplies.
- Budgeting for advertising or offering incentives to ensure a steady flow of new clients.
- Paying for all continuing education.
- Working in an independent atmosphere where teamwork usually does not exist and where salon standards are interpreted on an individual basis.
- Adhering to state laws and regulations. To date, one state (Pennsylvania) does not allow booth rental at all; others may require that each renter in an establishment hold his or her own establishment license and carry individual liability insurance. Always check with your state regulatory agency.

? DID YOU KNOW?

Currently, booth rental is legal in every state except Pennsylvania, where there is a law prohibiting it. In New Jersey, the state board does not recognize booth rental as an acceptable method of doing business.

As a booth renter, you will not enjoy the same benefits as an employee of a salon would, such as paid days off or vacation time. Remember, as a booth renter, when you do not work, you do not get paid. Perhaps most importantly, you must continually attract new clients and maintain the ones you have, which means working the hours your clients need you to be available. For more information on booth rental as a business option, reference Milady's: *Booth Renting 101: A Guide for the Independent Stylist*.

After reading the next few sections, you will be able to:

LO **7** Distinguish the elements of successful salon operations.

LO **8** Validate why selling services and products is a vital aspect of a salon's success.

Elements of a Successful Salon

The only way to guarantee that you will stay in business and have a prosperous salon is to take excellent care of your clients. Clients visiting your salon should feel that they are being well taken care of, and they should always have reason to look forward to their next visit. To accomplish this, your salon must be physically attractive, well organized, smoothly run, and, above all, sparkling clean.

Planning the Salon's Layout

One of the most exciting opportunities ahead of you is planning and constructing the best physical layout for the type of salon you envision. Maximum efficiency should be the primary concern. For example, if you are opening a low-budget salon offering quick service, you will need several stations and a small- to medium-sized reception area because clients will be moving in and out of the salon fairly quickly. Retail sales are essential to a profitable salon business. Make sure the products you carry and the space you design reflect the importance of high retail sales (**figure 32-8**).

However, if you are opening a high-end salon or luxurious day spa where clients expect the quality of the service to be matched by the environment, you may want to plan for more room in the waiting area. In fact, you might choose to have several areas in which clients can lounge between services and enjoy beverages or light snacks. The spa area and quiet rooms should be separated from busy, noisy areas where hair services are performed. Some upscale salons feature small coffee bars that lend an air of sophistication to the environment. Others offer quiet, private areas where clients can pursue business activities, such as phone or laptop work between services. Most salons provide complimentary wifi access to their guests. The retail area should be spacious, inviting, and well lit. High-end salons and spas are extremely costly to design, construct, and maintain. Construction alone can be upward of $300 per square foot.

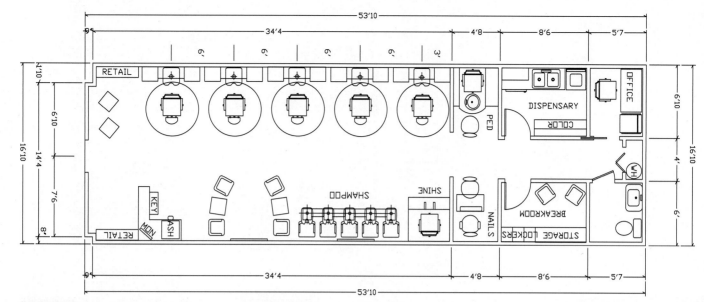

figure 32-8
Layout for a typical salon

Layout is crucial to the smooth operation of a salon. Once you have decided the type of salon that you wish to run, seek the advice of an architect with plenty of experience in designing salons. For renovations, a professional equipment and furniture supplier will be able to help you (**figure 32-9**).

Costs to create even a small salon in an existing space can range from $75 to $125 per square foot. Renovating existing space requires familiarity with building codes and the landlord's restrictions before you do anything. All the plumbing should be in the same area, and electrical wiring must be up to code. If they are not, you'll pay thousands extra. Before you begin, get everything in writing from contractors, design firms, equipment manufacturers, and architects. It is a good idea to get three quotes on everything from contractors and cleaning services to salon stations and equipment. Don't be afraid to negotiate whenever you can (**figure 32-10**).

Try to estimate how much each area in the salon will earn, so you can use space efficiently. An inviting retail display in your reception area is a good investment; on the other hand, an employee break area produces no income. In addition to start-up costs for creating your salon, you'll need financing for operational expenses. Realistically, you should plan to have at least several months and up to one year of expenses available to help get you up and running. It takes most new salons about six months to begin operating at full capacity

Personnel

Your **personnel** (PER-son-elle) is your staff or employees. The size of your salon will determine the size of your staff. Large salons and day spas require receptionists, hairstylists, colorists, nail technicians, assistants, massage therapists, estheticians, hair removal specialists, and housekeepers.

Smaller salons have some combination of these personnel who perform more than one type of service. For example, a stylist might also be the

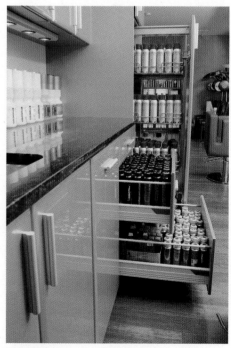

figure 32-9
Salon haircolor dispensary

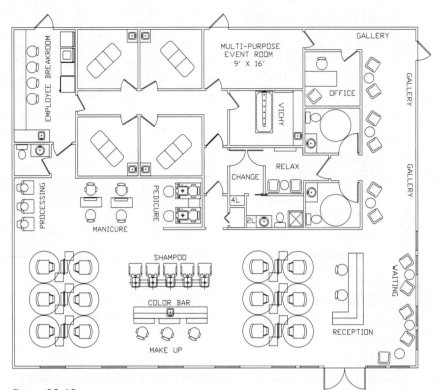

figure 32-10
A typical layout for a larger spa/salon

colorist and texture specialist. Ultimately, whether your salon is large or small, high end or economical, the success of a salon depends on the attitude and quality of work done by the staff.

When interviewing potential employees, consider the following:

- **Level of skill.** What is their educational background? When was the last time they attended an educational event? How long have they been in the industry? What can they bring to the organization beyond hairdressing or haircoloring?

- **Personal grooming.** Do they look like professionals you would consult for personal grooming advice?

- **Image as it relates to the salon.** Are they too progressive or too conservative for your environment? Does their image reflect the image of your business?

- **Overall attitude.** Are they mostly positive or mostly negative in their responses to your questions? Do they seem self motivated and self directed?

- **Communication skills.** Are they able to understand your questions? Can you understand their responses?

- **Work history.** Have they been at a previous salon for many years, or do they hop from salon to salon? Are they bringing a clientele, or do they expect you to build one for them?

Making good hiring decisions is crucial. Undoing bad hiring decisions is painful for all involved, and it can be more complicated than one might expect.

Payroll and Employee Benefits

In order to have a successful business, one in which everyone feels appreciated and is happy to work hard to service clients well, you must be willing to share your success with your staff whenever it is financially feasible to do so. You can do this in a number of ways.

- Make it your top priority to meet your payroll obligations. In the allotment of funds, this comes first. It will also be your largest expense.

- Whenever possible, offer hardworking and loyal employees as many benefits as possible. Either cover the cost of these benefits, or simply make them available to employees, who can decide if they can cover the cost themselves.

- Provide staff members with a schedule of employee evaluations. Make it clear what is expected of them if they are to receive pay increases.

- Create and stay with a tipping policy. It is a good idea both for your employees and your clients to know exactly what is expected. It is also important to be familiar with the tax laws around tipping.

- Put your entire pay plan in writing.

- Create incentives by giving your staff opportunities to earn more money, prizes, or tickets to educational events and trade shows; when there is a reward involved it can inspire employees to achieve more.

- Create salon policies and stick to them. Everyone in the salon should be governed by the same rules, including you!

Managing Personnel

As a new salon owner, one of your most challenging tasks will be managing your staff. At the same time, leading your team can also be very rewarding. If you are good at managing others, you can make a positive impact on their lives and their ability to earn a living. If managing people does not come naturally to you, don't despair. People can learn how to manage other people, just as they learn how to drive a car or perform hair services. Keep in mind that managing others is a serious job. Whether it comes naturally to you or not, it takes time to become comfortable with the role.

Human Resources, or HR, is an entire specialty in its own right. It not only covers how you manage employees, it also covers what you can and cannot say when hiring, managing, or firing. All employers must be familiar with various civil rights laws, including Equal Employment Opportunity Commission (EEOC) regulations, and the Americans with Disabilities Act (ADA), which pertains to hiring and firing, as well as business design for accessibility. Every business should have a written personnel policies and a procedures manual, and every employee must read and sign it. If you choose to use a payroll company, they can provide HR services and employee manuals for a nominal fee. The more documented systems you have for managing human resources, the better.

There are many excellent books, both within and outside the professional salon industry that you can use as resources for learning about managing employees and staff. Spend an afternoon online or at your local bookstore researching the topic and purchasing materials or registering for classes that will educate and inform you. Once you have a broad base of

ACTIVITY

What would your dream salon look like? Try your hand at designing a salon that would attract the kinds of clients you want, offer the services you would like to specialize in, and provide an efficient, comfortable working environment for cosmetology professionals.

Draw pictures, use word pictures, or try a combination of both. Pay attention to practical requirements, but feel free to dream a little, too. Skylights? Fountains? You name it. It's your dream (**figure 32-11**)!

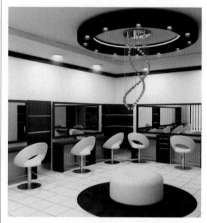

figure 32-11
What does your dream salon look like?

information, you will be able to select a technique or style that best suits your personality and that of your salon.

The Front Desk

Most salon owners believe that the quality and pricing of services are the most important elements of running a successful salon. Certainly these are crucial, but too often the front desk—the operations center—is overlooked. The best salons employ professional receptionists to handle the job of answering phones, scheduling appointments, greeting clients, and attending to the client's needs.

The Reception Area

First impressions count, and since the reception area is the first thing clients see, it needs to be attractive, appealing, and comfortable. This is your salon's nerve center, where your receptionist will stand, where retail merchandise will be on display, and where the phone system is centered.

Make sure that the reception area is stocked with business cards and a prominently displayed price list that shows at a glance what your clients should expect to pay for various services.

The Receptionist

When it comes to staffing, your receptionist is second in importance only to your licensed professionals. A well-trained receptionist is crucial because the receptionist is the first and last person the client contacts. The receptionist should have an image that reflects your brand, should be pleasant, should greet each client with a smile, and should address each client by name. Efficient, friendly, and consistent service fosters goodwill, confidence, and satisfaction.

In addition to filling the crucial role of greeter, the receptionist handles other important functions, including answering the phone, booking appointments, informing professionals that a client has arrived, preparing daily appointment information for the staff, and recommending additional services and products to clients. The receptionist should have a thorough knowledge of all retail products carried by the salon so that she or he can also serve as a salesperson and information source for clients (figure 32-12).

During slow periods, it is customary for the receptionist to perform certain other duties and activities, such as straightening up the reception area and maintaining inventory and daily reports. Personal calls or personal projects are done on personal time, not at work.

Booking Appointments

The key duty of the receptionist is booking appointments. This must be done with care because services are sold in terms of time on the appointment page. Appointments must be scheduled to make the most efficient use of everyone's time—both the client and the service provider.

Under ideal circumstances, a client should not have to wait for a service, and a professional should not have to wait for the next client.

Booking appointments is primarily the receptionist's job, but when he or she is not available, the salon owner or

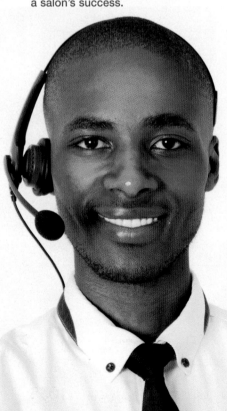

figure 32-12
A good receptionist is key to a salon's success.

manager or in small salons, or one of the other professionals can help with scheduling. It is important for each person involved in working the reception area to understand how to book an appointment and how much time is needed for each service. Regardless of who actually makes the appointment, anyone who answers the phone or deals with clients must have a pleasing voice and personality.

In addition, the receptionist must have the following qualities:

• Appearance that conveys your salon's image.

• Knowledge of the various services offered.

• Unlimited patience with both clients and salon personnel.

Appointment Book

The appointment book helps professionals arrange time to suit their clients' needs. It should accurately reflect what is taking place in the salon at any given time. In most salons, the receptionist prepares the appointment schedule for staff members; in smaller salons, each person may prepare his own schedule (figure 32-13).

Increasingly, the appointment book is a computerized book that is easily accessed through the salon's computer system. It may also be an actual hard copy book that is located on the reception desk. Some salons have websites with online booking systems, which tie in to salon management software.

Use of the Telephone in the Salon

An important part of the business is handled over the telephone. Good telephone habits and techniques make it possible for the salon owner and employees to increase business and improve relationships with clients and suppliers. With each call, a gracious, appropriate response will help build the salon's reputation. For example, "Thank you for calling Milady Salon, Shannon speaking. How may I help you?"

Good Planning

Because it can be noisy, business calls to clients and suppliers should be made at a quiet time of the day or from a quiet area of the salon.

When using the telephone, you should:

• Have a pleasant telephone voice, speak clearly, and use correct grammar. A smile on your face will be reflected in your voice and counts for a lot.

• Show interest and concern when talking with a client or a supplier.

• Be polite, respectful, and courteous to all, even though some people may test the limits of your patience.

• Be tactful. Do not say anything to irritate the person on the other end of the line.

Incoming Telephone Calls

Incoming phone calls are the lifeline of a salon. Oftentimes, an incoming call is your client's first impression of your business. Clients usually call

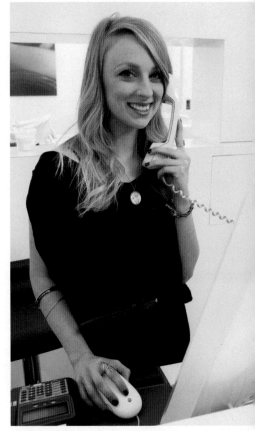

figure 32-13
Computerized appointment book

ahead for appointments with a preferred stylist, or they might call to cancel or reschedule an appointment. The person answering the phone should have the necessary telephone skills to handle these calls.

When you answer the phone, say, "Good morning (afternoon or evening), thank you for calling Milady Salon. How May I help you?" or "Thank you for calling Milady Salon. This is Jane speaking. How may I help you?" Some salons require that you give your name to the caller. The first words you say tell the caller something about your personality. Let callers know that you are glad to hear from them.

Answer the phone promptly. A good rule of thumb is to not let the phone ring more than three times. On a system with more than one line, if a call comes in while you are talking on another line, ask to put the first person on hold, answer the second call, and ask that person to hold while you complete the first call. Take calls in the order in which they are received.

If you do not have the information requested by a caller, either put the caller on hold and get the information, or offer to call the person back with the information as soon as you have it.

Do not talk with a client standing nearby while you are speaking with someone on the phone. Have one conversation at a time. You are doing a disservice to both clients.

Booking Appointments by Phone

When booking appointments, take down the client's first and last name, their phone number, their email address, and the service booked. Many salons call the client to confirm the appointment one or two days before it is scheduled. Automated systems can send an e-mail or even a text message confirmation.

You should be familiar with all the services and products available in the salon and their costs, as well as which cosmetology professionals perform specific services, such as color correction. Be fair when making assignments. Don't schedule six appointments for one professional and only two for another, unless it's necessary because you are working with specialists.

However, if someone calls to ask for an appointment with a particular cosmetology professional on a particular day and time, make every effort to accommodate the client's request. If the professional is not available when the client requests, there are several ways to handle the situation:

- Suggest other times that the professional is available.
- If the client cannot come in at any of those times, suggest another professional.
- If the client is unwilling to try another professional, offer to call the client if there is a cancellation at the desired time.

Handling Complaints by Telephone

Handling complaints, particularly over the phone, is a difficult task. The caller is probably upset and possibly short tempered. Respond with self-control, tact, and courtesy, no matter how trying the circumstances. Only then will the caller feel that he or she has been treated fairly.

The tone of your voice must be sympathetic and reassuring. Your manner of speaking should convince the caller that you are really concerned about the complaint. Do not interrupt the caller. After hearing the complaint in full, try to resolve the situation quickly and effectively.

Building Your Business

A new salon owner will want to get the business up and running as soon as possible to start earning some revenue and to begin paying off debts. The first area of opportunity for building your business is through social media.

Social Media

The term **social media** refers to a platform used to engage and communicate with groups of people by way of online communities, networks, websites or blogs, for personal or professional means. Social Media platforms such as Facebook, Twitter, YouTube, and Instagram are free to use and a great way to build awareness about your business and at the same time engage your audience in an interactive format. Some salons have one person in charge of their social media to control the content and ensure certain standards are met. Other salons allow the salon staff to post on their behalf.

Some guidelines to effectively using social media are:

• Have the same username for all accounts.

• Get permission from clients if you use their image in your posting.

• Post regularly so your followers pay attention.

• Respond to questions, comments, or "likes."

Another, more costly option the new salon owner should consider is advertising the salon. It is important to understand the many aspects of advertising.

Advertising

The term *advertising* encompasses promotional efforts that are paid for and are directly indeed to increase business.

Advertising includes all activities that promote the salon favorably, from newspaper ads to radio spots to charity events that the salon participates in, such as fashion shows. In order to create a desire for a service or product, advertising must attract and hold the attention of readers, listeners, or viewers.

A satisfied client is the very best form of advertising because he or she will refer your salon to friends and family. So make your clients happy (**figure 32-14**)! Then, have your clients work for you. Develop a referral program and a loyalty program in which the referring client reaps a reward.

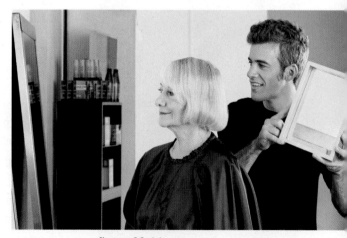

figure 32-14
Customer satisfaction is your best advertising.

If you have some experience developing ads, you may decide to do your own advertising. On the other hand, if you need help, you can hire an agency or ask a local newspaper or radio station to help you produce the ad. As a general rule, an advertising budget should not exceed three percent of your gross income. Make sure you plan well in advance for holidays and special yearly events, such as proms, New Year's Eve, or the wedding season.

Make certain you know what you are paying for. Get everything in writing. No form of advertising can promise that you'll get business. Sometimes, local circulars can work well. You must know your clientele, which types of media they use, and what kinds of messages attract them.

Here are some tools you may choose to use to attract customers to the salon:

- Newspaper ads and coupons (**figure 32-15**).

- Build a website. If you don't have a large budget now, buy your domain name and keep that ownership current. You can set up a site very inexpensively and as your business grows, you can build it to have many pages and features. A website is an easy way for new clients to find you through Internet searches or friends-sharing links.

- E-mail newsletters and discount offers to all clients who have agreed to receive such mailings (Always include an *Unsubscribe* link.) You can also purchase e-mail lists targeted to your demographic to help you build your subscriber list.

- Website offerings, including those on your own website, social networking websites, and blogs.

- Direct mail to mailing lists and your current salon client list.

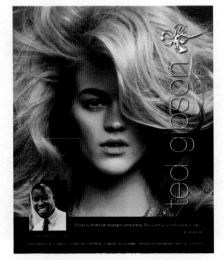

figure 32-15
Newspaper advertisement for services at the ted gibson salon.

Designed for ted gibson beauty by Laura Brill at 954 design.

- Classified advertising.
- Giveaway promotional items or retail packages, such as, "Buy a shampoo and conditioner, and get a hairbrush for free."
- Window displays that attract attention and feature the salon and your retail products.
- Radio advertising.
- Television advertising.
- Community outreach by volunteering at women's and men's clubs, church functions, political gatherings, charitable affairs, and on TV and radio talk shows.
- Make donations of services for local organizations like school fundraisers.
- Client referrals.
- In-salon videos that promote your services and products.
- Create an on-hold message featuring your salons best attributes.

Many of these vehicles can help you attract new clients, but the first goal of every business should be to maintain current clients. It takes at least three salon visits for a new client to become a loyal current client. Encourage your staff to have their guests pre-book their appointments: Just because a client has visited the salon 100 times doesn't mean he or she will come one more. By having a pre-booking system in place, you are guaranteeing future business. Once you have a loyal client base, it is far less expensive to market to that base. That is why you should follow up every visit to determine the client's satisfaction and why you should personally contact any client who has not been in the salon for more than eight weeks.

Selling in the Salon

An important aspect of the salon's financial success revolves around upselling (adding on additional services), cross promoting (encouraging a client who is booked for a haircut to also get a manicure or facial), and retailing (selling take-home or maintenance products). No matter the size or style of your business, adding services and retail sales to your service ticket means additional revenue. Remember—your client will spend money during his or her visit. It is your job to encourage your client to invest in retail and services that will keep him or her coming back for more but will help maintain to look you just gave them!

It is important that we as professionals feel confident in selling services and retail. Remove any negative feelings or stereotypes you have toward sales or sales people and start fresh. Helpful and knowledgeable professionals make customer care their top priority. These people play a major role in the lives of their customers and are very valuable to clients because they offer good advice. In fact, the successful salon owner, like the successful stylist, makes his or her living by giving complete beauty advice every day (figure 32-16).

ACTIVITY

All the planning in the world can't guarantee success as much as a happy client can. Great customer service and a fabulous customer experience are the most important aspects of salon success. What will your customer service look like? Imagine you are calling or walking into your dream salon. Write down everything about your ideal experience as a customer, from the way you are greeted to the actual service to checkout at the desk when you leave. Include all five senses.

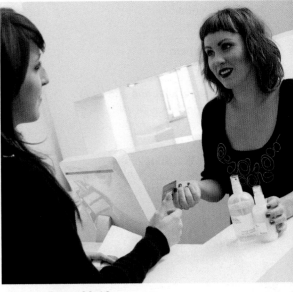

figure 32-16
Selling retail products benefits everyone.

REVIEW QUESTIONS

1. Name and describe the two most common options for going into business for yourself.

2. What responsibilities does a booth renter assume? What are the disadvantages of booth renting?

3. List at least three of the basic factors that potential salon owners should consider before opening their business.

4. How many types of salon ownership are there? Describe each.

5. List and describe the categories of information that should be included in a business plan.

6. Why is it important to keep good records? What types of records should be kept?

7. List and describe the five elements of a successful salon.

8. Why is selling services and products such a vital aspect of a salon's success?

STUDY TOOLS

- **Reinforce what you just learned:** Complete the activities and exercises in your Theory or Practical Workbook, or your Study Guide.

- **Expand your knowledge:** Search for websites about the topics in this chapter and make a list of additional resources.

- **Study and prepare for your quiz:** Take the chapter test in your Exam Review or your Milady U: Online Licensing Prep.

- **Re-Test your knowledge:** Take the Chapter 32 *Quizzes*!

- **Learn even more:** Look up in a dictionary or search the internet for the definitions of any additional terms you want to learn about.

CHAPTER GLOSSARY

booth rental BOO-th ren-tal	p. 1089	Also known as *chair rental*; renting a booth or station in a salon.
business plan BIZ-nez plahn	p. 1081	A written description of your business as you see it today and as you foresee it in the next five years (detailed by year).
business regulations and laws BIZ-nez reg-U-lay-shuns AND LAWZ	p. 1081	Any and all local, state, and federal regulations and laws that you must comply with when you decide to open your salon or rent a booth.
capital	p. 1083	Money needed to invest in a business.
consumption supplies KON-sump-shun sup-LYZ	p. 1088	Supplies used in the daily business operation.
corporation KOR-pour-aye-shun	p. 1083	An ownership structure controlled by one or more stockholders.
demographics dem-oh-graf-iks	p. 1081	Information about a specific population including data on race, age, income, and educational attainment.

goals	p. 1080	A set of benchmarks that, once achieved, help you to realize your mission and your vision.
insurance	p. 1082	Guarantees protection against financial loss from malpractice, property liability, fire, burglary and theft, and business interruption.
partnership	p. 1083	Business structure in which two or more people share ownership, although not necessarily equally.
personnel PER-son-elle	p. 1091	Your staff or employees.
record keeping	p. 1082	Maintaining accurate and complete records of all financial activities in your business.
retail supplies	p. 1088	Supplies sold to clients.
salon operation	p. 1082	The ongoing, recurring processes or activities involved in the running of a business for the purpose of producing income and value.
salon policies	p. 1082	The rules or regulations adopted by a salon to ensure that all clients and associates are being treated fairly and consistently.
social media	p. 1097	Social media refers to a platform used to engage and communicate with groups of people through online communities, networks, websites or blogs, for personal or professional means.
sole proprietor SOHL PRHO-pry-eh-tohr	p. 1082	Individual owner and, most often, the manager of a business.
vision statement	p. 1080	A long-term picture of what the business is to become and what it will look like when it gets there.
written agreements	p. 1081	Documents that govern the opening of a salon, including leases, vendor contracts, employee contracts, and more; all of which detail, usually for legal purposes, who does what and what is given in return.

Chapter 1

1. NYS Department of State Division of Licensing Services, Licensing of Nail Specialty, Natural Hair Styling, Waxing, Esthetics and Cosmetology Appearance Enhancement. (June 2013). General Business Law Article 27, Section 400. Retrieved from http://www.dos.ny.gov/licensing/lawbooks/APP-ENH.pdf

2. Bailey, D. (2014). *Milady Standard Natural Hair Care and Braiding: History and Career Opportunities.* Clifton Park, NY: Milady, a part of Cengage Learning.

3. Bell, H. (2012). Interview with Trevor Sorbie MBE. Retrieved from http://www.ukhairdressers.com/heather/interview%20with%20trevor%20sorbie.asp

4. Farouk Shami: Businessman and innovator. Retrieved from http://imeu.net/news/article006752.shtml

5. Professional Beauty Association. (2013). NAHA. Retrieved June 30, 2013, from http://probeauty.org/naha25/

Timeline (Table 1-1)

1. Bailey, D. (2014). *Milady Standard Natural Hair Care and Braiding: History and Career Opportunities.* (chap 1), 4-5. Clifton Park, NY: Milady, a part of Cengage Learning.

2. Professional Beauty Association. NAHA. (2013). NAHA. Retrieved June 30, 2013, from http://probeauty.org/naha25/

Chapter 5

1. United States Department of Labor. (n.d.) *Occupational Safety and Health Standards, Toxic and Hazardous Substances.* Retrieved from https://www.osha.gov

Chapter 12

1. Johnson, B. et. al. (2012). New silicone technologies for ethnic hair care. Dow Corning Corporation. Retrieved from http://www.dowcorning.com/content/publishedlit/27-1080.pdf

Chapter 29

1. MacFarlane, D.F., & Alonso, C.A. (2009). Arch Dermatol. *Occurrence of Nonmelanoma Skin Cancers on the Hands After UV Nail Light Exposure,* 145(4):447-449. doi: 10.1001/archdermatol.2008.622.

Chapter 30

1. Professional Beauty Association. (2013). *Economic Snapshot of the Salon and Spa Industry.* Retrieved from http://www.probeauty.org/docs/advocacy/2013_Economic_Snapshot_of_the_Salon_Industry.pdf

2. Ibid.

Anterior auricular artery, branch of the superficial temporal artery that supplies blood to the front part of the ear, 135

Anterior tibial artery, one of the popliteal arteries (the other is the posterior tibial artery) that supplies blood to the lower leg muscles and to the muscles and skin on the top of the foot and adjacent sides of the first and second toes. This artery continues to the to the foot where it becomes the dorsalis pedis artery, 136

Antiseptics, chemical germicide formulated for use on skin; registered and regulated by the Food and Drug Administration (FDA), 93

Aorta, the largest artery in the body, 133

Apex, also known as *arch;* the area of the nail that has all of the strength, 963

Apex, highest point on the top of the head, 359

Appearance enhancement, a term used to encompass a broad range of specialty areas, including hairstyling, nail technology, and esthetics, 6

Appointment book, 1096

Aromatherapy, the therapeutic use of plant aromas for beauty and health treatment, 795
in nail service, 875

Arrector pili muscles, small involuntary muscles in the base of the hair follicle that cause goose flesh, sometimes called *goose bumps,* and papillae, 157, 225

Arteries, thick-walled, muscular, flexible tubes that carry oxygenated blood away from the heart to the arterioles, 133

Arterioles, small arteries that deliver blood to capillaries, 133

Artistic director, 16

Associated Master Barbers and Beauticians of America (AMBBA), 10–11

Asymmetrical balance, is established when two imaginary halves of a hairstyle have an equal visual weight, but the two halves are positioned unevenly. Opposite sides of the hairstyle are different lengths or have a different volume. Asymmetry can be horizontal or diagonal, 304

Asymptomatic, showing no symptoms or signs of infection, 93

ATG. *See* Ammonium thioglycolate

Atoms, the smallest chemical components (often called particles) of an element; structures that make up the element and have the same properties of the element, 256

Attitudes, developing positive, 33–34, 41

Autonomic nervous system, abbreviated ANS; the part of the nervous system that controls the involuntary muscles, regulates the action of smooth muscles, glands, blood vessels, heart, and breathing, 128

Avicenna, 9, 15

B

Bacilli, singular: bacillus. Short, rod-shaped bacteria. They are the most common bacteria and produce diseases such as tetanus (lockjaw), typhoid fever, tuberculosis, and diphtheria, 77

Backbrushing, also known as *ruffing;* technique used to build a soft cushion or to mesh two or more curl patterns together for a uniform and smooth comb out, 454

Backcombing, also known as *teasing, ratting, matting,* or *French lacing;* combing small sections of hair from the ends toward the scalp, causing shorter hair to mat at the scalp and form a cushion or base, 454

Bacteria, one-celled microorganisms that have both plant and animal characteristics. Some are harmful; some are harmless, 76
classifications of pathogenic, 77
growth and reproduction, 78–79
infections, 79–80
movement of, 77–78
types of, 76–77

Bacterial spores, bacteria capable of producing a protective coating that allows them to withstand very harsh environments, and shed the coating when conditions become more favorable, 79

Bactericidal, capable of destroying bacteria, 76

Balance, establishing equal or appropriate proportions to create symmetry. In hairstyling, it is the relationship of height to width, 303

Balancing shampoo, shampoo designed to wash away excess oiliness while preventing the hair from drying out, 333

Baliage, also known as *free-form technique;* painting a lightener (usually a powdered off-the-scalp lightener) directly onto clean, styled hair, 700

Bang area, also known as *fringe area:* triangular section that begins at the apex, or high point of the head, and ends at the front corners, 316

Bantu knot or Nubian knots, the hair is double-strand twisted or coil twisted and wrapped around itself to make a knot. Knots are secured by bobby pins or elastic bands, 540

Bantu knot-out style, knots can be opened and released to create wavy and fuller loose curls, 540

Barrel curls, pin curls with large center openings, fastened to the head in a standing position on a rectangular base, 450

Barrier function, the complex of lipids between the cells that keep the skin moist by preventing water evaporation, and to guard against irritants penetrating the skin surface, 156

Basal cell carcinoma, most common and least severe type of skin cancer; often characterized by light or pearly nodules, 182

Basalt, a dark, fine-grained volcanic rock used in hot stone massage, 904

Base, stationary, or non-moving, foundation of a pin curl (the area closest to the scalp); the panel of hair on which a roller is placed, 451

Base color, predominant tone of a color, 675

Base control, position of the tool in relation to its base section, determined by the angle which the hair is wrapped, 614

Base cream, also known as *protective base cream;* oily cream used to protect the skin and scalp during hair relaxing, 621

Base direction, angle at which the rod is positioned on the head (horizontally, vertically, or diagonally); also, the directional pattern in which the hair is wrapped, 612

Base placement, refers to the position of the rod in relation to its base section; base placement is determined by the angle at which the hair is wrapped, 611

Base relaxers, relaxers that require the application of protective base cream to the entire scalp prior to the application of the relaxer, 621

Base sections, subsections of panels into which hair is divided for perm wrapping; one rod is normally placed on base section, 611

Basic permanent wrap, also known as *straight set wrap;* perm wrapping pattern in which all the rods within a panel move in the same direction and are positioned on equal-sized bases; all the base sections are horizontal and are the same length and width as the perm rod, 614

Beau's lines, sometimes called *furrows* or *corrugations;* visible depressions running across the width of the natural nail plate; usually a result of major illness or injury that has traumatized the body, 209

Bed epithelium, thin layer of tissue that attaches the nail plate and the nail bed, 199

Belly, the middle part of the muscle, 122

Beveling, haircutting technique using diagonal lines by cutting hair ends with a slight increase or decrease in length, 362

Contact dermatitis, an inflammation of the skin caused by having contact with certain chemicals or substances; many of these substances are used in cosmetology, 189

Contagious disease, also known as *communicable disease*; disease that is spread from one person to another person. Some of the more contagious diseases are the common cold, ringworm, conjunctivitis (pinkeye), viral infections, and natural nail or toe and foot infections, 80

Contamination, the presence, or the reasonably anticipated presence, of blood or other potentially infectious materials on an item's surface or visible debris or residues such as dust, hair, and skin, 81

Continuing education, education that is employment or license related; used to motivate, enrich, update skill sets, satisfy licensing requirements, or further your career, 12

Contour, an application technique that creates a shadow over an area, minimizing features, 823

Contraindication, condition that requires avoiding certain treatments, procedures, or products to prevent undesirable side effects, 767

Contrasting lines, horizontal and vertical lines that meet at a 90-degree angle and create a hard edge, 299

Contributing pigment, as known as *undertone*; the varying degrees of warmth exposed during a permanent color or lightening process, 673

Convex profile, curving outward; receding forehead and chin, 312

Cool colors, colors that suggest coolness and are dominated by blues, greens, violets, and blue-reds, 820

Cornrows, also known as *canerows*; narrow rows of visible braids that lie close to the scalp and are created with a three-strand, on-the-scalp braiding technique, 538, 552–554
  with extensions, 538–539

Corporation, an ownership structure controlled by one or more stockholders, 1083

Corrugator muscle, muscle located beneath the frontalis and orbicularis oculi muscles that draws the eyebrow down and wrinkles the forehead vertically, 124

Cortex, middle layer of the hair; a fibrous protein core formed by elongated cells containing melanin pigment, 227

Cosmetology, the art and science of beautifying and improving the skin, nails, and hair, and includes the study of cosmetics and their application, 6
  brief history, 7–12
  career paths, 13–17

timeline, 14–15

Cosmetology instructor, 16

Couperose, distended capillaries caused by weakening of the capillary walls, 774

Cowlick, tuft of hair that stands straight up, 119

Cranium, an oval, bony case that protects the brain, 119

Cream masks, masks often containing oils and emollients as well as humectants; have a strong moisturizing effect, 779

Creative director, 17

Creative Nail Design, 12, 14

Creativity
  enhancing, 24–25
  success and, 24

Croquignole perm wrap, perm in which the hair strands are wrapped from the ends to the scalp in overlapping concentric layers, 10, 11, 15, 612

Cross-checking, parting the haircut in the opposite way from which you cut it in order to check for precision of line and shape, 384

Crown, area of the head between the apex and back of the parietal ridge, 360

Crust, dead cells that form over a wound or blemish while it is healing; an accumulation of sebum and pus, sometimes mixed with epidermal material, 176

Cure, to harden, 990

Curette, a small scoop-shaped implement used for more efficient removal of debris from the nail folds, eponychium, and hyponychium areas, 905

Curl, also known as *circle*; the hair that is wrapped around the roller, 451

Curling iron manipulations, 463–464

Curl patterns, basic, 464–465

Curvature permanent wrap, perm wrap in which partings and bases radiate throughout the panels to follow the curvature of the head, 614

Curved lines, lines moving in a circular or semi-circular direction; used to soften a design, 298

Cuticle, dead, colorless tissue attached to the natural nail plate, 200

Cuticle removers, 863

Cutting line, angle at which the fingers are held when cutting, and, ultimately, the line that is cut; also known as *finger angle, finger position, cutting position, cutting angle*, 363

Cyanoacrylate, a specialized acrylic monomer that has excellent adhesion to the natural nail plate and polymerizes in seconds, 931

Cyst, closed, abnormally developed sac that contains fluid, pus, semifluid, or morbid matter above or below the skin, 174

Cysteine, an amino acid with a sulfur atom (S) that joins together two peptide strands, 228

Cystine, an amino acid formed when two cysteine amino acids (with single sulfur) are joined by their sulfur groups or disulfide bond, 228

Cytoplasm, the protoplasm of a cell, the watery fluid that surrounds the nucleus of the cell and is needed for growth, reproduction, and self-repair, 116

D

Damaged hair, 705

Dappen dish, special container that holds monomer liquid and polymer powder, 960

Day spas, 12, 14

DC. *See* Direct current

DeCaprio, Noel, 12, 15

Decontamination, the removal of blood and all other potentially infectious materials on an item's surface, and the removal of visible debris or residue such as dust, hair, and skin, 85

Deductive reasoning, the process of reaching logical conclusions by employing logical reasoning, 1029

Deep-conditioning treatment, also known as *hair mask* or *conditioning pack*; chemical mixture of concentrated protein and intensive moisturizer, 337

Deep peroneal nerve, also known as *anterior tibial nerve*; it extends down the front of the leg, behind the muscles. It supplies impulses to these muscles and also to the muscles and skin on the top of the foot and adjacent sides of the first and second toes, 132

Deionized water, water that has had impurities (such as calcium and magnesium and other metal ions that would make a product unstable) removed, 330

Deltoid, large triangular muscle covering the shoulder joint that allows the arm to extend outward and to the side of the body, 126

Demipermanent haircolor, also known as *no-lift deposit-only color*; formulated to deposit but not lift (lighten) natural hair color, 681, 693

Demographics, information about a specific population including data on race, age, income, and educational attainment, 1081

Depilatory, substance, usually a caustic alkali preparation, used for the temporary removal of superfluous hair by dissolving it at the skin surface level, 745

Depressor labii inferioris muscle, also known as *quadratus labii inferioris* muscle; muscle surrounding the lower lip; lowers the lower lip and draws it to one side, as in expressing sarcasm, 125

Dermal papillae, a small, cone-shaped elevation located at the base of the hair follicle that fits into the hair bulb, 157, 225

Dermatitis, inflammatory condition of the skin, 179

  recognizing contact, 189–190

Dermatologist, physician who specializes in disorders of the skin, hair, and nails, 154, 173

Dermatology, medical branch of science that deals with the study of skin and its nature, structure, functions, diseases, and treatment, 154

Dermis, also known as *derma, corium, cutis,* or *true skin;* underlying or inner layer of the skin, 156

Design texture, wave patterns that must be taken into consideration when designing a style, 300

Desincrustation, a form of anaphoresis; process used to soften and emulsify grease deposits (oil) and blackheads in the hair follicles, 281

Developers, also known as *oxidizing agents* or *catalysts;* when mixed with an oxidation haircolor, supplies the necessary oxygen gas to develop color molecules and create a change in hair color, 683

Diagnosis, determination of the nature of a disease from its symptoms and/or diagnostic tests. Federal regulations prohibit salon professionals from performing a diagnosis, 81

Diagonal back, a type of diagonal line that creates movement away from the face, 362

Diagonal forward, a type of diagonal line that creates movement toward the face, 362

Diagonal lines, lines positioned between horizontal and vertical lines. They are often used to emphasize or minimize facial features, 298

Diffuser, blowdryer attachment that causes the air to flow more softly and helps to accentuate or keep textual definition, 457, 495–496

Digestive system, also known as *gastrointestinal system;* the body system that is responsible for breaking down foods into nutrients and wastes; consists of the mouth, stomach, intestines, salivary and gastric glands, and other organs, 118

Digital nerve, sensory-motor nerve that, with its branches, supplies impulses to the fingers, 131

Dimethyl urea hardeners, a hardener that adds cross-links to the natural nail plate. Unlike others containing

formaldehyde, DMU does not cause adverse skin reactions, 865

Diplococci, spherical bacteria that grow in pairs and cause diseases such as pneumonia, 77

Direct current, abbreviated DC; constant, even-flowing current that travels in one direction only and is produced by chemical means, 275

Directional lines, lines with a definite forward or backward movement, 299

Direct transmission, transmission of blood or body fluids through touching (including shaking hands), kissing, coughing, sneezing, and talking, 78

Discolored nails, nails turn a variety of colors; may indicate surface staining, a systemic disorder, or poor blood circulation, 209

Disease, an abnormal condition of all or part of the body, or its systems or organs, which makes the body incapable of carrying on normal function, 74, 600

  preventing spread of, 84–93

  terms related to, 81

Disinfectants, chemical products approved by the EPA designed to destroy most bacteria (excluding spores), fungi, and viruses on surfaces, 73

  additives, powders, and tablets, 92

  choosing, 86–87

  dispensary for, 92

  hospital, 74

  proper use of, 87

  safety and, 89

  soaps and detergents, 92

  tuberculosis, 74

  types of, 88

Disinfection containers, 852–853

Disinfection (disinfecting), a chemical process that destroys most, but not necessarily all, harmful organisms on environmental surfaces. The pathogens of concern in the cosmetology industry are effectively destroyed by the disinfection process, which is required in all states, 70, 76

  disinfect *vs.* dispose, 89–90

  electrical tools and implements, 90

  foot spas and pedicure equipment, 91–92, 99–103

  logbooks for, 90

  nonelectrical tools and implements, 90, 97–98

  of towels, linens, and capes, 90–91

  work surfaces, 90

Distribution, where and how hair is moved over the head, 390

Distributor sales consultant, 16

Disulfide bond, strong chemical side bond that joins the sulfur atoms of two neighboring cysteine amino acids to create one cystine, which joins together two polypeptide strands like rungs on a ladder, 228

Dorsalis pedis artery, artery that supplies blood to the foot, 136

Dorsal nerve, also known as *dorsal cutaneous nerve;* a nerve that extends up from the toes and foot, just under the skin, supplying impulses to toes and foot, as well as the muscles and skin of the leg, where it becomes the superficial peroneal nerve, 132

Double flat wrap, perm wrap in which one end paper is placed under and another is placed over the strand of hair being wrapped, 610

Double press, technique of passing a hot curling iron through the hair before performing a hard press, 467

Double-process application, also known as *two-step coloring;* a coloring technique requiring two separate procedures in which the hair is pre-lightened before the depositing color is applied to the hair, 684

Double-rod wrap, also known as *piggyback wrap;* a wrap technique whereby extra-long hair is wrapped on one rod from the scalp to midway down the hair shaft, and another rod is used to wrap the remaining hair strand in the same direction, 613

Dry shampoo, also known as *powder shampoo;* shampoo that cleanses the hair without the use of soap and water, 333

Dyschromias, abnormal colorations of the skin that accompany skin disorders and are symptoms of many systemic disorders, 180

E

Eczema, an inflammatory, uncomfortable, and often chronic disease of the skin; characterized by moderate to severe inflammation, scaling, and sometimes severe itching, 179

Education director, 16

Effective communication, the act of sharing information between two people (or groups of people) so that the information is successfully understood, 50

  importance of, 50–54

Efficacy, the ability to produce an effect, 86

Effilating, also known as *slithering;* process of thinning the hair to graduated lengths with shears; cutting the hair with a sliding movement of the shears while keeping the blades partially opened, 396

Effleurage, light, continuous stroking movement applied with the fingers (digital) or the palms (palmar) in a slow, rhythmic manner, 781

Eggshell nails, noticeably thin, white nail plates that are more flexible than normal and can curve over the free edge, 210

Extensors, muscles that straighten the wrist, hand, and fingers to form a straight line, 126

External carotid artery, artery that supplies blood to the anterior (front) parts of the scalp, ear, face, neck, and sides of the head, 134

External jugular vein, vein located at the side of the neck that carries blood returning to the heart from the head, face, and neck, 136

Extraction, a procedure in which comedones are removed from the follicles by manual manipulation, 773

Extrinsic factors, primarily environmental factors that contribute to aging and the appearance of aging, 186

Eyebrow pencils, pencils used to add color and shape to the eyebrows, 814

Eyebrow powders, powders used to add color and shape to the eyebrows, 814

Eyelash adhesive, product used to make artificial eyelashes adhere, or stick, to the natural lash line, 834

Eyelashes, 834–835

Eyeliner, cosmetic used to outline and emphasize the eyes, 814

Eye makeup removers, special preparations for removing eye makeup, 816

Eye shadows, cosmetics applied on the eyelids to accentuate or contour, 814

F

Fabric wrap, nail wrap made of silk, linen, or fiberglass, 932

Face powder, cosmetic powder, sometimes tinted, that is used to add a matte or non-shiny finish to the face, 814

Facial, also known as *facial treatment;* a professional skin treatment that improves the condition and appearance of the skin, 766

Facial artery, also known as *external maxillary artery;* branch of the external carotid artery that supplies blood to the lower region of the face, mouth, and nose, 135

Facial makeup
  altering face shapes with, 823–828
  basic application procedure, 828–833, 837–839
  brushes and tools, 816–818
  check color, 815
  color theory and, 819–822
  concealers, 814
  eyebrow color, 814–815
  eyelashes, 834–835, 840–843
  eyeliners, 814
  eye shadow, 814
  face powders, 814
  foundation, 812–813
  lip color, 815
  mascara, 815–816
  single-use implements, 818
  special occasion, 835–836
  special preparations, 816

Facials
  acne-prone skin, 773, 793–794, 805–806
  aromatherapy and, 795
  basic application procedure, 792, 796–800
  chest, back, and neck manipulation, 787
  client consultation, 767–771
  contraindication grid, 767–768
  dry skin procedure, 801–802
  electrotherapy and light therapy, 788–792
  equipment, 787–788
  guidelines for, 792–793
  home care program, 794–795
  massage techniques and guidelines, 780–787
  for men, 794
  for oily skin with open comedones, 803–804
  record-keeping, 769–770
  skin analysis and consultation, 767–771
  skin types, determining, 771–774

Facial skeleton, the framework of the face; composed of 14 bones, 119

Factor, Max, 9, 14

Fallen hair, hair that has been shed from the head or gathered from a hairbrush, as opposed to hair that has been cut; the cuticles of the strands will move in different directions (opposite of turned or Remi hair), 576

Femur, heavy, long bone that forms the leg above the knee, 121

Ferrule, the metal part of the brush that attaches the glued bristles to the handle and adds a certain amount of strength to the bristles, 816

Fiberglass wraps, made from a very thin, synthetic mesh with a loose weave, 932

Fibula, smaller of the two bones that form the leg below the knee. The fibula may be visualized as a bump on the little-toe side of the ankle, 121

Fifth cranial nerve, also known as *trifacial nerve* or *trigeminal nerve;* the chief sensory nerve of the face that serves as the motor nerve of the muscles that control chewing, 129

Fillers, used to equalize porosity, 705

Film, theatrical, or editorial stylist, 17

Fine-grit abrasives, abrasives 240 grit and higher designed for buffing, polishing, and removing very fine scratches, 860

Finger bowls, 852

Finger waving, process of shaping and directing the hair into an S pattern through the use of the fingers, combs, and waving lotion, 445
  left-handed, 481–484
  right-handed, 477–480

Finger-waving lotion, also known as *liquid gel;* is a type of hair gel that makes the hair pliable enough to keep it in place during the finger-waving procedure, 446

Fishtail braid, simple two-strand braid in which the hair is picked up from the sides and added to the strands as they are crossed over each other, 536

Fissure, a crack in the skin that penetrates the dermis. Examples are severely cracked and/or chapped hands or lips, 176

Flagella, slender, hair-like extensions used by bacilli and spirilla for locomotion (moving about). May also be referred to as cilia, 78

Flat-twist, double-strand twists that are interwoven to lie flat on the scalp with various patterns with or without extensions, 540

Flexor, extensor muscle of the wrist involved in flexing the wrist, 126

Flexor digiti minimi, muscle that moves the little toe, 128

Flexor digitorum brevis, muscle that flexes the toes and helps maintain balance while walking and standing, 128

Foam, as known as *mousse;* a light, airy, whipped styling product that resembles shaving foam and builds moderate body and volume into the hair, 458

Foaming cleansers, cleansers containing surfactants (detergents) that cause the product to foam and rinse off easily, 775

Foil technique, highlighting technique that involves coloring selected strands of hair by slicing or weaving out sections, placing them on foil or plastic wrap, applying lightener or permanent haircolor, and then sealing them in the foil or plastic wrap, 699

Folliculitis barbae, synonym *tinea barbae.* Also known as *barbers itch,* inflammation of the hair follicles caused by a bacterial infection from ingrown hairs. The cause is typically from ingrown hairs due to shaving or other epilation methods, 83

Foot files, also known as *pedicure paddles;* large, abrasive files used to reduce and smooth thicker foot calluses, 906

Foot soaks, products containing gentle soaps, moisturizers, and other additives that are used in a pedicure bath to cleanse, deodorize, and soften the skin, 908

Foot spas, disinfection and cleaning of, 916–917

Forged, process of working metal to a finished shape by hammering or pressing, 372

Form, the mass of general outline of a hairstyle. It is three-dimensional and has length, width, and depth, 299

Foundation, also known as *base makeup;* a tinted cosmetic used to cover or even out the coloring of the skin, 812

Four corners, points on the head that signal change in the shape of the head, from flat to round or vice versa, 359

aromatherapy oils, botanical extracts, and other beneficial ingredients to cleanse, exfoliate, tighten, tone, hydrate, and nourish the skin, 778, 903

Massage, manual or mechanical manipulation of the body by rubbing, gently pinching, kneading, tapping, and other movements to increase metabolism and circulation, promote absorption, and relieve pain, 780, 871
pedicure, 914–915

Massage creams, lubricants used to make the skin slippery during massage, 778

Matching test format, 1030

Material Safety Data Sheet, abbreviated MSDS; replaced by *Safety Data Sheet*; information compiled by the manufacturer about product safety, including the names of hazardous ingredients, safe handling and use procedures, precautions to reduce the risk of accidental harm or overexposure, and flammability warnings, 72

Matrix, area where the nail plate cells are formed; this area is composed of matrix cells that produce the nail plate, 200

Matte, not shiny, 813

Matter, any substance that occupies space and has mass (weight), 255

Maxillae, singular: maxilla. Bones of the upper jaw, 120

Maxillary nerve, branch of the fifth cranial nerve that supplies impulses to the upper part of the face, 130

McDonough, Everett, 11

Mechanical exfoliants, methods used to physically remove dead cell buildup, 776

Median nerve, sensory–motor nerve that is smaller than the ulnar and radial nerves and that, with its branches, supplies the arm and hand, 131

Medicated scalp lotion, conditioner that promotes healing of the scalp, 336

Medicated shampoo, shampoo containing special chemicals or drugs that are very effective in reducing dandruff or relieving other scalp conditions, 332

Medium-grit abrasives, boards and buffers 150 to 180 grit that are used to smooth and refine surfaces and shorten natural nails, 860

Medium press, technique that removes 60 to 75 percent of the curl by applying a thermal pressing comb once on each side of the hair, using slightly more pressure than in the soft press, 467

Medulla, innermost layer of the hair that is composed of round cells; often absent in fine and naturally blond hair, 227

Melanin, tiny grains of pigment (coloring matter) that are produced by melanocytes and deposited into cells in the stratum germinativum layer of the epidermis and in the papillary layers of the dermis. There are two types of melanin: pheomelanin, which is red to yellow in color, and eumelanin, which is dark brown to black, 158, 230

Melanocytes, cells that produce the dark skin pigment called melanin, 156

Melanonychia, darkening of the fingernails or toenails; may be seen as a black band within the nail plate, extending from the base to the free edge, 210

Men
basic clipper cut, 434–437
basic nail shapes for, 870
facials for, 794
hairstyles for, 317
manicures for, 8770
permanent waving for, 616

Mentalis muscle, muscle that elevates the lower lip and raises and wrinkles the skin of the chin, 125

Metacarpus, bones of the palm of the hand; parts of the hand containing five bones between the carpus and phalanges, 121

Metal hydroxide relaxers, ionic compounds formed by a metal (sodium, potassium, or lithium) which is combined with oxygen and hydrogen, 620

Metallic haircolors, also known as *progressive haircolors;* haircolors containing metal salts that change hair color gradually by progressive buildup and exposure to air creating a dull, metallic appearance, 683

Metallic salts, 616–617

Metal pusher, a multiuse implement, made of stainless steel; used to push back the eponychium but can also be used to gently scrape cuticle tissue from the natural nail plate, 856

Metatarsal, one of three subdivisions of the foot; long and slender bones, similar to the metacarpal bones of the hand. The other two subdivisions are the tarsal and phalanges, 122

Methicillin-resistant Staphylococcus aureus, abbreviated MRSA; a type of infectious bacteria that is highly resistant to conventional treatments due to incorrect doses or choice of antibiotic, 79–80

Microcurrent, an extremely low level of electricity that mirrors the body's natural electrical impulses, 281, 790

Microdermabrasion, mechanical exfoliation that involves shooting aluminum oxide or other crystals at the skin with a hand-held device that exfoliates dead cells, 792

Microdermabrasion scrubs, scrubs that contain aluminum oxide crystals, 776

Microorganism, any organism of microscopic or submicroscopic size, 76

Microtrauma, the act of causing tiny, unseen openings in the skin that can allow entry by pathogenic microbes, 856

Middle Ages, 8–9

Middle temporal artery, branch of the superficial temporal artery that supplies blood to the temples, 135

Mildew, a type of fungus that affects plants or grows on inanimate objects, but does not cause human infections in the salon, 83

Milia, benign, keratin-filled cysts that can appear just under the epidermis and have no visible opening, 178

Miliaria rubra, also known as *prickly heat;* an acute inflammatory disorder of the sweat glands, characterized by the eruption of small, red vesicles and accompanied by burning, itching skin, 179

Milliampere, abbreviated mA; 1/1,000 of ampere, 277

Miscible, liquids that are mutually soluble, meaning that they can be mixed together to form stable solutions, 261

Mission statement, a statement that establishes the purpose and values for which an individual or institution lives and works by. It provides a sense of direction by defining guiding principles and clarifying goals, as well as how an organization operates, 25

Mitosis, the usual process of cell reproduction of human tissues that occurs when the cell divides into two identical cells called daughter cells, 116

Mixed melanin, combination of natural hair color that contains both pheomelanin and eumelanin, 673

Mix ratio, the amount of monomer liquid and polymer powder used to create a bead, 956

Modalities, currents used in electrical facial and scalp treatments, 280

Modelage masks, facial masks containing special crystals of gypsum, a plaster-like ingredient, 779

Moisturizer, product formulated to add moisture to dry hair or promote the retention of moisture, 331

Moisturizers, products that help increase the moisture content of the skin surface, 777

Mole, small brownish spot or blemish on the skin, ranging in color from pale tan to brown or bluish black, 181

Molecule, a chemical combination of two or more atoms in definite (fixed) proportions, 256

Money management, 1063–1067

compresses, contracts, puckers, and wrinkles the lips, 125

Organic chemistry, the study of substances that contain the element carbon, 254

Organs, structures composed of specialized tissues designed to perform specific functions in plants and animals, 117

Origin, the part of the muscle that does not move; attached closest to the skeleton, 122

Ostium, follicle opening, 773

Oval nail, a conservative nail shape that is thought to be attractive on most women's hands. It is similar to a squoval nail with even more rounded corners, 869

Overdirection, combing a section away from its natural falling position, rather than straight out from the head, toward a guideline; used to create increasing lengths in the interior perimeter, 366

Overhand technique, a technique in which the first side section goes over the middle one, then the other side section goes over the middle strand, 535

Overlay, a layer of any kind of nail enhancement product that is applied over the natural nail or nail and tip application for added strength, 929

Oxidation, a chemical reaction that combines a substance with oxygen to produce an oxide, 258

Oxidation-reduction, also known as *redox*; a chemical reaction in which the oxidizing agent is reduced (by losing oxygen) and the reducing agent is oxidized (by gaining oxygen), 258

Oxidizing agent, substance that releases oxygen, 259

P

Palm-to-palm, cutting position in which the palms of both hands are facing each other, 381

Paper wraps, temporary nail wraps made of very thin paper, 932

Papillary layer, outer layer of the dermis, directly beneath the epidermis, 157

Papule, also known as *pimple*; small elevation of the skin that contains no fluid but may develop pus, 161

Paraffin, a petroleum by-product that has excellent sealing properties (barrier qualities) to hold moisture in the skin, 854

Paraffin baths, 854, 904

Paraffin wax masks, specially prepared facial masks containing paraffin and other beneficial ingredients; typically used with treatment cream, 779

Paraffin wax treatments, 875–877

Parallel lines, repeating lines in a hairstyle; may be straight or curved, 299

Parasites, organisms that grow, feed, and shelter on or in another organism (referred to as the host), while contributing nothing to the survival of that organism. Parasites must have a host to survive, 84

Parasitic disease, disease caused by parasites, such as lice and mites, 81

Parietal artery, branch of the superficial temporal artery that supplies blood to the side and crown of the head, 135

Parietal bones, bones that form the sides and top of the cranium, 119

Parietal ridge, widest area of the head, usually starting at the temples and ending at the bottom of the crown, 359

Paronychia, bacterial inflammation of the tissues surrounding the nail. Redness, pus, and swelling are usually seen in the skin fold adjacent to the nail plate, 216

Partnership, business structure in which two or more people share ownership, although not necessarily equally, 1083

Part/parting, line dividing the hair at the scalp, separating one section of hair from another, creating subsections, 362

Patch test, also known as a *predisposition test*; test required by the Federal Food, Drug, and Cosmetic Act for identifying a possible allergy in a client, 691, 710–711

Patella, also known as *accessory bone* or *kneecap*; forms the kneecap joint, 121

Pathogenic, harmful microorganisms that cause disease or infection in humans when they invade the body, 77

Pathogenic disease, disease produced by organisms, including bacteria, viruses, fungi, and parasites, 81

Pectoralis major, muscles of the chest that assist the swinging movements of the arm, 125

Pectoralis minor, muscles of the chest that assist the swinging movements of the arm, 125

Pediculosis capitis, infestation of the hair and scalp with head lice, 241

Pedicure, a cosmetic service performed on the feet by a licensed cosmetologist or nail technician; can include exfoliating the skin and callus reduction, as well as trimming, shaping, and polishing toenails. A pedicure often includes foot massage, 900

basic procedure, 918–920

cleaning and disinfection of footspas, 916–917

disinfection procedures for, 916–917

elderly clients, 913

ergonomics, 916

interaction during service, 910–911

massage, 914–915, 921–923

pricing, 913–914

professional products, 907–909, 909–910

reflexology, 915–916

scheduling, 911–912

series pedicures, 912–913

service menu, 910

spa pedicure, 913

tools and materials for, 901–907

Pedicure carts, 903

Pedicure stations, 901–902

Pedicure stools/footrests, 902

Peptide bond, also known as an *end bond*; chemical bond that joins amino acids to each other, end-to-end, to form a polypeptide chain, 228, 600

Perfectionism, an unhealthy compulsion to do things perfectly, 24

Perimeter, outer line of a hairstyle, 364

Periodic strand testing, 622

Perionychium, the tissue bordering the root and sides of a fingernail or toenail, 201

Peripheral nervous system, abbreviated PNS; system of nerves that connects the peripheral (outer) parts of the body to the central nervous system; it has both sensory and motor nerves, 128

Permanent haircolors, lift and deposit color at the same time and in a single process because they are more alkaline than no-lift, deposit-only colors and are usually mixed with a higher-volume developer, 681

Permanent waving, a two-step process whereby the hair undergoes a physical change caused by wrapping the hair on perm rods; the hair then undergoes a chemical change caused by the application of permanent waving solution and neutralizer, 11, 601

base direction, 612

base placement, 611–612

basic permanent wrap, 631–634

bricklay permanent wrap, 638–639

categories, 606

chemistry of, 602

curl re-forming, 659–663

curvature permanent wrap, 635–637

end papers for, 610–611

hydroxide relaxer retouch, 656–658

hydroxide relaxer to virgin hair, 653–655

for men, 616

piggyback wrap, 613

procedures, 609

reduction reaction, 602–603

rod types for, 609

safety precautions, 616

sectioning for, 611

selecting right type, 605–609

spiral wrap technique, 644–646

thio relaxer retouch, 650–652

thio relaxer to virgin hair, 647–649

types of, 603–605

weave double-rod technique, 642–643

weave technique, 640–641

Retailing, the act of recommending and selling products to your clients for at-home use, 1067

Retail supplies, supplies sold to clients, 1088

Retention hyperkeratosis, the hereditary tendency for acne-prone skin to retain dead cells in the follicle, forming an obstruction that clogs follicles and exacerbates inflammatory acne lesions such as papules and pustules, 184

Reticular layer, deeper layer of the dermis that supplies the skin with oxygen and nutrients; contains fat cells, blood vessels, sudoriferous (sweat) glands, hair follicles, lymph vessels, arrector pili muscles, sebaceous (oil) glands, and nerve endings, 157

Reverse highlighting, also known as *lowlighting;* technique of coloring strands of hair darker than the natural color, 698

Revlon, 11, 15

Rhythm, a regular pulsation or recurrent pattern of movement in a design, 304

Ribboning, technique of forcing the hair between the thumb and the back of the comb to create tension, 449

Ribs, twelve pairs of bones forming the wall of the thorax, 121

Ridge curls, pin curls placed immediately behind or below a ridge to form a wave, 44

Ridges, vertical lines running through the length of the natural nail plate that are caused by uneven growth of the nails, usually the result of normal aging, 211

Ringed hair, variety of canities characterized by alternating bands of gray and pigmented hair throughout the length of the hair strand, 237

Risorius muscle, muscle of the mouth that draws the corner of the mouth out and back, as in grinning, 125

Rod, round, solid prong of a thermal iron, 461

Roller curls, 450–453, 485–486

Rolling, massage movement in which the tissues are pressed and twisted using a fast back-and-forth movement, 782

Romans, 8

Root curl, a curl pattern that creates volume of hair, movement, and a curl formation from roots to ends, 464

Rope braid, braid created with two strands that are twisted around each other, 536

Rosacea, chronic condition that appears primarily on the checks and nose, and is characterized by flushing (redness), telangiectasis (distended or dilated surface blood vessels), and, in some cases, the formation of papules and pustules, 178

Round nail, a slightly tapered nail shape; it usually extends just a bit past the fingertip, 869

S

Safety Data Sheet, abbreviated SDS; required by law for all products sold. SDSs include safety information about products compiled by the manufacturer, including hazardous ingredients, safe use and handling procedures, proper disposal guidelines, precautions to reduce the risk of accidental harm or overexposure, and more, 72

Salicylic acid, an organic acid that derives originally from the bark of willow trees, 909

Salon management, 17–18

Salon operation, the ongoing, recurring processes or activities involved in the running of a business for the purpose of producing income and value, 1082

  compensation plans, 1060–1062

  employee evaluation, 1062–1063

  teamwork, 1058

Salon polices, the rules or regulations adopted by a salon to ensure that all clients and associates are being treated fairly and consistently, 1082

Salon survey

  basic value-priced operations, 966

  booth rental establishments, 1036

  franchise salons, 1035

  high-end image salons/day spas, 1035

  independent salon chains, 1034

  large national salon chains, 1034

  mid-priced full-service salons, 1035

  small independent salons, 1033–1034

Salon trainer, 16

Salt bond, a weak, physical, cross-link side bond between adjacent polypeptide chains, 228

Sanitizers, waterless hand, 93

Sanitizing, a chemical process for reducing the number of disease-causing germs on cleaned surfaces to a safe level, 70

Saphenous nerve, nerve of the leg that supplies impulses to the skin of the inner side of the leg and foot, 132

Sassoon, Vidal, 11, 14

Scabies, a contagious skin disease that is caused by the itch mite, which burrows under the skin, 84

Scale, any thin, dry, or oily plate of epidermal flakes. An example is abnormal or excessive dandruff, 176

Scalp

  analysis, 242, 247

  disorders, 238–242

  massage, 352–353

Scalp astringent lotion, product used to remove oil accumulation from the scalp; used after a scalp treatment and before styling, 336

Scalp care procedures, 323–324

  antidandruff treatment, 325–326

  dry hair and scalp treatment, 325

  normal hair and scalp treatment, 324–325

  oily hair and scalp treatment, 325

Scalp conditioner, product, usually in a cream base, used to soften and improve the health of the scalp, 336

Scapula, also known as *shoulder blade;* large, flat, triangular bone of the shoulder. There are two scapulae, 121

Scar, also known as *cicatrix;* a lightly raised mark on the skin formed after an injury or lesion of the skin has healed, 177

Sciatic nerve, largest and longest nerve in the body; it passes through the gluteal region into the thigh, where it branches into smaller nerves. Pain from injury or compression of the sciatic nerve can radiate throughout the abdomen and be sensed in the lower back, hip, or lower abdomen, 131

Scissor-over-comb, also known as *shear-over-comb;* haircutting technique in which the hair is held in place with the comb while the tips of the shears are used to remove length, 393

Scope of practice, the list of services that you are legally allowed to perform in your specialty in your state, 850

Scutula, dry, sulfur-yellow, cuplike crusts on the scalp in tinea favosa or tinea favus, 240

Sebaceous cyst, a large, protruding pocket-like lesion filled with sebum. Sebaceous cysts are frequently seen on the scalp and the back and may be surgically removed by a dermatologist, 178

Sebaceous glands, also known as *oil glands;* glands connected to hair follicles. Sebum is the fatty or oily secretion of the sebaceous glands, 161

Seborrheic dermatitis, skin condition caused by an inflammation of the sebaceous glands. It is often characterized by redness, dry or oily scaling, crusting, and/or itchiness, 178

Sebum, a fatty or oily secretion that lubricates the skin and preserves the softness of the hair, 161, 225

Secondary color, color obtained by mixing equal parts of two primary colors, 676

Secondary skin lesions, characterized by piles of material on the skin surface, such as a crust or scab, or depressions in the skin surface, such as an ulcer, 175

Secretory coil, coiled base of the sudoriferous (sweat) gland, 160

Secretory nerve fibers, fibers of the secretory nerve that are distributed to the sudoriferous glands and sebaceous glands. Secretory nerves,

positioning the hair over the foil, and applying lightener or color, 699

Slicing, haircutting technique that removes weight and adds movement through the lengths of the hair; the shears are not completely closed, and only the portion of the blades near the pivot is used, 396

Slide cutting, method of cutting or layering the hair in which the fingers and shears glide along the edge of the hair to remove length, 393

Smile line, the curved line where the pink and the white meet each other on a French manicured nail, 877, 963

Soap cap, combination of equal parts of a prepared permanent color mixture and shampoo used the last five minutes and worked through the hair to refresh the ends, 682

Social media, the term—social media refers to a platform used to engage and communicate with groups of people by way of online communities, networks, websites or blogs, for personal or professional means, 1097

Sodium hypochlorite, common household bleach; an effective disinfectant for the salon, 88

Soft bender rods, tool about 12 inches long with a uniform diameter along the entire length, 610

Soft curl permanent, a thio based chemical service that reformats curly and wavy hair into looser and larger curls and waves, 627–628

Soft press, technique of pressing the hair to remove 50 to 60 percent of the curl by applying the thermal pressing comb once on each side of the hair, 467

Soft UV and LED gels, also known as *soakable gels;* these gels are removed by soaking in acetone, 1001

Soft water, rainwater or chemically softened water that contains only small amounts of minerals and, therefore, allows soap and shampoo to lather freely, 330

Sole proprietor, individual owner and, most often, the manager of a business, 1082

Soleus, muscle that originates at the upper portion of the fibula and bends the foot down, 127

Solute, the substance that is dissolved in a solution, 260

Solution, a stable physical mixture of two or more substances, 260

Solvent, the substance that dissolves the solute and makes a solution, 260

Sorbie, Trevor, 11–12, 15

Space, the area surrounding the form or the area the hairstyle occupies, 299

Special effects haircoloring, any technique that involves partial lightening or coloring, 698

Sphenoid bone, bone that joins all of the bones of the cranium together, 120

Spinal cord, portion of the central nervous system that originates in the brain and extends down to the lower extremity of the trunk. It is protected by the spinal column, 129

Spiral curl, method of curling the hair by winding a strand around the rod, 464

Spiral perm wrap, hair is wrapped at an angle other than perpendicular to the length of the rod, which causes the hair to spiral along the length of the rod, similar to the stripes on a candy cane, 612

Spiral rod set, this set can be done with rods, flexi-rods, or curl reformers of all sizes. Hair is wrapped around a vertical rod, moving up the rod in a spiral movement, 541

Spiral wrapping, 10

Spirilla, spiral or corkscrew-shaped bacteria that cause diseases such as syphilis and Lyme disease, 77

Splinter hemorrhage, hemorrhage caused by trauma or injury to the nail bed that damages the capillaries and allow small amounts of blood flow, 212

Spray-on thermal protector, product applied to hair prior to any thermal service to protect the hair from the harmful effects of blowdrying, thermal irons, or electric rollers, 336

Squamous cell carcinoma, type of skin cancer more serious than basal cell carcinoma; often characterized by scaly red papules or nodules, 182

Square nail, a nail shape completely straight across the free edge with no rounding at the outside edges, 869

Squoval nail, a nail shape with a square free edge that is rounded off at the corner edges, 869

Stain, abnormal brown-colored or wine-colored skin discoloration with a circular and/or irregular shape, 180

Standard Precautions, abbreviated SP; precautions such as wearing personal protective equipment to prevent skin and mucous membranes where contact with a client's blood, body fluids, secretions (except sweat), excretions, non-intact skin, and mucous membranes is likely. Workers must assume that all blood and body fluids are potential sources of infection, regardless of the perceived risk, 93–95

Staphylococci, pus-forming bacteria that grow in clusters like a bunch of grapes. They cause abscesses, pustules, and boils, 77

States of matter, the three different physical forms of matter: solid, liquid, and gas, 257

Stationary guideline, guideline that does not move, 364

Steam distillation, 9

Steamer, a facial machine that heats and produces a stream of warm steam that can be focused on the client's face or other areas of skin, 787

Steamer, used to deeply hydrate, moisturize, and condition the hair with water vapor; infuses water hydration, opening the cuticle layer of the hair shaft and enabling nourishing protein conditioners and botanical oils to penetrate deeply into the cortex layer, 533

Stem, section of the pin curl between the base and first arc (turn) of the circle that gives the curl its direction and movement; the hair between the scalp and the first turn of the roller, 451; the basic question or problem, 1029

Sterilization, the process that completely destroys all microbial life, including spores, 84

Sternocleidomastoideus, muscle of the neck that lowers and rotates the head, 123

Sternum, also known as *breastbone;* flat bone that forms the central (front) support of the ribs, 121

Straightening gel, styling product applied to damp hair that is wavy, curly, or extremely curly and then blown dry; relaxes the hair for a smooth, straight look, 459

Straight profile, neither convex nor concave; considered ideal, 312

Straight rods, perm rods that are equal in diameter along their entire length or curling area, 610

Strand bonding, bonding method with loose hair or wefts that are cut into very small sections, 590

Strand test, determines how the hair will react to the color formula and how long the formula should be left on the hair, 692

Stratum corneum, also known as *horny layer;* outer layer of the epidermis, 156

Stratum germinativum, more commonly called the basal cell layer; deepest, live layer of the epidermis that produces new epidermal skin cells and is responsible for growth, 156

Stratum granulosum, also known as *granular layer;* layer of the epidermis composed of cells that look like granules and are filled with keratin; replaces cells shed from the stratum corneum, 156

Stratum lucidum, clear, transparent layer of the epidermis under the stratum corneum, 156

Stratum spinosum, the spiny layer just above the stratum germinativum layer, 156

Strengthening shampoo, shampoo that contains a variety of strengthening and nourishing ingredients and is designed to repair damaged and brittle hair, 333

Streptococci, pus-forming bacteria arranged in curved lines resembling a string of beads. They cause infections such as strep throat and blood poisoning, 77

Stress area, the part of the nail enhancement where the natural nail grows beyond the finger and becomes the free edge. This area needs strength to support the nail extension, 963

Stress strip, strip of fabric cut to ⅛-inch (3.12 mm) in length and applied to the weak point of the nail during the four-week fabric wrap maintenance to repair or strengthen a weak point in a nail enhancement, 934

Strip lashes, eyelash hairs attached to a band that is applied with adhesive to the natural lash line, 834

Stylus, a tool with a solid handle with a rounded ball tip on each end that can range in size, used to create nail art, 878

Subcutaneous tissue, also known as *adipose* or *subcutis tissue;* fatty tissue found below the dermis that gives smoothness and contour to the body, contains fat for use as energy, and also acts as protective cushion for the outer skin, 157

Submental artery, branch of the facial artery that supplies blood to the chin and lower lip, 135

Subsections, smaller sections within a larger section of hair, used to maintain control of the hair while cutting, 362

Success
action steps for, 23–24
creativity and, 24

Sudoriferous glands, also known as *sweat glands;* excrete perspiration and detoxify the body by excreting excess salt and unwanted chemicals, 160

Sugaring, temporary hair removal method that involves the use of a thick, sugar-based paste, 747

Sulfate-free shampoo, shampoo that does not contain harsh soap detergents. They are formulated with little to no alkaline soap base; manufactured as wetting agents to be compatible with hair and soft water sources, and generally are known to be sensitive to artificial hair color and to maintaining the natural oils in the hair, 333

Sunscreens, 778, 866

Superficial peroneal nerve, also known as *musculocutaneous nerve;* extends down the leg, just under the skin, supplying impulses to the muscles and the skin of the leg, as well as to the skin and toes on the top of the foot, where it becomes the dorsal nerve, 132

Superficial temporal artery, a continuation of the external carotid nerve artery; supplies blood to the muscles of the front, side, and top of the head, 135

Superior labial artery, branch of the facial artery that supplies blood to the upper lip and region of the nose, 135

Supinator, muscle of the forearm that rotates the radius outward and the palm upward, 126

Supraorbital artery, branch of the internal carotid artery that supplies blood to the upper eyelid and forehead, 134

Sural nerve, nerve of the lower leg that supplies impulses to the skin on the outer side and back of the foot and leg, 132

Surfactants, a contraction of surface active agents; substances that allow oil and water to mix, or emulsify, 262

Suspensions, unstable physical mixtures of undissolved particles in a liquid, 261

Sweat glands, they excrete perspiration and detoxify the body by excreting excess salt and unwanted chemicals, 160

Symmetrical balance, two halves of a style; form a mirror image of one another, 304

Synthetic hair, 574–575

Systemic circulation, also known as *general circulation;* system that carries the oxygen-rich blood from the heart throughout the body and returns deoxygenated blood back to the heart, 132

Systemic infection, infection that affects the body as a whole, often due to under-functioning or over-functioning of internal glands or organs. This disease is carried through the blood stream or the lymphatic system, 79

T

Tactile corpuscles, small epidermal structures with nerve endings that are sensitive to touch and pressure, 157

Talus, also known as *ankle bone;* one of three bones that comprise the ankle joint. The other two bones are the tibia and fibula, 122

Tan, change in pigmentation of skin caused by exposure to the sun or ultraviolet light, 181

Taper, haircutting effect in which there is an even blend from very short at the hairline to longer lengths as you move up the head; *to taper* is to narrow progressively at one end, 400

Tapotement, also known as *percussion;* movements consisting of short quick tapping, slapping, and hacking movements, 782

Tarsal, one of the subdivisions of the foot. There are seven bones—talus, calcaneus, navicular, three cuneiform bones, and the cuboid. The other two subdivisions are the metatarsal and phalanges., 122

Teamwork, salon, 1058

Telangiectasis, distended or dilated surface blood vessels, 178

Telogen phase, also known as *resting phase;* the final phase in the hair cycle that lasts until the fully grown hair is shed, 233

Temper, a process used to condition a new brass pressing comb so that it heats evenly, 469

Temporal bones, bones that form the sides of the head in the ear region, 119

Temporal nerve, branch of the seventh cranial nerve that affects the muscles of the temple, side of the forehead, eyebrow, eyelid, and upper part of the cheek, 131

Temporary haircolor, nonpermanent color whose large pigment molecules prevent penetration of the cuticle layer, allowing only a coating action that may be removed by shampooing, 680

Tension, amount of pressure applied when combing and holding a section, created by stretching or pulling the section, 380

Terminal hair, long, coarse, pigmented hair found on the scalp, legs, arms, and bodies of males and females, 240

Terry cloth mitts, 854, 904

Tertiary color, intermediate color achieved by mixing a secondary color and its neighboring primary color on the color wheel in equal amounts, 676

Tesla high-frequency current, also known as *violet ray;* thermal or heat-producing current with a high rate of oscillation or vibration that is commonly used for scalp and facial treatments, 282

Test-wise, understanding the strategies for successful test taking, 1027

Textured hair, hair with a tight coil pattern, 531

Textured set and style, textured sets elongate the natural frizzy hair and make a smooth-silky curl, wavy or zig-zag pattern when the hair is set wet or dry on natural curly or coily hair textures, 540

Texture specialist, 13

Texturizing, haircutting technique designed to remove excess bulk without shortening the length; changing the appearance or behavior of the hair through specific haircutting techniques using shears, thinning shears, or a razor, 394
basic haircuts enhanced with, 399
razor, 397–398
shears, 395–398